Integrative Medicine

Integrative Medicine

David Rakel, M.D.
Assistant Professor
Department of Family Medicine
Medical Director, Integrative Medicine Program
University of Wisconsin Medical School
Madison, WI

SAUNDERS
An imprint of Elsevier Science
Philadelphia   London   New York   St. Louis   Sydney   Toronto

SAUNDERS
An Imprint of Elsevier Science

The Curtis Center
Independence Square West
Philadelphia, PA 19106

Integrative Medicine   ISBN 0-7216-9288-5

Notice

Medicine is an ever-changing field. Standard safety precautions must be followed, but as new research and clinical experience broaden our knowledge, changes in treatment and drug therapy may become necessary or appropriate. Readers are advised to check the most current product information provided by the manufacturer of each drug to be administered to verify the recommended dose, the method and duration of administration, and contraindications. It is the responsibility of the treating physician, relying on experience and knowledge of the patient, to determine dosages and the best treatment for each individual patient. Neither the Publisher nor the author assume any liability for any injury and/or damage to persons of property arising from this publication.

Library of Congress Cataloging-in-Publication Data

Integrative medicine/[edited by] David Rakel].-- 1st ed.
      p. cm.
      Includes index.
      ISBN 0-7216-9288-5
      1. Alternative medicine. 2. Medicine--Practice. I. Rakel, David.

   R733.I5755 2003
   615--dc21

                                                        2002066973

Acquisitions Editors: Lisette Bralow, Steven Merahn
Book Designer: Steven Stave

AB/MVB
Printed in the United States of America.
Last digit is the print number: 9 8 7 6 5 4 3 2 1

For my sister Cindy, whose memory continues to teach me about the beauty and challenges of life.

Contributors

Robert Abel, Jr., M.D.
Clinical Professor of Ophthalmology, Thomas Jefferson University, Philadelphia, PA; Senior Attending, Christiana Care Health System, Wilmington, DE
Preventing Cataracts; Preventing Age-Related Macular Degeneration

Patricia Ammon, M.D.
Clinical Faculty, Department of Family Medicine, University of Colorado School of Medicine, Denver, CO
Multiple Sclerosis

Louis J. Aronne, M.D., F.A.C.P.
Clinical Associate Professor of Medicine; Medical Director, Comprehensive Weight Control Program, Weill Medical College of Cornell University, New York, NY
Obesity

Iris R. Bell, M.D., Ph.D.
Associate Professor Psychiatry and Psychology; Director of Research, Program in Integrative Medicine, The University of Arizona College of Medicine, Tucson, AZ
Detoxification

William Benda, M.D.
Adjunct Associate Research Scientist, Institute for Children, Youth, and Families, The University of Arizona, Tucson, AZ
Integrative Approach to Cancer

Bhaswati Bhattacharya, M.D.H., M.D., M.A.
Attending Physician, Department of Family Practice and Community Medicine; Director of Research, Development, and Education, Wyckoff Heights Medical Center, New York-Presbyterian Health Care System, Brooklyn, NY
Prevention of Breast Cancer; Prevention of Urinary Tract Infections

Mary Martin Bunker, D.O.
Highland, MI
Therapeutic Homeopathy

Opher Caspi, M.D., M.A.
Research Assistant Professor, The University of Arizona, Tucson, AZ
Activating the Healing Response

Remy Coeytaux, M.D.
Assistant Professor of Family Medicine, University of North Carolina School of Medicine; Attending Physician, University of North Carolina Hospitals, Chapel Hill, NC
Migraine and Tension-Type Headache

Michael W. Cohen, M.D.
Clinical Professor of Pediatrics, The University of Arizona College of Medicine; Medical Consultant, The Attention Disorder Center of Tucson, Tucson, AZ
Attention Deficit Disorder

Alan M. Dattner, M.D.
Scientific Director, HealthDataLink.com; President, ImmunoClarity Research Associates, New Rochelle, NY
Seborrheic Dermatitis

Brian F. Degenhardt, D.O.
Associate Professor, Department of Osteopathic Manipulative Medicine, Assistant Vice-President for Osteopathic Research, Kirksville College of Osteopathic Medicine; Family Practice/ Osteopathic Neuromusculoskeletal Medicine Residency Co-Director, Northeast Regional Medical Center, Kirksville, MO
Low Back Pain Exercises

Phillip C. DeMio, M.D., F.A.C.E.P.
Ohio University Medical Faculty, Medina, OH
Gout

Vivian M. Dickerson, M.D.
Associate Clinical Professor, Director of General Obstetrics/Gynecology Division, University of California, Irvine, CA
Prevention of Skin Cancer

Raffaele Filice, M.D.
Medical Director, Tzu Chi Institute for Complementary and Alternative Medicine, Vancouver, BC, Canada
Prevention of Memory Loss

Susan Fleishman, B.A.
Integrative Medicine Resource Group, Tucson, AZ
The Integrative Assessment

Tracy Gaudet, M.D.
Assistant Clinical Professor of Clinical Obstetrics and Gynecology, Director, Duke Center for Integrative Medicine, Duke University Medical Center, Durham, NC
Integrative Approach to Pregnancy

Steffie Goodman, C.N.M., M.S.N.
Nurse Midwifery Faculty, School of Nursing, University of Colorado Health Sciences Center, Denver CO
Post-term Pregnancy; Labor Pain Management; Nausea and Vomiting in Pregnancy

Kathryn L. Grant, Pharm.D.
Assistant Professor, College of Pharmacy, The University of Arizona, Tucson, AZ
Integrative Approach to Cancer

Russell Greenfield, M.D.
Visiting Assistant Professor, The University of Arizona College of Medicine, Tucson, AZ; Medical Director, Carolinas Integrative Health, Charlotte, NC
Congestive Heart Failure; Prescribing Probiotics

Steven Gurgevich, M.D.
Clinical Assistant Professor of Medicine, Program in Integrative Medicine, The University of Arizona Health Sciences Center, Tucson, AZ
Self-Hypnosis Techniques

Susan Hadley, M.D.
Faculty, Family Practice Residency Program, Middlesex Hospital, Middletown, CT
Urinary Tract Infections; Hypothyroidism

Jane L. Hart, M.D.
Clinical Instructor, Case Western Reserve University School of Medicine, Cleveland, OH; Director, Preventive Medicine Consultations, Beachwood, OH
Preventing Hypertension

Michael J. Hewitt, M.S., Ph.D.
Director of Health and Healing, Exercise Physiologist, Canyon Ranch Health Resort, Tucson, AZ
Writing an Exercise Prescription

Catherine A. Hoffman, M.D.
Dermatology, Surgical and Medical Associates, Fresno, CA
Atopic Dermatitis; Psoriasis

Sharon K. Hull, M.D.
Assistant Professor, Clinical Family and Community Medicine, Assistant Dean of Student Affairs, Southern Illinois University School of Medicine; Consulting Staff, Memorial Hospital of Carbondale, Carbondale, IL
Acne Vulgaris and Acne Rosacea; Human Papillomavirus and Warts

David W. Infanger, B.A.
Microbiologist, Fermentation Research and Development, Cargill, Inc., Minneapolis, MN
Prevention of Atherosclerosis

Robert S. Ivker, D.O.
Littleton, CO
Chronic Sinusitis

Kathleen Johnson, M.S., R.D.
Nutrition Preceptor, Program in Integrative Medicine, The University of Arizona Health Sciences Center, Tucson, AZ
The Elimination Diet and Diagnosing Food Hypersensitivities; The Glycemic Index

Dharma Singh Kalsa, M.D.
President and Medical Director, Alzheimer's Prevention Foundation, Tucson, AZ
Alzheimer's Disease

Benjamin Kligler, M.D., M.P.H.
Assistant Professor of Family Medicine, Albert Einstein College of Medicine, Bronx, NY; Associate Medical Director, Co-Director, Fellowship Program in Integrative Medicine, Continuum/Beth Israel Center for Health and Healing, New York, NY
HIV Disease

Evan W. Kligman, M.D.
Professor of Public Health, Family and Community Medicine, and Medicine, Co-Director, University of Arizona Center on Aging, Colleges of Public Health and Medicine, The University of Arizona Health Sciences Center, Tucson, AZ
Prevention of Effects of Aging

Karen Koffler, M.D.
Associate Professor, Northwestern University, Healthcare Director of Integrative Medicine, Evanston Northwestern, Evanston, IL
The Integrative Assessment

Wendy G. Kohatsu, M.D.
Assistant Professor, East Tennessee State University, Johnson City, TN; Advisory Board, WomenHeart, Wellmont Holston Valley Hospital and Medical Center, Kingsport, TN
Low Back Pain

Judith Korner, M.D., Ph.D.
Assistant Professor of Clinical Medicine, Columbia University College of Physicians and Surgeons; Attending Physician, New York-Presbyterian Hospital, New York, NY
Obesity

Roberta A. Lee, M.D.
Assistant Clinical Professor, Albert Einstein Medical School; Medical Director, Co-Director, Integrative Medicine Fellowship, Center of Health and Healing, Beth Israel Medical Center, New York, NY
Anxiety

Alison Levitt, M.D.
Asheville, NC
Prevention of Osteoporosis

Lee D. Litvinas, M.D.
Physician, Martha Jefferson Hospital, Charlottesville, VA
Prevention of Stroke

Sheree Loftus, M.S.N., C.R.R.N., R.N.C.
New York, NY
Parkinson's Disease

Jay Lombard, D.O.
Assistant Clinical Professor of Neurology, Cornell University Medical College; Attending Physician, New York-Presbyterian Hospital, New York, NY
Parkinson's Disease

Tieraona Low Dog, M.D.
Assistant Clinical Professor, Department of Family and Community Medicine, University of New Mexico, Albuquerque, NM; Clinical Lecturer, Department of Medicine, The University of Arizona, Tucson, AZ; Chair, United States Pharmacopoeia Dietary Supplements/Botanicals Information Panel, Rockville, MD
Premenstrual Syndrome

Robert B. Lutz, M.D., M.P.H.
Coordinator, Medical Education and Medical Editor, Associate Fellowship, Program in Integrative Medicine, The University of Arizona, Tucson, AZ
Irritable Bowel Syndrome; Gastroesophageal Reflux Disease; Peptic Ulcer Disease; Inflammatory Bowel Disease

Victoria Maizes, M.D.
Executive Director, Program in Integrative Medicine, The University of Arizona, Tucson, AZ
The Integrative Assessment; Hypertension

Bill Manahan, M.D.
Assistant Professor, Department of Family Practice and Community Health, University of Minnesota Medical School, Minneapolis, MN
Food Allergy

Doug Mann, M.D.
Professor of Neurology, University of North Carolina School of Medicine; Director, Neurology Outpatient Services, University of North Carolina Hospitals, Chapel Hill, NC
Migraine and Tension-Type Headache

John D. Mark, M.D.
Assistant Professor of Clinical Pediatrics, Pediatric Pulmonary and Integrative Medicine, Department of Pediatrics, The University of Arizona, Tucson, AZ
Asthma

Ann L. Mattson, M.D., F.A.C.O.G.
Medical Director, Boulder Valley Women's Health Center, Boulder, CO
Post-term Pregnancy; Labor Pain Management; Nausea and Vomiting in Pregnancy

Mark McClure, M.D.
Active Staff, Rex Hospital, Raleigh Community Hospital, Wake Medical Center, Raleigh, NC; Western Wake Hospital, Cary, NC
Chronic Prostatitis; Preventing Prostate Cancer

Sharon I. McDonough-Means, M.D.
Research Assistant Professor, College of Nursing and Pediatrics, College of Medicine, The University of Arizona, Tucson, AZ; Integrative Developmental-Behavorial Pediatrician, Scottsdale, AZ
Attention Deficit Disorder; Detoxification

Shiraz I. Mishra, M.D., Ph.D.
Associate Professor of Medicine, Susan Samueli Center for Complementary and Alternative Medicine, Center for Health Policy and Research, Chao Comprehensive Cancer Center, University of California, Irvine, CA
Prevention of Lung Cancer

Jeffrey A. Morrison, M.D.
Clinical Director, Wellness Medical Center, New York, NY
The Prevention of Diabetes Mellitus

Daniel Muller, M.D., Ph.D.
Associate Professor of Medicine (Rheumatology) and Medical Microbiology and Immunology, University of Wisconsin Medical School, Madison, WI
Fibromyalgia Syndrome and Chronic Fatigue Syndrome; Rheumatoid Arthritis

Karen L. Mutter, D.O.
Medical Director, Integrative Medicine Healing Center, Clearwater, FL
Prescribing Antioxidants

Harmon L. Myers, D.O.
Preceptor in Manipulative Medicine, Program in Integrative Medicine, The University of Arizona, Tucson, AZ
Strain and Counterstrain Manipulation Technique

Wadie I. Najm, M.D.
Associate Clinical Professor, University of California, Irvine, CA
Prevention of Lung Cancer; Prevention of Skin Cancer

James P. Nicolai, M.D.
Fellow, Program in Integrative Medicine, The
    University of Arizona, Tucson, AZ
Upper Respiratory Infection

Sharon Norling, M.D., M.B.A.
Assistant Professor, Department of Obstetrics and
    Gynecology and Women's Health, University of
    Minnesota Medical School; Medical Director,
    Women's Health Center, Medical Director, Mind
    Body Spirit Clinic, University of Minnesota
    Academic Health Center, Minneapolis, MN
Osteoporosis

Brian Olshanksy, M.D.
Professor of Medicine, University of Iowa; Director of
    Cardiac Electrophysiology, University of Iowa
    Hospitals, Iowa City IA
Arrhythmias; Hyperlipidemia

Sunil Pai, M.D.
Associate Fellow of Integrative Medicine, The
    University of Arizona, Tucson, AZ; President and
    Medical Director, Sanjevani, Santa Fe, NM
Peripheral Neuropathy

Adam I. Perlman, M.D., M.P.H.
Assistant Clinical Professor, Mount Sinai School of
    Medicine, New York, NY; Director of Integrative
    Medicine, St. Barnabas Health Care System,
    Livingston, NJ
Osteoarthritis

Gregory A. Plotnikoff, M.D., M.T.S.
Associate Professor, Clinical Medicine and Pediatrics,
    University of Minnesota Medical School; Medical
    Director, Center for Spirituality and Healing,
    University of Minnesota Academic Health Center,
    Minneapolis, MN
*Osteoporosis; Prevention of Atherosclerosis; Spiritual
Assessment and Care*

Francine Rainone, Ph.D., D.O.
Assistant Professor, Albert Einstein College of
    Medicine; Director of Community Palliative Care,
    Department of Family Medicine, Montefiore
    Medical Center, Bronx, NY
Dysmenorrhea

David Rakel, M.D.
Assistant Professor, Department of Family Medicine;
    Medical Director, Integrative Medicine Program,
    University of Wisconsin Medical School, Madison,
    WI
*Philosophy of Integrative Medicine; Herpes Simplex Virus
Infection; Hepatitis; Insulin Resistance Syndrome;
Cholelithiasis; Benign Prostatic Hyperplasia; Neck Pain;
Recurrent Aphthous Ulceration; Preventing Prostate
Cancer; The Anti-Inflammatory Diet; The DASH Diet;
Breathing Exercises; Self-Hypnosis Techniques; Prescribing
Relaxation Techniques; Guided Imagery and Interactive
Guided Imagery; Journaling; Learning to Meditate;*

*Motivational Interviewing Techniques; Strain and
Counterstrain Manipulation Technique*

Malcolm Riley, B.D.S., F.D.S., M.R.D.
Tucson, AZ
*Recurrent Aphthous Ulceration; Acupuncture for
Headache; Acupuncture for Nausea and Vomiting*

J. Adam Rindfleisch, M.D.
Chief Resident, Department of Family Medicine,
    University of Wisconsin Medical School, Madison
    WI
Neck Pain

Jean Riquelme, M.D.
Medical Staff, Department of Family Medicine, St.
    Luke's Medical Center, Milwaukee, WI
Yeast Infections; Uterine Fibroids (Leiomyomata)

Martin L. Rossman, M.D.
Clinical Associate, Department of Medicine,
    University of California, San Francisco, CA; Co-
    Director, Academy for Guided Imagery, Mill Valley,
    CA
Guided Imagery and Interactive Guided Imagery

Craig Schneider, M.D.
Clinical Assistant Professor, College of Medicine,
    University of Vermont, Burlington, VT; Assistant
    Residency Director, Director of Integrative
    Medicine, Department of Family Practice, Maine
    Medical Center, Portland, ME
Depression

Marcey Shapiro, M.D.
Albany, CA
Otitis Media; Prevention of Otitis Media

Victor S. Sierpina, M.D.
Associate Professor, Department of Family Medicine,
    University of Texas Medical Branch, Galveston, TX
Diabetes Mellitus

William S. Silvers, M.D.
Clinical Professor of Medicine, Division of Allergy and
    Clinical Immunology, University of Colorado Health
    Sciences Center, Denver, CO
Allergic Rhinitis

Coleen M. Smith, D.O.
Johnson City Osteopathic Medicine, Johnson City, TN
Low Back Pain Exercises

Marnee Spierer, M.D.
Resident in Radiation Oncology, Memorial Sloane
    Kettering Cancer Center, New York, NY
Osteoarthritis

Monica J. Stokes, M.D., F.A.C.O.G.
Integrative Medicine Consultant, San Francisco, CA
Menopause

Benjamin M. Sucher, D.O., F.A.O.C.P.M.R., F.A.A.P.M.R.
Co-Principal Investigator, Department of Exercise Science, Arizona State University, Tempe, AZ; Medical Director, Center for Carpal Tunnel Studies, Scottsdale, AZ
Carpal Tunnel Syndrome

Steven Tenenbaum, M.D.
Integrative Medicine Specialist, The Celebration of Health Center, Bluffton, OH; Staff Physician, Department of Emergency Medicine, Wood County Hospital, Bowling Green, OH
Urticaria (Acute and Chronic)

Sue Towey, M.S., R.N., C.N.S., L.P.
Faculty, Center for Spirituality and Healing, University of Minnesota Academic Health Center; Clinical Nurse Specialist, Licensed Psychologist, Mind Body Spirit Clinic, Fairview-University Medical Center, Minneapolis, MN
Prevention of Atherosclerosis

Sara L. Warber, M.D.
Lecturer, Department of Family Medicine, University of Michigan Medical School; Co-Director, Complementary and Alternative Medicine Research Center, University of Michigan, Ann Arbor, MI
Coronary Artery Disease; Peripheral Vascular Disease

Don Warne, M.D., M.P.H., D.A.B.M.A.
Staff Clinician, National Institutes of Health, NIDDK, Phoenix, AZ
Alcoholism and Substance Abuse

R. W. Watkins, M.D., M.P.H.
Clinical Assistant Professor of Family Medicine, University of North Carolina School of Medicine, Chapel Hill, NC
Urolithiasis (Kidney and Bladder Stones)

Andrew Weil, M.D.
Director, Program in Integrative Medicine, The University of Arizona Health Sciences Center, Tucson, AZ
Philosophy of Integrative Medicine

Joy A. Weydert, M.D.
Fellow, Pediatric Integrative Medicine, The University of Arizona Health Sciences Center, Tucson, AZ
Recurring Abdominal Pain in Pediatrics

Hunter Yost, M.D.
Tucson, AZ
Functional Medicine

Melissa C. Young, M.D.
Fellow, Program in Integrative Medicine, The University of Arizona, Tucson, AZ
Prevention of Colon Cancer

Suzanna M. Zick, N.D., M.P.H.
Research Investigator, Department of Family Medicine, University of Michigan Medical School, Ann Arbor, MI
Coronary Artery Disease; Peripheral Vascular Disease

Foreword

It cannot be said too often that integrative medicine is not synonymous with complementary and alternative medicine (CAM). CAM is about modalities—treatments that are not currently taught in conventional schools of medicine and that are not part of conventional (allopathic) treatment protocols. Integrative medicine does try to incorporate the best CAM ideas and practices into comprehensive treatment plans, but it has more important goals than the simple substitution, say, of herbs for pharmaceutical drugs.

Above all, integrative medicine seeks to work with the body's natural potential for healing. It assumes that the organism has an array of mechanisms to maintain health and promote healing and that the aim of treatment should be to unblock or activate or enhance those mechanisms. In practice, it pays attention not only to the physical bodies of patients but also to their minds and emotions and their spiritual lives. It looks at their total lifestyles in order to suggest changes in routines that might favor healing, and it exhorts physicians to model healthy lifestyles for their patients. It also emphasizes the centrality of the doctor/patient relationship in the healing process.

Those in academic medicine who feel threatened by the rise of integrative medicine focus only on its promotion of CAM, which they view as unscientific or even anti-scientific. Integrative medicine is committed to scientific method and evidence-based practice. But it is important to keep these facts in mind: (1) most conventional medical scientists are unaware of the evidence that already exists for the safety and efficacy of many CAM treatments; (2) the evidence base for many widely used allopathic treatments is not very solid; and (3) most medical decision-making takes place in areas of scientific uncertainty, where physicians and patients must use good judgment and intuition in the absence of definitive evidence. With regard to this last point, it seems to me that we need to get in the habit of using a sliding scale of evidence—i.e., the greater the potential of treatment to cause harm, the stricter the standard of evidence it should be held to.

Many conventional treatments would not pass this review. Take the recent example of bone marrow transplant for patients with metastatic breast cancer. I know many patients who were persuaded to opt for this most invasive procedure, which is now acknowledged to be worthless. It is in this situation that both physicians and patients should really demand evidence for safety and efficacy.

Integrative medicine is here to stay and, I am confident, will influence the development of medical education and research as well as practice. A Consortium of Academic Health Centers for Integrative Medicine that includes deans and chancellors of a number of leading medical schools is already developing guidelines for new curriculums, research strategies, and healthcare policy. Nevertheless, for the average healthcare consumer integrative medicine is still hard to access for the simple reason that qualified practitioners are few and far between. Demand greatly exceeds supply for physicians trained in the new paradigm, and training opportunities are limited.

I meet many clinicians who are open to change. They realize their training did not prepare them to meet the expectations and needs of consumers today, and they are willing to learn about more natural, less harmful ways of treating disease and supporting health and healing. I believe this book will be helpful to them. My colleague and former fellow (at the University of Arizona's Program in Integrative Medicine) has assembled a stellar group of contributors to present the integrative perspective on the treatment of the commonest categories of disease. This is a very practical text that takes account of the best available scientific evidence as well as the accumulated experience of practitioners of many different systems of treatment.

It is a pleasure to introduce this book to readers. I hope it will lead to better treatment outcomes and improve the experience of clinical medicine for both doctors and patients.

Andrew Weil, MD
Director, Program in Integrative Medicine
Clinical Professor of Medicine
University of Arizona
Tucson, Arizona
July 2002

Preface

I began to conceptualize the format of this book four years ago, when in private practice, patients would ask how to incorporate nontraditional therapies into their medical care. Despite growing evidence, there was no reference to help integrate these therapies with my traditional Western methods of treatment. The available medical literature dealt mainly with pharmaceuticals and surgical therapies. Few offered guidance regarding complementary therapies that would honor the multifactorial, bio-psycho-social-spiritual influences on health. This motivated me to take the two-year fellowship program in Integrative Medicine at the University of Arizona where my colleagues and I learned to incorporate nontraditional tools with traditional methods to enhance health and healing. These tools included nutrition, botanicals, supplements, mind-body therapies, acupuncture, and manual therapies, among others.

We learned, however, that the magic is not in the tools, but in the process, the process of building relationships that help us understand the unique complexities of those we serve. This provides insight that, along with science, helps us pick the most appropriate combination of tools for each individual. Once we develop a holistic understanding of our patient, whatever tools we choose will likely work better. This text offers guidance on how to select and use these tools.

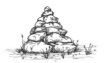

Throughout the text you will see a drawing of a cairn, a symbolic mound of stones that serves as a landmark to direct us along a path that may not be obvious. This text offers guidance to help integrate less familiar therapies, remove barriers to self-healing, and facilitate long-term health for our patients. An image of the cairn is placed at the end of each chapter to indicate a summary of important clinical information.

This book is divided into four main parts:

I. Philosophy of Integrative Medicine

This part covers the philosophy of the field and discusses an integrative patient evaluation.

II. Integrative Approach to Disease

This is the heart of the text, where specific disease states are discussed. These chapters are generally presented in the following format:

> *pathophysiology,*
> *integrative therapy,* which may include any of the following:
> *lifestyle choices,*
> *nutrition and nutritional supplements,*
> *botanicals,*
> *mind-body techniques,*
> *manual therapy,*
> *pharmaceuticals,*
> *constitutional therapies* (Traditional Chinese Medicine, homeopathy, etc.),
> *spirituality,*
> *surgery,*
> *therapies to consider* (discusses therapies that the authors have found beneficial but may lack scientific support at this time), and
> *therapeutic review,* a summary focusing on key clinical information that can be easily referenced.

Throughout each chapter you will see boxed "*notes*" that focus on clinical pearls, e.g.:

NOTE

St. Johns Wort enhances the hepatic metabolism of cytochrome P450 3A4 and can lower serum levels of medications taken concomitantly if this pathway clears them.

III. Disease Prevention

This part covers integrative therapies that can help prevent the most common disease conditions. It follows a format similar to that used in Part II, but also includes *etiology* and *screening*. It is summarized under the heading, *Prevention Prescription*. This is a summary of recommendations for patients that will help them avoid disease development and progression.

IV. Tools for Your Practice

This part focuses on specific therapeutic tools and how they can be used in everyday practice. Each chapter discusses practical applications involving nutrition, exercise, mind-body, biochemical, biomechanical, and bioenergetic influences on health. They are short and concise practical tips focused on helping you apply these complementary therapies in your practice. Patient instruction handouts are included.

This book was prepared with the busy clinician in mind. For this reason, topics were chosen that are most commonly encountered in the primary care setting. The information is organized for rapid retrieval. Dosages and precautions for using botanicals, dietary supplements, and pharmaceuticals are clearly outlined. All dosages have been carefully checked. Nevertheless, please always recheck before prescribing. Tables, graphs, and photographs are used throughout the book to enhance clarity.

This text is unique in that it integrates traditional and nontraditional therapies. The information is evidence based and referenced (positive and negative) to help guide selection of therapy. I had the pleasure of inviting experienced and talented clinicians to share their expertise, combining evidence with the wisdom of practice. To each of them I am eternally grateful.

Facilitating health in our patients is rarely as simple as following treatment guidelines based on the data. We need the evidence to tell us what works and what doesn't. It will continue to be the main source of information that guides us toward the most appropriate therapeutic decisions. The best therapy, though, comes when we can match the scientific evidence to the unique personality and beliefs of the individual. I hope this book empowers you to do this for your patients and, in the process, helps make your practice a little easier and more fulfilling.

Acknowledgments

I would like to thank Andy Weil and the faculty, fellows, and staff at the University of Arizona Program in Integrative Medicine for giving me the guidance and resources needed to put this text together. Without their support and expertise, this project would not have been possible. Thanks to the first four classes of fellows for being cofacilitators in helping explore and define our own balance of health. Thanks to Russ, Wendy, Karen, Robbie, Bill, Opher, Bob, Victoria, Raffaele, John, Sharon, Craig, Monica, Diane, Joy, Monica, Jim, and Melissa.

Thanks to Lisette Bralow and the editorial staff at W.B. Saunders for their guidance and education. Thanks to Steve Merahn for taking the baton and seeing this project through.

I greatly appreciate the time and expertise of all the contributing authors. They gave their time and knowledge with little in return. I am thankful we can all learn from them.

A special thanks to my father, Robert Rakel, for his advice and editorial pearls of wisdom. Thanks to my mother, Peggy Rakel, and my sisters, Barbara and Linda, and their families for their eternal support. Thanks to my wife Denise and children, Justin, Sarah, and Lucas, for making it all worthwhile.

David P. Rakel, M.D.
University of Wisconsin Medical School
Madison, Wisconsin

Contents

PART *I*

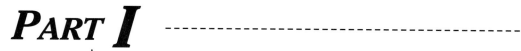

Integrative Medicine

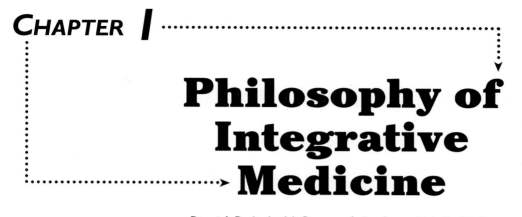

CHAPTER 1

Philosophy of Integrative Medicine

David Rakel, M.D., and Andrew Weil, M.D.

LEARNING ABOUT THE PRESENT FROM THE PAST

From Aristotle to the Flexner Report

Long before there were magnetic resonance imaging and computed tomography scanners, Aristotle (384 to 322 BC) was able to simply experience, observe, and reflect on the human condition. He was one of the first holistic physicians who believed that every person was a combination of both physical and spiritual properties with no separation between mind and body. It was not until the 1600s that a spiritual mathematician became worried that prevailing scientific materialistic thought would reduce the conscious mind to something that could be manipulated and controlled. René Descartes (1596 to 1650), respecting the great unknown, did his best to separate the mind and the body to protect the spirit from science. He believed that mind and spirit should be the focus of the church, leaving science to dissect the physical body. This philosophy lead to the "Cartesian split" that resulted in mind/body duality.

Shortly after, John Locke (1632 to 1704) and David Hume (1711 to 1776), were influential in the reductionistic movement that shaped our science and medical systems. The idea was that if we could reduce natural phenomena to greater simplicity, we could understand the larger whole. So, to learn about a clock, all we need to do is take it apart and study its parts. Reductionism facilitated great discoveries that helped humans gain control over their environment. Despite this progress, physicians had few tools to effectively treat disease. In the early 20th century, applied science started to transform medicine. In 1910, the Flexner report[1] had a significant impact on the development of allopathic academic institutions. These institutions were founded on the triad that prevails today: research, education, and medical practice. Reductionism and the scientific method produced the knowledge that encouraged the growth of these institutions.

The scientific model led to greater understanding of the pathophysiologic basis of disease and the development of tools to help combat its influence. Subspecialization of medical care was developed to help apply this explosion of information and to combat disease. We now have practitioners who focus on the pieces and a society that appreciates their abilities to fix problems. Unfortunately, this approach does not work well for chronic disease that involves more than just a single part. In fact, all body organs are interconnected, so that repairing only a part without addressing the underlying causes provides merely temporary relief and a false sense of security.

More Technology, Less Communication

The tremendous success of medical science of the 20th century was not without cost. The amount of money allocated to health during the 1990s has almost doubled from $391 billion to $668 billion. The healthcare market grows when more attention is focused on problems that can be treated with drugs or procedures. Financial rewards increase when there are more subtypes of disease to which treatments can be attached. The system encourages patients to believe that tools are the answer to their physical woes and discourages them from paying attention to the interplay of mind, community, and spirit. Technology is the golden calf in this scenario. We have become dependent on it, and overutilization has widened the barrier of communication between patient and provider. The old tools of the trade—rapport, gestalt, intuition, and laying on of hands—are used less and less as powerful drugs and high-technology interventions become available.

To help curtail costs, managed care and capitation were born. These new models reduced excessive costs and further eroded the patient-provider relationship—placing increased demands on physicians that did not involve patient care. Physician and patient unrest followed. Doctors are unhappy in part because of loss of autonomy in practicing medicine. Patients are unhappy in part because they feel they are not getting the attention they need. Most upset are those with chronic medical conditions whose diseases do not respond well to the treatments of specialized medicine. This comes at a time when the incidence of chronic and degenerative diseases is at an all-time high. Diseases such as irritable bowel syndrome, chronic fatigue, and chronic pain syndromes are very common. They require evaluation and treatment of much more than any one organ. The public has started to realize the limitations of Western medicine and wants more attention paid to health and healing of the whole person, especially when there is no "part" to be fixed.

Public Interest Influences Change

The deterioration of the patient-provider relationship, the overutilization of technology, and the inability of the medical system to adequately treat chronic disease has contributed to rising interest in complementary and alternative medicine (CAM). The public has sent its message with feet and pocketbooks. In fact, there were more visits to CAM providers in the early 1990s than to all primary care medical physicians, and patients paid for these visits out of pocket with an estimated expenditure of $13 billion.[2] This trend continued throughout the 1990s with 42% of the public using alternative therapies, increasing expenditures to $27 billion from 1990 to 1997.[3] Patients are also demanding less aggressive forms of therapy, and they are leery of the toxicity of pharmaceutical drugs. Adverse drug reactions were found to be the sixth leading cause of death,[4] and in 1994, botanicals were the largest growth area in retail pharmacy.[5] Research showed that people thought complementary approaches were more aligned with "their own values, beliefs, and philosophical orientations toward health and life."[6] The public, before the medical establishment, realized that health and healing involved more than pills and surgery. Less invasive, more traditional remedies—such as nutrition, botanicals, manipulation, meditation, and massage—that were neglected with the explosion of medical science and technology were now being rediscovered with great enthusiasm (Fig. 1–1).

Medicine Gets the Message

The popularity of CAM therapies created a need for research in these areas. In 1993, an Office of Alternative Medicine was started within the National Institutes of Health. The budget consisted of $2 million, a fraction of the $80 billion budget of the National Institutes of Health. The office was later upgraded to the National Center for Complementary

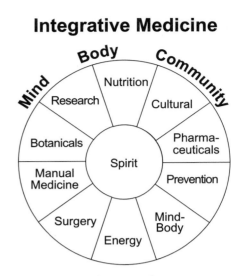

Integrative Medicine

Figure 1–1. Integrative medicine pie chart.

and Alternative Medicine (NCCAM) and the amount of money available for scholarly research kept pace with this growth. By the year 2000, the NCCAM budget grew to $68.7 million.[7] This allowed for needed research for exploration of how these areas of medicine could enhance healthcare delivery. At first, researchers tried to use traditional methods to learn about CAM therapies. These methods were sufficient for studying therapies such as botanicals. But the limitations of the reductionistic model became apparent when it was used to study more dynamic systems of healing such as homeopathy, traditional Chinese medicine, and energy medicine. New methods were required to understand the multiple influences involved. Outcome studies with attention to quality of life were initiated. Research grants in "frontier medicine" were created to help learn about fields such as energy medicine, homeopathy, magnet therapy, and therapeutic prayer. Interest grew in learning how to combine the successes of the scientific model with the potential of CAM to improve the delivery of healthcare.

EXPLORING OTHER PATHS TOWARD KNOWLEDGE

Since the mid-20th century, medical science has recognized only one source of knowledge, the double-blind, placebo-controlled study. With the complex interaction of human belief, culture, community, and spirit, this is the best tool we have to remove these disturbances that cloud our ability to see whether the part being studied has merit. As discussed, this method has brought great rewards but is not without limitations. These limitations are mainly related to ignoring factors that are commonly thought to be irrelevant.

Understanding how a tool such as a pharmaceutical or botanical can be used in the context of the consumer's belief system, culture, and community will enhance the effectiveness of the therapy chosen. Although this greater understanding does not get respect within the traditional scientific model, we use it daily in the artful practice of medicine. This art requires the inclusion of three other key sources of knowledge:

- Single-case study
- Experience and judgment
- Intuition

Single-Case Study

When Norman Cousins used laughter to help overcome ankylosing spondylitis, we were able to see how one individual used a mind-body technique to recover from what science taught us to be an incurable chronic disease. By learning from cases that are on the extreme edges of the bell-shaped curve, we are able to quickly advance our knowledge and understanding of beneficial influences on health. Studying only the cohort of people in the middle of the curve with the scientific model will limit understanding of those unique factors that can lead us to new discovery.

Experience and Judgment

"I have not failed 10,000 times. I have successfully found 10,000 ways that will not work."

Thomas Edison

It is through the experience of multiple single-case studies that one develops judgment. This accumulation of knowledge helps create wisdom that allows the experienced clinician to make better decisions. For this reason, clinical guidelines will never be followed universally because they ignore the wisdom of the clinician in matching the therapy to the unique individual. Research should help us to follow and improve our judgment. The assimilation of the information should be global whereas the implementation should be local. Experience and judgment allow us to use the research more efficiently. In fact, when asked what they would do when published data and "clinical experience" conflict, 53% of doctors said they would trust "my clinical experience."[8]

Intuition

Experience, knowledge, empathy, and energy are key factors involved in the process of developing intuition. Intuition relies on processing information from the five senses that organizes finite bits from many different sources into an understanding that is often without rationale and independent of linear reasoning. This understanding is strengthened when the experienced clinician combines it with a knowledge base of multiple case studies. Experienced or not, every physician has this ability and can strengthen it by developing close relationships with patients. Empathy and understanding of patients' culture and lifestyles increase the amount of available information that our brain is able to organize. The more information available, the more accurate the intuition. If we narrow our thought into one area of focus or limit our time with the patient, there will be less information for intuition to work with. Listening to our gut or having a "hunch" is involved in the everyday practice of medicine. It reaches beyond what we can currently explain and accesses a subtle energy than we can only feel. Many lives have been saved by the astute clinician who admits the patient with atypical chest pain when diagnostic studies are negative and risk factors few. Our system de-emphasizes this powerful human characteristic in medical decision-making. Instead, we need to learn how to maximize its ability to enhance patient care.

The scientific method has and will continue to be our primary source of knowledge. But in trying to understand the complex interactions of the human body that result in health, it alone will not have all the answers. We will improve our understanding if we integrate other sources of knowledge into the learning process, just as we integrate other forms of health and healing into the art of medicine.

NOTE

It is important to see the benefits and limitation of our current allopathic system and realize that science alone will not meet all the complex needs of our patients.[9]

INTEGRATIVE MEDICINE

Integrative medicine is healing oriented and emphasizes the centrality of the doctor-patient relationship. It focuses on the least invasive, least toxic, and least costly methods to help facilitate health by integrating both allopathic and complementary therapies. These are recommended based on an understanding of the physical, emotional, psychological, and spiritual aspects of the individual (Table 1–1).

Healing-Oriented Medicine

Health comes from the Old English word "Hal," which means wholeness, soundness, or spiritual wellness. "Health" is defined by the World Health Organization as "a state of complete physical, mental and social well being, and not merely the absence of disease or infirmity."[10] To "cure," conversely, refers to doing something (such as giving drugs or perform-

Table 1–1. Defining Integrative Medicine

Provides relationship centred care
Integrates conventional and complementary methods of treatment and prevention
Involves removing barrier to activate the body's healing response
Uses natural, less invasive intervention before costly, invasive ones when possible
Engages mind, body, spirit, and community to facilitate healing
Healing is always possible, even when cursing is not

ing surgery) that alleviates a troublesome condition or disease. Healing does not equal curing. We can cure a condition such as hypertension with a pharmaceutical without healing the condition. Healing would facilitate changes that reduce stress, improve diet, promote exercise, and increase the person's sense of community. In doing this, we help improve the balance of health of the body that may result in the ability to discontinue a pharmaceutical, reducing the need for the cure.

An example of this can be seen in Figure 1–2. Here we have two trees, A and B. Tree A is obviously in a better state of health than tree B. This is likely owing to its ability to be in balance with its environment. If a branch breaks on tree A, we can feel comfortable that if we mend the branch, it will likely heal very well or even heal itself. But if a branch breaks on tree B and we mend it, our intuition tells

us that even if we have a talented tree surgeon, that branch is not going to heal. The point here is that our focus in medicine has been on fixing the branch while neglecting the health of the tree. If we give more attention to helping tree B find health either by removing barriers that are blocking its own ability to heal or by improving areas of deficiency, the branch will heal itself. We will not need to spend as much time and energy fixing the parts. Cure and fix when able, but if we ignore healing, the cure will likely not last or will give way to another disease that may not have a cure.

Integrative medicine is about changing the focus in medicine to one of healing rather than disease. This involves an understanding of the influences of mind, spirit, and community as well as of the body. It entails developing insight into the patient's culture, beliefs, and lifestyle that will help the provider understand how to best trigger the necessary changes in behavior that will result in improved health. This cannot be done without a sound commitment to the doctor-patient relationship.

Relationship-Centered Care

"It is much more important to know what sort of patient has a disease than what sort of disease a patient has."
Sir William Osler

One of the authors (DR) started a fellowship in integrative medicine eager to learn tools and techniques that would help fill the void left by his allopathic training. After observing practitioners of various trades in fields such as manual medicine, Chinese medicine, and botanicals, he realized that some practitioners had better results with their chosen trade. Those with more success were able to develop rapport, understanding, and empathy that helped them facilitate healing with their therapy. The relationship fostered healing not only by allowing the practitioner to gain insight into the patient's situation but also by building trust and confidence that the patient had in the provider. This trust acted as a tool to activate the patient's natural healing response, supporting whatever technique the provider uses, whether it is acupuncture, botanicals, pharmaceuticals, or surgery.

Developing a holistic understanding and relationship with patients allows the practitioner to guide them more efficiently toward health. The integrative clinician can point out the way toward health while realizing that the patient will have to do the work to actually get there. This attitude does a great deal to remove pressure and guilt from providers who have been trained to think of themselves as failures when they cannot fix problems. In fact, relationship-centered care is a necessity when dealing with the many chronic conditions that do not have simple cures. Success is now defined as helping the patient find an inner peace that results in a better quality of life, whether the problem can be fixed or not.

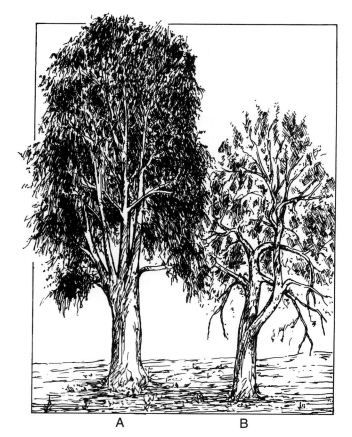

Figure 1–2. Healthy *(A)* and sickly *(B)* trees.

> **NOTE**
>
> *In conventional medicine, healing occurs outside the body-mind and is viewed as something done to the patient. In integrative medicine, healing occurs within the body-mind and requires active participation of the patient.*

Prevention

Integrative medicine encourages more time and effort on disease prevention instead of waiting to treat disease once it presents. Chronic disease now accounts for much of our healthcare costs and also causes significant morbidity and mortality. The incidence of heart disease, diabetes, and cancer could be significantly reduced with a change in lifestyle choices. Instead, they are affecting our health in epidemic proportions. Cardiologist Robert Elliot, M.D., said it well when describing our current medical situation: "We have a three trillion-dollar a year medical system waiting at the bottom of a cliff for people to fall off and injure themselves. When we suggest building a fence at the top of the cliff to prevent people from falling in the first place, the answer from the bottom is, 'We can't afford it. We're spending all our money down heeeeere.'"

The system needs a reallocation of resources. Unfortunately, this is a large ship to turn. In the meantime, integrative practitioners can use their broad understanding of the patient to make recommendations that will lead to disease prevention and slow or reverse disease progression.

Integration

Integrative medicine involves using the best possible treatments from both CAM and allopathic medicine, based on the patient's individual needs and condition. This selection should be based in good science and neither rejects conventional medicine nor uncritically accepts alternative practices. It integrates successes from both worlds and is tailored to the individual, using the safest, least invasive, most cost-effective approach while incorporating a holistic understanding of the individual.

CAM is not synonymous with integrative medicine. CAM is a collection of therapies, many of which have a similar holistic philosophy. Unfortunately, the Western system views these as tools that are simply added on to the current model, one that attempts to understand healing by studying the tools in the tool box. David Reilly said it well in an editorial in the *British Medical Journal*: "We are the artists hoping to emulate Michaelangelo's David only by studying the chisels that made it. Meantime, our statue is alive and struggling to get out of the stone."[11]

Integration involves a larger mission that calls for a restoration of the focus on health and healing based on the provider-patient relationship.

EDUCATION

The goal before us is to educate the system how to bring the art back to medicine. This will be done by studying not only the tools but also the process of healing. This involves emphasis on rapport building; history-taking that includes emotional, psychological, and spiritual aspects; and learning of the patient's belief system and culture. In providing education regarding integrative medicine, we need to divide the focus into two parts: foundational knowledge of how to facilitate health and healing, and critical assessment of the modalities that can help us do this (CAM). Once practitioners understand the art of healing, they will be able to use their relationships with patients to activate the healing response. For example, if we simply train a cardiologist to perform angioplasty, we have a technician. But if we teach the cardiologist to understand the process of healing, he or she is more likely to have better results with that tool. This foundation of knowledge requires education in some core areas (Table 1–2) that should be incorporated into every medical school curriculum.

Once the student has a good understanding of the "healing art" of medicine, focus can be turned to learning about areas of health and healing that are not usually covered in Western medical training (Table 1–3). In learning about them, the practitioner will be able to help build the bridge between the two worlds of conventional and complementary/alternative medicine, learning the language that will lead to integrative care.

Table 1–2. Core Concepts Regarding Education in Healing-Oriented Medicine

Healing-oriented medicine
Relationship-centered care
Philosophy of science
History of medicine
Cross-cultural medicine
Mind-body influences on health
Self-healing
Motivational interviewing
Spirituality

Table 1–3. Curricular Topics in Integrative Medicine

Systems of medicine such as traditional Chinese medicine, Ayurveda, and homeopathy
Nutritional medicine including dietary supplements
Manipulative medicine such as osteopathic and chiropractic
Energy medicine
Botanical medicine
Mind-body therapies such as hypnosis, guided imagery, and meditation
Physical activity/movement therapy
Functional medicine

Self-Care and Healing for the Provider

Unfortunately, our current medical system takes open-minded, idealistic, compassionate individuals and teaches them a narrow-minded way of life based on "scientific truth." Students come out of it burdened with a set of rules that set them up for failure and burnout. Little attention is focused on students' physical, emotional, and spiritual health. Even more, they become removed from their own feelings to better adapt to the training environment and workplace, leaving them less able to connect with those they serve. It is difficult to help someone along her or his path toward health if we have neglected looking at our own.

Integrative medicine provides space for this self-exploration, resulting in a balance and understanding that lead to health of the practitioner and a more rewarding professional career. We may never actually reach this balance, but it should always be consciously pursued. An excellent example of this can be learned from traditional Chinese medicine. Here the focus of therapy is based on returning the body to a state of balance that is health. Imagine you are in a sailboat starting at island A and you want to get to island B. As you set course, bad weather may push you astray. A traditional Chinese medicine practitioner would help you get back on course so you can reach your destination of island B (health). Until we look inward to help define our own balance, we will not understand what changes need to be made to reach the destination. Bad weather is inevitable, but the choices we make to adapt to it can result in better health.

Self-healing requires time for this process to unfold. At the University of Arizona Program in Integrative Medicine, physicians meet regularly with a facilitator to discuss and explore personal issues. This is accompanied by instruction in meditation that is used to decrease distracting thought, allowing deeper exploration of one's self. This process helps bring a better understanding of what is needed for the practitioner's own health so he or she can better help their patients with the same (see Chapter 94, Learning to Meditate).

COST SAVINGS FOR THE ECONOMY AND COMMUNITY

"One of the first duties of the physician is to educate the masses not to take medicine."

Sir William Osler

The benefits of pharmaceuticals, herbs, and supplements should not be understated. But our dependence on the "quick fix" has made us less self-reliant regarding matters of health. The focus in medicine should be on creating an environment in which the body needs as few of these fixes as possible, and people become less dependent on the medical system, not more. At the moment, there is much economic incentive for physicians to do the fixing and very little for them to do the lifestyle education that would reduce the need for expensive pills and procedures. Ornish and colleagues[12] showed how coronary heart disease can be reversed by incorporating lifestyle changes including nutrition, exercise, stress management, group psychosocial support, and smoking cessation. This is an excellent example of how an integrative approach can result in not only self-healing but also a great savings in morbidity and mortality and the money needed to treat them.

The beauty of the integrative concepts is that they transcend the examination room to include the community and society as a whole. The philosophy teaches us that health involves more than just ourselves but incorporates the community in which we live. Integrative medicine will succeed in improving not only monetary costs but also costs to society as a whole through its emphasis on these key areas.

• Healing-Oriented Approach

When the focus is on creating a balance of health and an improved quality of life, there is less need for expensive interventions owing to decreased incidence of disease. As described in Figure 1–2, barriers are removed so that the body can better fix itself. Helping the individual along this journey has a beneficial effect on those around them, creating a positive change throughout the community and the larger society.

• Relationship-Centered Care

Developing an understanding of the patient provides us with the information necessary to be better and more efficient diagnosticians. Allowing time and space to understand the patient's story decreases the need for expensive diagnostic tests when the problem may be better handled and understood with a compassionate ear. Medical providers and patients regain the joy and happiness that comes with more personalized care. The saying rings true that curing goes one way (provider to patient) while healing goes both ways.

• Using the Least Invasive and Least Toxic Therapies First

When able, the integrative practitioner uses the mildest therapy that will trigger positive change. In general, these therapies are less expensive and have less potential for toxic side effects.

• Matching Treatment Plan to the Patient's Beliefs and Culture

In our conventional medical system, we have traditionally pulled patients into our paradigm of thought, telling them what they need. This method is often necessary for acute illness, but for chronic conditions in which there is no "right" answer, we will be more effective by offering treatment plans that best match patients' belief systems. In this way, we can activate the internal healing response, a process that we know as the *placebo effect*. Instead of brushing this response off as a nuisance, the talented clinician uses it to enhance healing. The ability to integrate methods of healing from various cultures enables the clinician to better match the therapy to the individual. The art of medicine may lie in the clinician's ability to activate this response without deception, resulting in enhanced health and reduced cost.

• Use Integrative Philosophy to Strengthen Our Primary Care Model

Despite spending more on healthcare delivery than any nation in the world, the United States ranks 15th in quality among the top 25 industrialized countries, according to the 2000 World Health Report. Success of the higher-ranked countries comes from a strong primary care infrastructure.[13] White and Ernst[14] showed that those primary care providers that provided a range of CAM therapies had a reduced number of referrals and treatment costs. Unfortunately, not all CAM therapists are primary care providers, and the use of CAM without the direction and continuity of these clinicians will only further fragment care and increase costs. The key is to incorporate this integrative philosophy into medical education so that primary care is enhanced and CAM therapies can be used to better enable the provider to facilitate health.

THE FUTURE

The information age continues to increase the amount of data available regarding the variety of therapies available but also complicates how we apply them. Informed patients seek competent providers who can help them navigate the myriad of therapeutic options, particularly for conditions in which conventional approaches are not so effective. They demand scientifically trained providers who are knowledgeable about the body's innate healing mechanisms and who understand the role of lifestyle factors in creating health, including nutrition, the appropriate use of supplements, herbs, and other forms of treatment from osteopathic manipulation to Chinese and Ayurvedic practices. They seek providers who can understand the unique interplay of mind, body, and spirit to help them better understand what is needed to create their own balance of health. This requires a restructuring of medical training that involves more research and education regarding how the body heals and how the process can be facilitated.

The Consortium of Academic Health Centers for Integrative Medicine consists of leaders from a group of medical schools who meet annually to discuss ideas on how to foster the rational introduction of integrative medicine into medical education and practice. The goal is to admit new delegations until one fifth of the nation's 125 medical schools are represented. At this time, a significant voice will be organized to call for fundamental changes in the way physicians of the future are being trained (see Table 1–3).

There is also momentum to add a fourth year onto a primary care residency to allow further study of those curricular areas (discussed in Tables 1–2 and 1–3) that will respond to the public's demand for this type of care.

SUMMARY

The philosophy of health based on a balance of mind, body, and spirit is not new or unique to integrative medicine. This understanding has been around since the time of Aristotle. What we call it is not important but the underlying concepts are. It is time that the pendulum swings back to the middle where technology is used in the context of healing and focus is given to the complexity of the whole mind and body. One only needs to experience the beauty of a flower, a sunset, a poem, or a human being to appreciate that there is much more involved to being than a sum of the parts. Integrative medicine will provide the balance needed to create the best possible medicine for both the doctor and the patient. We will know that we are near this balance when the medicine of the future no longer needs the term *integrative* and is seen as simply "good medicine."

 ── *THERAPEUTIC REVIEW* ──────────────

Integrative medicine:
- *Emphasizes relationship-centered care.*
- *Develops an understanding of the patient's culture and beliefs to help facilitate the healing response.*
- *Focuses on the unique characteristics of the individual person based on the interaction of mind, body, spirit, and community.*

THERAPEUTIC REVIEW *continued*

- *Regards the patient as an active partner who takes personal responsibility for health.*
- *Focuses on prevention and maintenance of health with attention to lifestyle choices including nutrition, exercise, stress management, and emotional well-being.*
- *Encourages providers to explore their own balance of health that will allow them to better facilitate this change in their patients.*
- *Requires providers to act as educators, role models, and mentors to their patients.*
- *Uses natural, less invasive interventions before costly, invasive ones when possible.*
- *Uses an evidence-based approach from multiple sources of information to integrate the best therapy for the patient, be it conventional or complementary.*
- *Searches for and removes barriers that may be blocking the body's innate healing response.*
- *Sees compassion as always helpful, even when other therapies are not.*
- *Focuses on the research and understanding of the process of health and healing and how to facilitate it.*
- *Accepts that health and healing are unique to the individual and may differ for two people with the same disease.*
- *Works collaboratively with the patient and a team of interdisciplinary providers to improve the delivery of care.*
- *Maintains that healing is always possible, even when curing is not.*
- *Agrees that the job of the physician is to cure sometimes, heal often, support always (Hippocrates).*

References

1. Flexner A: Medical Education in the United States and Canada: A Report to the Carnegie Foundation for the Advancement of Teaching. New York, Carnegie Foundation, 1910.
2. Eisenberg DM, Kessler RC, Foster C, et al: Unconventional medicine in the United States—prevalence, costs and patterns of use. N Engl J Med 328:246–252, 1993.
3. Eisenberg D, Davis RB, Ettner SL, et al: Trends in alternative medicine use in the United States, 1990–1997: Results of a follow-up national survey. JAMA 280:1569–1575, 1998.
4. Lazarou J, Pomeranz BH, Corey PN: Incidence of adverse drug reactions in hospitalized patients. JAMA 279:1200–1205, 1998.
5. Brevoort P: The United States botanical market—an overview. Herbal Gram 36:49–57, 1996.
6. Astin JA: Why patients use alternative medicine: Results of a national study. JAMA 279:1548–1553, 1998.
7. National Center for Complementary and Alternative Medicine: http://NCCAM.nih.gov
8. Fallowfield LJ, Jenkins V, Brennan C, et al: Attitudes of patients to randomised clinical trial of cancer therapy. Eur J Cancer 34:1554–1559, 1998.
9. Snyderman R, Weil AT: Integrative Medicine: Bringing Medicine Back to its Roots. Unpublished, 2001.
10. Goldberg RM: What's happened to the healing process? Wall Street J, June 18, 1997, p A22.
11. Reilly D: Enhancing human healing. BMJ 322(7279):120–121, 2001.
12. Ornish D, Scherwitz LW, Billings JH, et al: Intensive lifestyle changes for reversal of coronary heart disease. JAMA 280:2001–2007, 1998.
13. Starfield B: Is US health really the best in the world? JAMA 284:483–485, 2000.
14. White AR, Ernst E: Economic analysis of complimentary medicine: A systemic review. Complement Ther Med 8:111–118, 2000.

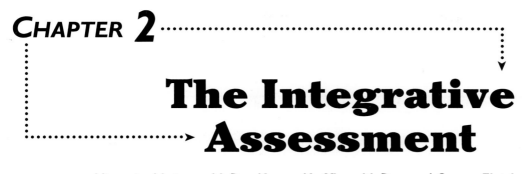

CHAPTER 2

The Integrative Assessment

Victoria Maizes, M.D., Karen Koffler, M.D., and Susan Fleishman, B.A.

DEVELOPING INSIGHT

An integrative medicine assessment serves as a prelude to understanding the whole human being—mind, body, and spirit. It is a complex "getting to know you" and is often initiated with just that beginning. We frequently open the visit by saying, "My goal is to get a sense of who you are as a person, to understand the important relationships and events in your life in addition to the medical condition that brings you in today." As physicians and healthcare professionals, we help patients to foster a deeper understanding of self. We believe that understanding can lead to real change, which can translate into physical, emotional, and spiritual healing.

Not surprisingly, given the breadth of integrative medicine, the questions we ask are far-reaching. Some of these questions have long been posed by psychiatrists and psychotherapists; others are asked by family doctors trained in behavioral medicine; and still others come from our work with ministers, Chinese medicine practitioners, and homeopaths.

Certain questions give people new insights.[1] Others help patients to recognize when their behaviors are consistent (or inconsistent) with their stated values and goals. When people become aware of discrepancies between their values and their behaviors it often catalyzes change (see Chapter 95, Motivational Interviewing Techniques). Evocative questions can reveal hidden truths and forgotten strengths. The process thus initiated may be useful in formulating a new approach to treatment and, indeed, a new approach to living.

Often, not all of the questions that follow are asked. In the flow of a history they often do not come out as a sequence. What commonly occurs is that by raising a particular issue, the patient becomes aware of underlying concerns, and the conversation follows that vein. It may be about relationship or work or exercise. And, of course, the questions are not really important. Rather, the answers evoked by the questions are important. Listening attentively, empathetically, and without interruption may be more valuable than raising particular questions.[2] Allowing patients to hear their own thoughts on intimate matters constitutes a potent medicine in itself.

These questions do not replace a conventional medical history. Rather, they augment traditional questions that focus on past medical, surgical, family, and social history. This expanded line of inquiry also serves to unearth information that is valuable for practitioners of alternative disciplines such as Chinese medicine and homeopathy. Thus, questions about vivid or recurrent dreams and reactions to heat and cold may elicit fears or phobias. By soliciting information that these practitioners use in the process of diagnosing and treating, we foster a more meaningful dialogue. Referrals become clearer.

In the interest of time efficiency, we use an intake form (Fig. 2–1), which is included here in abbreviated fashion. The actual form provides more room for the patient's answers.

> ### NOTE
> *The interview opens with three purposes: to gain an understanding of the person, the medical condition and the goals for the visit.*

We begin with broad questions such as: "Tell me about yourself. What have been pivotal events in your life? What are your roots? What are important features of your background?" These questions allow patients to begin to tell the story of themselves. Articulating one's story helps a person make connections. James Pennebaker, who has extensively studied the value of disclosure, describes this process as "organizing."[3] The story of an event often becomes shorter over time. The causes and effects become clearer, as do the implications. Expression of traumatic experiences by speaking or writing improves physical health, enhances immune function, and is associated with fewer medical visits.[4] The converse is true as well. Not sharing emotional experiences is a form of active inhibition that leads to long-term health problems.[5, 6]

HISTORY AND PRESENT ILLNESS

The interview proceeds to explore the medical

University of Arizona
Program in Integrative Medicine
Integrative Medicine Patient Intake Form

MR # _____

Name	Appointment Date	Appointment Time

○ ○ ○ **Please attach medical records as appropriate. Contact #** _____

Concern (Please rank by priority)	Onset	Frequency	Severity
Example: Headaches	June 1978	4 times/wk	mild/mod/severe
1.			
2.			
3.			
4.			
5.			
6.			

What are your goals for this visit?

_____

_____

_____

_____

_____

Illnesses

	Past	Present	List family members who have had these illnesses (siblings, parent, grandparent, children)
Heart Disease	○	○	_____
Hypertension	○	○	_____
Cancer	○	○	_____
Diabetes	○	○	_____
Lung Disease (asthma, etc.)	○	○	_____
Hepatitis	○	○	_____
Digestive	○	○	_____
Seizures	○	○	_____
Thyroid Disease	○	○	_____
Other _____	○	○	_____
Other _____	○	○	_____
Other _____	○	○	_____
Other _____	○	○	_____

Allergic reaction to medications

Medication	Reaction/Intolerances
_____	_____
_____	_____
_____	_____
_____	_____
_____	_____

Patient Intake Form 12 1 00

Figure 2–1 University of Arizona Program in Integrative Medicine Patient Intake Form (abbreviated). (© Program in Integrative Medicine, University of Arizona, June 2000.)

Operations		**Injuries**	
What	When	What	When
_____	_____	_____	_____
_____	_____	_____	_____
_____	_____	_____	_____
_____	_____	_____	_____

Comments

_____
_____
_____
_____

Occupation _____

What interests/hobbies do you have? _____

_____
_____

With whom do you live? (Include roommates, friends, partner, spouse, children, parents, relatives, pets)

Name	Age	Relationship	Name	Age	Relationship
_____	___	_____	_____	___	_____
_____	___	_____	_____	___	_____
_____	___	_____	_____	___	_____
_____	___	_____	_____	___	_____

What physical activity do you participate in? __

_____
_____
_____

What are the major stressors in your life? _____

_____
_____
_____

What do you do to relax? _____

_____
_____
_____

Religious affiliation, past and present _____

_____
_____
_____

What prior experiences have you had with alternative medicine? _____

_____
_____
_____

Patient Name _____   MRN _____
Patient Intake Form 12 1 00

Tobacco

○ Never used   ○ Smoked from age____ to ____ . ____ packs per day.

Alcohol

○ Never used   ○ Estimated drinks per day ____ .

Other drugs

○ Never used   ○ Frequency ____ .

What medications are you taking now? (Include prescription and over-the-counter drugs.)

Medication	Reason	When started	Dosage Per Day	Cost
_____	_____	_____	_____	_____
_____	_____	_____	_____	_____
_____	_____	_____	_____	_____
_____	_____	_____	_____	_____
_____	_____	_____	_____	_____

What vitamins/mineral/supplements are you taking now?

Brand or Other Name (Manufacturer) *Example: St. John's wort (Nature's Way)*	Reason *Feeling down*	When Started *2 months ago*	Dosage Per Day *3 caps*	Cost *15.00/30*
Brand or Other Name (Manufacturer)	Reason	When Started	Dosage Per Day	Cost
Brand or Other Name (Manufacturer)	Reason	When Started	Dosage Per Day	Cost
Brand or Other Name (Manufacturer)	Reason	When Started	Dosage Per Day	Cost
Brand or Other Name (Manufacturer)	Reason	When Started	Dosage Per Day	Cost
Brand or Other Name (Manufacturer)	Reason	When Started	Dosage Per Day	Cost
Brand or Other Name (Manufacturer)	Reason	When Started	Dosage Per Day	Cost
Brand or Other Name (Manufacturer)	Reason	When Started	Dosage Per Day	Cost
Brand or Other Name (Manufacturer)	Reason	When Started	Dosage Per Day	Cost
Brand or Other Name (Manufacturer)	Reason	When Started	Dosage Per Day	Cost
Brand or Other Name (Manufacturer)	Reason	When Started	Dosage Per Day	Cost
Brand or Other Name (Manufacturer)	Reason	When Started	Dosage Per Day	Cost
Brand or Other Name (Manufacturer)	Reason	When Started	Dosage Per Day	Cost
Brand or Other Name (Manufacturer)	Reason	When Started	Dosage Per Day	Cost
Brand or Other Name (Manufacturer)	Reason	When Started	Dosage Per Day	Cost
Brand or Other Name (Manufacturer)	Reason	When Started	Dosage Per Day	Cost
Brand or Other Name (Manufacturer)	Reason	When Started	Dosage Per Day	Cost

Patient Name _____   MRN _____

condition(s) for which the patient is seeking advice and the patient's goals for the visit. Understanding goals is critical. Is the patient hoping for a cure? Does the patient want to augment allopathic treatment or seek alternative approaches?

Social History

We inquire into the patient's social context. The goal is to gain a deeper understanding of the mesh of relationships that shape the patient's life. There may be issues that contribute intimately to the root of an illness. There may be wounds from the family of origin that need to be addressed. In addition, patterns of behavior are often uncovered. We ask: "Whom do you consider to be in your family? Is it your family of origin? Or is it a family that you have constructed from your church group, your neighbors, your coworkers, or your friends? What is (or was) the quality of your relationship with your parents? Similarly, what is the quality of your relationships with your siblings? How deeply involved are you in each other's lives? Has an illness of theirs affected you?"

Turning then to other relationships in the person's life, we explore the nature of those interactions. We learn whether there is a significant person in the patient's life. We ask: "What activities do you do together? (Do you do activities together?) Do you feel supported? Or, if you are alone, are you satisfied with that?" Similarly, we discover the nature of the parent-child relationship. We ask: "What type of relationship do you have with your children? How involved are you in their daily lives? Would you like that to change?" We ask, as well, about friendships: "What do your friendships mean to you? How do you acknowledge them?"

Occupational History

Working adults spend most of their waking time at work. There are people who love their work and who find in it a sense of fulfillment and purpose. We wonder what the cost to a person's health is when work is not a sustaining factor. The cost is likely to be magnified if one feels compromised by work in some way.[7] We ask: "Reflect for a moment on your job. To what extent are you defined by your job? Is your job an expression of who you are? If it is not, what would you like to be doing?"

Lifestyle

There are many subtle aspects to well-being that are not typically addressed in an allopathic interview. They involve the day-to-day experiences of our patients and reveal important clues in diagnosis, treatment, and referral. We ask: "Think about your energy levels. What times of day or what activities make you feel energized? What times of day or what activities make you feel depleted? When you feel depleted, what do you do? Do you nap? Eat? Are you satisfied with your levels of energy, or do you feel yourself dragging? What is your tendency toward illness? Do you get all your kids' colds? Do you have a fear of flying because you constantly pick up germs?" We inquire as well into patient sleeping patterns. We ask: "Do you sleep well? Do you wake up feeling refreshed and ready to go? If you nap, do you sleep briefly and feel refreshed?"

Preventive Health Care

Integrative medicine values prevention. This is broadly defined to include physical activity, nutrition, stress management, and spirituality, in addition to screening tests and immunizations. Begin to discover your patient's habits. "You are what you eat" is a homily. How you eat and with whom you eat may also be important. We ask: "What is your eating pattern? Do you graze throughout the day, or do you eat defined meals? Who prepares your food? Do you eat only when you are hungry? When you eat, what part of you are you feeding? Are you conscious of what you crave? Do you share your meals with someone?" Similarly, we discover the relationship with physical activity. We ask: "What kind of relationship do you have with your body? Does the word exercise make you cringe or feel guilty? Or is exercise something you enjoy? Do you exercise regularly? Do you hike, garden, or play golf? How has this activity benefited you?"

Stress and Coping Strategies

We live in a stressful society that does not support relaxation and relaxing behaviors. Dean Ornish has said that the hardest thing for patients to follow in his program is not the restrictive diet or the daily exercise but rather the relaxation program![8] We validate our patients' taking time to care for themselves in this way. We ask: "What are sources of stress in your life? Are they financial or job related or in your family? What are your coping strategies or practices to get through stress? How do you relax? How do you recharge? Do you meditate? Breathe? Exercise? Watch television? Do you take time regularly to recharge?"

Spirituality

Spiritual strength and religious connections help many patients get through a variety of difficult or stressful events. Religious bonds are a source of richness in many people's lives. The literature supports the connection between religion and mental and physical health.[9] Physicians have not historically addressed this aspect of patients' lives, although patients say they wish their doctors would do so. [10] We ask: "Where do you derive your strength during difficult times? How do you feel connected to the family of life? What gives your life purpose and meaning?" Other useful questions are: "What does spirituality imply to you? Were you ever involved in a faith community?"

Finally, we seek to discover and to allow our patients to articulate their feelings about things that give them real joy and pleasure. Patients shift as they discuss these things. They feel good about themselves. They remind themselves of who they are beyond their disease. Ask: "What is it that you love?[11] And how is that manifested regularly? If it is art, are you painting or sculpting or playing music? What do you do well? What are your strengths? What would your family and your friends say they find most wonderful about you? What is your personal gift that you bring to the world?" (See Chapter 102, Spiritual Assessment and Care.)

Past Medical History

The conventional past medical history (PMH) can be adapted with this approach as well. When we take the medication history, we ask: "How do you feel about taking pills? Is it an effort? Do you miss doses?" As you learn of the patient's medical diagnosis, ask: "What impact has it had on your life? What insight has it given you? What does your intuition tell you about what has contributed to this illness? What motivates you to fight? What are your expectations or hopes?" It is amazing how often patients have a sense of what has caused an illness and what they need to do to heal. As healthcare professionals we can validate their chosen path. And guided by in-depth questioning, patients can clarify what is really important to them.

Helpful Questions for Special Situations

When a patient is dying
How long do you expect to live?
How would you like to look back at your last months or years?
Have you ever taken the time to review your life? Would you like to do it together?

Questions that touch on the mind-body connection
What are you experiencing?
What words would help me to know what you are feeling?

When the answer is "pain like a knife in my back" or "a heavy weight on my head," ask:
How do these words fit into your life?

When a patient cries
If those tears could speak, what would they say?

We are struck by how often in an interview such as this, change happens. This may be due to the power of disclosure. Hearing oneself articulate powerful aspects of one's life story can lead to change. Empathic listening alone may be sufficient to create change.

We have found, as practitioners of integrative medicine, that this approach serves us in several important ways. It allows individuals a chance to reflect deeply on their lives; in so doing, the potential for them to make life changes is enhanced. It allows physicians to gain insight into the patients who seek their help and into how patients' responses can be used to facilitate healing. The method of inquiry translates directly to the treatment and lifestyle recommendations that we make and to our ability to reflect about the whole person—rather than simply arriving at a diagnosis. Dialogue with patients gives us fertile ground for communication with other practitioners. Finally, the integrative assessment serves us in a deeper level by restoring soul to our work. The connections we foster nourish who we are and what we have to offer as physicians and fellow human beings.

References

1. Rogers CR: On Becoming a Person. Boston, Houghton Mifflin, 1995.
2. Remen RN: Kitchen Table Wisdom. New York, Riverhead Books, 1996.
3. Dienstfrey H: Disclosure and health: An interview with James W. Pennebaker. Adv Mind-Body Med 1999; 15:161–195.
4. Berry DS, Pennebaker JW: Nonverbal and verbal emotional expression and health. Psychother Psychosom 1993; 59:11–19.
5. Cole SW, Kemeny ME, Taylor SE, Visscher BR. Elevated physical health risk among gay men who conceal their homosexual identity. Health Psychol 1996; 15: 243–251.
6. Kagan J, Reznick JS, Snidman N: Biological bases of childhood shyness. Science 1988; 24: 167–172.
7. Willich SN, Lowel H, Lewis M, et al: Weekly variation of acute myocardial infarction. Increased Monday risk in the working population. Circulation 1994; 90:87–93.
8. Ornish D: Oral communication, February 1998.
9. Ellison CG, Levin JS: The religion-health connection: Evidence, theory, and future directions. Health Ed Behav 1998; 25:700–720.
10. Ehman JW, Ott BB, Short TH, et al: Do patients want physicians to inquire about their spiritual or religious beliefs if they become gravely ill? Arch Intern Med 1999; 159:1803–1806.
11. Muller W: How Then Shall We Live? Four Simple Questions That Reveal the Beauty and Meaning of Our Lives. New York, Bantam Books, 1996.

PART *II*

Integrative Approach to Disease

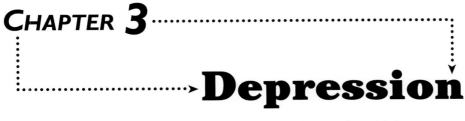

CHAPTER 3

Depression

Craig Schneider, M.D.

There are many subtypes of depressive disorders, yet studies suggest that the major subtypes of depression, including major depressive disorder, dysthymia, recurrent brief depression, and minor depression, are actually quite fluid, with patients moving from one subtype to another throughout the clinical course. Depression can thus more accurately be considered to represent a spectrum of disease, rather than to comprise discrete subtypes.[1] It is also important to recognize that many people seen in primary care settings do not meet the diagnostic criteria for many of the well-known depressive disorders set forth in the *Diagnostic and Statistical Manual of Mental Disorders,* edition 4 (DSM-IV), but rather fall under the DSM-IV category "depressive disorder not otherwise specified (NOS)."

PATHOPHYSIOLOGY

Despite the ubiquity of depression, we still do not fully understand what is probably a very complicated, multifactorial etiology. The *stress-diathesis* model of illness emphasizes that significant emotional, social, and environmental antecedents such as the loss of a family member or a romantic or professional disappointment, as well as genetic and acquired vulnerabilities, are clearly involved. Significant stressors appear to be more frequently involved with initial episodes. In recurrent depression, vulnerability appears to increase as episodes become less and less related to "stress" and more autonomous in a process known as *kindling*.[2] With repeated episodes of illness (kindling), central nervous system dysfunction evidently increases, as manifested by hypercortisolemia, decreased slow wave (restful) sleep, and increased rapid eye movement or REM (arousing) sleep. It is now hypothesized that the biochemical impact of states of depression may be "stored" in neurons via changes in the activity of gene transcription factors and neuronal growth factors.[3] The common final pathway (some investigators would say primary) is the biochemical imbalance of biogenic amines or neurotransmitters (i.e., serotonin, norepinephrine, gamma-aminobutyric acid [GABA], dopamine, and so on and their relationship to their respective receptors in the brain. Potential effects on neurotransmitters include impaired synthesis, increased breakdown, and increased pump uptake, with consequent alterations in neurotransmitter levels. Successful pharmaceutical approaches to treating depression involve correction of these altered neurotransmitter levels and of neurotransmitter receptor interactions.

Various psychological theories of depression exist to explain the illness, including *learned helplessness*, which sees depression as the result of habitual feelings of pessimism, and *helplessness*. Of interest with this regard, dogs taught to be helpless are noted to have alterations in neurotransmitter levels, which normalize on being re-educated in control.

PHYSICAL ACTIVITY

More than 1000 trials have examined the relationship between exercise and depression. Well designed trials demonstrate that regularly performed exercise is as effective an antidepressant as psychotherapy, which is as effective as pharmaceutical approaches are.[4] Both aerobic and anaerobic activities are effective.[5] Exactly why exercise relieves depression is not understood, but the explanation is probably multifactorial. Although exercise may increase levels of serotonin and endorphins, its benefits have been reported even when naloxone is administered to block endorphins. One important aspect may be that exercise requires that patients take an active role in their recovery and also generally leads to improved self-esteem and self-confidence as body strength and self-image improve. Exercise may also provide a "time out" period—an opportunity to leave troubles behind temporarily. It is of interest that participation in an exercise program, rather than the level of fitness attained, appears to be the most important condition for antidepressive effect.[6] According to Fox, "Moderate regular exercise should be considered as a viable means of treating depression and anxiety and improving mental well-being in the general public."[7] The combination of exercise and antidepressant pharmacotherapy is superior to exercise alone,[5] but exercise appears to be superior in maintaining therapeutic benefit.[8]

Because exercise is inexpensive, has proven benefits beyond the treatment of depression, with a low occurrence of side effects, and is available to everyone, I tend to think of it as the essential foundation on which other, more specific modalities may fit as the situation dictates.

The appropriate exercise prescription depends on the specific patient's health, level of fitness, and interests (see Chapter 86, Writing an Exercise Prescription). For more seriously depressed patients and those with significant psychomotor retardation, the exercise regimen should be started as adjunctive therapy as soon as symptoms begin to abate.

NUTRITION

Caffeine and Simple Sugars

A small controlled trial found that eliminating refined sucrose and caffeine from the diets of people experiencing unexplained depression resulted in improvements by 1 week, and symptoms worsened when patients were challenged with these substances but not with placebo challenge.[9] Regular high-level caffeine consumption (>750 mg daily) appears to be associated with depression.[10, 11] Examination of the diets of people suffering from depression reveals increased consumption of sucrose compared with the general population.[12]

A trial eliminating caffeine and simple sugars is warranted.

Alcohol

Although consumption of alcohol transiently increases the turnover of serotonin, the long-term result is diminished levels of serotonin and catecholamines.[13] Discontinuation of alcohol consumption is warranted.

Omega-3 Fatty Acids

Epidemiologic data suggest that a deficiency of omega-3 fatty acids or an imbalance in the ratio of omega-6 and omega-3 fatty acids correlates positively with increased rates of depression.[14] Because dietary polyunsaturated fatty acids (PUFAs) and cholesterol are the major determinants of membrane fluidity in synaptic membranes involved in the synthesis, binding, and uptake of neurotransmitters, it is hypothesized that alterations may lead to abnormalities contributing to increased rates of depression.[15] Clinical trials have not examined this possibility, but indirect evidence suggests that correction of the ratio of omega-6 and omega-3 fatty acids may be helpful. Because these substances are safe and have other demonstrated benefits (cardiovascular health), the level of evidence for recommending increased intake need not be high. Recommended consumption of cold water fish (herring, mackerel, salmon, sardines) is two to three servings each week. Vegetarian alternatives include flaxseed oil or ground flaxseed meal (2 tablespoons daily) and a small handful of walnuts each day (see Chapter 84, The Anti-Inflammatory Diet).

DIETARY SUPPLEMENTS

The B Vitamins

Folic acid and vitamin B_{12} are intimately linked with the synthesis of S-adenosyl methionine (SAMe), and each functions as a "methyl donor," carrying and donating methyl molecules to a variety of brain chemicals, including neurotransmitters. Although large-scale clinical studies are lacking, a trial of a B-complex vitamin is advisable, particularly for elderly patients, in whom B_{12} deficiency is common, and for persons with sub-optimal diets. Vitamin B_6 is essential in the manufacture of serotonin, and B_6 levels have been found to be low in many depressed patients, particularly those taking oral contraceptive pills or replacement estrogen (Premarin).[14]

Dosage. Vitamin B Complex 100, one tablet daily (contains approximately 100 mg each of the major B vitamins).

NOTE

Dosages of vitamin B_6 as low as 200 mg daily may result in neurotoxicity.

Folic Acid

Studies have shown borderline or low folate levels in 31% to 35% of depressed adults. A recent study identified a biosubgroup of depressed patients with folate deficiency and impaired methylation and monoamine neurotransmitter metabolism.[17] In fact, depression is the most common symptom of a folate deficiency.[18] Patients with low levels of folate also appear to respond more poorly to therapy with selective serotonin reuptake inhibitors (SSRIs).[18] Remember to check serum vitamin B_{12} levels and supplement as needed when giving folate, to avoid masking a vitamin B_{12} deficiency.

Dosage. Folate 400 to 800 μg daily is sufficient to prevent deficiency, although doses of 5 to 20 mg daily have been used in studies.

Precautions. High doses of folic acid have been reported to cause altered sleep patterns, vivid dreaming, irritability, exacerbation of seizure frequency, GI disturbances, and a bitter taste in the mouth.

S-Adenosyl Methionine

SAMe (see Fig. 3–1) is the major "methyl donor" in the body and is involved in the metabolism of norepinephrine, dopamine, and serotonin. Its synthesis

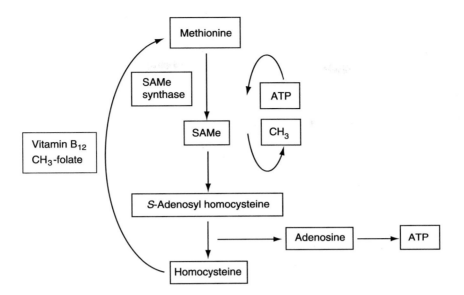

Figure 3–1. *S*-Adenosyl methionine (SAMe) metabolism. ATP, adenosine triphosphate; CH₃, methyl group.

is impaired in depression, and supplementation results in increased brain monoamine levels, enhanced binding of neurotransmitters to receptors, and increased brain cell membrane fluidity. Although larger trials are warranted, multiple open and randomized controlled trials suggest that SAMe is an effective natural antidepressant. It is generally well tolerated and has an onset of action more rapid than that of standard pharmaceutical antidepressants.[19] Because of this characteristic, it is sometimes useful to begin SAMe concurrently with another dietary supplement or pharmaceutical approach to therapy of depression that has been more thoroughly studied, and then taper the dosage of SAMe to zero as the other antidepressant begins to take effect. The most stable oral form appears to be 1,4-butanedisulfonate, which is stable for up to 2 years at room temperature (distributed by Nature Made [Pharmavite] and GNC). SAMe is relatively free of side effects and does not have known cardiac, anticholinergic, or orthostatic effects.

NOTE

SAMe may cause hypomania or mania in patients with bipolar disease and should be avoided in this population.

Dosage. Initial treatment of depression may require 1600 mg daily given in equal doses, followed by maintenance dosage of 200 mg twice daily. I recommend starting with 200 mg once or twice daily to minimize GI side effects, and then titrating upward to effect over 1 to 2 weeks.

Precautions. High dosages can cause nausea, vomiting, flatulence, and diarrhea.

Hydroxytryptophan

Hydroxytryptophan (5-HTP) is the intermediate in the metabolism of tryptophan to serotonin. A number of open and random controlled trials suggest that 5-HTP is as effective as standard antidepressants are.[16, 20] Tryptophan itself appeared promising as a treatment for insomnia and depression but was removed from the market when a contaminated batch was linked to an outbreak of eosinophilia myalgia syndrome (EMS) in people with abnormal activation of the kynurenin pathway. Although 5-HTP is not metabolized along this pathway, case reports now link 5-HTP to an EMS-like illness. The suspected culprit is a family of contaminants known as peak X that is commonly found in commercially available 5-HTP.[21] Because of the uncertainty surrounding 5-HTP at this time, it seems advisable to avoid recommending its use pending further information. Case reports of seizures in Down syndrome and of dermatomyositis in conjunction with the use of carbidopa have appeared in the literature. Use with other serotonin agonists is not recommended, to avoid serotonin syndrome.

Dosage. 100 to 200 mg three times daily, enteric-coated 5-HTP 20 minutes before meals.

BOTANICAL MEDICINE

St. John's Wort (*Hypericum perforatum*)

The exact mechanism of action of St. John's wort remains unknown, but this botanical affects serotonin, dopamine, norepinephrine, and GABA reuptake inhibition and also in vitro monoamine oxidase inhibition and L-glutamate.[22] It also appears to inhibit interleukin-6 and increase cortisol production, which may result in an additional indirect antidepressant effect.[23] Clinical effects are probably the result of a combined contribution of multiple mechanisms, each individually too weak to account for the action.[24] St. John's wort has been a licensed prescription medicine in Germany since 1984, and nearly twice the number of prescriptions are written for it as for all other antidepressants in that country. One recently published trial found that St. John's wort was not effective for treating severe major depression,[35] but as a whole, the body of evidence suggests that St. John's wort is as effective as conventional antidepressant medications are in the treatment of mild to moderate depression.[25] Longer trials and studies examining its use in severe depression are warranted.

Indication. Mild to moderate depression.

Dosage. St. John's wort 900 mg daily given in 3 equal doses. Choose a product standardized to a minimum of 2% to 5% hyperforin or 0.3% hypericin. I recommend Perika (Willmar Schwabe; imported by Nature's Way). Once clinical improvement has been obtained, consider twice-daily dosing. Up to 2 months may be required before full effects are noted.

Precautions. Although side effects are fewer than with current pharmacologic antidepressants, such effects can include gastrointestinal upset, allergic reaction, fatigue, dry mouth, restlessness, and constipation.

Caution. Probable cytochrome P450 induction by St. John's wort requires that care be taken when prescribing this in the setting of other drugs metabolized along this pathway. Reports of interactions with indinavir, cyclosporine, digoxin, theophylline, possibly oral contraceptives, and warfarin have been reported. The MAOI-inhibiting effect of St. John's wort appears to be clinically insignificant in vitro when this botanical is used in recommended doses.[22] Avoid use concurrently with SSRIs, and in pregnancy and lactation. High doses may predispose the patient to photodermatitis.

Ginkgo biloba

The most prescribed herb in Europe, ginkgo is considered "safe and effective" by the German Commission E for treatment of cerebral insufficiency. It also has been found to be useful in treating elderly patients with depression related to organic brain dysfunction. In a double-blinded placebo-controlled trial, 40 elderly patients (51 to 78 years of age) with depression were maintained on standard drug treatment to which they were unresponsive, and the treatment group was additionally given 240 mg of gingko daily. After 1 month, Hamilton Depression Scale scores of the treatment group dropped by 50%, whereas those of the control group dropped only 7%.[26] Ginkgo can be used as an adjunctive agent in selected elderly patients who are not responding satisfactorily to conventional therapy.

Indication. *Ginkgo biloba* is given as an adjunctive agent for treatment-resistant depression in patients older than 50 years.

Dosage. 40 to 80 mg three times daily of an extract standardized to 24% ginkgo flavonglycosides and 6% terpenoids. Many patients respond within 2 to 3 weeks, but it may take up to 3 months for full effects to be noted.

Precautions. Rare cases of mild gastrointestinal upset, headache, and allergic skin reactions have been reported. Ginkgo has an antiplatelet effect, so caution should be taken in prescribing this to patients on anticoagulants.

MIND-BODY MEDICINE

Psychotherapy

"Depression-specific" psychotherapies are designed to provide acute, time-limited interventions. They are present-oriented and pragmatic, focusing on depression and issues considered relevant to both its onset and its perpetuation.[27] The combination of psychotherapy and pharmacotherapy may be the most effective approach for treating mild to moderate depression that does not respond to other, more conservative approaches. Primary care physicians can certainly provide limited, supportive psychotherapy of this type at frequent visits necessary to monitor effectiveness of medications.[28]

Cognitive therapy (CT) is the most-studied psychotherapeutic approach to major depression. The physician or the therapist assists the patient in replacing negative patterns of thinking with a more positive, realistic approach. Multiple studies have demonstrated the equivalency of this modality to rigorous antidepressant medication regimens.[27] One controlled trial demonstrated that monthly CT was as effective as antidepressant medications were, for prophylaxis against recurrence over 6 months, but not all studies support this.

Interpersonal therapy (IPT) focuses on identifying and renegotiating interpersonal problem areas. It has also compared favorably with antidepressant medication in controlled trials, both as single-modality and combined therapy, as well as for prophylaxis against recurrence.[27]

Other Mind-Body Therapies

Although well-designed clinical studies investigating the role of meditation, hypnosis, and imagery in the treatment of depression have been limited, centuries of experience in traditional healing systems (e.g., Ayurvedic, Tibetan) support this kind of therapeutic approach. In my experience, these mind-body techniques are often extremely useful therapeutic adjuncts that appear to enhance the efficacy of other treatments. Emerging data suggest that relaxation therapy, including yoga involving breath work, also appears promising.[29] Recommend that interested patients explore one of these approaches (see Chapter 91, Prescribing Relaxation Techniques).

ACUPUNCTURE

Acupuncture has been used for centuries in Asia for the treatment of virtually all known disease states. The exact mechanism of action is unknown, but human and animal studies have demonstrated that the stimulation of certain acupuncture points can alter neurotransmitter levels.[30] The United Nations World Health Organization (WHO) recognizes acupuncture as effective in treating mild to moderate depression. Case series indicate that acupuncture is promising for treating depression; this finding is supported by several uncontrolled and controlled studies. Electroacupuncture has proved as effective as amitriptyline in two random controlled trials of 5 and 6 weeks' duration. Follow-up at 2 and 4 years revealed no difference in rates of recurrence.[31]

Appropriate use of acupuncture requires training. Referrals may be located by contacting the American Academy of Medical Acupuncture (AAMA) at www.medicalacupuncture.org, for medical and osteopathic trained acupuncturists, or the National Certification Commission for Acupuncture and Oriental Medicine (NCCAOM) at www.nccaom.org, which licenses other acupuncturists.

PHARMACEUTICALS

Antidepressants are believed to work by inhibiting the degradation and reuptake of neurotransmitters important in regulating psychological and neurovegetative function (i.e., serotonin, norepinephrine, dopamine), thus increasing their availability at the synaptic level. Newer theories suggest they may also mediate intracellular signaling systems affecting neurotrophic factors vital to the functioning of neuronal systems involved in mood regulation.

Selective Serotonin Reuptake Inhibitors and Mixed Reuptake Blockers

Safety in overdose and side effect profiles for SSRIs and mixed reuptake blockers are greatly improved over those for cyclics and monoamine oxidase inhibitors (MAOIs). Be aware that there is emerging concern over long-term effects of SSRIs, including uncommon but serious neurologic sequelae including seizures and extrapyramidal symptoms[32] and worsening of long-term outcomes despite effective short-term control.[33]

Precautions. Nausea, cramping, agitation, insomnia, headache, decreased libido, delayed ejaculation, erectile dysfunction, and anorgasmia have been reported in patients taking SSRIs. Gastrointestinal side effects are more pronounced with sertraline (Zoloft) but may be minimized by taking the drug with food and water. Fluoxetine (Prozac) is generally the most activating. Paroxetine (Paxil) has mild anticholinergic properties. Venlafaxine (Effexor) has side effects similar to those of the other SSRIs but may cause serious hypertension over time. Citalopram (Celexa) seems to have the fewest side effects and least impact on the cytochrome P450 enzyme system.

Tricyclic Antidepressants

Tricyclic antidepressants (TCAs) have significant side effects (anticholinergic effects, weight gain, and cardiac dysrhythmias) and can be lethal in overdoses as small as an average 10-day supply.

Heterocyclic Antidepressants

Heterocyclic antidepressants are much safer than TCAs in overdose and have side effect profiles that make them useful in specific clinical circumstances. Amoxapine (Asendin) is useful in treating psychotic depression. Trazodone (Desyrel) is highly sedating and is useful in low dosage (25 to 50 mg qhs) when used in combination with SSRIs. Bupropion (Wellbutrin) is highly stimulating and may be a good option for patients wishing to discontinue smoking tobacco; also has less effect on sexual function but is associated with seizures in underweight people. Nefazodone (Serzone) has anxiolytic properties and may be useful in patients who develop anxiety and insomnia while taking SSRIs. Mirtazapine (Remeron) increases appetite and tends to cause weight gain, which may be desirable in some cases.

Monoamine Oxidase Inhibitors

MAOIs have significant side effects and can be lethal in overdose. Orthostatic hypotension, weight gain, and sexual dysfunction are common. Tyramine-containing foods must be avoided, as the interaction results in headache and significant elevations in blood pressure. Patients should wait at least 2 weeks after discontinuing therapy with a drug from another class of antidepressant medication before starting MAOI therapy.

ELECTROCONVULSIVE THERAPY

Electroconvulsive therapy (ECT) reportedly is effective in achieving remission in 90% of patients

Table 3–1. Drugs and Supplements Used in Treatment of Depression

Drug/Supplement	Initial Dose (mg*)	Range (mg/d*)	Frequency
Vitamin B Complex 100	1 tablet		qd
Folic acid	400 μg	400–800 μg	qd
SAMe (1,4-butanedisulfonate)	200	200–800	bid
Hydroxytryptophan (5-HTP) (enteric-coated)	100	100–200	tid
St. John's wort (standardized to 5% hyperforin)	300		tid
Ginkgo biloba (standardized to 24% ginkgo flavonglycosides and 6% terpenoids)	40	40–80	tid
Selective Serotonin Reuptake Inhibitors and Mixed Reuptake Blockers			
Fluoxetine (Prozac)	20	20–80	qd (AM)
Sertraline (Zoloft)	50	50–200	qd
Paroxetine (Paxil)	20	20–50	qd (AM)
Fluvoxamine (Luvox)	50	50–300	qd (hs)
Citalopram (Celexa)	20	20–40	qd
Venlafaxine (Effexor)	75	75–375	bid
Extended-release	37.5	75–375	qd (hs)
Heterocyclic Antidepressants			
Nefazodone (Serzone)	200	200–600	bid
Bupropion (Wellbutrin)	200	200–450	tid†
Sustained-release	150	150–450	bid
Mirtazapine (Remeron)	15	15–60	qd (hs)

* Unless otherwise indicated.
† Initial dose: 100 mg bid for 3 days; then 100 mg tid.

with depression within 7 to 14 days. Generally, ECT is reserved for suicidal, psychotic, or catatonic patients. It is also helpful in cases refractory to other treatment modalities. Use with caution in patients with recent myocardial infarction, cardiac arrhythmia, or intracranial space-occupying lesions. Expect transient postictal confusion, and anterograde and retrograde memory impairment.

Dosage. ECT requires referral to an experienced treatment center but generally involves treatment 3 times weekly for up to 4 weeks, until symptoms abate.

OTHER THERAPIES TO CONSIDER

Transcranial magnetic stimulation uses topographically selective mild electrical stimulation to left anterolateral prefrontal cortex. It requires no general anesthesia and has minimal side effects. It is currently being studied as a promising alternative to ECT.

Phototherapy is commonly used for patients with seasonal affective disorder (SAD) but may be useful as an adjunctive modality added to pharmacotherapy in both unipolar and bipolar depression.[34] Consider recommending 30 minutes of bright, white (full-spectrum) light daily from special bulbs, lamps, or light-boxes. Therapeutic lights are available from a number of manufacturers (e.g., Bio-Brite, Inc., telephone 800 621-LITE [800 621-5483], www.biobriteinc.com, and The SunBox Co., telephone 800 548-3968, www.sunboxco.com).

Estrogen replacement has been demonstrated to reduce symptoms in perimenopausal and postmenopausal women with depression in a number of small studies. Consider recommending hormone replacement therapy (HRT).

THERAPEUTIC REVIEW

The following three steps are recommended for initial management of all patients with depressive symptoms:

1. Remove exacerbating factors.
   Review current medications and supplements that could be contributing to depression, and consider decreasing dosages or discontinuing drugs that are suspect if they are not vital to the patient's well-being.

2. Improve nutrition.
   Sharply decrease intake of refined sugar (sucrose), caffeine, and alcohol.
   Encourage a diet rich in omega-3 fatty acids. Recommend 2 to 3 servings of cold-water fish (salmon, herring, mackerel, sardines) each week, 2 tablespoons of ground flaxseed or flaxseed oil daily, or a small handful of walnuts each day.

3. Institute physical activity.

Encourage daily aerobic (e.g., walking, jogging, cycling) or anaerobic (weight lifting) exercise. Explore options and help patients select activities they feel might be enjoyable. Emphasize starting slowly and setting realistic short-term goals. Gradually increase to an ideal exercise prescription (see Chapter 86, Writing an Exercise Prescription).

Dietary Supplements and Botanicals

- *Vitamin B 100 Complex and 400 µg of additional folic acid daily.*
- *St. John's wort: 900 mg daily in 3 equal doses. Choose a product standardized to a minimum of 2% to 5% hyperforin or 0.3% hypericin. If no improvement is seen after 4 to 6 weeks, consider switching to SAMe or a pharmaceutical antidepressant. Concurrent psychotherapy is recommended if this approach is acceptable to the patient.*
- *SAMe: Start at 200 mg once or twice daily to minimize gastrointestinal side effects; then titrate upward to effect over 1 to 2 weeks. Initial treatment of depression may require 1600 mg daily given in 2 equal doses, followed by a maintenance dosage of 200 mg twice daily. If recommending a pharmaceutical antidepressant, consider using SAMe initially along with it to minimize the latency period. SAMe may be withdrawn after 4 to 6 weeks. If SAMe is given without a pharmaceutical antidepressant, consider switching to another agent if no resolution of symptoms is noted after 2 weeks. Concurrent psychotherapy is recommended if this approach is acceptable to the patient.*

Psychotherapy

The combination of supportive psychotherapy with antidepressant supplements or pharmacotherapy is generally recommended. Primary care physicians can provide limited psychotherapy at frequent visits to monitor lifestyle modifications, dietary supplements, or drug therapy. Alternatively, referral for cognitive or interpersonal therapy is recommended.

Pharmaceuticals

If no improvement is obtained with the use of lifestyle modification measures and dietary supplements, discontinue the supplements and start a pharmaceutical antidepressant. All currently approved antidepressant drugs are equally effective and exhibit similar latency periods.[28] Choice of an SSRI, mixed reuptake blocker, or heterocyclic antidepressant should be guided by matching the most appropriate side effect profile to each patient's symptoms. Continue treatment for at least 6 months after improvement and consider full dosage maintenance if there is a history of recurrent depression.

If only a partial response has occurred at 6 weeks, either change the class of antidepressant medication being used or continue the antidepressant and consider adding lithium carbonate 300 mg tid (necessitating experience in monitoring serum levels) or liothyronine sodium (Cytomel) 25 to 50 µg.

Consider referral to a psychiatrist if the patient remains refractory to treatment, is suicidal or psychotic, or requires psychiatric hospitalization and/or ECT.

References

1. Angst J, Sellaro R, Marikargas KR: Depressive spectrum diagnoses. Compr Psychiatry 41 (2 Suppl 1): 39–47, 2000.
2. Post RM: Transduction of psychosocial stress into the neurobiology of recurrent affective disorder. Am J Psychiatry 149:999–1010, 1992.
3. Duman R, Heninger G, Nestler E: A molecular and cellular theory of depression. Arch Gen Psychiatry 54:597–606, 1997.
4. Freemont J, Craighead LW: Aerobic exercise and cognitive therapy in the treatment of dysphoric moods. Cognit Ther Res 2:241–251, 1987.
5. Martinsen EW, Hoffart A, Solberg O: Comparing aerobic with nonaerobic forms of exercise in the treatment of clinical depression: a randomized trial. Compr Psychiatry 30:324–331, 1989.
6. Moore K: Exercise training as an alternative treatment for depression among older adults. Alternative Therapies 4(1):48–56, 1998.
7. Fox KR: The influence of physical activity on mental well-being. Public Health Nutrition 2(3A):411–418, 1999.
8. Babyak M, Blumenthal JA, Herman S, et al: Exercise treatment for major depression: maintenance of therapeutic benefit at 10 months. Psychosom Med 62:633–638, 2000.
9. Kreitsch K, et al: Prevalance, presenting symptoms, and psychological characteristics of individuals experiencing a diet-related mood disturbance. Behav Ther 19:593-604, 1988.
10. Gilliland K, Bullick W: Caffeine: A potential drug of abuse. Av Alcohol Subst Abuse 3(1–2):53–73, 1984.
11. Greden J: Caffeine and tobacco dependence. In Kaplan HI, Sadock BJ (eds): Comprehensive Textbook of Psychiatry. 4th ed. Baltimore, Williams & Wilkins, 1985, pp. 1026–1033.

12. Christensen L, Somers S: Comparison of nutrient intake among depressed and nondepressed individuals. Int J Eat Disord 20(1):105–109, 1996.

13. Goodwin FK: Alcoholism research: delivering on the promise. Public Health Rep 103(6):569–574, 1988.

14. Bruinsma KA, Taren DL: Dieting, essential fatty acid intake, and depression. Nutrition Reviews 58(4):98–108, 2000.

15. Maes M, et al: Fatty acid composition in major depression: decreased omega 3 fractions in cholesteryl esters and increased C20:4 omega 6/C20:5 omega 3 ratio in cholesteryl esters and phospholipids. J Affect Disord 38:35–46, 1996.

16. Murray M, Pizzorno J: Affective disorders. In Pizzorno J, Murray M (eds): Textbook of Natural Medicine. 2nd ed. New York, Churchill Livingstone, 1999, pp. 1039–1057.

17. Bottiglieri T, Laundy M, Crellin R, et al: Homocysteine, folate, methylation, and monoamine metabolism in depression. J Neurol Neurosurg Psychiatry 69:228–232, 2000.

18. Alpert JE, Fava M: Nutrition and depression: the role of folate. Nutrition Reviews 55(5):145–149, 1997.

19. Bressa GM: SAMe as antidepressant: meta-analysis of clinical studies. Acta Neurol Scand Suppl 154:7–14, 1994.

20. Meyers S: Use of neurotransmitter precursors for treatment of depression. Alternative Medicine Review 5(1):64–71, 2000.

21. Klarskov K, Johnson KL, Benson LM, et al: Eosinophilia-myalgia syndrome case–associated contaminants in commercially available 5-hydroxytryptophan. Adv Exp Med Biol 467:461–468, 1999.

22. Delle, et al: Abstract 90-56. Presented at the 6th World Congress of Biological Psychiatry, Nice, France, June 22–27, 1997.

23. Lake J: Psychotropic medications from natural products: a review of promising research and recommendations. Altern Ther 6:36–60, 2000.

24. Bennet DA Jr, Phun L, Polk JF, et al: Neuropharmacology of St. John's wort (Hypericum). Ann Pharmacother 32:1201–1208, 1998.

25. Linde K, Ramirez G, Mulrow CD, et al: St. John's wort for depression–an overview and meta-analysis of randomized clinical trials. BMJ 313:253–258, 1996.

26. Schubert H, Halama P: Depressive episode primarily unresponsive to therapy in elderly patients: Efficacy of *Ginkgo biloba* extract Egb 761 in combination with antidepressants. Geriatics Forsch 3:45–53.

27. Frank E, Thase ME: Natural history and preventative treatment of recurrent mood disorders. Ann Rev Med 50:453–458, 1999.

28. Rakel RE: Depression. Prim Care 26:211–224, 1999.

29. Janakiramaiah N, Gangadhar BN, Naga Venkatesha Murthy PJ, et al: Antidepressant efficacy of Sudarshan Kriya Yoga (SKY) in melancholia: a randomized comparison with electroconvulsive therapy (ECT) and imipramine. J Affect Disord 57:255–259, 2000.

30. Han J: Electroacupuncture: An alternative to antidepressants for treating affective diseases? Int J Neurosci 29:79–92, 1986.

31. Ernst E, Rand JI, Stevinson C: Complementary therapies for depression: An overview. Arch Gen Psych 55:1026–1032, 1998.

32. Gerber PE, Lynd LD: Selective serotonin-reuptake inhibitor-induced movement disorders. Ann Pharmacother 32:692–698, 1998.

33. Fava GA: Do antidepressants and antianxiety drugs increase chronicity in affective disorders? Psychother Psychosom 61:125–131, 1994.

34. Beauchemin KM, Hays P: Phototheraphy is a useful adjunct in the treatment of depressed in-patients. Acta Psychiatri Scand 95:424–427, 1997.

35. Shelton RC, Keller MB, Gelenberg A, et al: Effectiveness of St. John's wort in major depression: a randomized controlled trial. JAMA 285:1978–1986, 2001.

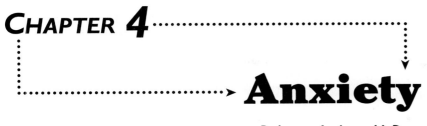

CHAPTER 4

Anxiety

Roberta A. Lee, M.D.

Anxiety disorders are one of the most commonly encountered medical conditions in primary care. According to the National Institute of Mental Health, the 1-year prevalence rate is 13.3% of the population, or 19.1 million people. Underdiagnosis is common; the average patient with an anxiety disorder consults 10 healthcare professionals before a definitive diagnosis is made.[1] Furthermore, patients who carry the diagnosis use primary care services three times as often as other patients.[2] In the past, when underdiagnosis was more common, patients received elaborate medical workups, but the definitive diagnosis remained elusive. These patients became categorized as the "worried well." Nevertheless, because anxiety can mask in numerous psychosomatic ways, practitioners must maintain a high index of suspicion for this disorder.

Anxiety disorders encompass a wide variety of subtypes, the most common being generalized anxiety disorder (GAD), obsessive-compulsive disorder (OCD), panic disorder, phobias, and post-traumatic stress disorder. All are marked by irrational, involuntary thoughts. One of the most defining diagnostic elements of anxiety disorders is the disruption of daily life by overt distress. Frequently, there is a significant reduction in the ability to carry out routine tasks, whether social, personal, or professional.[3] In this chapter the focus is on an integrative approach to the management of generalized anxiety (GAD), as defined in the *Diagnostic and Statistical Manual of Mental Disorders*, 4th edition (DSM-IV). In primary care practice, the prevalence of GAD can be as high as 10% to 15%.[2]

DEFINITION AND DIAGNOSTIC CRITERIA

Generalized anxiety involves unremitting excessive worry involving a variety of issues. These concerns may be related to family, health, money, or work. Once the initial concern subsides, another quickly takes its place. The practitioner observes over time that the concerns seem pervasive and repetitive. Additionally, the distress seems out of proportion to the actual life circumstance.

In order to meet the DSM-IV criteria for GAD, intense worrying must occur on a majority of days during a period of at least 6 continuous months.[3] In addition, three of the following signs and symptoms must be present: easy fatigability, difficulty concentrating, irritability, muscle tension, restlessness, and sleep disturbance. Patients usually present with physical complaints, failing to recognize the stress-related etiology. The most frequent signs and symptoms are diaphoresis, headache, and trembling.[4] There can be psychological manifestations of GAD as well. Patients often report impaired memory, or a diminished ability to concentrate or take directions, and frequently make statements such as "I can't seem to stop thinking of . . . ."

COMORBID CONDITIONS

Approximately 40% of people with GAD have no comorbid conditions, but many develop another disorder as time evolves.[5] In fact, concurrent or coexistent organic or psychiatric disease is the rule rather than the exception in patients with GAD.[5] For example, panic disorder is common among persons who have irritable bowel syndrome; a shared brain-gut mechanism incorporating a serotonin link has been theorized.[6] Psychiatric overlap is common. Anxiety disorders and depression frequently coincide—either can trigger the other. In the case of coexisting depression, especially of significant severity, treatment of the depression is the primary objective. Subsequent visits will reveal whether the anxiety is relieved simply by addressing depression. Many persons coping with anxiety use alcohol or drugs to mask their distress. About 30% of people with panic disorder abuse alcohol, and use of drugs occurs in 17%.[1]

PATHOPHYSIOLOGY

The pathophysiology of GAD is multifactorial and remains incompletely understood. Studies in animals and humans have attempted to pinpoint body structure and systems involved in the pathogenesis of anxiety. One that has been identified is the amygdala, a small structure deep inside the brain that communicates with the autonomic nervous system to relay perceived danger to other centers of the brain, which in turn ready the body for the perceived danger. Furthermore, the memory of these dangers stored in the amygdala appears to be indelible, thus creating a pathophysiologic phenomenon that may progress to GAD.

> **NOTE**
>
> *Although the pathophysiology of GAD is multifactorial, the amygdala in the brain appears to be a focus for stressful memories that stimulate the autonomic nervous system when the body and mind perceive danger.*

Other contributing factors may lie in the realm of cognitive phenomena. Research is currently under way to evaluate exposure to stress early in life and subsequent development of GAD.[7]

In post-traumatic stress disorder, a subtype of anxiety, studies have identified low cortisol levels (and high levels of corticotropin-releasing factor) and an overabundance of norepinephrine and epinephrine as contributing factors.[8]

Finally, genetics are thought to be another influence. Studies indicate genetic concordance with certain genetic loci that produce functional serotonin polymorphisms.[9]

RULING OUT ORGANIC DISEASE

The symptoms of anxiety disorders can resemble those of a variety of medical conditions, and a full medical workup is in order if the possibility of disease exists (see Table 4–1).

INTEGRATIVE THERAPY

Exercise

Numerous studies assessing the effects of exercise (both acute and chronic) on anxiety exist. The bulk of these studies have measured the effects of exercise by the presence of signs and symptoms of elevated anxiety rather than with use of a diagnostic system like that of the DSM.[10] Nonetheless, the results of most studies generally show a reduction in symptoms with increased physical activity.

Aerobic exercise programs seem to have produced a larger effect than that obtained with weight training and flexibility regimens, although both appear effective for improvement in mood.[10,11] The length of physical activity also seems important. In one study, programs exceeding 21 minutes for a minimum of 10 weeks were needed to achieve significant anxiety reduction.[12] The beneficial effect appeared to be maximal with 40 minutes per session.[10] Furthermore, the benefits seem to be lasting. In one study assessing the long-term effects of aerobic exercise, participants evaluated at 1-year follow-up examination were found to maintain the psychological benefits initially recorded. Their exercise routines over the 12-month follow-up were either the same as those in the original study design or less intensive.[13]

The exact reason for the improvement of mood with exercise is not completely known. However, increased physical activity has been correlated with changes in brain levels of monoamine—norepinephrine, dopamine, and serotonin—which may account for improved mood.[14] The endorphin hypothesis is another explanation for the beneficial effects of exercise on mood. Many studies have demonstrated significant endorphin secretion with increased exercise, with beneficial effects on state of mind. However, blockade of endorphin elevation with antagonists such as naloxone during exercise does not correlate with decreased mental health benefits.[14] Some investigators have argued that the latter finding reflects flaws in methodologic design.

> **NOTE**
>
> *Both length of the exercise session and duration of the physical activity program seem important in maximizing the beneficial effect of exercise on anxiety reduction.*

No matter what the hypothesis, the involvement of each patient in active recovery may confer a sense of independence, leading to increased self-confidence. In turn, the patient's ability to cope with challenging life events is increased. This is consistent with the integrative philosophy of healing. Furthermore, few side effects, low cost, and general availability all make exercise a crucial component of integrative management.

The level of exertion and specific exercise prescription should be determined by the patient's level of fitness, interests in specific physical activities, and health concerns (see Chapter 86, Writing an Exercise Prescription).

Table 4–1. Medical Conditions Often Associated with Symptoms of Anxiety
....

Cardiovascular
Acute myocardial infarction
Angina pectoris
Arrhythmias
Congestive heart failure
Hypertension
Ischemic heart disease
Mitral valve prolapse

Endocrine
Carcinoid syndrome
Cushing's disease
Hyperthyroidism
Hypothyroidism
Hypoglycemia
Parathyroid disease
Pheochromocytoma
Porphyria
Electrolyte imbalance

Gastrointestinal
Irritable bowel syndrome

Gynecologic
Menopause
Premenstrual syndrome

Hematologic
Anemia
Chronic immune diseases

Neurologic
Brain tumor
Delirium
Encephalopathy
Epilepsy
Parkinson's disease
Seizure disorder
Vertigo
Transient ischemic attack

Respiratory
Asthma
Chronic obstructive pulmonary disease
Pulmonary embolism
Dyspnea
Pulmonary edema

Nutrition

Caffeine

On average, Americans consume one or two cups of coffee a day, which represents approximately 150 to 300 mg of caffeine. Although most people can handle this amount with no effect on mood, some experience increased anxiety. People who are prone to feeling stress have reported that they experience increased anxiety from even these small amounts. With long-term use, caffeine has been linked with anxiety as well as depression. Discontinuation is warranted.[15]

Alcohol

With long-term use, alcohol has been found to diminish levels of serotonin and catecholamine. Discontinuation of alcohol consumption is therefore warranted.[16]

Omega-3 Fatty Acids

Epidemiologic data suggest that an omega-3 fatty acid deficiency or imbalance between the ratio of omega-6 and omega-3 fatty acids in the diet correlates with increased anxiety and depression. It is well documented in animal studies that levels of polyunsaturated fats (PUFAs) and cholesterol metabolism influence neuronal tissue synthesis, membrane fluidity, and serotonin metabolism.[17] Primarily indirect evidence, particularly in depression, suggests that correction of the ratio of omega-6 to omega-3 consumption may improve mood. Given the evidence concerning neuronal tissue synthesis and serotonin metabolism, increased supplementation with omega-3 fatty acids seems beneficial.[18] Recommending consumption of cold water fish (sardines, mackerel, tuna, salmon, herring) at least two or three times a week or flaxseed oil or freshly ground flaxseed (2 tablespoons daily) or as a supplement (1000–2000 mg) seems reasonable (see Chapter 84, The Anti-inflammatory [Omega-3] Diet).

Supplements

B Vitamins

A deficiency of a variety of nutrients can alter brain function and therefore lead to anxiety. Deficiency of a number of vitamins, including the B vitamins, has been linked with mood disorders. The B vitamins, including B_6 (pyridoxine) and B_{12}, are linked with the synthesis of S-adenosyl methionine (SAMe), which carries and donates methyl molecules to many chemicals in the brain including neurotransmitters. B_6 is essential for the production of serotonin and has been linked with improvement in a variety of mood disorders including anxiety when used as a supplement.[19] Although large-scale clinical studies are lacking, a trial of a B complex supplement seems advisable, especially in the elderly and persons taking medications that may deplete this vitamin (e.g., oral contraceptive or replacement estrogen [Premarin].[20])

Dosage. The dosage is a B complex 100 vitamin, one tablet daily (containing approximately 100 mg of each of the major B vitamins).

Folic Acid

Studies have shown that folic acid supplementation is helpful in persons who are depressed (see section on folic acid use in Chapter 3, Depression). Patients with low levels of folic acid also have been reported to respond less well to selective serotonin reuptake inhibitors (SSRIs).[21] Serum vitamin B_{12} levels should be checked if folic acid supplementation is used, especially if megaloblastic anemia is noted in laboratory tests, as B_{12} deficiency can be masked by folic acid supplementation.

Dosage. The recommended dose of folic acid for supplementation is 400 to 800 μg per day.

Precautions. High doses of folic acid have been reported to cause altered sleep patterns, exacerbation of seizure frequency, GI disturbances, and a bitter taste in the mouth.

Pharmaceuticals

Conventional options for initial therapy in GAD are based on a variety of factors and drug side effect profiles. Depression frequently coexists with GAD, so antidepressants are often considered. None of the SSRIs has a formal indication for the treatment of GAD, although some agents have been approved for panic disorder, social phobia, and post-traumatic stress disorder. Less cardiotoxicity is associated with SSRIs than with tricyclic antidepressants, so an SSRI may be a better choice for patients with heart disease. Other conventional options for treatment of GAD involve the use of multiple receptor agents. Venlafaxine (Effexor) is the only serotonin-norepinephrine reuptake inhibitor approved for GAD. The use of tricyclic antidepressants has always been a consideration, but the difficulty in using these medications is that they can have anticholinergic and cardiovascular side effects, as well as a more pronounced sedative effect. Most experts recommend a trial of at least 4 to 6 weeks to determine efficacy.

For acute treatment of GAD, the use of anxiolytics, especially benzodiazepines, has always been a consideration. However, the risk of abuse and habituation has made most primary care practitioners cautious in prescribing these medications. The nonbenzodiazepine anxiolytic buspirone (BuSpar) may

Table 4–2. Supplement and Drug Recommendations for Treatment of Anxiety

Drug/Supplement	Initial Dose (Range)	Frequency
Vitamin B Complex 100	1 tablet	qd
Folic acid	400–800 μg	qd
Kava	50–70 mg (of kava lactones)	tid
Valerian root	150–300 mg q AM and 300–600 mg qhs	
Selective Serotonin Reuptake Inhibitors and Mixed Reuptake Blockers		
Fluoxetine (Prozac)	10–20 mg (10–80)	qd
Fluvoxamine (Luvox)	50 mg (50–300)	qd
Paroxetine (Paxil)	10 mg (10–60)	qd
Sertraline (Zoloft)	50 mg (50–200)	qd
Others		
Venlafaxine (Effexor)	75 mg (75–375)	bid
Nefazodone (Serzone)	200 mg (200–600)	bid
Bupropion (Wellbutrin)	100 mg (200–450)	bid
Azapirones		
Buspirone (Buspar)	7.5 mg (15–60)	bid

be a conventional alternative lacking the problematic issue of drug dependence and excessive sedation.

Dosage. See Table 4–2.

Botanical Medicine

Kava (*Piper methysticum*)

In the realm of botanical pharmaceuticals, kava has become known as a botanical option for the treatment of GAD in the United States and Europe. It is derived from the pulverized lateral roots of a subspecies of a pepper plant, *Piper methysticum*, and is indigenous to many Pacific island cultures. In Europe it is recognized by health authorities as a relatively safe remedy for anxiety.[22] Seven small clinical trials have been done evaluating the efficacy of kava in GAD.[23] In all trials, kava was found to be superior to placebo in the symptomatic treatment of GAD.

The constituents considered to be most pharmacologically active are the kava lactones, which have a chemical structure similar to that of myristicin, found in nutmeg.[24] These lactone structures are present in the highest concentration in the lateral roots and are lipophilic. Of the 15 isolated kava lactone structures, 6 are concentrated maximally in the root and vary depending on the variety of *Piper methysticum*.[25] The mechanism of action of kava in GAD has not been completely elucidated, although the action seems similar to that of benzodiazepines, but results of studies in rats and cats are conflicting.

Benazodiazepines exert their actions by binding to the gamma-aminobutyric acid (GABA) site and benzodiazepine receptors in the brain; animal studies analyzing kava's anxiolytic action, however, show mixed and minor effects at both sides. Other studies indicate the kava constituents produce anxiolytic effects by altering the limbic system, especially at the amygdala and hippocampus.[26] Other documented uses of kava have been as a muscle relaxant, an anticonvulsant, an anesthetic, and an anti-inflammatory agent.

Indication. Mild to moderate generalized anxiety.

Dosage. Kava for anxiety 50 to 70 mg (of the purified extract, kava lactones) three times daily. For doses with a standardized kava lactone concentration of 30%, this would be equivalent to 100 to 250 mg of dried root.

Precautions. Anecdotal reports have noted excessive sedation when kava is combined with other sedative medications.[27] Extrapyramidal side effects in four patients using two different preparations of kava have been reported. Kava thus should be avoided in those with Parkinson's syndrome.[28] The effects diminished once the extract was discontinued. In high doses from heavy kava consumption, a yellow, ichthyosiform condition of the skin known as kava dermopathy has been observed. This condition is reversible with discontinuation of the kava.[29] The overdose potential appears to be low. In many cases, the rash, ataxia, redness of the eyes, visual accommodation difficulties, and yellowing of the skin reported in the literature from Australia and the Pacific region emerged after ingestion of up to 13 liters per day, equivalent to 300 to 400 g of dried root per week. It should be noted that this amount represents a dose 100 times that of the recommended therapeutic dose.[30]

Caution. There are insufficient data to determine teratogenicity; for this reason, it is wise to avoid use of kava during pregnancy. Kava is present in the milk of lactating mothers; therefore, use is discouraged during breastfeeding.[31] Avoid use with other sedative medications.

Kava has been reported to cause toxic hepatitis. To date all case reports (a total of 31) have been in patients from Europe using concentrated extracts manufactured in Germany or Switzerland. The exact cause for the effects is under investigation. Kava should not be used in individuals who have liver problems, nor should it be used concomitantly in patients who are on multiple medications that are metabolized in the liver or in individuals who drink alcohol on a daily basis.[41] Liver tests should be routinely done in individuals who use kava on a daily basis, and patients should be counseled on the signs and symptoms of hepatotoxicity (jaundice, malaise, and nausea). Furthermore, kava should be discontinued from daily use after approximately four months.

Valerian (*Valeriana officinalis*)

Valerian is another botanical alternative for the treatment of GAD. The clinical efficacy of valerian has been evaluated mostly for treating sleep disturbances; fewer clinical studies assessing its use in anxiety are available. Nevertheless, it has been used in Europe for over a thousand years as a tranquilizer and calmative.[32] The use of valerian in combination with either passionflower (*Passiflora incarnata*) or St. John's wort (*Hypericum perforatum*) for anxiety has been studied in small clinical trials. One study evaluated valerian root in combination with passionflower (100 mg of valerian root with 6.5 mg of passionflower extract) compared with chlorpromazine hydrochloride (Thorazine) (40 mg daily) over a period of 16 weeks. In this study, 20 patients were randomly assigned to the two treatment groups after being identified as suffering from irritation, unrest, depression, and insomnia. Electroencephalographic changes in both groups consistent with relaxation were comparable; two psychological scales measuring these qualities demonstrated scores consistent with reduction in anxiety.[33] Another study evaluated anxiety in 100 anxious persons receiving either a combination of 50 mg of valerian root plus 90 to 100 mg of standardized St. John's wort for 14 days or 2 mg of diazepam (Valium) twice daily in the first week and up to 2 capsules twice daily in the second week. The results showed reduction of anxiety in the phytomedicine treatment group to levels in healthy persons. Patients in the diazepam treatment group still had significant anxiety scores.[34]

Indication. Mild to moderate anxiety.

Dosage. For adults with anxiety, a dose of 150 to 300 mg in the morning and another dose of 300 to 600 mg in the evening, using a standardized product containing 3.3% valpotriates, can be taken. Combinations with lemon balm and hops (*Humulus lupulus*) may be considered. It should be noted that these additions are based on herbal tradition and empirical medicine; no clinical trials demonstrating efficacy are available.[35,36]

NOTE

Contrary to common belief, valerian is not suitable for acute treatment of anxiety or insomnia. It may take several weeks for a beneficial effect to occur.

Precautions. Valerian root is not suitable for the treatment of acute insomnia or nervousness, as it takes several weeks before a beneficial effect is obtained. An alternative that gives a more rapid response should be taken when valerian root is initiated.[13] Products with Indian and Mexican valerian should be avoided owing to the mutagenic risk associated with their high concentrations of valpotriates and baldrinals (up to 8%).[35] Adverse effects are rare with products that do not contain valpotriates. There are occasional reports of headache and gastrointestinal complaints.

Mind-Body Medicine

Psychotherapy

Psychotherapy has been shown to be effective as a therapeutic option in the treatment of GAD with or without medical intervention. Two clinically proven forms are used frequently: behavioral therapy and cognitive-behavioral therapy (CBT). Behavioral therapy focuses on changing the specific unwanted actions by using several techniques to stop the undesired behavior. In addition, both behavioral therapy and CBT help patients to understand and change their thinking patterns so that they can react differently to their anxiety.

Relaxation Techniques

Relaxation training, stress reduction techniques, and breath work are of proven benefit. In fact, imaginal exposure is used as a tactic for repeated exposure to induce anxiety (in a gradual way). Patients learn through repeated exposure to cope with and manage their anxiety rather than to eliminate it. Relaxation training paired with this interceptive therapy is useful. I often encounter patients who admit to their anxiety and are willing to confront and learn to cope with it but lack the ability to completely relax. Depending on their preferences, I help them choose a relaxation technique that reinforces a sense of calm. Therapies that can be used for this purpose are massage, sound therapy, aromatherapy, guided interactive imagery, and hypnosis. Because many patients have somatic sensations that accompany their anxiety, a complementary therapy that imparts a "remembrance" of a deeply relaxed state (see Chapter 91, Relaxation Techniques) should also be reinforced on a more somatic-kinesthetic level.

Therapies to Consider

Traditional medical systems (TMS) such as acupuncture and Ayurvedic medicine can be other options for the treatment of anxiety.[39] Several small trials assessing relaxation in an anxiety state showed reduction of anxiety in a normal patient population using auricular acupuncture.[40] Although the mechanisms are not well elucidated, these systems may somehow interface favorably to balance the autonomic nervous system.

— *THERAPEUTIC REVIEW*

The following four steps are recommended for initial management of patients with GAD.

1. *Remove exacerbating factors.*
   Review of current medications and supplements that could contribute to anxiety (especially botanical supplements such as ephedra and over-the-counter preparations that are stimulants). Supplements that are unnecessary should be discontinued.

2. *Screen for diseases that mimic anxiety.*
   Screening for underlying medical conditions that produce anxiety—for instance, hyperthyroidism or a withdrawal syndrome—should be done.

3. *Improve nutrition.*
   Nutritional support such as with omega-3 fatty acid supplementation (two to three servings of cold water fish per week, or flaxseed oil 2 tablespoons a day or 1000 mg of flaxseed oil in a capsule) is recommended. In addition, caffeine and alcohol consumption should be avoided.

4. *Institute physical activity.*
   Physical activity (aerobic or anaerobic) at least 5 days out of 7 should be encouraged. In order to ensure long-term compliance, an activity that is enjoyable to the patient is important. Futhermore, adherence to a regular exercise regimen and setting realistic short-term goals may need emphasis. Increases in exercise level and intensity should be gradual (see chapter 86, Writing an Exercise Prescription).

- *Supplements*
  - Vitamin B_6 included in vitamin B 100 complex preparation with the addition of folic acid (400 μg daily) should be considered.
- *Botanical medicine*
  - Kava 50 to 70 mg 3 times a day (of the purified kava lactones) can be given. Choose a standardized product with either a 30% or a 50% to 55%, kava lactone concentration. If no improvement is observed over 4 to 6 weeks, consider valerian or a valerian combination or a pharmaceutical anxiolytic (use for at least 6 weeks before evaluating efficacy). Concurrent psychotherapy is highly recommended if this approach is acceptable to the patient.
- *Mind-Body Therapies*
  - Psychotherapy: The combination of psychotherapy in conjunction with supplements, botanicals, or a pharmaceutical anxiolytic or antidepressant is highly recommended, especially in GAD, An integrative therapeutic approach is associated with higher success rates in cases of severe anxiety. Often, psychotherapy can provide the patient with skills for coping with anxiety, as opposed to extinguishing the symptoms. Primary care physicians can monitor lifestyle modification, dietary and supplement interventions, and drug therapy. However, referral to a psychotherapist is advised.
  - Relaxation training: Educate patient in relaxation techniques that will empower them to bring anxiety symptoms under control when needed.
  - Traditional medical systems: Use of traditional medicine is always somewhat problematic in that TMSs have historically been used to provide primary care for a variety of medical ailments (including anxiety). As an allopathic physician, I generally designate the use of TMSs as an adjunctive modality. However, for those patients who have strong feelings about the use of singular botanical preparations (mostly as being insufficient for treatment) or whose medical conditions appear mild, I am more than willing to be a medical partner and to consider use of a TMS (such as Chinese medicine or Ayurvedic medicine) as a primary therapeutic option, provided that the well-being of the patient is not in jeopardy.
  - Pharmaceuticals: If no improvement is obtained with lifestyle measures, dietary measures, and supplement interventions in conjunction with botanical supplements, use of a pharmaceutical anxiolytic or antidepressant

THERAPEUTIC REVIEW continued

should be considered. Depending on the severity of the anxiety and degree of lifestyle impairment, I often use a conventional prescriptive option with dietary and lifestyle interventions in combination with complementary therapy (e.g., acupuncture, mind-body therapy) to induce a sense of relaxation and then wean the patient off the prescriptive treatment (often a couple of months later). Depending on the severity, I may introduce a botanical supplement (such as kava).

Obviously, different clinical responses will be obtained with the various anxiolytics (and SSRIs). Optimal management may require a change of medication, depending on the patient's symptoms. For long-term therapy, I refrain from the use of benzodiazepines, as tolerance can be problematic.

Consider referral to a psychiatrist if the patient remains refractory to treatment, is suicidal or psychotic, or requires psychiatric stabilization in a hospital unit.

References

1. Pozuclo L, et al: The anxiety spectrum: Which disorder is it? Patient Care 1999; 33:13.
2. Goldberg RJ: Practical Guide to the Care of the Psychiatric Patient, 2nd. ed. St. Louis, CV Mosby, 1998.
3. American Psychiatric Association: Diagnostic and Statistical Manual of Mental Disorders, 4th ed—Primary Care Version. Washington, DC: American Psychiatric Association, 1995.
4. Kaplan H, et al: Anxiety disorders. In Kaplan and Sadock's Synopsis of Psyciatry, 8th ed. Baltimore, Williams & Wilkins, 1998.
5. Scheweitzer E: Generalized anxiety disorder: Longitudinal course and pharmacologic treatment. Psychiatric Clin North Am 1995; 18:843–857.
6. Lydiard RB: Anxiety and the irritable bowel syndrome: Psychological, medical, or both? J Clin Psychiatry 1997; 58(Supp 13):51–58.
7. Stewart SH, et al: Causal modeling of relations among learning history, anxiety sensitivity and panic attacks. Behav Res Ther 2001; 39:443–456.
8. Heim C, et al: The potential role of hypocortisolism in the pathophysiology of stress-related bodily disorders. Psychoneuroendocrinology 2000; 25:1–35.
9. Osher Y, et al: Association and linkage of anxiety related traits with a functional polymorphism of the serotonin transporter gene regulatory region in an Israeli sibling pair. Mol Psychiatry 2000; 5:216–219.
10. Paluska S, et al: Physical activity and mental health: Current conepts, Sports Med 2000; 29:167–180.
11. Martinsen EW, et al: Aerobic and non-aerobic forms of exercise in the treatment of anxiety disorders. Stress Med 1989; 115–120.
12. Moses J, et al: The effects of exercise training on mental well-being in the normal population: A controlled trial. J Psychosom Res 1989; 33:47–61.
13. DiLorenzo T, et al: Long-term effects of aerobic exercise on psychological outcomes. Prev Med 1999; 28:75–88.
14. Dunn AL, et al: Exercise and the neurobiology of depression. Exer Sport Sci Rev 1991; 19:41–98.
15. Bruce M, et al: Caffeine abstention in the management of anxiety disorders. Psychol Med 1989; 19: 211–241.
16. Goodwin FK: Alcoholism research: Delivering on the promise. Public Health Rep 1989; 103:569–574.
17. Maes M, et al: Lowered omega 3 polyunsaturated fatty acids in serum phospholipids and cholesteryl esters of depressed patients, Psychiatry Res 1999; 85: 275–291.
18. Bruinsma K, et al: Dieting, essential fatty acid intake, and depression. Nutr Rev 2000; 4: 98–108.
19. McCarty MF: High-dose pyridoxine in "anti-stress strategy." Med Hypotheses 2000; 54: 803–807.
20. Murray M, et al: Affective Disorders. In Pizzorno JE, Murray MT (eds): Textbook of Natural Medicine, 2nd ed. Churchill Livingstone, 1999.
21. Alpert JE, et al: Nutrition and depression: The role of folate, methylation and monoamine metabolism in depression. J Neurol Neurosurg Psychiatry 2000; 228–232.
22. Blumenthal M, et al: The Complete German Commission E Monographs: Therapeutic Guide to Herbal Medicines. Austin, Tex, American Botanical Council, 1998.
23. Pittler M, et al: Efficacy of kava extract for treating anxiety: Systematic review and meta-analysis. J Clin Psychopharmacology 2000; 20: 84–89.
24. Shulgin AT: The narcotic pepper: The chemistry and pharmacology of *Piper methysticum* and related species. Bull Narc 1973; 25: 59–74.
25. Lebot V, et al: Kava—the Pacific Drug. New Haven, Conn, Yale University Press, 1992.
26. Pepping J: Alternative therapies: Kava: *Piper methysticum*. Am J Health Syst Pharm 1999; 56: 957–960.
27. Almeida JC, et al: Coma from the health food store: Interaction between kava and alprazolam. Ann Intern Med 1996; 125: 940–941.
28. Schelosky L, et al: Kava and dopamine antagonism. J Neurol Neurosurg Psychiatry 1995; 58: 639–640.
29. Norton SA, et al: Kava dermopathy. J Am Acad Dermatol 1994; 31: 89-97.
30. Shultz V, et al: Kava as an anxiolytic. In Rational Phytotherapy: A Physicians' Guide to Herbal Medicine, Berlin, Springer-Verlag, 1998; 65–73.
31. Brinker F, et al: Herbal Contraindications and Drug Interactions, 2nd ed. Sandy, Ore, Eclectic Medical Publications, 1998.
32. Youngken, H: Textbook of Pharmacognosy, 6th ed. Philadelphia, Blakiston, 1948; 852–856.
33. Schellenberg R, et al: EEG—monitoring and psychometric evaluation of the therapeutic efficacy of Biral N in psychosomatic diseases. Naturamed 1994; 4:9.
34. Panijel M: The treatment of moderate states of anxiety: Randomized double-blind study comparing the clinical effectiveness of a phytomedicine with diazepam. Therapiwoche 1985; 41: 4659–4668.
35. Schultz V, et al: Rational Therapy: A Physicians' Guide to Herbal Medicine, Berlin, Springer-Verlag, 1998.
36. Reichert R: Valerian [clinical monograph]. Q Rev Nat Med 1998; Fall: 207–215.
37. Schweitzer E, et al: Strategies for treatment of generalized anxiety disorder in the primary care setting. J Clin Psychiatry 1997; 58(Suppl 3): 27–31.
38. Wang SM, et al: Auricular acupuncture: A potential treatment for anxiety. Anesth analg 2001; 92: 548–543.
39. Moyad MA, et al: Ear acupuncture in psychosomatic medicine: The importance of Sanjiao (triple heater) area. Acupunct Electrother Res 1993; 18: 185–194.
40. Breier A, et al: Controllable and uncontrollable stress in humans: Alterations in mood and neuroendocrine and psychophysiological function. Am J Psychiatry 1987; 244:11.
41. Blumental M: American Botanical Council announces new safety information on Kava. ABC Safety Release, December 20, 2001.

CHAPTER 5

Attention Deficit Disorder

Sharon I. McDonough-Means, M.D., F.A.A.P.,
and Michael W. Cohen, M.D., F.A.A.P.

Disorders of attention have been recognized since 1902, when George Still, a British physician, described a cluster of symptoms (aggression, defiance, emotionality, disinhibition, limited sustained attention and deficient rule) that governed behavior, with the core feature being "a defect in moral control"—a limitation in self-regulatory behavior.[1]

The most current term, *Attention Deficit/Hyperactivity Disorder,* is defined as a persistent pattern (greater than 6 months' duration with 6 or more symptoms in each category) of (1) inattention and/or (2) hyperactivity-impulsivity that is age-inappropriate, that had onset younger than age 7 years, that is present in more than two settings and disrupts developmentally appropriate social, academic, or occupational functioning. The diagnosis depends solely on clinical observation and assessment, which creates variance in terminology and criteria.

Attention span and level of behavioral activity are two categorical traits in human development that express along a continuum with a bell-shaped distribution and age-specific features.[2] Attention deficit disorder spectrum (ADD) affects persons throughout the life span with the functional difficulty profile shifting in focus: (1) preschool—motor behavior and completing daily tasks; (2) school age—academics and following directions; and (3) adolescence/adult—maintenance of social relationships and work placements. ADD is the most prevalent of the neurodevelopmental disorders: 3% to 17% of U.S. children are affected. The male-to-female ratio is 4:1 for the hyperactive-impulsive type and 2:1 for the inattentive type.[3] There is a high association of other diagnoses: 10% to 25% learning disorders and 42% to 53% axis I[4] (disorders of conduct and emotions) diagnoses. Symptoms persist into adulthood in up to 65%, although this population has been considerably less well studied.

The use of nonconventional therapies in studied populations with ADD is roughly two thirds whether or not they are taking pharmaceuticals at the same time.[5] However, nearly all (93%) physicians caring for patients with ADD will at some time have patients who ask about the use of nonconventional therapies.[6] An excellent theoretical framework for integration of nonconventional therapies into the care of ADD is provided.[7] Consistently, no matter the geographic location, the predominant form of nonconventional therapy since about 1990 has been nutrition and dietary supplements[5, 8]; and these are the most commonly used (75%) by those not using pharmaceuticals. Botanicals are now the second most commonly used nonconventional therapy.[5] The spectrum of nonconventional therapies with reported benefit for and being used in ADD is rapidly expanding, driven by consumer demand.

PATHOPHYSIOLOGY

"If only he would just pay attention!"

"Paying attention" sounds like a singular, simple function, but the reality is complex. Research in the structure and function of the central nervous system and the attentional process is abundant and burgeoning, facilitated by the recent advances in neuropsychology and neurobiology (neuroimaging, electroencephalography [EEG], epidemiology, and genetic) research.

Neuropsychology

Table 5–1[9] lists the components of attentional function and the associated dysfunctions in parentheses—common descriptors of those with ADD. This

Table 5–1. Components of "Attention" (Associated Dysfunction)* See Anatomical Locations in Fig. 5–1

[1] Stimulus detection *"focusing"*
[2] *Encoding*/processing detected information
[3] *Sustaining* attention to relevant stimulus and filtering out others
[4] *Shifting* attention when appropriate (perseveration)
[5] *Inhibiting* involuntary shifting (distractibility)
[6] *Organizing*/inhibiting *response* (impulsivity)

*Associated dysfunctions are in parentheses.
Mirsky AF: Disorder of attention. In Lyon GR, Krasnegor NA (eds): Attention, Memory, and Executive Function. Baltimore, PH Brookes, 1996, pp 71–95.

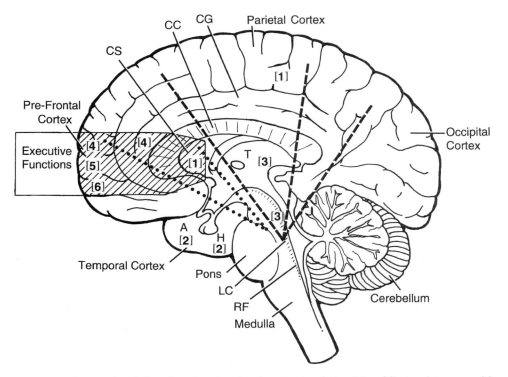

Figure 5–1. Primary processes in attentional disorders: functional and anatomic relationships. CG, cingulate gyrus; CC, corpus callosum; CS, cortical striatum; T, thalamic nuclei; H, hippocampus, A, amygdala; LC, locus ceruleus, RF, pontine reticular activating formation; [1] to [6], components of attention. Broken line, norepinephrine; dotted line, dopamine.

process occurs along a continuum from the initial step **[1]** of noting a stimulus (sensory observations, thoughts or emotions) through components **[2]** to **[6]**, the process of preparing to act (intention), to the final production of a response. Each of these components in the attentional process appears to require different portions of the brain working in concert with each other, as shown in Figure 5–1.

The latter components of the attentional process are embedded within the *Executive Functions*—uniquely human capacities that include self-regulation, sequencing of behavior, cognitive flexibility, response inhibition, planning, organization of behavior, and working memory. These functions primarily involve the frontostriatal circuitry including the prefrontal cortex. The prefrontal cortex has the most protracted course of development, undergoing myelinization into adolescence, thereby rendering it particularly sensitive to traumatic or toxic insult. Neurons from the locus ceruleus (norepinephrine) and the pontine reticular formation (dopamine) act to enhance the "signal-to-noise" ratio for components of the attention process.

In ADD, dysfunction may occur throughout the continuum of the attentional process, but the most significant and consistent abnormalities are in the organization and inhibition of a response **[6]**, the executive functions and working memory.[10] In ADD, the processing style tends to be *simultaneous,* thereby creating strengths in creativity,[11] sensitivity, and abundance of ideas and weakness in separating out the influence of both cognitive and

emotional information on intention and motor responses.

Neurobiology

Neurochemistry provided the first "window" into understanding ADD. Early studies of neurotransmitters in urine, blood, and cerebrospinal fluid provided inconsistent results. Currently, serotonin is thought to be primarily involved in impulsivity when associated with aggression but is not central to the primary symptoms of ADD. Current research indicates that:

NOTE

Dopamine and norepinephrine are the primary neurotransmitters associated with the task of attending. Both need to be enhanced to achieve sustained clinical benefit.

Transporters for norepinephrine and dopamine (DAT) remove neurotransmitter from the extracellular space of the neuronal synapse. The transporter for dopamine appears to be significantly increased in subjects with ADD. Methylphenidate (Ritalin) blocks these transporters, increasing the levels of the neurotransmitters, most specifically in the striatum.[12, 13] There appears to be an association between the expression of a specific form of dopamine transporter gene (DAT1 allele) and the scores for hyperactivity-impulsivity ratings in ADD children.[14]

NOTE

Neuroimaging and quantitative EEG (qEEG) research has shown that the primary area of functional alteration in ADD is the prefrontal–striatal/basal ganglia–cortical circuitry.

Neuroimaging research in ADD[15, 16] using volumetric analyses has shown variance in size, most consistently in basal ganglia, cerebellar vermis, and the right cerebral cortex, which tends to be diminished (also in reading disabilities and other conditions). ADD is a functional rather than a structural disorder, so development of specific functional techniques (single-photon emission computed tomography [SPECT], positron emission tomography [PET], and functional magnetic resonance imaging [fMRI] has allowed study of perfusion and metabolism of the frontostriatal circuitry and the cerebellar vermis. Recent research using a specific fMR1 technique has shown that in ADD basal state blood flow is significantly decreased solely in the right and left putamen (similar trend in the right caudate), which strongly correlates clinically with the capacity to sit still and accuracy on computerized test of attention (CPT). Treatment with methylphenidate appears to alter blood flow in the right and left putamen in a dose-dependent manner with the direction dependent on ADD subtype—increasing in the hyperactive and decreasing in the inattentive type[17]; the reverse occurs in the cerebellar vermis.[18] These techniques are not yet practical primary tools for differential diagnosis owing to cost and overlap with other developmental disorders.

Quantitative electroencephalography (qEEG) research appears to show reliable differences which discriminate ADD, specific developmental learning disorders, and subtypes of ADD from "normal" subjects with high sensitivity and specificity.[19] Study of specific wave forms after stimulation tend to show slow processing of information and selection of appropriate responses.[20] qEEG techniques may offer some support for clinical differential diagnosis but may not correlate with specific approaches to treatment.

The central nervous system structure and functions that control attention/intention are complex and have a protracted developmental course, thus making the process uniquely vulnerable to multiple influences and exquisitely sensitive to injury. Research in the 21st century holds significant promise because these powerful tools will allow us to further elucidate the complex mechanisms for ADD, support clarification of multifactorial individualized causation, and improve clinical care.

ETIOLOGY

It is estimated that at least 17% of children in the United States have more than one disorder of development, learning, or behavior.[21] In at least 25% of these children, determination of these neurocognitive traits is equally shared by *genetic* factors (genetic vulnerability, sensitive period of development) and *environment* (toxins [single and multiple] and infectious agents, social and cultural factors, and general health status, including nutrition). See Figure 5–2.

The neurodevelopmental process of "attending" is controlled by both genetic and environmental factors, which may be either enhancing or injurious.

Genetic

Family, twin, and adoption studies support the hereditary component of ADD; multiple genes are involved. Fifty percent of ADD parents will have an ADD child and 10% to 35% of ADD children have an ADD relative. Care of persons with ADD truly requires family-centered management.

Environmental

Social and Cultural. Environmental factors known to negatively affect neurodevelopment and behavior include violence,[22, 23] disorganization, chronic stress, and overstructuring/overscheduling.[24] Loss of traditional family and tribal structures has been associated with the expression of ADD.[25] Chronic maternal stress produces less organized and mature behavioral response to normal stimulation (light, noise, and vibration) in the fetus.[26] Chronic neonatal stress has been shown to alter brain structure and neurotransmitters that may result in permanent alterations in attention span and memory and spatial difficulties in later adult life.[27–29]

Chemical Environmental Toxins. For the first time in history, synthetic compound organic chemicals exist that are foreign to living systems, including our human physiology. A single compound may affect multiple systems with differing impact along the developmental spectrum. Parallel to this rise in environmental toxins, the incidence of developmental disorders, such as autism and ADD, is thought to be increasing.[30]

NOTE

Five major classes of chemical environmental developmental neurotoxicants: (1) heavy metals; (2) dioxins and PCBs—food chain bioaccumulators; (3) pesticides; (4) solvents; and (5) nicotine.

Table 5–2 provides a summary of environmental sources, routes of exposure, metabolism, exposure biomarkers, and developmental impact. Food addi-

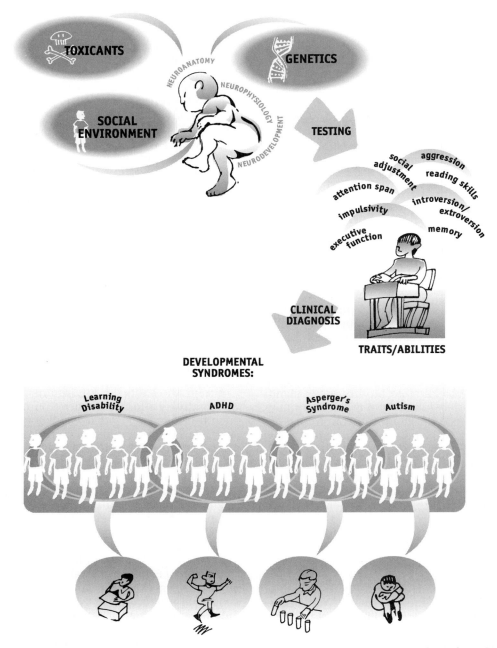

Figure 5–2. Framework for understanding learning, behavior, and developmental disabilities in children. (From Schettler T, Stein J, Reich F, Valenti M: In Harm's Way: Toxic Threats to Child Development. A report by Greater Boston Physicians for Social Responsibility and Clean Water Fund, May 2000. Design and illustration by Stephen Burdick, www.stephenburdickdesign.com)

tives and dyes are discussed later. Electromagnetic fields from specific sources may also be potential sources, but these are not covered in this text.

The manifestations of "attention deficit" are multiple, are individually variable with core common features, and occur in combination with other neurocognitive processes (such as learning disabilities or aggression). The cause of ADD is multifactorial, systemic (family), and contextual (social and cultural). Therefore, an integrated, multidisciplinary outcomes model for healthcare and research is required.

INTEGRATIVE THERAPY

All of the many therapeutic modalities presented here have a body of clinical experience supporting their use in ADD. Good research support is available in children with ADD for the pharmaceuticals, nutrition and dietary supplements (including food additives and allergens), and mind-body therapies (especially self-hypnosis and EEG biofeedback). Research is beginning in children with ADD with the use of botanicals, acupuncture, homeopathy and massage therapies.

Table 5–2. Environmental Developmental Neurotoxicants[80]

Source	Route	Metabolism	Effects
METALS			
Lead			
Gasoline: US—mostly gone	Air: Industrial products—	Physiologically normal levels =	0–2-year-olds: blood levels from
Developing countries—still present	production, handling, disposal/incineration	0; no biologic process requires lead; current "safe"	14.6–1.8 μg/dL; later effects— decreased attention span,
Paint: interior < 1978	• Paint dust	level < 10 μg/dL blood; likely	persistence, and ability to
Industrial products: 1990– 1997—increasing; primarily owing to PVC and coated wire products	• Gasoline exhaust Soil: paint flakes, air contaminant settlement Water: residential—pipe solder;	soon to be reduced Depends on delta ALA-D (aminolevulinic acid dehydratase); stored in	follow directions; learning disabilities; increased impulsivity and externalizing behaviors (older ages); effects
Industrial on-site emissions: point source (monitored) and fugitive (nonmonitored)	open bodies of water—air settlement, goes into food supply	tissue, including hair and bone; remobilized with stress/ pregnancy	of exposure from fetal age to 2 years last into later childhood/adult
		Crosses placenta and blood- brain barrier in fetus (immature < 6 mo)	Fetus: alters CNS cellular structure and chemistry; alters neurotransmitters— acetylcholine, dopamine, and glutamate; decreases dopamine receptors (different parts of brain) and inhibits glutamate receptors
Mercury			
Industrial: coal-fired power plant emissions	Air: long distances as elemental metal	No physiologic process requires mercury; normal level = 0;	Fetal CNS: alters neuronal migration, disrupts synaptic
Product disposal/incineration: municipal and medical	Soil: air sediment → methyl mercury	current "safe" level = 1 μg/kg/ day; may be reduced	transmission, and lowers dopamine levels
Food chain: bioaccumulation in fish—primarily flesh; often in combination with dioxin and PCBs (fat) → synergy of negative effects	Fish: fresh water and large predator ocean; Tuna (0.2 ppm): 7 oz = 0.09 μg/kg for a 130 lb person	Binds to proteins throughout body; inhibits protein synthesis, reactive O_2 species form, damage DNA and disrupt cell division Fetal exposure: cord blood and maternal hair levels	Fetal exposure: high (hair 10–20 ppm)—infant: seizures, mental retardation, and disturbed gait, vision and hearing; maternal hair (3–20 ppm)—school age: impaired language, attention, memory, and visual recognition correlated with prenatal level of exposure; effects occur even without maternal symptoms

Pharmacotherapy

Stimulant medications have been the primary class of drugs for treatment of ADD since their initial use in the late 1930s. Although varying opinions exist regarding effectiveness of specific stimulant preparations, short-term clinical benefits have been noted in at least 70% to 75% of treated individuals appropriately diagnosed with ADD.[31] In general, there is less beneficial effect on academic and social performance than on the core ADD symptoms. There is marked variability in individual response to medication. A trial of more than one stimulant is indicated before presuming that this class of drugs will not be helpful or tolerated.[32]

The stimulants used primarily, methylphenidate and amphetamines, are available in short-acting and sustained-release forms (see Table 5–3). New preparations, which have extended the duration of action, include an amphetamine preparation (Adderall) that incorporates four different salts and a methylphenidate preparation (Concerta) that utilizes an osmotic delivery system; both have similar benefits and adverse effects as their predecessors. Pemoline (Cylert), a long-acting nonamphetamine

stimulant, has demonstrated benefits in ADD. However, owing to the potential for chemical hepatitis and hepatic failure, current recommendations are that liver function tests be monitored every 2 weeks and pemoline not be used as a first-line drug.[33] Tables 5–3 and 5–4 list the available stimulants, dosages, benefits, and adverse effects.[34] *General guideline:* Start with a low dose and gradually increase to clinical benefit; decrease with occurrence of side effects.

Concern regarding long-term adverse effects of stimulant medications has focused on growth suppression and abuse/addiction potential. Adult height and weight, as expected by family history, are achieved regardless of dose or length of treatment; a mild delay in the onset of the adolescent growth spurt may occur in some patients. Appropriately diagnosed and properly treated children are actually less likely to abuse drugs as adolescents. However, stimulant drugs *do* have the potential for abuse—as long as they are being prescribed and therefore are readily available—and for addiction—only when taken by the nonoral route.[31] Other agents have been used in the treatment of ADD; none are as efficacious as the stimulants for the core ADD symp-

Table 5–2 (Continued). Environmental Developmental Neurotoxicants

Source	Route	Metabolism	Effects
Cadmium Industrial: (1) fuel burned; (2) production: batteries, paint pigments, plastic stabilizers, metal plating; (3) sewage sludge Mining: other metals Fertilizers (phosphate) Product incineration: medical and municipal Cigarette smoke	Soil: most significant—sewage sludge, air sediment and fertilizers → foods: grains and leafy green vegetables Water: industrial waste; concentrates in shellfish of coastal waters Air: industrial, cigarettes	No physiologic process requires cadmium; normal body level = 0; absorbed with other metals, gastrointestinal into blood; rapid removal/storage—kidneys, liver, adrenal glands and pancreas; interferes with normal processes, body and brain; produces secondary deficiencies: e.g., zinc and other metals Chronic exposure: induces binding protein—metalothionen; acute exposure does not, so ↑ toxicity* Best indicator of body burden: hair levels, not blood†	Exposure coexists with lead; difficult to individualize effects; general: ↓ weight gain; hyperactivity and hypoactivity ↓ IQ: cadmium ~ verbal skills; lead ~ performance skills Fetal exposure: (1) alters neurotransmitters—dopamine, serotonin, norepinephrine, and acetylcholine; (2) ↑ free radicals → cell membrane damage and altered physiologic function;* (3) ↑ maternal and neonatal hair levels: at age 6 yr—decreased IQ, perceptual, motor and quantitative functions†
Manganese Normal: foods—tea, legumes, nuts, grains; breast milk—6 μg/L; formula—77–200 μg/L Toxic: Industrial—metals production and welding Mining: with other metals—copper (US); manganese mines (outside US)	Air: metal products, esp. welding; emissions from industrial plants; mining of metals Waters: mining → soil, open water bodies, ground water and wells Soil: around mining or industrial sites	Biologically required: catalyst in critical enzymatic processes in body and brain. *Oral intake* (Mn^{2+}): intestinal absorption (1–11%) and excretion liver/bile (70%)—depends on body stores and other nutrients in diet. Liver—$Mn^{2+} \rightarrow Mn^{3+}$/transferrin, this ↑ tissue absorption. Bone—40% total body Mn. Brain—slow accumulation and release; liver, kidney, pancreas and hair. *Air* (Mn^{2+}): → lungs → systemic (Mn^{3+}) → nose/olfactory nerve → brain; *Infant*: ↑ absorption and ↓ excretion. *Fetus*: crosses placenta and blood-brain barrier	Toxic: chronic air. *Adults*—high-level = "manganism" Parkinson-like movement disorder, pneumonia, and bronchitis; lower level = ↓ response speed, motor function, balance, and memory *Children*: probable deficits in short-term memory, visual spatial frequency (low-to-mid range), visual memory, balance, and fine-motor dexterity; hair levels (↑ + other metals)—associated with LD/ADD.[81, 82] *Brain*: first to transferrin-rich receptor sites → accumulate in pallidum, thalamic nuclei, and substantia nigra (MRI) *Exposure markers*: ↑ chronic oral—urine(?); tissue (best); ↑ acute air—blood
DIOXINS Industrial production, solely a by-product: copper smelting; paper—chlorinated pulp and bleaching processes; PVC manufacturing Product disposal and incineration: • municipal and medical • hazardous waste	Air: Long-range transport in air into water and soil (retained many years) Dietary: Bioconcentrates in fat and moves up the food chain—plant to animal; greatest in beef, dairy, pork, and fish; breast milk (34–53× the 1 pg/kg/day recommended lifetime exposure)	Fetal neurotoxicity: coexist in fat tissue with PCBs; bind to cellular Ah receptor → cell nucleus, binds to DNA, acts on variety of growth factors, hormones, and hormone receptors; readily passed transplacentally	Co-exist with PCBs; effects difficult to differentiate; exposure marker: **blood levels**: At ambient environmental levels, primary impact on brain is during fetal life/maternal fat stores and diet Animal fetal exposure studies: impact on reproduction, learning and social behavior; less known from human study.
POLYCHLORINATED BIPHENYLS (PCBs) Industrial chemicals: lubricants, coatings, electrical transformer insulation Banned now Future two thirds of products remain for disposal—? incineration—in landfills, hazardous waste sites, and electrical transformers	As above; plus dermal absorption from the soil Breast milk = significant concentrations; readily passed transplacentally Dietary: as above, owing to dietary preferences, child 0–4 yr consumes a markedly disproportionate share of life-time exposure	Neurotoxicity as above; also, nonattach to Ah receptor → thyroid hormone function: interfere in TBG-thyroxine binding; ↑ turnover of thyroxine and ? gene transcription; also interferes in neurotransmitter levels	Prenatal exposure effects = permanent Large human study populations of prenatal exposure at ambient environmental levels: deficits in child's play behavior, psychomotor development, attention, and IQ; maternal blood levels (2–15 ppm), last third of pregnancy, show significant >> impact on cognition than lactational exposure.[83]

Table 5–2 (Continued). Environmental Developmental Neurotoxicants

Source	Route	Metabolism	Effects
SOLVENTS			
Industrial: toluene, xylene, styrene, trichloroethylene Ethanol Gasoline and products: toluene and xylene	Air: primary, as all are volatile Waste into water and soil Oral beverage: transplacental Waste into water and soil	Neurotoxicity: all likely similar to ethanol: reduction of placental transport of nutrients; disruption of cell-cell interactions and synaptic transmission	Other than ethanol: Adult exposure—peripheral and CNS effects; birth defects in offspring. Fetal exposure (not well studied in humans): large impact with toluene: growth retardation, persistent deficits in cognition, speech, and motor skills. Likely that small exposures, as with ethanol, have subtle neurocognitive effects
PESTICIDES			
Organophosphates			
General use of pesticides in US: no required reporting Agriculture Industrial and residential (home, yard, schools, and play areas) ~ ¼ of total use in US. Chlorpyrifos (Dursban): home use (recently banned); still used in lawn and garden and commercial food supply Diazinon: residential	Primary: food, esp. fruits and vegetables (children consume >> volume/weight than adults) Air and skin; also accumulates in carpets in home	Thirty-seven of pesticides registered for food use = neurotoxic; urine levels of TCP (metabolite of chlorpyrifos), detectable in adults (82%) and in children (92%) Inhibits acetylcholinesterase = ↑ levels of acetylcholine which results in (1) overstimulation of cholinergic function; and (2) ↓ in neurite outgrowth in developing brain*	Dursban: in utero exposure from home use, consistent pattern of defects: growth retardation, mental retardation, hypotonia, external genitalia, structure of palate and eye (with blindness) and brain[84] †↓ DNA synthesis in developing brain; results in ↓ cell numbers, at or below levels in some home use *Hyperactivity, motor dysfunction and behavior disorders
Organochlorines			
Agriculture; DDT—banned in US; used in developing countries; mixtures—used in Mexico	Air, food and skin	Exposure on critical day of brain development, ↓ in muscarinic cholinergic neurotransmitter receptors*	Toxic to wildlife; persist and bioaccumulate in environment †Hyperactivity, ↓ in stamina, coordination, memory, and ability to draw familiar objects/people
Pyrethroids and Pyrethrins			
Common household	Air, food and skin	Interfere with electrical activity of nerve cells by altering cell permeability	*Fetal exposure using *small doses* on critical day resulted in hyperactivity and ↓ muscarinic cholinergic receptor levels in brain cortex; permanent effect
NICOTINE			
Maternal (pregnancy) smoking—active or passive	Maternal bloodstream to fetus	Nicotine and other chemicals—carbon monoxide and cyanide Fetal/neonatal exposure; ↓ DNA synthesis in brain in areas of rapid cell division; ↑ cholinergic receptor sites; ↓ levels of norepinephrine and dopamine; persist in brain as adult	Placental abnormalities; IUGR secondary to ↓ O₂ delivery; RDS and prematurity *Fetal exposure, low chronic*—newborn hyperactivity, ↑ tremors, ↓ auditory responsiveness; *>10 cigarettes/day*—↓ general IQ; *passive smoke* (fetus or early childhood)—↓information processing and ADD—persist as adult

* Animal studies; all tables.
† Human studies; all tables.
ADD, attention deficit disorder; CNS, central nervous system; LD, learning disability; PCB, polychlorinated biphenyls; PVC, polyvinyl chloride; TBG, thyroid-binding globulin; TCP, trichloro-z-phyridinol; pg, picogram; ppt, parts per trillion; ppm, parts per million.

toms. Tricyclic antidepressants, alpha-adrenergic antagonists, and bupropion (Wellbutrin) may have a role when comorbid conditions are present and require simultaneous pharmacologic treatment.[35]

The use of psychoactive medications in children needs to be approached with great respect, care, and caution. Children, prior to late school age, do not have the cognitive ability to verbally express the effects (such as difficulty with short-term memory or mental sluggishness) that the psychoactive med-

Table 5–3. Stimulant Medication

Methylphenidate	Dosaging	Onset/Duration of Action	Amphetamines	Dosaging	Onset/Duration of Action
Short-Acting					
Ritalin tabs, 5, 10, 20 mg Methylin 5, 10, 20 mg	Variable Generally 2 or 3 times/day	30–45 min/3–5 hr	Dextroamphet-amines Dexedrine 5 mg	Variable Generally 2 or 3 times/day	30–45 min/3–5 hr
Sustained Release					
Ritalin SR 20 mg Metadate ER 10, 20 mg Methylin ER 10, 20 mg	Variable Generally 1 or 2 times/day	30–90 min/4–8 hr	Dexedrine SP 5, 10, 15 mg Dextroamphet-amines and racemic amphetamine (Adderall) 10, 20, 30 mg	Variable Generally 1 or 2 times/day	45–60 min/4–8 hr
Longest-Acting					
Concerta 18, 36, 54 mg	Variable Single daily dose	30–45 min/10–12 hr			

ications may exert on their internal neurocognitive and affective processes—other than in simple terms such as mad, sad, glad, or scared. The most reliable indicators are observed behavior, affect, and physical symptoms, which require input from those in the child's life. This makes management with these medications a more lengthy and uncertain process.

Recent landmark research in the treatment of ADD is the National Institute of Mental Health Collaborative Multisite Multimodal Treatment Study of Children with Attention-Deficit/Hyperactivity Disorder (MTA study).[36] A total of 579 subjects (7- to 9-year-olds) were randomized to one of four *treatment strategy groups* for 14 months. Many clinical recommendations have resulted.[37–39] For the core ADD symptoms (hyperactivity, inattention, and impulsivity), **medication alone** (group 1) and **combined therapy** (group 3) were equivalent and significantly better than **behavioral alone** (group 2) and **community-based** treatment (group 4). Use of medication

Table 5–4. Stimulants Benefits/Adverse Effects

Benefits	Adverse Effects	
Short-Term	**Common**	**Uncommon**
Increased attention	Appetite suppression	Tics
Decreased distractibility	Initial insomnia	Overfocusing
Decreased overactivity	Abdominal pain	Compulsiveness
Decreased impulsivity	Headaches	Decreased social interaction
Improved social interaction	Tachycardia	Stereotypic behavior
Increased compliance	Rebound irritability	Reduced spontaneity
Long-Term		**Rare**
No proven benefit as an exclusive treatment		Acute hallucinations

was more successful when dosage and choice of medication were individualized and optimized and monitored consistently. Combined therapy was equal to medication alone on all outcome measures, superior for parent-child relations/opposition and aggression. So behavioral treatments are specifically effective with some of the comorbidities, allow for effective management when an alternative to medication is preferred or medication fails, and allow for reduction in medication dose and therefore side effects. This creates a logical niche for the very reasonable consideration of nonconventional therapeutic modalities—either singly or in combination with pharmacotherapy.

Botanicals

Herbs are complex systems of bioactive chemicals that change with plant maturation, are uniquely affected by the soil and environment in which they are grown, act bioenergetically because they contain the subtle energy of the plant living system, and originally may even have been adapted to suit the genetics of the population within which they were grown. Herbs used for ADD[8] in children primarily focus on associated disturbances and potential mechanisms for efficacy—sleep disturbance, neuroprotection (antioxidants), and cognition/memory enhancement—based on research done in adults.

St. John's Wort. St. John's Wort is the single most studied herb for mild-to-moderate depression, which is a comorbidity in adolescents and adults with ADD.[40, 41] Hyperforin is thought to be the principal active ingredient (more so than hypericin), but the efficacy—whether owing to a single constituent (e.g., hyperforin) or to the whole herb (combinations of the chemical constituents)—is being actively researched. The herb is believed to act on metabolism of neurotransmitters—serotonin, norepinephrine, and dopamine—and does appear to act in the striatum on qEEG. The efficacy of St. John's Wort therapy is equal to that of imipramine and tricyclics, without adverse cardiac effects, and has a significantly lower dropout rate owing to less frequent and severe side effects (half as likely to occur).

Dosage. Recommended adult: 300 mg three times daily—(standardized to 3% minimum hyperforin). Companies that make reputable products include Eclectic and Nature's Way.

Precautions. Photosensitivity can occur but is generally mild and transient. Herb-drug interactions do occur secondary to induction of P-glycoprotein or cytochrome P450 enzyme system; this enhances drug metabolism of digoxin, cyclosporine, indinavir, warfarin, and others and potentiates the action of oral steroids and selective serotonin reuptake inhibitors.

Herbs Used for Sleep Disturbance

Melatonin Supplements. Research in children with neurodevelopmental disorders, including ADD, demonstrated significant health, behavior, and social benefits without side effects with the use of melatonin.[42]

Dosage. For children, 2 to 10 mg (5 mg most often) at bedtime for 4 weeks.

Precautions. Side effects may occur with high doses (decreased daytime alertness and fatigue) and may affect seizure frequency.[43] Extended use may inhibit gonadotropin and thus suppress puberty.

Chamomile (Manzanea). Chamomile is a good gastrointestinal antispasmodic and mild sedative with little if any side effects; is a member of the aster family (alcohol preparation denatures the potential allergenic protein); is safe for use in pregnancy, lactation, and young children.

Dosage. Dried herb, steeped as a tea (>2 tea bags) covered, for 15 minutes; 2 capsules three times daily in adults. Tincture—alcoholic or glycerite—start with 3 to 5 mL per dose (taken in liquid or plain) and increase until the sedative effect is obtained.

Lemon Balm (*Melissa officianalis*). Lemon balm blunts the stress response by direct action on the limbic system. It is very effective for calming/sedation in those who overreact to stimulation or in "the worrier."

Dosage. Dried herb—tea prepared by cold infusion (steeped overnight in room temperature or cooler water) or three capsules three times daily in adults; tincture—alcoholic or glycerite—start with 1 mL three times daily and increase to effect.

Valerian (*Valeriana officianalis*). Compared with benzodiazepams, valerian binds to the same gamma-aminobutyric acid receptor sites, is a bit slower in onset of action but lacks addictive potential and "hungover" feeling the next day.

Dosage. 450 to 900 mg at bedtime in adults. Both valerian and lemon balm are considered generally safe by the U.S. Food and Drug Administration.

Kava Kava. Kava kava is an anxiolytic, muscle relaxant, and analgesic. It is best used in those who do not sleep owing to muscle pain; it does not quiet the mind but may be mood altering in higher doses. Variability in components of preparations likely accounts for variable effects.

Dosage. 100 to 200 mg of standardized extract two to three times daily in adults.

Precaution. Kava kava should not be used with other sedatives. It is potentially hepatotoxic.

Herbs Used for Their Neuroprotective Effects

Ginkgo biloba—increases blood flow, increases cognitive activation/attending by enhancing alpha waves on EEG and decreasing slow waves and protects neurons from oxidative damage with potential improvement in memory via improved dopamine transport.

Chinese herbals (includes ginseng, biota, schizandra)—enhance memory and antioxidant.

Pycnogenol (50 mg/100 lb)—a bioflavonoid antioxidant, contains pine bark or grapeseed extract. There is no research in children for ADD.

Aromatherapy

The essential oils of plants function as the plant's immune system and in human use act bioenergetically and as complex chemicals that have neurohormonal, vitamin, anti-inflammatory, and antiseptic properties. They are used in oils on the skin (may be part of massage therapy) or volatilized (use infusor of any type) and act directly on the limbic system of the brain to modulate mood, memory, and other mental functions—for example, lavender for sedation and balancing, clary sage for anxiety, tea tree as antiseptic, and rosemary for memory enhancement. They may also be prescribed constitutionally. Use of the volatilized form does not require a child's direct cooperation, and the general environment of a family system can be enhanced.

Nutrition and Dietary Supplements

Avoidance of Neurotoxic or Irritant Substances

Since Feingold published his work in 1975, the relationship between food—additives, naturally occurring salicylates, and allergens—and behavior, especially ADD, has generated much controversy and research (Table 5–5).

Research studies[44] support a clear relationship between whole foods or substances within (usually multiple) and behavior. The "gold standard" for assessment involves a 1- to 3-month trial on an elimination diet with behavioral improvement followed by behavioral deterioration with challenges (see Chapter 82, The Elimination Diet and Diagnosing Food Sensitivities). Using this design, a critical study[45] evaluated 2- to 14-year-old children—34 with behavioral symptoms in response to dyes, "responders," and 20 "normal." All had normal behavior ratings on a tartrazine-free diet for 1 to 6 months (tartrazine is a base for common food dyes such as yellow dye No. 5). Tartrazine was reintroduced and symptoms (irritability, sleep disturbance, restlessness, aggression, and decreased attention span) were induced in a dose-dependent response in two thirds of the original "responders" and 10% of the original "normals." The tartrazine doses were 1 to 50 mg, whereas the level of mixed dyes in the routine daily diet of 5- to 12-year-olds is 76 mg/day. Behavioral disturbances were notably more severe in the 2- to 6-year-olds and tended to disrupt the whole family, especially for sleep.

Refined Sugar. Sugar has been found to be a nonspecific cause for symptoms of ADD; in general, a high intake of refined carbohydrate causes an increase in serotonin (produces sleepiness) and may also cause reactive hypoglycemia with release of catecholamines (produces restlessness and anxiety).

Provision of Essential Nutrients

Vitamins and Minerals. Dietary imbalances in vitamins and minerals most commonly are multiple. Relying on laboratory biomarkers to reflect the nutritional status of vitamins and minerals in the brain is problematic—cost, availability of an accurate test procedure, availability of a sample that truly reflects tissue-fluid balance, and the need for serial measures.[46] Currently, for trace minerals, the most reliable is atomic absorption spectroscopy (AAS)—serum magnesium and plasma zinc and possibly red cell levels as more reflective of brain levels. The critical factor is assessment of competing nutrient balance—for example, copper-to-zinc ratio (normal is 1:1). The gold standard remains clinical replacement with monitoring for improvement in clinical symptoms, because normal blood values may not reflect tissue deficiency. Serum iron values can be relied on to accurately reflect body nutrient status. Hair levels of trace minerals have been studied (including in children with learning and attention

disorders[47]); in general, results are unreliable but may be used for heavy metal exposure.

Iron. Iron is the mineral most commonly low in marginally nourished infants and toddlers; deficiency results in decreased arousal, attending, social responsiveness, and persistence.

Zinc. Zinc is a key cofactor in metabolism of essential fatty acids (EFAs). One study showed those with low serum levels may be less responsive to stimulant medications.

One approach in current clinical work indicates that increased levels of copper (Cu:Zn > 1) predominate in the profile of children with ADD.[48] Therapeutic supplementation avoids copper, includes zinc along with other nutrients, and is based on the individual profile.

Magnesium. Magnesium is often lost in food processing and may be deficient in a significant number of normally nourished people. Magnesium supplementation in two populations resulted in (1) improved behavior rating (non-blinded) for hyperactivity and distractibility in a diagnosed ADD population compared with the control ADD group[49] (200 mg/day) and (2) significantly increased nonverbal IQ (positive correlation with attention span) and reduced antisocial, impulsive, violent behavior in a well-controlled, double-blind study in a large general school age (7- to 12-year-olds) population[50, 51] using a multivitamin/mineral tablet (50% RDA) for 3 to 4 months.

Vitamin B$_6$. Vitamin B$_6$ supplementation (10 to 15 mg/kg/day) was compared with placebo and with Ritalin in one study of ADD subjects; there was a nonsignificant trend in favor of the impact of B$_6$ on behavior.

Megavitamins. Two percent of those on megavitamin therapy had elevated liver enzymes and 25% had more disruptive behavior on therapy than those administered placebo. However, more rational pharmacologic doses (one to two times RDA) of zinc, magnesium, and vitamin C and B$_{6,1}$ and folate for a school year in learning disabled/ADD children resulted in significant academic improvements that persisted for 1 year after discontinuation.[52]

Essential Fatty Acids. *EFAs,* especially omega-6 and omega-3, are an area of active current research because they pertain to mental health. They are essential for brain structure (60% is lipid), as precursors for the eicosanoids (mediators/modulators of nerve transmission), and for metabolism into specific long-chain polyunsaturated fatty acids (LCPUFAs)—eicosapentaenoic acid (EPA) (more associated with adult mental illness) and docosahexaenoic acid (DHA) (most associated with neuronal membranes and retina)—which are neurotransmitter precursors and components of neuronal membranes. The EFAs need an ω6-to-ω3 ratio in the range of 4:1; however, the current average diet in the U.S. culture is skewed toward saturated fats and a ω6-to-ω3 ratio of 25:1. Adequate levels are a significant factor (along with antioxidant protection of vitamin E) in vulnerability of fetal brain to insult (including

Table 5–5. Neurotoxic or Irritant Substances in Foods

Additives	Salicylate-containing	Common Allergens
Anticaking compounds	Strawberries	Milk and dairy products
Antioxidants	Plums	Eggs
Bleaching agents	Raspberries	Soy
Emulsifiers	Chicory	Wheat
Preservatives	Almonds	Corn
Thickeners	Peanuts	Citrus fruits
Artificial flavorings	Tomatoes	Peanuts
Colorings	Honey	Tree nuts
	White vinegar	Fish and shellfish

hypoxia) and resultant developmental disabilities such as ADD. Research shows correlation between levels of LCPUFAs in plasma and red cell membranes and the presence of mental illness[53]; supplementation with a 2:1 ratio of EPA-to-DHA produces significant improvement in bipolar disorder.[54]

A study by Teicher and Polcari is now under way evaluating clinical response in a general ADD population to supplementation with an ω3 EPA-to-DHA ratio of 7:1 (OmegaBrite). In a subset of ADD patients with EFA deficiency signs and symptoms (increased thirst and urination, dry hair/skin), a clear relationship exists with alterations in specific fatty acids (absolute decrease in omega 3 LCPUFAs and increased ω6-to-ω3 ratio).[55] This subset, two fifths of a general group of ADD boys, had increased water intake, somewhat *increased* total fatty acid intake (specific polyunsaturated fatty acids [PUFAs] not calculated), and significantly greater incidence of allergic rhinitis, temper tantrums, and problems getting to sleep. The other three fifths of the ADD boys had low EFA deficiency symptoms and PUFAs similar to those of non-ADD boys. Supplementation with a 5:1 ratio of DHA-to-EPA (Efalex Focus), in a total PUFA ω6-to-ω3 ratio of 3:2, correlated significantly with improved EFA deficiency symptoms, blood EFA values, and attention span.[56] In Walsh's[48] clinical and chemical database, the majority of children with ADD have low ω3 PUFAs, have an increased ω6-to-ω3 ratio, and benefit from high-dose oral ω3 EFA replacement. The cause for EFA alterations in ADD is not yet clear, is probably multifactorial (dietary deficiency, altered metabolism, genetics or environmental toxins), and may have significant specificity in some individuals. Numerous EFA preparations are available; and although no single one will likely prove effective for all those with ADD, the ratio of the ω6-to-ω3 LCPUFAs is probably a key factor. (See Table 5–7 for food sources of essential fatty acids.)

Lifestyle: Exercise and Spirituality

Exercise

Done on a regular basis, exercise enhances the body physically, creates mental and physiologic relaxation, improves mood, and develops mind-body coordination. Individuals with ADD often have relative weakness in coordination, so the emphasis should be on individual strengths and self-improvement rather than competition. The habit established early in childhood has the strongest influence on behavior as an adult.

Spirituality

The best support for dealing with the adversity that often accompanies ADD is a strong spiritual foundation of love and ultimate trust. Children learn best from their parents' behavior and sharing of their own beliefs rather than verbal directives.

Children are born with a spiritual dimension that begins with a clear connection with the nonvisible realm and that undergoes a normal sequence of development.[57] Parental practice of seeking sustenance from a spiritual source is key in creating a hopeful, loving home environment in which the child is valued and positive support and guidance are provided.

Mind-Body

As a group, these therapies promote physiologic and psychological self-regulation and are highly effective for increasing a sense of self-mastery and control, self-esteem, and competence; reducing stress; and positively affecting emotional problems.

Relaxation and Meditation

Relaxation training in grade-school children positively affects the core behaviors in ADD and is at least as effective as other therapies.[58] However, locus of control is significantly more internal with the use of the group techniques; individual electromyographic (EMG) training may become boring after the first few sessions.[59] Increase in internal locus of control consistently associates with enhanced academic achievement and behavioral control. The meditative state can be attained through a sitting practice or movement practice (tai chi, yoga postures, or asanas), which is particularly well suited for children; both are coordinated with breathing patterns. These provide both mind-body connection and experience with seeking direction from internal resources (rather than external distractions).

Guided Imagery: A Way of Thinking That Has Sensory Qualities

Children (especially those younger than age 5 years) are inherently more magical and imaginative; so the imagery process is short, moves quickly, and may be done while moving about or with eyes open. For persons with ADD, this therapy allows the use and amplification of a strength (creativity) to gain insight and mastery over the difficult areas of life—performance in social or school/work settings or thoughts and feelings. Imagery can be used to help the child create a safe and relaxing place. A wisdom figure or guide can then be recruited to help the child with problem solving or to empower the child in difficult situations (see Chapter 92, Guided Imagery and Interactive Guided Imagery). Parents can easily facilitate their child, and it is creative and fun!

Self-Hypnosis[60]

Self-hypnosis (hypnotherapy used by the person himself or herself) combines the creativity of imagery with self-regulation. Specific suggestion[s] are provided during an altered state of consciousness/ mental relaxation to achieve improved behavior and learning. It does not directly address the core neurocognitive processes of attention; rather, it decreases anxiety and increases recognition capacity for associated difficulties, development of coping strategies, and changed attitudes. The height of hypnotic suggestibility occurs in school-age children before they reach adolescence; and preschool children informally experience self-hypnosis with activities such as being read a story. Whereas induction techniques vary considerably by age and by child, self-hypnosis provides an excellent therapeutic option for ADD in the child who is imaginative and for whom the family environment is supportive.

Neurotherapy (EEG Biofeedback)

In ADD, EEG biofeedback counterbalances genetic and environmental tendencies with the learned skill of altering brain wave patterns to gain specific benefits. An excellent review of the research conducted since about 1990[61] shows (1) 60% or more of those treated develop either decreased theta or increased beta or both during task performance and improve on the TOVA (Test of Variables of Attention) continuous performance task; (2) all (90%+) improve significantly on behavior ratings (of attention but not of aggression/defiance) by nonblinded observers; (3) effects may be more global as IQ tends to increase; and (4) improved attention on the TOVA is as strong as with stimulant medication. Treatment sessions are individually structured with task performance reinforcement and coupled with behavioral reinforcement in home and school environments. Further research is required to sort out specific from nonspecific factors in the effectiveness of this modality.

Dosage. Thirty to 40 sessions, 20 to 40 minutes each, twice weekly (may also be intensified and done daily) over a 5- to 6-month period; cost is $1000 to $2000.

Behavior Management and Other Psychological Supports

Parents have a pivotal emotional role with their children because most youngsters truly want to be successful and to satisfy parental expectations. Because youngsters with ADD are more different than they are alike, the recommendations for behavioral management noted in Table 5–6 are general in nature. This approach has enormous therapeutic impact on maintenance of self-esteem, academic functioning, social interaction, and fostering effective communication within families. Successful intervention requires intensive strategies throughout the child's day. However, most parents find that successful strategies require no greater expenditure of energy or time than their previous attempts to manage, which generally did not work.[62] For parent

resources, see "Professional Resources," later in this chapter.

Biomechanical

Massage Therapy

Field and coworkers[63] have consistently shown benefits of massage therapy in differing populations: stable preterm and term infants, preschoolers, and children with chronic conditions such as asthma, cancer, and diabetes, and adults with fibromyalgia and depression. Results include improved physical growth, learning, mood, and relaxation and decreased pain. In one study of adolescents with ADD in a self-contained classroom, blinded teacher behavior ratings for hyperactivity (Conners) and time on task improved significantly (came within the normal range) after 10 days of 15 minutes of massage to neck, shoulders, and back compared with subjects with an identical time of guided relaxation of the same areas.[64] The same authors have shown similar improved teacher ratings of behavior after 1 month of twice-weekly massage.

Osteopathic Manipulative Therapy: Craniosacral Most Pertinent for ADD

The musculoskeletal system is a key element of health; manipulative osteopathy restores subtle structural-functional relationships, both biomechanically and bioenergetically. Craniosacral osteopathy concentrates on the cranial bones' subtle articular mobility, the interrelationships of the central nervous system membranes (dura, falx cerebri, and tentorium), and their attachments to specific cranial bones and to the sacrum. The integrity of the craniosacral system influences not only neurochemical function but also neural structure (e.g., cranial nerves that pass through these membranes/bones). These relationships are of particular interest in the newborn whose skull is highly mobile. Sphenobasilar and occipital condyle alignment patterns were

Table 5-6. Recommendations for Behavior Management in Attention Deficit Disorder
....

1. Provide **structure** with flexible boundaries
2. Define **expectations** regularly and consistently
3. **Subdivide** tasks into their component parts
4. Teach by **modeling**
5. Use **multisensory communication**: provide simultaneous visual and auditory input
6. **Reward** effort in addition to outcomes or product
7. Provide **frequent positive reinforcement** even for behaviors generally taken for granted
8. Respond specifically to a youngster's **behavior**, not to the child's self-worth or value
9. Be **consistent**
10. Learn to **accept** the child for who he or she is
11. Remain **emotionally neutral** as much as possible
12. Be **patient** with the child; results from behavioral efforts may not be seen for months or years

studied in a series of 1250 newborns[65]; some disturbance of the patterns occurred in greater than 60% of symptom-free infants. In infants with symptoms, there were associations between the type of symptoms and the specific alignment patterns found: respiratory and circulatory symptoms with torsion of the sphenobasilar; behavioral/feeding symptoms with bilateral occipital condylar compression and flexion of the sphenobasilar. Craniosacral osteopathic treatment of the abnormal patterns in the newborn may have a role in the prevention of developmental disorders, including ADD. It can be used to treat acute symptoms such as colic, sleeplessness, or increased muscle tone as well. In a study of preschool and early school-age children, treated with 6 to 12 individualized osteopathic treatments, those with neurologic problems (learning, behavior, or neuromotor function) showed an increased velocity of development.[66]

Bioenergetic

Homeopathy: Constitutionally Prescribed

Homeopathy is the healing system based on "like cures like"—*homeo,* same; *pathos,* suffering. This principle of the Law of Similars governs the selection of a remedy that most closely resembles the totality of the patient's symptoms (the constitutional remedy)[67]—the essential nature of the child, the disturbance from the child's perspective. Symptoms result from an imbalance or disorganization in the subtle energy system; the remedy "coaxes back that energy by conveying information about what sort of adaptive response is needed."[68] Similar reasoning is seen in allergy desensitization therapy. Homeopathy is most applicable to the neuropsychological disorders such as ADD, working from "inside out" (i.e., spirit, mind, emotions, then the physical body)—the most profound reorganization of the organism as a whole.

Constitutional prescription necessitates a whole range of remedies as potential in ADD. Children tend to be less diverse in their constitutions. Therefore, a few remedies seem to be most common for ADD: tuberculinum, stramonium, hyoscyamus, tarentula, lycopodium, and perhaps medorrhinum—although sources differ. Little cooperation or energy for compliance is required; a single dose is given, occasionally with follow-up doses. In a single double-blind, partial crossover study of 43 children with the *Diagnostic and Statistical Manual of Mental Disorders,* fourth edition (DSM IV), criteria for ADD and significant comorbid diagnoses, there was statistically significant improvement (P = .05 to .01) using a constitutional remedy compared with placebo for all conditions (initial remedy to placebo, best remedy to placebo, and placebo crossed over to remedy).[69] Related treatments include tissue salts (potassium phosphate or combination 5 phosphate salts) and flower essences (chamomile, impatiens, and clematis are common examples), both constitutionally prescribed.[68] Tissue salts ($6\times$ preparation) address more physical disturbances, which is particularly needed with pervasive exposure to environmental toxic chemicals and quite appropriate for the less complex system of children. In general, flower essences address emotional disturbances.

Therapeutic Touch/Healing Touch

Therapeutic touch/healing touch is a gentle therapeutic approach to healing that employs both touch and energy, using the hands of a practitioner to create a state of balance and relaxation, thus supporting the body's own ability to heal. There are reports of clinical efficacy in ADD but no published research to date.

Movement Therapies: Yoga, Tai Chi, Qi Gong

Movement therapies are practices that exert their effect primarily on the flow and balance of the body's subtle energy system and, to a greater or lesser extent, on the biomechanics of the body—flexibility, coordination, balance, and strength. The control of the flow and rhythm of the breath (generally diaphragmatic) connects body and mind, modulates neurochemistry (activates parasympathetic tone and the limbic system), and facilitates energy flow (likely along fascial planes) throughout the body. The attention is drawn inward, concentrating the mind on body movement or postures in coordination with the cycle of the breath—"moving meditation." Most cultural traditions (including American Indian) select postures and movements to simulate the qualities and actions of living beings within their experience, providing connection with the spiritual dimension. These practices are particularly good for those with ADD, because they combine movement, creativity in imagery, and inward focusing rather than the more outward focusing associated with the patient's own "distractibility" or that of performance and competition in sports or exercise.

Whole System Therapies

Traditional Chinese Medicine

Traditional Chinese medicine (TCM) understands infants and young children to be not yet strong or well integrated. They can accumulate fetal toxins from the mother through imbalance of her own diet and lifestyle. These cause eruptions or remain latent in the body to become manifest disease when triggered later in life; *diet is the key cause of children's diseases.*[71] Ancient thought, yet so applicable to the developmental disorders of present-day children! Loo correlates the cognitive and psychoemotional developmental stages of children (Piaget and Freud) with TCM five-element theory (specific energetic systems are vulnerable at certain ages) into an integrated evaluation and treatment of children with developmental disorders, including ADD (see "Professional Resources").

TCM has reported efficacy in children with ADD; three major patterns are described as occurring in ADD.[71, 72] Each has recommended treatment with a combination of Chinese herbs and acupuncture points. Research shows potential benefit on behavior (comparable with that of methylphenidate) with the use of a Chinese herbal mixture and, preliminarily, with the use of laser acupuncture.[73–75] Loo[76] recommends combined treatment with diet, herbs, acupuncture, and home management with acupressure as the most successful. Tui Na, the TCM practice of therapeutic massage and manipulation, is adapted for the developing energy system of the infant and child. The techniques can be taught to parents for use with their child and considered in the difficult-to-console, night-crying (colicky) infant—sometimes an early behavior associated with later ADD.[77]

Detoxification

The impact of environmental toxins—chemical (see Table 5–2) and social/cultural—deserves special attention, because ADD is a common sequela. Prevention and treatment may have a significantly positive impact on central nervous system development during the critically formative period—fetal[78] through age 5 years. A primary focus then is the health of the pre-pregnant woman—a uniquely available niche for the family practitioner. All toxins impact central nervous system reparative and neurotransmitter functions throughout life, thereby affecting expression of ADD characteristics during school age. Adolescents are another population of focus; the myelinization of the prefrontal cortex does not complete until adolescence, and elective exposure to environmental toxins may increase at this age.

Therapies to Consider

Ayurvedic Medicine

Ayurvedic medicine utilizes a framework of constitutional types (prakruti) and current balance of principal forces (doshas) that are the foundation for prescription of diet, herbs, spices, and daily life to create balance in the mind, body, and spirit. Specific herbs have been identified as clinically useful in treating ADD.

Tomatis Method

The Tomatis method[79] (http://www.tomatis.com) utilizes individualized sound therapy to improve attention through auditory integration and listening. This may be most applicable for those with an accompanying learning disorder in auditory processing.

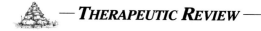 *THERAPEUTIC REVIEW*

Multiple, integrated strategies are most effective. Choose one or more interventions from each of the following categories and implement gradually across the developmental age span. Consider the level of energy and motivation of the child and the family. If it is low, start with those therapies that provide energy to the patient and are less dependent on motivation for compliance (e.g., biochemical, bioenergetic, and biomechanical).

Women in Childbearing Years: Prevention

Nutrition
- General: Instruct in dietary sources of B vitamins/folate (B_6), magnesium, zinc, and iron. If at risk for undernutrition (based on diet history), supplement with vitamin-mineral (zinc, magnesium) preparation. Use laboratory values to guide supplementation for iron.
- Balance dietary fatty acid intake with a ratio of less than 6:1 ω6-to-ω3 EFAs by decreasing saturated fats and ω6 oils and increasing ω3 oils and sources. (For specifics, see "Older Preschool-Age" section, below.)
- Avoid food and water sources of environmental toxins.

Detoxification—Environmental Neurotoxicants
- Take environmental chemical and social toxin exposure history on all patients.
- Know practice community sources of air and water pollution (active industry) and soil (former and active industrial sites). See "Professional Resources."
- Provide herbal supplement support for liver metabolism and

follow recommendations for active detoxification if pre-pregnant (see Chapter 98, Detoxification).

- *Avoidance of exposure*: Excellent guidelines for pesticides, lead, foods, household products, building materials, solvents, alcohol and tobacco, and breast-feeding on www.igc.org/psr/protect-child.htm

Therapeutic/Sustaining Practices

- Relaxation, meditation, guided imagery, and breath work are used for chronic stress reduction (see Chapter 92, Guided Imagery and Interactive Guided Imagery). Enhance with energy healing modalities—for example, healing touch or biomechanical techniques such as massage.
- Provide support with regular exercise and spiritual practice.

Infant/Toddler: Prevention/Treatment

Nutrition

- Breast-Feeding: Please DO! The benefits outweigh the risks in the current research in the U.S. population.[78] Breast milk can contain lipophilic neurotoxic chemicals; however, the amounts and the central nervous system impact are significantly less than during pregnancy.
- Whole, fresh foods organically grown: particularly cost-effective in this age group. Avoid food additives (e.g., dyes, preservatives) and refined sugars completely or as much as possible. Use single-item pureed foods rather than mixtures for infant feeding. If family history of allergy: avoid the highly allergenic foods—wheat, corn, soy, cow's milk, citrus, and peanut. If physical or behavioral symptoms require treatment, try an oligoantigenic elimination diet (see later). Essential nutrients: assure adequate intake of EFAs (especially $\omega 3$), B vitamins (B_6), magnesium, iron, and zinc (see "Older Preschool and School-Age" section, below).

Daily Routine—Parent Practices

- Behavior management is critical at this age of discovering limits! Consistency in family routine is important from birth.
- *Bedtime*: Quiet period for the whole family along with guided imagery (one example is the traditional ritual of the bedtime story) is excellent. Herbs, aromatherapy with lavender, and relaxing music may be added.

Therapeutic/Sustaining Practices

- Herbs: Chamomile—use a small quantity of very concentrated tea or a tincture. Start with 1 to 3 mL of tincture (dissipate alcohol with heat or use glycerite preparation) in small amount of liquid, one to four times daily, for soothing or antispasmodic effect. Other herbs not recommended.
- Infant Massage: Preterm, stable infant—all benefit; especially good for behavioral regulatory control. Term infant, irritable, overly active—may add pediatric Chinese acupressure or Tui Na. Use in 5- to 15-minute periods, one to three times daily or as needed.
- Healing touch, therapeutic touch, and prayer (bioenergetic forms of healing)—may be the preferred method of enhancing neuroregulatory development in the ill premature infant; this remains to be researched.

Therapeutic Interventions

- Craniosacral osteopathy as prevention. Essential for birth trauma (prolonged labor/forceps delivery); may also be helpful for feeding difficulties, fussiness, or behavior difficulties. Infant: 1 to 4 treatments; toddler: 4 to 10.

Older Preschool and School-Age: Treatment

Nutrition
In the exhausted family and child, diet change may not be the first intervention; in that case, rely on supplementation.

Level I: *All children with ADD symptoms:*
- Assure adequate intake of essential neurocognitive nutrients, preferably in the diet. Switch the balance of EFAs by decreasing the intake of saturated and omega-6 fats and increasing omega-3 sources (Table 5–7; see also Chapter 84, The Anti-Inflammatory Diet).
- Use whole, nonprocessed food (avoid additives and dyes); use organically grown foods (avoid chemical toxins), primarily for foods consumed in greatest quantity; avoid animal fat when consuming meat or use organically fed sources. Cold water fish: mackerel, sardines, herring, albacore tuna, and some fresh water fish—risk of mercury; salmon—mercury-free.
- When there is risk of undernutrition, supplement 50% to 100% RDA of vitamins and minerals for age—see "Professional Resources," later.
- *Supplement:* (1) Multivitamin: B_6 (0.1 to 1.0 mg/day) in B complex, C, A, and E. (2) Minerals: magnesium 30 to 200 mg/day, zinc and copper (ratio of 10:1), and iron based on laboratory values. (3) EFAs: Use black currant oil, fish body oil preparation (purified for toxins), or balanced $\omega6$-to-$\omega3$ preparation—*Attention Focus* ($\omega6$-to-$\omega3$ ratio is 3:2 of both short-chain and long-chain PUFAs from tuna, evening primrose oil, and thyme oil) by Nature's Way. Trial for 3 months. Monitor behavior—blinded teacher ratings (Conners or ACTeRS).

Level II: *Nonresponders to therapies previously discussed and those with ADD symptoms and fatty acid deficiency (increased thirst, dry skin and allergy):*
- Supplement guided by laboratory assessment: (1) iron: blood levels (Fe, total iron-binding capacity [TIBC], ferritin). (2) Trace minerals/AAS: serum magnesium and copper and plasma zinc—normal values do NOT rule out abnormality; serial measures necessary. May use doses above RDA but not above upper limits for safety. Ratio of copper-to-zinc (1:1 is normal)—avoid copper in supplementation if ratio is increased because it may aggravate ADD. (3) EFA levels (serum/red blood cells): need *specific* omega-3, 6 PUFAs, totals, and ratios. May also use clinical trial alone. Supplement trial (>3 months) with LCPUFAs to bypass weakness in converting to EFAs.
- Use predominantly omega 3 preparations (although a few may require predominately $\omega6$), containing EPA and DHA (exact amounts and ratios likely variable). Options: neuromins (several brands)—DHA (algae) only; OmegaBrite—EPA-to-DHA ratio 7:1; and Children's DHA chewables by Nordic Naturals. All are safe for environmental neurotoxins.

Table 5–7. Food Sources of Essential Neurocognitive Nutrients

B_6	Iron	Magnesium	Zinc	Fatty Acids	
				Omega 6	*Omega 3*
Eggs	Beef	Whole grains	Whole grains	Seeds	Nuts: walnuts
Beans	Pork	Potassium-rich fruits and vegetables		Oils—corn, soy, safflower	Leafy green vegetables
Beef	Blackstrap molasses			Borage	Oils: flax, canola
Pork	Dried prunes			Evening primrose oil [arachidonic acid]	Fish oils [EPA/DHA]
Broccoli	Raisins and apricots				Fish, algae
Spinach	Leafy green vegetables			Red meats	
Banana					

EFA, essential fatty acid; EPA/DHA, eicosapentaenoic acid/docosahexaenoic acid.

- Use blinded teacher behavior ratings as guide.
- *ADD with allergies*/allergic family history or severe ADD: Treat with an oligoantigenic diet (lamb, chicken, potato, rice, banana, apple, pear, cabbage, broccoli, celery, carrot, and cucumber) + elimination of any specific allergenic item + organic foods for 1 month.

If behavior improves, then re-introduce potential allergenic foods (see Chapter 82, The Elimination Diet and Diagnosing Food Hypersensitivities).

Level III: *Pharmacologic Nutrient Therapy.*
- Referral to nutritionist or naturopathic physician or a center that specializes in nutritional management of ADD. See Appendix A for referral sources. Obtain specific nutrient laboratory analysis followed by individualized supplementation and blinded monitoring of behavior; may require longer than 3 months. Avoid megavitamin therapy.

Daily Routine—Parent and child practices. Behavior management and bedtime: see previously.

"Chemical" Interventions
- Pharmaceuticals: (1) A bridge to initiate treatment; most immediate and potent intervention. Especially helpful when family/child are in crisis and resources are exhausted. (2) Consider deferring use until other forms of intervention with fewer side effects have been tried. (3) Always use in combination with other interventions—allows lower dose and fewer side effects. (4) Long-term use may be necessary. Use can be considered after age 5 years (see Tables 5–2 and 5–3).
- Herbs: *Chamomile* (see earlier): as antispasmodic or for sedation; start with 3 to 5 mL, may safely increase to efficacy. *Lemon balm*: for the overreactor or anxiety; use as tincture (alcohol dissipated with heat) or the glycerite, start with 1 mL and increase to efficacy; or as a cold infusion tea. Both may be used at bedtime or three times daily. *Melatonin* may be tried—2 to 10 mg at bedtime to improve sleep. All may be used along with the stimulants and amphetamines. Other herbs are generally not recommended in this age group.
- Homeopathy—constitutional prescription: the preferred therapy for general treatment (ideally in lieu of pharmaceuticals) owing to depth of therapeutic effect, lack of side effects, simplicity of treatment, low dependence on compliance for efficacy, and low cost; may include tissue salts and flower essences. Support with nutritional and other therapies.

Therapeutic/Sustaining Practices
- Exercise and spirituality: regular practice begun at this age, before the resistance of adolescence, is particularly important—and fun. Sports/activities should emphasize individual skill development rather than competition.
- Guided imagery and self-hypnosis—best when family environment is supportive; utilizes the child's inner resources to develop coping strategies.
- Meditation, most often a moving practice (tai chi, yoga) at this age, is fun and also well-suited for family involvement—others may also be ADD! Tae kwon do strengthens the mind-body connection and appropriately channels physical energy or aggression.
- *Massage*, of many varieties including tui na and acupressure, is effective for ADD behavioral symptoms when given twice weekly; it may incorporate aromatherapy.
- *Therapeutic touch/healing touch* is especially beneficial for those who do not tolerate physical touch and for physical or emotional discomfort.

Therapeutic Interventions

- Osteopathic manipulation (include craniosacral): particularly indicated with history of birth trauma. For attention and behavior, provides periodic support (every 4 to 6 weeks).
- EEG biofeedback: efficacy requires significant motivation by the child and commitment of resources. Excellent for concrete reinforcement and structure external to school/family.

Adolescent and Adult
Nutrition—Daily Routine

- General guidelines (see earlier): Reliance on supplements may increase owing to irregularity of routine and greater independence in eating—emphasize use of mobile whole foods.

Therapeutic/Sustaining Practices

- Relaxation, meditation (includes sitting, movement, and breathing practices), imagery, self-hypnosis, spiritual exploration, and exercise/sports.
- These mature, become self-initiated, and increasingly provide structure and key support for self-esteem, as daily routine becomes less predictable.
- Therapeutic interventions (massage, craniosacral osteopathy, and acupuncture) may become less utilized; these may have specific benefit for the mood disorders seen comorbidly at this age.

"Chemical" Interventions

- Herbs: *St. Johns Wort* may be tried for depression. Recommended adult dose: 300 mg three times daily—standardized (3% minimum hyperforin), or the stabilized hydroalcoholic extract (Eclectic and Nature's Way). *Valerian* (450 to 900 mg) or *kava kava* (100 to 200 mg) standardized extract—two to three times daily or at bedtime may be beneficial for anxiety and sleep.
- Pharmaceuticals: medication may still be needed. See previous guidelines.
- Homeopathy may be particularly well accepted by the adolescent; its theoretical base (energy healing) may be especially appealing and interference in daily life is significantly less than with pharmacotherapy or herbs.
- Detoxification: the focus now shifts to the workplace; owing to drug exposure and often declining nutrition, there may be a greater need for periodic treatment.

PROFESSIONAL RESOURCES

Physician Information

1. Elkind D: The Hurried Child: Growing Up Too Fast Too Soon, 3rd ed. Perseus, 2001.
2. Loo May: East West Healing. New York, John Wiley & Sons, 2001.

   An integrated approach [Western and Chinese medicine] to various disorders for patient and family, incorporates home management strategies. Specific energetic systems are vulnerable during each developmental stage in children. Author is a physician trained in both traditions.

3. The Health Research Institute and Pfeiffer Treatment Center http://www.hriptc.org 1804 Centre Point Circle, Suite 102, Naperville, IL 60563. community@hriptc.com

   Referral source for nutrient assessment and treatment with large-dose vitamin-mineral and EFA supplementation. Less than $1000 for complete initial evaluation and first supply of supplements. Directed by Ph.D. biochemist, pharmacist, nutritionists, and physicians.

4. Nutritional information: (1) Murray M, Pizzorno J: Textbook of Natural Medicine, 2 vols. New York, Churchill Livingstone. (2) www.nal.usda.gov/fnic/etext/fnic.html and go to Dietary Reference Intakes.
5. Environmental toxins information: (1) Sources by geographic location: state and county, including Superfund sites—Environmental Defense Fund Scorecard: www.scorecard.org Also: www.imapdata.com/health-track. (2) Background and updates: www.igc.org/psr/ and www.ourstolenfuture.org
6. Rapp DJ: Is This Your Child's World? Bantam, 1996. Hyperactivity, learning disabilities, allergies, and school environment.

Patient Material

1. Greenfield RH, Ditchek SH: Healthy Child, Whole Child. HarperCollins, 2001.
2. Jones CB: Parent Articles About ADHD. San Antonio, TX, Communication Skill Builders, 1999.
3. The Association of Birth Defect Children, Betty Mekdeci, Executive Director; 930 Woodcock Road, Suite 225, Orlando, FL 32803. (407) 895–0802. www.birthdefects.org

Advocacy and exposure information expertise; birth defects epidemiologic database. A nongovernmental organization; funded by private contributions and research grants.

4. ADD Information: Research; family and legal issues; support groups
National Attention Deficit Disorder Association: www.add.org
CHADD: national support organization with local chapters www.chadd.org

Discipline Information: Education, Credentialing, Licensure, and Location of Practitioners

1. National Center for Homeopathy (703) 548–7790 nch@igc.apc.org 801 N. Fairfax Street, Suite 306, Alexandria, VA 22314.
2. The Cranial Academy (317) 594–0411; (317) 594–9299 (Fax) 8202 Clearvista Pkwy, Bldg #9, Suite D, Indianapolis, IN 46256.
3. American Academy of Medical Acupuncture (213) 957–5514; 5820 Wilshire Blvd, Suite 500, Los Angeles, CA 90036.
4. American Association of Naturopathic Physicians 2366 Eastlake Avenue East, Suite 322, Seattle, WA 98102; (206) 323–7610 http://infinity.dorsai.org/Naturopathic.Physician
5. Academy for Guided Imagery, PO Box 2070, Mill Valley, CA 94942 (415) 389–9324 (800) 726–2070 http://www.interactive-imagery.com
6. American Massage Therapy Association, 820 Davis Street, Suite 100, Evanston, IL 60201.
7. International Association of Yoga Therapists, Larry Payne, Ph.D., and Jnani Chapman, R.N., 20 Sunnyside Avenue, Suite A-243, Mill Valley, CA 94941–1928.

References

1. Still GF: Some abnormal physical conditions in childhood. Lancet 1:1008, 1902.
2. Wolraich ML, Felice ME, Drotar D (eds): The Classification of Child and Adolescent Mental Diagnoses in Primary Care (DSM-PC). Elk Grove Village, Ill, American Academy of Pediatrics, 1996.
3. Richters JE, Arnold LE, Jensen PS, et al: NIMH Collaborative Multisite Multimodal Treatment Study of Children with ADHD: I. Background and rationale. J Am Acad Child Adolesc Psychiatry 34:987–1000, 1995.
4. AACAP Policy Statement: Practice parameters for the assessment and treatment of children, adolescents, and adults with attention-deficit/hyperactivity disorder. J Am Acad Child Adolesc Psychiatry 36(10 Suppl):85S–121S, 1997.
5. Stubberfield TG, Wray JA, Parry TS: Utilization of alternative therapies in attention-deficit hyperactivity disorder. J Paediatr Child Health 35:450–453, 1999.
6. ACQIP: Monitoring Children with Attention Deficit Hyperactivity Disorder. Ambulatory Care Quality Improvement Program. Elk Grove, Ill, American Academy of Pediatrics, 1997.
7. AAP Committee on Children with Disabilities: Counseling families who choose complementary and alternative medicine for their child with chronic illness or disability. Pediatrics 107:598–601, 2001.
8. Chan E, Gardiner P, Kemper KJ: "At least it's natural . . .": Herbs and dietary supplements in ADHD. Contemp Pediatr 17(9):116–130, 2000.
9. Mirsky AF: Disorder of attention. In Lyon GR, Krasnegor NA (eds): Attention, Memory, and Executive Function. Baltimore, PH Brookes, 1996, pp 71–95.
10. Mercugliano M: What is attention-deficit/hyperactivity disorder? In Morgan AM (ed): Attention-Deficit/Hyperactivity Disorder. Pediatr Clin North Am 6:831–843, 1999.
11. Low CB: Attention deficit hyperactivity disorder: Dissociation and adaptation. Am J Clin Hypnosis 41:253–261, 1999.
12. Krause K, Dresel SH, Krause J, et al: Increased striatal dopamine transporter in adult patients with attention deficit hyperactivity disorder: Effects of methylphenidate as measured by single photon emission computed tomography. Neurosci Lett 285:107–110, 2000.
13. Volkow ND, Wang G-J, Fowler JS, et al: Therapeutic doses of oral methylphenidate significantly increase extracellular dopamine in the human brain. J Neurosci 21:RC121:1–5, 2001.
14. Waldman ID, Rowe DC, Abramowitz A, et al: Association and linkage of the dopamine transporter gene and attention-deficit hyperactivity disorder in children: Heterogeneity owing to diagnostic subtype and severity. Am J Hum Genet 63:1767–1776, 1998.
15. Castellanos FX: Neuroimaging of attention-deficit hyperactivity disorder. Child Adolesc Psychiatr Clin N Am 6:383–411, 1997.
16. Zametkin AJ, Ernst M: Problems in the management of attention-deficit-hyperactivity disorder. N Engl J Med 340:40–46, 1999.
17. Teicher MH, Anderson CM, Polcari A, et al: Functional deficits in basal ganglia of children with attention-deficit/hyperactivity disorder shown with functional magnetic resonance imaging relaxometry. Nat Med 6:470–473, 2000.
18. Anderson CM, Polcari, Lowen SB, et al: Rate- and dose-dependent effects of methylphenidate on functional magnetic resonance relaxometry of the cerebellar vermis in children with ADHD. Submitted for publication March 2001.
19. Hughes JR, John ER: Conventional and quantitative electroencephalography in psychiatry [review]. J Neuropsychiatry Clin Neurosci 11:190–208, 1999.
20. Tannock R: Attention deficit hyperactivity disorder: Advances in cognitive, neurobiological and genetic research. J Child Psychol Psychiatry 39:65–99, 1998.
21. Boyle CA, Decoufle P, Yeargin-Allsopp M: Prevalence and health impact of developmental disabilities in US children. Pediatrics 93:399–403, 1994.
22. Cook DE, Kestenbaum C, Honaker LM, Anderson ER: Joint statement on the impact of entertainment violence on children: Congressional Public Health Summit, July 26, 2000. Available: www.AAP.org/advocacy/releases
23. AAP Policy Statement: Media violence (RE9526). Pediatrics 95:949–951, 1995.
24. Elkind D: The Hurried Child: Growing Up Too Fast Too Soon, 3rd ed. Cambridge, Mass, Perseus, 2001.
25. Biederman J, Milberger S, Faraone S, et al: Family-environment risk factors for ADHD: A test of Rutter's indicators of adversity. Arch Gen Psychiatr 52:464–470, 1995.
26. Brazelton TB: Fetal observations: Could they relate to another modality, such as touch? In Field TM (ed): Touch in Early Development. Mahwah, NJ, Lawrence Erlbaum Associates, 1995, pp 53–65.
27. Gunnar MR, Connors J, Isensee J, Wall L: Adrenocortical activity and behavioral distress in newborns. Dev Psychobiol 21:279–310, 1988.
28. Meaney MJ, Aitken D, et al: Neonatal handling and the development of the adrenocortical response. In Gunzenhauser N (ed): Advances in Touch: New Implications in Human Development. Skillman, NJ: Johnson & Johnson, 1990, pp 80–89.
29. Greenfield RH, Ditchek SH: Healthy Child, Whole Child. New York, HarperCollins, 2001.
30. Polluting Our Future: Chemical Pollution in the US That Affects Child Development and Learning. National Environmental Trust (NET), Physicians for Social Responsibility (PSR), and Learning Disabilities Association of America (LDA). September 2000.
31. Bennett FC: Stimulant medication for the child with attention deficit hyperactivity disorder. In Morgan AM (ed): Attention-Deficit/Hyperactivity Disorder. Pediatr Clin North Am 6:929, 1999.
32. Adesman AR, Morgan AM: Management of stimulant medication in children with attention deficit/hyperactivity disorder. In Morgan AM (ed): Attention-Deficit/Hyperactivity Disorder. Pediatr Clin North Am 6:945, 1999.
33. 2001 Physicians' Desk Reference. Montvale, NJ, Medical Economics, 2001.
34. Cohen MW: The Attention Zone: A Parents' Guide to Attention Deficit/Hyperactivity Disorder. New York, Bruner Mazel, 1998.

35. Silver LB: Alternative (nonstimulant) medication in the treatment of attention deficit hyperactivity disorder in children. In Morgan AM (ed): Attention-Deficit/Hyperactivity Disorder. Pediatr Clin North Am 6:965, 1999.

36. Jensen PS, et al, for the MTA Cooperative Group: A 14 month RCT of treatment strategies for A-D/HD. Arch Gen Psychiatry 56:1073–1086, 1999.

37. Swanson JM, Kraemer HC, Hinshaw SP, et al: Clinical relevance of the primary findings of the MTA: Success rates based on the severity of ADHD and ODD symptoms at the end of treatment. J Am Acad Child Adolesc Psychiatry 40:168, 2001.

38. Pelham WE: Implication of the MTA study for behavioral and combined treatment. The ADHD Report 8:4, 2000.

39. Jensen PS, Hinshaw SP, Kraemer HC, et al: ADHD comorbidity findings from the MTA study: Comparing comorbid sub groups. J Am Acad Child Adolesc Psychiatry 40:147, 2001.

40. St. John's Wort. Pharmacopsychiatry 30 and 31 (Suppl), 1997 & 1998.

41. McIntyre M: A review of the benefits, adverse events, drug interactions and safety of St. John's Wort (Hypericum perforatum): The implications with regard to the regulation of herbal medicines. J Altern Complement Med 6:115–124, 2000.

42. Smits M, Nagtegaal E, Valentijn S, et al: Melatonin for chronic sleep onset insomnia in children with attention deficit hyperactivity disorder: Randomized placebo controlled trial. J Neurol Neurosurg Psychiatry 67:840, 1999.

43. Sheldon SH: Pro-convulsant effects of oral melatonin in neurologically disabled children [letter]. Lancet 351:1254, 1998.

44. Breakey J: The role of diet and behavior in childhood [review]. J Paediatr Child Health 33:190–194, 1997.

45. Rowe KS, Rowe KJ: Synthetic food coloring and behavior: A dose response effect in a double-blind, placebo-controlled, repeated-measures study. J Pediatr 125:691–698, 1994.

46. Underwood BA: Evaluating the nutritional status of individuals: A critique of approaches. Nutr Rev 44(Suppl):213–224, 1986.

47. Phil RO, Parkes M: Hair element content in learning disabled children. Science 198:204–206, 1977.

48. Walsh WJ, et al: Biochemical therapy and behavior outcomes [abstract accepted for publication]. Physiol Behav 2001 www.hriptc.org

49. Starobrat-Hermelin B, Kozielec T: The effects of magnesium physiological supplementation on hyperactivity in children with attention deficit hyperactivity disorder (ADHD): Positive response to magnesium oral loading test. Magnes Res 10:149–156, 1997.

50. Schoenthaler SJ, Bier ID: The effect of vitamin-mineral supplementation on juvenile delinquency among American schoolchildren: A randomized, double-blind placebo-controlled trial [see comments]. J Altern Complement Med 6:7–17, 2000.

51. Schoenthaler SJ, Bier ID: The effect of vitamin-mineral supplementation on the intelligence of American schoolchildren: A randomized, double-blind placebo-controlled trial [see comments]. J Altern Complement Med 6:19–29, 2000.

52. Carlton RM, Ente G, Blum L, et al: Rational dosages of nutrients have a prolonged effect on learning disabilities. Altern Ther Health Med 6:85–91, 2000.

53. Cott J: Omega-3 fatty acids and psychiatric disorders. Altern Ther Women's Health 97–104, December 1999.

54. Stoll AL, Severus WE, Freeman MP, et al: Omega 3 fatty acids in bipolar disorder: A preliminary double-blind, placebo-controlled trial. Arch Gen Psychiatry 56:407–412, 1999.

55. Stevens LJ, Zentall SS, Deck JL, et al: Essential fatty acid metabolism in boys with attention-deficit hyperactivity disorder. Am J Clin Nutr 62:761–768, 1995.

56. Burgess JR, Stevens L, Zhang W, et al: Long-chain polyunsaturated fatty acids in children with attention-deficit hyperactivity disorder. Am J Clin Nutr 71(1 Suppl):327S–330S, 2000.

57. Coles R: The Spiritual Life of Children. Boston, Houghton Mifflin, 1991.

58. Richter NC: The efficacy of relaxation training with children [review]. J Abnorm Child Psychol 12:319–344, 1984.

59. Denkowski KM, Denkowski GC: Is group progressive relaxation training as effective with hyperactive children as individual EMG biofeedback treatment? Biofeedback Self Regul 9:353–364, 1984.

60. Olness K, Kohen D: Hypnosis and Hypnotherapy with Children, 3rd ed. New York, Guilford, 1996.

61. Nash JK: Treatment of attention deficit hyperactivity disorder with neurotherapy [review]. Clin Electroencephalogr 31:30–37, 2000.

62. Jones CB: Parent Articles About ADHD. San Antonio, Tex, Communication Skill Builders, 1999.

63. Field T: Massage therapy effects. Am Psychol 53:1270–1281, 1998.

64. Field T, Quintino O, Hernandez-Reif M, Koslovsky G: Adolescents with attention deficit hyperactivity disorder benefit from massage therapy. Adolescence 33:103–108, 1998.

65. Frymann VM: Relation of disturbances of craniosacral mechanism to symptomatology of the newborn: Study of 1250 infants. J Am Osteopath Assoc 65:1059–1075, 1966.

66. Frymann VM: Effect of osteopathic medical management on neurologic development in children. J Am Osteopath Assoc 92:729–744, 1992.

67. Hahnemann S: Organon of the Medical Art, 6th ed. Redmond, Wash, Birdcage Books, 1996, pp 5, 62–63.

68. Ballentine R: Radical Healing. New York, Harmony Books, 1999, pp 62–63.

69. Lamont J: Homeopathic Treatment of ADHD: A controlled study. Biomed Ther 16:219–222, 1998.

71. Flaws B: A Handbook of TCM Pediatrics. Boulder, Colo, Blue Poppy, 1997.

72. Scott J: Acupuncture in the Treatment of Children, rev. ed. Seattle, Wash, Eastland, 1992.

73. Sun Y: Clinical observation and treatment of hyperkinesia in children by traditional Chinese medicine. J Tradit Chin Med 14:105–109, 1994.

74. Zhang H, Huang J: Preliminary study of traditional Chinese medicine treatment of minimal brain dysfunction: Analysis of 100 cases [Chinese]. Zheng Xi Yi Jie He Za Zhi 10:278–279, 1990.

75. Loo M, Naeser MA, Hinshaw S, Bay RB: Laser acupuncture treatment for ADHD. NIH grant #1 R03 MH56009–01. Presentation, 1998 American Academy of Medical Acupuncture Symposium, San Diego, Calif.

76. Loo M: Attention Deficit Disorder. In Loo M (ed): East West Healing. New York, John Wiley & Sons, 2001, pp 154–157.

77. Fan Y: Chinese Pediatric Massage Therapy: A Parent's and Practitioner's Guide to Treatment and Prevention of Childhood Disease. Boulder, Colo, Blue Poppy, 1994.

78. Darvill T, Londy E, Reihman J, et al: Prenatal exposure to PCBs and infant performance on the Fagan test of infant intelligence. Neurotoxicology 21:1029–1038, 2000.

79. Leeds J: Therapeutic music and sound in health care, part 2: The Tomatis method—frequency medicine for the 21st century. Am J Acupunct 25:299–305, 1997.

80. Schettler T, Stein J, Reich F, Valenti M: In Harm's Way: Toxic Threats to Child Development. A report by Greater Boston Physicians for Social Responsibility and Clean Water Fund, May 2000.

81. Collipp PJ, Chen SY, Maitinsky S: Manganese in infant formulas and learning disability. Ann Nut Metab 27:488–494, 1983.

82. Phil RO, Parkes M. Hair element content in learning disabled children. Science 198:204–206, 1977.

83. Darvill T, Lonky E, Reihman J, Stewart P, Pagano J: Prenatal exposure to PCBs and infant performance on the Fagan Test of Infant Intelligence. NeuroToxicology 21:1029–1038, 2000.

84. Sherman JD: Chlorpyrifos (DURSBAN)-associated birth defects: report of four cases. Arch Environmental Health, 51:5–8, 1996.

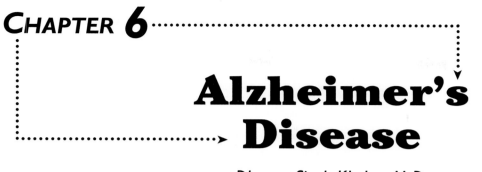

CHAPTER 6

Alzheimer's Disease

Dharma Singh Khalsa, M.D.

The integrative medical model is based on good science and good sense. Conventionalists, who focus narrowly on this gene or that neurotransmitter, often overlook the fact that the brain is a flesh and blood organ. Because the brain is flesh and blood, like the heart for example, it responds to health-promoting interventions such as improved blood flow, good nutrition, stress reduction, and exercise. Because an integrative approach brings surviving neurons to their optimal potential, using it can reverse many of the symptoms of Alzheimer's disease and slow its progression.

Like many degenerative diseases associated with aging, memory loss spans a spectrum of signs, symptoms, etiologies, pathogenesis, and prognosis. Although the term "memory loss" does not imply a specific cause, it signifies a clinical syndrome characterized by the acquired loss of cognitive and emotional abilities that is severe enough to interfere with daily functioning and quality of life.

The best known of the dementias is Alzheimer's disease (AD), which affects more than 4 million Americans at an annual cost of $155 billion. These figures are expected to rise dramatically as the population ages: As many as 16 million people may suffer from the disease by the year 2025. Alzheimer's disease is the third most expensive healthcare problem in the country.[1]

PATHOPHYSIOLOGY

Age-associated memory impairment (AAMI) was initially used to describe the minor memory difficulties that were previously believed to accompany the aging process. This impairment is now known to exist in patients as young as 50 years of age. An at-risk population with mild cognitive impairment (MCI) that converts to AD at a rate of approximately 12% per year has been identified and is discussed later in the chapter.[2] Moreover, Lupien[3] has noted a conversion to AD in subjects with cortisol-induced, stress-related memory loss. This chapter includes the emerging etiology for cognitive dysfunction in the discussion on chronic stress.

Neuroscientists now agree that memory loss is a disease that begins to attack the brain 30 to 40 years before symptoms appear. Snowden[4] showed that nuns who displayed linguistic difficulties in their 20s had a higher incidence of AD later in life. Using positron emission tomographic scans, Reiman and colleagues[5] noted that patients can have lesions consistent with severe cognitive decline years before symptoms are seen. It is becoming increasingly clear, therefore, that AD is an insidious process similar to other chronic diseases such as heart disease, and, therefore, AD has lifestyle management implications.

PLAQUES OR TANGLES?

For a century, scientists have wondered which of the brain lesions associated with AD are more important—the plaques that litter the empty spaces between nerve cells or the stringy tangles that erupt from within the cell. An enzyme called secretase on the surface of the brain cell makes a protein called beta amyloid (BAP). Patients with AD have too much amyloid, which forms the so-called plaques on the outside of brain cells. These plaques grow so dense that they trigger an inflammatory reaction from the brain's immune system that kills nerve cells. Among the powerful weapons the immune system brings to bear are oxygen-free radicals, which help to explain why antioxidants such as vitamin E are helpful.

A strong piece of evidence supporting the beta amyloid theory is that a significant number of mice genetically engineered to develop plaques remained plaque free compared with controls after vaccination with a fragment of beta amyloid. Researchers then vaccinated year-old mice whose brains were riddled with plaques. These mice became plaque free. There are now plans to test this vaccine in humans.

The second major school of thought among neuroscientists concerns Tau, a molecule that acts much like the ties on a railroad track. Tau assembles microtubules that support the structure of the nerve cell. Chemical changes in the nerve cell cause the Tau molecules to change shape so that they no longer hold the microtubule in place. The "railroad ties" begin to twist and tangle, causing neuronal cell death.

Many questions remain. Are the plaques and tangles seen in AD causative or simply tombstones? Is there some still unknown biochemical event that precedes the formation of plaques and tangles and causes the inflammatory death knell? AD, no less than heart disease, certainly has multiple causes. Like aging itself, there are risk factors in the development of AD, which means that lifestyle choices, especially relating to stress management, are critically important.

RISK FACTORS FOR MEMORY LOSS

Hard Risk Factors:

- *Increased age*: This is the most important risk factor. Ten percent of persons aged 65 years develop AD. The incidence at age 85 is 50%.
- *Family history*: The risk of developing AD is increased threefold to fourfold if a first-degree relative has the disease.
- *Genetic factors*: Individuals with two APOE4 genes on chromosome 19 are at least eight times more likely to develop AD. Gatz and associates[6] noted that the APOE4 gene exerts its maximal effect on people in their 60s and is a strong predictor of AD. The APOE4 gene is also a strong predictor for heart disease.
- *Head injury*: AD risk doubles in patients who have suffered traumatic brain injuries early in life. Moderate head injury increased the risk of AD by two to three times, whereas severe head injury more than quadrupled the risk of dementia.
- *Gender*: Because women have longer life spans than men, they have a higher incidence of AD. Lower estrogen levels may also play an important role in AD.[7]
- *Educational level*: The risk of developing AD decreases with the number of years of formal education. This fact highlights research suggesting that mental activity throughout life is neuroprotective.[8]

Warning signs for AD are shown in Table 6–1.

Table 6–1. Warning Signs for Alzheimer's Disease
....

Recent memory loss that affects job skill
Difficulty performing familiar tasks
Problems with language
Disorientation to time and space
Poor or decreased judgment
Problems with abstract thinking
Misplacing objects of importance
Changes in mood or behavior
Changes in personality
Loss of initiative

Lifestyle Risk Factors That Can Be Influenced by Integrative Medicine:

Mild Cognitive Impairment

Mild cognitive impairment (MCI) is characterized primarily by recent memory loss. It is the "transitional state" that can occur between normal aging, AAMI, and dementia. People with MCI are at an increased risk of developing AD, at a rate of 12% to 15% per year. Symptoms of MCI are distinguished from normal aging by recent memory loss. For example, people with MCI suffer frequently from forgetfulness and may visibly have difficulty learning new information and recalling previously learned information. The primary distinction between people with MCI and those with AD appears to be in the areas of cognition outside of memory. Unlike people with AD, those with MCI are able to function normally in daily activities requiring other cognitive abilities such as thinking, understanding, and decision-making.[9]

Nutrition

Ethnic Americans, who consume a high-calorie, high-fat American diet, have a much higher incidence of AD than those living in countries where a relatively low-fat diet is eaten. A high-fat and high-calorie intake leads to oxidative stress, which contributes to the onset and progression of cognitive decline.

The dietary consumption of fish—especially salmon and tuna, which contain docosahexaenoic acid, an omega-3, long chain, polyunsaturated fatty acid—is considered beneficial to cognitive health.

Researchers at New York University's Nathan Kline Institute put transgenic mice on high-fat diets and then observed an increase in the rate at which beta amyloid built up in their brains. Cholesterol-lowering medication slowed the rate of plaque formation.[10, 11]

Mind-Body

Innovative neurobiologic research has shown that chronic, unbalanced stress exerts a powerful negative effect on the development and progression of cognitive decline. In response to chronic stress, the adrenal gland releases cortisol, which has an inhibitory effect on human learning and memory.[12]

Lupien has shown that subjects (median age equals 70) with the highest level of cortisol elevation at the end of a 4-year study period had a marked deficit in explicit memory, a hippocampus-dependent memory function. The group with the lowest cortisol levels displayed no deficit.

In an extension of this work, Lupien observed that without intervention, subjects in the high cortisol group could progress to AD. Magnetic resonance imaging scans also disclosed hippocampal atrophy among this group. Subjects consistently reported morning stress, tension, and anxiety.

Cortisol produces memory dysfunction by (1) preventing the uptake of glucose by the hippocampus, (2) by inhibiting synaptic transmission, and (3) by causing neuron injury and cellular death.[13]

Because of these events, brain cells react abnormally with the excitatory neurotransmitter glutamic acid, creating an intracellular flood of calcium that leads to increased free radical production. Free radicals injure the mitochondria, microtubules, and even the nucleus itself, resulting in dendritic atrophy and neuron death.[14] McEwen[15] showed that this arborization of dendritic spines is reversible.

Stress-relieving techniques such as meditation have been shown to reduce cortisol levels and enhance cognitive function in patients with MCI and AD.[16]

This review suggests that lifestyle modification, including nutrition, stress management, and cardiovascular disease risk reduction, may play a strong role in the reversal of AD.

Diagnosis.
1. *Patient history*: Family history is important because of the correlation between AD in patients and their first-degree relatives. A personal history of illnesses, especially cardiovascular disease, and metabolic disorders is also useful. Other areas of concern include medication usage and a history of head trauma. In general, the diagnosis of MCI can be made if an individual has a memory complaint and an abnormal memory for his/her age and education. Moreover, the person demonstrates normal activities of daily living and a normal level of general cognitive function. The patient with MCI is not demented.
2. *Cognitive assessment*: I have found the Mini-Mental State Examination (MMSE) to be valuable in an office setting. This test offers a relatively rapid and reliable means of assessing cognitive function, memory, and visual/spatial skills (Fig 6–1). Individuals with low levels of education, however, tend to do more poorly on the test, independent of any effects of cognitive function. Moreover, the test is less sensitive in individuals with higher educational levels; they may have a normal score on the MMSE yet have early signs of dementia. Repeated MMSE testing offers a good means of tracking disease progression and monitoring the effects of treatment.
3. *Physical examination and laboratory tests:* The physical examination and standard neurological evaluation may reveal evidence of a stroke. Focal findings of hemiparesis, sensory loss, cranial nerve deficits, and ataxia are not consistent with a diagnosis of AD. Conventional laboratory testing should include a complete blood count, electrolyte and metabolic panels, a thyroid function test, vitamin B_{12} levels, and tests for syphilis and HIV. Beyond that, the integrative medical practitioner also tests for certain hormone levels. Measuring

DHEA has proved clinically useful. In my experience, patients with AD have markedly low levels of DHEA. I also measure levels of free testosterone in men and estrogen in women. Although full hormone replacement therapy is not a regular part of my work, I do order an insulin-like growth factor (IGF-1) level. Urinalysis, electrocardiogram, chest radiograph, and determination of folate levels are no longer recommended.
4. *Neuroimaging:* The time to use neuroimaging is somewhat controversial, but I have found this modality useful in identifying lesions such as hippocampal and cerebral atrophy that are consistent with AD. I believe neuroimaging can help in determining the stage of dementia and the patient's prognosis.

   Some experts suggest computed tomography or magnetic resonance imaging for all patients with suspected AD. Others consider positron emission tomography more useful when the diagnosis is uncertain. The latter imaging modality can be used to identify a declining metabolic rate in the parietal/temporal lobe, which is characteristic of AD.
5. *Genetic testing:* Determining APOE-4 status can contribute to diagnostic accuracy in patients who already have a clinical diagnosis of AD. It is most commonly used in academic medicine.

INTEGRATIVE THERAPY

A true integrative medical model combines evidence from therapies based on nutrition, stress reduction, exercise, and pharmaceuticals into a total synergistic program. Ornish[17] showed that this type of program can reverse coronary artery disease, and I have had compelling success in my own practice involving patients with AD.

At this juncture, there is a large difference of opinion between the conventionalist who only prescribes a cholinesterase inhibitor such as donezapil (Aricept) and perhaps vitamin E in the treatment of MCI or AD and the forward-thinking clinician who practices integrative medicine. The integrative medicine practitioner understands by virtue of experience and knowledge that there is much that can be done in patients with MCI and AD to slow the progression and, in many cases, reverse the symptoms. What follows is an organized and scientific approach to the treatment of cognitive decline.

Lifestyle Factors

Physical Exercise

Aerobic conditioning has been shown to improve some aspects of mental function by 20% to 30%. Smith and Fredlund have demonstrated that physical exercise has a retardant effect on the develop-

One point for each answer.

1. Orientation

	Correct	Incorrect
What is the year we are in?	1	0
What season is it?	1	0
What is today's date?	1	0
What day of the week is today?	1	0
What month are we in?	1	0
What state are we in?	1	0
What country are we in?	1	0
What town are we in?	1	0
Can you tell me the name of this place?	1	0
What floor of the building are we on?	1	0

Subtotal Correct. [   ]

2. Registration

Ask the patient if you may test his/her memory. Then say the names of 3 unrelated objects, clearly and slowly, about one second for each. After you have said all 3, ask him/her to repeat them. This first repetition determines his/her score (0–3), but keep saying them until he/she can repeat all 3, up to 6 trials. If he/she does not eventually learn all 3, recall cannot be meaningfully tested.

Score   0   1   2   3

3. Attention And Calculation

Ask the patient to begin with 100 and count backwards by 7. Stop after 5 subtractions (93, 86, 79, 72, 65). Score the total number of correct answers.

If the patient cannot perform this task, ask him/her to spell the word world backwards. The score is the number of letters in correct order (e.g., dlrow = 5, dlrow = 3)

Score   0   1   2   3   4

4. Recall

Ask the patient if he/she can recall the 3 words you previously asked him/her to remember. Score 0–3.

Score   0   1   2   3

5. Naming

a. Show the patient a wrist watch and ask him/her what it is.
b. Repeat for a pencil.

Score   0   1   2

6. Repetition

Ask the patient to repeat this sentence after you—"No If's, And's, or But's."

Score   0   1

7. 3-Stage Command

Have the patient follow this command—"Take a paper in your hand, fold it in half, and put it on the floor."

Score   0   1   2   3

8. Reacting

On a blank piece of paper print the sentence "Close your eyes" in letters large enough for the patient to see clearly. Ask him/her to read it and do what it says. Score 1 point only if he/she actually closes his/her eyes.

Score   0   1

9. Writing

Give the patient a blank piece of paper and ask him/her to write a sentence for you. Do not dictate a sentence; it is to be written spontaneously. It must contain a subject and a verb and be sensible. Correct grammar and punctuation are not necessary.

Score   0   1

10. Copying

On a clean piece of paper, draw intersecting pentagons, each side about one inch, and ask him/her to copy it exactly as it is. All 10 angles must be present and 2 must intersect to score 1 point. Tremor and rotation are ignored.

Score   0   1

Total Score [   ]

Total Possible Score = 30

Score suggesting dementia ≤ 23

* Using a cut-off score of 23, the MMSE has a sensitivity of 87% and a specificity of 82%

Figure 6–1. Mini-Mental State Examination.

ment of AD. In a retrospective analysis of subjects aged 40 to 60 years, those with a regular exercise program did not develop AD as frequently as those who followed no exercise program. Exercise increases cerebral blood flow and the production of nerve growth factors.[18]

Cognitive Exercise

Based on research by Diamond and coworkers, an integrative medical program that includes cognitive stimulation such as headline discussion, crossword puzzles, music, or art could help to maintain cognitive ability.[19] Mental training increases dendritic sprouting and enhances central nervous system plasticity.[20] In addition to inducing positive medical benefits, cognitive exercise allows patients and their spouses to spend quality time together.

Nutrition

The key points are to reduce dietary fat and cholesterol, add omega-3 rich foods such as salmon or tuna, and lower caloric consumption.

A number of studies have shown that a diet restricted in calories and consisting of 15% to 20% fat can help prevent and treat AD. This approach extends the life expectancy of animals and enhances health and cognitive ability of humans. In my consultation practice, my nutritionist works to create a 15% to 20% fat diet based on patient preferences. This has proved beneficial.[21–23]

Results of the Biosphere II experiment on caloric restriction and reduced fat show reductions in triglyceride and cholesterol levels, which are important in the treatment of AD.[24]

Supplements

The most important supplements to consider are the B complex vitamins, antioxidants such as vitamin E, and the nutrients phosphatidyl serine, and coenzyme Q10.

The B Vitamins
The B complex vitamins are critical for neurotransmitter control and carbohydrate energy metabolism. Niacin itself (B_3) has been shown to have memory-improving benefits.[25] Folate reduces homocysteine, high levels of which have been implicated in heart disease and AD. An integrative brain program should also contain adequate antioxidants and vitamin C in the diet as well as through supplementation.[26]

Vitamin E
Vitamin E at a dose of 2000 IU has been shown to slow the progression of mid-stage AD primarily because it protects cell membranes from oxidative damage.[27]

Additional brain-specific nutrients that play a part in the prevention and treatment of AD are phosphatidyl-serine (PS), with an intake of up to 300 mg per day, ubiquinone (co-enzyme Q10) up to 100 mg per day, ginkgo biloba at a dose up to 240 mg per day, and the omega-3 fatty acid DHA, 50 to 100 mg per day. Newer nutrients that hold great promise are huperzine-A, at a dose of 100 to 200 μg a day and vinpocetine at 2.5 to 10 mg a day.

Phosphatidyl Serine
Phosphatidyl serine (PS) is a negatively charged phospholipid that is almost exclusively located in cell membranes. It has a set of unique physiologic properties that are important to neuronal functions, including stimulation of neurotransmitter release, activation of ion-transport mechanism and an increase in glucose and cyclic adenosine monophosphate levels in the brain. In the aging brain, a decline in these functions is associated with memory impairment and deficits in cognitive abilities.

Phosphatidyl serine has been the subject of 23 studies, 12 of which were double blinded. The findings indicate that PS improves short-term memory, mood, concentration, and activities of daily living.[28, 75, 76, 77] Although early research utilized bovine PS, concern over possible slow viral infection prompted the search for an alternative plant source. A novel PS product made by enzymatic conversion of soy lecithin has now been developed and has been shown to be beneficial in patients with memory loss, including those with AD.[29] In my experience PS is highly effective, especially at improving the recall of names and objects, both of which are symptoms of AD. For some reason, conventionalists have decided not to include PS in their armamentarium against AD.

Dosage. 100–300 mg a day
Precautions. None known.

Co-Enzyme Q10 (Ubiquinone)

Ubiquinone, a powerful neuroprotective agent, works as a dynamic antioxidant and is present throughout the brain cell membrane and mitochondria, where it is involved in the production of high-energy phosphate compounds.[30]

Dosage. 100 mg a day
Precautions. Can lead to gastritis, loss of appetite, nausea, and diarrhea when taken in doses greater than 300 mg a day. Can also elevate serum aminotransferases.

Botanicals

Ginkgo Biloba
Ginkgo biloba increases microvascular circulation, scavenges free radicals, and helps improve concen-

tration and short-term memory in patients with AAMI and AD. A recent 52-week, randomized, double-blinded, placebo-controlled, parallel-group, multi-centered study showed that in 309 patients with mild to severe AD or multi-infarct dementia, there were modest although significant improvements. These changes were equal to those of drugs with a higher side-effect profile and were of a sufficient magnitude to be recognized by the patient's care-givers.[31]

Dosage. Up to 240 mg per day

Precautions. Reports in the medical and lay media have emphasized the need to exercise caution when combining vitamin E and ginkgo, especially in patients taking anticoagulants. In patients taking Coumadin, for example, I measure the appropriate coagulation parameters and perhaps lower the dose of all the compounds. I believe it is a disservice to the AD patient, however, to automatically withhold compounds with a proven benefit in fighting AD because of a purely theoretical concern. If the patient is not on Coumadin, I do not believe there is a danger of excessive bleeding. In my clinical experience I have not seen it, nor have I heard of it from any practitioner of integrative medicine.

Huperzine-A

Huperzine-A is a natural anticholinesterase inhibitor derived from Chinese club moss. Many studies, most of which were done in China, show that huperzine-A surpassed donepazil (Aricept) in reversing memory deficits in aging animals. Huperzine's activity is also reportedly long lasting. What makes huperzine attractive is its apparent lack of serious side effects and low toxicity.

Dosage. I use 50 μg once or twice daily depending on the severity of symptoms.

Precautions. Can cause nausea, sweating, blurred vision, and fasciculations, but less often than with prescription anticholinesterase inhibitors.

Vinpocetine

A nutrient derived from the periwinkle plant has been shown to increase cerebral blood flow and enhance neuronal metabolism.

Dosage. I find the dose of 2.5 to 5 mg twice daily is less stimulating and hence more effective than higher doses recommended by others.

Precautions. Gastrointestinal distress, dry mouth, low blood pressure, and rash are rare. Avoid in pregnancy.

Mind-Body

Meditation

Because of the effects of chronic, unbalanced stress and cortisol secretion on memory, it is beneficial to suppress elevated glucocorticoid levels or normalize their release. Because age increases the vulnerability to stress and cortisol-induced hippocampal damage, stress-relieving meditation is highly recommended for patients of all ages to reduce cortisol and limit the loss of hippocampal neurons.

Meditation has consistently been found to decrease cortisol levels and promote normalization of adaptive mechanisms.[32] Practitioners of meditation also displayed lower levels of lipid peroxidase, a marker of free radical production and higher levels of the hormone dehydroepiandrosterone (DHEA), which I consider important for optimal brain function. Wallace[33] reviewed studies that noted the positive health benefits of meditation on cognition. In a landmark study in the elderly, it was found that meditators had a greater life expectancy than nonmeditators[34] (see Chapter 9, Recommending Meditation).

Kriyas

Specific brain exercises called kriyas are derived from the science of Kundalini yoga as taught by Yogi Bhajan. They combine breathing, finger movements, and regenerating sound currents. The practice of these exercises serves a dual purpose. They induce a meditative state and stimulate the central nervous system. Kriyas have been clinically shown be very useful in increasing global brain energy. Positron emission tomography scans demonstrate that these types of exercises enhance regional cerebral blood flow, oxygen delivery, and glucose use. Beyond that, recent research at Harvard proved that what I call medical meditation, based on kriyas, is quite specific

---

NOTE

Method of a Kriya

This exercise is called kirtan kriya. This kriya involves the chanting of the primal sounds. Say each of these words repeatedly, in order: Sa Ta Na Ma. The a in these words is pronounced as a soft a, or ah. Repeat this mantra while sitting with your spine straight and your mental energy focused on the area of your brow, or forebrain. Yogis believe that this stimulates your pituitary. You can find this spot by rolling your eyes to the top, or root, of your nose. For 2 minutes, chant in your normal voice. For the next 2 minutes, chant in a whisper. For the middle 3 minutes, chant silently, while still touching the fingertips. Then reverse the order, whispering for 2 minutes and chanting the mantra out loud for the last 2 minutes. The total time is 11 minutes. The mudras, or finger positions, are very important in this kriya. On Sa, touch the index fingers of each hand to your thumbs. On Ta, touch your middle fingers to your thumbs. On Na, touch your ring fingers to your thumbs. On Ma, touch your little fingers to your thumbs. At the end, inhale very deeply, stretch your hands above your head, and then bring them down in a sweeping motion as you exhale.

in increasing activity to the hippocampus compared with basic meditation. Moreover, this same research group is studying the effect of meditation on cortisol levels and grades in school-aged children.[35]

Pharmaceuticals

Acetyl-Cholinesterase Inhibitors

There are currently three drugs approved by the FDA to treat early Alzheimer's disease. These are acetyl-cholinesterase inhibitors, which act to increase the level of the neurotransmitter acetylcholine (Ach). Ach is critically important for memory formation and retrieval.

The first, tacrine (Cognex), is minimally effective and has poor patient compliance because of its side effects. It is no longer used. The second, donepezil HCl (Aricept), is moderately effective in improving short-term memory in patients with early AD. Neither has any effect on the progression of the disease. Rivastigmine (Exelon) is slightly more effective than the others and has the best side-effect profile of the available cholinesterase-inhibiting drugs.[36]

MAO-B Inhibitors

Deprenyl (selegiline), an MAO-B inhibitor, was shown to limit degeneration of patients with AD in a 5-year double-blinded study at a dose of 10 mg per day.[37] The drug also slowed the progression of Alzheimer's disease as part of a large-scale, multicenter trial. Deprenyl acts to increase the level of important catecholamines, especially dopamine, which are decreased in AD. It also inhibits oxidative deamination, thereby reducing neuronal damage.

Hormones

DHEA and/or pregnenolone, both neurospecific hormones and precursors to estrogen, are also useful. An animal study demonstrated that DHEA affected excitability in the hippocampus, thereby enhancing memory function at dosages of 50 mg per day. Another study showed that DHEA enhanced acetyl choline release from hippocampal neurons in the rat brain. DHEA has been shown to be consistently low in patients with AD.[38]

Pregnenolone has been the subject of research in both animals and humans. It has been found to be a powerful memory enhancer. A study has demonstrated improved memory with pregnenolone use in the elderly.[39]

As noted earlier, estrogen deficiency in postmenopausal women is a factor in the development of Alzheimer's disease. Observational studies indicate that estrogen replacement delays the expression of AD by 40% to 70%, enhances hippocampal plasticity, and increases nerve growth factor. Estrogen has antioxidant properties that protect the neuron from oxidative stress. Estrogen also enhances glucose transport in neuronal tissue, which may be impaired in AD. Finally, estrogen stimulates the production of several neurotransmitters whose deficiency characterizes AD.[40]

The hormone melatonin is a reasonable alternative to use of benzodiazepines in patients with AD. Melatonin restores circadian rhythm and may help to prevent wandering.

Dosage. A good starting dose is 3 mg at bedtime.

Spirituality

Beyond reported improvements in memory, concentration, learning ability, and activities of daily living, patients enrolled in an integrative medical program also note positive changes in what can be described as personal awareness. This awareness sometimes appears as a sense of increased self-knowledge or spirituality and leads to a feeling of connectedness. Some patients report that this spiritual connection leads to a profound level of wisdom: the combination of age, intelligence, and experience. This wisdom, or maturity, brings greater life satisfaction. These changes are consistent with the work of Benson, Larson, and Matthews, who established that after an integrative medical program, including mind-body interactions, enhances spirituality.[41] Spirituality was expressed as experiencing the close presence of a higher power. Furthermore, spirituality, faith, belief, and religion are now well known to be associated with fewer medical symptoms and better outcomes when medical interventions are needed.

As the population ages, cognitive decline, including AAMI, MCI, and AD, is expected to rise. An integrative medical program can have a powerful impact on these diseases.

 THERAPEUTIC REVIEW

Treatment of MCI and AD:

Nutrition
- *Recommend a diet containing 15% to 20% fat based on patient preferences. Include organic fruits and vegetables, fish or seeds rich in omega-3 fatty acid, such as salmon, and flaxseed oil.*

THERAPEUTIC REVIEW continued

Supplements

- *Vitamin E, 2000 IU per day; coenzyme Q10, 100 to 300 mg per day; ginkgo biloba, 240 mg per day; phosphatidyl-serine, 100 to 300 mg per day; DHA EPA (fish oil), 500 to 1000 mg per day; huperzine-A, 50 to 100 μm per day; and vinpocetine, 2.5 to 10 mg per day.*

NOTE

Be aware of the rare possibility of increased clotting time in patients taking maximum doses of ginkgo, vitamin E, and DHA, especially with Coumadin and ASA.

Mind Body

- *Control stress: Perform daily morning meditation for at least 15 minutes.*
- *Exercise: Physical, mental and mind/body exercise should be part of the integrative prescription.*

NOTE

Caution: Do not use deprenyl with antidepressant medication because fatal reactions can occur. Deprenyl can be used in conjunction with anticholinesterase drugs.

Pharmaceuticals

- *Deprenyl, 5 mg twice daily, slows progression.*
- *Rivastigmine is the most effective acetylcholinesterase inhibitor available. Others are under development. Start with 2.5 mg twice daily and work up as per package insert.*

Hormone Replacement Therapy

- *DHEA, 25 to 100 mg per day, depending on sex and blood level; pregnenolone, 10 to 100 mg per day; melatonin, 3 mg per day at bedtime. Proper dose allows a complete night's sleep without AM grogginess.*

NOTE

When using DHEA in men, measure and follow the PSA level. If elevated, do not use DHEA. Also consider using saw palmetto with DHEA.

References

1. Ernst R, Hay J: The US economic and social cost of Alzheimer's disease revisited. Am J Pub Health 84:1261–1264, 1991.
2. Thal LJ: Trials to Prevent Alzheimer's Disease in a Population at Risk. Abstracts of the Fourth International Nice/Springfield Symposium on Advances in Alzheimer Therapy. p 86, 1996.
3. Lupien S: Personal communication, 1999.
4. Snowdon DA, Kemper SJ, Mortimer JA, et al: Linguistic ability in early life and cognitive function and Alzheimer's disease in late life: Findings from the nun study. JAMA, 275:528–532, 1996.
5. Reimen EM, Caselli RJ, Yun L, et al: Preclinical evidence of Alzheimer's disease in persons homozygous for the e 4 allele for apolipoprotein E. N Engl J Med 334:752–758, 1996.
6. Gatz M, Lowe B, Berg S, et al: Dementia: Not Just a Search for the Gene. The Gerontologist 34:251–255, 1994.
7. Birge SJ, Mortel KF: Estrogen and the treatment of Alzheimer's disease. Am J Med 103:36S-45S, 1997.
8. Katzman R, Kawas C: The epidemiology of dementia and Alzheimer's disease. In Jerry RD, Katzman R, Bich KL (eds): Alzheimer Disease. New York, Raven Press, 1994, pp 105–122.
9. Shah Y, Tangalos E, Petersen R: Mild cognitive impairment. When is it a precursor to Alzheimer's disease? Geriatrics 55:62–68, 2000.
10. Grant WB: Dietary links to Alzheimer's disease. Alz Dis Rev 2:42–45, 1997.
11. Hendrie HC, Ogunniyi A, Hall KS, et al: Incidence of dementia and Alzheimer disease in two communities. JAMA 285:739–747, 2001.
12. Lupien S, Lecour SA, Lussier I, et al: Basal cerebral cortisol levels and cognitive deficits in human aging. J Neurosci. 14:2893–2903, 1994.
13. Stein-Behrens BA, Sapolsky RM: Stress, glucocorticoids and aging. (Milano) 4:197–210, 1992.
14. Sapolsky RM, McEwen BS: Stress, glucocorticoids and their role in degenerative changes in the aging hippocampus. In Crook T, Bartus R (eds): Treatment Development Strategies for Alzheimer's disease. Madison, Conn, MPA Press, 1986.
15. McEwen BS, Sapolsky RM: Stress and cognitive functions. Curr Opin Neurobiol 5:205–206, 1995.
16. Khalsa DS, Stauth C: Meditation as Medicine: Activate the Power of Your Natural Healing Force. New York, Pocket Books, 2001.
17. Gould LK, Ornish D, Scherwitz L, et al: Changes in myocardial perfusion abnormalities by positron emission tomography

after long-term, intense risk factor modification. JAMA 274:894–901, 1995.

18. Smith AL, Fredlund R, et al: The protective effects of physical exercise on the development of Alzheimer's disease. Neurology 50:A89-A90, 1998.

19. Diamond MC, Lindner B, Johnson R, Bennett EL: Differences in occipital corticol synapses from environmentally enriched, impoverished and standard colony rats. J Neurosci Res 1:109–119, 1975.

20. Cotman C: Synaptic Plasticity, Neurotrophic Factors and Transplantation in the Aged Brain. Handbook of the Biology of Aging. Academic Press 1990, pp 255–274.

21. Walford RL, Spindler SR: The response to caloric restriction in mammals shows features also common to hibernation: A cross-adaptation hypothesis. J Gerontol 52A, B: 179–183, 1997.

22. Weindruch R: Caloric restriction and aging. Sci Am 274:46–52, 1996.

23. Weindruch R, Walford RL: The retardation of aging and disease by dietary restriction. Springfield, Ill., Charles C Thomas, 1998.

24. Verdery R, Walford R: Caloric restriction in biosphere II: Effects of energy restriction on lipid and lipoprotein levels and HDL subfractions. 1996 American Aging Association Annual Meeting [abstract # 75], p. 37.

25. Zhang X, Zhand BZ, Zhang WW: Protective effects of nicotinic acid on disturbance of memory induced by cerebral ischemia-reperfusion in rats. Clin J Pharm Toxicol 10:178–180, 1996.

26. Peetot GJ, Cole R, Conaway C, et al: Adult lifetime dietary patterns of antioxidant vitamin and carotenoid consumption in a case control study of risk factors for Alzheimer's disease. 1996 American Aging Association Annual Meeting [abstract # 78], p. 38.

27. Sano M, et al. A controlled trial of selegiline, alpha-tocopherol, or both as treatment for Alzheimer's disease. N Engl J Med 336:1216–1222, 1997.

28. Crook TN, et al: Effects of phosphatidylserine in Alzheimer's disease. Psychopharmacol Bull 28:61–66, 1992.

29. Gindin J, Nouikov D, Kedar A, et al: The effect of plant phosphatidyl serine on age-associated memory impairment and mood in the functional elderly. An unpublished paper from The Geriatric Institute for education and research, and Department of Geriatrics, Kaplan Hospital, Rehovot, Israel, 1995.

30. Beal FM: Cell Death by Oxidants: Neuroprotective Antioxidant Therapies. Fourth International Nice/Springfield Symposium on Advances in Alzheimer's Therapy.

31. LeBars PL, Katz MM, et al: A placebo-controlled, double-blind, randomized trial of an extract of ginkgo biloba for dementia. JAMA 278:1327–1332, 1997.

32. Jevening R, Wilson AF, Davidson JM: Adrenocortical activity during meditation. Horm Behav 10:54–60, 1978.

33. Wallace RR: The Physiology of Consciousness. A joint publication of the Institute of Science, Technology and Public Policy and Maharishi International University Press.

34. Alexander CN, Langer EJ, Newman RI: Transcendental meditation. Mindfulness and longevity in experimental studies in the elderly. J Pers Soc Psychol 6:950–964, 1989.

35. Khalsa DS, Stauth C: Meditation As Medicine. New York, Pocket Books, 2001.

36. Khalsa DS: Exelon: A new drug for Alzheimer's disease. Int J Anti-Aging Med 1:10–12; 1998.

37. Riekhman, Pasio. Rationale to treat AD with selegiline. Presented at the Fourth International Nice/Springfield Symposium on Advances in Alzheimer Therapy, April 1996.

38. Rhodes ME, Li PK, Flood JF, Johnson DA: Enhancement of hippocampal acetylcholine release by the neurosteroid. Dehydroepiandrosterone sulfate: An in vivo microdialysis study. Brain Res 733:284–286, 1996.

39. Flood JF, Morley JE, Roberts E: Memory-enhancing effects in male mice of pregnenolone and steroids metabolically derived from it. Proc Natl Acad Sci U S A 89:1567–1571, 1992.

40. Berge SJ, Mortel KF: Estrogen and the treatment of Alzheimer's disease. Am J Med 103:36S-45S, 1997.

41. Larson DB: Scientific research on spirituality and health: The consensus report. National Institute for Healthcare Research, 1997.

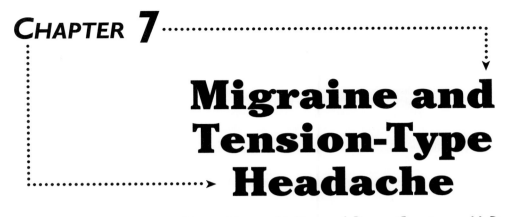

CHAPTER 7

Migraine and Tension-Type Headache

Doug Mann, M.D., and Remy Coeytaux, M.D.

Headache is one of the most common complaints that brings a patient to the attention of health care providers. The majority of headaches are benign in the sense of being symptomatic of treatable or non-disabling disorders. Ninety percent of all headaches are either vascular headaches, tension type headaches (TTH), or a mixture of the two. The remaining 10% are largely secondary to disorders of the cervical spine, the sinuses, the temporomandibular joints, the dental structures, or trauma, with tumors or other masses constituting a small fraction of the group of possible causes.

Symptoms of more serious disorders of the head and neck include early morning headaches that awaken the patient (suggestive of increased intracranial pressure), visual dimming or double vision, headaches that increase in frequency or severity over a period of weeks to months, headaches made significantly worse by postural changes, explosive onset of severe head pain, and headaches associated with mental status changes, focal motor or sensory deficits, syncope, seizures, fever, or stiff neck. Headache in the setting of systemic symptoms (e.g., weight loss, human immunodeficiency virus infection, or known malignancy) require thorough investigation. Findings on examination that prompt further diagnostic workup include focal neurologic signs, tender temporal arteries, papilledema, and evidence of local or systemic infection or malignancy.

This chapter is limited to integrative therapies that are effective in the treatment of the two most common types of headache: migraine and tension headache.

MIGRAINE

Pathophysiology

Clinical characteristics typical of migraine include the rapid onset of throbbing head pain (unilateral or bilateral), often associated with nausea and vomiting, photophobia, and sonophobia. Headache may or may not be heralded by a visual or other type of aura. Duration is usually greater than 6 hours and may last several days with fluctuating intensity. Precipitating factors include menses, certain foods, stress or letdown following stress, weather changes, infection, fatigue, and sunlight.

The final event leading to the pain of migraine is release of inflammatory vasodilators by peripheral nerve endings of cranial nerve V on blood vessels in the scalp and meninges. A major enhancer of that process is the release of serotonin by circulating platelets. The presence of a headache generator in the brainstem is supported by findings from positron emission tomographic studies obtained during migraine attacks. Genetic influences are evident in a majority of patients, with multiple family members exhibiting full or partial symptoms. Variants are common, and comorbid TTH is frequent.

The following sections describe currently available complementary approaches that are useful for integration with conventional therapies (Table 7–1). Conventional approaches rely heavily on pharmaceutical interventions to prevent or abort a headache, along with a variety of standard analgesics and antiemetics. Although these measures are effective in management of symptoms, they are often expensive and fail to address the underlying physical, psychological, and energetic issues that lead to headache in the first place.

NOTE

Patients with migraine often suffer from more than one kind of headache. A carefully recorded history uncovers distinctions to guide therapy based on symptom characteristics.

Lifestyle

Effective management of headache requires a careful assessment of lifestyle patterns as they relate to sleep, nutrition, exercise, and stress management.

Table 7–1. Summary of Migraine Therapies

Preventive Therapies	Specific Examples/Comments
Lifestyle	Sleep hygiene, exercise, stress reduction
Nutrition	Avoidance of food triggers
Dietary supplements	Magnesium, riboflavin
Botanicals	Feverfew, herbal remedies for sleep
Pharmaceuticals	Tricyclic antidepressants, beta blockers, calcium channel blockers, anticonvulsants, nonsteroidal anti-inflammatory drugs, botulinum toxin
Abortive and Acute Therapies	
Pharmaceuticals	Nonsteroidal anti-inflammatory drugs, ergot alkaloids, isometheptene, intranasal lidocaine, triptans
Biofeedback	Requires motivation on the part of the patient
Relaxation	Includes progressive muscular relaxation, focused breathing exercises, and guided imagery
Cognitive-behaviour therapy	Especially useful in conjunction with other approaches
Neurolinguistic programming	Alters the subjective experience of pain, modifies expectations
Hypnosis	May be especially useful during pregnancy
Mindfulness meditation	Improvement in mood, blood pressure, muscle tone, reaction to pain, and possibly pain perception
Chiropractic	May be especially useful for headaches associated with neck discomfort
Acupuncture	Appropriate for severe acute attacks, in lieu of a visit to an urgent care center

Regularization of eating and sleeping habits can have a significant, beneficial effect on headache frequency. A sleep hygiene program can improve the quality and quantity of sleep, thereby reducing fatigue and raising the threshold for migraine. Simply providing instructions on how to improve sleep hygiene can lead to a decrease in duration and frequency of migraine attacks.[1] Our experience is that a 30-minute exercise program undertaken three times per week at aerobic levels has a similar effect on pain intensity and a milder effect on frequency.

Nutrition

Dietary triggers are found in 8% to 20% of patients with migraine.[2] Patients usually know their own sensitivities and which foods to avoid. Wine, dark beer, aged cheese, cashews, onions, chocolate, and processed meats such as hot dogs, bologna, and pepperoni are common offenders. Caffeine withdrawal can precipitate headache of the vascular or tension type but does not directly cause migraine.[2] Caffeine alleviates migraine acutely in some patients, possibly owing to its vasoconstrictive effects on scalp vessels. Chronic daily headache can be caused by excessive use of caffeine (more than 1200 mg, or 5 to 6 cups of coffee per day). It is important to raise the possibility of dietary triggers when educating patients about migraine. Although specific mechanisms remain unknown, diet does influence migraine and represents an important avenue for improving outcomes. (See Chapter 81, Food Allergies.)

Supplements

Magnesium. The level of ionized magnesium has been found to be low in a significant percentage of those with classic or common migraine.[3] Determination of standard serum magnesium levels is unreliable in detecting those with deficiency, and measurement of biologically active ionized magnesium is costly and usually not routinely available. A single trial of an orally administered magnesium supplement (magnesium dicitrate, 600 mg/day in a single dose) showed significant benefit in the prevention of migraine compared with placebo.[4] Another study showed that administration of 360 mg of pyrrolidone carboxylic acid magnesium daily for 2 months was associated with greater pain relief than was placebo in women with menstrual migraine.[5] In general, patients with menstrual migraine should be encouraged to continue magnesium for at least 3 months, because the beneficial effects may be delayed for several cycles.

Preventive benefit can also be achieved with oral magnesium aspartate (1000 mg/day at bedtime). Supplemental magnesium is well tolerated but causes diarrhea in some patients. Magnesium oxide is more readily available and cheaper than the aspartate version but is poorly absorbed, especially when given with calcium. The mechanism of action of magnesium in migraine may be stabilization of neural excitability and vascular tone. We find that a variation of a published method for intravenous magnesium administration (2 g in 50 mL of saline solution given over 15 minutes) is very effective for acute migraine attacks treated in the office.[6]

Dosage. Magnesium aspartate, 1000 mg at bedtime.

Precautions. High doses may cause diarrhea. If needed, magnesium gluconate is a form that has been found to cause less diarrhea.

Riboflavin (Vitamin B$_2$). Riboflavin was shown to have preventive effects in migraine in a small prospective, randomized, placebo-controlled study.[7] One hypothesis for the mechanism of action of riboflavin is that it improves mitochondrial energy reserves without changing neuronal excitability.[8] It may have a synergistic preventive effect when used concurrently with a beta blocker.[8] There are no head-to-head studies comparing riboflavin with other preventive measures.

Dosage. The recommended dose is 200 mg twice daily with meals.

Precautions. Riboflavin is well tolerated and does not influence metabolism of other agents. Patients may notice that their urine turns an intense yellow with daily use.

Botanicals

Feverfew (*Tanacetum parthenium*). Feverfew is the only botanical with demonstrated preventive effects in migraine. Johnson and associates showed that there was a significant increase in migraine severity and frequency when feverfew was stopped in a cohort taking it for prevention.[9] In one well-designed study, a 70% reduction in headache frequency and severity was shown in 270 patients with migraine.[10] Another study with a different concentration of the marker molecule parthenolide was negative for migraine prevention, however. Variations in the standardization of the dried leaf constituents confound comparison studies of this herb. There are no long-term studies documenting safety and no head-to-head trials with other preventive medications. The mechanism of action in migraine may be related to its inhibiting effects on platelet aggregation and inflammatory promoters such as serotonin and prostaglandins or its effect in dampening vascular reactivity to amine regulators of blood flow.

Dosage. Recommendations include oral administration of up to 125 mg/day of the dried leaf standardized to 0.2% parthenolide.[11] Beneficial effects may take weeks to develop.

Precautions. Aphthous ulcers and gastrointestinal side effects develop in 5% to 15% of users. Abrupt cessation of feverfew occasionally results in agitation and increased headache. It is not recommended during pregnancy because it prolongs bleeding time.

Herbals in Sleep Management

Sleep management is a major therapeutic strategy in helping patients gain control over their headaches. Melatonin, valerian, and kava kava can be safely used on a temporary basis to improve sleep.

Melatonin. Melatonin is used in a comprehensive management program for migraine to improve sleep and circadian rhythms. Sleep induction is not influenced by melatonin, but maintenance is improved. Melatonin is used nightly for 4 to 6 weeks and then tapered. Over that period of time, a sleep hygiene program can be put into place to reduce the need for the drug. We find that it is well tolerated with minimal side effects and is best used as a temporary measure, repeated at intervals as needed. Additionally, Leone and colleagues demonstrated that daily intake of 10 mg of melatonin for 14 days significantly reduced headache frequency.[12]

Dosage. A standard regimen is 4 to 8 mg per night 1 to 2 hours before anticipated sleep.

Precautions. Fatigue, drowsiness, dizziness, abdominal cramps, and irritability may occur.

Valerian (*Valeriana officinalis*). Valerian root is an alternative to melatonin for sleep. It does not cause daytime drowsiness and is nonaddictive. It is useful as an anxiolytic when given during the daytime (up to 250 mg three times per day). The mechanism of action includes stimulation of gamma-aminobutyric acid receptors in the central nervous system along with enhanced release and inhibition of reuptake of gamma-aminobutyric acid at the synapse. Interactions with other medications are not well documented. It is well tolerated, with gastrointestinal upset as the most common side effect.

Dosage. The dosage is 100 to 300 mg of the extract standardized to 0.8% valerenate at bedtime or 250 mg every 8 hours for anxiety.

Precautions. Valerian has a strong smell that may aggravate nausea during a migraine attack. It may sometimes cause worsening of TTH if taken regularly during the daytime for anxiety for longer than 3 months. It should not be used during pregnancy.

Kava kava (*Piper methysticum*). Kava kava may be used for insomnia as another option when sleep management is an issue. Its effects are primarily on the gamma-aminobutyric acid system and are similar to those of valerian root.[11]

Dosage. The usual bedtime dose is 150 or 200 mg 1 hour before sleep.

Precautions. Side effects are dose related and include scaly dermatitis when doses of more than 400 mg per day are used for extended periods. Hepatic toxicity has been noted in some cases. It is nonaddictive but should not be used during pregnancy or breast-feeding.

Pharmaceuticals

Conventional pharmacologic approaches are centered on preventive and abortive medications, which have the appeal of efficiency and symptom relief but are associated with significant expense, major side effects, and masking of underlying problems that lead to headache. There is no inherent difficulty in the integration of conventional and complementary techniques in treatment of headache. The pharmaceutical approaches discussed here are the ones for which there is greatest evidence of efficacy and clinical usefulness, according to the United States Headache Consortium's clinical guidelines published in 2000.[13]

Preventive Pharmaceutical Therapies

Application of conventional preventive therapies in practice is typically organized around classes of medications, such as tricyclic antidepressants, beta blockers, calcium channel blockers, anticonvulsants, and other miscellaneous agents. The goals are reduction in headache frequency or severity, improved function, and better responsiveness to abortive agents.

A decision to start preventive therapy is based on (1) headache frequency of more than two per month or more than 3 days per month lost to headache; (2) willingness of the patient to take a medication on a long-term basis; and (3) ability to keep a headache calendar. Medications are taken on a daily basis and are administered according to both their half-life and a schedule that minimizes side effects. Effectiveness is best measured by having the patient keep a calendar, noting headache frequency and intensity as well as significant life events such as stressful situations, menses, and vacations. Patients may respond to any of several beta blockers (such as propranolol, atenolol, or timolol), making the choice of an agent highly individualized. It is not possible to predict who will respond to a given agent in advance, although the history of a family member who achieved effective prevention with a given agent may guide initial choices. Comorbid depression, asthma, or thyroid disease limits use of beta blockers, whereas obesity limits use of tricyclic antidepressants and valproate.

NOTE

Patients with migraine often suffer from more than one kind of headache. A carefully recorded history uncovers distinctions to guide therapy based on symptom characteristics.

Agents are prescribed one at a time for at least a 6-week period at maximal dosing. Most agents are started at less than half the predicted maximum dose, and the dose is increased slowly with pauses at 2-week intervals to assess effectiveness. Many times, patients achieve satisfactory results at doses well below the maximum, particularly with the tricyclic antidepressants. On the other hand, verapamil usually has to be given at doses of at least 320 mg/day. Combinations of magnesium, vitamin B$_2$, and daily aspirin mix well with conventional preventive agents, sometimes ameliorating side effects such as constipation.

Once improvement is achieved, the medication is continued for periods of 3 months with periodic gradual reductions to determine the minimum effective dose. Preventive agents, when effective, allow time for patients to work on lifestyle issues including stress, sleep, diet, and exercise as well as to develop skills such as relaxation, biofeedback, and self-hypnosis techniques. Preventive agents are chosen in part to facilitate treatment of comorbid depression and sleep dysfunction. As patients improve, calendars that focus attention on pain are best discontinued, and a positive scale is substituted that draws attention to improvement in lifestyle and wellness in its various dimensions.

Tricyclic Antidepressants. The best data support use of amitriptyline in doses of up to 150 mg at bedtime, starting as low as 25 mg. If the patient cannot tolerate even 25 mg per day, it is worth going even lower to a single evening dose of 10 mg. Other useful medications in this group include nortriptyline, up to 100 mg at bedtime. Sleep may be improved, which tends to reduce migraine frequency. Dry mouth, drowsiness, and constipation are significant side effects.

Beta Blockers. Generally well tolerated, medications in this class shown to be effective for migraine include propranolol, nadolol, timolol, atenolol, and metoprolol. Long-acting formulations have not been studied. Side effects include fatigue, depression, insomnia, dizziness, and nausea. Rebound headaches may occur if beta blockers are withdrawn suddenly. The typical dose of propranolol in migraine prevention ranges from 80 to 240 mg per day in two or three divided doses. It is available in 10-, 20-, 40-, 60-, and 80-mg tablets.

Calcium Channel Blockers. Calcium channel blockers shown to be effective in some trials include verapamil, nimodipine, flunarizine, and nifedipine. Delayed onset of effectiveness is typical, and side effects such as abdominal pain, bloating, weight gain, constipation, and even headache are not uncommon. A typical dose of verapamil is 180 mg twice daily.

Anticonvulsants. The major members of this group are sodium valproate (Depakote) and gabapentin (Neurontin), with weaker evidence supporting carbamazepine (Tegretol) for the prevention of migraine. A typical dose for sodium valproate for prevention is 1500 mg/day with a starting dose of 250 mg twice daily. Side effects include weight gain, alopecia, tremor, nausea, and somnolence. Sodium valproate is available in 125-, 250-, and 500-mg capsules.

Nonsteroidal Anti-inflammatory Drugs. Trends toward reduction in migraine frequency have been seen with daily use of aspirin, naproxen, ketoprofen (Orudis), and tolfenamic acid for prevention. Gastric side effects are common, and patient compliance is a limiting factor. Dosing for naproxen is 500 mg twice daily, whereas that for aspirin is 350 to 975 mg/day. For ketoprofen, the dose is 150 mg/day.

Botulinum Toxin. Botulinum toxin has been found to prevent migraine when injected in small quantities at multiple sites into the muscles of the forehead and the temples.[14, 15] Effects last 2 to 4 months on average with few side effects. It has been reported to be effective in TTH as well, suggesting a common pathophysiology or a nonspecific effect.[16]

Homeopathy. One recent study of homeopathy in a group of 98 patients with mixed headaches found that in the group as a whole, there was a 20% overall improvement rate, which was stable at 1 year. Half the patients continued homeopathic treatments with or without conventional therapy. The investigators concluded that the patients who had the most improvement suffered from both TTH and migraine and had a disease history of 25 years on average.[17] Other studies suffer from limitations of methods. Individuality of approach is the heart of homeopathic therapy, which makes group comparison studies difficult to interpret. Integration with conventional treatments is sometimes difficult because of differences in conventional and homeopathic models of healing. Our experience is that side effects of homeopathic remedies are minimal and that the positive effects achieved make integrative efforts worthwhile.

Abortive Pharmaceutical Therapies

Migraine is often associated with warning symptoms, which may include a visual or somatic aura. Medication taken in these early phases of migraine can be remarkably effective in blocking the full expression of symptoms.

Nonsteroidal Anti-inflammatory Drugs. Ibuprofen (800 mg) and naproxen sodium (200 to 400 mg) can be very effective in blocking headache when given during the first few hours. Ibuprofen in liquid form (200 to 400 mg) is recommended when nausea occurs early in the headache. Variability in responsiveness to nonsteroidal anti-inflammatory drugs that are used in this way is high, but they are worth exploring for most patients.

Ergot Alkaloids. Now largely supplanted by the triptans, these agents can be useful in those who cannot tolerate other abortive methods. A typical dose is ergotamine tartrate, 1 mg orally, 2 mg sublingually, or 2 mg per rectum every hour for up to three doses.

Isometheptene (Midrin). Isometheptene has a low side-effect profile and modest cost. It acts as a weak vasoconstrictor of scalp vessels. The dosing should be two or three capsules at the start of a headache, then one every 45 minutes for three more doses as needed.

Intranasal Lidocaine. Several studies support the use of intranasal lidocaine, which is effective for all forms of migraine and is particularly useful during the aura phase. It is also indicated for those with significant nausea and vomiting early in the headache.[13] We use 4% lidocaine liquid, applied with a dropper, 0.25 mL in each nostril with the patient supine and the neck hyperextended. Side effects include a transient burning sensation and numbness in the throat. The nasal spray form of lidocaine is not usually effective.

5-Hydroxytyramine$_{1B/1D}$ Agonists (Triptans). The triptans are among the most effective agents available for migraine. They act by blocking the release of inflammatory substances from the distal nerve endings in the trigeminal system on scalp vessels and by direct vasoconstriction. Multiple forms are now available, most of them in oral or sublingual form, with sumatriptan additionally available as a 6-mg injection and a 20-mg intranasal formulation. Efficacy is 60% to 80% in terms of pain and nausea relief with a 25% to 30% recurrence rate necessitating more than one dose. Choice of triptan depends on patient response, side effect profile, and route of administration.

Dosage. Usual dosing is at 2-hour intervals if necessary for a maximum of three doses in 24 hours.

Sumatriptan (Imitrex): Available in 25- or 50-mg tablets, 5- or 20-mg spray, and 6 mg/0.5 mL injection.

Naratriptan (Amerge): Available in 1- or 2.5-mg tablets.

Rizatriptan (Maxalt): Available in 5- or 10-mg regular tablets or 5- or 10-mg disintegrating tablets (MLT).

Zolmitriptan (Zomig): Available in 2.5- or 5-mg tablets.

Precautions. These agents are contraindicated during pregnancy and in those with cardiovascular disease. Cost is a major limiting factor for some patients. Side effects include a sensation of pressure in the chest, the neck, and the head.

Mind-Body Techniques

Biofeedback. Biofeedback as part of a stress management program can provide significant benefit in regard to migraine and TTH without major side effects. Thermal biofeedback, in which patients learn to increase the temperature of their fingertips through the use of imagery and relaxation, is a commonly employed technique. The combination of thermal biofeedback and relaxation training has been shown to improve migraine symptoms significantly.[18] A meta-analysis of 25 controlled studies revealed that the efficacy of biofeedback is comparable with that of prophylactic pharmacotherapy.[19] Another meta-analysis of five studies revealed a 37% improvement in headache symptoms associated with thermal biofeedback training.[20] There are no reliable criteria for predicting benefit, and the training requires a significant time commitment. Pharmacotherapy in combination with biofeedback has not been studied for interactive therapeutic effects. This is an important point because vascular reactivity (a major target in biofeedback training) may be influenced by medications used in prevention of migraine, potentially impairing the training process itself in some situations. With a qualified trainer, biofeedback is ideal for patients intolerant to medications, for those oriented toward self-efficacy in pain management, for women who are pregnant, and especially for those willing to practice the techniques regularly.

Relaxation. In this category, we include progressive muscular relaxation, focused breathing exercises, and guided imagery. Holroyd and Penzien in a meta-analysis found that these techniques are as effective as biofeedback.[19] Treatment effects were enhanced by beta blockers and some other preventive agents, making integration both feasible and effective. Some patients are able to identify the very early stages of a headache in time to deploy focused relaxation or guided imagery sufficiently early to abort the full development of pain. These techniques can be taught in groups or on a one-on-one basis and then continued by the individual at home using audiotapes. Relaxation appeals to those with an internal locus of control and above-average motivation. (See also Chapter 91, Relaxation Exercises.)

Cognitive-Behavioral Therapy. Cognitive-behavioral therapy is a stress management approach designed to help patients identify maladaptive thought patterns (e.g., self-blame, hopelessness, helplessness, worthlessness, and "catastrophising") and suppressed anger or anxiety that contribute to headache. There is an emphasis on identification of emotional states, modification of physiologic responses, and shifting of habitual thought patterns. We recommend that it be combined with other behavioral therapies, but it has shown to be effective alone.[21] One advantage is that it can be combined with group therapy. A meta-analysis of seven studies revealed a 49% improvement in headache activity with this approach.[20] Trials of combined cognitive-behavioral and biofeedback training have also revealed improvement in migraine headache symptoms.

Neurolinguistic Programming. Neurolinguistic programming relies on establishing solid rapport between provider and patient; developing an agreed-upon, positively stated, and well-formed set of therapeutic goals; and skillful application of a set of linguistic techniques, providing the patient with tools to deal with pain. Therapeutic approaches include reframing the meaning of headache, shifting the sensory coding of the pain, using guided dissociation techniques, modifying expectations, accessing resources, and anchoring resource states during and between episodes of pain. Patients often respond favorably because it provides them with specific methods for pain management that are not medication based, are easily learned, and are readily accessible.[22, 23]

Hypnosis. The use of hypnosis in the treatment of headache is based on modification of sensory processing of peripheral pain signals. Hypnosis has been shown to reduce the number of headache days and to decrease headache intensity among patients with chronic TTH.[24] For abortive therapy, hypnosis has been found to be useful in helping patients identify the very early stages of migraine so that they can initiate a relaxation response or a self-hypnosis routine. Regular practice of self-hypnotic techniques is a vital part of this strategy, and patient motivation needs to be carefully assessed beforehand. Hypnosis is also useful in resetting expectations, reducing rumination about the future, and modifying patterns of negative thought. (See also Chapter 89, Self-Hypnosis.)

Mindfulness Meditation. Meditation has been shown to have positive effects on mood, cardiac function, blood pressure, and muscle tone when practiced regularly. Effects are felt to be mediated in part by a rebalancing of the sympathetic and parasympathetic systems with reduction in sympathetic dominance.[25] We recommend an 8-week course of training, including 2 hours of formal training each week combined with daily practice of at least half an hour. Patients report improved sleep and less anticipatory anxiety relating to headache as well as reduction in headache intensity.

Biomechanical Techniques

Physical Therapy. Physical therapy alone does not appear to be effective in the treatment of migraine, but it can be useful as an adjunct to biofeedback and relaxation training.[18]

Chiropractic and Other Manipulative Techniques. A recently published randomized controlled trial of chiropractic spinal manipulative therapy for migraine revealed improvement in frequency, duration, disability, and medication use compared with a control group. Another study, published in 1978, revealed moderate improvement of symptoms among those with migraine who received either chiropractic manipulation or mobilization (one of two control groups) compared with medical care only. There are few other data derived from clinical trials pertaining to the efficacy of manipulative techniques for the treatment of migraine. We find it useful as adjunctive therapy when guided by patient reports of significant neck discomfort during and between headaches. Biofeedback using muscle end points is often prescribed simultaneously.

Bioenergetics

Acupuncture. A systematic review and meta-analysis of randomized clinical trials of acupuncture for the treatment of recurrent headache was published in 1999.[26] Twenty-two studies met the authors' inclusion criteria: 15 involved patients with migraine, 6 involved patients with TTH, and 1 involved patients with mixed diagnoses. Ten of these studies reported sufficient information to be included in a meta-analysis. Based on these 10 studies, a pooled responder rate of 1.53 (95% confidence interval, 1.11 to 2.11) was calculated, suggesting that acupuncture is effective compared with the control groups used. This result must be interpreted with caution, however; the patient populations, acupuncture treatments, control groups, and outcome measures of these 10 studies were very heterogeneous. Most of the studies employed "formulaic" acupuncture point combinations such that all the patients in a given arm of the study received identical treatments. The problem with this approach is that it is widely believed by acupuncturists that an individualized approach to acupuncture point selection is generally more effective. The clinical trials may therefore have underestimated the true effectiveness of acupuncture. Furthermore, there is good evidence to suggest that the "sham" acupuncture procedures (the insertion of needles in non–acupuncture point locations) employed as a placebo in the majority of these studies are associated with greater clinical benefit than might be expected from the placebo effect alone. These two methodologic problems raise the distinct possibility that acupuncture is more effective in practice for the treatment of migraine than is suggested by the findings of the clinical trials published to date.

> ### NOTE
> *The triad of acupuncture, biofeedback, and exercise works synergistically by optimizing the body's homeostatic physiology and healing systems of energy flow.*

Therapies to Consider

Although evidence of benefit is limited, our experience supports the use of the following additional methods in patients who are open to using alternative models of healing in an integrated treatment plan: craniosacral therapy, Reiki, therapeutic touch, Tai Chi, yoga, aromatherapy, traditional Chinese medicine, naturopathy, and distance healing.

 ── *THERAPEUTIC REVIEW* ───────────────

Migraine Prevention
- *Level one: Fewer than two headaches per month.*
  Lifestyle review and management
  Stress management, sleep, hygiene, regular aerobic exercise
  Drug detoxification
  Nutrition
  Restriction of specific foods: wine, dark beer, aged cheese, cashews, onions, chocolate, processed meats
  Caffeine reduction
  Biofeedback
  Six- to eight-week training + practice
- *Level two: Two to four headaches per month. Use level one approach plus:*
  Supplements/Botanicals
  Magnesium aspartate, 1000 mg qhs
  Riboflavin (vitamin B_2), 200 mg twice a day
  Botanicals
  Headache prophylaxis:
  Feverfew, 125 mg two to three times daily
  Improve sleep cycle:
  Valerian, 100 to 300 mg at bedtime
  Melatonin, 6 to 10 mg at bedtime
  Kava kava, 150 to 200 at bedtime
  Acupuncture
  Four sessions
  Mind-Body
  Cognitive behavioral therapy, neurolinguistic programming
  Two to four sessions per month
  Mindfulness meditation
  Eight-week course + daily practice
  Pharmaceuticals
  Nonsteroidal anti-inflammatory drugs
  Aspirin, 325 to 975 mg every day
  Tricyclics
  Amitriptyline, 10 to 100 mg at bedtime
  Beta blockers
  Propranolol, 60 to 180 mg at bedtime
  Alternative approaches
  Homeopathy, massage, aromatherapy, yoga

THERAPEUTIC REVIEW *continued*

- *Level three: More than four headaches per month. Use same approach as for levels one and two plus:*
Acupuncture
Allergy testing
Herbalist consultation
Mind-Body
Hypnosis
Four training sessions, minimum
Pharmaceuticals
Anticonvulsants
Valproate (Depakote), 500 to 1500 mg three times daily
Gabapentin (Neurontin), start at 300 mg orally qhs and increase by 300 mg each day to usual dose of 900 to 2400 mg given three times daily
Calcium channel blockers
Verapamil, 180 to 480 mg daily
Botulinum toxin, subcutaneous 25 IU every 3 months
Alternative approaches
Craniosacral therapy, Reiki, Tai Chi, traditional Chinese medicine, Ayurvedic medicine, distance healing

Acute migraine management
Abortive measures are considered in terms of combined factors of efficacy, cost, side effects, and ease of administration.
Acupuncture
Aromatherapy
Peppermint, eucalyptus
Relaxation, visualization, and self-hypnosis
Cue- and aura-initiated
Naproxen sodium
250 to 500 mg every 4 hours
Ibuprofen liquid
200 to 400 mg every 2 hours for three doses
Lidocaine 4% liquid
0.25 mL in each nostril every 2 hours
Isometheptene (Midrin)
Two tablets at onset, then one every 45 minutes for three doses
Triptans (prototype, others available)
Sumatriptan, 25 to 100 mg every 2 hours for three doses
Sumatriptan, 6.0 mg subcutaneously every 2 hours for three doses

TENSION-TYPE HEADACHE

Pathophysiology

The mechanisms underlying TTH are largely unknown, making it likely that it is a syndrome rather than a specific entity. It may exist in a spectrum with migraine, as shown by positive responses to antimigraine agents in patients with TTH and coexisting migraine. A benefit from migraine medications such as the triptans is not commonly seen in those with TTH alone, however. History and physical examination suggest intermittent muscle traction on pain-sensitive tendons and attachments of connective tissue to the skull. Pain is often bilateral, nonthrobbing, and bandlike, with intensification at the base of the skull and neck, the temples, and the forehead. The slow onset and intermittent nature of symptoms, the lack of autonomic features, the limited family history, and positive responses to nonsteroidal anti-inflammatory drugs suggest that inflammatory and myofascial influences dominate, with modest secondary contributions from blood vessels and nerves.

One critical factor in the approach to TTH is diagnosis. Organic disease of the head and neck often presents with pain that is highly localized, with characteristics that lead directly to a diagnosis. Certain pericranial conditions, however, including tumor and infection, can present with features of TTH and little else. It is rare for a vascular headache pattern to be the presenting complaint for such conditions. Warning symptoms and signs that should suggest further workup are listed in the first section of this chapter.

Therapeutic Overview

There is considerable overlap with migraine in an integrated treatment approach to TTH. Lifestyle issues of stress, sleep, exercise, and diet are central to effective management and need to be reviewed carefully. The caregiver in this setting can guide the patient through a meticulous review of these issues in both work and home environments. It is important to remember that individuals with baseline TTH may develop aggravating conditions that suddenly amplify the pain. Examples include sinus or tooth infection, head or neck trauma, refraction errors, glaucoma, cervical disk disease, and hypertension.

A thorough physical examination may lead to discovery of tender areas and trigger points in the head, the neck, or the shoulders that promote or sustain head pain. Observation of the patient while sitting, walking, and lying down can provide useful clues to therapy. Careful examination of temporomandibular joints is important in all patients because bruxism and associated problems can contribute to TTH. Dental, sinus, and ophthalmologic assessment is critical in looking for contributing conditions.

Patient education in ergonomics, upper body posture, and breathing is often central to relief of TTH. Mind-body approaches are often equally effective in migraine and TTH and need to be integrated into a treatment plan from the onset. The effectiveness of biofeedback, stress management, guided imagery, and self-hypnosis is well documented in TTH. Biofeedback, for instance, is effective for young adolescents with TTH.[27] Time-contingent and limited use of analgesics is the rule along with education about the risks of analgesic rebound headache. Our opinion is that a headache calendar, because of a possible reinforcing effect, is useful only until the pain is reduced by more than half of baseline.

We have found that a combination of sleep hygiene strategies, dietary timing, and regularization of daily schedules is effective in reducing pain in motivated and compliant patients. The botanicals for sleep described previously for migraine can be equally effective for those with TTH when sleep is an issue. We strongly encourage patients to reduce sugar, caffeine, and other stimulant intake along with increasing omega-3 fatty acid consumption to reduce sympathetic nervous system stimulation and to enhance production of anti-inflammatory prostaglandins. (See also Chapter 84, The Anti-inflammatory [Omega-3] Diet.) Detoxification from unneeded drugs is a vital part of TTH management.

Pharmaceuticals have a limited role because of the risk of rebound and also because they tend to reduce the patient's motivation to attend to the lifestyle changes needed to prevent headache. Nonsteroidal anti-inflammatory drugs should be medium- to long-acting and strictly limited in number per week. Although muscle relaxants might be expected to work, our experience is that they are of only short-term benefit and tend to lead to psychological dependency and rebound headache. Triptans work rarely in TTH and only in those with concurrent migraine.

When TTH occurs daily or almost daily without evidence of an underlying organic condition, analgesic rebound headache is considered, especially when supported by a history of use of more than 20 analgesic tablets a week of all kinds for pain. Treatment of chronic daily headache relies on the elimination of caffeine (over a period of 2 to 3 weeks) as well as the use of short-acting analgesics (over-the-counter and prescription), opioids, nasal decongestants and steroids, ergots, and benzodiazepines. Pain is managed with patient education, nonsteroidal anti-inflammatory drugs and muscle relaxants with a long half-life, massage, biofeedback, and slow stretch exercises.

NOTE

Chronic daily headache is often caused by excessive use of medications, including over-the-counter analgesics. Integrating nonpharmacologic approaches early in the course of treatment for migraine can help prevent development of difficult-to-treat chronic headaches.

Biomechanical

Chiropractic and Other Manipulative Techniques. We identified only four clinical trials in the published literature pertaining to spinal manipulation for TTH. One study demonstrated a 50% reduction of headache severity after a single, 10-minute cervical manipulation session.[28] Another study demonstrated a 57% reduction in pain intensity and a 64% reduction in analgesic medicine use over a 2-week period after two cervical spine manipulation treatments, compared with treatment with ice packs.[29] The third study found no differences between chiropractic stimulation and amitriptyline use on completion of a 6-week course of treatment, but patients who received chiropractic stimulation had fewer headaches on follow-up 6 weeks later (after discontinuation of treatment).[30] Finally, a randomized, controlled trial, published in 1998, which compared soft tissue therapy and spinal manipulation with soft tissue therapy and placebo laser treatment for episodic TTH, did not show any statistically significant difference in outcome between the two study arms.[31]

Bioenergetics

Acupuncture. The recent systematic review of acupuncture for recurrent headache by Melchart and associates[26] included only six clinical trials involving patients with TTH.[32, 33] Four studies compared true acupuncture to sham acupuncture, whereas two studies used physiotherapy control groups. Results of these studies suggest but do not prove that acupuncture may be useful in the treatment of TTH.

Therapies to Consider

In general, therapies that promote mind-body connections have the potential to reduce TTH pain. Our working model of TTH is based on the idea that the pain is in some part due to a failure to address imbalances that arise from disconnection between mind and body. Hence, the following approaches may prove useful to some patients suffering from this condition who are open to alternative models of health and healing: mindfulness meditation, Reiki, healing touch, magnet therapy, aromatherapy, Tai Chi, yoga, polarity therapy, traditional Chinese medicine, Ayurvedic medicine, and naturopathy.

THERAPEUTIC REVIEW

Tension-Type Headache
Emphasis is placed on lifestyle and self-management techniques with reduced reliance on medication.
Lifestyle
Stress management, sleep hygiene, nutrition, ergonomics, regular aerobic exercise
Nutrition
Increase omega-3 fatty acid intake
Reduce sugar, caffeine, tobacco, alcohol intake
Sleep and exercise
Sleep hygiene program; melatonin, 6–10 mg at bedtime; valerian, 100–300 mg at bedtime
Exercise three times per week at an aerobic level
Mind-Body
Biofeedback and relaxation
Specific muscle relaxation training, electromyographically guided
Stress management
Cognitive-behavioral approaches to managing stress, neurolinguistic programming
Mindfulness meditation
Biomechanical
Acupuncture
Four to six sessions with additional follow-up
Massage
Every 2 weeks for 3 months
Pharmaceuticals
Time-contingent nonsteroidal anti-inflammatory drugs; limit to less than 15 tablets per week
Alternative approaches integrated at any level
Yoga, Reiki, Tai Chi, traditional Chinese medicine, naturopathy, herbalist consultation, detoxification, homeopathy

Acknowledgment

We gratefully acknowledge Ms. Heidi Soeters' research assistance.

References

1. Bruni O, Galli F, Guidetti V: Sleep hygiene and migraine in children and adolescents. Cephalalgia 25(suppl):57–59, 1999.
2. Constantine LM, Scott S: Migraine: The Complete Guide. New York, Dell Publishing, 1994.
3. Mazzotta G, Sarchielli P, Alberti A, Gallai V: Electromyographical ischemic test and intracellular and extracellular magnesium concentration in migraine and tension-type headache patients. Headache 36:357–361, 1996.
4. Peikert A, Wilimzig C, Kohne-Volland R: Prophylaxis of migraine with oral magnesium: Results from a prospective, multi-center, placebo-controlled and double-blind randomized study. Cephalalgia 16:257–263, 1996.
5. Facchinetti F, Sances G, Borella P, et al: Magnesium prophylaxis of menstrual migraine: Effects on intracellular magnesium. Headache 31:298–301, 1991.
6. Mauskop A, Altura BT, Cracco RQ, Altura BM: Intravenous magnesium sulfate rapidly alleviates headaches of various types. Headache 36:154–160, 1996.
7. Schoenen J, Jacquy J, Lenaerts M: Effectiveness of high-dose riboflavin in migraine prophylaxis. A randomized controlled trial. Neurology 50:466–470, 1998.
8. Sandor PS, Afra J, Ambrosini A, Schoenen J: Prophylactic treatment of migraine with beta-blockers and riboflavin: Differential effects on the intensity dependence of auditory evoked cortical potentials. Headache 40:30–35, 2000.
9. Johnson ES, Kadam NP, Hylands DM, Hylands PJ: Efficacy of feverfew as prophylactic treatment of migraine. BMJ 291:569–573, 1985.

10. Murphy JJ, Heptinstall S, Mitchell JRA: Randomised double-blind placebo-controlled trial of feverfew in migraine prevention. Lancet 2:189–192, 1988.
11. Murry M, Pizzorno J: Encyclopedia of Natural Medicine. Rocklin, Calif, Prima Publishing, 1998.
12. Leone M, D'Amico D, Moschiano F, et al: Melatonin versus placebo in the prophylaxis of cluster headache: A double-blind pilot study with parallel groups. Cephalalgia 16:494–496, 1996.
13. Matchar DB, Young WB, Rosenberg JH, et al: Evidence-based guidelines for migraine headache in the primary care setting: Pharmacological management of acute attacks. http://www.aan.com/public/practiceguidelines/03.pdf.
14. Klapper JA, Klapper A: Use of botulinum toxin in chronic daily headaches associated with migraine. Headache Q 10:141–143, 1999.
15. Wheeler AH: Botulinum toxin A, adjunctive therapy for refractory headache associated with pericranial muscle tension. Headache 38:468–471, 1998.
16. Rollnik JD, Tannenberger O, Schubert M, et al: Treatment of tension-type headache with botulinum toxin type A: A double-blind, placebo controlled study. Headache 40:300–305, 2000.
17. Walach H, Lowes T, Mussbach D, et al: The long-term effects of homeopathic treatment of chronic headaches: 1 year follow-up. Cephalalgia 20:835–837, 2000.
18. Marcus DA, Scharff L, Mercer S, Turk DC: Nonpharmacological treatment for migraine: Incremental utility of physical therapy with relaxation and thermal biofeedback. Cephalalgia 18:266–272, 1998.
19. Holroyd KA, Penzien DB: Pharmacological versus non-pharmacological prophylaxis of recurrent migraine headache: A meta-analytic review of clinical trials. Pain 42:1–13, 1990.
20. Campbell JK, Penzien DB, Wall EM: Evidence-based guidelines for migraine headache: Behavioral and physical treatments. http://www.aan.com/public/practiceguidelines/04.pdf.
21. Bogaards MC, ter Kuile MM: Treatment of recurrent tension headache: A meta-analytic review. Clin J Pain 10:174–181, 1994.
22. Dilts R, Hallbom T, Smith S: Beliefs: Pathways to Health and Well-Being. Portland, Ore, Metamorphous Press, 1990.
23. McDermott I, O'Conner J: Neurolinguistic Programming and Health. San Francisco, Harper Collins, 1996.
24. Melis PML, Rooilans W, Spierings ELH, Hoogguin CAL: Treatment of chronic tension-type headache with hypnotherapy: A single-blind time controlled study. Headache 31:686–689, 1991.
25. Murphy M, Donovan S: The Physical and Psychological Effects of Meditation. Sausalito, Calif, Institute of Noetic Sciences, 1997.
26. Melchart D, Linde K, Fischer P, et al: Acupuncture for recurrent headaches: A systematic review of randomized controlled trials. Cephalalgia 19:779–786, 1999.
27. Bussone G, Grazzi L, D'Amico D, et al: Biofeedback-assisted relaxation training for young adolescents with tension-type headache: A controlled study. Cephalalgia 18:463–467, 1998.
28. Hoyt WH, Shaffer F, Bard DA, et al: Osteopathic manipulation in the treatment of muscle contraction headache. J Am Osteopath Assoc 78:322–325, 1979.
29. Jensen OK, Nielsen FF, Vosmar L: An open study comparing manual therapy with the use of cold packs in the treatment of post-traumatic headache. Cephalalgia 10:241–250, 1990.
30. Boline PD, Kassak K, Bronfort G, et al: Spinal manipulation vs. amitriptyline for the treatment of chronic tension-type headaches: A randomized clinical trial. J Manipulative Physiol Ther 18:148–154, 1995.
31. Bove G, Nilsson N: Spinal manipulation in the treatment of episodic tension-type headache. JAMA 280:1576–1579, 1998.
32. Hansen E, Hansen JH: Acupuncture treatment of chronic tension headache: A controlled cross-over trial. Cephalalgia 5:137–142, 1985.
33. Tavola T, Gala C, Conte G, Invernizzi G: Traditional Chinese acupuncture in tension-type headache: A controlled study. Pain 48:325–329, 1976.

CHAPTER 8

Peripheral Neuropathy

Sunil Pai, M.D.

PATHOPHYSIOLOGY

Peripheral neuropathy, or peripheral neuritis, is a common neurologic disorder resulting from damage to the peripheral nerves. It may be caused by diseases of the nerves or may be the result of systemic illnesses. There are a variety of causes including toxic trauma (Table 8–1), certain medications and chemotherapeutic agents (Table 8–2), or mechanical injury causing compression or entrapment, as with carpal tunnel syndrome (see Chapter 55, Carpal Tunnel Syndrome). Even simple pressure on superficial nerves such as with prolonged use of crutches or from sitting in the same position for too long can be a cause. Nutritional deficiencies can cause peripheral neuropathy, as with vitamin B deficiency (i.e., from alcoholism, pernicious anemia, isonazid-induced pyridoxine deficiency, malabsorption syndromes). Other causes include viral and bacterial infections and other infectious diseases (e.g., HIV infection, Lyme disease), autoimmune reactions (e.g., in Guillain-Barré syndrome), cancer (e.g., lymphoma, multiple myeloma), collagen-vascular disorders (e.g., systematic lupus erythematosus, rheumatoid arthritis, polyarteritis nodosa, Sjögren's syndrome), endocrinopathies (e.g., hypothyroidism, acromegaly), and rare inherited genetic abnormalities.

One of the most common causes is diabetes; peripheral neuropathy is estimated to be present in about 40% to 60% of persons with diabetes of 25 years', duration.[1] Diabetic neuropathy is now thought to be the most common form of peripheral neuropathy that afflicts humankind.[2] Although the exact pathophysiology of diabetic neuropathy has not yet been clearly identified, the etiology is multifactorial, with persistent hyperglycemia and autoimmune and microvascular mechanisms being important factors.

Persistent hyperglycemia is the most common primary factor responsible for the development of diabetic neuropathy. It is thought that persistent hyperglycemia increases the activity of the polyol pathway, which results in the intraneural accumulation of fructose and sorbitol, which causes damage to the nerves.[3] Persistent hyperglycemia alone, however, cannot account for the development of nerve damage, because diabetic neuropathy also occurs in patients with well-controlled disease whereas others with poorly controlled disease have no evidence of neuropathy.[1]

Table 8–1. Agents Causing Symptoms Associated with Toxic Neuropathy

Acrylamide (truncal ataxia)
Allyl chloride
Arsenic (sensory alterations, brown skin, Mees' lines)
Buckthorn toxin
Carbon disulfide
Cyanide
Dimethylaminopropionitrile (urinary complaints)
Biologic toxin in diphtheritic neuropathy (pharyngeal neuropathy)
Ethylene oxide
n-Hexane
Lead (wrist drop, abdominal colic)
Lucel-7 (cataracts)
Mercury
Methyl bromide
Organophosphates (cholinergic symptoms, neuropathy of delayed onset)
Thallium (pain, alopecia, Mees' lines)
Trichloroethylene (facial numbness)
Vacor

From Wyngaarden JB, Smith LH Jr, Benne HJC (eds): Cecil Textbook of Medicine, 19th ed. Philadelphia, WB Saunders, 1992; 2246.

Table 8–2. Pharmaceutical Agents Associated with Generalized Neuropathy

Chloramphenicol	Nucleosides (ddC, ddI)
Dapsone*	Nitrofurantoin*
Disulfiram	Nitrous oxide
Ethionamide	Phenytoin
Gold	Platinum (cisplatin)†
Glutethimide	Pyridoxine†
Hydralazine	Sodium cyanate
Isoniazid†	Paclitaxel (Taxol)
Metronidazole, misonidazole	Thalidomide†
Vincristine	

* Predominantly motor.
† Predominantly sensory.
From Wyngaarden JB, Smith LH Jr, Benne HJC (eds): Cecil Textbook of Medicine, 19th ed. Philadelphia, WB Saunders, 1992; 2247.
ddC, dideoxycytidine (zalcitabine); ddI, dideoxyinosine (didanosine).

In addition to accumulation of intraneural fructose and sorbitol, other factors in the development of diabetic neuropathy are immunologic mechanisms. This damage is caused by antineural autoantibodies that circulate in the serum of some diabetic patients. Antiphospholipid antibodies may also be present and may contribute to nerve damage in combination with vascular abnormalities.[4]

Finally, endoneural vascular insufficiency has been found to be a primary cause of diabetic neuropathy.[4] It is postulated that ischemia due to endoneural and epineural vascular changes causes nerve damage by thickening the blood vessel wall. Eventually, occlusion of the vessel may occur, leading to vascular permeability and compromise of endoneural blood flow.

Other multifactorial mechanisms implicated in the development of diabetic neuropathy are body habitus, environmental factors (including alcohol, smoking, and exposure to heavy metals), and genetic predisposition.

By these mechanisms, the sensory, autonomic, and motor nerves all may be affected, beginning with the distal lower extremities and spreading to involve the upper extremities as the diabetes continues.[3] Diabetic neuropathy usually presents in a "stocking and glove" distribution, with sensory loss, dysesthesias, and painful paresthesias, most commonly in the lower extremities. Common symptoms include tingling, prickling, or numbness; burning or freezing pain; sharp, stabbing, or electric pain; extreme sensitivity to touch; muscle weakness; and loss of balance and coordination.

INTEGRATIVE THERAPY

Because diabetic neuropathy is the most common peripheral neuropathy encountered in clinical practice, and its symptoms consist primarily of pain, the management of neuropathy involves not only prevention and control of underlying disease—in this case, diabetes—but also alleviation of the painful symptoms that result.

Lifestyle

Nutrition and Exercise

It has been adequately demonstrated that strict glycemic control may reduce the incidence of diabetic neuropathy by up to 64%.[5] Thus, maintaining diabetic control and avoiding environmental toxins such as heavy metals, cigarettes, alcohol, and pollution, are of the utmost importance. Healthy eating habits should be established (see Chapter 27, Diabetes mellitus). Because body habitus can play an important role in control of glycemia, regular exercise of walking for a minimum of 30 minutes per day 3 times a week should be implemented. An optimal regimen would be daily walks for 30 minutes to 1 hour as tolerated.

Mind-Body Therapy

Biofeedback

Biofeedback may be used to reduce stress and improve coping skills, which may aid in improving compliance, thereby promoting better glycemic control and reducing pain associated with diabetic neuropathy.[6, 7] The patient can be referred to a behavioral therapist or a psychologist who teaches biofeedback techniques. Recommendation is for a minimum of six 1-hour biofeedback sessions at approximately 1-week intervals. Usually, treatments include sessions of guided imagery or relaxation techniques. During these sessions, the patient wears a biofeedback device that indicates physiologic responses, such as electromyographic or electrodermal response, and a vital sign monitor (typically for blood pressure, pulse, or oxygen saturation). The monitoring enables the patient to conceptualize how emotion, anxiety, stress, and pain can affect physiologic status.

Once patients gain the ability to alter their physiologic state, they are taught to perform the relaxation biofeedback techniques at home with the use of audio tapes or guided imagery exercises (10 to 20 minutes each day) to attain the same result without the monitoring equipment. Thus, biofeedback is a tool the patient can use to control certain physiologic parameters during times of stress or pain, to help alleviate symptoms.

Bioenergetics

Bioelectromagnetics

In 1999, a study on the use of biomagnetics in pain management reported positive outcomes in 90% of patients suffering from diabetic neuropathy.[8] Magnetic footpad insole devices (Magstep) with a 475-gauss steep field gradient were worn for 24 hours of direct contact, for up to 4 months. This research speculates that magnets may lessen the sensation of pain by altering nerve C-fiber firing frequency, possibly by stimulating K^+ internal rectifying channels to repolarize or hyperpolarize. More research is needed before the results can be considered conclusive.

Acupuncture

Acupuncture and electroacupuncture have been found to be useful in neuropathic pain. Because beta-endorphins have been found to be involved in the pathogenesis of both painful and painless neuropathy,[9] acupuncture may exert its well-known effect by stimulating the production of endorphins in the central nervous system.[10] Acupuncture reduces primary or secondary symptoms of peripheral neuropathy in up to 77% of patients, in some cases (67%) enabling patients to reduce or stop their pain medications.[11]

Patients can receive six courses of classical acupuncture analgesia[12, 13] to both lower limbs over a 10-week period. The traditional Chinese acupuncture points of liver 3, spleen 6, spleen 9, and stomach 39 can be used. These points are located, respectively, at the heads of the fibula and the upper tibia, above the medial malleolus, and in the web of the big toe.

In addition to classical acupuncture, electroacupuncture may have a positive influence on nerve conduction velocity and may also relieve neuropathic pain.[12] This benefit has been demonstrated with use of the following protocol. Electroacupuncture is performed in two cycles of 5 sittings each (10 sessions) at 2-day intervals. Electrostimulation is given through the needles introduced at points along 5 of the 6 meridians traversing the shanks—namely, the gallbladder, liver, stomach, pancreas, and kidney meridians. The frequency of the impulse is slow (2 to 6 hertz), with a mean stimulation duration of 10 to 15 minutes, with the intensity adapted to individual sensitivity, between 200 and 900 μA. The stimulation wave (from negative pole to positive pole) is applied in the direction of energy circulation in the stimulated meridians in an attempt to obtain a stimulating effect.[12] Before such therapies can be recommended, a constitutional evaluation by a practitioner trained in acupuncture should be considered because each modality is prescribed on the basis of the unique symptoms and physical characteristics of the patient.

Botanical Medicine

Although there are no botanicals that directly affect neuropathy, there are many that may prevent diabetic neuropathy by controlling blood glucose levels (see Chapter 27, Diabetes Mellitus).

Supplements

Supplements can be helpful in diabetes control (see Chapter 27, Diabetes Mellitus), but only a few are directly used for neuropathy.

Alpha-Lipoic Acid

Alpha-lipoic acid (thiotic acid) works as a constituent of the body—that is, it is a vital substance that the organism itself produces. Alpha-lipoic acid increases muscle cell glucose uptake and also enhances insulin sensitivity.[14] A deficiency of alpha-lipoic acid causes, among other things, a restricted gain in energy for the cells, cell damage, and far-reaching disturbances in the breakdown of sugar. The cellular changes are particularly enduring in the peripheral nerve cells. Alpha-lipoic acid has been found to increase neuronal blood flow, to reduce oxidative stress, and to improve distal nerve conduction.[15] It is thought to act by chelating copper ions[16]; thus, it works as an antioxidant. Alpha-lipoic acid also has a favorable effect worthy of mention: It protects vitamin E, vitamin C, glutathione, and coenzyme Q10, thereby reducing the consequences of deficiency of these vitamins.

Reduction in chief symptoms with use of a dosage of 600 mg three times a day will take at least 3 weeks, but research has not tested beyond this end point.[17] Administration of 800 mg (in divided doses given 4 times a day) for 4 to 7 months appears to ameliorate neuropathic deficits and cardiac autonomic neuropathy and to improve motor and sensory nerve conduction over the long term.[18] No toxicity was reported in human studies (at doses of 800 mg a day for 4 months and 600 mg three times a day for 3 weeks), but too much alpha-lipoic acid may cause problems not yet identified.[19]

Dosage. The initial dose of alpha-lipoic acid is 100 mg twice daily which may be increased to 400 mg twice daily as tolerated for long-term use. Short-term treatment can be tried, using a higher dose of 600 mg three times daily for 3 weeks only. Although these dosages have yielded better results, I do not recommend increases above 400 mg twice daily until further trials with larger sample sizes and longer-term results have been completed.

Precautions. Use with caution in person who may be predisposed to hypoglycemia (including those receiving hypoglycemic agents, in whom blood sugar levels should be monitored closely). Gastrointestinal upset may occur at higher doses. Rarely, this supplement may cause skin rash.

B Vitamins

Vitamins B_1 (thiamine), B_6 (pyridoxine), and B_{12} (cobalamin) play an important role in the pathogenesis of peripheral neuropathy in deficiency syndromes such as those due to alcoholism or pernicious anemia, isoniazid-induced pyridoxine deficiency, and malabsorption syndromes. Recommendations are B-100 B-complex (a multivitamin which usually contains 100 mg of each B vitamin and also may include other vitamins such as folate) for ease of administration and intake of all B vitamins. Benfothiamine (Millgamma) 100 mg is a lipid-soluble vitamin B_1 analogue. It is thought that its lipid solubility allows it to penetrate the nerves more readily. It has been found to give higher bioavailability of thiamine than that for its water-soluble counterparts[20] and to significantly reduce neuropathy scores.[21, 22]

Dosage. Vitamin B complex (B-100), one tablet twice daily.

NOTE

In prescribing B-complex vitamins, make sure that the patient is not already taking another vitamin supplement that may contain B vitamins. Vitamin B_3 (niacin) in doses greater than 300 mg per day may cause headache, nausea, skin tingling, and flushing. Vitamin B_6 in doses greater than 250 mg per day may cause reversible nerve damage.

Vitamin E

As with alpha-lipoic acid, the effects of vitamin E may be a result of its antioxidant activity. Research trials appear to indicate that vitamin E preparations given in daily doses of 900 mg per day (1 mg is roughly equivalent to 1 international unit [1U] of vitamin E) for a period of 6 months significantly improved nerve conduction velocity measurements.[23] In general, the *d*-alpha tocopheryl (the natural type of vitamin E) has better antioxidant effects than those of the *dl*-alpha tocopheryl (the synthetic type).

Dosage. 400 to 800 IU of vitamin E daily.

Precautions. Vitamin E is relatively nontoxic. Because this vitamin can result in impairment of hemostasis, it should be stopped 1 week before surgical or dental procedures. Toxicity can occur if vitamin E (in doses greater than 200 IU equivalent) is taken with anticoagulants, resulting in prolongation of the prothrombin time. It is not to be given to patients taking the antiviral HIV medication amprenavir (which has vitamin E as a component).

Pharmaceuticals

Capsaicin

Capsaicin is an extract of chili peppers thought to relieve neuropathic pain, when applied topically, by depleting substance P.[24] Capsaicin does not reverse, stabilize, or lesser neuropathy but decreases the pain that occurs from it.

Dosage. Capsaicin cream 0.025% (Zostrix) 45 g, 90 g, or 0.075% (Zostrix-HP) 30 g or 60 g, applied to the affected area up to three or four times daily. Wash the hands immediately after application.

Precautions. Patients may experience burning, erythema, or contact dermatitis. Burning occurs in greater than 30% of patients but diminishes with continued use. Pain more commonly occurs when capsaicin is applied less often than three times a day.

Antidepressants

Tricyclic antidepressants (TCAs) such as amitriptyline (Elavil, Endep), nortriptyline (Aventyl, Pamelor) and desipramine (Norpramin) have been the mainstay in the palliation of pain secondary to diabetic neuropathy.[25] TCAs work by increasing the postsynaptic concentration of norepinephrine (NE). Because the inhibitory pathways in the spinal cord use NE as a neurotransmitter, TCAs are believed to increase the inhibitory influence on nociceptive transmitting neurons.[26] The selective serotonin reuptake inhibitors (SSRIs) such as fluoxetine have also been used; although better tolerated than the tricyclics, they appear to be less efficacious.

Dosage.

- Amitriptyline (Elavil, Endep)
- Nortriptyline (Aventyl, Pamelor)

In order to minimize side effects and to encourage compliance, start therapy with amitriptyline or nortriptyline at a dose of 10 mg at bedtime. Titrate this dose upward to 25 mg at bedtime as side effects allow, in 25-mg increments. Even at lower doses, patients will generally report rapid improvement in sleeping and will begin to experience some pain relief in 10 to 14 days. If no relief of pain is obtained with increased doses (usual range, 50 to 300 mg per day), the addition of gabapentin alone or in combination with nerve blocks with local anesthetics is recommended.[27]

Precautions. Significant anticholinergic side effects, including dry mouth, constipation, sedation, and urinary retention, are common. TCAs may also cause orthostatic hypotension and arrhythmias. These agents are not to be used with monoamine oxidase inhibitors (MAOIs).

Anticonvulsants

- Phenytoin (Dilantin)
- Carbamazepine (Tegretol)
- Gabapentin (Neurontin): First-line choice

Phenytoin and carbamazepine have been used with varying degrees of success whether alone or in combination with antidepressants. Gabapentin has been shown to be highly efficacious in the treatment of a variety of painful neuropathic conditions including postherpetic neuralgia and diabetic neuropathy.[28] Gabapentin has a favorable side effect profile compared with phenytoin and carbamazepine and thus should be considered a first-line agent for treatment of neuropathic pain.[29] I recommend using only gabapentin instead of phenytoin and carbamazepine, because patients experience fewer side effects and demonstrate a better therapeutic response. It is unknown precisely which mechanisms of action of anticonvulsants account for their analgesic efficacy. Some research indicates that the primary effect of anticonvulsants on *N*-

methyl-D-aspartate (NMDA) receptors is inhibition of high-frequency firing in neurons, which reduces ion flow. As a result, there is a reduction in excitatory synaptic transmission, which can lead to an increase in the refractory period for the cell membrane. These changes eventuate in a slower rate of firing of action potentials in the damaged neuron.[30]

- Gabapentin

Dosage. A single bedtime dose of 300 mg of gabapentin for 2 nights can be followed by 300 mg given twice daily for an additional 2 days. If the patient tolerates this twice-daily dosage, it can be increased to 300 mg three times a day.

Additional titration upward can be carried out in 300-mg increments as side effects allow. Total daily doses greater than 3600 mg are not currently recommended.[27]

Precautions. Multiple drug interactions with phenytoin and carbamazepine have been reported. A complete blood count and platelet count should be performed and repeated periodically in patients receiving carbamazepine, to watch for aplastic anemia and agranulocytosis; Stevens-Johnson syndrome and hepatitis may also occur. Thus, only gabapentin is recommended; with this drug, the dose should be decreased in patients with renal dysfunction.

Antiarrhythmics

- Mexiletine (Mexitil)

Mexiletine is an antiarrhythmic compound that may be effective in the management of diabetic neuropathy, especially for sharp lancinating or burning pain.[31] Unfortunately, this drug is poorly tolerated by patients and has severe side effects; therefore, it should be reserved for those who fail to respond to first-line agents such as gabapentin or amitriptyline alone or in combination with neural blockade. Various studies have used dosages ranging from 225 to 1200 mg per day. Because a standard dose has not been established, consultation with a cardiologist is recommended to help with monitoring and dosage.

Analgesics

Simple analgesics such as acetaminophen, aspirin, and other nonsteroidal anti-inflammatory drugs (NSAIDs) may be used in conjunction with anticonvulsants and antidepressants but have very poor response. Caution must be taken not to exceed the recommended daily dose because of the risk of renal and hepatic toxicity, particularly in diabetics. The role of cyclo-oxygenase-2 (COX-2) inhibitors in the palliation of neuropathic pain has not been adequately studied.

Narcotic analgesics also are suboptimal agents for pain control. Owing to their significant central nervous system and gastrointestinal side effects coupled with problems of tolerance, dependence, and addiction, these agents should rarely if ever be used. If a narcotic analgesic is being considered, the analgesic tramadol (Ultram), which binds weakly to opioid receptors, may provide some symptomatic relief.

Dosage. Tramadol (Ultram) 50 to 100 mg PO every 6 hours as needed for pain. Maximum dose 400 mg per day.

NOTE

Caution should be used with the combination of tramadol (Ultram), antidepressants, and anticonvulsants, owing to increased seizure risk.

Biomechanical Modalities

Electrical Stimulation

Electrical stimulation modalities such as transcutaneous electrical nerve stimulation (TENS)[32] and application of spinal cord stimulators[33] have been used successfully to alleviate the pain and discomfort associated with peripheral neuropathy. TENS portable units that generate a biphasic, exponentially decaying wave form (pulse width 4 ms, 25 to 35 volts, >2 hertz) should be used for 30 minutes daily for 4 weeks. A recent study showed that percutaneous electrical nerve stimulation (PENS), in addition to decreasing pain, improves patients' capacity for physical activity, sense of well-being, and quality of sleep while reducing the need for oral nonopioid analgesic medication.[34] PENS is similar to electroacupuncture in that electrical stimulation is given via disposable acupuncture-type needles, but differs in that it is delivered along the peripheral nerves innervating the region of neuropathic pain rather than being delivered at acupuncture points or along meridians. Although use of alternating low and high frequencies of 15 and 30 Hz at 30-minute intervals 3 times a week is recommended, the patient should be evaluated by a healthcare professional familiar with electrical stimulation techniques for adjustment of frequencies and time intervals as tolerated.

Neural Blockade

Local anesthetic peripheral and sympathetic blocks provide useful diagnostic information but tend to confer only temporary therapeutic benefit in patients with peripheral neuropathy.[35]

Surgery

Entrapment neuropathies such as carpal tunnel syndrome may be relieved by surgical decompression (see Chapter 55, Carpal Tunnel Syndrome). Also, compression or entrapment from cancers may also be addressed by removal of the tumor directly.

Upcoming Treatments

Research continues to find more effective therapies for peripheral neuropathy. Promising early results have been obtained with several agents. One group of such agents is nerve growth factors, substances that are manufactured forms of naturally produced chemicals that signal the body to repair small nerve fibers. Other agents such calcium channel blockers and drugs to treat Parkinson's disease may help slow nerve damage. For treatment of diabetic neuropathy, two classes of drugs—new selective serotonin reuptake inhibiters (SSRIs) and aldose reductase inhibiters—may offer hope.

OTHER THERAPIES TO CONSIDER

Traditional Chinese Medicine

In a preliminary experiment, reinforced tianma (*Rhizoma gastrodiae*) duzhong (*Cortex eucommiae*) capsules were found to be useful in treating limb discomfort due to diabetic peripheral neuropathy.[36] A review of the advances in treatment of diabetic neuropathy by traditional Chinese medicine (TCM) shows that this modality acts to promote blood circulation and correct blood stasis, with significant effects of anticoagulation, thrombolysis, dilatation of blood vessels, cardiotonic activity, decrease in blood platelet aggregation and fibrinogen, improvement in microcirculation, and increase in vascular permeability.[37] Before these therapies are recommended, a constitutional evaluation by an experienced TCM practitioner should be considered, because each preparation is prescribed on the basis of the unique symptoms of the patient.

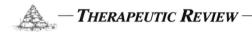 *THERAPEUTIC REVIEW*

- *Lifestyle and nutrition*
  - Daily exercise of walking at least 30 minutes per day three times per week should be implemented. Healthy eating habits with strict glycemic control should be encouraged. Environmental and other toxins such as heavy metals, cigarette smoke, alcohol, and pollution should be avoided.

- *Mind-body therapy*
  - Biofeedback: Recommendation is for at least six 1-hour biofeedback sessions at approximately 1-week intervals. Thereafter, relaxation biofeedback techniques can be performed at home with the use of audio tapes or guided imagery exercises (for 10 to 20 minutes each day).

- *Bioenergetics*
  - Bioelectromagnetics: Magnetic footpad insole devices (Magstep) with a 475-gauss steep field gradient can be worn for up to 24 hours of direct contact, and for up to 4 months, to obtain symptomatic relief.
  - Acupuncture: Patients can receive six courses of classical acupuncture analgesia to both lower limbs over a 10-week period.
  - Electroacupuncture: This treatment can be performed in two cycles of 5 sittings each (10 sessions) at 2-day intervals.

- *Supplements*
  - Alpha-lipoic acid: 100 mg twice daily; dose may be increased to 400 mg twice daily as tolerated.
  - Vitamin B complex (B-100): one tablet twice a day.
  - Vitamin E: 400 to 800 IU daily

- *Pharmaceuticals*
  For topical relief:
  - Capsaicin cream 0.025% (Zostrix), 45 g or 90 g, or 0.075% (Zostrix-HP), 30 g or 60 g. Apply to affected area 3 or 4 times daily.
  For acute pain management, consider:
  - Analgesics: Acetaminophen and NSAIDs as usually prescribed for pain, as well as narcotics.

THERAPEUTIC REVIEW *continued*

For chronic pain management, consider:

- Antidepressants

    Amitriptyline (Elavil, Endep) or nortriptyline (Aventyl, Pamelor): 10 mg at bedtime; titrate dose upward to 25 mg at bedtime as side effects allow (usual range: 50 to 300 mg per day)

- Anticonvulsants

    Gabapentin (first-line choice): 300 mg PO at bedtime for 2 days, then 300 mg twice daily for 2 days; can be increased to 300 mg 3 times a day as tolerated, with increases in 300-mg increments as side effects allow; maximum daily dose: 3600 mg.

- *Biomechanical*

    - Transcutaneous electrical nerve stimulation (TENS): Use of a TENS portable unit for 30 minutes daily for 4 weeks is recommended.
    - Percutaneous electrical nerve stimulation (PENS): This modality can be used 3 times a week; stimulation is delivered along the peripheral nerves innervating the region of neuropathic pain.
    - Neural blockade: Of only temporary therapeutic benefit.
    - Surgery: Surgical decompression may relieve symptoms in carpal tunnel syndrome; with neuronal entrapment from cancer, removal of the tumor itself may also be helpful.

References

1. Hamberg H: Diseases of the peripheral nervous system. In Wyngaarden JB, et al. (eds): Cecil Textbook of Medicine, 19th ed. Philadelphia, WB Saunders, 2240–2247, 1992.
2. O'rian SP, Schwedler M, Kerstein MD: Peripheral neuropathies in diabetes. Surg Clin North Am 1998; 78:393–408.
3. Vinik AL: Diagnosis and management of diabetic neuropathy. Clin Geriatr Med 1999; 15: 294–303.
4. Vinik AL: Diabetic neuropathy: Pathogenesis and therapy. Am J Med 1999; 107[Suppl]:17S–18S.
5. Diabetes Control and Complications Trial Research Group: The effect of intensive treatment of diabetes on the development and progression of neuropathy. Ann Intern Med 1995; 122:561–568.
6. Jablon SL, Nalifboff BD, Gilmore SL, Rosenthal MJ: Effects of relaxation training on glucose tolerance and diabetic control in type II diabetes. Appl Psychophysiol Biofeedback 1997; 22:155–169.
7. Rosenbaum L: Biofeedback-assisted stress management for insulin-treated diabetes mellitus. Biofeedback Self-Regul 1983; 8:519–532.
8. Weintraub MI: Magnetic bio-stimulation in painful diabetic neuropathy: A novel intervention—a randomized, double-placebo crossover study. Am J Pain Manage 1999; 9:8–17.
9. Tsigos C: Cerebrospinal fluid levels of beta endorphin in painful and painless diabetic polyneuropathy. J Diabetes Complications 1995; 9:92–96.
10. Han JS, Ding XZ, Fan SG: Cholecystokinin octapeptide (CCK-8) antagonism to electroacupuncture analgesia and a possible role in electroacupuncture tolerance. Pain 1986; 27:101–115.
11. Abuaisha BB, Costanzi JB, Boulton AJM: Acupuncture for the treatment of chronic painful peripheral neuropathy: A long-term study. Diabetes Res Clin Pract 1998; 39:115–121.
12. Ionescu-Targoviste C, Phleck-Khhayan A, Danciu V, et al: The treatment of peripheral polyneuritis by electroacupuncture. Am J Acupunct 1981; 9:92–96.
13. O'Connor J, Bensky D: Acupuncture: A comprehensive text. Chicago, Ill, Shanghai College of Traditional Medicine/Eastland Press, 1981.
14. Kishi Y, Schmelzer JD, Yao JK, et al: Alpha lipoic acid: Effect on glucose uptake, sorbitol pathway, and energy metabolism in experimental diabetic neuropathy. Diabetes 1999; 48:2045–2051.
15. Nagamatsu M, Nicklander KK, Schmelzer JD, et al: Lipoic acid improves nerve blood flow, reduces oxidative stress, and improves distal nerve conduction in experimental diabetic neuropathy. Diabetes Care 1995; 18:1160–1167.
16. Ou P, Tritschler HJ, Wolff SP: Thiotic (lipoic) acid: A therapeutic metal-chelating antioxidant? Biochem Pharmacol 1995; 50:123–126.
17. Ruhnau KJ, Meissner HP, Finn JR, et al: Effects of 3-week oral treatment with the antioxidant thiotic acid (alpha-lipoic acid) in symptomatic diabetic polyneuropathy. Diabet Med 1999; 16:1040–1043.
18. Ziegler D, Schatz H, Conrad F, et al: Effects of treatment with the anti-oxidant alpha-lipoic acid on cardiac autonomic neuropathy in NIDDM patients. A 4-month randomized controlled multicenter trial (DEKAN study). Diabetes Care 1997; 20:369–373.
19. Ziegler D, Reljanovic M, Mehnert H, Gries FA: Alpha-lipoic acid in the treatment of diabetic polyneuropathy in Germany: Current evidence in clinical trials. Exp Clin Endocrinol Diabetes 1999; 107:421–430.
20. Schreeb KH, Freudenthaler S, Vormfelde SV, et al: Comparative bioavailability of two vitamin B$_1$ preparations: benfotiamine and thiamine mononitrate. Eur J Clin Pharmacol 1997; 52:319–320.
21. Haupt E, Ledermann H, Kopcke W: Benfothiamine in treatment of diabetic polyneuropathy. Paper presented at the 4th International Symposium on Diabetic Neuropathy, July 15–19, 1997.
22. Barkai L, Kempler P, Kadar E, Feher A: Benfothiamine treatment for peripheral sensory nerve dysfunction in diabetic adolescents. Paper presented at the 4th international Symposium on Diabetic Neuropathy, July 15–19, 1997.
23. Tutuncu NB, Bayractar M, Varli K: Reversal of defective nerve conduction with vitamin E supplementation in type 2 diabetes: A preliminary study. Diabetes Care 1998; 21:1915–1918.
24. Lynn B: Capsaicin: Actions on nociceptive C-fibers and therapeutic potential. Pain 1990; 41:61–69.
25. Joss JD: Tricyclic antidepressant use in diabetic neuropathy. Ann Pharmacol 1999; 33:996–1000.
26. Ross E: The evolving role of antiepileptic drugs in treating neuropathic pain. Neurology 2000; 55(5 Suppl 1):S41–S46.
27. Waldman SD: Diabetic neuropathy: Diagnosis and treatment for the pain management specialist. Curr Rev Pain 2000; 4:383–387.
28. Backonja M, Beydon A, Edwards KR, et al: Gabapentin for the symptomatic treatment of painful neuropathy in patients with diabetes mellitus. JAMA 1998; 280:1831–1836.
29. Backonja MM: Anticonvulsants (antineuropathics) for neuropathic pain syndromes. Clin J Pain 2000; 16:S67–S72.
30. Bennett GJ, Dworkin RH, Nicholson B: Anticonvulsant therapy

in the treatment of neuropathic pain. Available at: http://www.medscape.com/Medscape/Neurology/TreatmentUpdate/1999/tu04/public/toc-tu04.html.

31. Jarvis B, Coukell AJ: Mexiletine: A review of its therapeutic use in painful diabetic neuropathy. Drug 1999; 56:691–707.
32. Kumar D, Marshall H: Diabetic peripheral neuropathy: Amelioration of pain with transcutaneous electrostimulation. Diabetes Care 1997; 20:1702–1705.
33. Tesfaye S, Watt J, Benbow SJ, et al: Electrical spinal-cord stimulation for painful diabetic peripheral neuropathy. Lancet 1996; 348:1696–1701.
34. Hamza M, et al: Percutaneous electrical nerve stimulation: A novel analgesic therapy for diabetic neuropathic pain. Diabetes Care 2000; 23:365–370.
35. Abram S: Neural blockade for neuropathic pain. Clin J Pain 2000; 16:S56–S61.
36. Mingrui L, Xiang W: Clinical observation on treatment of diabetic peripheral neuropathy with reinforced tianma duzhong capsule. J Tradit Chin Med 1999; 19:182–184.
37. Farong Z: Advances in treatment of diabetic neuropathy by traditional Chinese medicine. J Tradit Chin Med 1998; 18:146–152.

CHAPTER 9

Multiple Sclerosis

Patricia Ammon, M.D.

PATHOPHYSIOLOGY AND DIAGNOSIS

Multiple sclerosis (MS) is the most common cause of chronic neurologic disability in young adults, with a prevalence of about 1 in 1000. It is characterized by demyelination of the central nervous system with subsequent plaque formation. Despite decades of research, the cause of MS remains unknown. The onset of MS is typically in the third or fourth decade of life but may be as early as 2 years of age[1] or as late as 70 years of age. The course of the disease is unpredictable, with mild forms occurring in approximately 20% of patients. Because of the wide variability in the disease presentation, it has been found useful to categorize patients with MS into four groups.[2] *Relapsing-remitting* (RR) *disease* occurs at onset in 80% of cases and is characterized by acute attacks followed by remissions with a steady baseline between attacks. In 50% to 80% of patients with RR disease, progressive deterioration with less marked attacks occurs within 10 years of onset; the disease in these patients is called *secondary progressive phase MS* (SP-MS). *Primary progressive disease* (PP-MS) occurs in 10% to 15% of patients and is characterized by progressive deterioration from the outset without superimposed relapses. Approximately 6% of patients with PP-MS also experience relapses in parallel with their disease progression and are said to have *progressive-relapsing MS* (PR-MS).

The diagnosis is based on established clinical and laboratory criteria. The hallmark of MS is neurologic dysfunction manifested clinically in different body systems and varying in severity over time. On magnetic resonance imaging, the finding of lesions involving the periventricular white matter supports the clinical diagnosis.

ETIOLOGY

The search for the cause of MS is made difficult by the marked variation in disease expression. It is not clear whether MS is one disease with variable symptoms or whether the different subtypes represent unique causes.[3]

At present, there are four major theories of the cause of MS: immunologic, environmental, infectious agent, and genetic (Fig. 9–1).

Immunologic Factors

The theory that MS is an organ-specific autoimmune disease is, although unproven, widely accepted. Antibodies against antigens located on the surface of the myelin sheath cause demyelination either directly or by complement-mediated processes.[4] Activation of autoreactive T lymphocytes in the systemic circulation may enhance their movement through the blood-brain barrier.

Environmental Factors

For several decades, the geographic distribution of MS has promoted studies of the environmental influence on the incidence of MS. For at least three decades, it has been documented that the incidence of MS increases with increasing distance from the equator. Possible explanations for this finding include genetic predisposition in population groups, dietary factors, and levels of the active form of vitamin D. Epidemiologic studies have shown that people who are born in an area of the world with a high risk of developing MS, and who move to an area with a lower risk, acquire the risk for the geographic location of their new home, if the move occurs before adolescence.[5] This finding suggests that exposure to some environmental agent encountered before puberty may predispose a person to develop MS later in life.

The dietary influence on MS was first reported by Swank in 1952. This investigator noted that people living in colder climates tend to consume diets higher in fat compared with those living in more tropical regions, and he made the observation that there was a direct correlation between the incidence of MS and the amount of dairy products consumed.[6] The relationship between mercury from dental fillings and MS is one of extreme controversy, with some studies concluding a clear relationship between mercury and MS[7] and other studies showing a relationship between the extent of dental caries and MS but no association between MS and the number of mercury fillings.[8] At present, there are too many connections

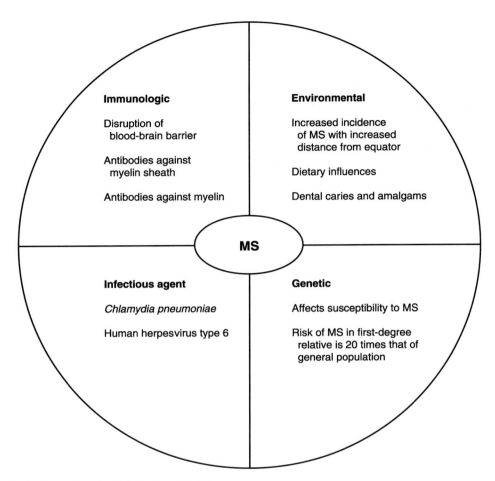

Figure 9-1. Theories for the cause of multiple sclerosis (MS).

between mercury toxicity and MS to be ignored. Further research may clarify this relationship.

Infectious Agent(s)

At least 16 different infectious agents have been identified as possible causes of MS; however, none has been definitely proved to cause MS. The two infectious agents receiving the most attention at present are human herpesvirus 6 (HHV-6) and *Chlamydia pneumoniae*. HHV-6 is a known neurotropic virus, with HHV-6 clearly identified in case reports as the pathogen in fulminant demyelinating disease.[9] Evidence from more recent research describing the possible relationship between MS and *C. pneumoniae* is quite compelling,[10] and unlike viruses, *C. pneumoniae* is susceptible to specific antimicrobial agents.

Genetic Factors

Although most cases of MS are sporadic, susceptibility to develop MS is substantially affected by genetic factors. A first-degree relative of a person with MS is 10 to 20 times more likely to develop MS than someone in the general population. The pre-

sence of the HLA-DR2 allele increases the risk of MS.[11] Although gene mapping is continuing, it is likely that no single gene exerts a strong effect on the development of MS.

INTEGRATIVE THERAPY

Nutrition

Although a relationship between MS and dietary fat intake was described a half-century ago, the concept that diet plays a role in MS has not been widely accepted by conventional medicine. However, more contemporary research continues to show a direct relationship between dietary saturated fat, animal fat, and MS.[12]

A review of the role of dietary fats, essential fatty acids (EFAs), and prostaglandins (PG-1, PG-2, and PG-3) in the inflammatory response will help to elucidate the importance of diet in the etiology of MS. Dietary fats affect prostaglandins by a pathway of chemical reactions (Fig. 9-2). Prostaglandins direct lymphocytes either to modulate their response (decreased inflammation) or to become more active (increased inflammation). PG-1 and PG-3 modulate the immune

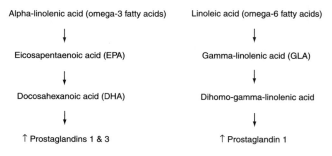

Figure 9–2. Pathway by which dietary fats are converted to prostaglandins.

response, and PG-2 signals the lymphocytes to become more active in the immune response.

Many studies have found a lower level of these fatty acids, particularly gamma-linolenic acid (GLA) and docosahexanoic acid (DHA), in MS patients.[13] One hypothesis to explain the low level of fatty acids in people with MS is the possibility of an abnormality in the enzymatic conversion of eicosapentaenoic acid (EPA) to DHA. Low dietary intake of polyunsaturated fats by people with MS is another theory to explain the deficiency. An omega-3 EFA preparation (flaxseed oil or fish oil) that supplies DHA 500 mg per day and of an omega-6 EFA preparation (evening primrose oil, borage oil, or black currant oil) that supplies GLA 300 mg per day should be added to the diet of persons with MS. To keep the fatty acids from degrading, EFA supplements should always be refrigerated and taken with a daily dose of vitamin E of 200 IU.

PG-2 production, which increases inflammation and immune activity, is triggered by dietary saturated fat, cholesterol, and alcohol. Adherence to a primarily vegetarian diet, with protein sources including cold water fish and soy products, should be recommended for patients with MS. Alcohol should be eliminated.

Supplements

Antioxidants

The inflammation caused by the immune reaction directed against myelin in MS leads to excessive free radical activity, damaging the mitochondria and leading to further breakdown of the myelin sheath.[14] Increased free radical formation and decreased antioxidant defense in the central nervous system have been implicated as causal factors in MS in several studies.[15]

Alpha-Lipoic Acid

Alpha-lipoic acid is rapidly absorbed from the gut, crosses the blood-brain barrier, and has powerful antioxidant activity.

Dosage. Alpha-lipoic acid 100 mg per day.

Glutathione and N-Acetylcysteine

Endogenous glutathione provides the primary cellular defense against free radicals, but supplemental glutathione cannot be given orally. A qualified health care practitioner can give glutathione intravenously (IV). An alternative to intravenous methods of raising glutathione levels is oral administration of N-acetylcysteine (NAC). NAC produces an increase in blood glutathione levels.

Dosage. Glutathione 600 to 800 mg IV diluted in 10 ml of normal saline over a 15- to 20-minute period, given two or three times per week for optimal benefit, or NAC 200 mg PO per day.

Precautions. Nausea, vomiting, urticaria, stomatitis, rhinorrhea, drowsiness, and elevation of liver enzymes have been reported in patients taking these supplements.

Vitamin D

Vitamin D, in a mouse model, has been shown to prevent the development of an MS-like disease.[16] Decreased formation of the active form of vitamin D secondary to decreased sun exposure may be one reason why MS is more prevalent in northern latitudes.

Dosage. Vitamin D 200 international units (IU) per day.

Ginkgo biloba

Ginkgo biloba will, in addition to its antioxidant effects, also enhance neurotransmission.

Dosage. 120 to 240 mg per day.

Energy for Cells

Vitamin B$_{12}$

Deficiency of vitamin B$_{12}$ and errors in B$_{12}$ metabolism are known to cause demyelination of the central nervous system.[17] During an MS attack, B$_{12}$ deficiency can enhance the destruction of myelin and compromise the body's ability to repair the myelin sheath after the attack has subsided.

Because serum B$_{12}$ levels do not always correspond with cerebrospinal fluid levels of B$_{12}$,[18] it is not sufficient to simply measure the serum B$_{12}$ level in evaluating a patient for a B$_{12}$ deficiency. One way to test for a functional B$_{12}$ deficiency is to measure serum homocysteine levels. Homocysteine is converted to methionine in a reaction that requires B$_{12}$ as a cofactor. The possible explanation for B$_{12}$ deficiency in MS focuses on B$_{12}$ binding or transport, as most patients do not have a deficiency of intrinsic factor.[18]

Although there are no controlled reports of neurologic benefit from B$_{12}$ injections, my patients have almost universally improved with B$_{12}$ injections. Teaching patients self-injection of B$_{12}$ can be a cost-effective way of improving overall well-being.

Dosage. Vitamin B$_{12}$ 1000 μg IM daily for 5 days, then twice weekly for 4 weeks, and then twice monthly.

Phosphatidylserine

Phosphatidylserine plays a crucial role in preserving function of the cell membrane. When compromised, energy production can be decreased to the point of damage to the neuron.

Dosage. Phosphatidylserine 50 mg per day.

Coenzyme Q10

Coenzyme Q10 is an essential component of the electron transport chain and functions as a fat-soluble antioxidant. Deficiencies of coenzyme Q10 can enhance the damaging effects of naturally occurring free radicals.

Dosage. Coenzyme Q10 60 mg twice a day.

Other Nutrients

Vitamins B$_3$, B$_6$, and C and the minerals zinc and magnesium can reduce the production of PG-2.

Dosage. B$_3$ 50 mg, B$_6$ 50 mg, zinc 20 mg, and magnesium 200 mg daily.

Hormones

A role for hormonal factors in the etiology and pathophysiology of MS has long been suspected, with the incidence of MS in women twice that in men. Evidence for the role of sex hormones includes the alteration of disease symptomatology with change in sex hormones during pregnancy and menopause and with the use of hormone replacement therapy and use of oral contraceptives.[19] In the majority of patients, symptoms of MS disappear with pregnancy, but there is an increased rate of relapse during the postpartum period. Women often report premenstrual worsening of symptoms with return to baseline levels of severity during menses. How sex hormones exert their effect is quite complex, but research indicates these hormones inactivate proinflammatory cytokines.[20] The paradox of why women—who produce these hormones—have an increased prevalence of MS can be explained by a biphasic effect of estrogen on immune function. At low concentrations of estrogens, the proinflammatory cytokines are activated, whereas at high concentrations consistent with pregnancy, use of oral contraceptives, or postmenopausal hormone replacement therapy, activation of these cytokines is inhibited. Estrogen's effect on cognitive function in MS patients has been detailed in studies.[21] These findings suggest that prescribing estrogen to menopausal and postmenopausal women with MS may prevent cognitive deterioration. Estriol, the form of estrogen formed by the fetal-placental unit and sig-nificantly elevated in the last trimester of pregnancy, has been shown in animal models to ameliorate symptoms of cell-mediated autoimmune disease.[19] Progesterone, again at concentrations consistent with late pregnancy, has also been shown to decrease activation of proinflammatory cytokines.

Dosage. Estriol, available through compounding pharmacies, may be given in a dose of 4 to 8 mg per day to menopausal and postmenopausal women. Progesterone may be given in a dose of 100 mg twice a day (see Chapter 44, Menopause).

Anti-infective Treatments

Chlamydia pneumoniae Infection

On the basis of the research linking *C. pneumoniae* to MS,[10] it is not unreasonable for patients with MS to be given presumptive treatment for *C. pneumoniae* infection. There are no protocols developed as yet, but use of antibiotics effective against *C. pneumoniae* is reasonable. Although doxycycline and tetracycline are both effective against *C. pneumoniae*, doxycycline may penetrate the blood-brain barrier more effectively.

Dosage. Doxycycline 100 mg twice a day for 14 days.

Human Herpesvirus-6 Infection

Further investigations into the role of HHV-6 in MS is needed before general use of antiviral agents can be recommended. If such treatment is to be initiated, determining the subclass of HHV-6 will be important owing to differences in sensitivity to antiviral agents.

Pharmaceuticals

Treatment for Relapses

Steroids

There is evidence that the administration of glucocorticosteroids, with their potent anti-inflammatory effects, shortens the duration of acute relapses. Generally, methylprednisolone 500 to 1000 mg IV per day for 3 to 5 days is the pharmaceutical used, however, there is evidence that similar efficacy can be achieved with oral administration.[22] There is no evidence that glucocorticosteroids affect the overall degree of recovery or long-term course of the disease. Side effects of steroids are numerous and can be severe. Some of the more severe side effects include congestive heart failure, hypertension, osteoporosis, peptic ulcer with possible perforation, immune suppression with increased susceptibility to infection, and decreased carbohydrate tolerance.

Disease-Modifying Agents

The goal of these medications is to reduce the frequency and severity of relapses as well as to prevent or delay the onset of progressive disease.

Interferon Beta-1b

Interferon beta-1b (Betaseron) was approved by the U.S. Food and Drug Administration (FDA) in 1993 for use in relapsing-remitting MS. The precise method of how interferon beta-1b decreases the frequency of relapses is not known, but its activity as an antiviral and immunoregulatory agent is what prompted the initial research on this medication. Although studies show a decrease in the number of exacerbations with use of interferon beta-1b, it should be noted that patients in the placebo treatment group of these studies also show a decrease in the number of exacerbations.

Interferon beta-1b is injected subcutaneously every other day. It comes as a powder that must be mixed with saline immediately before injection. Adverse reactions are quite common and include injection site reaction, headache, fever, flulike symptoms, pain, diarrhea, constipation, decrease in lymphocytes, elevation of liver enzymes, lowering of glucose levels to less than 55 mg/dL, myalgias, dizziness, anxiety, sinusitis, dysmenorrhea, and conjunctivitis. The cost is about $10,000 per year.

Interferon Beta-1a

Interferon Beta-1a (Avonex) has also been found to reduce the frequency of relapses, with efficiency similar to that of interferon beta-1b. The percentage of patients receiving interferon beta-1a who were exacerbation-free at the end of 2 years of treatment was 38%; the percentage of exacerbation-free patients in the placebo treatment group was 26%.[23] Interferon beta-1a is injected intramuscularly once a week and has the same side effect profile as for interferon beta-1b. The cost is similarly about $10,000 per year.

Glatiramer Acetate

Glatiramer acetate (Copaxone) was the third agent approved for use in relapsing-remitting MS by the FDA. This drug is thought to mimic myelin basic protein (MBP) and to block T cell responses to MBP. Studies show slightly less improvement with glatiramer than with the interferons, but also far fewer side effects are noted with this drug. Glatiramer is injected subcutaneously once daily, and the prominent side effect is local injection site reactions. The cost is approximately $7000 per year.

All three of the so-called ABC drugs—Avonex, Betaseron, and Copaxone—are quite expensive and have significant side effects, and although they have been shown to be somewhat effective for the short term, they have a relatively modest impact on overall disease course, with no long-term use information available. Before these medications are prescribed it seems important to consider whether they have a favorable impact on quality of life for the MS patient. Studies so far have not provided solid evidence for improvement in quality of life when these drugs are used and, in fact, studies have demonstrated that treatment with interferon beta has a high cost per quality-adjusted life years gained.[24]

With recent observations of axonal damage and increasing disability despite optimal anti-inflammatory treatment, perhaps the optimal approach to this aspect of MS lies not in attempts at controlling inflammation but in identifying factors influencing demyelination and injury to axons.

NOTE

Until research identifies treatments that are more rational (i.e., address the underlying degenerative process), less costly, and have fewer side effects, it makes sense to this author to use nutrition and specific supplements to decrease free radical damage to the axons and optimize the patient's own healing system.

Mind-Body Therapies

Many body-based systems of treatment are used with MS. These treatments include craniosacral therapies, Feldenkrais, massage, Pilates method, reflexology, and Tragerwork. All of these therapies have been shown to reduce anxiety, to improve self-image and self-esteem, possibly to reduce spasticity, and to relieve different types of pain. Generally, these therapies are very well tolerated, with few if any side effects.

Combining counseling with body work therapies is a very effective way to counter the major depression that affects about 50% of all MS patients. Encouraging patients to learn some form of stress reduction (meditation, relaxation exercises, breathing techniques) is imperative in the overall treatment plan.

Yoga can be a very effective form of relaxation while providing exercise and stretching. I generally recommend yoga or the traditional Chinese exercise Qi gong to all patients with MS. These two forms of gentle exercise can be very calming and centering.

Other Therapies To Consider

4-Aminopyridine

4-Aminopyridine is a potassium channel blocker that improves nerve conduction, reducing motor and visual symptoms and decreasing fatigue.[25] The dose must be increased gradually to reduce side effects, with optimal results not seen until the dose reaches 30 mg per day. The effects are short-lived and the medication must be taken frequently, (i.e., 3 times a day). Side effects include seizure, dizziness, nausea and vomiting, and nervousness. This medication can be obtained from compounding pharmacies and costs approximately $90 per month.

Bee Sting Therapy

Bee sting therapy (apitherapy) was first advocated for treating MS in the 1930s. Studies are under way to evaluate this therapy, but thousands of people with MS are already using this approach and reporting good results. As bee venom contains many different substances, it appears that actually undergoing the "sting" is important to achieve the beneficial effects. Therapy usually consists of 30 stings three times a week. Obviously, a person allergic to bees should not undergo this therapy.

Hyperbaric Oxygen Therapy

In many European countries, hyperbaric oxygen (HBO) therapy is consistently used in any MS treatment program. Studies have demonstrated a slowing of the deterioration of the cerebellum, resulting in improved coordination. This therapy can be very expensive, and the number of HBO chambers available in the United States is limited.

Procarin

Procarin is a transdermal agent containing histamine and caffeine. This novel agent was developed by a nurse with MS to control her own symptoms. There are no studies using Procarin as yet, but reported results include better balance, improved bladder control, less fatigue, increased heat tolerance, enhanced cognitive function, and increased extremity strength. This agent is available by prescription through compounding pharmacies at a cost of approximately $240 per month.

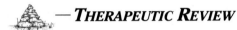 *THERAPEUTIC REVIEW*

Nutrition
- *Recommend a primarily vegetarian diet with little to no dairy or saturated fat.*
- *Increase intake of foods rich in omega-3 fatty acids (salmon, walnuts, or flaxseed) or take an omega-3 EFA preparation that supplies 500 mg per day of DHA (fish oil) and an omega-6 EFA preparation that supplies 300 mg per day of GLA (evening primrose oil).*

Supplements
- *Alpha-lipoic acid 100 mg per day*
- *Glutathione 600 to 800 mg IV 2 or 3 times per week, or N-acetylcysteine 200 mg per day*
- *Vitamin D 200 IU per day*
- *Vitamin B_{12} 1000 μg IM daily for 5 days, then twice per week, then twice per month*
- *Phosphatidylserine 50 mg per day*
- *Coenzyme Q10 60 mg twice per day*
- *Vitamin B_3 50 mg per day*
- *Vitamin B_6 50 mg per day*
- *Zinc 20 mg per day*
- *Magnesium 200 mg per day*

Botanical medician
- *Ginkgo biloba 120 to 240 mg per day*

Pharmaceuticals
- *Estriol 4 to 8 mg per day in perimenopausal or postmenopausal women, with progesterone 200 mg per day*
- *Doxycycline 100 mg twice daily for 14 days if C. pneumoniae suspected*
- *"ABC" drugs if patient desires, only after careful explanation of limitations, risks, and side effects of these medications*

References

1. Bejar JM, Zieglar DK: Onset of multiple sclerosis in a 24-month child. Arch Neurol 1984; 41:881–882.
2. Weinstock-Guttman B, Jacobs LD: What is new in the treatment of multiple sclerosis? Drugs 2000; 59:401–410.
3. Willer CJ, Ebers GC: Susceptibility to multiple sclerosis: Interplay between genes and environment. Curr Opin Neurol 2000; 13: 241–247.
4. Noseworthy JH, Lucchinetti C, Rodriguez M, Weinshenker BG: Multiple sclerosis. N Engl J Med 2000; 343:938–952.
5. Visscher BR, Detels R, Coulson AH, et al: Latitude, migration,

and the prevalence of multiple sclerosis. Am J Epidemiol 1977; 106: 470–475.

6. Swank RL, Lerstad O, Strom A: Multiple sclerosis in rural Norway: Its geographical and occupational incidence in relation to nutrition. N Engl J Med 1952; 246:721–728.

7. Huggins HA, Levy TL: Cerebrospinal fluid protein changes in multiple sclerosis after dental amalgam removal. Altern Med Rev 1998: 3:295–300.

8. McGrother CW, Dugmore C, Phillips MJ, et al: Multiple sclerosis, dental caries and fillings: A case-control study. Br Det J 1999; 187:261–264.

9. Greenlee JE, Rose JW: Controversies in neurological infectious diseases. Semin Neurol 2000; 20: 375–386.

10. Sriram S, Stratton CW, Yao S, et al: *Chlamydia pneumoniae* infection of the central nervous system in multiple sclerosis. Ann Neurol 1999; 46:6–14.

11. Jersild C, Fog T, Hansen GS, et al: Histocompatibility determinants in multiple sclerosis, with special reference to clinical course. Lancet 1973; 2:1221–1225.

12. Esparza ML, Sasaki S, Kesteloot H: Nutrition, latitude and multiple sclerosis mortality: An ecologic study. A J Epidemiol 1995; 142:733–777.

13. Mayer M: Essential fatty acids and related molecular and cellular mechanisms in multiple sclerosis: New looks at old concepts. Folia Bio (Praha) 1999; 45:133–141.

14. Karg E, Klivenyi P, Nemeth I, et al: Nonenzymatic antioxidants of blood in multiple sclerosis. J Neurol 1999; 246:533–539.

15. Hunter MIS, Nlemadim BC, Davidson DLW: Lipid peroxidation products and antioxidant proteins in plasma and cerebrospinal fluid from multiple sclerosis patients. J Neurochem Res 1985; 10:1645–1652.

16. Hayes CE, Cantorna MT, DeLuca HF: Vitamin D and multiple sclerosis: Proc Soc Exp Biol Med 1997: 216:121–127.

17. Kira J, Tobimatsu S, Goto I: Vitamin B_{12} metabolism and massive-dose methyl vitamin B_{12} therapy in Japanese patients with multiple sclerosis. Inter Med 1994; 33:82–86.

18. Reynolds EH: Multiple sclerosis and vitamin B_{12} metabolism. J Neuroimmunol 1992; 40:225–230.

19. Kim S, Liva SM, Dalal MA, et al: Estriol ameliorates autoimmune demyelinating disease: Implications for multiple sclerosis. Neurology 1999; 52:1230–1238.

20. Drew PD, Chavis JA: Female sex steroids: Effects upon microglial cell activation. J Neuroimmunol 2000; 111:77–85.

21. Sandyk R: Estrogen's impact on cognitive functions in multiple sclerosis. Intern J Neurosci 1996; 86:23–31.

22. Barnes D, Hughes RAC, Morris R, et al: Randomized trial of oral and intravenous methylprednisolone in acute relapses of multiple sclerosis. Lancet 1997; 349:902–906.

23. Jacobs LD, Cookfair DL, Rudick RA, et al: Intramuscular interferon beta-la for disease progression in relapsing multiple sclerosis. Ann Neurol 1996; 39:285–294.

24. Parkin D, Jacoby A, McNamee P, et al: Treatment of multiple sclerosis with interferon beta: An appraisal of cost-effectiveness and quality of life. J Neurol Neurosurg Psychiatry 2000; 68:144–149.

25. Stefoski D, Davis FA, Fitzsimmons WE, et al: 4-Aminopyridine in multiple sclerosis: Prolonged administration. Neurology 1991; 41:1344–1348.

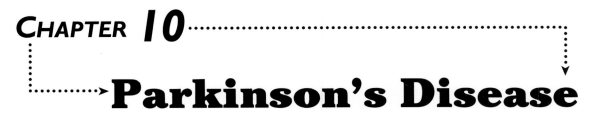

CHAPTER 10

Parkinson's Disease

Jay Lombard, D.O., and Sheree L. Loftus, M.S.N., C.R.R.N., R.N.C.

PATHOPHYSIOLOGY

The pathophysiology of Parkinson's disease involves a variety of factors that contribute to the loss of dopamine-containing neurons in the substantia nigra. These include genetic factors that impair cellular detoxification pathways, environmental exposure to mitochondrial toxins, mitochondrial complex I deficiency, oxidative stress in association with excessive iron deposition, and reduced levels of tyrosine hydroxylase.

Environmental Toxins

Many epidemiologic studies have demonstrated an association among pesticide exposure, mitochondrial injury, and the risk of developing Parkinson's disease. Rotenone is a complex I inhibitor and a common environmental pesticide that induces neuronal cell death and produces a Parkinson-like syndrome in experimental animal models.[1] The neurotoxin (MPTP) also inhibits complex I and selectively destroys dopamine neurons of the substantia nigra in humans and other primates.[2] Diminished complex I activity has been detected in both platelets and brain tissue of Parkinson's patients.[3]

Oxidative Stress

The free radical hypothesis of Parkinson's disease is supported by the findings of reduced levels of glutathione in the substantia nigra of Parkinson's disease patients.[4] Additional markers of oxidative stress in Parkinson's patients include reduced levels of polyunsaturated fatty acids and an increase in the levels of malondialdehyde in the central nervous system.[5] Free radicals can injure DNA, proteins, and lipids of neuronal cell membranes and may induce apoptotic changes consistent with neurodegeneration.

Abnormalities of iron metabolism and increased iron levels in the substantia nigra of Parkinson's patients have also been demonstrated by researchers.[6] Intracellular iron is normally sequestered as an inorganic material complexed with ferritin. Recently, it has been observed that there are decreased levels of ferritin in the brains of patients with Parkinson's disease.[7] A consequence of decreased ferritin is the liberation of iron from its carrier molecule into the cytoplasm with excessive free radical production.

Tyrosine Hydroxylase Deficiency

In the production of dopamine, the amino acid tyrosine acts as a precursor in catecholamine synthesis. L-Tyrosine is converted to L-dihydroxyphenylalanine (L-dopa) by the enzyme tyrosine hydroxylase; this is the rate-limiting step in dopamine biosynthesis.

Tyrosine $\rightarrow$ L-Dopa $\rightarrow$ L-Dopamine
Tyrosine hydroxylase   L-Aminoacid decarboxylase

Tyrosine hydroxylase is significantly reduced in the brains of Parkinson's patients compared with age-matched controls. In the caudate and putamen of Parkinson's patients, tyrosine hydroxylase levels are 83% less than in age-matched controls.[8]

INTEGRATIVE TREATMENT APPROACHES

Nutrition

Isothiocyanates

Isothiocyanates are widely distributed in plants and induce cellular antioxidant defenses, including glutathione transferase activity. Isothiocyanates include the cruciferous vegetables such as broccoli and cauliflower. Isothiocyanates can augment brain antioxidant defense activity because of their relatively small size and ability to cross the blood-brain barrier.[9] Patients should be advised that 3 to 5 servings of cruciferous vegetables per day provide approximately 100 mg of isothiocyanates.

Exercise

Exercise is essential in the management of Parkinson's disease. Daily exercise can maintain and improve muscle tone (strength), normal range of motion in the joints (flexibility), and balance and posture. Specific exercises may also prevent constipation and urinary incontinence, and may help maintain vision. An exercise prescription must be provided when the patient is diagnosed. Lifelong participation in an exercise program is recommended regardless of patient age at disease onset. (See Chapter 86, Writing an Exercise Prescription.)

Occupational, physical, and speech therapy all provide exercise instruction, but such instruction may be limited by reimbursement. Occupational therapy emphasizes fine motor coordination, home safety, and patient evaluation for use of adaptive equipment; physical therapy focuses on fall prevention, flexibility, posture, balance, gait, and ambulation. Speech therapy uses specific techniques to prevent aspiration and improve voice volume and clarity.

Complementary movement modalities may be employed indefinitely, and most can be done anywhere, usually without equipment. Alexander, Bobath, Feldenkrais, Laban, massage, tai chi, Trager, and yoga may all provide benefit. Additional studies are needed to assess the therapeutic effectiveness of each technique. Massage offers relaxation and relief from rigidity and dystonias common to Parkinson's disease. Tai chi, an ancient Chinese martial art form, reinforces balance, coordination, flexibility, body awareness, relaxation, and mental concentration; with its slow movements, it is known to reduce falls in older adults and is currently being studied for use in Parkinson's disease patients.

Supplements

Lipoic Acid

Lipoic acid is a thiol-based antioxidant that acts as a free radical scavenger as well as a potential metal chelator. It stimulates glutathione transferase activity, which enhances glutathione production.[10] Lipoic acid supplementation has been demonstrated to increase liver and plasma glutathione levels and to protect against lipid peroxidation in a variety of animal studies.[11] In one human study, oral administration of lipoic acid in doses of 500 mg per day increased brain mitochondrial activity measured by magnetic resonance spectroscopy.[12] Dihydrolipoic acid, a reduced form of lipoic acid, was demonstrated to prevent some pathologic changes in postmortem brains of Parkinson's disease patients.[13]

Dosage. Lipoic acid, 400 to 800 mg daily. (Because of the short half-life of lipoic acid, a sustained-release formulation is preferable.)

Precautions. Lipoic acid is generally safe orally. It may cause skin rash, and high doses can lead to thiamine deficiency.

Reduced Nicotinamide Adenine Dinucleotide (NADH)

The use of reduced nicotinamide adenine dinucleotide (NADH) for Parkinson's disease was first suggested by Birkmayer and associates, who demonstrated modest improvement in an open-label study involving more than 800 patients.[14] NADH may increase complex I activity and stimulate tyrosine hydroxylase, the rate-limiting step in dopamine biosynthesis. Follow-up studies of NADH in Parkinson's disease have been equivocal, however, including a study by researchers in Sweden who found no significant benefit derived from treating patients with intravenous NADH.[15] This may be accounted for by the finding that NADH has been demonstrated to increase dopamine production in vitro but not in vivo.[16] Clearly, more follow-up studies are required regarding the use of NADH in Parkinson's disease.

Dosage. NADH, 5 to 10 mg daily.

Precautions. None known.

Coenzyme Q₁₀ (Ubiquinone)

Coenzyme Q_{10} is a fat-soluble quinone that is responsible for assisting in the mitochondrial electron transport chain. In addition to its role in the use of energy, coenzyme Q_{10} may also function as a free radical scavenger, exerting beneficial effects on cell membrane stability. Oral coenzyme Q_{10} increases complex I activity and protects mitochondria from free radical damage. Oral coenzyme Q_{10} has been found to be protective to dopamine-manufacturing neurons and is neuroprotective in animal models of Parkinson's disease.[17] Multicenter studies are currently being conducted by the Parkinson's Study Group to evaluate the usefulness of coenzyme Q_{10} in Parkinson's patients.

Dosage. Patient should take 200 mg daily.

Precautions. Coenzyme Q_{10} can cause gastritis, loss of appetite, nausea, and diarrhea. It can elevate serum aminotransferase at doses greater than 300 mg per day.

Tea Polyphenols

Iron-chelating phytochemicals hold significant promise as a neuroprotective strategy in Parkinson's disease. Despite the fact that iron is essential for cell viability, free iron is highly toxic to cells. Reduced iron catalyzes free radical–generated processes and participates in neurodegeneration.[18] This has prompted interest in iron chelators as a potential neuroprotective strategy. Naturally occurring iron-chelating molecules include tea polyphenols from black and green teas. Tannic acid, a plant polyphenol, chelates iron and inhibits hydroxyl radical formation.[19] Furthermore, theanine, one of the major components of Japanese green tea, causes significant increases in brain dopamine concentrations, especially in the corpus striatum.[20] Whether green tea and black tea can prevent the progression of Parkinson's disease is currently unknown. However, their beneficial effects in iron metabolism may support such a role.

Dosage. 100 to 200 mg per day.

Glutathione

Oral use of glutathione for Parkinson's disease is limited owing to its poor absorption. Intravenous glutathione has been recommended by some physicians. An open-label study in a small sample of Parkinson's patients demonstrated a small but significant decline in disability scores in patients treated with 600 mg of IV glutathione daily.[21]

Tetrahydrobioptrein

Inhibition of tetrahydrobioptrein synthesis increases the susceptibility of dopamine neurons to glutathione depletion; changes in tetrahydrobioptrein levels may correlate with the pathogenesis of Parkinson's disease.

Tetrahydrobioptrein, also referred to as BH4, is a cofactor for tyrosine hydroxylase, the rate-limiting step in the production of L-dopa from tyrosine. Because the levels of tyrosine in the brain are relatively high, it is normally not possible to augment dopamine synthesis by increasing dietary intake of tyrosine. However, because tyrosine hydroxylase is the rate-limiting step in the biosynthesis of dopamine, this enzyme is subject to nutritional or pharmacologic manipulation. Tetrahydrobioptrein increases tyrosine hydroxylase activity and promotes the conversion of tyrosine to L-dopa.[22] Tetrahydrobioptrein is currently used for investigation only.

Pharmaceuticals

Carbidopa-Levodopa (Sinemet)

Carbidopa-levodopa is regarded as the most effective symptomatic management of Parkinson's disease, but controversy surrounds its use. It has been speculated that levodopa damages dopamine-containing neurons via its contribution to the formation of free radicals.[23] Furthermore, early treatment with levodopa may lead to a late complication of therapy known as *on-off phenomena*. In this condition, patients fluctuate from severe dyskinesia to hypokinesia at various unpredictable times of the day. This complication may be secondary to drug-induced changes in dopamine receptor sensitivity.

Dosage. Starting dose is usually 25/100 three times per day. This dose is titrated to achieve maximal symptomatic benefit. Doses of levodopa greater than 1000 mg per day usually are not recommended.

Precautions. Dyskinesia, nausea, and hallucinations, as well as sporadic cases of neuroleptic malignant syndrome, have been reported in association with abrupt withdrawal of carbidopa-levodopa.

Sinemet CR

Sinemet CR is a sustained-release combination of carbidopa and levodopa in which there is less variation in plasma levodopa levels; thus, its use may prevent motor fluctuations.

Dopamine Agonists

Dopamine agonists include amantadine, pergolide, bromocriptine, pramipexole, and ropinirole. Although the use of dopamine agonists results in less symptomatic improvement than is noted with levodopa therapy, they may exhibit additional neuroprotective effects. Dopamine agonists have the potential to stimulate autoreceptors on dopamine neurons, thereby decreasing dopamine synthesis and reducing the potential for formation of reactive oxygen species. Bromocriptine scavenges hydroxyl radicals and superoxide radicals and inhibits lipid peroxidation.[24] Pergolide scavenges nitric oxide radicals and increases superoxide dismutase levels in the substantia nigra.[25] Pramipexole protects against levodopa-induced damage in cultured neurons; this effect may be mediated by pramipexole-induced production of a trophic-like protein.[26] A number of clinical studies are under way to determine whether dopamine agonists clinically exhibit neuroprotective effects.

Dosage. Dopamine agonists need to be started at low doses and slowly titrated, usually at weekly intervals, to avoid significant adverse effects. An exception is amantadine, which is started at its maintenance dose. Starting doses are listed below:

Bromocriptine (Parlodel)—1.25 mg twice daily with meals
Pergolide (Permax)—.05 mg per day
Ropinirole (Requip) and pramipexole (Mirapex)—.125 mg 3 times per day
Amantadine (Symmetrel)—100 mg PO twice daily

Precautions. Monitor patient for hypotension, hallucinations, confusion, nausea, somnolence or insomnia, and headache.

Selegiline (Eldepryl)

Selegiline is considered to be a neuroprotective agent in the treatment of Parkinson's disease. As a selective inhibitor of monoamine oxidase B, selegiline may prevent the oxidative metabolism of dopamine, thereby inhibiting degradation-induced production of free radicals. Several studies have suggested that patients treated with selegiline demonstrate less deterioration over time than do patients treated with placebo, but it is unclear if this is a symptomatic effect rather than the result of a direct neuroprotective influence.[27]

Dosage. 5 mg twice daily with meals

Precautions. Patient should be monitored for confusion, vivid dreams, hallucinations, headache, nausea, and dizziness.

Mirtazapine (Remeron)

Remeron is a novel antidepressant that enhances noradrenergic and serotonergic neurotransmission. Anecdotal evidence suggests that this agent may be effective in reducing both tremors and dyskinesia.

Dosage. 15 to 30 mg at night

Precautions. Patient should be monitored for sedation and weight gain.

Surgery

Recently, surgical treatments for Parkinson's disease, including ablative procedures and deep brain stimulation, have gained wider acceptance. These procedures alleviate Parkinson's symptoms by creating a compensatory blockage in neuronal circuits that are abnormally active in Parkinson's disease. Deep brain stimulation may be preferable to surgery because it can induce reversible changes in the brain that are physiologic rather than structural.[28]

THERAPEUTIC REVIEW

Following is a summary of therapeutic options for Parkinson's disease. The goal of symptomatic therapy is to ameliorate functional impairments. Several classes of pharmacologic agents are currently in use, including carbidopa-levodopa, dopamine agonists, and anticholinergics. Symptomatic therapy should be initiated when there is clear functional impairment in an individual. Dopamine agonists are regarded as front-line agents for treatment of younger patients because they may have an additional benefit of being neuroprotective.

Diet
Encourage foods rich in isothiocyanates such as cruciferous vegetables like broccoli and cauliflower. Currently, isothiocyanates are not found in supplement form owing to their relative instability.

Supplements
Lipoic acid—400 to 800 mg per day (preferably in sustained-release formulation)
Glutathione—600 mg per day (owing to its poor oral bioavailability, intravenous administration of glutathione is preferable)
NADH—5 to 10 mg per day
Coenzyme Q_{10}—200 mg per day
Tea polyphenols—100 to 200 mg per day

Exercise
Modalities include occupational therapy, physical therapy, yoga, and tai chi.

Pharmaceuticals
Initiate carbidopa-levodopa when functional impairments are present.
Dopamine agonists such as amantadine, pergolide, bromocriptine, ropinirole, and pramipexole may be used as first-line agents owing to their combined symptomatic and neuroprotective effects.
Selegiline may be used in combination with any of the previously discussed medications but dose adjustments may be necessary.

Surgery
Deep brain stimulation is becoming a widely accepted procedure for patients with advanced Parkinson's disease. Electrical stimulation of thalamic regions is especially effective for treatment of drug-resistant tremors.

References

1. Greenamyre JR, Betarbet R, Sherer T, et al: Chronic systemic complex-I inhibition by a pesticide causes selective nigrostriatal degeneration with cytoplasmic inclusions [abstract]. Soc Neurosci 26:1026, 2000.
2. Singer TP, Castagnoli N, Ramsay R, et al. Biochemical events in the development of Parkinsonism induced by MPTP. J Neurochem 49:1–8, 1987.
3. Schapira AHV, Cooper JM, Dexter D, et al: Mitochondrial complex-I deficiency in Parkinson's disease. Lancet 1:1269, 1989.
4. Perry TL, Godin DV, Hansen S: Parkinson's disease: A disorder due to nigral glutathione deficiency. Neurosci Lett 33:305, 1982.

5. Dexter DT, Carter CJ, Wells FR, et al: Basal lipid peroxidation in substantia nigra is increased in Parkinson's disease. J Neurochem 52:381, 1989.

6. Dexter DT, Carayon A, Vidailhet M, et al: Decreased ferritin levels in brain in Parkinson's disease. J Neurochem 55:16, 1909.

7. Dexter DT, Carayon A, Vidailhet M, et al: Decreased ferritin levels in brain in Parkinson's disease. J Neurochem 55:16, 1909.

8. Hornykiewicz O: Biochemical aspects of Parkinson's disease. Neurology 51:S2, 1998.

9. Ratan R: Antioxidants in the treatment of neurological disease. In Koliatsos V, Ratan (eds): Cell Death and Diseases of the Nervous System. Unana Press, 1999, p 649.

10. Khanna S, Atalay M, Laaksonen DE, et al: Alpha lipoic acid supplementation: Tissue glutathione homeostasis at rest and after exercise. J Appl Physiol 86:1191, 1999.

11. Obrosova IG, Fathallah L, Greene DA: Early changes in lipid peroxidation and antioxidant defense in diabetic retina: effect of alpha lipoic acid. Eur J Pharmacol 398:139, 2000.

12. Barbiroli B, Medori R, Tritschler HJ, et al: Lipoic acid increased brain energy availability and skeletal muscle performance as shown by in vivo 31PMRS in a patient with mitochondrial cytopathy. J Neurol 242:471, 1995.

13. Spencer JP, Genna P, Daniel SE, et al: Conjugates of catecholamines with cystine and GSH in Parkinson's disease: Possible mechanism of formation involving reactive oxygen species. J Neurochem 5:2112, 1998.

14. Birkmayer JG, Vreko C, Volc D, et al: Nicotinamide adenine dinucleotide (NADH)—a new therapeutic approach to Parkinson's disease. Comparison of oral and parenteral application. Acta Neurol Scand Suppl 146:32, 1993.

15. Dizdar N, Kagedal B, Lindvall B: Treatment of Parkinson's disease with NADH. Acta Neurol Scand 90:345, 1994.

16. Pearl SM, Antion MD, Stanwood GP, et al: Effects of NADH on dopamine release in rat striatum. Synapse 36:95, 2000.

17. Beal MF: Co-enzyme Q10 administration in a potential for treatment in neurodegenerative disease. Biofactors 9:261, 1999.

18. Sayre LM, Perry G, Smith MA: Redox metals and neurodegenerative disease. Curr Opin Chem Biol 3:220, 1999.

19. Lopes GK, Schulman HM, Hermes-Lima M: Polyphenol tannic acid inhibits hydroxyl radical formation from Fenton reaction by complexing ferrous ions. Biochim Biophys Acta 1472:142, 1999.

20. Okogoshi H, Kobayashi M, Mochizuki M, et al: Effect of theanine on brain monoamines and striatal dopamine release in conscious rats. Neurochem Res 232:667, 1998.

21. Sechi G, Deledda MG, Bua G, et al: Reduced intravenous glutathione in the treatment of early Parkinson's disease. Prog Neuropsychopharmacol 7:1159, 1996.

22. Nakamura K, Wright DA, Wiatr T: Inhibition of tetrahydrobioptrein synthesis increases the susceptibility of dopaminergic neurons to glutathione depletion. J Neurochem 74:2305, 2000.

23. Blin J, Bonnet AM, Agid Y: Does levodopa aggravate Parkinson's disease? Neurology 38:1410, 1998.

24. Ogawa N. Tanaka K, Asanuma M, et al: Bromocriptine protects mice against 6 hydroxydopamine and scavenges hydroxy free radicals in vitro. Brain Res 657:207, 1994.

25. Nishibayashi S, Asanuma M, Kohno M, et al: Scavenging effects of dopamine agonists on nitric oxide radicals. J Neurochem 67:2208, 1996.

26. Olanow CW, Jenner P, Brooks D: Dopamine agonists and neuroprotection in Parkinson's disease. Ann Neurol 44:S167, 1998.

27. Shoulson I: Datatop: A decade of neuroprotective inquiry. Ann Neurol 44:S160, 1998.

28. Bakay R, Kordower J: Restorative surgical therapies for Parkinson's disease. In Tuszynski M, Kordower J (eds): CNS Regeneration. San Diego, Academic Press, 1999, p 389.

CHAPTER 11

Otitis Media

Marcey Shapiro, M.D.

PATHOPHYSIOLOGY AND NATURAL HISTORY OF OTITIS MEDIA

The term *otitis media* refers to middle ear effusion, or the presence of fluid in the middle ear space. In *acute otitis media*, acute inflammatory symptoms, such as pain, fever, and malaise, are also present. Often, a viral or bacterial pathogen that has tracked from the nasopharynx during an acute upper respiratory infection is the culprit in such infections. *Serous otitis media*, or otitis media with effusion, refers to the presence of fluid in the middle ear without inflammatory symptoms. Serous otitis media may be a sequela of acute otitis or may occur idiopathically.

Common bacterial pathogens implicated in acute otitis media include *Haemophilus influenzae*, *Streptococcus pneumoniae*, and *Branhamella catarrhalis*.[1] However, some studies have shown no bacterial pathogen in up to 62% of the cases.

In children, otitis media is especially common because the eustachian tube is small and narrow.[2] It is easily closed in the presence of inflammation, preventing drainage of fluids. Otitis media is the most frequently diagnosed illness in children under 15 years of age. In fact, otitis media is the second most common reason for a child to visit a physician, after well-child checkups.

A review of the literature indicates that regardless of treatment approach, otitis media tends to have a benign natural history with resolution of signs and symptoms including effusion.[3]

NOTE

Acute illness resolves in 24 hours, without any treatment, in up to 80% of cases of otitis media.

Serous fluid may remain for up to 12 weeks after an episode of acute otitis. The evidence for this conclusion is based both on observational research and on the results of placebo controls in clinical trials. In one review, it was found that children with acute otitis media who received treatment with placebo only had a 70% to 90% rate of complete resolution at 7 to 14 days, whereas children with serous otitis media following the acute disease who received only placebo showed a 60% cure rate at 1 month and a 90% cure rate at 3 months.

ANTIBIOTICS AND OTITIS MEDIA

Numerous articles and meta-analyses, both in the United States and abroad, have questioned the wisdom and value of routine treatment with antibiotics in uncomplicated otitis media. A review of the evidence indicates that the benefit of antibiotic treatment of all cases of acute otitis media is minimal; in fact, 17 children must receive early antibiotic treatment to prevent just one child from experiencing pain at 2 to 7 days.[4] In other countries, such as the Netherlands, Denmark, and Sweden, most children who present with routine otitis media do not initially receive antibiotic treatment.[5] The Netherlands has the lowest overall use of antibiotics; only 31% of the patients in that country will eventually receive them.[6] German physicians who practice complementary and alternative medicine (CAM) typically treat only 5% to 10% of cases of otitis media with antibiotics.[7] The British medical literature now encourages practitioners to avoid prescribing antibiotics for treatment of routine upper respiratory tract ailments, including otitis media.[8, 9] Nonetheless, in the United States, and also in Australia, up to 98% of cases are treated with antibiotics—perhaps because providers feel that they have no viable alternatives to offer patients or parents seeking treatment for their children.

Overuse of antibiotics in otitis is believed to be a major cause of antibiotic resistance. In some countries, from 50% to 80% of strains of *Streptococcus*, including the majority of strains responsible for disease in children, are resistant to penicillin.[10] There is an alarming frequency of multiple drug–resistant strains as well.[11]

Antibiotics also kill beneficial flora in other mucosal areas such as the gastrointestinal tract. Repeated and prolonged courses of antibiotics in childhood are associated with overgrowth of yeast (*Candida*) in the gastrointestinal tract and may also be associated with increased risk of allergies. Immediate consequences of the use of antibiotics include the occurrence of diarrhea, vomiting, and rashes at twice the usual rates.[12] Of interest, the

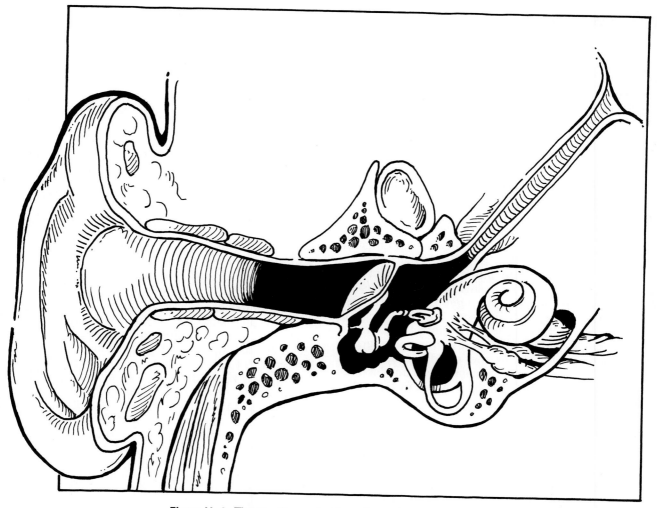

Figure 11–1. The ear. The eustachian tube in children is small.

most common reason cited for giving antibiotics is for prophylaxis of meningitis, a rare complication of otitis media.[13]

ANATOMIC CONSIDERATIONS

The eustachian tube of infants and small children is small and narrow (Fig. 11–1), causing poor drainage. As the child grows, the tube also grows and becomes less narrow, allowing better drainage, and with less fluid retained, pathogens have less opportunity to cause infection.

COMPLICATIONS OF OTITIS MEDIA

Severe complications arising from untreated or poorly managed cases of otitis media are rare but may occur (Table 11–1).

Table 11–1. Complications of Otitis Media

Complication	Comment
Meningitis	Although rare, the most common reason cited for giving antibiotics
Mastoiditis/ periosteitis	Look for retroauricular swelling and tenderness
Hearing loss	A result of recurring or persistent fluid collection in the middle ear
Speech delay	A result of long-standing hearing loss

INTEGRATIVE THERAPY OF OTITIS MEDIA

CAM fortunately offers many promising treatments for otitis media. Among the most widely used approaches are nutritional and dietary modifications, osteopathy and manual medicine, acupuncture and traditional Chinese medicine including use of Chinese herbs, Western herbal medicine, and homeopathy. Lymphatic drainage therapies are also of benefit.

Table 11-2. Clinical Manifestations of Uncomplicated versus Complicated Otitis Media

Uncomplicated Otitis Media

Unilateral
Mild fever or no fever
No perforation of eardrum
Little or no bulge in tympanic membrane
Little or no erythema of tympanic membrane
Some movement of tympanic membrane with insufflation
Well appearance
Mild pain

Complicated Otitis Media

Perforation of tympanic membrane
Suppuration
Mastoiditis
High fever
Ill appearance
Severe pain

The numerous CAM modalities used for management of otitis media have not been studied as extensively as conventional treatments. Nonetheless, given the favorable natural history of uncomplicated otitis media, there is generally no harm and much potential benefit in beginning with a CAM treatment.

As an alternative to routine use of antibiotics to treat all cases of otitis media, the decision to treat otitis media initially with CAM should be based on severity of the illness and level of complication. Accordingly, mild to moderate uncomplicated acute otitis media or serous otitis media should be treated first with CAM or supportive measures, whereas complicated or severe acute otitis media is treated initially with antibiotics. Antibiotics are thus reserved for initial treatment of only the more severe cases, or the cases that fail to improve with CAM (Table 11-2).

Botanicals

Chamomile (Matricaria chamomilla)

Chamomile may be used in the initial management of otitis in all persons who are not sensitive to it. It is also safe to use in conjuction with pharmaceuticals including antibiotics. Chamomile is a herb with which children and adults throughout the world are familiar. It is a versatile and gentle herb, effective as an antiviral and anti-infective. It also helps with infant colic, digestive upsets, and diarrhea.

Several fractions including the essential oils, flavonoids, and sesquiterpene lactones contribute to chamomile's medicinal activity. The essential oil fraction is particularly responsible for the anti-infective properties, and several of the flavonoids have shown significant anti-inflammatory activity. Chamomile can be used at any time in the course of otitis media.

Significant Constituents. These include essential oils: chamazulene, matricin, bisbaloxides A, B, and C, and spiroethers; esters: bisbalol; sesquiterpenes: matricin, matricarin; flavonoids: apigenin, luteolin, quercitrin, and several others; coumarins: herniarin, umbelliferone; and polyacetylenes, phenols, choline, and mucilage.

Dosage. Chamomile tea is popular with children. It is made by pouring 1 cup of boiling water over 1 heaping tablespoon of flowers. This tea is steeped, covered, for 10 minutes or longer and then strained and drunk. Chamomile tincture or glycerinate can also be taken orally. Tincture 1 to 3 mL three times daily is often used for children. For infants, 1 to 3 drops per pound of body weight three times daily can be used.

Precautions. Occasional allergic reactions may be observed in susceptible persons, most commonly those allergic to asters and chrysanthemums.

Echinacea (Echinacea angustifolia, Echinacea purpurea)

This native North American plant is one of the most popular and widely used herbs in the United States. Its medicinal activity is believed to invoke nonspecific activation of the immune system, but knowledge about its pharmacology is incomplete. Echinacea has a number of activities: it activates natural killer cells and macrophages and increases circulating levels of alpha-interferon. The caffeic esters of echinacea are antibacterial and antiviral, and the polyacetylenes probably also contribute to bacteriostatic activity of the herb. Echinacea is used for prevention and treatment of all sorts of upper respiratory infections but has been studied most in treatment and prevention of the common cold.[14-16] For otitis media, it is best selected at the onset of acute symptoms but may be used throughout the course of treatment, and it is an excellent choice when lymphatic congestion is present as it activates the nonspecific immune system to clear debris.

Significant Constituents. These include polysaccharides; caffeic esters: echinoside, cichoric acid, cynarin; anthocyanins; alkylamides: echinaceine; and essential oil.

Dosage. Both the tincture (in a 1:5 dilution) and the glycerinate preparation are available. Usually for small children and babies, glycerinates are preferred. Dosage varies; 1 to 5 mL of tincture three to five times daily is often used for children. For infants, 1 or 2 drops per pound of body weight three times daily may be used. Tablets, capsules, and whole herb taken as a tea or an infusion are also used orally.

Precautions. Use of echinacea is to be avoided in persons with autoimmune disorders such as systemic lupus erythematosus.

Marshmallow (Althea officinalis)

Marshmallow is a safe, gentle herb, used for soothing inflamed mucous membranes. It is a mucilaginous demulcent and will help to loosen and moisten thick mucus in sinusitis, colds, and bronchitis. Marshmallow also settles a queasy stomach and intestinal tract. It is safe for long-term use but may have mild diuretic effects.

Significant Constituents. Mucilage, 5% to 10%, found in the leaves and roots (leaves have the highest concentration just before flowering); phytosterols.

Dosage. Tincture: 1 drop per 2 pounds of body weight (up to 2 mL) three to six times daily. Decoction: 1 tablespoon of root simmered in 1 cup of water for 10 minutes; 1 to 3 tablespoons of the strained liquid is taken two to six times daily.

Precautions. If the patient is also taking prescription medications, these agents should be taken at least 1 hour before or 2 hours after taking marshmallow root, as the herb may decrease absorption of drugs.

NOTE

The mucus-thinning properties of marshmallow and mullein have been found to be very helpful in opening the eustachian tube in patients with otitis media.

Mullein (*Verbascum thapsus*)

Mullein decreases phlegm and strengthens the respiratory mucosa. It is safely used with other herbs and pharmaceuticals for treating numerous respiratory tract problems. Mullein also acts topically as a local anti-inflammatory and is often advised as an ear oil for treating otitis externa. It should *not be instilled in the ear* during otitis media. For otitis media, it is chosen to unblock the eustachian tube and to decrease inflammation.

Significant Constituents. These include mucilage; phytosterols; digiprolactone; iridoids: aucubincatalpol, isocatalpol and others; flavonoids: apigenin, luteolin, kaempferol, rutin; phenol, carboxylic acids: caffeic, ferulic, protocatechuic; saponins: verbascosaponin.

Dosage. Tea: 1 to 2 teaspoons per cup of boiling water, steeped, covered, 10 to 15 minutes and strained. From 1 to 4 cups per day of this liquid is given for older children, 1/4 to 3/4 cup per day for babies. Tincture: For babies and children, 1 drop per 2 pounds of body weight can be given every 4 hours.

Precautions. None known.

Other Herbs

Cleavers (Galium aparine)

This botanical is used to assist lymphatic clearance of debris during AOM or with serous OM.

Tincture: 1/2 to 2 mL 3 times daily is the dose. Tea: Tea made from the fresh herb is also useful; 1 cup is taken two or three times per day.

Elder flower/Elder berry (Sambucus nigra), European Alder, (Sambucus Canadensis), American Elder (Caprifoliaceae)

These botanicals are used to dry excessive nasal secretions; they also have antiviral activity. They are used mostly during acute otitis media, especially if an upper respiratory infection is present. Tincture 1/2 to 3 mL three times daily is the dose in children; tea or infusion of the fresh herb is also useful in a dose of 1 cup two or three times per day.

Elecampane Root (Inula helenium)

Elecampane is a camphorous root taken for its bacteriostatic and antiviral activity. It is also felt to strengthen resistance and tone mucosal tissues. It is used during AOM or with serous OM. Tincture (1/2 to 2 mL) three times daily is the dose. Tea and infusion are not used, as the medicinal constituents of the plant do not extract well into water.

Eyebright (Euphrasia officinalis)

Eyebright is used especially when allergies are present, as it decreases histamine response. Taken orally, it is especially helpful for eye irritation accompanying allergy. It is used especially if allergies trigger acute otitis media or serous otitis media. Tincture 1/4 to 1 mL six times daily is the dose; tea of fresh herb is also useful in a dose of 1/4 cup two to six times per day.

Eucalyptus (Myristicus globulus)

Eucalyptus is administered most often as a steam inhalation, as it is used to open clogged nasal or bronchial passages. A drop or two of essential oil can be applied directly to the skin in adults, if they have been patch-tested and are not sensitive to this herb. However, eucalyptus essential oil should *never* be applied directly to the skin of children under 5 years of age because their skin is too delicate, and inflammation and vesiculation may occur. Eucalyptus is used mostly late in the course of acute otitis media.

Goldenseal (Hydrastis canadensis)

This botanical is best used only in cases with green or yellow phlegm, and not for a routine cold. There is some disagreement among herbalists whether this herb is even absorbed orally, or if it can be of benefit only on mucosal surfaces with which the berberine alkaloids present in the herb come in contact. Goldenseal is used only during acute otitis media when there is evidence of purulence. Tincture 1/2 to 2 mL three times daily is the dose. Use in pregnancy is contraindicated.

Usnea (Usnea barbata)

Usnea is an effective herbal antiviral and antibacterial agent, used during acute episodes of otitis media. Tincture $1/2$ to 5 mL three times daily is the dose. The tea and the infusion are not used, as the medicinal constituents of the plant do not extract well into water.

Pharmaceuticals

Antibiotics

In the United States, antibiotics are chosen as a first-line treatment for all cases of otitis media including uncomplicated otitis media. Most often amoxicillin is prescribed, but erythromycin and amoxicillin–clavulanate potassium (Augmentin) are used frequently as well. As bacterial resistance progresses, a wider range of antibiotics may be used routinely.

Decongestants and Secretolytics

A number of antihistamines and decongestants such as diphenhydramine and ephedrine are normally prescribed as adjunctive agents in uncomplicated otitis media. These agents dry secretions in the nasal passages and provide symptomatic relief of accompanying upper respiratory tract infection symptoms. Side effects of these agents may include sedation or excess stimulation. Also, uncomfortable dryness of mucosa is common. The efficacy of these agents is not greater than that of placebo; therefore, use of these agents is not advised.[3]

Analgesics and Anti-Inflammatory Agents

Acetaminophen or ibuprofen is usually advised for symptomatic relief of pain, and to reduce fever. Potential side effects include irritation or toxicity in the gastrointestinal tract, liver, or kidneys, as well as the loss of the physiologic benefits of a low-grade fever in assisting the immune system in naturally clearing a pathogen.

Cranial Osteopathy

Osteopathic practitioners commonly treat otitis media with manual medicine. It is noted that common patterns of cervical and cranial osteopathic restrictions are found in children with otitis. These restrictions are noted particularly in the movement of the temporal bones, but other cranial bone movement restrictions may be found as well. Cervical osteopathic restrictions of movement in the upper and middle cervical regions are also common. Although all doctors of osteopathy (DOs) are trained in the rudimentary diagnosis of these conditions, DOs, medical doctors, and physical therapists who regularly or exclusively include manual medicine in clinical practice are most proficient in treating these restrictions.

Treatment in children is done gently. In fact, it may appear to parents as if the practitioner is merely placing the hands on the child's head or neck, with minimal motion. Usually, the younger a child is who is treated in this manner for otitis media, or any cranial bone restriction that may be present, the quicker and easier is the resolution of the problem. Also, the improvements obtained are likely to be long-lasting, and early treatment may prevent later problems with allergies, sinus conditions, and other ailments.

Surgery

Myringotomy

When multiple courses of antibiotics have failed to clear repeated episodes of otitis media, myringotomy, or surgical placement of drainage tubes through the tympanic membrane, is often performed. Myringotomy is often advised in children in whom persistent middle ear effusion is interfering with hearing and thus language development. Side effects are risks associated with anesthesia and with a major surgical procedure. It should be noted that the incidence of recurrence of otitis media is significant despite placement of drainage tubes. The tubes can become clogged or can be expelled by the healing tympanic membrane. Occasionally, tubes will lodge behind the tympanic membrane, and a second procedure will be required to extract them.

Acupuncture and Traditional Chinese Medicine

Traditional Chinese medicine (TCM) encompasses a number of techniques including acupuncture and herbology. These modalities are quite effective for treating otitis media, both in the acute setting and when there is persistent effusion. Typically with an acute infection, herbs are given along with acupuncture treatment, although either herbs or acupuncture can be administered alone. Both acupuncture and Chinese herbal medicine are approved by the World Health Organization (WHO) as therapies to treat acute or chronic otitis. A trained acupuncturist or herbalist should administer the treatment.

Diagnosis in TCM relies on symptom presentation as well as on examination of pulses, tongue, and general appearance of the patient. An otoscopic examination should be performed as well. The practitioner attempts to ascertain the unique pattern of disharmony implicated in the patient's illness at that time. If acupuncture is selected, the selection of points will vary with the configuration of the illness.

There is much leeway in therapeutic choice, both in acupuncture point selection and in herbal formula selection. Thus, otitis media in a specific patient may not necessarily be treated in the same manner by two different practitioners, and variance in the treatment of different patients with the same disorder, even with the same practitioners, is to be expected.

Most commonly, acupuncture and Chinese herbs, alone or in combination, are used in treatment. If the patient is a child, it is good to remember that although the idea of needles may be frightening, the needles themselves are usually well tolerated. Otitis media in anxious children may also be treated in some cases with acupressure, adhesive magnets on acupuncture points, or laser acupuncture.

In Chinese herbal medicine, typically formulas are used rather than individual herbs. Bulk herbs that are decocted at home are often selected by traditionally trained practitioners. It can be difficult to get children and some adults to ingest these formulas, so tinctures, powders, and capsules are preferred by some Western providers.

Kanpo is traditional Japanese medicine. It is similar to Chinese medicine in employing acupuncture, herbs, and physical manipulation. Usually, needles are not inserted as deeply in Kanpo acupuncture as in TCM; this difference may make the acupuncture component easier for children to accept.

Homeopathy

Typically in homeopathy, the more closely an illness matches the characterization of a remedy, the more likely it is to be an appropriate remedy. Usually, acute otitis is treated with low potencies such as 6 c or 30 c of most remedies. Only brief and general guidelines for selected homeopathic remedies commonly used to treat otitis media are presented here. Training in homeopathy is desirable before any of these remedies are prescribed, although all of these remedies are commonly available over the counter, and many persons self-prescribe common homeopathic medicines. Nonetheless, these synopses are included for informational purposes only, and not to provide instruction in homeopathy. A reading of these synopses does not constitute training in homeopathy.

The following section lists some of the most frequently used homeopathic remedies for otitis media, along with some of the considerations that direct the use of these remedies.

Common Remedies Based on Presenting Signs and Symptoms

- Aconite (*Aconitum napellus*): for acute pain, heat, fever; ear is hot and painful; redness at auricle or tympanic membrane may be noted; hot compresses can relieve pain; this form of otitis media usually occurs after exposure to wind or draft
- Belladonna: for otitis media, especially in the right ear; may accompany a cold with fever; scant thirst, photophobia, restlessness, facial flushing, noise sensitivity
- Capsicum: for heat and inflammation, with significant pain
- Chamomile: for otitis media with irritability; children are fussy cannot be appeased for long; hot compresses exacerbate pain; one cheek may be red while the other is pale
- Ferrum phosphoricum: in early otitis media, the most common remedy used; gradual onset of symptoms, facial flushing, sensitivity to noise; patient wants to lie still
- Hepar sulphuris: for pain in the ears, especially with swallowing, aggravation of pain by wind or draft; patient wants to be covered and still; irritability, pain
- Kali muraticum: used when popping and crackling sounds are heard in ear during swallowing and with nose blowing; hearing may be decreased; earache, feeling of fullness and congestion in the ear; also used to clear eustachian tubes when fluid persists after acute otitis media
- Magnesia phosphorica: for earache, especially after exposure to cold wind and drafts; pathologic process may be nerve irritation rather than infection; right ear affected more often than left; use of cold water to wash face worsens pain; pain is always relieved by heat; ear feels better with rubbing
- Mercuris vivus: for earaches with colds, "swollen glands"; earache tends to occur in damp or foggy conditions or with weather changes; hyper salivation, sweating; excessive purulence
- Pulsatilla: for earaches with colds, especially with whitish nasal drainage; throbbing pain in ears; also a main remedy for external otitis with redness and inflammation in the external canal; patient wants consolation and can be clingy, weepy, or fidgety or experience rapid mood changes; insomnia may be reported; heat aggravates pain; thirst is decreased; symptoms are usually worse in the evenings or at night; fresh air relievers symptoms
- Verbascum: especially for left-sided otitis media, with possible cough or laryngitis

Lifestyle Interventions

Smoking Cessation

In acute otitis media, it is important for the patient to avoid cigarette smoke. Family members who smoke should do so outdoors only, as smoking can aggravate the condition and prolong illness. Smoke from wood fires can also exacerbate the illness. Smoke from wood-burning stoves and fireplaces is a major source of indoor air pollution.

Nutrition

Avoiding mucus-forming foods will shorten recovery time in acute otitis media. Foods commonly accepted to be mucus-forming are dairy products including milk and cheese, orange juice, and wheat products such as bread and noodles made with refined or bleached flour. Consumption of these foods should be minimized during the illness.

Lymphatic Drainage

Lymphatic drainage therapy is an important adjunct in treatment of otitis. In persons including children, for whom this gentle technique is most appropriate, palpation of anterior, posterior cervical, or posterior auricular lymph nodes will reveal congestion or "shotty" adenopathy. If employed early in the course of an acute otitis, lymphatic drainage can hasten recovery and minimize the risk of recurrence. More detail about the applications of lymphatic drainage can be found in the chapter on prevention of otitis (see Chapter 77, Prevention of Otitis Media).

Other Therapies to Consider

In a short overview it is not possible to discuss in detail all of the CAM modalities that may be of benefit

Table 11–3. Dosages for Botanicals Used in the Treatment of Otitis Media

Echinacea Tincture

Children:	1–5 mL 3–5 times daily
Infants:	1 or 2 drops per 1b of body weight 3 times daily

Chamomile Tincture

Children:	1–3 mL 3 times daily
Infants:	1–3 drops per 1b of body weight 3 times daily

Mullein Tea

1–2 tsp/cup of boiling water, steeped covered for 10 minutes and strained

Children:	1–4 cups per day
Infants:	$^1/_4$–$^3/_4$ cup per day

Tincture: 1 drop per 2 1b of body weight every 4 hours

Marshmallow Tincture

One drop per 2 1b of body weight (up to 2 mL) 3–6 times daily

in treatment of otitis media. For example, naturopathy, or treatment with natural methods, administered by a naturopathic doctor (ND) would probably employ many of the aforementioned modalities. If interested, practitioners should also investigate aromatherapy, Ayurveda, and chiropractic.

An allergy rotation diet may be tried in patients who experience recurrent otitis media (see Chapter 87, Food Allergy).

 — *THERAPEUTIC REVIEW*

Single or First Acute Episode of Otitis Media

- *No smoking, or no smoking in the environment of the patient*
- *Eliminate mucus-forming foods such as milk and dairy products, wheat, and orange juice*
- *Evaluate the complexity and the severity of the case. If the illness is complex, or severe, antibiotics are prescribed. If the illness is simple and mild to moderate in severity, botanicals, osteopathic manipulation, acupuncture, or homeopathic medicines may be considered, depending on the client level of comfort with these modalities.*
  - *Botanicals such as echinacea, chamomile, mullein, and marshmallow may be used depending on symptoms (Table 11–3).*
  - *Consider a course of treatment with lymphatic drainage techniques if the lymphatics are congested.*

Serous Otitis Media (Otitis Media with Effusion)

- *Smoking cessation in the adult patient, or prohibiting smoking in the environment of children with recurrent otitis media is crucial.*
- *Cranial osteopathy: Refer the patient to a cranial osteopathy practitioner with the appropriate training.*
- *Evaluate lymph nodes; if they are full or "shotty," treat with lymphatic drainage.*
- *Consider evaluation and treatment for food and environmental allergies.*

Recurrent Otitis Media

- *Treat acute OM as described; then follow up with the treatment guidelines presented in the section on secondary prevention in Chapter 77, Prevention of Otitis Media.*

References

1. Bluestone CD, Stephenson JS, Martin LM: Ten year review of otitis media pathogens. Pediatr Infect Dis J, 1992; 11 (Suppl):7.
2. Suzuki C, Balaban C, Sando I, et al: Postnatal development of eustachian tube: A computer-aided 3-D reconstruction and measurement study. Acta Otolaryngol (Stockh) 1998; 118:837–843.
3. Rosenfeld R: An evidence based approach to treating otitis media. Pediatr Otolaryngol 1996; 43:1165–118.
4. Del Mar C, Glasziou P, Hayem M: Are antibiotics indicated as initial treatment for children with acute otitis media? A meta-analysis. BMJ 1997; 314:1526–1529.
5. Jensen PM, Louis J: Treatment of acute otitis media in Danish general practice. Abstracts of the Sixth International Symposium on Recent Advances in Otitis Media. Fort Lauderdale, Fla, 1995; 123.
6. Glasziou PP, Hayem M, Del Mar CB: Antibiotics for otitis media in children. Cochrane Database Syst Review 2000; 2:CD000219.
7. Lohman M: Treatment of otitis media: An interdisciplinary interview of experts. Ear Nose Throat J, Germany, October 1998; 1–4.
8. Butler CC, Rollnick S, et al: Reducing antibiotics for respiratory tract symptoms in primary care: Consolidating "why" and considering "how." Br J Gen Pract 1998; 48:1865–1870.
9. Damoiseaux RA, van Balen FA, Hoes AW, de Melker RA: Antibiotic treatment of acute otitis media in children under two years of age: Evidence based? Br J Gen Pract 1998; 48:1861–1864.
10. Crook DW, Spratt BG: Multiple antibiotic resistance in Streptococcus pneumoniae. Br Med Bull 1998; 54:595–610.
11. Reichler MR, Allphin AA, Breiman RF, et al: The spread of multiply resistant streptococcus pneumoniae at a day care center in Ohio. J Infect Dis 1992; 166:1346.
12. Vartiainen E: Changes in the clinical presentation of chronic otitis media from the 1970's to the 1990's. Journal of Laryngol Otol 1998; 112(11):1034–1037.
13. Niv A, Nash M, Peiser J, et al: Outpatient management of acute mastoiditis with periosteitis in children. Int J Pediatr Otorhinolaryngol 1998; 46(1–2):9–13.
14. Melchart D, Linde K, Worku F, et al: Immunomodulation with Echinacea—a systematic review of controlled clinical trials. Phytomed 1994; 1:245–254.
15. Braunig B, Dorn M, Limburg E, Knick E: Echinacea purpurea root for strengthening the immune response in flu-like infections. Zeitschr Phytother 1992; 13:7–13.
16. Schoneberger D: The influence of immune stimulating effects of pressed juice of Echinacea purpurea on the course and severity of colds. Forum Immunol 1992; 8:2–12.

CHAPTER 12

Chronic Sinusitis

Robert S. Ivker, D.O.

PREVALENCE AND PATHOPHYSIOLOGY

Since 1981, chronic sinusitis has been the most common chronic disease in the United States. According to the most recent survey from the National Center for Health Statistics (a division of the Centers for Disease Control and Prevention [CDC]), about 40 million Americans of all age groups suffer from this ailment.[1] It affects nearly 15% of the population or 1 out of every 7 people. Twenty-two percent of all women between the ages of 45 and 64 years have chronic sinusitis (15% of men in this age group have it)—an incidence about equal to that of hypertension. Sinusitis is second only to arthritis among the most common chronic diseases for women in this age group. In men in this age group, it ranks fourth, behind hypertension, hearing impairment, and arthritis. It was the primary reason for nearly 12 million physician office visits in 1995,[2, 3] and over 200,000 sinus surgical procedures were performed in 1998.[4]

When sinusitis is considered together with allergic rhinitis (the fourth most common chronic condition), asthma,[8] and chronic bronchitis,[9] respiratory disease due to these ailments affects over 90 million people—nearly 1 out of every 3 Americans—and thus constitutes our first environmental epidemic. In the 1960s, not one of these four conditions was among the top ten chronic health problems. The modern-day plague of air pollution is insidiously destroying the respiratory tract of those breathing polluted air. According to the Environmental Protection Agency (EPA), 60% of Americans currently live in areas where the air quality makes breathing a risk to their health. A 1993 study performed by the EPA and the Harvard School of Public Health reported that 50,000 to 60,000 deaths a year are caused by particulate air pollution.[5] A subsequent study in 1995 bolstered the earlier findings while concluding that people who live in highly polluted cities die earlier (about 10 years sooner — a 15% decrease in life expectancy) than they would have if they had been breathing healthier air. In addition to particulates, other components of toxic air include carbon monoxide, ozone, sulfur dioxide, nitrogen dioxide, hydrocarbons, and lead.

The nose and sinuses are lined by the respiratory epithelium and by virtue of the histologic and physiologic characteristics of its outermost lining, the *ciliated mucous membrane* or *mucosa*—serve as the body's primary *air filter, humidifier,* and *temperature regulator,* as well as *protector of the lungs.* This continuous mucous membrane that extends from just inside the nostrils to the alveolar sacs in the lungs is a connected porous protective shield for the body's air portal. The respiratory epithelial mucosa serves as a vital component of the immune system and acts as the first line of defense against bacteria, viruses, pollen, animal dander, cigarette smoke, dust, chemicals, automobile exhaust, and other potentially harmful air pollutants. The bulk of its job of filtration, humidification, and temperature regulation occurs in the nose and in the four pairs of paranasal sinuses (maxillary, ethmoid, frontal, and sphenoid) comprising the entrance and vestibule of the respiratory tract. If the membrane is weakened from chronic irritation or inflammation, the immediate consequence may be a cold or sinus infection.

Nothing is more important to optimal physical well-being than the quality of the air breathed and the ability to breathe it. Pollutant-laden air, which often has far less than the optimal 20% oxygen or negative ion content (3000 to 6000 ions per cm^3), acts as a chronic irritant that can create inflamed and hypersensitive mucous membranes. These conditions can lead to increased mucus secretion, obstruction of the ostia, and/or nasal allergy.

ETIOLOGY

Risk Factors for Acute and Chronic Sinusitis

- Air pollution (both indoor and outdoor) and pollen
- Emotional stress (especially repressed anger)
- The common cold and cigarette smoke (both can paralyze the cilia)
- Fungal and Candida organisms
- Food allergies and sensitivities
- Dry air and cold air
- Fumes
- Occupational hazards (as in automobile mechanics, construction workers, painters, cosmetologists)
- Dental infection
- Immunodeficiency
- Malformations (polyps, cysts, deviated septum)
- Gastroesophageal Reflux Disease (GERD)

These factors have the potential to adversely affect even the healthiest sinus. However, a person who has a compromised or imbalanced immune system, especially from fungal or *Candida* organisms, has had previous sinus infections, or in whom the mucosa has been weakened for any of the aforementioned reasons is at especially high risk for developing chronic sinusitis.

Fungus and Sinusitis

A landmark Mayo Clinic study[7] in 1999 reported that an immune system response to fungus rather than to bacterial infection is the cause of most cases of chronic sinusitis. The investigators reached this conclusion after studying 210 patients with chronic sinusitis and finding 40 different kinds of fungus, including *Candida*, in the mucus of 96%. In a control group of normal healthy volunteers, very similar organisms were found. The investigators concluded that the immune system response to these fungi in patients with chronic sinusitis is markedly different from that in healthy people, and that this unusual immune reaction is responsible for the chronic inflammation, pain, and swelling of the mucous membranes associated with sinusitis. They called the condition "allergic fungal sinusitis." However, the investigators failed to speculate on the possible impact of previous multiple courses of broad-spectrum antibiotics on the immune response to the fungal organisms in these patients. The resultant profound disruption of the normal bacterial flora of the mucosa likely contributed to the immune response observed. However, this issue was not addressed, and this study concluded simply by stating that "We must begin looking at chronic sinusitis as more than simply a bacteriological and/or anatomical problem, but as a dysfunction of the immune system mediated by a fungus."

NOTE

An allergic inflammatory response to fungal organisms is an important etiologic factor in chronic sinusitis.

The Common Cold and Sinusitis

Anything that causes obstruction of the flow of mucus through the ostia can trigger a sinus infection. A lifetime of sinus problems most often begins with the common cold. The cold that persists beyond 7 to 10 days is most likely symptomatic of acute sinusitis. In a 1993 study at the University of Virginia, college students and university employees who thought they had the common cold underwent computed tomography (CT) scanning of the sinus. Eighty seven percent of the study objects were found to have sinus infections.[35]

SYMPTOMS AND DIAGNOSIS

Chronic sinusitis is defined as persistent or recurrent episodes of infection and/or inflammation of one or more sinus cavities producing most or all of the following symptoms and signs: headache, facial pain, head congestion, purulent postnasal drainage or rhinorrhea, and fatigue.[8] Although most otolaryngologists rely on the CT scan for a definitive diagnosis of sinusitis, in a primary care setting I have found that a good history and physical examination to detect the presence of most or all of the defining manifestations can provide a reliable diagnosis of acute sinusitis.

INTEGRATIVE THERAPY FOR CHRONIC SINUSITIS

A Holistic Medical Treatment Program for Chronic Sinusitis: The "Sinus Survival Program"

The primary goals in holistic treatment of chronic sinusitis are as follows:

- To heal the chronically inflamed mucous membrane lining the nose and sinuses
- To strengthen and restore balance to a dysfunctional immune system while promoting overall balance of the patient's life
- To greatly reduce *Candida* or fungal organisms in the mucous membranes, if applicable

The holistic medical treatment for any chronic disease involves the practitioner's guiding the patient in a healing process of self-love directed at body, mind, and spirit. The patient is initially directed toward nurturing the dysfunctional part of the body. Beyond simply fixing the broken part, however, patients also commit to healing their lives—that is, increasing their energy, vitality, peace of mind, self-awareness, self-acceptance, and capacity for intimacy with a loved one and for meaningful spiritual practices. There is no quick fix in this lifetime process of optimizing health. Because each person is a unique individual, the prescription for healing is based on the degree of the patient's *self-awareness*. However, the patient with sinus disease can promote the healing process by closely adhering to specific physical and environmental health recommendations, based on clinical experience, presented in the next section of this chapter.

It will usually take only 1 to 2 months before the patient experiences significant improvement with the physical and environmental health components of the Sinus Survival Program. But to effect life healing, and to cure chronic sinusitis and prevent subsequent episodes of acute sinusitis, the entire holistic medical treatment program must be practiced on a regular basis. Practice must include the *mind* (mental and emotional health) and *spirit* (spiritual and social health) components, as discussed later under Mind-Body Medicine.

Physical and Environmental Health Recommendations

Air Quality (see Table 12–1)

Ideal air quality is rated by clarity (freedom from pollutants), humidity (between 35% and 55%), temperature (between 65° and 85° F), oxygen content (21% of total volume and 100% saturation), and negative ion content (3000 to 6000 .001-μ ions per cm^3). Air that is clean, moist, warm, oxygen-rich, and high in negative ions is the healthiest air a human being can breathe. To create optimal indoor air I recommend the following:

- Use of a negative ion generator[9–11]: used as an air cleaner, it should be placed in the room(s) in which the patients spend the bulk of their time, especially the bedroom and office
- Furnace filter: an electrostatic or a pleated filter (e.g., Filtrete by 3M)
- Furnace cleaning
- Carpet cleaning
- Use of a humidifier: a warm-mist room unit, especially during the winter months

- Plants, especially those that can remove formaldehyde (Boston fern, chrysanthemums, striped *Dracaena*, dwarf date palm) and carbon monoxide (spider plant)

Water, Moisture, and Nasal Hygiene
(see Table 12–1)

- Bottled or filtered water: Patient should drink $\frac{1}{2}$ ounce of water per pound of body weight on days without exercise and $\frac{2}{3}$ ounce per pound on exercise days when the patient exercises for at least 20 to 30 minutes aerobically.
- Saline nasal spray: Use daily every 2 to 3 hours.
- Steam inhaler[12]: Use this device for 15 to 20 minutes two or three times daily. A medicinal eucalyptus oil should be added to the steam for optimal benefit.
- Nasal irrigation[13, 14]: There are several effective methods for nasal irrigation.[34] Perform two to three times daily. This modality is most effective following steam inhalation therapy.

Another solution that has been effective in irrigation is called Alkalol. It is a mucus solvent and cleaner and can be used with the saline solution in a 1:1 ratio (one-half saline, one-half Alkalol) with all of the methods described in the accompanying box. The patient may have to ask the pharmacist to order Alkalol, as it is not usually available, but it is very inexpensive.

Table 12–1. Physical and Environmental Health Components of "Sinus Survival Program" for Preventing and Treating Sinusitis

Program Stage*	Measure	Preventive Maintenance	Treatment
1	Sleep	7–9 hr; no alarm clock	8–10+ hr/day
1	Negative ions or air cleaner	Continuous operation; use ions especially with air conditioning	Continuous operation
1	Room humidifier, warm mist	Use during dry conditions, especially in winter if heat is on and in summer if air conditioner is on	Continuous operation
3	Central humidifier		
1	Saline nasal spray (SS spray)	Use daily, especially with dirty and/or dry air	Use daily every 2–3 hr
1	Steam inhaler	Use as needed with dirty and/or dry air	Use daily, 2–4/d; add eucalyptus oil
1	Nasal irrigation	Use as needed with dirty and/or dry air	Use daily, bid–qid after steam
1	Water, bottled or filtered	Drink $\frac{1}{2}$ oz/lb body weight; with exercise, drink 2–3 oz/lb	$\frac{1}{2}$–$\frac{1}{3}$ oz/lb of body weight
1	Diet	Emphasize fresh fruit and vegetables, whole grains, fiber; limit sugar, dairy, caffeine, and alcohol	No sugar, dairy
1	Exercise, preferably aerobic	Minimum of 20–30 min 3–5 × week; avoid outdoors with high pollution and/or pollen levels, and extremely cold temperatures	No aerobic; moderate walking OK Avoid outdoors with high pollution and/or pollen levels and cold temperatures

*Stage 1 of program: begin with these measures; stage 2: add these after 3 weeks into the program; stage 3: add these 6 weeks into the program.
From Ivker RS: Sinus Survival, 4th ed. New York, Tarcher/Putnam, 2000.

METHOD

Nasal Irrigation Options

Method 1. I recommend use of the Neti Pot or SinuCleanse for nasal irrigation. The Neti Pot is a small porcelain pot with a narrow spout; Sinu-Cleanse is plastic with a very similar shape and size. Use of either of these devices is probably the most gentle and convenient method for irrigation. Therefore, people with chronic sinusitis are much more apt to use this method on a regular basis, both therapeutically in treating an infection and preventively. SinuCleanse (available through Thriving Health Products, telephone: 888 434–0033) is sold with packets of hypertonic saline to mix with water, making this method even more convenient. The Neti Pot (made by the Himalayan Institute in Honesdale, PA) is available in many health food stores.

Method 2. Use an angled nasal irrigator attachment (the Grossan nasal irrigator is available at some pharmacies or through Thriving Health Products) on an oral irrigation appliance (e.g., Water Pik). Set the irrigator at the lowest possible pressure and insert the irrigator tip just inside one nostril, pinching the nostril to form a seal. Irrigate with the mouth open, allowing the fluid to drain out either the mouth or nose. Repeat the procedure in the other nostril.

Method 3. Completely fill a large all-rubber ear syringe (available at most pharmacies) with saline solution. Lean over the sink and insert the syringe tip just inside one nostril, so that it forms a comfortable seal. *Gently* squeeze and release the bulb several times to swish the solution around the inside of the nose. The solution will run out both nostrils and may also run out of the mouth. Repeat this for each nostril until 1 cup of saline solution is used, or until the solution is clear.

Method 4. For very small children, irrigate with 10 to 20 drops of saline solution per nostril from an eyedropper.

If a decongestant nasal spray or a corticosteriod nasal spray is used, apply only *after* the salt-water nasal irrigations.

These methods obviously require more effort than required by the saline nasal sprays, but many patients comment on how much more helpful they are.

Exercise (see Table 12–1)

The recommended intensity of aerobic exercise is based on maintaining the patient's target heart rate, which is calculated as follows: 220 − age × 60% (mild intensity), 70% (moderate intensity), or 85% (strenuous). Although exercise can be an effective immunostimulator,[27] people with chronic sinusitis should begin exercising at a heart rate below the mild intensity level and work their way up *very gradually*. Doing too much too soon can easily weaken immunity to an even greater extent.

For chronic sinusitis sufferers, and for those practicing respiratory preventive medicine, air quality is a crucial factor in determining where and when to exercise. Ozone, a very harmful air pollutant, is created by the combination of nitrogen oxides, hydrocarbons, and sunlight. On a bright sunny day in the downtown area of most large cities, high concentrations of ozone will be produced. Exercise should be scheduled around the rise and fall of pollution levels. In the summer, ozone builds up during the morning, reaches maximal levels late in the afternoon, and then ebbs in the evening. In the winter, ozone is less of a problem, but cold night air can trap a layer of carbon monoxide, nitrogen dioxide, sulfur dioxide, and particulates that can linger into the early morning. A good general practice is to do outdoor exercise in the morning during the summer and in the evening during the winter.

Sleep and Rest

Although diet, the use of supplements, and exercise all can benefit physical health and improve immune function, perhaps the most powerful and most often overlooked key to overall physical well-being is *sleep*. Lack of sleep and the resulting depression of the immune system can be a factor in many chronic health conditions and is a common cause of colds and sinus infections. Additional sleep is, therefore, an essential component in the holistic treatment of such conditions.

Diet, Supplements, and Botanicals
(See Table 12–2)

Diet

The patient should avoid milk and dairy products, sugar, wheat, caffeine, and alcohol[15–20] and should increase intake of fresh organic vegetables and fruits, whole grains, fiber, and protein. If candidiasis is suspected (history of multiple antibiotics), strict adherence to a *Candida*-control diet[7] is recommended. This diet avoids yeast-containing foods such as breads, and foods that promote yeast growth such as processed foods, refined sugars, cheeses, peanuts, vinegar, and alcoholic beverages.

Antioxidant Vitamins, Minerals, and Herbs

Vitamin C
Vitamin C[21] is a natural antihistamine and anti-inflammatory that enhances immune response and white blood cell activity. Foods highest in vitamin C are guavas, oranges, cantaloupe, strawberries, red

Table 12–2. Vitamins and Supplements used in "Sinus Survival Program" for Preventing and Treating Sinusitis

		Adults		Children (Age > 3 yr)		Pregnant WOMEN	
Program stage		Preventive Maintenance*	Treatment	Prevention	Treatment	Prevention	Treatment
Antioxidant Vitamins and Supplements							
1	Vitamin C (polyascorbate or ester C)	1000–2000 mg tid	3000–5000 mg tid	100–200 mg tid	500–1000 mg tid	1000 mg bid	1000 mg qd
1	Vitamin E	400 IU qd/bid	400 IU bid	50 IU bid	200 IU bid	200 IU qd	200 IU bid
	Proanthocyanidin (grape seed extract)	100 mg qd/bid (on an empty stomach)	100 mg tid (on an empty stomach)	—	100 mg qd	—	100 mg/d
2	Beta carotene	25,000 IU qd/bid	25,000 IU tid‡	5000 IU of qd/bid	10,000 IU bid	25,000 IU qd	25,000 IU bid
3	Vitamin B$_6$	50 mg bid	200 mg bid	10 mg qd	25 mg of d	25 mg qd	25 mg bid
Other Supplements							
1	Multivitamin§	qd (1/n) tid	qd (1/n) tid	Pediatric multivitamin		Prenatal multivitamin with 800 mg folic acid	
2	Selenium	100–200 μg/d	200 μg/d	—	100 μg/d	25 μg/d	100 μg bid
2	Zinc picolinate	20–40 mg/d	40–60 mg/d	10 mg/d	10 mg bid	25 mg/d	40 mg/d
2	Magnesium citrate, aspartate, or glycinate	500 mg/d	500 mg/d	150–250 mg/d	300 mg/d	500 mg/d	500 mg/d
2	Calcium (citrate or hydroxyapatite)	1000 mg/d; menopause: 1500 mg/d	1000 mg/d; menopause: 1500 mg/d	600–800 mg/d from diet		1200 mg/d	1200 mg/d
3	Chromium picolinate	200 μg/d	200 μg/d	—	—	In prenatal multivitamin	
Botanicals/Herbs							
1	Garlic	1200 mg/d	1200–2000 mg 3 ×/d	—	1000 mg tid	—	1200 mg 3 ×/d
1	Echinacea	200 mg bid or 25 drops bid/tid (allergy prevention)	200 mg tid or 25 drops 4–5 ×/d	—	100 mg tid or 7–10 drops	—	200 μg tid or 25 drops 4 ×/d
1	Grapefruit (citrus) seed extract	—	100 mg tid or 10 drops in water tid	—	4 drops in water bid	—	100 mg tid or 10 drops in water tid
2	Berberis or goldenseal‖	—	200 mg tid or 20 drops 4–5 ×/d	—	100 mg tid or 7–10 drops tid	—	—
3	Bee propolis	—	500 mg tid	—	200 mg tid or 500 mg qd	—	500 mg tid
Essential Fatty Acids							
2	Flaxseed oil (or omega-3 fatty acids in fish oil)	2 tbsp/d	2 tbsp/d	1 tbsp/d	1 tbsp/d	2 tbsp/d	2 tbsp/d
	Antibiotics¶						

* Use the higher dosage on days of higher stress, less sleep, and increased air pollution.

† Stage 1: begin the program with these; stage 2: start these after 3 weeks into the program, or earlier if desired; stage 3: start these 6 weeks into the program, or sooner if patient/practitioner is comfortable with doing so.

‡ Use this dosage for a maximum of 1 month.

§ Dosage depends on brand.

‖ Some people with ragweed allergy are sensitive to goldenseal.

¶ Antibiotics—an option for sinusitis if taken infrequently. Once or twice per year, or if no improvement is obtained with this program after 2 weeks.

Modified from Ivker RS: Sinus Survival, 4th ed. New York, Tarcher/Putnam, 2000.

chili peppers, red and green sweet peppers, kale, parsley, broccoli, and cauliflower.

Dosage. 1000 to 2000 mg three times daily

Precautions. Diarrhea, nausea, vomiting, esophagitis, abdominal cramping, and insomnia may be experienced by persons taking vitamin C in these doses. These side-effects can be minimized if it is taken in the form of *Ester C.*

Vitamin E

Vitamin E[22] is a strong antioxidant that helps to minimize effects of air pollution. Foods highest in vitamin E are crude and unrefined soybean oil and wheat germ oil, fresh wheat germ, whole grains, raw nuts (most varieties), and all green leafy vegetables.

Dosage. 400 international units (IU) twice daily

Grape Seed Extract

Grape seed extract (proanthocyanidin)[23] is a type of bioflavonoid. Multiple studies have shown it to be an extremely potent antioxidant—50 times more powerful than vitamin E and 20 times more powerful than vitamin C. It has been used for prevention of infections, as an anti-inflammatory, and for anti-aging, and is widely used in Europe for treating allergic rhinitis and asthma.

Dosage. 100 mg one or two times daily

Selenium

Selenium is an antioxidant that breaks down leukotrienes, which are allergy-related inflammatory substances. Foods highest in selenium are whole wheat products, fish, whole grains, mushrooms, beans, garlic, and liver.

Dosage. 100 to 200 μg daily

Medicinal Herbs and Botanicals

Garlic

Garlic[24] can be effective used as an antibacterial, antiviral, antifungal, and anti-inflammatory agent.

Dosage. 1200 mg daily

Precautions. Gastrointestinal irritation and contact dermatitis are possible adverse effects.

Caution. When used with antocoagulants, garlic may enhance their effect.

Echinacea

Echinacea[25] is a powerful immunostimulator and anti-inflammatory.

Dosage. 200 mg twice daily, or 25 drops of tincture 2 or 3 times daily

Precautions. Avoid long-term use.

Grapefruit Seed Extract

Grapefruit seed extract is an excellent antifungal botanical.

Dosage. 100 mg 3 times daily

Precautions. This botanical may slow hepatic metabolism of some drugs (e.g., statins).

Essential Fatty Acids

Essential fatty acids[26] both nourish the mucous membranes and have a potent anti-inflammatory effect. They should be taken in the form of omega-3 oils, eicosapentaenoic acid (EPA) and docosahexaenoic acid (DHA), from cold water fish (salmon, sardines, tuna, sole, mackerel) and flaxseed oil (flaxseed contains almost twice as much omega-3 as in fish oils). Other food sources of omega-3 fatty acids include wild game, canola oil, walnuts, pumpkin seeds, soybeans, fresh sea vegetables, and leafy greens.

Dosage. 2 tablespoons a day of flaxseed oil or 1–3 gms DHA/EPA fish oil

Mind-Body Medicine

Mental and Emotional Health Recommendations for Chronic Sinusitis

Most sufferers of chronic sinusitis have repeatedly heard the message, "You're going to have to live with it" from their physician, or have come to this conclusion themselves. This belief often adds to already existing feelings of anger, sadness, fear, and possibly hopelessness. Modifying beliefs and attitudes through *affirmations* and *visualizations;* creating a *goal list* and an *ideal life vision* (developing clarity about personal and professional objectives); undergoing *counseling, psychotherapy,* or *biofeedback training;* learning to express painful emotions, especially through the *safe release of anger, journaling,* and finding more *humor, optimism,* and *play* in life are all essential mental and emotional components of the Sinus Survival Program.

Physical problems with the nose and sinuses bioenergetically correspond with mental and emotional issues associated with self-evaluation, truth, intellectual abilities, openness to the ideas of others, the ability to learn from experience, emotional intelligence (the ability to identify, experience, and express feelings) and feelings of adequacy. These issues are all associated with the sixth ("third eye") chakra in Ayurvedic medicine. I have found the majority of chronic sinusitis patients to be high achievers, perfectionistic with a strong need for control, and unforgiving of themselves and others. This personality trait is often associated with a great deal of anger. Assisting the patient to self-awareness of these possible contributing factors can help to begin the process of healing.

Mental and Emotional Health Practices
- Affirmations
- Visualizations[28]
- Goal or ideal vision list

These first three should be practiced daily for 10 to 20 minutes. Affirmations are most effective when written, recited, and visualized.

- Anger release (safely): punching (a punching bag, sofa, or pillow), screaming, stamping — this is highly therapeutic for chronic sinusitis
- Journaling[29] (see also Chapter 93, Journaling)
- Optimism
- Humor
- Biofeedback
- Psychotherapy: cognitive therapy and family therapy
- Play
- Energy medicine modalities: healing touch, therapeutic touch, reiki, Qi gong, or craniosacral therapy

Conventional Medical Treatment

Antibiotics have been the mainstay of conventional medical treatment for chronic sinusitis, often followed by sinus surgery if the problem has not resolved. However, to an increasing extent these therapeutic modalities are offering only temporary relief and have failed to resolve or cure the problem of chronic sinusitis. In a recent study[33] of 161 children with acute sinusitis, researchers concluded that "antimicrobial treatment offered *no benefit* in overall symptom resolution, duration of symptoms, recovery to usual functional status, days missed from school or child care, or relapse and recurrence of sinus symptoms." For the growing number of patients who have failed to respond to repeated courses of broad-spectrum antibiotics and surgery, for the postoperative patient, and for the growing number of people who elect not to have (or are not candidates for) surgery or to take antibiotics, the Sinus Survival Program has consistently produced successful outcomes.

The vast majority of the more severe and unresponsive (to conventional treatment) cases of chronic sinusitis require anti–*Candida*/fungal treat-

ment (see Table 12–3). An antifungal medication such as fluconazole (Diflucan), itraconazole (Sporanox) or ketoconazole (Nizoral), along with adherence to a hypoallergenic *Candida* diet, is often necessary to restore the patient to a state of good health. Although antifungal homeopathic remedies and special strains of bacteria, (e.g., *Bacillus laterosporus* B.O.D [Latero-Flora]) can also achieve a similar result, they usually do not act as quickly or quite as effectively as the prescription drugs. However, they do not have the liver toxicity associated with these medications.

In March 2000, in collaboration with William Silvers, M.D., a Denver allergist, the first Sinus Survival Program study was completed. Each of the participants had a long-term history of moderate to severe chronic sinusitis. Every one of these patients scored above 180 on a "*Candida* questionnaire and scoresheet" (adapted from Dr. William Crook's book *The Yeast Connection*), and each was treated with fluconazole (200 mg daily for 1 month and then every other day for another 2 weeks), in addition to the rest of the Sinus Survival Program as described (plus the mental/emotional and spiritual/social components of the program). After 4 months on the program, including 6 weeks on fluconazole therapy, all but one of the participants (who had severe asthma and was placed on a course of antibiotic and prednisone during the study) experienced a very significant improvement in their condition. The majority of the patients reported feeling better than they had in years. Following statistical analysis of the 1 year follow-up, publication of the study results is anticipated and the therapeutic benefits of a holistic integrative approach to treating chronic sinusitis are expected to be confirmed.

Spiritual and Social Health Recommendations

Healing the spirit is by far the most powerfully therapeutic component of the Sinus Survival Program. The ultimate outcome of healing the self

Table 12–3. *Candida* Treatment Program
....

- *Candida* diet (see section under diet)
- Antifungal medication (prescription pharmaceuticals) Diflucan, Sporanox, or Nizoral*
- Antifungal homeopathic remedy: Mycocan Combo, Aqua Flora, Candida-Away, and several others—an alternative to conventional antifungal medication
- Latero-Flora (found in health food stores as Flora Balance): 2 capsules 20 minutes before breakfast†
- *Acidophilus* (*Lactobacillus acidophilus* and *Lactobacillus bifidus*): $^1/_2$ teaspoon or 2 capsules tid for adults and during pregnancy; $^1/_4$ teaspoon tid for children older than 3 years of age‡
- Colon hydrotherapy (colonic treatments)§

---

*Expect some "die-off" effect, with possible worsening of symptoms within the first 2 weeks after beginning antifungal medication. Recommended dosage is 200 mg daily for 4 to 6 weeks, then every other day for 3 to 4 weeks.

†A beneficial bacterium that is effective in killing *Candida*. Usual dosage is 2 capsules daily for 2 or 3 months, then 1 capsule 20 minutes before breakfast for an additional 2 to 3 months.

‡Patient should begin taking acidophilus along with antifungal medication, and Latero-Flora.

§Not absolutely necessary, but can speed clinical progress, especially during the first month of treatment. To find a colon hydrotherapist, call the office of a holistic (M.D. or D.O.) or naturopathic (N.D.) physician, or a chiropractor.

From Ivker RS: Sinus Survival, 4th ed. New York, Tarcher/Putnam, 2000.

holistically is the recognition that we are truly spiritual beings, and the heightened awareness of the transcend power known as God or Spirit. By making the commitment to become spiritually healthy, we open ourselves to the underlying life force energy to which all religions refer, known in holistic medicine as *unconditional love.* Learning to love the self in body, mind, and spirit is also the simplest and most effective way to develop spiritually. To heal the self spiritually involves relating to the aforementioned transcendent Spirit in a personal way and becoming attuned to its presence in all aspects of daily existence. By doing so, patients will begin to experience a profound reduction in feelings of fear and a greater capacity for unconditional love of self and of others. Patients will also become better able to identify special talents and gifts and to use them to fulfill life's purpose, while fully experiencing the power of the present moment. The spiritual practices I recommend most are *prayer, meditation, gratitude,* and *spending time in nature.*

Relationship with others is the crucible that most strongly determines the spiritual health of each person. Optimal *social health* consists of a strong positive connection to others in community and family, and intimacy with one or more people. It is often much easier to feel a connection with Spirit during moments of solitude than it is to express that connection through interactions with others. At the same time, relationships offer the greatest opportunities for spiritual growth and for learning how to receive and impart unconditional love. *True spiritual health is a balance between the autonomy of the self and intimacy with others.*

The importance of social relationships with respect to health is documented in a growing number of studies demonstrating the benefits of the diversity and depth of connection to community, family, and spouse. Lack of healthy social relationships is a common denominator among patients with heart disease, particularly when accompanied by feelings of hostility and a sense of isolation. Conversely, the longevity of terminal cancer patients with long-term survival rates has been attributed to a relatively high degree of social involvement. On the basis of a growing number of relationship studies, researchers have concluded that social isolation is statistically just as dangerous as smoking, high blood pressure, high cholesterol, obesity, or lack of exercise.

The primary opportunities available to each person for improving social health include *forgiveness, friendships, selfless acts and altruism, support groups,* and especially *marriage, committed relationships,* and *parenting.* Practicing forgiveness is particularly challenging for and most helpful to the typical patient with chronic sinusitis. Much of the patient's anger, which often precipitates a sinus infection, is ultimately self-directed for making mistakes. In learning to forgive themselves, such patients are able to expand their capacity to forgive others and thereby heighten intimacy in their relationships.

Spiritual and Social Health Practices

- Prayer
- Meditation[30]
- Gratitude
- Intuition
- Spiritual practices: observing a sabbath, fasting, earth/air/fire/water
- Forgiveness
- Communication exercises: shared vision, attentive listening,[31] requests
- Parenting
- Selflessness and altruism
- Support groups[32]

Other Therapies to Consider

Homeopathy

The homeopathic remedies Kali bichromium 30c 3 times daily and Kali sulphuricum 30c 3 times daily, but not at the same time, can be highly effective in treating acute sinusitis.

THERAPEUTIC REVIEW

As presented in Tables 12–1 and 12–2, stage 1 of the sinusitis treatment regimen incorporates the lifestyle measures, vitamins, and supplements that should be started at the outset. Other measures and medicines are added in stage 2, which begins 3 weeks later. Still other measures and medicines are added in stage 3, which begins after another 3 weeks. The patient may, however, use any or all of the recommended treatment elements at the beginning of the program or at any time later on.

After about 2 months of incorporating most of the physical and environmental health measures into the patient's daily routine, addition of the mental and emotional health components of the program should be recommended, followed in another 1 to 2 months by the spiritual and social health components. With the addition of each component, factors that have contributed to causing the sinus condition, or that have triggered most of the patient's colds, will be uncovered.

THERAPEUTIC REVIEW   *continued*

It may prove valuable to also add *a Candida* treatment program (see Table 12–3) to the therapeutic regimen if the patient shows evidence of serious infection.

Many of the products listed in the tables that are not readily available at most health food stores can be obtained by referring to the Sinus Survival Program web site: www.sinussurvival.com

References

1. Centers for Disease Control and Prevention/National Center for Health Statistics: Vital and health statistics. Current estimates from the National Health Interview survey, 1995.
2. Kaliner M, Oguthorpe J, Fireman P, et al: Sinusitis: Bench to bedside—current findings, future directions. Otolaryngol 1997; 116(Suppl):S1–S20.
3. Anon J: Report of the Rhinosinusitis Task Force committee meeting. Otolaryngol Head Neck Surg 1997; 117(Suppl):S1–S68.
4. Terris M, Davidson T: Review of published results for endoscopic sinus surgery. Ear Nose Throat J 1994; 73:574–580.
5. Dockery DW, Pope CA, et al: An association between air pollution and mortality in six U.S. cities. N Engl J Med 1993; 329(24):1753–1759.
6. Adinoff A: Difficult asthma? Look for sinusitis. National Jewish Center for Immunology and Respiratory Medicine Medical/Scientific Update 1987 (February); 6(2).
7. Ponikau JV, Sherris DA, Kern EB, et al: The diagnosis and incidence of allergic fungal sinusitis. Mayo Clin Proc 1999; 74:877–884.
8. Middleton E, et al: Allergy: Principles and Practice, 5th ed.
9. Ben-Dov I, et al: Effect of negative ionization of inspired air on the response of asthmatic children to exercise and inhaled histamine. Thorax 1983; 38:584–588.
10. Warner JA, Marchant JL, Warner JO: Double-blind trial of ionizers in children with asthma sensitive to the house dust mite. Thorax 1993; 48:330–333.
11. Kornblueh I: Artificial ionization of the air and its biological significance. Clin Med 1962; 68(8).
12. Ophir D, Elad, Y: Effects of steam inhalation on nasal patency and nasal symptoms in patients with the common cold. Am J Otolaryngol 1987; 8:149–153.
13. Talbot AR, Herr TM, Parsons DS: Mucociliary clearance and buffered hypertonic saline solution. Laryngoscope 1997; 107:500–503.
14. Georgitis JW: Nasal hyperthermia and simple saline irrigation for perennial rhinitis. Changes in inflammatory mediators. Chest 1994; 106:1487–1482.
15. Nanda R, James R, Smith H, et al: Food intolerance and the irritable bowel syndrome. Gut 1989; 30(8):1099–1104.
16. Antibiotics in milk. Br Med J 1963; 1(5344):1491–1492.
17. Ogle KA, Bullock JD: Children with allergic rhinitis and/or bronchial asthma treated with elimination diet. Ann Allergy 1977; 39(1):8–11.
18. Sanchez A: Role of sugars in human neutrophilic phagocytosis. Am J Clin Nutr 1973; 26(11):1180–1184.
19. Shirakawa T, Morimoto K: Lifestyle effect on total IgE. Lifestyles have a cumulative impact on controlling total IgE levels. Allergy 1991; 46(8):561–569.
20. Bell IR, Schwartz GE, Peterson JM, et al: Symptom and personality profiles of young adults from a college student population with self-reported illness from foods and chemicals. J Am Coll of Nutr 1993; 12(6):693–702.
21. Vojdani A, Ghoneum M: In vivo effect of ascorbic acid on enhancement of human natural killer cell activity. Nutr Resource 1993; 13(7):753–764.
22. Meydani SN, Barklund MP, Liu S, et al: Vitamin E supplementation enhances cell-mediated immunity in healthy elderly subjects. Am J Clin Nutr 1990; 52(3):557–563.
23. Agache P. Mise en evidence d'un effet-dose l'antagonisme visa vis de la papule histaminique. La Vie Medicale. 16 pp. 1153–1154.
24. Garlic in cryptococcal meningitis: a preliminary report of 21 cases. Chin Med J 1980; 93(2):123–126.
25. Bauer VR, Juric K, Puhlmann J, et al: Immunologic in vivo and in vitro studies on Echinacea extracts. Arzneimittelforschung 1988; 38(2):276–281.
26. Meydani SN, Lichtenstein AH, White PJ, et al: Food use and health effects of soybean and sunflower oils. J Amer Coll Nutr 1991; 10(5):406–428.
27. LaPierre A, Fletcher MA, Antoni MH, et al: Aerobic exercise training in an AIDS risk group. Int J Sports Med 1991; 12(supplement 1):S53–S57.
28. Ornish D, Brown SE, Scherwitz LW, et al: Can lifestyle changes reverse coronary heart disease? The Lifestyle Heart Trial. Lancet 1990; 336(8704):129–133.
29. Smyth JM, Stone AA, Hurewitz A, Kaell A: Effects of writing about stressful experiences on symptom reduction in patients with asthma or rheumatoid arthritis. A Randomized Trial. JAMA 1999; 281(14):1304–1309.
30. Solberg EE, Halvorsen R, Sundgot-Borgen J, et al: Meditation: a modulator of the immune response to physical stress? A brief report. Br J Sports Med 1995; 29(4):255–257.
31. Kiecolt-Glaser JK, Malarky WB, Chee M, et al: Negative behavior during marital conflict is associated with immunological down-regulation. Psychosom Med 1993; 55(5):395–409.
32. Spiegel D, Bloom JR, et al: Effect of psychosocial treatment on survival of patients with metastatic breast cancer. Lancet 1989;888–891.
33. Garbutt JM, Goldstein M, Gellman E, et al: A randomized, placebo-controlled trial of antimicrobial treatment for children with clinically diagnosed acute sinusitis. Pediatrics 2001; 107(4) April: 619–625.
34. Heatley DG, McConnell KE, et al: Nasal irrigation for the alleviation of sinonasal symptoms. Otolaryngol Head Neck Surg 2001; 125(1):44–48.
35. Gwaltney JM, Phillips CD, Miller RD, Riker DK: Computed tomographic study of the common cold. N Engl J Med 1994; 330(1):25–30.

CHAPTER 13

Upper Respiratory Infection

James P. Nicolai, M.D.

UPPER RESPIRATORY INFECTION

Upper respiratory infection (URI) has the highest incidence of acute illness in the developed world, accounting for at least half of all human illnesses.[1] No acute illness is more prevalent in the United States than the common cold.[2] According to estimates, the average adult has 2 to 4 colds per year, and the average school-age child has 6 to 10.[3] The economic impact is substantial, with an estimated $1.5 billion spent annually on caring for these patients in physicians' offices and nearly $2 billion on nonprescription cough and cold treatments.[4] Forty percent of time lost from jobs and 30% of school absences can be attributed to colds.[2]

Uncomplicated URIs have been shown to be usually viral in nature. Although patients with complications such as bacterial sinusitis, otitis media, streptococcal pharyngitis, bronchospasm, or pneumonia may benefit from antibiotics or inhaler treatment, medical science has little to offer for uncomplicated infections. Nevertheless, antibiotics are often prescribed despite convincing evidence of little or no benefit.[5] The widespread use of antibiotics for primarily viral self-limited respiratory infections has become a cause of great concern.[6] Investigators report that resistance to common respiratory pathogens is positively correlated with exposure to antibiotic treatment.[7-9] Because treatment of uncomplicated URI focuses primarily on relief of symptoms, and because physicians feel somewhat pressured to prescribe medicines that are not necessarily indicated, it is important to be aware of interventions that are not only effective but also deal with the overuse of antibiotics and its input on cost, adverse reactions, and resistance.

PATHOPHYSIOLOGY

The etiology of the common cold is known to be viral, with over 200 possible serologically different viruses known to cause cold-type symptoms (Table 13–1). These viruses are transmitted in respiratory droplets from sneezing, by hand-to-hand contact, or by touching contaminated objects. Risk factors include attendance at day care centers and crowded conditions, poor hygiene, and stress.

Table 13–1. Most Common Pathogens Causing Upper Respiratory Infections

Rhinovirus
Coronavirus
Adenovirus
Echoviruses
Coxsackievirus
Respiratory syncytial virus
Parainfluenza virus

Various organisms cause colds. The single-stranded rhinovirus is the most common agent, causing 10% to 40% of colds, with over 100 serotypes. Coronavirus is the second most common etiologic agent, accounting for 10% to 20% of colds, with three specific subgroups. Other causative viruses are adenoviruses, echoviruses, coxsackieviruses, respiratory syncytial virus, and parainfluenza viruses. Colds due to rhinovirus are most prevalent in early fall and late spring, whereas coronavirus strains seem to be most prevalent during winter months in the United States.[10]

Infection begins in the posterior adenoidal region of the nasopharynx, which contains receptor sites for the rhinovirus.[11] Viral replication peaks in 48 hours and then declines, but viral shedding may go on for up to 3 weeks.[11] With infection, an inflammatory response ensues, including the recruitment of neutrophils, lymphocytes, plasma cells, and eosinophils. The mucosa becomes edematous and hyperemic, with hyperactive mucous glands, which translates to the characteristic nasal congestion (discharge, sneezing, stuffiness), pharyngeal irritation (sore, scratchy throat), lower respiratory problems (cough, hoarseness), and constitutional symptoms (headache, low-grade fever, myalgias) of the URI.[10]

INTEGRATIVE THERAPY

Lifestyle Modification

Prevention

To prevent "catching a cold," the best measure is to avoid exposure to aerosol particles or airborne droplets. Self-inoculation of secretions transferred by hand is another common mode of infection. Careful hand washing and avoiding contact with the mucous membranes of the eyes, nose, and mouth are the best ways to avert nonaerosol contamination. Interferon intranasal sprays are moderately prophylactic for prevention of rhinovirus infection but may cause localized nasal irritation (oxymetazoline 0.05%, two sprays to each nostril twice daily for 5 days).[12, 13] High doses of vitamin C (4 to 5 g daily) and zinc lozenges may be no more effective than placebo in preventing a cold,[14, 15] Results of studies on *echinacea* and URIs support the use of this botanical for treatment of these infections but not as a preventative.[16]

Pharmaceuticals

Antihistamines

Antihistamines seem to give the most favorable results in reducing rhinorrhea, sneezing, and nasal secretions, although they have minimal effects on other symptoms. These agents have an atropine-type drying effect, which may actually exacerbate symptoms of congestion and cause upper airway obstruction by impairing flow of mucus.[17] Drowsiness is a common side effect; therefore, taking the antihistamine at bedtime may be of benefit to patients whose cold symptoms disturb their sleep. Long-acting antihistamines are not as effective, probably owing to their limited anticholinergic activity.[18]

Alpha-Adrenergic Agonists

Decongestants (such as phenylpropanolamine and pseudoephedrine) are used not only to provide symptomatic relief but to also prevent sinus and eustachian tube obstruction, which can lead to sinusitis or otitis media. The most common decongestants are the α-adrenergic agents, which come in both oral and nasal forms. They work by causing generalized vasoconstriction, thereby reducing formation of excess nasal secretions; however, they are not without potentially dangerous side effects. Prolonged use of nasal decongestants can lead to rebound congestion (rhinitis medicamentosa), which may lead to abuse of the spray. In addition, because oral adrenergic agents are not selective, they may raise blood pressure when used in doses sufficient to alleviate nasal congestion. Care must be taken in patients with borderline or clinical hypertension because of the sympathomimetic effects of these drugs.

Nonsteroidal Anti-inflammatory Drugs

Analgesics are useful in treating the headache and myalgias brought on by viral infection. However, both aspirin and acetaminophen have been found to be capable of delaying the immune response in experimental rhinovirus infection. In addition, these nonsteroidal anti-inflammatory drugs (NSAIDs) may cause a slight increase in nasal congestion, as well as increasing viral shedding.[19, 20] More recently, the cyclo-oxygenase inhibitor naproxen was found to alleviate pain without the promotion of viral shedding or reduction of antibody responses.[21]

Cough Suppressants and Expectorants

Drugs that act to suppress cough, which include narcotic as well as non-narcotic preparations, are effective for symptomatic relief, especially in promoting sleep uninterrupted by coughing. Narcotic suspensions may be more potent antitussives but also carry with them the potential for abuse, the ability to interfere with delta wave sleep, and the risk of rebound insomnia. Their use in the short term is efficacious, but the physician should proceed with caution when the duration of symptoms exceeds 10 to 14 days. Cough suppressants may not work completely, as the cough stimulus can be brought about by other factors, such as postnasal drip. With regard to expectorants, these agents are included in many preparations and are thought to stimulate the flow of mucus. There has been no evidence to verify this claim, even though combinations of cough suppressants (dextromethorphan) coupled with an expectorant (e.g., guaifenesin) are common preparations in over-the-counter cold remedies.

Antibiotics

A 1997 survey showed that approximately 21% of all antibiotic prescriptions for adults by ambulatory care physicians were for URIs.[22] Another survey found that 60% of patients seen by primary care practitioners for the common cold received a prescription for an antibiotic.[23] A conservative estimate of the annual cost of prescription of antibiotics for the common cold in the United States in 1994 was $37.5 million.[24] In addition, there is a growing debate regarding the pathogenesis of acute sinusitis, acute bronchitis, and uncomplicated URI. The etiology of uncomplicated URI is known to be viral, and some researchers have proposed that the common cold, acute sinusitis, and acute bronchitis all should be considered to be forms of URI, as it is difficult to distinguish among these entities owing to significant overlap of symptoms.[25] Researchers have suggested that diagnoses of "acute sinusitis" and "acute bronchitis" are made to justify antibiotic prescriptions, when in fact the effectiveness of antibiotics in these disorders has been shown to be minimal at best. In analyzing the reasons why doctors prescribe antibiotics in these instances, such issues as patient expectations, physician perceptions of these expectations, patient education, and physician communication all play a role in the decision-making process. Preservation of the physician-patient relationship is not dependent on the patient's walking out of the examination room with a prescription for antibiotics; patients are satisfied when they understand their illness, have their questions answered, and feel that the physician spent enough time with them.[26, 27] In addition, research suggests that many patients do not know what an antibiotic is and use the word to indicate any prescription medication. They may not be seeking an antibiotic agent per se; rather, their perception of an antibiotic may be one of "powerful medicine"—perhaps the most powerful one they know of existing in the conventional physician's arsenal.[28] If the patient wants the best treatment the physician has to offer, it is in the best interest of patient and physician alike to be aware of alternatives to antibiotics that not only are available but have also been shown to be safe and effective. Moreover, the Centers for Disease Control and Prevention (CDC) has recently published guidelines for more judicious use of antibiotics in the treatment of URIs. This information is readily available, as it can be downloaded off the Internet and then provided as a "handout" for educating patients about why antibiotics should not be prescribed indiscriminately (for more information, contact the CDC at www.cdc.gov).

NOTE

The CDC guidelines promote two principles for judicious use of antimicrobial medications in patients with URIs: (1) an antimicrobial should not be given for the common cold, and (2) mucopurulent rhinitis (thick, opaque, or discolored nasal discharge) is not an indication for treatment unless it persists for more than 10 to 14 days.[29]

General Measures

Rest

The immune system requires energy to fight viral infection. Reducing activity not only allows energy conservation to be maximized but also decreases exposure to potential other challenges to immunity and helps to avoid complications.

Adequate Hydration

Water is needed to maintain good balance with body tissues. The body's supply of water must be constantly replenished as it is used up in the processes of life. Moreover, during illness, the rate of metabolic processes is increased, leading to augmented utilization of water in the body. Other mechanics of infection such as increased respirations, coughing, and fever all lead to depletion of body water. Getting plenty of fluids aids in keeping blood flow optimal, avoiding strain on the heart and kidneys, and helping to loosen secretions. At least 64 ounces (eight 8-oz. glasses of water) daily is recommended—more so with fever or frequent coughing.

Steam Inhalation

Steam inhalation is useful for patients with chest congestion or productive cough, as the heat and moisture generated act to increase the rate of mucus flow. Research in the United Kingdom showed that nasal hyperthermia resulted in subjective relief of symptoms and in objective nasal patency in patients with naturally acquired or experimentally induced colds.[30] For steam inhalation treatments in the home, a pot of water is brought to boil on the stove; the patient then holds a towel over both the head and the pot and breathes deeply through the nose or mouth with pursed lips for several minutes. The effects of steam can be enhanced by adding aromatic herbs to the water, such as sage or eucalyptus, which are thought to halt bacterial growth and reduce the chance of getting secondary infections. Herbs can be bought in bulk, or essential oils can be purchased. Add a handful of herbs or 1 or 2 drops of oil to water that has stopped boiling.

Gargling

Gargling with a simple saline solution made by mixing $1/4$ teaspoon of salt with 1 cup of the warmest water tolerable can alleviate the pain and irritation of a sore throat and can open up congested ears. Gargling works to increase blood flow to the irritated area while bathing it with a restorative solution. The solution can be combined with a powder made from the herbal disinfectant goldenseal and red pepper to taste. The patient with tonsillitis may want to consider gargling with hydrogen peroxide mixed with an equal amount of water. The patient should gargle four times daily for a few minutes each with whichever solution has been compounded.[31]

Supplements

Vitamin C

Since the 1970s, studies have been done to assess the effectiveness of vitamin C on the common cold. The role of vitamin C in the prevention and treatment of colds remains controversial. A meta-anlaysis of the available literature suggested that although vitamin C may not prevent colds, it may significantly decrease the duration of episodes and severity, by an average of 23%.[32] There was no clear indication of the optimal dosage; however, in trials that tested use of vitamin C after cold symptoms appeared, results suggested that higher doses were of greater benefit than that obtained with lower doses. Megadoses of vitamin C consisting of 1000 mg each hour for the first 6 hours, and then three times daily thereafter, were reported to be associated with a significant decrease in symptoms and in duration of illness.[33]

Dosage. 1000 mg three to six times daily

Precautions. Nausea, abdominal distention, flatulence, and diarrhea have been reported in patients taking vitamin C in these doses.

Zinc

The mechanism by which zinc affects the clinical course of the common cold has yet to be determined. Various hypotheses explaining its action range from the prevention of viral binding to respiratory tract epithelium and stabilization of epithelial cell membranes, to inhibition of viral protein synthesis, to inhibition of prostaglandin metabolites, to increasing interferon production. Eight trials have been published on the effects of zinc in the treatment of the common cold. All eight were double-blinded, placebo-controlled studies, but different formulations and doses of zinc were used in each. Four of the studies showed a benefit and four did not.[34, 35] Of the four studies not showing beneficial effects, three have been criticized for using a formulation that inactivated the zinc, and the fourth study was thought to use an ineffective dose.[35] The best data available are from studies replicating similar treatment models; doses used were well above the minimal daily requirements.

The zinc preparation that seems to be most effective is zinc acetate in the form of lozenges containing 23 mg of zinc (13-mg lozenges have also been used and shown to be effective). Zinc gluconate is also common but may be less biologically active. Lozenges should be taken at the first sign of cold symptoms. For optimal effectiveness, treatment should be started within at least 24 hours of symptom onset. Zinc lozenges should then be taken every 2 hours while the patient is awake until symptoms abate. Studies have not shown prophylactic treatment with high-dose zinc to be effective in preventing cold symptoms. There is also a newer form of zinc, a nasal spray gel called Zycam (discussed later in "Other Therapies to Consider").

Dosage. Zinc, 23-mg lozenges every 2 hours while the patient is awake.

Precautions. Lozenges may cause nausea and leave a disagreeable taste.

Herbal Therapies

Echinacea

Reviews of the medical literature have shown several studies that provide evidence of the efficacy of echinacea in the treatment of URI. Although there is a moderate degree of methodologic deficiency in all of the reviewed studies, the published evidence supports the ability of echinacea to decrease the severity and duration of acute URI.[37] However, although the consensus of studies has indeed shown echinacea to be effective in the treatment of colds, interpretation of existing literature does not suggest its effectiveness in prevention of illness.

Echinacea is an herbal medicine that has been used for centuries, especially by Native Americans, in the treatment of colds and URIs, burns and other inflammatory conditions, and even snakebite. Although many of the active compounds of echinacea have been identified, the complete mechanism of action is still unknown. The plant and its active components are thought to affect the phagocytic immune system and modulate immunity on a cellular level, as opposed to affecting the acquired humoral immune response. Echinacea is also thought to increase T cell (natural killer cell) activity and the production of interferon.[38]

Confusion exists regarding which echinacea preparation to use in treatment of the common cold. Approval has been given for the use of specific types of echinacea but not for others. Three species of *Echinacea* are used for medicinal purposes: *E. purpurea* (the purple coneflower), *E. angustifolia*, and *E. pallida*. Each is purported to have different properties, but little has been done to analyze the effectiveness of each species.[39] Moreover, extracts from roots, leaves, and flowers of each species are also claimed to have varying medicinal value but have not been completely distinguished from each other in terms of apparent beneficial activity. For example, the German Commission E has approved the oral use of *E. purpurea* herb, specifically the above ground parts for colds and respiratory tract infections, whereas the *E. pallida* root has been approved for use in the treatment of flu-like illnesses.[39] The fact that other preparations have not been approved does not necessarily mean that they are not efficacious; either research has not been adequately verified with these preparations, or there has not been proper identification of species types in each respective study. Recommendations for treatment are that echinacea, in any form, should be started early in the course of the cold, used several times daily, and then discontinued when symptoms subside.

Dosage. Because of the confusion regarding different preparations and the lack of a known standardized active constituent, it is difficult to offer specific recommendations. A reasonable dosage is 2 to 3 mL of *E. purpurea* juice or 1 to 2 mL of an extract taken 3 or 4 times a day in juice or water or sublingually. For the encapsulated form of *E. purpurea,* the dosage is 150 to 300 mg of a 6.5:1 powdered extract preparation. A recommended dosage for a tincture of 1:5 (45% ethanol) is 1 to 2 mL every 2 hours on the first day of symptoms and then 4 times a day for 5 days or until symptoms abate. For children younger than 10 years, half of the adult dose is recommended.

Precautions. Echinacea is not recommended for routine, chronic use, as evidence does not support its effectiveness in the prevention of URIs.[36] It may also be contraindicated in pregnant or lactating women, or in persons suffering from serious autoimmune disorders or chronic diseases or those taking immunosuppressive agents or with HIV infection. Echinacea appears to be well tolerated, with a low frequency of adverse effects, which include dyspepsia, headache, and dizziness. No drug interactions with echinacea have been reported. Although serious anaphylactic reactions are rare, echinacea has been linked with allergies in some people with history of asthma or allergic rhinitis. Caution is advised for anyone who is hypersensitive to plants, especially those of the daisy family (sunflower, seeds, ragweed).[38]

OTHER THERAPIES TO CONSIDER

Mast Cell Stabilizers

Drugs such as sodium cromoglycate (Cromolyn sodium) administered intranasally or via nebulizer have been shown to reduce the severity of upper respiratory infections.[40] These drugs prevent release of chemical mediators in response to infection as well as down-regulating the receptor site where rhinovirus particles attach in the respiratory epithelium. Although these drugs are classified as being very safe, epidemiologic data documenting their effectiveness in treating the common cold are insufficient thus far.

Zycam

Zycam is a specific preparation of zinc in the form of a nasal gel. A recent pilot study showed that the use of Zycam was able to significantly shorten the duration of cold symptoms from 9 days to 2. The apparent mechanism of action focuses on zinc's impairment of viral attachment to epithelium lining the nasal passages. The product works best when started within 24 hours of symptom onset.

Dosage. One spray per nostril every 2 to 4 hours while the patient is awake until symptoms subside and then for an additional 48 hours.

Astragalus

Astragalus is a Chinese herb that has been traditionally used for treating cold and flu symptoms. It comes from the root of a plant in the pea family (*Astragalus membranaceus*), and has a reputation for enhancing the immune system by stimulating white blood cell activity and the production of useful antibodies. It also increases interferon in the body and is therefore used as an antiviral remedy; consequently, it acts to shorten the duration of an upper respiratory infection. Astragalus comes in capsule and tincture forms.

Dosage. Two capsules or one dropperful of tincture twice daily until symptoms resolve.

Elderberry

A product made from elderberries (*Sambucus nigra*) is also thought to have antiviral properties. This botanical is available as Sambucol, which was developed by an Israeli doctor who claims it as a specific remedy for the flu; however, it can also be used for cold-type symptoms. It seems both safe and effective. It is available in the form of syrup as well as lozenges.

Dosage. One teaspoon or one lozenge 4 times daily until resolution of symptoms.

Homeopathy

An experienced homeopathic physician should assess individual constitutional types and severity of disease to select the correct remedy and potency. For acute cases, use 3 to 5 pellets of a 12X to 30C remedy every 1 to 4 hours until symptoms resolve. The following four remedies are available for the treatment of the common cold in its various forms[41] (see Chapter 103, Therapeutic Homeopathy):

- *Allium cepa,* for colds with profuse watery discharge that burns or irritates the nostrils
- *Euphrasia,* for colds with profuse watery discharge that is irritating to the eyes
- *Aconite,* for colds that come on suddenly with fever and anxiety
- *Mercurius,* for profuse discharge associated with generalized irritation and accompanied by weakness

THERAPEUTIC REVIEW

Following is a summary of therapeutic options for the common cold. As noted previously, the best advice is to start treatment within 24 hours of symptom onset.

Prevention
- Careful hand washing
- Avoiding contact with mucous membranes of eyes, nose, and mouth

General measures
- Rest
- Adequate hydration
- Steam inhalation, sweating, gargling
- Pharmaceuticals

Antihistamines (may cause drowsiness)
- Decongestants (may cause rebound congestion, hypertension)
- Cough suppressants (may cause drowsiness)
- Analgesics

Supplements
- Vitamin C: 1000 mg 3 to 6 times/day
- Zinc: zinc acetate or gluconate lozenges 23 mg one every 2 hours while patient is awake; Zycam nasal gel one spray per nostril every 2 to 4 hours until symptoms subside

Botanicals
- Echinacea purpurea: 2 to 3 mL of juice or 1 to 2 mL of extract three to four times daily in juice or water, or sublingually; 150 to 300 mg powdered extract three to four times daily or 1 to 5 mL of tincture 1:5 (ethanol) three times daily

References

1. Campbell H: Acute respiratory infection: A global challenge. Arch Dis Childhood 73:281–283, 1995.
2. Kirkpatrick GL: The common cold. Primary Care 23: 657–675, 1996.
3. Spector SL: The common cold: Current therapy and natural history. J Allergy Clin Immunol 95:1133–1138, 1995.
4. Turner RB: Epidemiology, pathogenesis, and treatment of the common cold. Ann Allergy Asthma Immunol 78:531–539, 1997.
5. Dosh SA, et al: Predictors of antibiotic prescribing for non-specific upper respiratory infections, acute bronchitis, and acute sinusitis. J Fam Pract 49:407–414, 2000.
6. Schwartz B, Mainous AG III, Marcy SM: Why do physicians prescribe antibiotics for children with upper respiratory infections? JAMA 279:881–882, 1998.
7. Arason VA, et al: Do antimicrobials increase the carriage rate of penicillin-resistant pneumococci in children? Cross sectional prevalence study. BMJ 313:387–391, 1996.
8. Henning C, Bengtsson L, Jorup C, Enquist S: Antibiotic resistance in Streptococcus pneumoniae, Haemophilus influenzae and Streptococcus pyogenes in respiratory tract infections in outpatients. Scand J Infect Dis 29:559–563, 1997.
9. Wang EE, Kellner JD, Arnold S: Antibiotic-resistant Streptococcus pneumonia: Implications for medical practice. Can Fam Physician 44:1881–1888, 1998.
10. Lorber B: The common cold. J. Gen Intern Med 11:229–236, 1996.
11. Gwaltney JM Jr: Rhinovirus infection of the normal human airway. Am J Respir Crit Care Med 152:S36–S39, 1995.
12. Farr MB, Gwaltney JM Jr, Adams KF, Hayden FG: Intranasal interferon-α2 for prevention of natural rhinovirus colds. Antimicrob Agents Chemother 26: 31–34, 1984.
13. Samo TC, Greenberg SB, Couch RB, et al: Efficacy and tolerance of intranasally applied recombinant leukocyte A interferon in normal volunteers. J Infect Dis 148:535–542, 1983.
14. Garland ML, Hagmeyer KO: The role of zinc lozenges in the treatment of the common cold. Ann Pharmacother 32: 63–69, 1998.
15. Douglass RM, Chalker EB, Tracy B: Vitamin C for preventing and treating the common cold. Cochrane Database Syst Rev 2: CD000980, 2000.
16. Melchart D, Walther E, Linde K, et al: Echinacea root extracts for the prevention of upper respiratory tract infections. Arch Fam Med 7: 541–545, 1998.
17. Simon HB: Management of the common cold. In Groll AH et al (eds): Primary Care Medicine: Office Evaluation and Management of the Adult Patient, 3rd ed. Philadelphia, Pa, JB Lippincott, 1995.
18. Gaffey MJ, Kaiser DL, Hayden FG: Ineffectiveness of oral terfenadine in natural colds: Evidence against histamine as a mediator of common cold symptoms. Pediatr Infect Dis J 7:223–228, 1998.
19. Stanley ED, Jackson CG, Panusarn C, et al: Increased virus shedding with aspirin treatment of rhinovirus infection. JAMA 231:1248–1251, 1975.
20. Graham NMH, Burrel CJ, Douglas RM, et al: Adverse effects of aspirin, acetaminophen and ibuprofen on immune function, viral shedding and clinical status in rhinovirus infected volunteers. J Infect Dis 162: 1277–1282, 1990.
21. Sperber SJ, Hendley O, Hayden FG, et al: Effects of naproxen on experimental rhinovirus colds: A randomized, double blind, controlled trial, Ann Intern Med 117:37–41, 1992.
22. Gonzalez R, Steiner JF, Sande MA: Antibiotic prescribing for adults with colds, upper respiratory infections, and bronchitis by ambulatory care physicians. JAMA 278:901–904, 1997.
23. Mainous AG III, Hueston WJ, Clark JR: Antibiotics and upper respiratory infection: Do some folks think there is a cure for the common cold? J Fam Pract 42:357–361, 1996.
24. Mossad SB: Treatment of the common cold. BMJ, 317:33–36, 1998.
25. Dosh SA, Hickner JM, Mainous AG III, Ebell MH. Predictors of antibiotic prescribing for nonspecific upper respiratory infec-

tions, acute bronchitis, and acute sinusitis. J Fam Pract 49:407–414, 2000.

26. Mangione Smith R, McGlynn EA, Elliott MN, et al: The relationship between perceived parental expectations and pediatrician antimicrobial prescribing behavior. Pediatrics 103:711–718, 1999.

27. Hamm RM, Hicks RI, Bemben DA: Antibiotics and respiratory infections: Are patients more satisfied when expectations are met? J Fam Pract 43:56–62, 1996.

28. Gonzalez R, Corbett K: The culture of antibiotics. Am J Med 107:525–526, 1999.

29. Rosentein N, Phillips WR, Gerber MA, et al. The common cold–principles of judicious use of antimicrobial agents. Pediatrics 101(Suppl 1): 181–184, 1998.

30. Tyrrell D, Barrow I, Arthur J: Local hyperthermia benefits natural and experimental common colds. BMJ 289:1280–1283, 1989.

31. Weil A: Three Easy Cold Remedies. Dr. Andrew Weil's Self Healing [newsletter], vol 1. Watertown, Mass, Thorne Communications, 1996, pp. 2–3.

32. Hemila H, Herman ZS: Vitamin C and the common cold: A retrospective analysis of Chalmers' review. J Am Coll Nutr 14:116–123, 1995.

33. Gorton HC, Jarvis K: The effectiveness of vitamin C in preventing and relieving the symptoms of virus induced respiratory infections. J Manipulative Physiol Ther 22:530–535, 1999.

34. Potter YJ, Hart LL: Zinc lozenges for treatment of common colds. Ann Pharmacother 27:589–592, 1993.

35. Mossad SB, Macknin ML, Medendorp SV, Mason P: Zinc gluconate lozenges for treating the common cold. Ann Intern Med 125:81–88, 1996.

36. Melchart D, Linde K, Fischer P, Kaesmayr J: Echinacea for preventing and treating the common cold. Cochrane Database Syst Rev 1:CD001218, 2001.

37. Giles JT, Cuthbert TP, Chien SH, et al: Evaluation of echinacea for treatment of the common cold. Pharmocotherapy 20:690–697, 2000.

38. Barrett B. Vohmann M, Calabrese C: Echinacea for upper respiratory infection. J Fam Pract 48:628–635, 1999.

39. Percival SS: Use of echinacea in medicine. Biochem Pharmacol 60:155–158, 2000.

40. Aberg N, Aberg B, Alestig K: The effect of inhaled and intranasal sodium cromoglycate on symptoms of upper respiratory tract infections. Clin Exp Allergy 26:1045–1050, 1996.

41. Cummings S, Ullman D: Homeopathic Medicines. Los Angeles, Calif, Jeremy P. Tarcher, 1984.

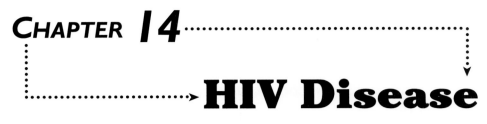

CHAPTER 14

HIV Disease

Benjamin Kligler, M.D., M.P.H.

PATHOPHYSIOLOGY

Acquired immunodeficiency syndrome (AIDS) is a potentially life-threatening disease caused by the human immunodeficiency virus (HIV). The virus, which is transmitted by sexual contact and contact with blood and certain other body fluids, attacks a class of T lymphocytes called CD4$^+$ cells, resulting in severe declines in both number and effective function of this arm of the immune system. The result is a dramatically weakened immune system and a host at risk for life-threatening opportunistic infections including *Pneumocystis carinii* pneumonia (PCP), *Mycobacterium avium-intracellulare* (MAI) sepsis, cerebral toxoplasmosis, and Kaposi's sarcoma. Before the advent of effective antiretroviral medications, AIDS was a slowly progressive but almost universally fatal condition.

In recent years, AIDS has been transformed by the widespread use of antiretroviral medications into a serious but manageable chronic illness. Many of the current challenges in the management of the HIV-positive patient in developed nations pertain to minimizing the possibility of developing viral resistance while maximizing quality of life by preventing or controlling the adverse effects associated with long-term use of antiretrovirals. In the developing world, where the HIV epidemic continues to spread, the cost of antiretroviral medications is prohibitive, and deaths from AIDS continue to mount.

ROLE OF ALTERNATIVE APPROACHES TO TREATMENT

People with HIV disease typically use alternative approaches for several reasons. First is to promote healthier functioning of the immune system; this approach can apply both to patients very early in the course of HIV infection and not yet on antiretroviral medications and to those with more advanced disease who are receiving conventional medications. Second is for a claimed antiviral effect of the therapy, as in the use of intravenous vitamin C infusions. Third is to treat an HIV-associated symptom or condition. Fourth is to mitigate one or more of the side effects of conventional antiretroviral medica-

tions, as in the use of glutamine supplements for protease inhibitor–associated diarrhea.

INTEGRATIVE THERAPY

Pharmaceuticals

Two general categories of pharmaceutical are widely used in the treatment of HIV disease. The first category is the antiretrovirals, used for their specific activity against HIV. These agents are currently divided into three groups: the nucleoside reverse transcriptase inhibitors (NRTIs), which include zidovudine (azidothymidine [AZT]) (Retrovir), didanosine (dideoxyinoside [ddI]) (Hivid), stavudine (Zerit), and lamivudine (Epivir); the protease inhibitors (PIs), which include indinavir (Crixivan), nelfinavir (Viracept), and numerous others; and the non-nucleoside reverse transcriptase inhibitors (NNRTIs), which include efavirenz (Sustiva) and nevirapine (Virammune), among others. The most widely used approach over the past five years has been to use these agents in combinations of at least three drugs—usually two NRTIs and either one PI or one NNRTI—to reduce the possibility of viral resistance. Recent research is looking at the possibility that antiviral medications should be withheld during the early stages of HIV infection to minimize the problems with long-term toxicity of these agents. Other investigators are examining the risk-benefit analysis of "drug holidays"—planned periods off medication to minimize toxicity.

The second category of pharmaceuticals, used less widely now since the advent of effective antiretroviral medications, comprises the prophylactic agents used for prevention of specific HIV-related opportunistic infections. These drugs include trimethoprim-sulfamethoxazole (Septra, Bactrim) for PCP and toxoplasmosis prophylaxis and azithromycin and rifabutin for prophylaxis of *Mycobacterium avium* infection.

NOTE

Studies have shown that if CD4$^+$ counts rise and remain above 250, it is safe to discontinue prophylaxis for HIV-related opportunistic infections.

Nutrition

Early research in the 1980s showed that decreases in body weight, body mass index, and body fat percentage may be the first signs of declining nutritional status due to HIV disease and may begin even during the early asymptomatic phase of HIV infection. Many patients with HIV infection or AIDS experience HIV-associated wasting and lose body mass despite nutritional intake that should be adequate for their height and weight. In a study of nutritional status in 108 HIV-positive patients, some with and some without AIDS, body weight, serum cholesterol level, and CD4+ level progressively decreased over a 6-month period, and HIV-associated wasting persisted.[1] This study also found a significant relationship between low serum cholesterol—a marker for poor nutrition—and adverse patient outcome.

Nutrition counseling and intervention in the early stages of HIV disease constitute an important component of a prevention-oriented treatment plan, as these measures may help to forestall adverse nutritional changes in HIV-positive patients. Although definitive data supporting specific nutritional recommendations are scarce, reasonable suggestions include a diet high in omega-3 essential fatty acids (EFAs) such as flaxseed and fish oils; small frequent meals to ensure intake of adequate calories and to reduce the likelihood of malabsorption; avoidance of simple sugars, which some studies show may inhibit immune function on a short-term basis; and avoiding large amounts of alcohol and caffeine.

Another role for which nutritional interventions are widely utilized is to address the problems with malabsorption experienced by many HIV-positive patients. Common recommendations include the use of *Lactobacillus, Bifidobacterium,* and other "friendly bacteria" to maintain proper balance of intestinal flora (see Chapter 97, Prescribing Probiotics); the use of a multivitamin supplement to prevent the development of subclinical vitamin deficiencies even in patients eating a well-balanced diet; and the use of glutamine supplements to promote the health of colonic mucosa. Although these recommendations to date have not been shown to affect the course of HIV disease progression, all are safe and reasonable to include in an integrative treatment plan.

Supplements

Vitamin A

Vitamin A supplementation has been extensively studied for ameliorating infection with HIV in adults, and for possibly reducing the likelihood of vertical HIV transmission. An association between lower vitamin A levels, lower CD4+ counts, and higher risk of progression to AIDS has been reported.[2] A study in African women demonstrated a connection between vitamin A deficiency and increased maternal-fetal transmission of HIV.[3] However, other pro-

spective trials, including one with 341 HIV-positive patients followed over 9 years, have demonstrated no significant difference in risk of AIDS progression with vitamin A levels.[4] Trials of high-dose vitamin A supplementation have also failed to show an effect on CD4+ or CD8+ counts, viral loads, lymphocyte responsiveness to mitogens, or progression of disease.[5] The association between vitamin A deficiency and increased vertical transmission of HIV initially reported in Kenya has not been borne out in subsequent U.S. studies. The Women and Infants Transmission Study (WITS), a large prospective ongoing cohort study, has found that vitamin A level does not correlate with increased risk of HIV vertical transmission in North America.[6] The investigators suggested that vitamin A supplementation in addition to prenatal vitamins is not necessary.

Vitamin B₁₂

Supplementation with a B-complex vitamin may be beneficial in HIV-infected patients. Lack of vitamin B_{12} has been associated with peripheral neuropathy and myelopathy; a 9-year prospective cohort study in 310 patients found vitamin B_{12} levels to be an early and independent marker of HIV disease progression, and time to development of AIDS was found to be 4 years less on average in persons observed to have lower B_{12} levels.[7] Results of intervention trials using B_{12} supplementation have been equivocal. Nevertheless, vitamin B_{12} supplementation continues to be widely used in HIV disease.

Antioxidants: Vitamins C and E, Selenium, and Alpha-Lipoic Acid

Vitamin C and vitamin E both have been explored for a role in treatment of HIV disease owing to their antioxidant properties. Other substances including selenium and alpha-lipoic acid are commonly used for the same purpose. In addition, vitamin C has been shown in vitro to inhibit viral replication at high doses.[8] On the basis of this finding, intravenous vitamin C has been widely used to achieve the high serum levels necessary for antiviral activity. There is no evidence to support this aggressive approach, although anecdotally it has not been proved to be as dangerous as was initially feared.

The role of antioxidant supplements in general in HIV disease requires further study. Vitamin E and vitamin C at more standard doses are safe and may decrease lipid peroxidation and enhance the immune system; however, conclusive evidence on the effects of these vitamins in HIV disease is still lacking.

Dosage. Vitamin E 400 international units (IU) daily, vitamin C 500 to 2000 mg 3 times daily

N-Acetylcysteine

Because of the strong evidence that depletion of glutathione levels correlates with progression of HIV infection,[9] a great deal of interest has focused on use of the nutritional supplement *N*-acetylcysteine (NAC) as a means to replete intracellular glutathione levels. Despite its early promise, however, NAC has not been proved beneficial in treatment of HIV disease. One randomized controlled trial[10] failed to show any influence of NAC on T cell counts or disease progression. Despite the lack of evidence supporting its use, this is a very commonly used supplement. There are no reported adverse effects of NAC supplementation.

L-Carnitine

L-Carnitine may be helpful in mitigating some of the adverse effects of antiretroviral medications, including peripheral neuropathy and dyslipidemia. Acetylcarnitine acts to facilitate transport of essential fatty acids across cell membranes and thus may have a role in normalizing intracellular lipid metabolism and regulating peripheral nerve function and regeneration. Decreased levels of carnitine have been found in HIV-positive people; in addition, AIDS patients experiencing neuropathy with AZT or ddI therapy had significantly lower levels of acetylcarnitine than those in patients without neuropathy.[11] An increased proliferation of peripheral blood mononuclear cells in vitro was noted after oral supplementation with L-carnitine; a significant decrease in triglyceride levels was also noted.[12] No significant adverse effects of or interactions with L-carnitine have been demonstrated to date; further study of this supplement is needed to substantiate these possible benefits.

Dosage. L-Carnitine 2000 mg orally daily for HIV-positive patients with peripheral neuropathy or high triglyceride levels.

Glutamine

L-Glutamine supplementation has been shown in animal models to speed proliferation of colonocytes. Glutamine deficiency is also hypothesized to play a role in the process of HIV-associated wasting.[13] Many patients taking protease inhibitors experience chronic diarrhea as a medication side effect. Anecdotally, many patients find glutamine to be helpful in mitigating this particular side effect.

Dosage. L-Glutamine 2000 mg daily in 2 or 3 divided doses.

Botanical Medicine

Chinese Herbal Approaches

In the traditional practice of Chinese medicine, herbal formulas are typically individualized to suit a given patient's condition rather than standardized as a treatment for a given "disease." However, in the United States, the use of standardized formulas for certain conditions has become quite popular. Randomized controlled trials of two such Chinese herbal formulas (Enhance and Clear Heat, formulated by Health Concerns in California) showed a trend (statistically nonsignificant) toward fewer symptoms in the treatment group than in the placebo group.[14] Well-controlled long-term follow-up studies of use of these Chinese herbal preparations are needed before Western practitioners can recommend them with confidence. Significant concerns remain regarding possible herb-drug interactions, given the large number of herbs in most Chinese formulas, especially in those patients concurrently taking conventional antiretroviral medications.

Boxwood

An extract of the boxwood plant (*Buxus sempervirens*), SPV 30, has been studied in one small randomized trial, which showed possibly delayed progression in asymptomatic HIV-positive subjects when compared with that in patients given placebo.[15] In keeping with the preliminary nature of these data, an appropriate application for this botanical may be early in the course of HIV infection in patients for whom antiretroviral medications are not yet clearly indicated.

Dosage. 990 mg per day was the lowest effective dose of boxwood extract studied.

Mistletoe

The herb mistletoe (*Viscum album*) may be useful in treating HIV disease.[16] This herb has been investigated for its possible role as an immunomodulator in cancer treatment. In HIV disease, mistletoe has been shown to cause proliferation of granulocytes, natural killer cells, and CD4$^+$ cells and to stimulate T cell activity. Limited studies have shown increased appetite, weight gain, and decreased pain in HIV-positive patients. Mistletoe is administered subcutaneously.

Dosage. The dosage studied was 1 to 2 mg *Viscum album* extract subcutaneously biweekly, starting gradually with 0.01 mg for the first week with increases to 1 to 2 mg by week 4.

Precautions. An induration at the site of injection, usually less than 5 cm in diameter, is a common side effect. Other side effects can include fever, flu-like symptoms, fatigue, and headache.

Milk Thistle

Milk thistle extract (silymarin) may help to normalize liver function tests in patients on antiretroviral therapies, especially if they are co-infected with hepatitis C. Numerous in vitro studies have found that silymarin speeds regeneration of hepatocytes after chemical injury.[17] A significant improvement in liver function in patients with alcoholic hepatitis was noted after treatment with milk thistle extract.[18] At present, no firm evidence exists specifically linking the hepatoprotective function of silymarin with liver damage from antiretrovirals. However, clinical experience suggests that milk thistle may be useful in this situation. There are no reported contraindications or adverse effects of silymarin. It is important to note that contrary to a widely held popular belief among patients with HIV disease and many practitioners, milk thistle has no documented antiviral effect either in HIV disease or in hepatitis C.

Dosage. 240 mg twice daily of standardized milk thistle (silymarin) extract.

Red Rice Yeast Extract

Hyperlipidemia is a common side effect of treatment with protease inhibitors. A standardized extract of Chinese red rice yeast can reduce cholesterol levels by up to 20% in certain patients. One recent randomized controlled trial showed a significant decrease in lipids with use of this supplement, with no significant toxicity.[19] Red rice yeast has not been tested specifically in protease inhibitor–related hyperlipidemia. No significant adverse effects have been reported to date in patients using this supplement.

Dosage. 1200 mg orally twice daily. Red rice yeast extract is marketed in the United States as Cholestin.

Precaution. Because this supplement contains statin-like compounds, it is probably prudent to periodically monitor liver function in patients taking red rice yeast extract over the long term.

Mind-Body Therapies

Research in psychoneuroimmunology (PNI) has clearly linked psychological stress to impaired immune function. Although a specific link between T cell count or function and stress reduction in HIV disease has not been clearly established, one study did find a trend toward increased T cell count in persons practicing a mind-body approach, and other studies have found improvement in natural killer cell function and other immune parameters. Stress reduction approaches studied to date in HIV-positive patients include biofeedback, meditation, systematic relaxation, hypnosis, and cognitive behavioral stress management training. A review of several mind-body applications from the literature follows.

Ten HIV-positive men who were asymptomatic but had T cell counts below 400 were enrolled in a randomized 10-week study in which the experimental group received a 1-hour training session twice weekly in progressive muscle relaxation and biofeedback-assisted relaxation.[20] The subjects were expected to practice the techniques daily. Follow-up at 1 month after the intervention was completed showed decreased anxiety and improved mood and self-esteem, and increased T cell counts, as shown by the State Anxiety Inventory, the Profile of Mood States, and the Self-Esteem Inventory and by a basic T cell count. The extremely small sample size limits the generalizability of these findings, however.

A correlation between stress management and titers of antibody to herpes simplex virus types 1 and 2 (HSV-1 and HSV-2) was the subject of a 10-week study including 33 participants.[21] Subjects participated in 135-minute weekly sessions in cognitive-behavioral stress management. Overall, the frequency of practice, rather than the total number of times practiced, produced positive results over the period of intervention. Again, anxiety was reduced in the intervention group; however, dysphoria and HSV-2 antibody titers also decreased. There was no change in HSV-1 or CD4+ or CD8+ antibody titers. Further questions that arise with these results are in the exploration of the difference between effects on HSV-1 and HSV-2 antibody titers, and the reason for the differential effects of cognitive-behavioral techniques on levels of each.

A third study[22] focused on both CD4+ counts and quality of life measurements in 45 HIV-infected and AIDS patients (30 in the intervention group and 15 in the control group). This study found a lower mean stress level and a trend toward higher CD4+ counts in the intervention group. The intervention led to immediate increase in emotional well-being and perceived quality of life, but these outcomes were not sustained at a 6-month follow-up. The presence of illness-related intrusive thinking was higher in the control group at follow-up, whereas that of the intervention group actually decreased.

The differing effects of guided imagery, progressive muscle relaxation, and no intervention were tested on 69 participants in an uncontrolled study over a span of 6 weeks.[23] Subjects were instructed in their particular intervention and then expected to continue daily practice for the duration of the study. The outcome showed improved quality of life scores for the guided imagery group but no change in the group practicing progressive muscle relaxation.

Further studies are needed to distinguish whether any one of the mind-body approaches is more effective than others in patients with HIV disease. Generally, these strategies are considered extremely safe. The one exception to this general rule is that patients with a history of psychosis or unstable behavior should avoid hypnosis and should undertake other deep relaxation approaches with caution, as these practices may increase the risk of relapse in certain patients (see Chapter 91, Relaxation Techniques).

Other Therapies to Consider

Acupuncture

Acupuncture has been widely used both to enhance immune function and general well-being in HIV-positive patients and to treat specific HIV- or medication-related symptoms. One randomized controlled trial that examined amitriptyline plus acupuncture found no benefit of standardized acupuncture over sham ("placebo") acupuncture[24] in the treatment of HIV disease–related peripheral neuropathy. Methodologic challenges in studying acupuncture make it very difficult to demonstrate a small positive effect of an acupuncture intervention. Specifically, it is difficult to construct a valid placebo intervention (i.e., "sham" acupuncture) that does not in itself carry a therapeutic benefit beyond that of placebo. In addition, individualized strategies both for specific symptoms and for overall health may have higher efficacy than that of standardized treatment protocols more amenable to study in such trials; however, these individualized strategies are extremely difficult to study in blinded trials. Thus, a trial such as this one examining standardized acupuncture treatment versus individualized choice of points may fail to show efficacy because of the lesser efficacy of the standardized approach.

With regard to neuropathy in particular, it is important to note that many acupuncturists believe that in order for this modality to be effective in treating peripheral neuropathy, the treatment must be initiated as soon as possible after onset of symptoms. Perhaps future acupuncture trials in HIV disease should focus on efficacy in treating new-onset neuropathies.

Massage Therapy

Massage therapy has been definitively shown to produce a reduction in anxiety levels. The ability of massage to produce significant effects in the treatment of patients with HIV disease or AIDS in particular requires further study. A randomized trial of massage therapy in HIV-exposed neonates showed a significant benefit;[25] other evidence is all anecdotal. Although massage therapy has not been proved to affect $CD4^+$ levels per se, there is evidence showing that daily massage in HIV-positive men improves natural killer cell function and increases $CD8^+$ cell counts.[26] The benefits in terms of mood and decreased anxiety and the lack of adverse effects make massage therapy a reasonable choice for the HIV-positive patient.

 — *THERAPEUTIC REVIEW* —————————————

If viral load exceeds 30,000, or if $CD4^+$ counts fall below 500, or if patients are in any way symptomatic of HIV disease, good practice requires that they be offered combination antiretroviral medication as the mainstay of their treatment. This approach does not preclude the use of integrative strategies as supportive adjuncts and to alleviate certain disease-related or medication-related symptoms.

Pharmaceuticals
- *Consultation with a physician familiar with the rapidly changing range of medication options is recommended for proper choice of pharmaceutical approaches.*

Nutrition
- *Nutritional consultation early in the course of HIV infection should be recommended.*
- *Adequate calories and an emphasis on high intake of omega 3 essential fatty acids are important elements.*
- *Absorption issues should be considered as well.*

Supplements
- *Multivitamin daily*
- *Additional vitamin B, C, and E supplements*
- *L-Carnitine 2000 mg daily, especially in peripheral neuropathy or lipid disturbance*
- *L-Glutamine 2000 mg daily, especially in chronic diarrhea or malabsorption syndromes*

Botanicals
- *Milk thistle extract, 240 mg twice daily, with elevated values on liver function tests or with coinfection with hepatitis C*
- *Red rice yeast (cholestin) 1200 mg twice daily for hyperlipidemia*
- *Use of Chinese herbal formulas in patients not meeting criteria for pharmaceutical treatment*

THERAPEUTIC REVIEW *continued*

Mind-Body Approaches

- *Biofeedback, deep relaxation therapy, visualization, cognitive-behavioral stress reduction training, or another mind-body strategy*

Other Therapies

- *Acupuncture and massage therapy for promoting healthy immune function*

References

1. Guenter P, Muurahainen N, Simons G, et al. Relationships among nutritional status, disease progression, and survival in HIV infection. J Acquir Immune Defic Syndr 6:1130–1138, 1993.
2. Beach R, Mantero-Atienza E, Shor-Posner G, et al. Specific nutrient abnormalities in asymptomatic HIV-1 infection. AIDS 6:701–708, 1992.
3. Semba R, Miotti P, Chiphangwi J, et al. Maternal vitamin A deficiency and mother-to-child transmission of HIV-1. Lancet 172:1461–1468, 1994.
4. Tang A, Graham N, Semba R, et al. Association between serum vitamin A and E levels and HIV-1 disease progression. AIDS 11:613–620, 1997.
5. Humphrey J, Quinn T, Fine D, et al. Short-term effects of large-dose vitamin A supplementation on viral load and immune response in HIV-infected women. J Acquir Immune Defic Syndr Hum Retroviral 20:44–51, 1999.
6. Burns DN, FitzGerald G, Semb R, et al.: Vitamin A deficiency and other nutritional indices during pregnancy in human immunodeficiency virus infection: prevalence, clinical correlates, and outcome. Women and infants transmission study group. Clin Infect Dis 29:328–334, 1999.
7. Tang A, Graham N, Chandra R, et al. Low serum vitamin B-12 concentrations are associated with faster human immunodeficiency virus type 1 (HIV-1) disease progression. J Nutr 127:345–351, 1997.
8. Jariwalla RJ, et al. HIV suppression by ascorbate and its enhancement by glutathione precursor. In Proceedings of the Eighth International Conference on AIDS. Amsterdam 1992; 2:B207.
9. Buhl R, Jaffe HA, Holroyd KJ, et al. Systemic glutathione deficiency in symptom-free HIV seropositive individuals. Lancet 2: 1294–1298, 1989.
10. Akerlund B, Jarstrand C, Lindeke B, et al. Effect of *N*-acetylcysteine treatment on HIV-1 infection: A double-blind placebo controlled trial. Eur J Clin Pharmacol 50:457–461, 1996.
11. Famularo G, Moretti S, Marcellini S, et al. Acetyl-carnitine deficiency in AIDS patients with neurotoxicity on treatment with antiretroviral nucleoside analogues. AIDS 11:185–190, 1997.
12. De Simone C, Tzantzoglou S, Famularo G, et al. High dose L-carnitine improves immunologic and metabolic parameters in AIDS patients. Immunopharmacol Immunotoxicol 15:1–12, 1993.
13. Shabert JK, Wilmore DW. Glutamine deficiency as a cause of human immunodeficiency virus wasting. Med Hypotheses 46:252–256, 1996.
14. Burack J, Cohen MR, Hahn JA, Abrams DI: Pilot randomized controlled trials of Chinese herbal treatments for HIV-associated symptoms. J Acquir Immune Defic Syndr Hum Retrovirol 12:386–393, 1996.
15. Durant J, et al. A multicenter, randomized, double-blind, placebo-controlled trial of efficacy and safety of *Buxus sempervirens* L. preparations (SPV-30) in HIV-infected asymptomatic patients. In Proceedings of the Eleventh International Conference on AIDS (abstract B6040) 1996.
16. Stoss M, Van Wely M, Musielsky H, et al. Study on local inflammatory reactions and other parameters during subcutaneous mistletoe application in HIV-positive patients and HIV-negative subjects over a period of eighteen weeks. Arzneimittelforschung 49:366–373, 1999.
17. Blumenthal M, et al. (ed.). "Milk thistle fruit" in herbal medicine (Expanded Commission E Monographs). Integrative Medicine Communications 257–263, 2000.
18. Flora K, et al. Milk thistle for the therapy of liver disease. Am J Gastroenterol 93:139–143, 1998.
19. Heber D, et al. Cholesterol-lowering effects of a proprietary Chinese red-yeast-rice dietary supplement. Am J Clin Nutr 69:231–236, 1999.
20. Taylor D: Effects of behavioral stress management program on anxiety, mood, self esteem, and T-cell count in HIV-positive men. Psycholog Rep 76:451–457, 1995.
21. Fletcher M, Schneiderman N. Cognitive behavioral stress management decreases dysphoric mood and herpes simplex virus-type 2 antibody titers in symptomatic HIV-seropositive gay men. J Consul Clin Psychol 65:31–43, 1997.
22. McCain NL, et al. The influence of stress management training in HIV disease. Nurs Res 45:246–253, 1996.
23. Sanzero L. Effects of cognitive-behavioral interventions on quality of life in persons with HIV. Int J Nurs Stud 36:223–233, 1999.
24. Shlay CJ, et al. Acupuncture and amitriptyline for pain due to HIV-related peripheral neuropathy. JAMA 280:1590–1595, 1998.
25. Scafidi F, Field T. Massage therapy improves behavior in neonates born to HIV-positive mothers. J Pediatr Psychol 21:889–897, 1996.
26. Ironsen G, Field T: Massage therapy is associated with enhancement of the immune system's cytotoxic capacity. Int J Neurosci 84:205–217, 1996.

Additional Reading

Allard J, Aghdassi E, Chau J, et al. Effects of vitamin E and C supplementation on oxidative stress and viral load in HIV-infected subjects. AIDS 12:1653–1659, 1998.

Constants J, Delmas Beauvieux MC, Sergeant C, et al. One year antioxidant supplementation with beta-carotene or selenium for patients infected with human immunodeficiency virus: A pilot study. Clin Infect Dis 23:654–656, 1996.

Coodley G, Coodley M, Lusk R, et al. Beta-carotene in HIV infection: An extended evaluation. AIDS 10:967–973, 1996.

Elion RA, Cohen C: Complementary medicine and HIV infection. Primary Care 24:905–919, 1997.

Ernst E: Complementary AIDS therapies: The good, the bad and the ugly. Int J STD AIDS 8:281–285, 1997.

Garewal S, Ampel N, Watson R, et al. A preliminary trial of beta-carotene in subjects infected with the human immunodeficiency virus. J Nutr 122:728–732, 1992.

Gorter R, Van Wely M, Reif M, et al. Tolerability of an extract of European mistletoe among immunocompromised and healthy individuals. Altern Ther 5:37–48, 1999.

Nimmagadda A, Burri B, Neidlinger T, et al. Effect of oral beta-carotene supplementation on plasma HIV RNA levels and CD4$^+$ cell counts in HIV-infected patients. Clin Infect Dis 27:1311–1313, 1998.

Ozsoy M, Ernst E: How effective are complementary therapies for HIV and AIDS? A systematic review. Int J STD AIDS 10:629–635, 1999.

Robinson F, Mathews H, Witek-Janusek L. Stress reduction and HIV disease: A review of intervention studies using a psychoneuroimmunology framework. J Assoc Nurses AIDS Care 11:87-96, 2000.

Tang A, Graham N, Humphrey J, et al. Dietary micronutrient intake and risk of progression to AIDS in HIV-infected homosexual men. Am J Epidemiol 138:937–951, 1993.

Weber R, Christen L, Loy M, et al. Randomized placebo-controlled trial of Chinese herb therapy for HIV-1 infected individuals. J Acquir Immune Defic Syndr 22:56–64, 1999.

Wu B: Recent developments of studies on traditional Chinese medicine in prophylaxis and treatment of AIDS. J Tradit Chin Med 12:10–20, 1992.

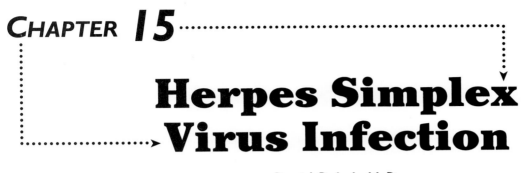

CHAPTER 15

Herpes Simplex Virus Infection

David Rakel, M.D.

PATHOPHYSIOLOGY

Herpes simplex virus (HSV), a member of the family Herpesviridae, has troubled the human race for more than 2000 years. The term *herpes* comes from the Greek language meaning "to creep or crawl." Two types of virus most commonly cause these creeping eruptions: herpes simplex virus type 1 (HSV-1) and herpes simplex virus type 2 (HSV-2). HSV infection can cause symptoms anywhere on the body, but HSV-1 is generally associated with outbreaks above the waist, particularly around the lips in the form of cold sores, and HSV-2 with symptoms below the waist, specifically the genital area. HSV infection preferentially affects these mucous membranes, where the skin is thin. Other common dermal areas of infection are those that are overly moist or where the natural protection has been compromised by injury or disease.

The first episode of HSV infection (primary herpes) is usually the most severe and starts after an incubation period of 4 to 6 days, but onset may be seen 1 to 26 days after exposure. The classic progression of symptoms involves pain, inflammation, and erythema followed by the formation of clear vesicles on an erythematous base. The clear fluid may then become pustular, followed by scab formation. Scarring is rare. Healing occurs over a 1- to 6-week period. After the primary infection, HSV has a unique ability to migrate up the peripheral sensory nerve to the dorsal root ganglia, where it lies dormant until reactivated (Fig. 15–1). How the virus is triggered to reactivate is unknown, but clinical correlation can be seen with a number of different stimuli (Table 15–1).

The function of the immune system plays an important role in the severity of disease and the frequency of recurrences. Persons with immune deficiency are at higher risk for complications. It is interesting to observe that many more people have been exposed to HSV than show symptoms or recurrences. In one study, 72% of persons with antibodies to HSV-2 shed virus when they were without symptoms.[1] What makes some people more or less susceptible to the potential effects of this virus is a point for further study and invites an integrative therapeutic approach to reduce the severity of the disease once exposure has occurred.

INTEGRATIVE THERAPY

Lifestyle Considerations

Personal Contact

Avoiding exposure to persons experiencing outbreaks of either HSV-1 or HSV-2 infection is warranted but does not ensure against contracting the disease. Use of condoms while limiting the number of sexual partners will help reduce the prevalence of infection. Oral sex should also be avoided because genital herpes can cause oral lesions, and vice versa.

NOTE

As many as 90% of persons infected with genital herpes are unaware of their infection and may unknowingly shed virus and transmit infection.[2]

Autoinoculation

The patient should be educated on how to prevent transmission to other parts of the body during an outbreak. For example, after bathing, patting dry with a towel instead of rubbing should be encouraged. The transmission of vesicular fluid to other parts of the body must be avoided.

Trauma to the Skin

HSV is more prone to causing recurrence and primary infection if the skin is traumatized or exposed to ultraviolet radiation. The patient should be encouraged to use sun protection to help prevent recurrence of HSV-1 infection, should avoid traumatic intercourse, and should prevent chapping of the lips. Using zinc ointment on the lips not only protects against ultraviolet light exposure but may also help to suppress HSV growth.

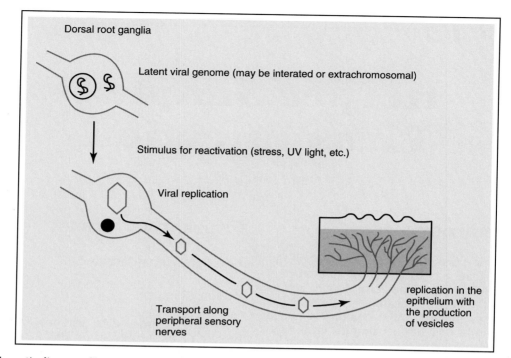

Figure 15–1. Schematic diagram of herpes simplex virus latency and reactivation. UV, ultraviolet. (From Whitley RJ: Herpes simplex virus infections. In Goldman L, Bennett JC [eds]: Cecil Textbook of Medicine, 21st ed. Philadelphia, WB Saunders, 2001; 1810–1814.)

Table 15–1. Potential Triggering Factors for Reactivation of Herpes

HSV-1–Specific Triggers
Ultraviolet light
Immunodeficiency
Stress, depression, anxiety (chronic)
Poor sleep
Trauma to mucosa
Cold, windy, or dry weather
Hot food or lip biting
Food allergy
Fever

HSV-2–Specific Triggers
Immunodeficiency
Stress, depression, anxiety (chronic)
Poor sleep
Food allergy
Trauma to genital mucosa
Menses (usually 5–12 days before onset)

Sleep

Poor sleep hygiene can result in fatigue, which may lead to an increased frequency of recurrence. The clinician should specifically inquire about sleep habits to help the patient make changes that will result in an improved sleep cycle.

Nutrition

Lysine- and Arginine-Containing Foods

A diet that promotes lysine-rich foods and reduces arginine-containing foods has become a popular recommendation for helping patients reduce recurrence of HSV infections. Evidence from in vitro studies supports this approach. The replication of the virus requires proteins rich in arginine, and arginine itself may be a stimulator of HSV replication. Lysine exerts antiviral effects by blocking the activity of arginine.[3] Clinical studies show mixed results.[4, 5] One argument is that inadequate doses of lysine were used. In one study, 52 people with recurring oral and genital HSV infections were assigned to receive either L-lysine 1 g 3 times daily or placebo; they also avoided nuts, chocolate, and gelatin (arginine-rich foods). After 6 months, 74% of persons receiving lysine reported their treatment as either effective or very effective, versus 28% of those receiving placebo. The mean number of outbreaks was 3.1 in the lysine group, compared with 4.2 in those taking placebo.[6]

There is some concern that taking supplemental lysine for prolonged periods of time may increase the risk of atherosclerosis, possibly by increasing levels of low-density lipoproteins.[7] Accordingly, adjusting

Table 15–2. Arginine-Containing and Lysine-Rich Foods: Dietary Recommendations for Prophylaxis of Herpes Simplex Virus Infection Recurrence

Foods to Avoid (High Arginine Content)	Foods to Include (High Lysine Content)
Chocolate	Vegetables
Peanuts	Beans
Almonds	Fish
Cashews	Turkey
Sunflower seeds	Chicken
Gelatin	

the amount of arginine in the diet by reducing arginine-rich foods may be the safer approach (see Table 15–2).

Food Allergy

Although there is limited research to back the claim that food allergies trigger recurrences of HSV infection, a trial of an elimination diet should be offered to persons with frequent recurrences (see Chapter 82, on elimination diets).

Good Nutrition

The most important nutritional factor in prevention of HSV infection is a balanced diet with 7 or 8 servings of fruits and vegetables a day, to help support a healthy immune system.

Mind-Body Medicine

It has been a common belief that isolated stressful events may lead to recurrent HSV outbreaks, although research has not supported this association. One study of 64 people with HSV infection found no correlation between acute stressful events and a later outbreak.[8] On the other hand, chronic or persistent stressors have been found to correlate with an increased frequency of recurrence.[9] This correlation is consistent with findings showing a decrease in HSV immunity in caregivers of dementia sufferers[10] and a decrease in herpes zoster immunity in persons with depression.[11] Therapeutic focus should be on helping the patient find a balance of lifestyle demands and on learning techniques to reduce day-to-day stress in persons with frequent recurrences.

NOTE

Chronic rather than isolated stress has been found to result in more frequent HSV outbreaks.

Relaxation Exercises

Teaching the patient a simple relaxation exercise that can be used on a regular basis or when needed for recurring stressful events can empower the patient to learn how to reduce stress (see Chapter 91, Prescribing Relaxation Techniques).

Meditation

For persons with chronic recurring stress, practice of meditation can help to reduce the stimulation of

the adrenal gland. Overactivity of the adrenals can lead to suppression of the immune response and increase susceptibility to recurrent HSV infection (see Chapter 94, Learning to Meditate).

Supplements

Vitamin C

When used early in the prodrome of an outbreak, vitamin C 1000 mg with the addition of 1000 mg bioflavonoids taken 5 times a day for 3 days after recognition of symptoms was found to reduce blister healing time in herpes labialis, from 10 days in the placebo group to 4.4 days in the treatment group.[12]

Zinc

Zinc has been found to inhibit HSV replication in vitro and enhances cell-mediated immunity to help reduce HSV infection recurrence. Oral compound of 25 mg of zinc with 250 mg of vitamin C was given twice a day for 6 weeks, which resulted in either complete suppression of an outbreak or resolution of HSV-1 eruptions within 24 hours.[13] Topical application of a zinc sulfate solution of 0.01% to 0.025% concentration has also been found to be helpful in healing HSV-1 lesions and in inhibiting recurrence.[14] Use of zinc and vitamin C supplementation constitutes an inexpensive option for the patient with frequent recurrences.

Dosage. Zinc 25 mg a day with vitamin C 250 mg a day for recurrence prophylaxis.

Precautions. In prescribing zinc supplementation, the clinician should be aware that zinc competes with copper, calcium, and iron absorption. The patient should not take more than the recommended dose and should not take calcium and iron supplements with zinc. Doses greater than 50 mg per day have been found to be associated with reduction in serum copper levels.

Lysine

As discussed previously under "Nutrition," lysine exerts antiviral effects by blocking the activity of arginine, which promotes HSV replication. Although the results of research are mixed, a trial of 1 g of lysine daily to prevent recurrences, increased to 1 g 3 times a day during an outbreak, seems reasonable.

Dosage. L-Lysine 1 g daily for prevention, 1 g 3 times a day for acute outbreaks.

Precautions. Diarrhea and abdominal pain have been reported in persons taking doses of more than 10 g a day. There has been a single case documented of tubulointerstitial nephritis progressing to renal failure.[15] Lysine may cause a modest rise in low-density lipoprotein levels.

Vitamin E Oil

Topical application of vitamin E oil has been found to help reduce the pain of oral herpetic lesions within 8 hours and to result in more rapid healing.[16, 17]

Dosage. Squeeze the contents of a vitamin E capsule (*d*-alpha-tocopherol) onto a cotton swab and apply directly to the lesion every 8 hours as needed.

Precautions. Local skin reaction is possible but is rare.

Botanicals

Lemon Balm

Lemon balm (*Melissa officinalis*) is the most common botanical used for treatment of herpes infections. Lemon balm ointment consists of a 70:1 lemon extract concentrate. The preparation has been found to be helpful for the treatment of active HSV outbreaks. In one large study involving three German hospitals and a dermatology clinic, when lemon balm was used to treat the primary infection of HSV-1, not a single recurrence was noted. This finding suggests that lemon balm may help to prevent recurrences if used during an initial infection. The cream has also been found to reduce the healing time for both genital and oral herpes lesions.[18]

Dosage. 70:1 lemon extract cream, applied fairly thickly (1 mm) to herpetic lesions 2 to 4 times a day.

Precautions. Toxicology studies have found lemon balm to be safe and suitable for long-term use.

Licorice Root

Licorice (*Glycyrrhiza glabra*) is well known for its anti-inflammatory properties and has also been found to be of benefit in inhibiting both the growth and cytopathic effects of HSV.[19] Topical application of licorice root preparations is an option to help reduce duration of outbreaks and severity of oral herpes lesions.

Dosage. Apply tincture of licorice with a cotton swab, or drop directly onto the lesions, three times a day until resolution.

Precautions. Local allergic reaction may be seen with topical application.

Tea Bags

A folk remedy that has been found to be an inexpensive and easy-to-prepare treatment for oral HSV lesions is to steep an ordinary tea bag (preferably Earl Gray tea), cool, and then apply to lesions. This measure is thought to speed healing and to prevent recurrence, although there are no studies to support this. Tea contains catechins that have been found to enhance the immune function and may be a component of its therapeutic benefit.

Dosage. Steep a tea bag, cool, and apply directly to lesions for 20 minutes 1 to 3 times a day.

Pharmaceuticals

Antiviral medications effective against HSV work by inactivating DNA polymerase, which inhibits viral replication. In order for these medications to be effective, they need to be started soon after symptoms appear because viral replication may end as early as 48 hours into an infection.

Oral antiviral medications should be used with caution in persons with underlying kidney disease or when given with other nephrotoxic drugs. As with any antimicrobial, regular use can result in viral resistance.

Treatment for Primary Genital Herpes Infection

- Acyclovir (Zovirax) 200 mg 5 times daily for 10 days
- Famciclovir (Famvir) 250 mg 3 times daily for 10 days
- Valacyclovir (Valtrex) 1 g twice daily for 10 days

Although more expensive, valacyclovir has the advantage of reduced frequency of dosing.

Treatment for Episodic Recurrences

Research has shown only a minimal benefit with treatment of recurrences with antiviral medications, and some experts may question the need for episodic treatment. Best results are obtained if the drug is started at the prodrome of the recurrence, when the patient notices itching, burning, or erythema.

- Acyclovir (Zovirax) 800 mg twice daily for 5 days
- Famciclovir (Famvir) 125 mg twice daily for 5 days
- Valacyclovir (Valtrex) 500 mg twice daily for 5 days

Pharmaceutical Prophylaxis

Prophylaxis is generally reserved for persons who have more than 6 outbreaks in a year. For patients with frequent recurrences, the practitioner should look holistically at other potential factors such as chronic stress, suboptimal nutrition, and decrease in perceived level of well-being before simply prescribing prophylactic antiviral medication. If pharmaceutical prophylaxis is started, therapy should be discontinued once a year to see whether continuation is necessary, and the patient should be encouraged to titrate down to the lowest effective dose.

Short-term prophylactic therapy for oral herpes

has been shown to reduce severity but not recurrence following ultraviolet light exposure in skiers.[20]

- Acyclovir (Zovirax) 400 mg twice daily
- Famciclovir (Famvir) 250 mg twice daily
- Valacyclovir (Valtrex) 1 g once daily
- Aspirin 125 mg daily

In a small pilot study, aspirin was found to reduce the rate of active infection by nearly 50%.[2] This inexpensive therapy may prove fruitful if more research supports this claim.

NOTE

Topical acyclovir is generally not highly effective for the treatment or prevention of oral herpes infections. Topical application of acyclovir every 2 hours was found to reduce healing time by just 1 day.[22]

Other Therapies to Consider

Monolaurin

Monolaurin (Laricidin) is a monoglycerol ester of lauric acid, a saturated fatty acid found in breast milk and coconut oil. It has been found to destroy the fatty coating of certain viruses that allows them to adhere to cells, causing infection. It is thought to help protect breast-feeding infants from viral infection. Monolaurin is currently being studied for its potential use in treating infections due to lipid-coated viruses including HIV. There is a lack of evidence to recommend its use at this time, but patients have reported clinical benefit from this inexpensive therapy.

Dosage. At the first sign of infection, the patient should take 1800 to 3600 mg (6 to 12 300-mg capsules) daily for 4 days and then reduce the dose to 600 to 1200 mg (2 to 4 300-mg capsules) daily until lesions have resolved.

Precautions. Animals fed monolaurin in amounts up to 25% of their diet showed no signs of harm after 6 weeks.[23] Human studies are limited.

Homeopathy

Homeopathic remedies are given until resolution of lesions occurs. Examples of remedies used for genital HSV infection are sepia, graphites, rhus (toxicodendron), and dulcamara. Hylands #27 is a common homeopathic remedy for oral HSV infection.

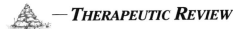 **THERAPEUTIC REVIEW**

Prevention of HSV Infection Recurrences

Lifestyle
- *Avoid trauma to genital and oral mucosa.*
- *Use sun protection.*
- *Encourage 7 to 8 hours of sleep a night.*

Nutrition
- *Encourage 7 or 8 servings of fruits and vegetables a day while increasing lysine-rich foods and reducing arginine-rich foods (see Table 15–2).*
- *Consider an elimination diet (see Chapter 82).*

Mind-Body Medicine
- *Make lifestyle changes to reduce chronic stress and anxiety.*
- *Educate regarding relaxation techniques such as breathing exercises and meditation.*

Supplements
- *Zinc 25 mg and vitamin C 250 mg a day*
- *If no reduction in frequency of recurrences is obtained after 3 months, consider replacing with or adding lysine 1 g daily.*

Botanical Medicine
- *Apply lemon balm extract cream 2 to 4 times a day for primary outbreaks of HSV infection*

Pharmaceuticals
- *Prophylactic therapy is reserved for persons who have not responded to a holistic therapeutic approach and who experience more than 6 outbreaks in a year.*
- *Acyclovir (Zovirax) 400 mg twice daily*
- *Valacyclovir (Valtrex) 1 g once daily*

THERAPEUTIC REVIEW continued

Acute Treatment of HSV Infection

Supplements

- *L-Lysine 1 g 3 times a day until resolution*
- *Topical vitamin E oil: Apply oil from capsule to oral HSV lesion 3 times a day.*

Botanicals

- *Lemon balm (70:1 lemon extract cream): Apply to herpetic outbreak 2 to 4 times a day.*
- *Licorice root tincture: Apply to lesions 3 times daily until resolution.*
- *Tea bag: Steep tea bag, cool, and apply directly to oral lesions for 20 minutes 1 to 3 times a day.*

Pharmaceuticals

For primary infection:

- *Acyclovir (Zovirax) 200 mg 5 times daily for 10 days*
- *Famciclovir (Famvir) 250 mg 3 times daily for 10 days*
- *Valacyclovir (Valtrex) 1 g twice daily for 10 days*

Efficacy of treating episodic recurrences remains to be established, but the following can be tried:

- *Acyclovir (Zovirax) 800 mg twice daily for 5 days*

References

1. Wald A, Zeh J, Selke S, et al: Reactivation of genital herpes simplex virus type 2 infection in asymptomatic seropositive persons. N Engl J Med 342:844–850, 2000.
2. Mertz GJ: Epidemiology of genital herpes infection. Infect Dis Clin North Am 7:825–839, 1993.
3. Griffith R, DeLong D, Nelson J: Relation of arginine-lysine antagonism to herpes simplex growth in tissue culture. Chemotherapy 27:209–213, 1981.
4. DiGiovanna J, Blank H: Failure of lysine in frequently recurrent herpes simplex infection. Arch Dermatol 120:48–51, 1984.
5. McCune MA, Perry HO, Muller SA: Treatment of recurrent herpes simplex infections with L-lysine monohydrochlorite. Cutis 34:366–373, 1984.
6. Griffith RS, Walsh DE, Myrmel KH: Success of L-lysine therapy in frequently recurrent herpes simplex infection. Dermatologica 175:183–190, 1987.
7. Sanchez A: Nutr RE Int 28:497, 1983.
8. Rand KH, Hoon EF, Massey JK, et al: Daily stress and recurrence of genital herpes simplex. Arch Intern Med 150:1889–1893, 1990.
9. Cohen F, Kemeny ME, Kearney KA, et al: Persistent stress as a predictor of genital herpes recurrence. Arch Intern Med 159:2430–2436, 1999.
10. Glaser R, Kiecolt-Glaser JK: Chronic stress modulates the virus-specific immune response to latent herpes simplex virus type 1. Ann Behav Med 19:78–82, 1997.
11. Irwin M, Costlow C, Williams H, et al: Cellular immunity to varicella-zoster virus in patients with major depression. J Infect Dis 178 (Suppl 1):S104–S108, 1998.
12. Terzhalmy G, Bottomley W, Pelleu G: The use of water-soluble bioflavonoid-ascorbic acid complex in the treatment of recurrent herpes labialis. Oral Surg 45:56–62, 1978.
13. Fitzherbert J: Genital herpes and zinc. Med J Aust 1:399, 1979.
14. Brody I: Topical treatment of recurrent herpes simplex and post-herpetic erythema multiforme with low concentrations of zinc sulphate solution. Br J Dermatol 104:191–213, 1981.
15. Lo JC, et al: Fanconi's syndrome and tubulointerstitial nephritis in association with L-lysine ingestion. Am J Kidney Dis 28:614–617, 1996.
16. Fink M, Fink J: Treatment of herpes simplex by alpha-tocopherol (vitamin E). Br Dent J 148:246, 1980.
17. Starasoler S, Haber GS: Use of vitamin E oil in primary herpes gingivostomatitis in an adult. N Y State Dent J 44:382–383, 1978.
18. Wolbing R, Leonhardt K: Local therapy of herpes simplex with dried extract from Melissa officinalis. Phytomed 1:25–31, 1994.
19. Pompei R, Pant A, Flore O, et al: Antiviral activity of glycerrhizic acid. Experientia 36:304, 1980.

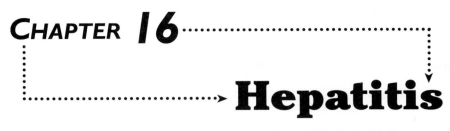

CHAPTER 16

Hepatitis

David Rakel, M.D.

PATHOPHYSIOLOGY

Hepatitis implies inflammation that, if present over extended periods, can result in fibrosis and scarring that may lead to cirrhosis or even hepatocellular carcinoma. The etiology of chronic hepatitis can be multifactorial (Table 16–1), but the clinician is most often confronted with the asymptomatic patient with hepatitis C virus (HCV) who wants to learn how best to prevent the progression of this inflammatory process. HCV is the focus of this chapter, but general guidelines for this integrative approach would also apply to most chronic forms of liver inflammation.

Chronic hepatitis is defined as liver cell necrosis with inflammation that lasts longer than 6 months. This process involves infiltration of mononuclear cells (lymphocytes and plasma cells) in the hepatic portal areas. As the inflammation progresses, these areas bridge from one portal area to the next, resulting in "bridging necrosis." Over time, fibrosis and nodular regeneration can result in cirrhosis. There does not appear to be a correlation between the amount of virus present (viral load) and the histologic injury of liver cells. This damage may be more related to an immune reaction to the virus that leads to inflammation.

NOTE

Even though the absence of virus (and normal ALT) in the serum is a marker for defining response to pharmacologic treatment, there does not appear to be a correlation between the amount of virus present and hepatocyte injury.[1]

The diagnosis of chronic hepatitis cannot be confirmed without a biopsy. The results of this test can also be very helpful in decision making about modes of treatment. For example, the 10-year risk for cirrhosis is less than 10% among those with mild to minimal hepatitis, 44% among those with moderate hepatitis, and 100% in those with severe hepatitis with bridging necrosis.

A majority of the patients infected with HCV have minimal inflammation and are not candidates for aggressive pharmaceutical therapy but would benefit from an integrative approach. Those with more severe inflammation should be considered for therapy that may include alpha interferon and ribavirin. A paradox arises when one considers the type of patient who "responds" best to treatment versus the type who is at higher risk of progressing to severe disease without it (Table 16–2). Treatment works best in those with minimal inflammation, but this group is least likely to have future problems. Treatment does not appear to work as well in those with more severe inflammation despite their higher risk for complications from the disease. The question is whether the patient with mild inflammation should be given a treatment with significant adverse effects and cost to treat a condition that has a natural history of a disease-free life.

This question can be approached with open discussion involving the individual, the primary care provider, and the gastrointestinal consultant. Whatever course is taken, the primary care provider can have a positive influence regarding the many other measures that can be taken to promote health.

Table 16–1. Etiology of Chronic Hepatitis

Autoimmune diseases
Hepatitis viruses
Drugs and toxins
Wilson's disease
α_1-Antitrypsin deficiency
Cryptogenic (nonimmunologic) causes

Table 16–2.

Patients who respond best to interferon plus ribavirin therapy
- Age <40 years
- Female
- No evidence of portal fibrosis
- HCV genotype 2 or 3 (majority [70%–80%] are type 1)
- HCV RNA viral load <3.5 million copies/mL
- Short duration of infection
- White or Asian ethnicity

Patients at high risk for end-stage liver disease who should consider interferon treatment
- Age >40 years
- HCV genotype 2 or 3
- Moderate to severe inflammation on biopsy with portal fibrosis
- Coexisting illness (e.g., HIV)

Liver Detoxification

Before therapy for hepatitis is discussed, it would be helpful to review how the liver performs its job of detoxification. The liver does this by filtering the blood, expelling toxic substances through the production and excretion of bile, and eliminating and neutralizing chemicals through a two-step process, called phase I and phase II detoxification.

Phase I Detoxification

This step neutralizes chemicals and many pharmaceutical agents through a series of enzymes grouped under the heading of the cytochrome P-450 system. Approximately 50 to 100 enzymes are involved. They transform a toxin to a more chemically reactive form that is then more easily metabolized by the phase II enzymes. When a toxin is neutralized by the P-450 enzymes, free radicals are produced that are removed by many of the antioxidants of the liver. One of the most important is glutathione. When the liver is exposed to high levels of toxins, the glutathione level (which is also used in phase II) can become depleted, resulting in an inability of phase II detoxification to further clear the toxins. This process may explain why exposing the body to high or prolonged levels of toxins may result in an imbalance of the body's ability to clear them.

Phase II Detoxification

This step generally involves a conjugation reaction whereby the liver changes the composition of the toxin so that it can be excreted through the urine or bile. The six detoxification pathways include glutathione conjugation, amino acid conjugation, methylation, sulfation, acetylation, and glucuronidation[2] (Table 16–3). Glutathione conjugation, for example, takes a fat-soluble toxin and makes it a water-soluble toxin so that it can be excreted through the urine. This system also acts as a powerful mechanism for protecting the body against carcinogenesis, mutagenesis, xenobiotics, and reactive forms of oxygen.

For the liver to function optimally, an environment must be created that encourages efficient functioning of these two systems. This is influenced by multiple factors that can be addressed when the practitioner focuses on the best approach to treating chronic hepatitis. There are three goals in treating the hepatitis patient:

1. Enhance the liver's detoxification ability.
2. Decrease inflammation of the liver that can result in further damage that leads to cirrhosis.
3. Prevent progression to hepatocellular carcinoma that can arise within fibrosis and scarring.

INTEGRATIVE THERAPY

Lifestyle

Reduce Exposure to Toxins

If the liver is inflamed or injured, its workload must be reduced. Reducing toxins or products that require metabolism by the liver prevents buildup that may cause further progression of the disease process.

Eating organically grown foods and drinking filtered water can also reduce the number of hepatotoxins. The patient should also avoid any unnecessary drugs or supplements that require liver metabolism.

Avoid Alcohol and Tobacco Products

Alcohol intake in patients with HCV has been associated with increased fibrosis, risk of cirrhosis, and mortality rate, as well as reduced response to interferon.[3]

Smoking reduces glutathione levels both by detoxifying nicotine and by neutralizing the free radicals produced by the toxins in the smoke. Smoking increases the risk of hepatocellular carcinoma.[4]

Exercise Regularly

Regular exercise enhances blood flow through the liver and results in improvement in fatigue and well-being. Encourage a realistic exercise program that meets patients at their current ability and encourages gradual progression. (See Chapter 86, Writing an Exercise Prescription.)

Obtain Vaccination

Anyone with documented viral hepatitis or chronic liver disease should be vaccinated for both hepatitis A and B. Coinfection with more than one

Table 16–3. Nutrients Needed by Phase II Detoxification Enzymes

Phase II System	Required Nutrients
Glutathione conjugation	Glutathione, vitamin B_6
Amino acid conjugation	Glycine
Methylation	S-adenosylmethionine (SAMe)
Sulfation	Cysteine, methionine, molybdenum
Acetylation	Acetyl-CoA
Glucuronidation	Glucuronic acid

Borrowed from Pizzorno and Murray.[2]

virus type is common and worsens prognosis in those who have contracted more than one hepatitis virus.

Nutrition

Cruciferous Vegetables

This term comes from the word *cruc* meaning "to cross." These plants in the cabbage family have four-petaled flowers or leaves that form a cross; these include Brussels sprouts, broccoli, cauliflower, kale, mustard greens, radish, and bok choy. They have been found to activate the cytochrome P-450 enzymes as well as the phase II system.

Cruciferous vegetables have also been found to have cancer-preventing effects. One of many components of these vegetables, indol-3-carbinol, stimulates detoxifying enzymes in the gut as well as the liver.[5, 6] Encourage regular consumption of these vegetables.

Oranges and Tangerines

These fruits contain a phytochemical called *limonene* that has been found to be a strong inducer of both phase I and II detoxification systems.[7] Orange juice may be a good product to recommend because of its high folate content, which may also have beneficial effects in chronic hepatitis. One glass of orange juice has approximately 60 mg of vitamin C and 60 μg of folate.

Grapefruit

Many foods can inhibit phase I detoxification; grapefruit is one of the more potent of these. Others include curcumin, the compound that gives tumeric its yellow color (but stimulates phase II), capsaicin from red chili pepper, and quercetin from onions. Grapefruit contains naringenin, which is thought to inhibit the cytochrome P-450 3A4 system by up to 30%. This can make toxins potentially more damaging because they remain in the body longer before they are metabolized.[8] Some healthcare providers even use this to their advantage by having patients take their cholesterol-lowering medicine (statin) with a glass of grapefruit juice, resulting in the need for lower doses and a financial savings. Unfortunately, this can also increase the potential for toxicity.

Dietary Fat

The goal here is to reduce the intake of unsaturated fats (particularly omega-6 fatty acids). Unsaturated fats are more prone to oxidation, which can be dangerous to a damaged liver. Heating omega-6–rich oils that have been partially hydrogenated, such as vegetable oil, sunflower oil, and soybean oils that are rich in trans-fatty acids, can produce even more free radicals. The patient should be instructed to use monounsaturated oils such as olive and canola oils for cooking, to reduce the total amount of fat intake,[9] and to replace omega-6 fatty acids with omega-3 fatty acids to help reduce inflammation. Omega-3 fatty acids from fish oils are known to reduce tumor necrosis factor that is involved in stimulating inflammation of the liver.[10] (See Chapter 84, The Anti-Inflammatory Diet.)

Dietary Fiber

Fiber has been found to help bind toxins in the intestines, resulting in the prevention of absorption and excretion through the bowel. Encourage a diet rich in fruits and vegetables and consider supplementing with a soluble fiber such as methylcellulose (Citrucel) or psyllium (Metamucil). A breakfast muesli originated by Milliman, Lamson, and Brignall at Bastyr University can be recommended for regular use (Table 16–4).

Green Tea

Research has shown that the polyphenols in green tea have preventative and inhibitory effects against tumor formation and growth.[11] One study of 124 patients with viral hepatitis treated with 3 g of catechins (found in green tea) versus placebo resulted in significantly lower levels of aspartate transaminase (AST), alanine transaminase (ALT), and serum bilirubin. Compared with other types of acute viral hepatitis, HCV had the best response.[12] Decaffeinated green tea would make for a nice beverage substitute. Encourage 2 to 3 cups daily.

Table 16–4. Breakfast Muesli

Rolled oats	4 lb
Oat bran	2 lb
Fresh ground flax	1 lb
Granulated lecithin	1 lb
Fresh ground milk thistle seed	1 lb
Whole raw almonds	½ lb
Whole raw sunflower seeds	½ lb
Wheat germ	1 lb

Instructions: Grind the flax and milk thistle seeds. Mix all ingredients together. Refrigerate the mixture until ready to use. Eat 4 oz every morning for breakfast served with dilute fruit juice and live yogurt. Recipe makes a 40-day supply.

From Milliman et al.[40]

NOTE

For patients with end-stage liver disease, a nutrition consult is warranted to help organize a diet based on individualized needs that would include protein requirements.

Supplements

Glutathione

Although dietary glutathione is well absorbed into the blood through dietary sources such as fresh fruits, vegetables, and cooked fish and meat, glutathione in supplements does not appear to do the same. One study found that giving up to 3000 mg of oral glutathione supplement did not result in increased circulating levels.[13] But there are other ways to increase serum glutathione, including vitamin E, vitamin C, N-acetylcysteine, and milk thistle.

Vitamin C

Vitamin C raises glutathione levels by increasing its rate of synthesis. This effect is not dose dependent. A dose of 500 mg per day has been found to raise red blood cell glutathione concentration by nearly 50%, but raising the dose to 2000 mg did not result in higher levels.[14]

Dosage. 200 to 250 mg twice daily

Vitamin E

Vitamin E also increases glutathione levels and has antioxidant effects. It has been found to reduce liver enzymes in patients with hepatitis C at a dose of 800 IU per day.[15] Vitamin E has also resulted in greater response to interferon therapy with reduced viral load in one small pilot trial.[16]

Dosage. *d*-alpha tocopherol 800 IU daily

N-Acetylcysteine

N-Acetylcysteine (NAC; Mucomyst) is used as a mucolytic for lung disease and to help protect the liver in acetaminophen poisoning. This poisoning is thought to occur by depletion of glutathione in the liver, a mechanism prevented by NAC. It is available over the counter as a dietary supplement and is commonly used as an antioxidant. It is a precursor to the production of glutathione and has been found to raise serum levels, although not by as much as they are raised by vitamin C.[17] The long-term safety of this product in otherwise healthy people is yet to be proved. In fact, one study showed that doses greater than 1.2 g per day resulted in increased damage secondary to its pro-oxidant effect.[18] Because of the questionable safety and high cost of N-acetylcysteine, the clinician would do better to recommend vitamin E, vitamin C, and milk thistle for raising glutathione levels at this time.

Dosage. 800 mg per day

Precautions. Doses higher than 1.2 g per day can result in a pro-oxidant effect.

N-Acetylcysteine can cause nausea, vomiting, urticaria, stomatitis, drowsiness, runny nose, chest tightness, bronchoconstriction, and even elevation of liver enzymes.

Selenium

We get selenium by eating plants that incorporate selenium from the soil into their structure. If plants are eaten from soil that is selenium-poor, supplementation may be needed. In the United States, the Eastern Coastal Plain and the Pacific Northwest have the lowest soil selenium levels. The main benefit of selenium for treatment of chronic hepatitis is its property of protecting the body from cancer. In one study, a group of 4800 patients with serum markers for hepatitis were followed over 5.3 years. Seventy-three cases of hepatocellular cancer were inversely related to mean selenium levels. Those with higher levels were found to have a 60% reduction in their chance of developing the cancer.[19]

Dosage. 200 μg per day

Precautions. When selenium is taken at recommended doses, adverse effects are rare. Some patients may acutely experience nausea, vomiting, fatigue, and irritability. Toxicity can occur with chronic elevated exposure. Serum levels greater than 2000 mcg/L can result in hepatorenal dysfunction and thrombocytopenia.

S-Adenosylmethionine

This naturally occurring molecule is found in virtually all body tissues and plays an essential role in transmethylation (donation of methyl groups), which is one of the key methods of detoxification in the phase II system. Methionine, an essential amino acid, needs to be activated to S-adenosylmethionine (SAMe), a process that is impaired in liver disease. Supplementing the patient with SAMe may aid this process. A placebo-controlled study showed that 400 mg tid for 2 years in patients with alcoholic cirrhosis resulted in improved survival and a delay in the need for liver transplantation.[20] The high cost of this supplement and the lack of clinical data regarding its use in viral hepatitis do not warrant regular use. But supplementation may be recommended for patients with alcoholic liver cirrhosis.

Dosage. Typical dose for liver disease is 800 mg twice daily.

Precautions. SAMe can cause flatulence, vomiting,

diarrhea, and headache, as well as anxiety in those with depression, and hypomania in those with bipolar disorder.

Iron Supplements

Elevated serum iron levels are associated with an increase in the severity of viral hepatitis infection.[21] In patients with reduced iron levels treated with interferon, response was improved and ALT levels were lowered.[22] Iron supplements should be avoided except in cases of documented deficiency. Supplements that bind iron and reduce its load on the liver may be beneficial. One of these is thiamine (vitamin B_1). Thiamine at 100 mg per day was associated with reduced ALT levels and a decline in hepatitis B virus (HBV) DNA to undetectable levels in three patients with chronic HBV.[23] Thiamine can be obtained by having the patient take a B-complex vitamin.

Botanicals

Milk Thistle (*Silybum marianum*)

This herb dates back 2000 years to the Roman empire, where it was mixed with honey and used for "carrying off bile" for liver obstruction. Today, much about this plant remains undiscovered, but research has found it to work through at least three mechanisms.

1. Protection of the hepatocyte cell membrane from toxins

    Silymarin is the treatment of choice for Deathcap mushroom *(Amanita phalloides)* poisoning, which provides an excellent example of how this protection takes place. Deathcap, when ingested, causes severe damage to the liver. One part of silymarin, silibinin, binds to the cell wall, preventing penetration of this toxin. Milk thistle has been found to be protective against other toxins as well, such as pesticides, drugs, and halogenated cyclic hydrocarbons.
2. Antioxidant activity

    Silymarin is a potent antioxidant that is 10 times greater than that of vitamin E. It has been found to raise glutathione levels by 50% in the liver and intestines in animal studies.[24] It increases the levels of the antioxidant superoxide dismutase in red blood cells and lymphocytes.
3. Regeneration of hepatocytes

    Silymarin stimulates DNA protein synthesis and accelerates regeneration of injured or damaged hepatocytes. One might think that this could promote growth of hepatocarcinoma, but an animal study showed that this did not promote cancer growth.[25]

Clinically, silymarin has been found to reduce liver transaminase levels and result in improvement of both acute and chronic viral hepatitis. Twelve months of therapy with 420 mg of silymarin in a double-blinded trial resulted in evidence on biopsy of a reversal in liver cell damage, improved serum protein levels, improved liver enzymes, and improved symptoms in the treatment group.[26]

Silymarin has also been found to prolong survival in patients with cirrhosis (58% in the treatment group and 39% in controls) after 4 years.[27]

Dosage. Patient should take 300 mg tid (210 mg silymarin tid) The standard dose of milk thistle is based on the silymarin content, which is 70% of the bulk herb; therefore, 300 mg of milk thistle = 210 mg of silymarin.

Recommend brands wherein the herb is bound to phosphatidylcholine. This improves absorption, is more effective, and reduces the frequency of dosing, which improves compliance. The dose is 120 mg twice daily for prophylaxis and 240 mg twice daily for active treatment.

Precautions. Adverse effects are rare, and there are no known drug interactions. Milk thistle can have a laxative effect, and allergic reactions may occur in those allergic to ragweed or plants in the daisy family. Avoid alcohol extracts of this herb during treatment of hepatitis.

NOTE

Milk thistle not only protects the liver when administered prophylactically but also acts curatively to promote the regeneration of cells that are already damaged.

Licorice Root (*Glycyrrhiza glabra*)

Licorice has been an accepted treatment for hepatitis in Japan for more than 20 years. It has been found to have antiviral activity and is thought to work by preventing the virus from entering the liver cell by altering the cell membrane permeability.[28] Glycyrrhizin also works as a free radical scavenger that potentiates hepatic immune activity.

Most clinical studies showing benefit have been done using a form of intravenous glycyrrhizin called Stronger Neo Minophagen C (SNMC), which has shown results comparable to those of interferon monotherapy (which is not great—~18%). Oral formulations are well absorbed and also appear to have hepatoprotective properties. Eighty subjects with acute or chronic hepatitis B were given 750 mg glycyrrhizin (30 days for the acute group, 90 days for the chronic group) compared with a control group. Eighty-five percent of the acute hepatitis group and 75% of those in the chronic hepatitis group had significant improvement of indicators of liver function compared with 35% and 10%, respectively, in the control group.[29]

Dosage. The dose is 250 to 500 mg three times daily of the solid dry powder, 1 to 2 g three times daily of the powdered root, or 2 to 4 mL three times daily of the fluid extract.

Precautions. If taken in high doses, this botanical can lead to an aldosterone effect, causing salt retention, potassium loss, and subsequent high blood pressure. Thus while taking it, one should eat a diet high in potassium-rich foods (vegetables) and low in salt. Blood pressure and potassium levels should be monitored.

Schisandra (*Schisandra chinensis*)

This herb has been used in China for more than 1000 years to treat hepatitis, cirrhosis, and stress. The medicinal value is in the fruit. It has been found to improve bile flow, metabolism, hepatic blood flow, and hepatic cell proliferation and regeneration. It contains an antioxidant (gomisin A) that appears to be specific to the liver and has been found to decrease inflammation. It prevents the release of arachidonic acid in macrophages, thus inhibiting leukotrienes that trigger this cascade.[30] This anti-inflammatory effect may support its success in Asian medicine.

Dosage. 100 mg of the extract twice daily

Precautions. *Schisandra* has been found to enhance phase I drug metabolism in the rat model.[31] If given with drugs metabolized in the P-450 system, it may lower serum levels. Possible adverse effects include decreased appetite, stomach upset, urticaria, and CNS depression.

Astragalus (*Astragalus membranaceus*)

Astragalus is promoted for its beneficial effect on the immune system. It may cause antiviral effects by potentiating the effect of interferon and has been found to increase antibody levels of immunoglobulin A (IgA) and immunoglobulin G (IgG) in nasal secretions.[32] It also acts as a strong antioxidant by increasing superoxide dismutase and decreasing lipid peroxide.[32] This may play a role in its protective effect from hepatic toxins in animal models.[33] Although low doses have been found to enhance the immune system, high doses (>28 g) may suppress it. Caution should be used not to exceed this daily amount. In summary, *Astragalus* benefits hepatitis through its immune-enhancing, antiviral properties.

Dosage. The dose is 4 to 7 g of *Astragalus* powder daily (*Astragalus* is most commonly used in combination with other herbs).

Precautions. Doses greater than 28 g per day may cause immune suppression. Adverse effects from this herb are uncommon. Owing to its immune-stimulating properties, long-term use should be avoided in those with autoimmune disease.

Traditional Chinese Medicine

Owing to the high incidence of viral hepatitis in China, traditional Chinese medicine (TCM) has had a long history of treating chronic hepatitis using regimens based on the individual's constitutional presentation. This method of treatment is more difficult to research from the Western model because not everyone with the same disease will receive the same treatment. It is likely to provide a more efficient model of delivery of a number of different herbs that often include those discussed earlier in this chapter.

Acupuncture is not a primary therapy for chronic hepatitis but may be added depending on the practitioner's evaluation. It may be helpful in treating some of the adverse effects seen with conventional treatment, including headaches, nausea, and insomnia.

Consider a TCM referral for those patients who are not candidates for, or who choose not to undergo, conventional therapy.

Mind–Body

Clinical experience has taught us that inflammation of the liver is correlated with psychological stress. In fact, the extent of hepatic fibrosis and inflammation has been found to be associated with the degree of psychological stress in those with alcoholic hepatitis.[34] How this actually takes place needs further study, but a good example of the mind–body connection can be seen in one of the most common treatments of hepatitis—interferon.

Interferon is a natural chemical of the immune system that helps inhibit viral replication. When given as a medicine, its main adverse effects are depression and fatigue. It would make sense that when our body is infected by a virus and interferon is secreted, it would want to produce these symptoms to conserve energy while our body heals. If this can happen with just one of many cytokines of the immune system, it is not a great stretch to appreciate how stress and depression may exacerbate symptoms or quicken the progression of the disease in this mind–body model.

The two chemicals that have received the most study in relation to stress and disease are glucocorticoids and catecholamines. These communicate with cytokines that influence inflammation through the more central hypothalamic-pituitary axis (HPA). Stress has been found to induce both interleukin-6 (IL-6) and tumor necrosis factor-alpha (TNF-α) within the liver and to trigger inflammation.[35] It appears that the influence on inflammation through this mechanism is more pronounced with chronic stress versus acute stress, which warrants a therapeutic mind–body regimen.[36]

Focusing on lifestyle changes that create more balance and increase the patient's sense of control, meaning, and purpose has a positive influence on this process. As the mind finds peace, the body is more likely to follow (and vice versa). This may involve a number of different modalities based on the individual and can include counseling, journaling, behavior therapy, support groups, hypnosis, and guided imagery. Relaxation techniques that the patient can use are also worth discussing. When recommending one of these or a meditative technique, tailor it to the patient's culture and belief system. For example, you may worsen anxiety if you encourage a goal-oriented type A individual to sit and meditate daily. This person may respond better to a more active technique such as imagery, walking/jogging meditation, tai chi, or yoga. (See Chapter 91, Prescribing Relaxation Techniques.)

Pharmaceuticals

The choice of whether to start pharmaceutical agents for the treatment of viral hepatitis is controversial owing to their poor response rate, high cost, and significant adverse effect profile. Current research shows that they are best used for those patients with moderate fibrosis on liver biopsy. Those with minimal or no fibrosis are not candidates, and those with end-stage disease with cirrhosis should be considered for liver transplant. Some gastroenterologists are encouraging therapy based on serum liver markers and ultrasound. The concern about this approach is whether aggressive treatment is warranted for a disease (HCV) that most often lies dormant without progression.

Interferon alpha-2b

Interferon is one of a group of cytokines that possess antiviral and immune-modulating activities and are produced in response to viral and other antigens. Interferon inhibits viral replication and promotes viral clearance from cells. Pegylation technology links the drug to a water-soluble polymer called *polyethylene glycol (PEG)* that cloaks the drug from degradation by the immune system. This allows for better efficacy and less frequent dosing. Instead of three times weekly, it can be given just once. This formulation may slightly increase the risk of bone marrow suppression.

Dosing. PEG-Intron, 1.0 mcg/kg SC weekly. Cost is more than $1000 per month.

Interferon and Ribavirin (*Rebetron*)

Combining interferon with ribavirin has resulted in better response rates to therapy. Ribavirin works by inhibiting viral replication of both RNA and DNA viruses. Sustained response to therapy is defined as normal ALT level and/or undetectable HCV RNA 6 months after completion of therapy, which is an

Table 16–5. Contraindications to Interferon with Ribavirin Therapy

Anemia (Hgb <12 g/dL women, <13 g/dL men)
Leukocytopenia (<1500 × $10^3/\mu$L)
Thrombocytopenia (<100× $10^3/\mu$L)
Depression or other severe psychiatric illness
Cardiovascular disease
Autoimmune disease
End-stage liver disease with cirrhosis
Seizure disorder
Normal ALT level
Poorly controlled diabetes mellitus
Pregnant or unable to practice contraception

interesting criterion when we have not found any correlation between HCV viral load and disease severity. A sustained response has been found to last up to 4 years in 96% of patients in one study.[37] The response rates to various drug therapies are as follows:

> Interferon monotherapy—18%
> Interferon PEG monotherapy—30%
> Interferon/Ribavirin therapy—40% (Table 16–5)
> Interferon PEG/Ribavirin therapy—~50% (needs further study)

Dosage. The dose is interferon alpha-2b, 3 million units SC three times weekly and ribavirin, 600 mg PO twice daily if greater than or equal to 75 kg; 400 mg q AM and 600 mg q PM if less than 75 kg. Get CBC at baseline and at weeks 2 and 4. Reduce dose if hemoglobin drops below 10 g/dL. Cost exceeds $1500 per month.

Precautions. Injection site inflammation and reaction can occur. Neuropsychiatric symptoms, including depression, anxiety, suicidal ideation, insomnia, and irritability, may be noted. Flulike symptoms with fatigue, myalgias, fever, and headache are associated as well. Gastrointestinal disorders, including dyspepsia, nausea, vomiting, and anorexia, may result, as may respiratory tract symptoms, including cough and shortness of breath. Hemolytic anemia, autoimmune disease, hair loss, thyroid disease, and skin disorders can occur.

Therapies to Consider

Hepatocyte regeneration can lead to hepatocellular carcinoma (HCC) if there is active necrosis with lymphocytic infiltration. Agents that act to delay this necrosis may be useful in delaying the progression to cirrhosis or HCC.

Colchicine (*Colchicum autumnale*)

An alkaloid isolated from the autumn crocus, colchicine has been found to reduce fibrosis during hepatocyte regeneration in animal studies. One study showed that in a group of cirrhotic patients, survival was three times greater in those taking colchicine versus placebo over 11 years.[38] To limit gastrointestinal adverse effects, it is given at 1 mg daily for a 5-day cycle followed by 2 days off.

Ursodeoxycholic Acid (UDCA or Actigall)

Ursodeoxycholic acid has been found to be cytoprotective owing to its ability to displace toxic hydrophobic bile acids in the liver and intestines. Additional studies are needed in the treatment of viral hepatitis.

Ayurvedic Medicine

Ayurveda means "the science of life" and consists of a constitutional approach (similar to traditional Chinese medicine) that treats the patient based on an individual balance of three doshas: pitta, kapha, and vata. A herbal combination that has been used in India for many years for the treatment of liver disease is Liv-52.

Liv-52

Although lacking good evidence in the treatment of viral hepatitis, Liv-52 has been found to inhibit TNF-α in animal studies. It consists of a combination of six herbs: *Capparis spinosa, Cichorium intybus, Solanum nigrum, Terminalia millefolium, Cassia occidentalis,* and *Tamarix gallica.*

THERAPEUTIC REVIEW

Patient with Normal ALT and No Hepatic Fibrosis

Laboratory	Get baseline ultrasound and monitor serial ALT levels. If ALT begins to rise, refer for consultation and/or biopsy.
Lifestyle	Reduce toxin exposure by avoiding unnecessary drugs or supplements. Use organic produce and drink filtered water. Avoid alcohol and tobacco. Participate in a regular aerobic exercise program. Give hepatitis A and hepatitis B vaccinations.
Nutrition	Consume cruciferous vegetables (broccoli, cauliflower, brussels sprouts), oranges, orange juice, and tangerines. Eat 6 or 7 servings of fruits and vegetables daily. Avoid grapefruit. Decrease fat intake. Avoid *trans* fats and partially hydrogenated oils. Cook with olive or canola oil; increase omega-3–rich foods (cold water fish, nuts, and flax) and decrease omega-6–rich foods (vegetable oils, processed foods). Increase fiber intake. Consider adding soluble fiber such as methylcellulose (Citrucel) or psyllium (Metamucil). Or, eat breakfast muesli (see Table 16–4) each morning. Green tea, 2 to 3 cups daily.
Supplements	Vitamin C, 200 to 250 mg twice daily Vitamin E, *d*-Alpha tocopherol, 800 IU daily Selenium, 200 μg daily B-100 complex (that includes thiamine), once daily Avoid iron supplements.
Botanicals	Milk thistle *(Silymarin marianum)* bound to phosphatidylcholine to improve absorption, 120 mg twice daily.
Mind–body connection	Help make lifestyle choices that result in less stress and anxiety. Encourage exploration and regular practice of a tailored relaxation exercise or meditation

Patient with Elevated ALT and Moderate Fibrosis

All previous, *plus,*

Laboratory	Consider liver biopsy.
Pharmaceuticals	Interferon/ribavirin therapy for 12 months for those with genotype 1, and for 6 months for those with genotypes 2 and 3.

If drugs are contraindicated, not tolerated, or ineffective, consider the following:

Botanicals	Increase dose of milk thistle to 240 mg twice daily (phosphatidylcholine-bound). Licorice root, 250 to 500 mg three times daily of the dry powder, or 2 to 4 mL three times daily of the fluid extract. *Schisandra* extract, 100 mg twice daily. *Astragalus* powder, 4 to 7 g daily.
Traditional Chinese Medicine	Consider referral to a TCM practitioner for individualized herbal therapy.

Formula	A small study showed significant results for three patients with active hepatitis.[39] It may take 6 months before an effect is noted, and the cost of the supplements is substantial. Owing to the favorable safety profile, the clinician may want to cautiously experiment with this approach for the patient who has limited options until further research is completed.
	   Milk thistle, 300 mg three times daily.
	   Selenium, 400 μg daily.
	   B-100 complex, one twice daily.
	   Vitamin C, 2 g daily.
	   Vitamin E (*d*-alpha tocopherol), 800 IU daily.
	   Coenzyme Q10, 300 mg daily.
	   Alpha-lipoic acid, 300 mg twice daily.
	   A mineral supplement.

Patients with Severe Hepatic Fibrosis with Cirrhosis

Laboratory	Check hepatic ultrasound and serum alpha-fetoprotein (AFP) levels every 6 months to 1 year to screen for hepatocellular carcinoma.
Surgery	Refer for determination of candidacy for liver transplant.
Nutrition	Consider referral to nutritionist for evaluation and calculation of protein needs.
Supplements	All previous, plus SAMe, 800 mg twice daily.
Botanicals	Consider adding *Schisandra* extract, 100 mg twice daily to milk thistle, 240 mg twice daily (phosphatidylcholine bound).

References

1. Rodriguez-Inigo E, Bartolome J, deLucas S, et al: Histological damage in chronic hepatitis C is not related to the extent of infection in the liver. Am J Pathol 154:1877–1881, 1999.
2. Pizzorno JE, Murray MT: Textbook of Natural Medicine: Detoxification, 2nd ed. Edinburgh, Churchill/Livingstone, 1999.
3. Regev A, Jeffers LJ: Hepatitis C and alcohol. Alcohol Clin Exp Res 23:1543–1551, 1999.
4. Mori M, Hara M, Wada I, et al: Prospective study of hepatitis B and C viral infections, cigarette smoking, alcohol consumption, and other factors associated with hepatocellular carcinoma risk in Japan. Am J Epidemiol 151:131–139, 2000.
5. Fahey JW, Zhang Y, Talalay P: Broccoli sprouts: An exceptionally rich source of inducers of enzymes that protect against chemical carcinogens. Proc Natl Acad Sci U S A 94:10367–10372, 1997.
6. Beecher CWW: Cancer preventive properties of varieties of *Brassica oleracea*. A review. Am J Clin Nutr 59(Suppl):1166S–1170S, 1994.
7. Crowell PL, Gould MN: Chemoprevention and therapy of cancer by d-limonene. Crit Rev Oncog 5:1–22, 1994.
8. Yee GC, Stanley DL, Pessa LJ, et al: Effect of grapefruit juice on blood cyclosporin concentration. Lancet 345:955–956, 1995.
9. Corrao G, Ferrari PA: Exploring the role of diet in modifying the effect of known disease determinants: Application to risk factors of liver cirrhosis. Am J Epidemiol 142:1136–1146, 1995.
10. Caughey GE, Mantzioris E, Gibson RA, et al: The effect of human necrosis factor alpha and interleuken 1-beta production of diets enriched in n-3 fatty acids from vegetable oil or fish oil. Am J Clin Nutr 63:116–122, 1996.
11. Katiyar SK, Mukhtar J: Tea antioxidants in cancer chemoprevention. J Cell Biochem 27:S59–S67, 1997.
12. Piazza M, Guadagnino V, Picciotto G, et al: Effect of (+)-Cyanidanol-3 in acute HAV, HBV and non-A, non-B viral hepatitis. Hepatology 3:45–49, 1983.
13. Witschi A, Reddy S, Stofer B, Lauterburg BH: The systemic availability of oral glutathione. Eur J Clin Pharmacol 43:667–669, 1992.
14. Johnston CJ, Meyer CG, Srilakshmi JC: Vitamin C elevates red blood cell glutathione in healthy adults. Am J Clin Nutr 58:103–105, 1993.
15. Von Herbay A, et al: Vitamin E improves the aminotransferase status of patients suffering from viral hepatitis C: A rando-

mized, double-blind, placebo controlled study. Free Radic Res 27:599–605, 1997.

16. Look MP, Gerard A, Rao GS, et al: Interferon/antioxidant combination therapy for chronic hepatitis C—A controlled pilot trial. Antiviral Res 43:113–122, 1999.

17. Jain A, Buist NR, Kennaway NG, et al: Effect of ascorbate or N-acetylcysteine treatment in a patient with hereditary glutathione synthetase deficiency. J Pediatr 124:229–233, 1994.

18. Kleinveld HA, Demacker PNM, Stalenhoef AFH: Failure of N-acetylcysteine to reduce low-density lipoprotein oxidizability in healthy subjects. Eur J Clin Pharmacol 43:639–642, 1992.

19. Yu MW, Horng IS, Hsu KH, et al: Plasma selenium levels and risk for hepatocellular carcinoma among men with chronic hepatitis virus infection. Am J Epidemiol 150:367–374, 1999.

20. Mato JM, Camara J, Fernandez de Paz J, et al: S-Adenosyl-methionine in alcoholic liver cirrhosis: A randomized, placebo-controlled, double-blind, multicenter clinical trial. J Hepatol 30:1081–1089, 1999.

21. Cotler SJ, Emond MJ, Gretch DR, et al: Relationship between iron concentration and hepatitis C virus RNA level in liver tissue. J Clin Gastroenterol 29:322–326, 1999.

22. Fontanan RJ, Israel J, LeClair P, et al: Iron reduction before and during interferon therapy of chronic hepatitis C: Results of a multicenter, randomized, controlled trial. Hepatology 31:730–736, 2000.

23. Wallace AE, Weeks WB: Thiamine treatment of chronic hepatitis B infection. Am J Gastroenterol 96:864–868, 2001.

24. Valenzuela A, Aspillaga M, Vial S, et al: Selectivity of silymarin on the increase of the glutathione content in different tissues of the rat. Planta Med 55:420–422, 1989.

25. Sonnenbichler J, Zetl I: Stimulating effect of silybin on the DNA-synthesis in partially hepatectomized rat livers: Non-response in hepatoma and other malignant cell lines. Biochem Pharmacol 35:538–541, 1986.

26. Berenguer J, Carrasco D: Double-blind trial of silymarin versus placebo in the treatment of chronic hepatitis. Munch Med Wochenschr 119:240–260, 1977.

27. Ferenci P, Dragosic SB, Dittrich H: Randomized controlled trial of silymarin treatment in patients with cirrhosis of the liver. J Hepatol 9:105–113, 1989.

28. Crance JM, Leveque F, Biziagos E, et al: Studies on the mechanism of action of glycyrrhizin against hepatitis A virus replication. Antiviral Res 23:63–76, 1994.

29. Xianshi S, Huiming C, Lizhuang W, et al: Clinical and laboratory observation on the effect of glycyrrhizin in acute and chronic viral hepatitis. J Tradit Chin Med 4:127–132, 1984.

30. Ohkura Y, Mizoguchi Y, Morisawa S, et al: Effect of gomisin A (TJN-101) on the arachidonic acid cascade in macrophages. Jpn J Pharmacol 52:331–336, 1990.

31. Zhu M, Yeung RY, Lin KF, et al: Improvement of phase I drug metabolism with *Schisandra chinensis* against CCl4 hepatotoxicity in a rat model. Planta Med 66:521–525, 2000.

32. Upton R: Astragalus Root: Analytical, Quality Control, and Therapeutic Monograph. Santa Cruz, CA, American Herbal Pharmacopoeia, 1999.

33. Zhang YD, Shen JP, Zhu SH, et al: Effects of astragalus (ASI, SK) on experimental liver injury. Yao Hsueh Hsueh Pao 27:401–406, 1992.

34. Fukudo S, Suzuki J, Tanaka Y, et al: Impact of stress on alcoholic liver injury: A histopathological study. J Psychosom Res 33:515–521, 1989.

35. Swain MG: Stress and the gastrointestinal tract: Stress and hepatic inflammation. Am J Physiol 279:G1135–G1138, 2000.

36. Stausbaugh HJ, Dallman MF, Levine JK: Repeated, but not acute, stress suppresses inflammatory plasma extravasation. Proc Natl Acad Sci U S A 96:14629–14634, 1999.

37. Marcellin P, Boyer N, Gervais A, et al: Long-term histologic improvement and loss of detectable intrahepatic HCV RNA in patients with chronic hepatitis C and sustained response to interferon-alpha therapy. Ann Intern Med 127:875–881, 1997.

38. Adhami JE, Baho J: Treatment with colchicine and survival of patients with ascitic cirrhosis: A double-blind randomized trial. Panminerva Med 40:75–81, 1998.

39. Berkson BM: A conservative triple antioxidant approach to the treatment of hepatitis C. Combination of alpha lipoic acid (thioctic acid), silymarin and selenium: Three case histories. Med Klin 94:84–89, 1999.

40. Milliman BW, Lamson DW, Brignall MS: Hepatitis C: A retrospective study, literature review, and naturopathic protocol. Altern Med Rev 5(4):355–370, 2000.

CHAPTER 17

Urinary Tract Infections

Susan Hadley, M.D.

PATHOPHYSIOLOGY

The urinary tract consists of the urethra, bladder, kidneys, and prostate, all of which are infection-prone. The microorganisms most often responsible for urinary tract infections are gram-negative bacilli, with *Escherichia coli (E. coli)* the causative agent in 80% of acute infections in patients without catheters, stones, or urologic abnormalities. The microorganisms gain access to the bladder via the urethra and may ascend to the renal parenchyma. Females, for anatomic reasons, are more susceptible than males to urinary tract infection (UTI). Colonization of the vaginal area and distal introitus by gram-negative bacilli gives the microorganisms access to the urinary tract.

Factors that predispose to periurethral colonization are poorly understood but may include (1) change in the normal perineal flora, which may be induced by antibiotics, other genital infections, sexual intercourse, or use of spermicides, diaphragms, tampons, or feminine hygiene products; (2) pregnancy, which is associated with decreased ureteral tone, decreased ureteral peristalsis, and incompetence of vesicoureteral valves; (3) obstruction, which is any impediment to free flow of urine, such as by tumor or stone; (4) in men, prostate hypertrophy; (5) neurogenic bladder dysfunction, in which neurologic impairment leads to stasis of urine; (6) bladder irritants such as condoms, tampons, or soaps, (7) vesicoureteral reflux, which facilitates reflux of bacteria; (8) foreign bodies; and (9) genetic factors. Typically, bacteria that gain access to the bladder are rapidly cleared by dilution, with voiding, and by the antibacterial properties of urine and bladder mucosa. Polymorphonuclear cells present in the bladder wall and prostate secretions possess antibacterial properties. Whether infection ensues depends on interacting effects of the pathogenicity of the strain, the inoculum size, and local and systemic host defense mechanisms.

INTEGRATIVE THERAPY

Nutrition

Removal of Bladder Irritants

Dietary bladder irritants such as caffeine, refined sugar, white flour, alcohol, and nicotine should be avoided.

Garlic

Allicin is a sulfur-containing component of garlic; in vitro analysis has demonstrated its antibacterial effect against gram-positive and gram-negative bacteria (including *E. coli*).[1–3]

Onion

Onion, a relative of garlic, contains alliin (which is broken down to allicin by the enzyme alliinase) and similar sulfur-containing compounds also noted to have antibacterial effects.[4]

Fluids

Water diuresis reduces bacterial counts in urine.

Flaxseed

Flaxseed contains abundant mucilage, which soothes the lining of the urinary tract. Flaxseed may also have anti-inflammatory effects.

There is a mild fishy taste to flaxseed that is mitigated by adding the ground seed directly to food. Ground flaxseed and flaxseed oil spoil quickly, and this nutrient should be stored only in the seed form.

Dosage. From 1 to 3 tablespoons of ground fresh flaxseed can be taken with food.

Supplements

Vitamin C

Vitamin C is recommended for patients susceptible to UTI because of its acidifying effect on the urine. Urine specimens from healthy subjects and from subjects with nitrite-positive urine were studied after acidification, by measuring nitrous oxide. The release of nitrous oxide was found to be potentiated by the presence of vitamin C.[5] Vitamin C is best absorbed from the powdered form, calcium ascorbate.

Dosage. No general dosing guidelines are available for vitamin C. A dose of 1 to 2 g can be taken until "loose bowels" are experienced and then decreased slightly.

Acidophilus

Acidophilus is recommended after meals to promote digestive tract health. It may be taken in yogurt or capsule form. Acidophilus may be found in probiotic formulas. In choosing a probiotic formula, the capsule form is most often recommended; it should be refrigerated. The probiotic formula should contain lactobacillus acidophilus, *Bifidobacterium* and frocto-oliga saccharides (FOS).

Acidophilus is indicated both for UTI prevention and for prevention and treatment of yeast infections if antibiotics are indicated.

Dosage. Dosage recommendations include 2 capsules of a probiotic daily between meals, 1 tablespoon of a liquid probiotic daily between meals, or yogurt (with acidophilus) at least 6 ounces.

Botanicals

Cranberry

Several studies have shown cranberry's effectiveness in the treatment and prevention of UTIs. Initially it was thought that the antimicrobial action of cranberry was due to increased urine acidity or its organic component hippuric acid. Subsequent studies have demonstrated that cranberry's role in the treatment and prevention of UTIs is due to its antiadherence properties. A 6-month placebo-controlled large-scale trial demonstrated reduction of bacteriuria in elderly women using 300 mL per day of a standard cranberry beverage. Voided samples were collected once a month from women receiving cranberry juice and women receiving placebo. The study demonstrated a statistically significant reduction in bacteriuria.[6] A subsequent study using cranberry concentrate (*Vaccinium macrocarpum*) and CFA medium with *E. coli* replicated the previous results. It has been determined that the mechanism of action is due to immediate inhibition of agglutination and loss of fimbrial adhesion of type I and P-fimbriated *E. coli* to the bladder wall.[7] (Bacterial adherence to mucosal surfaces is a prerequisite for the development of infection.) Further studies have suggested that the proanthocyanidins (condensed tannins, a component of cranberry) prevent adherence of *E. coli*.[8] The antiadherence properties of cranberry are also believed to play a role in prevention of UTIs. In one study, using daily consumption of powdered cranberry extract versus placebo, cranberry was found to decrease the occurrence of UTIs.[9]

Dosage. Sixteen ounces of **unsweetened** juice a day, diluted with water or sparkling water or 1 or 2 capsules of dried cranberry powder two to four times a day.

Precautions. None known.

NOTE

Unsweetened cranberry juice is recommended. Cranberry Juice Cocktail is 33% juice with fructose and artificial sweeteners added and is not recommended in the treatment of urinary tract infections.

Uva Ursi

Key constituents of uva ursi are arbutin and hydroquinone. Arbutin has demonstrated antimicrobial activity against gram-positive and gram-negative bacteria, including *E. coli*.[10] Arbutin is absorbed from the gastrointestinal tract and hydrolyzed to hydroquinone in alkaline urine.[11,12] One study demonstrated a decreased incidence of recurrent cystitis in patients using uva ursi.[13] The whole plant is suggested, because other components of the herb make the urine more alkaline.

Dosage. 3 g of the dried herb or 400 to 800 mg of hydroquinone derivatives four times a day.[12]

Precautions. Gastrointestinal discomfort and discoloration of the urine may occur with use of high doses.

Contraindications. This herb should not be used during pregnancy and lactation or in children younger than 12 years. This herb is not recommended to be given with other substances that cause acidic urine (which may reduce the antibacterial effect). It is recommended to keep the urine pH about 8 through dietary measures.[12]

Because of the large amount of tannins present in this herb, it is not recommended for use beyond a 1-week period and no more than five times a year. Prolonged tannin exposure may lead to gastrointestinal intolerance and hepatotoxicity. If symptoms do not abate within 48 hours, another source of treatment should be recommended.

NOTE

Uva ursi is not recommended for the treatment of urinary tract infections during pregnancy or lactation or in children. It is not recommended for use beyond 7 days.

NOTE

Recommended sources of botanical products for treatment of urinary tract infections:
- *Dried herbs: Frontier*
- *Capsules: Nature's Way, Eclectic Institute, Pure Encapsulations, Enzymatic Therapies*
- *Tinctures: Gaia; investigate locally produced tinctures*

Goldenseal

Berberine is one of the alkaloids in goldenseal and is believed to have antibacterial properties against gram-positive and gram-negative bacteria, including *E. coli*.[14]

More studies are needed to demonstrate effectiveness in UTI treatment.

Dosage. Recommend a standardized extract with berberine as the main component, 2 to 4 g of dried root or solid extract (4:1, or 8%–12% alkaloid content) 250 to 500 mg daily.

Precautions. Avoid goldenseal in pregnancy, as high doses may interfere with vitamin B metabolism.

This herb increases stomach acid, so it may interfere with the effectiveness of antacids and proton pump inhibitors.

Pharmaceuticals

Several different classes of antibiotics are effective in the treatment of UTIs. The combination agent trimethoprim-sulfamethoxazole (Bactrim, Septra) is typically the first choice, given its activity against *E. coli*. Cephalosporins and fluoroquinolones are also frequently used in the treament of UTIs. Several studies have compared different classes of antibiotics as well as duration of dosing. For example, one study compared ciprofloxacin, ofloxacillin, and trimethoprim-sulfamethoxazole and demonstrated similar efficacy for these three agents when they were given for 3 days to treat acute symptomatic uncomplicated lower UTI in women.[15] In pregnancy, the first choice for treatment is amoxicillin or cephalexin (Keflex). For antibiotic prophylactic treament in pregnancy, nitrofurantoin (Macrodantin) is recommended.

Pyridium (200 mg three times daily for 2 days) may be given for pain relief of dysuria and bladder spasm associated with UTIs. Red-orange discoloration of the urine is noted with Pyridium.

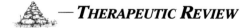 **THERAPEUTIC REVIEW**

Following is a summary of treatment options for patients with uncomplicated UTIs. If a patient presents with fever and there is suspicion of renal involvement, immediate aggressive therapy with antibiotics (possibly intravenous antibiotics, requiring hospitalization) is warranted. At the first signs of a UTI, it is possible to recommend fluids, cranberry juice, and/or uva ursi. If the patient has any evidence of flank pain, any immunosuppressant illness, or a chronic condition such as diabetes mellitus, or is pregnant, antibiotic treatment should not be delayed. If symptoms are unchanged after a 24-hour treatment period, a urine specimen for culture and sensitivity testing should be obtained.

Avoidance of Irritant Factors
- *Elimination of sugar and caffeine from diet*
- *Urination after intercourse*

Nutrition
- *Increase intake of garlic and onions.*
- *Increase fluid intake.*
- *Eat fresh whole foods.*

Supplements
- *Vitamin C (powder form to bowel tolerance)*
- *Acidophilus in yogurt daily or 2 capsules of a probiotic between meals*

THERAPEUTIC REVIEW *continued*

Botanicals

- *Start with cranberry juice, unsweetened, several glasses (16 ounces) daily, or dried powder in capsules (1 or 2, two to four times a day).*
- *Uva ursi: 3 g of the dried herb or 400 to 800 mg of hydroquinone derivatives four times a day: tincture (1:5), 4 to 6 mL (1–1.5 teaspoons or 1–1½ droppersful) three times a day*
- *Goldenseal: 2 to 4 g of dried root or solid extract (4:1 dilution, or 8% to 12% alkaloid content) 250 to 500 mg daily in divided doses; tincture (1:5), 4 to 6 mL three times a day*

Pharmaceuticals

- *Antibiotic therapy is the treatment of choice; trimethoprim-sulfamethoxazole (Bactrim, Septra) or a more broad-spectrum antimicrobial is selected as indicated by symptoms and/or culture results.*
- *Pyridium 200 mg three times daily for 2 days may be given for pain relief.*

References

1. Cavalitto CJ, Bailey JH: Allicin, the antibacterial principle of *Allium sativum*. Isolation, physical properties, and antibacterial action. J Am Chem Soc 66: 1959–1951, 1994.
2. Blumenthal M, et al (ed): The Complete German Commission E Monographs: Therapeutic Guide to Herbal Medicines. Austin, Tex, The American Botanical Council, 1998, pp 176–177.
3. Farbman KS, et al: Antibacterial activity of garlic and onions: A historical perspective. Pediatr Infect Dis 12:613–614, 1993.
4. Lundberg JO, et al: Urinary nitrite: More than a marker of infection. Urology 50: 189–191, 1997.
5. Avorn J, et al: Reduction of bacteriuria and pyuria after ingestion of cranberry juice. JAMA 271:751–754, 1994.
6. Ahuja S, Kaack B, Roberts J: Loss of fimbrial adhesion with the addition of *Vaccinium macrocarpum* to the growth medium of P-fimbriated *Escherichia coli*. J Urol 159:559–562, 1998.
7. Howell AB, Vorsa N, Marderosian AD, Foo LY: Inhibition of adherence of P-fimbriated *Escherichia coli* to uroepithelial surfaces by proanthocyanidin extracts from cranberries. N Engl J Med 339:1085–1086, 1998.
8. Walker EB et al: Cranberry concentrate: UTI prophylaxis. J Fam Pract 1997; 45:167–168.
9. Jellin JM, et al: Pharmacist's Letter/Prescriber's Letter: Natural Medicines Comprehensive Database, 3rd ed. Stockton, Calif, Therapeutic Research Faculty, 2000, pp 10549–10550.
10. Schulz V, Hansel R, Tyler VE: Rational Phytotherapy: A Physician's Guide to Herbal Medicine. Berlin, Springer-Verlag, 1998, pp 222–223.
11. Larsson B, Jonasson A, Fianu S: Prophylactic effect of Uva-E in women with recurrent cystitis: A preliminary report. Curr Therap Res 53:441–443, 1993.
12. Murray M: The Healing Power of Herbs, 2nd ed. Rocklin, Calif, Prima, 1995, pp 162–172.
13. McCarty JM, et al: A randomized trial of short-course ciprofloxacin, ofloxacin, or trimethoprim-sulfamethoxazole for the treatment of acute urinary tract infection in women. Ciprofloxacin Urinary Tract Infection Group. Am J Med 106:292–299, 1999.

CHAPTER 18

Yeast Infections

Jean Riquelme, M.D.

PATHOPHYSIOLOGY

Vulvovaginal candidiasis (yeast infection) appears to affect about half of all women over 25 years of age.[1] Because in many cases the disease is self-diagnosed and self-treated, however, its actual incidence is unknown. African American women are more frequently affected.[2] The most common organism cultured from symptomatic women is *Candida albicans,* although other organisms are increasingly implicated.[3] Symptomatology depends strongly on host response and does not appear to be related to yeast burden.

At a recent multidisciplinary conference,[4] a classification scheme for vulvovaginal candidiasis was suggested. As shown in Table 18–1, this classification is based on whether the infection is complicated or uncomplicated. Uncomplicated yeast vulvovaginitis usually responds to short courses of conventional therapy. Complicated yeast vulvovaginitis is more likely to benefit from an approach integrating conventional drug treatment with complementary modalities, nutritional modification, and risk factor reduction.

UNCOMPLICATED VULVOVAGINAL CANDIDIASIS

A woman's first vaginal yeast infection often occurs with the initiation of or an increase in vaginal sexual activity. Antibiotic use is also a precedent to acute, uncomplicated infections but is less likely to be a factor in recurrent vulvovaginal candidiasis.[5] Patients may complain of vulvovaginal pruritus,

Table 18–1. Classification of Vulvovaginal Candidiasis

Uncomplicated
Sporadic or infrequent vulvovaginal candidiasis
Mild to moderate vulvovaginal candidiasis
Causative agent likely to be *Candida albicans*
Normal, nonpregnant woman

Complicated
Recurrent vulvovaginal candidiasis
Severe vulvovaginal candidiasis
Non-*albicans* candidiasis
Abnormal host (e.g., with uncontrolled diabetes, debilitation, or immunosuppression)

irritation or pain, a vaginal discharge, dysuria, or dyspareunia. No symptom is pathognomonic of yeast vulvovaginitis. Potassium hydroxide preparation of a vaginal secretion specimen is negative for fungal elements in 30% of *C. albicans* infections, so diagnosis is often made on clinical grounds.

INTEGRATIVE THERAPY

Risk Factor Reduction

Nutrition

Studies about the influence of diet on vulvovaginal yeast have yielded mixed results. One case control recall study reported that *Candida* vulvovaginitis was associated with increased caloric intake, daily carbohydrate ingestion greater than 223 g, and consumption of some forms of fiber.[6] A similar study of college students found no dietary associations.[7]

NOTE

In a case control study, ingestion of saccharin, nitrites, calcium, iron, and zinc was neither a risk factor for nor protective against vulvovaginal candidiasis.[6]

Sex Practices

In young women, daily vaginal intercourse is associated with increased risk of vulvovaginal candidiasis, but the risk is not necessarily increased in older women. In a case control study,[8] engaging in cunnilingus more than five times per month was associated with increased risk of *Candida* vulvovaginitis. However, masturbation using saliva did not increase risk. The use of sex toys as a risk factor has not been studied, but trauma and irritation of the vulva and vagina may increase risk of incurring a candidal infection.

Pharmaceuticals

A short course of conventional medication is often the most cost-effective and efficacious approach in uncomplicated yeast infections.

The most commonly used conventional agents are the azoles, such as clotrimazole or ketoconazole. Systematic analysis[9] has shown that both oral and topical antifungals are effective in treating uncomplicated vaginal candidiasis. Patients seem to prefer oral medications, which may affect compliance, although oral agents also have the potential to cause more systemic side effects such as nausea and headache. There are also significant drug-drug interactions between azoles and other medications, including oral contraceptives and warfarin.

Topical Creams

Clotrimazole (Gyne-Lotrimin) 1% cream 5 g intravaginally for 7 to 14 days may be used. Other agents are miconazole (Monistat) 2% cream 5 g intravaginally for 7 days and terconazole (Terazol) 0.8% cream 5 g intravaginally for 3 days.

Vaginal Suppositories or Tablets

Clotrimazole (Lotrimin) 500-mg vaginal tablet may be given as a single dose. Alternatively, econazole (Spectazole), a 150-mg vaginal tablet for 3 days, or miconazole (Monistat), a 1200-mg vaginal suppository given as a single dose, may be used.

Oral Agents

Fluconazole (Diflucan) 150 mg orally may be given in a single dose; an alternative is ketoconazole (Nizoral) 400 mg daily orally for 5 days, or itraconazole (Sporanox) 200 mg twice daily in a single day.

NOTE

The selection of oral agent, topical cream, or vaginal suppository depends mostly on patient preference. Oral agents are available by prescription only in the United States.

COMPLICATED VULVOVAGINAL CANDIDIASIS

Complicated vulvovaginal yeast infections are caused not by more virulent organisms but by host factors that change susceptibility and treatment response. For this reason, additional diagnostic testing may be indicated. Recurrent vulvovaginal candidiasis is associated with compromise of the immune system, uncontrolled diabetes mellitus, oral contraceptive use, and infection with *Candida* species other than *C. albicans*. In recurrent disease, up to 50% of infections may be due to other *Candida* species, and fungal culture rather than microscopic examination of potassium hydroxide preparations should be performed.[10] The presence of symptoms despite negative cultures should prompt a search for nonyeast causes of vulvovaginitis, such as bacterial vaginosis, *Trichomonas*, contact dermatitis, or drug reaction.

INTEGRATIVE THERAPY

Nutrition

Yogurt Ingestion

Yogurt taken as food or applied topically has been a traditional treatment for yeast infections. The therapeutic ingredient appears to be live lactic acid–producing bacilli (LAB), which transiently colonize the gut and modulate its microecology and immune function.[11] The acidic metabolic byproducts of LAB inhibit growth of pathogenic bacteria. Cell wall components of LAB contain immunostimulants such as alpha-teichoic acid. The effect of yogurt on the human immune system has been studied mostly in ex vivo systems. Yogurt appears to increase cytokine production, macrophage activity, and lymphocytic mitogenic response. Theoretically, it may decrease intestinal yeast colonization and thus reduce vulvovaginal candidiasis, although this effect has not been proved.

One 12-month crossover trial[12] studied daily ingestion of yogurt containing *Lactobacillus acidophilus* as prophylaxis for candidal vaginitis. Patients who consumed 8 ounces of the yogurt daily had fewer infections. The utility of topical yogurt application remains unproved.

NOTE

Yogurt is defined as a coagulated milk product that results from fermentation of acid in milk by Lactobacillus bulgaricus *and* Streptococcus thermophilus.[14] *Yogurt is more likely than supplements to contain active lactic acid–producing bacteria and is usually less expensive for the patient to purchase.*

Patients who cannot tolerate yogurt often turn to supplements such as freeze-dried *Lactobacillus* or products labeled "probiotics." Probiotic therapy is an interesting approach to consider (see later), but such products are often expensive, and their effectiveness remains theoretical. A group of investigators in the United Kingdom[13] cultured products labeled "probiotic" and found discrepancies between labeling and contents.

Dosage. 8 ounces of yogurt with active *Lactobacillus* cultures consumed daily

Botanicals

Tea Tree Oil

Melaleuca alternifolia, the tea tree, is native to the continent of Australia, where its oil has a long history of use in traditional healing. It has gained popularity as a topical antibiotic and antifungal agent. The active ingredient appears to be terpin-4-ol, the content of which varies from preparation to preparation. A systematic review of tea tree oil in randomized clinical trials failed to endorse the use of tea tree oil for dermatologic conditions.[15] In vitro studies show tea tree oil to be equal in antifungal activity to ketoconazole, econazole, and miconazole.[16]

Dosage. 5% to 10% tea tree oil applied topically daily (after negative result on skin patch test). Discontinue if irritation occurs.

Precautions. Adverse reactions to topical tea tree oil, mostly allergic dermatitis, have been reported and occur in about 5% of users. A skin patch test is recommended before use. Allergic reactions are more common in oxidized or outdated preparations.

Pharmaceuticals

In complicated vulvovaginal candidiasis, long-term pharmacologic therapy is indicated, often for weeks or months. Correction of exogenous factors, such as those referable to diabetes, decreases post-treatment recurrence.

Boric Acid

Boric acid applied intravaginally is as effective as imidazoles in the treatment of vulvovaginal candidiasis.[17] It is especially useful in azole-resistant cases.[18] High doses of boric acid (equivalent to 3.3 kg daily for a 60-kg woman) caused fetal anomalies in rats. It should be stopped 2 weeks before conception and avoided in pregnancy.[18]

Dosage. For 2 weeks, 600 mg in a gelatin capsule should be inserted vaginally daily. For resistant infection, this regimen may be repeated every 2 weeks.

NOTE

Patients may wish to make their own boric acid capsules for home use. Size 0 gelatin capsules can be filled with pharmacy-grade boric acid and used as directed. Boric acid should not be taken internally.

Imidazoles

Patients with recurrent or complicated vulvovaginal candidiasis require longer treatment than those with uncomplicated infection, regardless of route of administration of azole antifungals. Duration of treatment should be doubled.[4] Symptom relief can be expected in 24 to 48 hours. Low-potency topical corticosteroids may provide rapid symptom relief in severe vulvitis.

Other Therapies to Consider

Probiotic and Prebiotic Therapy

A promising field of study is the use of probiotics and prebiotics to influence health and disease. Probiotics are food supplements that contain live microbes. They transiently colonize the gut and must be reingested on a regular basis to have consistent effects. Commercial probiotic products contain *Lactobacillus acidophilus, Bifidobacterium bifidum, Saccharomyces bouardii,* or other microbes. As described earlier in the chapter, lactobacilli have antibiotic and immunostimulatory effects. Bifidobacteria produce vitamins and participate in carbohydrate metabolism of the host. A placebo-controlled trial showed that probiotic administration reduced diarrhea in patients taking antibiotics.[20]

Prebiotics are nondigestible food ingredients, usually oligosaccharides, that stimulate growth or activity of beneficial gut bacteria. They are also called fructo-oligosaccharides (FOSs). Inulin, lactulose, and raffinose are examples of prebiotics. These oligosaccharides occur naturally in onions, leeks, garlic, artichokes, and chicory.[21]

Industry standards for these products vary, although European preparations seem more reliable.[13] Dosages and treatment regimens have not been established. Patients who wish to normalize intestinal flora using probiotics and prebiotics may find it more reliable to do so using whole foods, such as yogurt and onions, rather than expensive commercial products (see also Chapter 97, Prescribing Prebiotics).

THERAPEUTIC REVIEW

Vulvovaginal candidiasis may be complicated or uncomplicated. Uncomplicated cases are most effectively treated with conventional medicines. Complicated cases benefit from an approach integrating nutrition, risk factor reduction, and longer term pharmacotherapy.

Exacerbating Factors
- *Consider discontinuation of oral contraceptives and antibiotics.*
- *Control diabetes and minimize immunosuppression.*
- *Counsel patients to refrain from engaging in cunnilingus.*

Nutrition
- *Patients with complicated vulvovaginal candidiasis may benefit from eating 8 ounces daily of yogurt containing active lactobacilli.*

Botanicals
- *Topical tea tree oil may be useful in patients who are not sensitive or allergic to it.*

Pharmaceuticals
- *Oral and topical azoles are equally effective. Treatment times should be doubled for complicated cases.*
- *Boric acid can be used intravaginally for azole-resistant cases.*

References

1. Geiger, et al: The epidemiology of vulvovaginal candidiasis among university students. Am J Public Health 85:1146–1148, 1995.
2. Horowitz, et al: Sexual transmission of *Candida*. Obstet Gynecol 69:883–886, 1987.
3. Spinillo A, et al: Prevalence and risk factors for fungal vaginitis caused by non-*albicans* species. Am J Obstet Gynecol 176:138–141, 1997.
4. Sobel JD, et al: Vulvovaginal candidiasis: Epidemiologic, diagnostic and therapeutic considerations. Am J Obstet Gynecol 178:203–211, 1998.
5. Spinillo A, et al: Effect of antibiotic use on the prevalence of symptomatic vulvovaginal candidiasis. Am J Obstet Gynecol 180:14–17, 1999.
6. Reed BD, et al: The association between dietary intake and reported history of *Candida* vulvovaginitis. J Fam Pract 29:509–515, 1989.
7. Foxman B: The epidemiology of vulvovaginal candidiasis: Risk factors. Am J Public Health 80:329–331, 1990.
8. Reed BD, et al: Sexual behaviors and other risk factors for *Candida* vulvovaginitis. J Womens Health Gender Based Med 9:645–655, 2000.
9. Watson MC, et al: Oral versus intra-vaginal imidazole and triazole anti-fungal treatment of uncomplicated vulvovaginal candidiasis (thrush). Cochrane Database Syst Rev 1: CD002845, 2001.
10. Handa VL, Stice CW: Fungal findings in cyclic vulvitis. Obstet Gynecol 96:301–303, 2000.
11. Meydani SN, Hu W-K: Immunologic effects of yogurt. Am J Clin Nut 71:861–872, 2000.
12. Hilton E, et al: Ingestion of yogurt containing *Lactobacillus acidophilus* as prophylaxis for candidal vaginitis. Ann Intern Med 116:353–357, 1992.
13. Hamilton-Miller JM, et al: Public health issues arising from microbiological and labeling quality of foods and supplements containing probiotic microorganisms. Public Health Nutr 2:223–229, 1999.
14. Bourlioux P, Pochart P: Nutritional and health properties of yogurt. World Rev Nutr Diet 56:217–258, 1988.
15. Ernst E, Huntley A: Tea tree oil: A systematic review of randomized clinical trials. Fortschr Komplementarmed Klass Naturheilk 7:17–20, 2000.
16. Hammer KA, et al: In vitro activities of ketoconazole, econazole, miconazole and *Melaleuca alternifolia* (tea tree) oil against *Malassezia* species. Antimicrob Agents Chemother 44:467–469, 2000.
17. Rein MF: Current therapy of vulvovaginitis. Sex Transm Dis 8:316–320, 1981.
18. Sobel JD, Chaim W: Treatment of *Torulopsis glabrata* vaginitis: Retrospective review of boric acid therapy. Clin Infect Dis 24:649–652, 1997.
19. Culver BD: Vaginitis [letter]. N Engl J Med 338:1548–1549, 1998.
20. Elmer GW, et al: Biotherapeutic agents: A neglected modality for the treatment and prevention of selected intestinal and vaginal infection. JAMA 275:870–876, 1996.
21. Macfarlane GT, Cummings JH: Probiotics and prebiotics: Can regulating the activities of intestinal bacteria benefit health? B M J 318:999–1003, 1999.

CHAPTER 19

Hypertension

Victoria Maizes, M.D.

At least 50 million adult Americans have hypertension. The prevalence increases with age and is higher among African Americans compared with other ethnic groups. Ninety-five percent of diagnosed cases are classified as essential hypertension—yet there is epidemiologic evidence that hypertension exists almost entirely in developed countries. Much of what we call *essential* is likely due to diet, obesity, inactivity, stress, and alcohol consumption.

Conventional hypertension treatment fits well with the philosophies of integrative medicine. Conventional treatment stresses lifestyle modification and a stepwise approach to treatment. The Sixth Joint National Commission on Hypertension (JNC VI) guidelines for hypertension released in November 1997 placed increased emphasis on lifestyle modification. In patients with blood pressure measurement above 140/90 mm Hg (stage 1) with no other risk factors, lifestyle interventions are indicated as initial treatment. These lifestyle changes include weight loss, sodium restriction, moderate exercise regimens, and moderation of alcohol intake. They can be continued for as long as 1 year before drug treatment is initiated. However, drug therapy should be started immediately if comorbid conditions such as dyslipidemia or diabetes are present. There is now strong evidence that the greatest benefit of antihypertensive drug treatment occurs in patients with hypertension who have additional risk factors for cardiovascular disease.

ASSESSMENT

Assessment of the patient begins by exploring the patient's experience of hypertension. This is done by asking a series of questions, such as:

What does it mean to you to have high blood pressure?
How has it impacted your life?
What insight has it given you?
How do you feel about taking medication?
What are your fears or concerns about having hypertension?

INTEGRATIVE THERAPY

Lifestyle Modification

Nutrition

Vegetarian Diet

Vegetarians have lower blood pressure and a lower incidence of hypertension and other cardiovascular diseases than do nonvegetarians. Although there is no significant difference in sodium consumption between the two groups, vegetarian diets contain more potassium, complex carbohydrates, essential fatty acids, fiber, calcium, magnesium, and vitamin C, and less saturated fat and refined carbohydrate.

The Hypertension Control Program

The Hypertension Control Program (HCP) tested a nutritional intervention program that focused on three main factors: weight, excess dietary sodium, and excess alcohol intake. This 4-year trial explored whether individuals with hypertension could successfully discontinue their medications. Thirty-nine percent of individuals in the nutritional intervention group were able to maintain normal blood pressure when they were off medications compared with 5% in the control group. The changes were relatively modest: mean weight loss of 4 pounds, compared with a 4-pound weight gain in the control groups; reduction of daily sodium output of 36%, compared with a 13% increase in controls; and a reduction in mean alcohol intake of 13 g per day compared with a reduction of 7 g per day in the control group.[1]

This study was integrative in looking at several nutritional changes and not attempting to separate out which change was responsible. The behavioral changes made were not huge, yet the cumulative effect on blood pressure was substantial.

The DASH Diet

The Dietary Approaches to Stop Hypertension (DASH) trial was an 11-week multicenter randomized feeding trial that tested the effects of dietary patterns on blood pressure. Subjects (459) were divided into three groups: control, increased fruit and vegetables, and a combination diet (rich in fruits, vegetables, low-fat dairy, and reduced saturated fat). In hypertensive subjects, the combination diet led to a

157

mean reduction in blood pressure of −11.4 systolic and −5.5 diastolic. Blood pressure reductions occurred in the setting of stable weight and a sodium intake of approximately 3 g per day.[2] One positive aspect of DASH is that subjects ate whole foods, not supplements. The study was limited in that it lasted only 8 weeks and subjects were given all the food they were asked to eat. This study is currently being repeated to address these concerns. (See Chapter 85, The DASH Diet, for dietary recommendations for patients.)

NOTE

For many Americans, switching to a vegetarian diet is too radical a change. The positive messages from the DASH and HCP studies are that small, doable changes can lead to significant reductions in blood pressure, including reduction or elimination of the need for medications. In my clinical experience, patients with hypertension who switched to low-fat vegetarian diets were often able to discontinue their medications.

Alcohol

Decreasing alcohol intake has repeatedly been shown to reduce blood pressure.

Potassium-to-Sodium Ratio

The current ratio of potassium to sodium (K/Na) in a typical American diet is 1:2. The ideal ratio of K/Na is probably closer to 5:1. Most fruits and vegetables have a K/Na ratio of at least 50:1. Sodium restriction may be especially important in elderly whites, African Americans, and Latin Americans. Recommend to individuals with hypertension that they limit their Na intake to less than 2.4 g per day (1 tsp).

Olive Oil

The Mediterranean diet, which is rich in olive oil, has been found to be associated with lower levels of serum lipids and lower blood pressure compared with the typical American diet. Ferrara and colleagues[3] undertook a double-blind randomized controlled trial in which 23 individuals with hypertension were assigned to a diet of monounsaturated fatty acids (MUFAs) or polyunsaturated fatty acids (PUFAs) for 6 months, and then were crossed over to the other diet. Systolic and diastolic blood pressures were significantly lower after the MUFA than after the PUFA diet (127 vs 135 mm Hg systolic and 84 vs 90 mm Hg diastolic), and medication dosage was significantly reduced during the MUFA but not the PUFA diet. The mechanism for the blood pressure reduction induced by olive oil is not known. The antioxidant polyphenols may be a contributor. There may be as much as 5 mg of phenols in 10 g of extra virgin

olive oil. MUFAs have been shown to increase high-density lipoprotein (HDL) levels and to produce oleate-enriched low-density lipoprotein (LDL) cholesterol, which is more resistant to oxidative modifications.

NOTE

In the study, the MUFA used was extra virgin olive oil and the PUFA was sunflower oil. Sources of MUFAs include olive oil, canola oil, olives, nuts, and avocados. Sources of omega-3 PUFAs include flaxseed and flaxseed oil, pumpkin seed and oil, walnuts and walnut oil, hemp seed and oil, purslane and other leafy greens, canola oil, soy oil, and coldwater fish.

Sources of omega-6 PUFAs to be limited include seed oils like corn and safflower; margarines made from these oils; crackers, chips, and other snack foods; cookies, cakes, pastries, and other commercially baked goods; fast food fried foods; doughnuts; and anything containing hydrogenated or partially hydrogenated oil.

Soy

A significant reduction in diastolic blood pressure was observed in a study of 51 nonhypertensive perimenopausal women. The women took a soy protein supplement twice daily as part of a placebo-controlled trial.[4] However, an RCT of individuals with high normal blood pressure did not show reduction of blood pressure with soy.[5]

Fiber

There is an inverse relationship between fiber intake and blood pressure. This has been seen in both men[6] and women.[7]

Exercise

Exercise is a longstanding recommendation to patients who need to reduce blood pressure. In addition, exercise has a favorable effect on stress, lipids, diabetes, weight, and other cardiovascular disease risks. Mean changes in blood pressure with mild (50% maximum O_2 uptake) intensity cycle ergometer (60 min × 3 times per week × 10 weeks) in controlled studies were −11 mm Hg systolic and −6 mm Hg diastolic. The American College of Sports Medicine recommends endurance training, 20 to 60 minutes 3 to 5 days per week at 50% to 85% maximal oxygen uptake.[8]

Weight Loss

Modest weight loss of approximately 10% of body weight can normalize blood pressure.

Supplements

Omega-3 Fatty Acids

Sixty double-blind studies have shown that fish oil supplements or flaxseed oil is effective in lowering blood pressure. The fat found in fish is omega-3 fatty acid, mainly eicosapentaenoic acid (EPA) and docosahexaenoic acid (DHA). EPA competitively inhibits synthesis of thromboxane A_2, a vasoconstrictor that promotes platelet aggregation. Both EPA and DHA interfere with prostaglandin synthesis in platelets and blood vessels.[9]

NOTE

In general, eating four 4- to 6-ounce servings of northern coldwater fish per week is preferable to taking fish oil supplements. There is some concern that fish oil supplements may have high levels of toxic contamination. If fish oil is used, doses up to 9 gms per day have been used.

Coenzyme Q_{10}

Thirty-nine percent of people with hypertension have been shown to be CoQ_{10} deficient. There is evidence that, over 4- to 12-week periods, CoQ_{10} lowers blood pressure in people with hypertension. A small randomized controlled trial revealed improvement in blood pressure in patients treated with 60 mg CoQ_{10} bid for 8 weeks.[10] An intervention study including 109 patients with hypertension revealed that overall New York Heart Association (NYHA) functional class improved from a mean of 2.40 to 1.36 ($P < .001$), and 51% of patients were able to discontinue between one and three antihypertensive drugs 4.4 months after starting CoQ_{10}.[11] Another small intervention study of 26 people with World Health Organization (WHO) level 1 or 2 hypertension were given 50 mg bid of CoQ_{10}. This led to reductions in blood pressure from 167 to 148.9 mm Hg systolic, and from 98.9 to 88.6 mm Hg diastolic.[12]

The mechanism of action for CoQ_{10} appears to be a decrease in total peripheral resistance achieved via the direct impact of CoQ_{10} on the vascular wall.

Dosage. Recommend Q gel 60 to 120 mg. (Doses over 100 mg/day should be divided.) To maximize absorption, CoQ_{10} should be taken with meals that contain some fat.

Precautions. Adverse effects include anorexia, diarrhea, epigastric discomfort, mild nausea, and ischemic tissue damage (during acute exercise). CoQ_{10} has been reported to decrease the effect of warfarin.

Calcium

The effect of calcium on blood pressure is controversial. Calcium may reduce blood pressure in African Americans, pregnant women, and salt-sensitive people. For women with a calcium intake of at least 800 mg/day, the relative risk of hypertension was .78 when compared with that found with an intake of less than 400 mg/day.[13] Leanness may be a predictor of response to calcium supplementation in men who have a low baseline calcium intake.[14] In trials of calcium supplementation, blood pressure was reduced in individuals with hypertension, although in some studies, this was seen only in a subset. A 1996 meta-analysis[15] that pooled the data showed a very small effect size.

Dosage. Recommend at least 800–1200 mg per day of calcium carbonate or calcium citrate.

Precautions. Adverse effects include constipation and hypercalcemia.

Magnesium

There is a highly significant inverse relationship between magnesium and both systolic and diastolic blood pressures. Low dietary magnesium was found to be the dietary factor most strongly associated with high blood pressure in the Honolulu Heart Study and the Nurse's Health Study.[16] For women with a magnesium intake of at least 300 mg/day, the relative risk of hypertension was .77 compared with that found in women whose intake was less than 200 mg/day.[17] Supplementing magnesium has led to mixed results in studies. There may be a subgroup of responders. It may also be that the impact of long-term dietary intake is different than that of short-term supplementation.

Dosage. Recommend 6 mg/kg weight (approximately 420 mg for a 154-pound person).

Precautions. Adverse effects include diarrhea, renal stones, and, in patients with chronic renal failure, hypermagnesemia.

Potassium

A meta-analysis of 19 studies has revealed that oral potassium supplements significantly decrease blood pressure. The magnitude of this effect is greater in patients with hypertension—on average, −8.2 systolic and −4.5 diastolic.[18] Ideally, potassium supplementation is avoided by increasing intake of potassium-rich foods such as bananas, grapefruit, dried beans, peas, broccoli, spinach, pumpkins, and squash.

Dosage (if supplementation via food is not possible). Recommend 1.5 to 3 g (20–33 meq) per day as potassium chloride. Every gram of potassium chloride has 13.4 meq potassium.

Precautions. Monitor serum potassium levels. Adverse effects can include nausea, vomiting, diarrhea, and ulcers.

Vitamin C

Population studies reveal the higher the vitamin C intake, the lower the blood pressure. Preliminary studies show a modest blood pressure–lowering effect from vitamin C supplementation. This may occur because the excretion of lead is enhanced.[19]

Vitamin B₆

One small study of 20 people revealed reductions in systolic and diastolic blood pressures when B_6 was supplemented at 5 mg/kg.[20]

Mind-Body Approaches

Biofeedback, the relaxation response, meditation, deep breathing, yoga, progressive muscle relaxation, autogenic training, imagery, hypnosis, and stress management have all been shown to have a modest effect on lowering blood pressure. A wealth of published literature supports the use of biofeedback in the treatment of high blood pressure. Unfortunately, many of the studies were poorly designed or had small numbers of participants. Taken as a whole, there is good evidence that biofeedback may be useful in some people with high blood pressure, but exactly what biofeedback techniques are best and which people are most likely to respond are not as clear.[21] A meta-analysis by Eisenberg and co-workers[22] reviews the methodologic limitations of the studies and concludes that these interventions are superior to no therapy but not to credible sham techniques.

Botanicals

Garlic (*Allium sativum*)

A meta-analysis of eight clinical trials that included 415 subjects, most of whom received a dried powdered extract with standardized allicin, showed a "moderate benefit" on lowering blood pressure.[23] The optimal dose of garlic for treating hypertension has not been established. Garlic is also effective for reducing cholesterol by approximately 9%.

Dosage. Recommend ½ to 2 cloves daily of raw garlic, or Garlicin 350-mg capsules by Nature's Way, daily bid.

Precautions. Adverse effects include diaphoresis; dizziness; mouth, esophagus, and stomach irritation; nausea; and vomiting. Allergic reactions are rare. Garlic may increase the risk of bleeding if taken with anticoagulants or antiplatelet agents.

Hawthorn (*Crataegus monogyna*)

Hawthorn is used widely by physicians in Europe for treatment of hypertension, angina, arrhythmias, and congestive heart failure. It is considered a cardiovascular tonic. However, the blood pressure–lowering effect of hawthorn is mild.

Dosage. Recommend the liquid extract of the flower—.5 to 1 mL tid (1:1 in 25% alcohol).

Precautions. Adverse effects include fatigue, nausea, sweating, hypotension, arrhythmias, and sedation.

Herbs to Avoid in the Treatment of Hypertension

Contraindicated herbs in the treatment of patients with hypertension include licorice, ephedra, caffeine, and Panax ginseng. These can all raise blood pressure.

Pharmaceuticals

Treatment with a diuretic or a beta blocker has been the usual initial medication, particularly as these are the only agents that have been proven to reduce mortality. However, other effective antihypertensives have not yet been tested in similar trials. Angiotensin-converting enzyme (ACE) inhibitors are also often used as first-line treatments because of their low adverse effect profile, longer duration of action, and increased adherence rates.[24] With concomitant diseases, advanced age, or African American ancestry, the following medications are recommended:

Diabetes: ACE inhibitors
Heart failure: ACE inhibitors or diuretics
Myocardial infarction: Beta blockers or ACE inhibitors if left ventricular dysfunction present
Isolated systolic hypertension (elderly): Diuretics
African Americans: Diuretics or calcium channel blockers.

Communication

Because lifestyle change is such an important option for normalizing blood pressure, attention to motivating patients is critical. Communication style comes into play when one is presenting options, giving feedback, and enhancing motivation for change.

The key elements of communication include:

Keep the information or feedback simple, clear, and succinct.
Compare the patient's personalized feedback with norms and standards.
Elicit the patient's response to, and interpretation of, the information or feedback.

For example:
"Your blood pressure is 150/100. On your last visit, it was 155/100. The time before that, it was 150/98. A normal blood pressure for someone your age is 140/80 or less."
Pause and let person respond. (It is more effective

if the patient makes the interpretation.) If the patient does not respond, ask: "What do you make of that?"

Give feedback in general language—"Elevated blood pressure has been linked to an increased risk of heart attack and stroke. For most people, bringing blood pressure readings below 140/90 reduces that risk." (As opposed to: "You will have a stroke if you don't get your blood pressure down.")

"There are a number of things that people can do to lower blood pressure. These include decreasing alcohol consumption, reducing sodium intake, increasing exercise, taking medication, taking herbs or supplements, developing a relaxation practice, following a special diet, and so forth. Is one of these options something you would be interested in doing? Or, is there something else that you would like to explore?"

"On a scale of 1 to 10, how interested are you in _____ (e.g., reducing your alcohol consumption)?"

"On a scale of 1 to 10, how confident are you that you can _____ (e.g., eat a vegetarian diet)?"

THERAPIES TO CONSIDER

Chinese Medicine

A 1991 study by Wong and associates[25] compared the efficacy of Chinese traditional treatment with that of the Western medical regimen in 50 matched patients with hypertension. The 26 patients in the Chinese medicine group were treated according to gyan yan kan or sing yin shu diagnoses. The authors followed the patients for 23 days; they concluded that both treatments were effective and that Western treatment was more effective. Given that many herbal therapies can take up to 2 months to have their full effect, the duration of treatment may not have been adequate to fully compare the therapies.

Acupuncture may be useful in the treatment of mild and recent-onset hypertension owing to its autonomic regulating properties. Eight to ten visits over 2 months are recommended to determine whether the hypertension will respond to acupuncture.

Homeopathy

According to homeopathic principles, hypertension is a reflection of an individual's overall state of health and therefore is amenable to treatment. The efficacy of homeopathic treatment depends on the individual's age and the duration of the disease. A constitutional remedy chosen by an experienced prescriber is the most appropriate way to treat hypertension.

The following remedies are sometimes used:

- *Argentum nitricum* is used if blood pressure rises with anxiety and nervousness.
- *Aurum metallicum* is sometimes indicated for serious people who are focused on career and accomplishment.
- *Calcarea carbonica* is often helpful for people with high blood pressure who easily tire and have poor stamina.

A German randomized double-blind crossover study of ten patients comparing the effects of antihypertensive pharmaceuticals with the outcomes of homeopathic treatment revealed that the blood pressure–lowering effect of the pharmaceuticals was clearly superior to that of homeopathy; effectiveness of homeopathy was negligible and was statistically not significant. Interestingly, the subjective complaints of patients resolved equally well with pharmacotherapy and homeopathic treatment.[26]

Ayurveda

Ayurvedic herbal medicines are used to treat hypertension. *Terminalia arjuna* and *Inula racemosa* have both been found to have therapeutic benefit in the treatment of cardiovascular disease.[27]

THERAPEUTIC REVIEW

Mild to moderate hypertension is well treated with an integrative approach. Assessing your patient's motivation to make changes and understanding in what area her confidence is greatest helps you to tailor your recommendations. For severe hypertension, especially in the presence of concomitant disease, pharmaceuticals should be used first, along with encouragement that with lifestyle change, this may be modified in the future.

Nutritional Recommendations

- *Recommend to your patient increasing intake of fruits and vegetables (rich in potassium), substituting olive oil for other oils, increasing low-fat dairy products or following the DASH diet, substituting soy and fatty fish for other proteins, and increasing fiber intake.*
- *Recommend a reduction in sodium, caffeine, and alcohol consumption.*

THERAPEUTIC REVIEW *continued*

Exercise

- *Encourage 30 minutes daily of aerobic exercise.*

Weight Loss

- *Encourage 10% weight loss if obese.*

Mind-Body Advice

- *Develop a relaxation strategy such as breathwork, meditation, yoga, progressive muscle relaxation, or self-hypnosis; encourage daily practice.*

Supplement Advice

- *Consider addition of CoQ_{10}. Use Q gel, 60 to 120 mg daily.*
- *Consider trial of fish oil. Use 1–3 gm EPA/DHA per day.*
- *Consider trial of calcium. Use 800 mg per day of calcium citrate or carbonate.*
- *Consider trial of magnesium. Use 6 mg/kg.*

Botanical Advice

- *A trial of garlic is worthwhile, either taken raw or as Garlicin (product of Nature's Way), 350 mg bid daily.*
- *As a cardiovascular tonic, try Hawthorn liquid extract .5 to 1 mL tid.*

Patients who are particularly interested in alternative systems can be seen by a practitioner of Chinese medicine, homeopathy, or Ayurveda. Their blood pressure should be assessed regularly.

References

1. Stamler R, Stamler J, Grimm R, et al: Nutritional therapy for high blood pressure: Final report of a four-year randomized controlled trial—the hypertension control program. JAMA 257:1484–1491, 1987.
2. Appel LJ, Moore TJ, Obarzanek E, et al: A clinical trial of the effects of dietary patterns on blood pressure. DASH Collaborative Research Group. N Engl J Med 336:1117–1124, 1997.
3. Ferrara L, Raimondi AS, d'Episcopo L, et al: Olive oil and reduced need for antihypertensive medications. Arch Intern Med 160:837–842, 2000.
4. Washburn S, Burke GL, Morgan T, Anthony M: Effect of soy protein supplementation on serum lipoproteins, blood pressure and menopausal symptoms in perimenopausal women. Menopause 6:7–13, 1999.
5. Hodgson JM, Puddey IB, Beilin LJ, et al: Effects of isoflavonoids on blood pressure in subjects with high-normal ambulatory blood pressure levels: A randomized controlled trial. Am J Hypertens 12(1 Pt 1):47–53, 1999.
6. Ascherio A, Rimm EB, Giovannucci EL, et al: A prospective study of nutritional factors and hypertension among US men. Circulation 86:1475–1484, 1992.
7. Witteman JCM, Willett WC, Stampfer MJ, et al: A prospective study of nutritional factors and hypertension among US women. Circulation 80:1320–1327, 1989.
8. Arakawa K: Effects of exercise on hypertension and associated complications [review]. Hypertens Res 19(Suppl):S87–S91, 1996.
9. Fish oil for the heart (no authors given). Med Lett Drugs Ther 29(731):7–9, 1987.
10. Singh RB, Niaz MA, Rastogi SS, et al: Effect of hydrosoluble coenzyme Q10 on blood pressures and insulin resistance in hypertensive patients with coronary artery disease. J Hum Hypertens 13:203–208, 1999.
11. Langsjoen P, Langsjoen P, Willis R, Folkers K: Treatment of essential hypertension with coenzyme Q10. Mol Aspects Med 15(Suppl):S265–S272, 1994.
12. Digiesi V, Cantini F, Oradei A, et al: Coenzyme Q10 in essential hypertension. Mol Aspects Med 15(Suppl):S257–S263, 1994.
13. Witteman JCM, Willett WC, Stampfer MJ, et al: A prospective study of nutritional factors and hypertension among US women. Circulation 80:1320–1327, 1989.
14. Ascherio A, Rimm EB, Giovannucci EL, et al: A prospective study of nutritional factors and hypertension among US men. Circulation 86:1475–1484, 1992.
15. Allendar PC, Cutler JA, Follmann D, et al: Dietary calcium and blood pressure: A meta-analysis of randomized clinical trials. Ann Intern Med 124:825–831, 1996.
16. Ascherio A, Rimm EB, Giovannucci EL, et al: A prospective study of nutritional factors and hypertension among US men. Circulation 86:1475–1484, 1992.
17. Witteman JCM, Willett WC, Stampfer MJ, et al: A prospective study of nutritional factors and hypertension among US women. Circulation 80:1320–1327, 1989.
18. Cappuccio FP, MacGregor GA: Does potassium supplementation lower blood pressure? A meta-analysis of published trials. J Hypertens 9:465–473, 1991.
19. Simon JA: Vitamin C and cardiovascular disease: A review. J Am Coll Nutr 11:107–125, 1992.
20. Ayback M, et al: Effect of oral pyridoxine hydrochloride supplementation on arterial blood pressure in patients with essential hypertension. Arzneimittelforschung 45:1271–1273, 1995.
21. Patel C, Marmot MG, Terry DJ: Controlled trial of biofeedback-aided behavioural methods in reducing mild hypertension. Br Med J (Clin Res Ed) 282(6281):2005–2008, 1981.
22. Eisenberg DM, Delbanco TL, Berkey CS, et al: Cognitive behavior techniques for hypertension: Are they effective? Ann Intern Med 118:964–972, 1993.
23. Silagy CA, Neil HA: A meta-analysis of the effect of garlic on blood pressure. J Hypertens 12:463–468, 1994.
24. Available at http://www.harrisonsonline.com.
25. Wong ND, Ming S, Zhou HY, Black HR: A comparison of Chinese traditional and Western medical approaches for the treatment of mild hypertension. Yale J Biol Med 64(1):79–87, 1991.
26. Hitzenberger G, Korn A, Dorcsi M, et al: Controlled randomized double-blind study for the comparison of the treatment of patients with essential hypertension with homeopathic and with pharmacologically effective drugs [German]. Wien Klin Wochenschr 94:665–670, 1982.
27. Miller AL: Botanical influences on cardiovascular disease [review]. Altern Med Rev 3:422–431, 1998.

CHAPTER 20

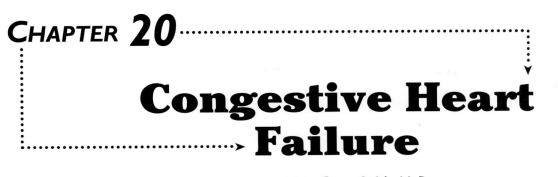

Congestive Heart Failure

Russell H. Greenfield, M.D.

The pharmacologic and technologic advances of recent decades have resulted in a marked improvement in the overall prognosis of heart disease, but morbidity and mortality associated with heart failure remain high, and people's quality of life suffers even when medical therapy is maximized. All signs point to the need for a shift in emphasis. As practitioners, we must focus on means of helping to *prevent* the onset of heart failure in our patients. In those people who have already developed heart failure, we must strive to slow the inexorable progression of the disease with the early institution of means both gentle and effective. Finally, we must not turn our backs on the proven benefits of specific Western medical approaches to this very common malady.

PATHOPHYSIOLOGY

Heart failure statistics in the United States are frightening. Considering that most experts believe the incidence of chronic left ventricular dysfunction will continue to grow as the population ages and as more people survive heart attacks, it is clear why those same experts equate the war on heart failure with the war on cancer. At present, heart failure contributes in some way to 3 million hospitalizations and 250,000 deaths each year.[1, 8, 10, 11] Heart dysrhythmias and sudden death occur with increased frequency, and half of all people with heart failure die within 5 years of receiving the diagnosis.

Heart failure most commonly develops as a consequence of long-standing cardiovascular disease, especially high blood pressure or coronary artery disease (Table 20–1). Whereas it was once believed that the syndrome merely involved the inability of the heart to adequately pump blood to the rest of the body, we now recognize the pathophysiology to be both complex and multifactorial. Initially positive compensatory mechanisms ultimately contribute to the deterioration of clinical status (Table 20–2). In its most severe form, pulmonary edema, backward pressure is so high within congested capillaries that fluid leaks into lung tissue and compromises gas exchange, creating a life-threatening situation for the patient.

Classification systems have been proposed owing to the myriad clinical presentations possible with heart failure. The commonly accepted schema of heart failure severity as put forth by the New York Heart Association (NYHA) defines levels of illness by functional capability (Table 20–3).

INTEGRATIVE THERAPY

The management of acute cardiac decompensation, as seen with cardiogenic pulmonary edema, initially falls squarely under the umbrella of conventional Western medical therapy. Once the patient has been stabilized, other options may be entertained, but during the acute emergency, there is no rationale for forgoing the benefits of rapid institution of IV access, pharmacologic support, and aggressive airway management (Fig. 20–1).

For a person with stable heart failure, as with most forms of significant chronic disease, the approach must be multidisciplinary. Whereas conventional Western pharmaceutical intervention remains the cornerstone of management, there exist many poten-

Table 20–1. Identifiable Causes of Heart Failure

Hypertension
Coronary artery disease
Valvular heart disease
Alcohol abuse
Diabetes mellitus
Chemotherapeutic agents
Chronic anemia
Hypothyroidism or hyperthyroidism
Toxic exposures

Table 20–2. Pathophysiologic Features Present in Heart Failure

Left ventricular dilatation and structural remodeling
Reduced wall motion
Systemic vasoconstriction
Sodium retention and circulatory congestion
Neurohormonal activation

Data from references 4, 12–14.

Table 20–3. The New York Heart Association Functional Classification System for Chronic Heart Failure
....

NYHA I—physical activity is not limited by symptoms like shortness of breath, fatigue or palpitations

NYHA II—physical exertion is mildly limited, with symptoms of shortness of breath, fatigue, or palpitations developing with typical daily activities

NYHA III—physical activity is severely curtailed as symptoms of shortness of breath, fatigue, or palpitations develop with any kind of activity

NYHA IV—symptoms and physical discomfort are present even at rest

tially beneficial complementary approaches that can be instituted easily and inexpensively (Fig. 20–2).

Lifestyle

The primary focus should be on prevention of disorders that ultimately lead to the development of heart failure, especially high blood pressure and coronary artery disease. Community education regarding the adverse effects of smoking and excessive alcohol intake must continue, and assistance with cessation should be made readily available.

Advise people to get adequate amounts of exercise, aiming for 30 to 45 minutes of physical activity appropriate for the individual three to five times weekly. The combination of physical exertion and a healthy diet can help maintain optimal body weight (excess weight puts a strain on the heart). Getting sufficient rest is also important, and asking people to get at least 7 to 8 hours of sleep each night is prudent. Numerous studies have likewise suggested that adequate means of stress reduction are impor-

tant when considering ways to lower the risk of cardiovascular disease.[34–44] Have a plan in mind to help individuals manage stress in their lives. Regular participation in spiritual or religious practices may also help fend off heart disease.[45–48]

Associated maladies, such as diabetes mellitus, kidney disease, or liver disease, should be managed aggressively, and the use of medications that might adversely affect heart function (such as nonsteroidal anti-inflammatory drugs, calcium channel blockers, and certain antidysrhythmic agents) minimized. People who have established problems related to atherosclerosis, such as coronary artery disease, hyperlipidemia, or high blood pressure, should also be informed of comprehensive management programs already in existence.[49, 50]

Nutrition

Give patients appropriate recommendations regarding limiting the intake of saturated fats, partially hydrogenated (trans) fats, polyunsaturated oils, fast foods, and salt.[15–18] People who fall into the NYHA functional class II require additional means to keep the illness in check. Sodium (salt) restriction has clearly been shown to positively affect cardiac function and symptoms in this situation. In the early stages of heart failure, the degree of restriction need not be severe, and avoiding added salt should be sufficient. With worsening heart function, it may be necessary to limit sodium intake to 2 to 3 g/day and daily ingestion of water to 1.5 to 2.0 L. Advice to increase the use of monounsaturated oils, such as extra virgin olive oil,[19] and foods high in essential fatty acids,[20–24] and an added emphasis on fruit, vegetable,[25–27] and fiber intake[28] are also well

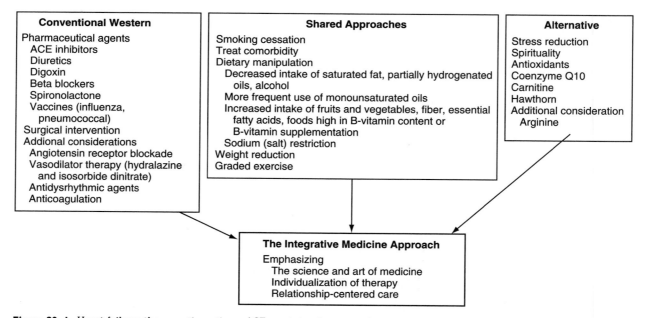

Conventional Western	Shared Approaches	Alternative

Pharmaceutical agents
  ACE inhibitors
  Diuretics
  Digoxin
  Beta blockers
  Spironolactone
  Vaccines (influenza,
    pneumococcal)
Surgical intervention
Addional considerations
  Angiotensin receptor blockade
  Vasodilator therapy (hydralazine
    and isosorbide dinitrate)
  Antidysrhythmic agents
  Anticoagulation
	Smoking cessation
	Treat comorbidity
	Dietary manipulation
	  Decreased intake of saturated fat, partially hydrogenated
	    oils, alcohol
	  More frequent use of monounsaturated oils
	  Increased intake of fruits and vegetables, fiber, essential
	    fatty acids, foods high in B-vitamin content or
	    B-vitamin supplementation
	  Sodium (salt) restriction
	Weight reduction
	Graded exercise
		Stress reduction
		Spirituality
		Antioxidants
		Coenzyme Q10
		Carnitine
		Hawthorn
		Additional consideration
		  Arginine

The Integrative Medicine Approach
Emphasizing
  The science and art of medicine
  Individualization of therapy
  Relationship-centered care

Figure 20–1. Heart failure: therapeutic options. ACE, angiotensin-converting enzyme.

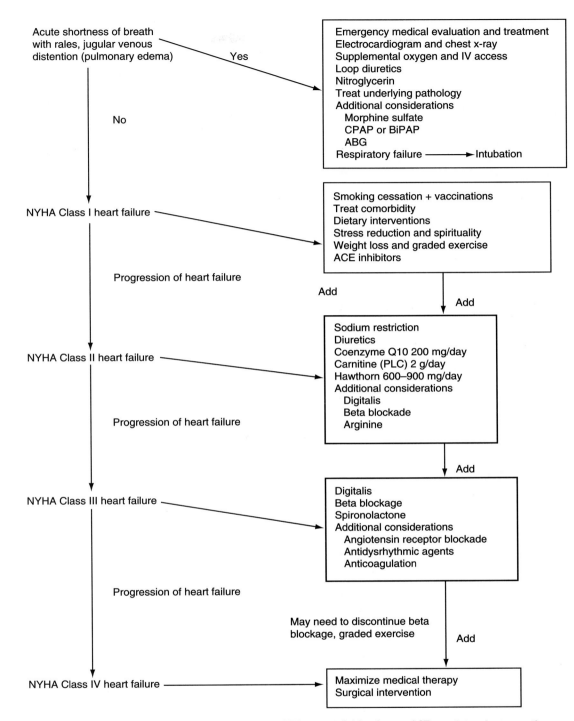

Figure 20–2. Clinical pathway: management of heart failure. ABG, arterial blood gas; ACE, angiotensin-converting enzyme; CPAP, continuous positive airway pressure; NYHA, New York Heart Association.

within the purview of the practitioner. People with elevated total and low-density lipoprotein cholesterol levels should try to eat more soy protein.[7] Antioxidant vitamins should be considered,[29–31] as should B vitamin supplements,[32, 33] especially when the diet is not meeting or cannot easily meet (as with vitamin E) the recommended daily intake.

NOTE

Once a person has developed signs and symptoms of heart failure, and has undergone an appropriate evaluation to secure the diagnosis, conventional Western pharmaceutical intervention should begin.

Pharmaceuticals

Angiotensin-Converting Enzyme Inhibitors

Numerous studies[51–53] have shown that early and maximal use of angiotensin-converting enzyme (ACE) inhibitors not only can slow the progression of heart failure but also can improve quality of life and long-term prognosis. Perhaps the biggest problem surrounding use of this class of agents is that most patients are not receiving the maximal beneficial dosage. Such undertreatment stymies therapeutic benefits. Many physicians are wary of potential side effects, such as hypotension and kidney and electrolyte problems. Starting with a low dosage, increasing the dosage slowly, and periodically checking electrolyte panels has been shown to be a safe and effective course. Anyone who has received the diagnosis of heart failure and can tolerate ACE inhibitors should be taking them, and the dosage should be appropriately maximized. Some people develop a chronic, dry cough with ACE inhibitor use that may limit the drug's utility. In this instance, angiotensin receptor blockade and vasodilator therapy are considered appropriate therapeutic options.

Dosage
Captopril (Capoten) 25 to 150 mg PO two to three times daily
Enalapril (Vasotec) 2.5 to 40 mg PO daily or divided twice daily
Lisinopril (Prinivil) 5 to 40 mg PO daily

Diuretics

Diuretics help to lessen cardiac workload by decreasing preload. The most commonly used diuretics in the setting of heart failure are the so-called loop diuretics, such as furosemide (Lasix), but thiazide diuretics can be used in milder forms of heart failure. Loop diuretics are especially beneficial once congestion has developed, but periodic blood tests are necessary to evaluate electrolyte balance, especially potassium levels.

Studies addressing the use of spironolactone, a diuretic and aldosterone antagonist, reveal that the agent reduces both the need for hospitalization and the risk of sudden death when added to standard conventional Western medical therapy.[54–57] Spironolactone is known to promote potassium and magnesium retention. Thus, be sure to document adequate kidney function before starting patients on spironolactone and monitor electrolyte levels frequently. It appears to be especially useful in those patients falling into NYHA classes III to IV.

Dosage
Hydrochlorothiazide 50 to 100 mg PO daily or divided twice daily

Furosemide (Lasix) 20 to 200 mg PO daily
Spironolactone (Aldactone) 12.5 to 50 mg PO daily or divided twice daily

Cardiac Glycosides (Digoxin)

Digoxin has been a mainstay of the conventional Western medical armamentarium since the days of William Withering, who first explored the benefit derived from the use of leaves of the common foxglove plant *(Digitalis purpurea)* over 100 years ago. It is most commonly employed in the treatment of supraventricular dysrhythmias and heart failure, especially when the latter is associated with hypertension, cardiac valvular disease, or coronary artery disease.

Digoxin has long been known to be a positive inotrope (increase the pumping efficiency of the heart), but recent work has shown it to possess beneficial neurohormonal activity as well. Although its administration does not appear to affect overall mortality, when added to the standard regimen of ACE inhibitors and diuretics, digoxin has been shown to improve symptoms, enhance exercise capacity, improve patients' quality of life and clinical status, and reduce hospitalization rates.[58–61]

Although digoxin is a useful drug, it has a very narrow therapeutic range, and toxicity is not uncommon. Some physicians initiate digoxin therapy early in the course of illness, and others prescribe it only in moderate-to-severe heart failure. It can be used both in the setting of acute cardiac decompensation and for chronic maintenance therapy. Do not prescribe digoxin as monotherapy—people with heart failure should almost always be taking an ACE inhibitor and utilizing other interventions, as described previously. A lowered dosage of digoxin is often necessary for patients with significant renal insufficiency.

Dosage. Digoxin (Lanoxin) 0.125 to 0.25 mg PO daily

Beta Blockers

Once contraindicated in the setting of heart failure, beta blockade has clearly been shown to benefit all but the most severe functional classes of heart failure.[62–64] The beta blockers not only affect the mechanical pump of the heart (improving ventricular function) and provide autonomic balance but also counteract specific neurohormonal processes that contribute to progressively worsening heart function. Appropriate use of beta blockade has been associated with enhanced left ventricular ejection fraction, a reduced hospitalization rate, and a decreased incidence of sudden death.[64] Cardiologists are now promoting early (NYHA class II) institution of beta blockade for patients with heart failure.

Dosage

Carvedilol (Coreg) 50 to 100 mg, start dose 6.25 mg 1/2 PO twice daily with food; double the dose every 2 weeks as tolerated up to a maximum of 25 mg twice daily (if the patient weighs < 85 kg) or 50 mg twice daily (if the patient weighs > 85 kg)

Metoprolol (Lopressor, Toprol) titrate up to 100 to 200 mg divided twice daily or daily in the extended release form (Toprol XL)

Angiotensin Receptor Blockers

Whereas ACE inhibitors help to modify the pathophysiologic changes associated with heart failure owing to activation of the renin-angiotensin system, blockage of the renin-angiotensin system remains incomplete, and progression of the disease is still the rule rather than the exception. Angiotensin II subtype I receptor blockers provide more complete blockade of the renin-angiotensin system than do ACE inhibitors, and may be of added benefit when combined with ACE inhibitors as part of the standard therapeutic regimen.[65–67] This group of drugs may also be helpful to patients who cannot tolerate ACE inhibitor therapy.

Dosage

Losartan (Cozaar) 50 to 100 daily or divided twice daily

Irbesartan (Avapro) 150 to 300 mg daily
Candesartan (Atacand) 16 to 32 mg daily

Herbs, Vitamins, and Supplements

Be sure to advise patients that the agents discussed in the following paragraphs do not act quickly, that 4 to 6 weeks may pass before clinical benefit is evident, and that these agents are most effective in people with less severe disease (NYHA classes II to III). Thus, their use is not appropriate for acute worsening of heart failure.

Botanicals

Hawthorn (Crataegus laevigata or monogyna)

Long a favored herbal remedy in Europe, hawthorn is a slow-acting cardiac tonic whose active constituents are considered to be flavonoids, like vitexin and rutin, and oligomeric proanthocyanidins. The German Commission E specifically recommends hawthorn leaf and flower as the plant parts to be used therapeutically.

Numerous beneficial effects have been ascribed to hawthorn based on both animal and human studies,[68–70] including:

Increased coronary artery blood flow

Enhanced pumping efficiency of the heart (improved contractility)
Antioxidant activity
Phosphodiesterase inhibition
ACE inhibition
Antidysrhythmic effects (lengthens the effective refractory period, unlike many cardiac drugs)
Mild reduction in systemic vascular resistance (lowered blood pressure)

Reviews of placebo-controlled trials have reported both subjective and objective improvement in patients with mild forms of heart failure (NYHA classes I to II).[69, 71] In one study, hawthorn was pitted against the ACE inhibitor captopril in comparable groups of people with heart failure. At trial's end, both groups had improved exercise capacity compared with baseline measurements, with no statistically significant differences between the two treatment arms. It should be noted, however, that the investigators employed a relatively low dosage of captopril.[72] Other studies of hawthorn in people with heart failure have revealed improvement in clinical symptoms, pressure-rate product, left ventricular ejection fraction, and patients' subjective sense of well-being.[73–76]

Dosage. Hawthorn is usually standardized to its content of flavonoids (2.2%) or oligomeric proanthocyanidins (18.75%). The recommended daily dosage as reflected in the literature ranges from 160 to 900 mg, but most practitioners believe there is greater therapeutic efficacy with higher dosages (600 to 900 mg/day). Again, there may be no noticeable improvement for 4 to 6 weeks.

Precautions. Although few side effects are associated with the use of hawthorn, one drug interaction is important to keep in mind. The existing data suggest that hawthorn can enhance the activity of digitalis glycosides, thus increasing the risk of side effects even though the plant does not contain digitalis-like substances itself. Most conventional Western medical practitioners would reflexively state that hawthorn should thus not be given to people taking digitalis for heart failure. A far more integrative perspective would be one considering the possibility of lowering the therapeutically effective dosage of digitalis, thereby minimizing the side effects associated with its use, by combining it with hawthorn.

Supplements

Coenzyme Q10

Coenzyme Q10, or CoQ10, has been used for decades as a nutritional supplement for cardiovascular disease, becoming one of the top six pharmaceuticals consumed in Japan under the name ubidecarenone.[77] In contrast, it remains relatively unknown in the United States, even though a significant amount of research examining its potential role in disease management has been published over a span of 30 years. A naturally occurring substance that behaves like a vitamin, CoQ10 is present in small amounts in most diets. CoQ10 is also synthesized within the body from tyrosine, partially through a common pathway shared with cholesterol synthesis. It is found in highest concentrations within the mitochondrial membranes of organs that have significant energy requirements, especially the heart, where it acts as a carrier of both electrons and protons, interacting with enzymes intricately involved with energy production.[78–81] CoQ10 exerts antioxidant[82] and membrane stabilizing[83] effects as well.

The concentration of CoQ10 within the plasma and myocardium is lower in subjects experiencing cardiac failure when compared with controls, regardless of etiology.[84–86] The more severe the degree of heart failure as reflected by the NYHA functional classification system, the greater is the deficiency of CoQ10.[87–90] It is unclear whether a decreased CoQ10 concentration is causal, as might be the case with idiopathic dilated cardiomyopathy, or secondary in nature, as is likely with ischemic cardiomyopathy. Regardless, a demonstrated myocardial deficiency of CoQ10, the knowledge that exogenous administration can correct the deficiency,[86, 91] and an appreciation of its necessity for adequate myocardial energy provision together formed the initial rationale for CoQ10 administration in the broad setting of heart failure.

The first clinical application of CoQ10 in cardiovascular disease was reported in 1967.[92] Since that time, numerous studies evaluating CoQ10 use for chronic heart failure have been published. As with many existing vitamin and supplement trials, unfortunately, the studies are of highly variable quality. Some of the trials were uncontrolled or of short duration (weeks to a few months); examined only a small number of subjects; were performed before the widespread use of ACE inhibitors, beta blockers, and aldosterone antagonists; or measured only functional parameters. Nonetheless, the majority of the published data do suggest a supportive role for CoQ10 with beneficial effects on ejection fraction,[93–95] end-diastolic volume index,[94, 96] development of pulmonary edema and hospitalization rate,[97] and symptoms.[95, 98, 99] Research has shown that withdrawal of CoQ10 supplementation results in worsening cardiac function and symptoms,[100] and two studies suggest a survival benefit when CoQ10 is added to a conventional therapeutic regimen.[101, 102] Two recent studies, however, failed to show clinical efficacy.[103, 104] Hopefully, increased awareness of CoQ10 will stimulate the performance of large, multicenter trials to determine its true efficacy in the setting of heart failure.

Dosage. The optimum dosage of CoQ10 in the setting of heart failure is as yet undetermined. Studies have utilized dosages ranging from 30 to 600 mg/day, but most practitioners initially prescribe 100 to 200 mg daily taken with a small amount of fat to aid in absorption. The most common commercially available formulations of CoQ10 are powder-filled, hard-shell capsules or oil-based suspensions; however, softgel capsules of CoQ10 appear to provide superior bioavailability.[110]

Precautions. CoQ10 has been found to be remarkably free of significant side effects. The most common adverse reaction is gastrointestinal upset (epigastric discomfort, loss of appetite, nausea, and diarrhea), occurring in fewer than 1% of all subjects.[105] Case reports exist of possible procoagulant activity in patients taking warfarin.[106] Patients taking 3-hydroxy-3-methyl-glutaryl-coenzyme A (HMG-CoA) reductase inhibitors (statin drugs) might benefit from supplementation with CoQ10. As alluded to earlier, cholesterol and CoQ10 partially share the mevalonate pathway, the same biosynthetic pathway disrupted by statin drugs. Cholesterol production and the endogenous pathways for CoQ10 production are thus both compromised by HMG-CoA reductase inhibition (statins).[107–109]

Carnitine

Carnitine, another vitamin-like substance, acts as a specific carrier of the fatty acids required for energy production, moving them from the cytoplasm into the mitochondria. Carnitine is synthesized from the amino acid lysine, but it is also available in small amounts in foods such as red meat. Unfortunately, the organs in which carnitine is most highly concentrated (those with high levels of fatty acid metabolism, including the heart and skeletal muscle) are incapable of synthesizing carnitine themselves.[111] Myocardial carnitine is most highly concentrated within the left ventricle.[112, 113] Levels of carnitine have been found to be low in patients with heart failure,[114, 115] and depletion of myocardial L-carnitine appears to adversely affect cell membrane function, translating into impaired myocardial contractility.[116–118]

Only the L-form of carnitine should be used therapeutically, and propionyl L-carnitine (PLC [created through the esterification of L-carnitine]) appears to be most effective in heart disease because it is reportedly highly lipophilic and thus readily available to myocardial cells.[119] PLC has been shown to improve muscle metabolism,[120] to stimulate the Krebs cycle,[121] and to improve heart contractility[122] in animal models. Studies using L-carnitine in humans with ischemic heart disease or peripheral vascular disease reveal enhanced cardiac performance and increased exercise tolerance.[123, 124]

Human trials using PLC in the setting of heart failure have provided promising results. Chronic administration of PLC has been shown to improve ventricular function, reduce systemic vascular resistance, and increase exercise tolerance.[125, 126] Administration acutely lowered pulmonary artery and capillary wedge pressure in one study.[127] Another reported a statistically significant reduced 3-year mortality rate in patients taking PLC.[128] In a well-done study that reported no significant benefit of PLC use in heart failure, there was a trend toward beneficial effects for those people with somewhat preserved heart function (ejection fraction between 30% and 40%), and the safety of the agent was confirmed.[129]

Dosage. The dosage used in most studies is 2 g/day (range, 1 to 3 g).

Precautions. The existing literature strongly suggests that the use of PLC is safe for patients with heart failure. L-Carnitine has been reported to cause an unpleasant body odor in very high doses. The majority of studies that used PLC, however, reveal no side effects, and no major toxicity has been reported.[130]

L-*Arginine*

L-Arginine is an essential amino acid possessing vasodilatory effects, which may enhance coronary artery blood flow and lessen the work of the heart by decreasing vascular resistance. Whereas further research is indicated, the existing data are promising. The use of L-arginine has been associated with improved hemodynamics and decreased endothelial dysfunction,[131-135] improved exercise tolerance,[131] and improved kidney function.[136]

Dosage. The typical dosage used in heart failure is 2 to 5 g three times daily.

Precautions. L-Arginine increases potassium levels when used with other potassium-sparing drugs[137] and may increase the incidence of recurrent herpetic lesions.

Surgery

People with the most severe forms of heart failure are considered for surgical intervention, including placement of implantable defibrillators, left ventricular assistance devices, cardiomyoplasty, and heart transplantation. Most people with this degree of cardiac insufficiency are unable to exercise or tolerate beta blockade.

— THERAPEUTIC REVIEW

Every patient with heart failure is singularly different from any other patient with the same malady and must be treated as such. The best combination of preventive measures, conventional therapeutics, and alternative medicines for a given individual is often not uncovered until after a number of patient visits have occurred, and even then the dynamic nature of health makes change inevitable. The healing relationship that can develop between patient and practitioner supports all parties through the dynamics of change in healthcare status, and enables individualization of therapy to take place in partnership. Clearly, conventional medical therapy must maintain a central role in the care of people with established heart failure, but specific complementary measures also offer proven medical benefits in some instances and at least the promise of benefit in others (see Figs. 20–1 and 20–2).

References

1. Ghali JK, Cooper R, Ford E: Trends in hospitalization rates for heart failure in the United States 1973–1986. Arch Intern Med 150:769–773, 1990.
2. Schocken DD, Arrieta MI, Leaverton PE, et al: Prevalence and mortality rates of congestive heart failure in the United States. J Am Coll Cardiol 20:301–306, 1992.
3. American Heart Association: 1998 Heart and Stroke Statistical Update. Dallas, American Heart Association, 1997.
4. Young JB: Contemporary management of patients with heart failure. Med Clin North Am 79:1171–1190, 1995.
5. Nagendran T: The syndrome of heart failure. Hosp Phys 37(4):46–57, 2001.
6. Carson PE: Management of congestive heart failure. Fed Practit Suppl, pp 4–29, 1995.
7. Krauss RM, Eckel RH, Howard B, et al: AHA dietary guidelines. Circulation 102:2284, 2000.
8. Massie BM, Shah NB: Evolving trends in the epidemiologic factors of heart failure: Rationale for preventive strategies and comprehensive disease management. Am Heart J 133:703–712, 1997.
9. O'Connell JB, Bristow MR: Economic impact of heart failure in the United States: Time for a different approach. J Heart Lung Transplant 13:S107–S112, 1994.
10. Graves EJ: National Hospital Discharge Survey: Annual summary, 1993. Vital and Health Statistics. Series 13: Data from National Health Survey, vol. 121. Washington, DC: U.S. Government Printing Office, 1995, pp. 1–63.
11. Centers for Disease Control and Prevention: Cerebrovascular disease mortality and Medicare hospitalization—United States, 1980–1990. MMWR Morb Mortal Wkly Rep 41:477–480, 1992.
12. Packer M: How should physicians view heart failure? The philosophical and physiological evolution of three conceptual models of the disease. Am J Cardiol 71(Suppl):3C–11C, 1993.
13. Francis GS, Goldsmith SR, Levine TB, et al: The neurohormonal axis in congestive heart failure. Ann Intern Med 101:370–377, 1984.
14. Packer M: The neurohormonal hypothesis: A theory to explain the mechanism of disease progression in heart failure. J Am Coll Cardiol 20:248–254, 1992.
15. Zock PL, Katan MB: Trans fatty acids, lipoproteins, and coronary risk. Can J Physiol Pharmacol 75:211–216, 1997.
16. Ascherio A, Willett W: Health effects of trans fatty acids. Am J Clin Nutr 66(Suppl):1006S, 1997.
17. Williams MJA, Sutherland WH, McCormick MP, et al: Impaired endothelial function following a meal rich in used cooking fat. J Am Coll Cardiol 33:1050, 1999.
18. Kotchen TA, McCarron DA: Dietary electrolytes and blood pressure: A statement for healthcare professionals from the American Heart Association Nutrition Committee. Circulation 98:613–617, 1998.

19. de Lorgeril M, Salen P, Martin JL, et al: Mediterranean diet, traditional risk factors, and the rate of cardiovascular complications after myocardial infarction: Final report of the Lyon Diet Heart Study. Circulation 99:779, 1999.

20. von Schacky C, Angerer P, Kothny W, et al: The effect of dietary omega-3 fatty acids on coronary atherosclerosis. A randomized, double-blind, placebo-controlled trial. Ann Intern Med 130:554, 1999.

21. Hu FB, Stampfer MJ, Manson JE, et al: Dietary intake of alpha-linolenic acid and risk of fatal ischemic heart disease among women. Am J Clin Nutr 69:890, 1999.

22. Daviglus ML, Stamler J, Orencia AJ, et al: Fish consumption and the 30-year risk of fatal myocardial infarction. N Engl J Med 336:1046–1053, 1997.

23. Connor WE: Do the n-3 fatty acids from fish prevent deaths from cardiovascular disease? Am J Clin Nutr 66:188–189, 1997.

24. Albert CM, Hennekens CH, O'Donnell CJ, et al: Fish consumption and risk of sudden cardiac death (The US Physicians' Health Study). JAMA 279:23–28, 1998.

25. McCarron DA, Oparil S, Chait A, et al: Nutritional management of cardiovascular risk factors. Arch Intern Med 157:169–177, 1997.

26. Ness AR, Powles JW: Fruit and vegetables, and cardiovascular disease: A review. Int J Epidemiol 26:1–13, 1997.

27. McDougall J, Litzau K, Haver E, et al: Rapid reduction of serum cholesterol and blood pressure by a twelve-day, very low fat, strictly vegetarian diet. J Am Coll Nutr 14:491, 1995.

28. Wolk A, Manson JE, Stampfer MJ, et al: Long-term intake of dietary fiber and decreased risk of coronary heart disease among women (The Nurses' Health Study). JAMA 281:1998–2004, 1999.

29. Tribble D: AHA Science Advisory. Antioxidant consumption and risk of coronary heart disease: Emphasis on vitamin C, vitamin E, and beta-carotene: A statement for healthcare professionals from the American Heart Association. Circulation 99:591, 1999.

30. Spencer AP, Carson DS, Crouch MA: Vitamin E and coronary artery disease. Arch Intern Med 159:1313, 1999.

31. Diaz MN, Frei B, Vita JA, et al: Antioxidants and atherosclerotic heart disease. N Engl J Med 337:408–416, 1997.

32. Rimm EB, Willett WC, Hu FB, et al: Folate and vitamin B6 from diet and supplements in relation to risk of coronary heart disease among women (The Nurses' Health Study). JAMA 279:359–364, 1998.

33. Malinow MR, Bostom AG, Krauss RM: Homocyst(e)ine, diet, and cardiovascular diseases: A statement for healthcare professionals from the Nutrition Committee, American Heart Association. Circulation 99:178, 1999.

34. Mann SJ: The mind/body link in essential hypertension: Time for a new paradigm. Altern Ther Health Med 6(2):39–45, 2000.

35. Alexander CN, Schneider RH, Staggers F, et al: Trial of stress reduction for hypertension in older African Americans. II. Sex and Risk Subgroup Analysis.

36. Barnes VA, Treiber FA, Turner JR, et al: Acute effects of transcendental meditation on hemodynamic functioning in middle-aged adults. Psychosom Med 61:525, 1999.

37. Castillo-Richmond A, Schneider RH, Alexander CN, et al: Effects of stress reduction on carotid atherosclerosis in hypertensive African Americans. Stroke 31:568–573, 2000.

38. Luskin FM, Newell KA, Griffith M, et al: A review of mind-body therapies in the treatment of cardiovascular disease. Part 1: Implications for the elderly. Altern Ther Health Med 4(3):46, 1998.

39. Spence JD, Barnett PA, Linden W, et al: Lifestyle modifications to prevent and control hypertension. 7. Recommendations on stress management. CMAJ 160(9 Suppl):S46–S50, 1999.

40. Ortho-Gomer K, Horsten M, Wamala SP, et al: Social relations and extent and severity of coronary artery disease. Eur Heart J 19:1648–1656, 1998.

41. Kulkarni S, O'Farrell I, Erasi M, et al: Stress and hypertension. WMJ 97(11):34–38, 1998.

42. Jain D, Shaker SM, Burg M, et al: Effects of mental stress on left ventricular and peripheral vascular performance in patients with coronary artery disease. J Am Coll Cardiol 31:1314–1322, 1998.

43. Dembroski TM, MacDougall JM, Costa PT Jr, et al: Components of hostility as predictors of sudden death and myocardial infarction in the Multiple Risk Factor Intervention Trial. Psychosom Med 51:514–522, 1989.

44. Gallacher JE, Yarnell JW, Sweetnam PM, et al: Anger and incident heart disease in the Caerphilly study. Psychosom Med 61:446, 1999.

45. Koenig HG, Cohen HJ, George LK, et al: Attendance at religious services, interleukin-6, and other biological parameters of immune function in older adults. Int J Psychiatry Med 27:233–250, 1997.

46. Levin J: How prayer heals: A theoretical model. Altern Ther Health Med 2:66–73, 1996.

47. Oman D, Reed D: Religion and mortality among the community-dwelling elderly. Am J Public Health 88:1469–1475, 1998.

48. Waldfogel S: Spirituality in medicine. Prim Care 24:963, 1997.

49. Ornish D, Scherwitz LW, Billings JH, et al: Intensive lifestyle changes for reversal of coronary heart disease. JAMA 280:2001–2007, 1998.

50. Kolasa KM: Dietary Approaches to Stop Hypertension (DASH) in clinical practice: A primary care experience. Clin Cardiol 22(7 Suppl):III16–III22, 1999.

51. SOLVD Investigators: Effect of enalapril on survival in patients with reduced left ventricular ejection fractions and congestive heart failure. N Engl J Med 325:293–302, 1991.

52. The CONSENSUS Trial Study Group: Effects of enalapril on mortality in severe congestive heart failure. N Engl J Med 316:1429–1435, 1987.

53. Collaborative Group on ACE Inhibitor Trials: Overview of randomized trials of angiotensin-converting enzyme inhibitors on mortality and morbidity in patients with heart failure. JAMA 273:1450–1456, 1995.

54. Dahlstrom U, Karlsson E: Captopril and spironolactone therapy in patients with refractory congestive heart failure. Curr Ther Res 51:235–248, 1992.

55. The RALES Investigators: Effectiveness of spironolactone added to an angiotensin-converting enzyme inhibitor and a loop diuretic for severe chronic congestive heart failure (the Randomized Aldactone Evaluation Study [RALES]). Am J Cardiol 78:902–907, 1996.

56. Pitt B, Zannad F, Remme WJ, et al: The effect of spironolactone on morbidity and mortality in patients with severe heart failure. Randomized Aldactone Evaluation Study Investigators. N Engl J Med 341:709–717, 1999.

57. Soberman JE, Weber KT: Spironolactone in congestive heart failure. Curr Hypertens Rep 2:451–456, 2000.

58. Haji SA, Movahed A: Update on digoxin therapy in congestive heart failure. Am Fam Physician 62:409–416, 2000.

59. Riaz K, Forker AD: Digoxin use in congestive heart failure. Current status. Drugs 55:747–758, 1998.

60. Hauptman PJ, Kelly RA: Digitalis. Circulation 99:1265–1270, 1999.

61. The Digitalis Investigation Group: The effect of digoxin on mortality and morbidity in patients with heart failure. N Engl J Med 336:525–533, 1997.

62. Constant J: A review of why and how we may use beta-blockers in congestive heart failure. Chest 113:800–808, 1998.

63. Packer M: Do beta-blockers prolong survival in chronic heart failure? A review of the experimental and clinical evidence. Eur Heart J 19(Suppl B):B40–B46, 1998.

64. Frantz RP: Beta blockade in patients with congestive heart failure. Why, who and how. Postgrad Med 108:103–118, 2000.

65. Carson PE: Rationale for the use of combination angiotensin-converting enzyme inhibitor/angiotensin II receptor blocker therapy in heart failure. Am Heart J 140:361–366, 2000.

66. Pitt B, Poole-Wilson PA, Segal R, et al: Effects of losartan compared with captopril on mortality in patients with symptomatic heart failure: Randomized trial—the Losartan Heart Failure Survival Study ELITE II. Lancet 355:1582–1587, 2000.

67. McKelvie RS, Yusuf S, Pericak D, et al: Comparison of candesartan, enalapril, and their combination in congestive heart failure. Randomized Evaluation of Strategies for Left Ventricular Dysfunction (RESOLVD) pilot study. Circulation 100:1056–1064, 1999.

68. Graham JDP: *Crataegus oxycantha* in hypertension. BMJ 951, 1993.

69. Busse W: Standardized *Crataegus* extract clinical monograph. Q Rev Nat Med Fall:189–197, 1996.

70. Schussler M, Holzl J, Fricke U: Myocardial effects of flavonoids from *Crataegus* species. Arzneimittelforschung 45:842–845, 1995.

71. Weihmayr T, Ernst E: Therapeutic effectiveness of *Crataegus*. Fortschr Med 114:27–29, 1996.

72. Tauchert M, et al: Effectiveness of hawthorn extract LI 132 compared with the ACE inhibitor captopril: Multicenter double-blind study with 132 NYHA stage II patients. Munch Med 136(Suppl 1):S27–S33, 1994.

73. Schmidt U, et al: Efficacy of the hawthorn (*Crataegus*) preparation LI 132 in 78 patients with chronic congestive heart failure defined as NYHA functional class II. Phytomedicine 1:17–24, 1994.

74. Weikl A, Assmus KD, Neukum-Schmidt A, et al: *Crataegus* Special Extract WS 1442. Assessment of objective effectiveness in patients with heart failure. Fortschr Med 114:291–296, 1996.

75. Leuchtgens H: *Crataegus* Special Extract WS 1442 in NYHA II heart failure. A placebo controlled randomized double-blind study. Fortschr Med 111:352–354, 1993.

76. Tauchert M, Gildor A, Lipinski J: High-dose *Crataegus* extract WS 1442 in the treatment of NYHA stage II heart failure. Herz24:465–474, 1999.

77. Bagchi D: A review of the clinical benefits of co-enzyme Q10. J Adv Med 10:139–148, 1997.

78. Nayler WG: The use of coenzyme Q10 to protect ischaemic heart muscle. In Yamamura Y, Folkers K, Ito Y (eds): Biomedical and Clinical Aspects of Coenzyme Q, vol. 2. Amsterdam, Elsevier-North Holland Biomedical, 1980, pp. 409–425.

79. Awata N, et al: The effects of coenzyme Q10 on ischemic heart disease evaluated by dynamic exercise test. In Yamamura Y, Folkers K, Ito Y (eds): Biochemical and Clinical Aspects of Coenzyme Q10, vol. 2. Amsterdam, Elsevier-North Holland Biomedical, 1980, pp. 247–254.

80. Nakamura Y, Takahashi M, Hayashi J, et al: Protection of ischaemic myocardium with coenzyme Q10. Cardiovasc Res 16:132–137, 1982.

81. Crane FL, Navas P: The diversity of coenzyme Q function. Mol Aspects Med 18(Suppl):S1–S6, 1997.

82. Frei B, Kim MC, Ames BN: Ubiquinol-10 is an effective lipid-soluble antioxidant at physiological concentrations. Proc Natl Acad Sci U S A 87:4879–4883, 1990.

83. Ondarroa M, Quinn P: Proton magnetic resonance spectroscopic studies of the interaction of ubiquinone-10 with phospholipid membranes. Int J Biochem 155:353, 1986.

84. Folkers K, Vadhanavikit S, Mortensen SA: Biochemical rationale and myocardial tissue data on the effective therapy of cardiomyopathy with coenzyme Q10. Proc Natl Acad Sci U S A 82:901–904, 1985.

85. Littarru GP, Ho L, Folkers K: Deficiency of coenzyme Q10 in human heart disease. Part II. Int J Vitam Nutr Res 42:413–434, 1972.

86. Mortensen SA, Kondrup J, Folkers K: Myocardial deficiency of coenzyme Q10 and carnitine in cardiomyopathy. Biochemical rationale for concomitant coenzyme Q10 and carnitine supplementation. In Folkers K, Littarru GP, Yamagami T (eds): Biomedical and Clinical Aspects of CoEnzyme Q10, vol. 6. Amsterdam, Elsevier, 1991, pp. 269–281.

87. Mortensen SA: Endomyocardial biopsy. Technical aspects and indications. Thesis, 1989, pp. 3–36.

88. Mortensen SA, Vadhanavikit S, Folkers K: Deficiency of coenzyme Q10 in myocardial failure. Drugs Exp Clin Res 10:497–502, 1984.

89. Kitamura N, et al: Myocardial tissue level of coenzyme Q10 in patients with cardiac failure. In Folkers K, Yamamura Y (eds): Biomedical and Clinical Aspects of Coenzyme Q, vol. 4. Amsterdam, Elsevier Science, 1984, pp. 243–252.

90. Mortensen SA: Perspectives on therapy of cardiovascular disease with coenzyme Q10. Clin Invest 71:116–123, 1993.

91. Langsjoen PH, Vadhanavikit S, Folkers K: Response of patients in classes III and IV of cardiomyopathy to therapy in a blind and crossover trial with coenzyme Q10. Proc Natl Acad Sci U S A 82:4240–4244, 1985.

92. Yamamura Y, et al: Clinical use of coenzyme Q for treatment of cardiovascular disease. Jpn Circ J 31:168, 1967.

93. Langsjoen PH, Langsjoen PH, Folkers K: Long-term efficacy and safety of coenzyme Q10 therapy for idiopathic dilated cardiomyopathy. Am J Cardiol 65:521–523, 1990.

94. Judy WV, et al: Double blind double crossover study of coenzyme Q10 in heart failure. In Folkers K, Yamamura Y (eds): Biomedical and Clinical Aspects of Coenzyme Q, vol. 5. Amsterdam, Elsevier, 1986, pp. 315–322.

95. Langsjoen PH, Langsjoen AM: Overview of the use of CoQ10 in cardiovascular disease. Biofactors 9:273–284, 1999.

96. Soja Am, Mortensen SA: Treatment of congestive heart failure with coenzyme Q10 illuminated by meta-analyses of clinical trials. Mol Aspects Med 18(Suppl):S159–S168, 1997.

97. Morisco C, Trimarco B, Condorelli M: Effect of coenzyme Q10 therapy in patients with congestive heart failure: A long-term multicenter randomized study. Clin Invest 71(Suppl):S34–S36, 1993.

98. Baggio E, Gandini R, Plancher AC, et al: Italian multicenter study on the safety and efficacy of coenzyme Q10 as adjunctive therapy in heart failure. Mol Aspects Med 15:287–294, 1994.

99. Langsjoen PH, Langsjoen AM: Coenzyme Q10 in cardiovascular disease with emphasis on heart failure and myocardial ischemia. Asia Pac Heart J 7:160–168, 1998.

100. Judy WV, Hall JH, Folkers K: Coenzyme Q10 withdrawal—clinical relapse in congestive heart failure patients. In Folkers K, Littaru GP, Yamagami T (eds): Biomedical and Clinical Aspects of Coenzyme Q. Amsterdam, Elsevier Science, 1991, pp. 283–298.

101. Langsjoen PH, Folkers K, Lyson K, et al: Pronounced increase of survival of patients with cardiomyopathy when treated with coenzyme Q10 and conventional therapy. Int J Tissue React 12:163–168, 1990.

102. Judy WV, Folkers K, Hall JH: Improved long-term survival in coenzyme Q10 treated chronic heart failure patients compared to conventionally treated patients. In Folkers K, Littarru GP, Yamagami T (eds): Biomedical and Clinical Aspects of Coenzyme Q, vol. 4. Amsterdam, Elsevier Science, 1991, pp. 291–298.

103. Watson PS, Scalia GM, Galbraith A, et al: Lack of effect of coenzyme Q10 on left ventricular function in patients with congestive heart failure. J Am Coll Cardiol 33:1549–1552, 1999.

104. Khatta M, Alexander BS, Krichten CM, et al: The effect of coenzyme Q10 in patients with congestive heart failure. Ann Intern Med 132:636–640, 2000.

105. Greenberg S, Frishman WH: Co-enzyme Q10: A new drug for cardiovascular disease. J Clin Pharmacol 30:596–608, 1990.

106. Spigset O: Reduced effect of warfarin caused by ubidecarenone [letter]. Lancet 344:1372–1373, 1994.

107. Folkers K, Langsjoen P, Willis R, et al: Lovastatin decreases coenzyme Q10 levels in humans. Proc Natl Acad Sci U S A 87:8931–8934, 1990.

108. Mortensen SA, Leth A, Agner E, et al: Dose-related decrease of serum coenzyme Q10 during treatment with HMG-CoA reductase inhibitors. Mol Aspects Med 18(Suppl):S137–S144, 1997.

109. Ghirlanda G, Oradei A, Manto A, et al: Evidence of plasma CoQ10-lowering effect by HMG-CoA reductase inhibitors: A double-blind, placebo-controlled study. J Clin Pharmacol 3:226–229, 1993.

110. Chopra RK, Goldman R, Sinatra ST, et al: Relative bioavailability of coenzyme Q10 formulations in human subjects. Int J Vitam Nutr Res 68:109–113, 1998.

111. Arsenian MA: Carnitine and its derivatives in cardiovascular disease. Prog Cardiovasc Dis 40:265–286, 1997.

112. Nakagawa T, Sunamori M, Suzuki A: The myocardial distribution and plasma concentration of carnitine in patients with mitral valve disease. Surg Today 24:313–317, 1994.

113. Pierpoint ME, Judd D, Goldenberg I, et al: Myocardial carnitine in end-stage congestive heart failure. Am J Cardiol 64:56–60, 1989.

114. Suzuki Y, Masumura Y, Kobayashi A, et al: Myocardial carnitine deficiency in congestive heart failure. Lancet 1:116, 1982.

115. Regitz V, Shug AL, Fleck E: Defective myocardial metabolism in congestive heart failure secondary to dilated cardiomyopathy and coronary, hypertensive and valvular heart disease. Am J Cardiol 65:755–760, 1990.

116. Corr PB, Gross RW, Sobel BE: Amphipathic metabolites and membrane dysfunction in ischemic myocardium. Circ Res 55:135–154, 1984.

117. Shug AL, Subramanian R: Modulation of adenine nucleotide translocase activity during myocardial ischemia. Z Kardiol 76(Suppl 5):26–33, 1987.

118. Siliprandi N, Di Lisa F, Pivetta A, et al: Transport and function of L-carnitine and L-propionylcarnitine: Relevance to some cardiomyopathies and cardiac ischemia. Z Kardiol 76(Suppl 5):3–40, 1987.

119. Paulson DJ, Traxler J, Schmidt M, et al: Protection of the ischaemic myocardium by L-propionyl-carnitine: Effects on the recovery of cardiac output after ischaemia and reperfusion, carnitine transport and fatty acid oxidation. Cardiovasc Res 20:536–541, 1986.

120. Tassani V, Cattapan F, Magnanimi L, Peschechera A: Anaplerotic effect of propionyl carnitine in rat heart mitochondria. Biochem Biophys Res Commun 199:949–953, 1994.

121. Di Lisa F, Menabo R, Siliprandi N: L-Propionyl-carnitine protection of mitochondria in ischemic rat hearts. Mol Cell Biochem 88:169–173, 1989.

122. Ferrari R, Di Lisa F, de Jong JW, et al: Prolonged propionyl-L-carnitine pretreatment of rabbit: Biochemical, hemodynamic and electrophysiological effects on myocardium. J Mol Cell Cardiol 24:219–232, 1992.

123. Cherchi A, Lai C, Angelino F, et al: Effects of L-carnitine on exercise tolerance in chronic stable angina: A multicenter, double-blind, randomized, placebo controlled crossover study. Int J Clin Pharmacol Ther Toxicol 23:569–572, 1985.

124. Brevetti G, Chiariello M, Ferulano G, et al: Increases in walking distance in patients with peripheral vascular disease treated with L-carnitine: A double-blind, cross-over study. Circulation 77:767–783, 1988.

125. Mancini M, Rengo F, Lingetti M, et al: Controlled study on the therapeutic efficacy of propionyl-L-carnitine in patients with congestive heart failure. Arzneimittelforschung 42:1101–1104, 1992.

126. Caponnetto S, Canale C, Masperone MA, et al: Efficacy of L-propionyl-carnitine treatment in patients with left ventricular dysfunction. Eur Heart J 15:1267–1273, 1994.

127. Anand I, Chandrashekhan Y, De Giuli F, et al: Acute and chronic effects of propionyl-L-carnitine on the hemodynamics, exercise capacity, and hormones in patients with congestive heart failure. Cardiovasc Drugs Ther 12:291–299, 1998.

128. Rizos I: Three-year survival of patients with heart failure caused by dilated cardiomyopathy and L-carnitine administration. Am Heart J 139:S120–S123, 2000.

129. Anand I, Chandrashekhan Y, De Giuli F, et al: Study on propionyl-L-carnitine in chronic heart failure. The Investigators of the Study on Propionyl-L-Carnitine in Chronic Heart Failure. Eur Heart J 19:70–76, 1999.

130. Arsenian MA: Carnitine and its derivatives in cardiovascular disease. Prog Cardiovasc Dis 40:265–286, 1997.

131. Rector TS, Bank AJ, Mullen KA, et al: Randomized, double-blind, placebo-controlled study of supplemental oral L-arginine in patients with heart failure. Circulation 93:2135–2141, 1996.

132. Hambrecht R, Hilbrich L, Erbs S, et al: Correction of endothelial dysfunction in chronic heart failure: Additional effects of exercise training and oral L-arginine supplementation. J Am Coll Cardiol 35:706–713, 2000.

133. Lerman A, Burnett JC Jr, Higano ST, et al: Long-term L-arginine supplementation improves small-vessel coronary endothelial function in humans. Circulation 97:2123–2128, 1998.

134. Adams MR, McCredie R, Jessup W, et al: Oral L-arginine improves endothelium-dependent dilatation and reduces monocyte adhesion to endothelial cells in young men with coronary artery disease. Atherosclerosis 129:261–269, 1997.

135. Bocchi EA, Vilella de Moraes AV, Esteves-Filho A, et al: L-Arginine reduces heart rate and improves hemodynamics in severe congestive heart failure. Clin Cardiol 23:205–210, 2000.

136. Watanabe G, Tomiyama H, Doba N: Effects of oral administration of L-arginine on renal function in patients with heart failure. J Hypertens 18:229–234, 2000.

137. McKevoy GK (ed): AHFS Drug Information. Bethesda, Md, American Society of Health-System Pharmacists, 1998.

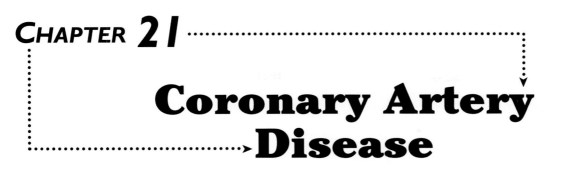

CHAPTER 21

Coronary Artery Disease

Sara L. Warber, M.D., and Suzanna M. Zick, N.D., M.P.H.

This chapter focuses on coronary artery disease (CAD), which is part of a larger picture of atherosclerotic disease that affects many areas of the vasculature and causes 42% of all deaths in the United States. Primary prevention is accomplished by making interventions with asymptomatic individuals at risk for CAD owing to increasing age, male sex, elevated low-density lipoprotein (LDL) cholesterol, elevated blood pressure, smoking, diabetes, family history of cardiovascular disease, obesity, and/or sedentary lifestyle. Examples of clinically overt CAD include acute myocardial infarction (MI), angina (stable or unstable), or a history of invasive coronary procedures. The long-term prognosis in individuals with overt CAD depends on the degree of left ventricular dysfunction, the presence of residual ischemia, and the extent of electrical instability. The therapeutic emphasis in these individuals is on long-term secondary prevention of recurrent MI, unstable angina, left ventricular dysfunction, heart failure, and sudden cardiac death. Further aims of secondary prevention are to promote a return to normal activities, improve quality of life, and improve long-term survival[1] (see Chapter 70, Prevention of Atherosclerosis).

PATHOPHYSIOLOGY

The etiologic factors in CAD include the presence of atheromatous plaques lining the coronary arteries, plaque rupture, and coronary artery spasm. The resultant ischemia, if transient, causes angina or, if more permanent, can cause myocardial cell death and/or electrical dysfunction. What are the factors that cause the plaque to be there in the first place? What are the factors that influence plaque stability? And what are the contributors to vasospasm?

The current theories of atherogenesis are represented in Figure 21–1. The "response to injury" of the endothelium hypothesis is not well supported at this time. However, the "response to retention" of LDL theory and the "LDL oxidation" theory enjoy more evidentiary support. Both hypotheses are related to various potential integrative approaches to treatment. The "response to retention" theory

suggests that increased concentrations of LDL in the lumen of the vessel readily enter the vascular wall extracellular spaces, but are unable to leave at the same rate and therefore accumulate, aggregate, and promote their own uptake by macrophages. The "LDL oxidation" theory postulates that LDL in the cell wall becomes oxidized via a variety of possible mechanisms and that this oxidized LDL is preferentially taken up by macrophages. LDL oxidation is thought to occur via some or all of the following mechanisms:

1. Cellular production of superoxides (inflammatory cells and vascular wall cells)
2. Reactive nitrogen species (from combination of nitric oxide [NO] and superoxide)
3. Glycoxidation (possible mechanism in diabetic vasculopathy)
4. Myeloperoxidase (oxidative enzyme secreted by macrophages)
5. Metal ions such as copper (although it is unknown whether this occurs in vivo)
6. Intracellular lipoxygenase (less likely because LDL oxidation is an extracellular process)

The net result is the accumulation of foam cells (lipid-laden macrophages) and atherogenesis.

Once the plaque is formed, it is relatively stable and may not cause problems for its owner for many years. The plaque consists of a "lipid core" of foam cells, extracellular cholesterol, and necrotic material overlaid by a "fibrous cap" of extracellular matrix, smooth muscle cells, and collagen. In order for atherosclerosis to become clinically overt, the plaque must become "activated" and rupture (Fig. 21–2). The process is thought to proceed in this manner. In areas of inflammation, activated T cells produce interferon-gamma. Interferon-gamma induces apoptosis (programmed cell death) in smooth muscle cells as well as decreased collagen synthesis. In the fibrous cap, the ratio of macrophages to smooth muscle cells begins to change in favor of macrophages. The macrophages secrete metalloproteinase enzymes that begin to degrade the extracellular matrix of the fibrous cap. The fibrous cap weakens, and in the shoulder region, it is most susceptible to mechanical sheer forces. This is often where rupture occurs. Rupture exposes the

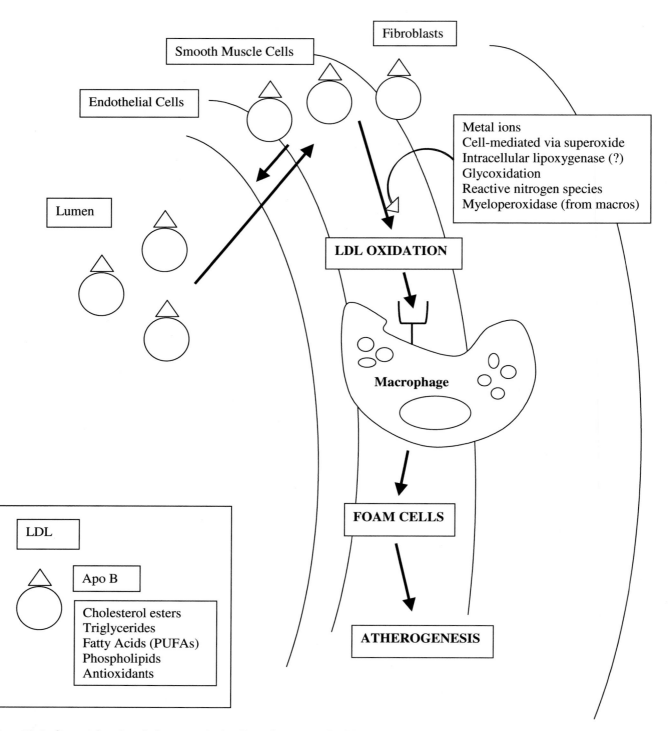

Figure 21–1. Current theories of atherogenesis. Apo B, apolipoprotein B; LDL, low-density lipoprotein; PUFAs, polyunsaturated fatty acids.

lipid core to blood in the lumen. The lipid core contents, including abundant tissue factor, activate the clotting cascade. This can rapidly fill the arterial lumen with thrombus, causing the overt manifestations of acute coronary events.

Lesion activation also involves a fundamental lapse in vasoregulation, including control of vascular tone and blood flow and inhibition of thrombosis.

The endothelium is the critical component of the vessel wall controlling these factors. Through several products, the endothelium maintains a state that favors fibrinolysis over thrombosis. One important product is NO, synthesized in the endothelial cells by nitric oxide synthase (eNOS). NO is particularly responsible for vasorelaxation, as well as smooth muscle cell phenotype, inhibition of platelet adhe-

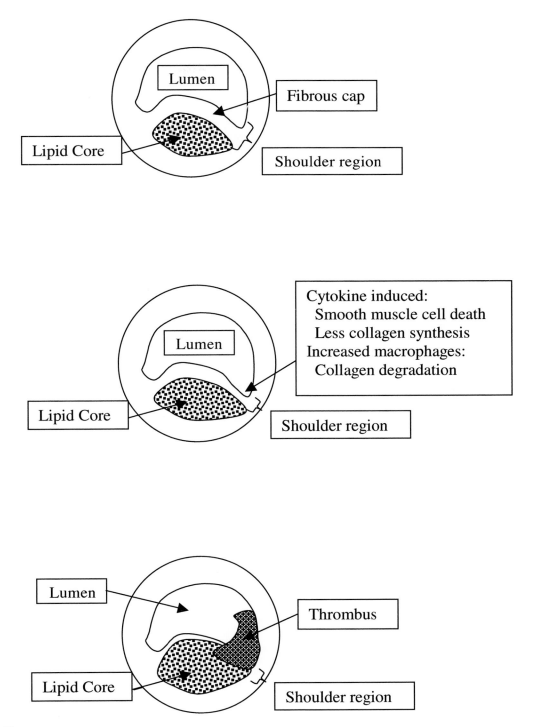

Figure 21-2. Plaque rupture.

sion, and leukocyte recruitment. Several integrative medicine treatments influence the bioactivity of NO. For example, when oxidants outnumber antioxidants (i.e., oxidative stress), NO activity is impaired. In particular, superoxide produced by endothelial cells, adventitial cells, xanthine oxidase, and eNOS itself inhibits the ability of NO to relax the arterial walls. Water-soluble antioxidants—glutathione and ascorbic acid—reach high concentrations in the cytosol of endothelial cells and stimulate NO synthesis and/or scavenge superoxide. Oxidized LDL can quench NO bioactivity; however, lipid-soluble antioxidants such as vitamin E, beta-carotene, and probucol preserve NO activity, possibly through interaction with oxidized LDL or its byproducts. Likewise, lipid-lowering improves endothelial functioning. Supplementation of L-arginine, a substrate of eNOS, and BH_4, a cofactor of eNOS, improves NO activity. Estrogen and angiotensin-converting enzyme (ACE) inhibitors also improve endothelial function, although the mechanism is not yet known.[2]

We have seen how the three elements of atherogenesis, plaque activation/rupture, and vasoregulation interrelate to create atherosclerotic disease and its sequelae. We now turn to various interventions that can be applied in an integrative manner for primary and/or secondary prevention of CAD.

LIFESTYLE

Very Low-Fat Diet

Very low-fat diets (<10%) are extremely challenging for patients to undertake but, for the exceptionally motivated individual, may provide important benefits owing to reduction of available LDL. Research done by Dean Ornish, using a very low-fat, whole-food, vegetarian diet high in complex carbohydrates and low in simple sugars along with walking, smoking cessation, and stress management techniques, demonstrated a 91% reduction in the frequency of angina and in regression of coronary atherosclerosis after only 1 year[3] and even more regression after 5 years.[4] This was in contrast to a control group of patients who followed a step 2 diet yet showed both increased coronary atherosclerosis and increased angina after 1 year and even more stenosis after 5 years. There were twice as many cardiac events in the control group compared with those patients following the Ornish program, whereas the experimental group was able to avoid revascularization for at least 3 years.[5, 6]

The Ornish program has been criticized because patients on the diet tend to have increased triglycerides and decreased high-density lipoprotein (HDL) serum levels. However, Dr. Ornish contends that increases in triglycerides can be minimized or eliminated by increasing exercise, avoiding or minimizing simple carbohydrates, and supplementing the diet with 3 to 4 g/day of flaxseed oil or fish oil. Further, he points to epidemiologic studies that show that populations eating a low-fat, primarily vegetarian, diet have lower serum HDLs, but also a lower prevalence of CAD.[7]

Smoking Cessation

See Chapter 22, Peripheral Vascular Disease, for a discussion of aids to smoking cessation, including abstinence, nicotine replacement, bupropion, acupuncture, and hypnosis.

Exercise

See Chapter 22, Peripheral Vascular Disease, for a discussion of the importance of exercise. (see Chapter 86, Writing an Exercise Prescription).

MIND-BODY THERAPIES

Depression is common among patients with heart disease and is associated with adverse outcomes and increased long-term mortality. In addition, the cost of treating cardiac patients with mild to moderate depression is 41% higher in the first year after MI. Type A behavior is also thought to predispose to heart disease. Hostility and anger are associated with increased risk of acute coronary events, as are anxiety, panic symptoms, and, perhaps, vital exhaustion. Social isolation and lack of social support are more powerful risk factors than some traditional risk factors like smoking.[8] The autonomic nervous system is exquisitely sensitive to thoughts and emotions, with negative reactions creating disorder and imbalance in the autonomic nervous system and positive feelings, such as appreciation, creating order and balance.[9] Sympathetic stimulation is one of the proposed mechanisms underlying the mind-heart connection. In addition, chronic stress elevates basal cortisol and impairs the body's ability to respond to acute stressors and can precipitate illness. Thus, many mind-body therapies have potential utility in both primary and secondary prevention of coronary heart disease manifestations.

Meditation, hypnosis, biofeedback, yoga, qi gong, tai chi, religious practice, cognitive behavior treatment, and music therapy have been looked at as possible mind-body interventions for heart disease. Transcendental meditation decreases basal cortisol and improves carotid atherosclerosis, a surrogate marker for CAD.[10, 11] Hypnosis and biofeedback are particularly useful for decreasing both heart rate and high blood pressure. The increasingly popular practice of yoga—which includes focused control of the mind, breath, and body—decreases sympathetic tone, improves blood pressure, decreases heart rate, and decreases oxygen requirement without affecting work. Qi gong, a traditional Chinese practice of breathing, meditation, and movement, has beneficial effects on hypertension, depression, anxiety, and CAD. Tai chi, another mind, breath, and movement discipline, improves exercise endurance, reduces stress, and enhances positive mood.[12] Religious practice, belief, and the related social support appear to play a positive role in various aspects of cardiac health. Cognitive behavioral treatment has been applied to reducing risk factors such as obesity, blood pressure, exercise, and type A behavior. Music therapy (i.e., singing, playing instruments, and listening to music) has the ability to directly alter heart rate, stress levels, and anxiety in heart patients.[13] Each of these approaches brings the mind, spirit, and emotions into balance with the body, thus enhancing a variety of mechanisms that promote optimal health. No one approach will be good for all patients. It is important to work with individuals to identify mind-body approaches that are consistent with their beliefs and interests. With a wide array available, all patients will be able to benefit from these approaches.

NOTE

Mind-body therapies are not entirely free of complications. Vertebral artery occlusion, acute cerebellar infarction, and acute medullary infarction have been reported in people practicing yoga.[12] Acute psychosis has been associated with qi gong practice.[14] Psychological problems may emerge during other mind-body work, and practitioners to whom you refer should be skillful in handling these issues or have a backup plan. In addition, the philosophy underlying meditation, yoga, tai chi, or qi gong may conflict with the belief systems of some individuals.[15]

SUPPLEMENTS

Antioxidants (Alpha-Lipoic Acid, Vitamins C and E, Beta-Carotene)

Because oxidation likely plays an important role in the development of atherosclerosis, it seems logical that antioxidants such as alpha-lipoic acid, vitamins C and E, beta-carotene, and coenzyme Q10 (CoQ10) may be protective. There are two proposed mechanisms of how antioxidants may inhibit atherogenesis and improve vascular function: disposing of reactive oxygen species and improving the biologic activity of endothelium-derived NO. However, epidemiologic and prospective clinical trials examining the effect of ingesting vitamins E and C and beta-carotene have been promising but inconclusive.

The Nurses' Health Study, a large epidemiologic trial, found that individuals with the highest dietary intake of vitamin E had about a 40% reduction in cardiovascular disease risk.[16] In addition, the Cambridge Heart Antioxidant Study (CHAOS), a prospective clinical trial, found that vitamin E reduced the risk of nonfatal MI in patients suffering from established CAD.[17] However, the α-Tocopherol, β-Carotene Cancer Prevention Study Group Trial, also a prospective clinical trial, found that there was no reduction in the incidence of CAD over an 8-year period in the Finnish men who participated in the study despite the high prevalence of CAD in the population.[18] The Physicians' Health Study also found no reduction in the incidence of CAD in physicians taking 50 mg of beta-carotene every other day.[19] A trial examining the effect of vitamins E and C in preventing restenosis in patients undergoing coronary angioplasty found that both vitamins failed to prevent restenosis from occurring.[20]

Dosage. Alpha-lipoic acid, 20 to 50 mg/day; vitamin E, 400 to 800 IU/day; vitamin C, 500 mg/day.

Precautions. There is an increased risk of bleeding owing to vitamin E interference with vitamin K–dependent clotting factors.

Arginine

Arginine is a semiessential amino acid that is synthesized in the liver and kidneys. During periods of physical or emotional stress, the endogenous production of arginine is insufficient and dietary sources of arginine are needed to avoid a relative deficiency. L-Arginine is the precursor to endothelium-derived NO and appears to enhance NO production when taken as a supplement.

In animal studies, L-arginine has been found to prevent the formation of endothelial lesions, prevent restenosis after percutaneous transluminal angioplasty (PTCA), and ameliorate ischemic and reperfusion injury during acute MIs. Moreover, in human studies, despite a small number of experimental subjects, oral L-arginine was found to decrease episodes of angina, increase exercise capacity in patients with both obstructive and nonobstructive CAD, and possibly, prevent the development of atherosclerosis.[21, 22]

Dosage. Lowest effective dose: L-arginine 6 to 8 g/day given orally; 18 to 20 g/day provides maximal benefit.

Precautions. There is a potential for increases in diarrhea, constipation, nausea, vomiting, and headache.

NOTE

Patients who have renal or hepatic failure or who are using potassium-sparing diuretics should avoid L-arginine supplementation, because it can lead to hyperkalemia. Oral L-arginine supplementation may increase the frequency of herpes simple outbreaks.

L-Carnitine

Carnitine is an amino acid made from lysine or derived from eating meat and dairy products. Carnitine is responsible for transporting long-chain fatty acids into the mitochondria. Without carnitine, there would be decreased concentrations of fatty acids in the mitochondria and, thus, decreased overall energy production. It is important to recall that the myocardium's primary energy source is fatty acids, not glucose. It is, therefore, not surprising that specific active transport proteins allow the heart to concentrate carnitine at 10 times the levels found in the plasma. See Chapter 22, Peripheral Vascular Disease, for further discussion of the use of carnitine in atherosclerosis.

Dosage. 1500 to 4000 mg, divided, twice daily.

Precautions. There may be episodes of transient nausea, vomiting, abdominal cramps, and diarrhea, which are rare in doses less than 6 g/day.

Vitamins B$_6$ and B$_{12}$ and Folic Acid

Recent evidence suggests that homocysteine may interact with physiologic mediators of the endothelial matrix. Oxidative mechanisms and decreased biologic activity of endothelium-derived NO may also contribute to homocysteine-associated endothelial dysfunction. B vitamins are essential cofactors in the metabolism of homocysteine to methionine via the remethylation pathway (vitamin B$_{12}$, folic acid) and to cystathionine via the transsulfuration pathway (vitamin B$_6$). Dietary deficiencies of folic acid and vitamins B$_{12}$ and B$_6$ appear to be common, especially among elderly people in the Western world, and represent one pathogenic factor related to the incidence of hyperhomocysteinemia.[23]

Whereas current evidence supports the link between hyperhomocysteinemia and endothelial cell damage, the progression toward cardiovascular disease is unclear. Currently, there are no completed randomized clinical trials that assess CAD end points; however, in small trials, patients given vitamins B$_6$ and B$_{12}$ and folate have experienced lower serum levels of homocysteine with limited side effects.[24, 25]

Dosage. Vitamin B$_6$, 50 to 100 mg/day in divided doses; vitamin B$_{12}$, 2000 μg/day; and folate, 400 μg/day.

Coenzyme Q10

CoQ10, also known as ubiquinone, is thought to benefit patients with CAD in two ways. First, CoQ10 is a coenzyme for the inner mitochondrial enzyme complexes involved in oxidative phosphorylation and, thus, the production of adenosine triphosphate. CoQ10's central role in energy production makes it particularly important for providing the needs of high-energy tissue such as the myocardium. Second, CoQ10 is a lipid-soluble antioxidant that appears to work synergistically with vitamin E to reduce low-density lipoprotein (LDL) oxidation.

Clinical research including numerous controlled trials has shown that supplementation with CoQ10 appears to benefit patients with CAD in several ways. Controlled trials in patients with angina showed an increase in exercise tolerance and time, fewer episodes of angina, less ST-segment depression with exercise, and decreased nitroglycerin consumption.[26-28] In randomized controlled trials, patients who underwent coronary artery bypass grafting (CABG) and were pretreated for at least 1 week with CoQ10 showed significant improvement in postoperative cardiac index, left ventricular ejection fractions, recovery time, ventricular arrhythmias, and markers of oxidative stress.[29-31]

Dosage. 100 to 300 mg/day in divided doses.

Precautions. CoQ10 can rarely cause gastritis, loss of appetite, nausea, and diarrhea. It can cause a reversible rise in serum aminotransferases when doses exceed 300 mg/day.

Omega-3 Fatty Acids (Fish Oil and Flaxseed Oil)

See Chapter 22, Peripheral Vascular Disease, and Chapter 84, The Anti-Inflammatory Diet, for a discussion of omega-3 fatty acids.

HERBS FOR CORONARY ARTERY DISEASE

Artichoke Leaf (*Cynara scolymus*)

Animal studies have shown that artichoke leaf inhibits cholesterol synthesis. In humans, this results in a 10% improvement in total cholesterol and a 17% improvement in LDL cholesterol compared with placebo.[32]

Dosage. 2 g dry powder three times per day.

NOTE

Allergy is common to Compositae, that is, the ragweed family, usually producing dermatitis. **Contraindications:** *obstruction of bile ducts, gallstones.*

Curcumin (*Curcuma longa*)

In vitro studies have shown that curcumin inhibits platelet aggregation.[33] In rabbits and in humans, it also decreases lipid peroxidation and lipid levels, thus possibly protecting against both atherogenesis and thrombotic sequelae.[34, 35]

Dosage. 1.5 to 3 g root powder/day.

Precautions. Curcumin may cause allergic reactions or contact dermatitis.

Fenugreek Seed (*Trigonella foenum-graecum*)

In rats and dogs, fenugreek seed has hypoglycemic effects. Glycoxidation is thought to be one of the mechanisms contributing to oxidized LDL cholesterol and atherogenesis. A single study in human diabetics reported decreased cholesterol when taking fenugreek seed.[36]

Dosage. 6 g/day crushed seeds.

Precautions. Fenugreek seed may produce allergic reactions, diarrhea, flatulence, and hypoglycemia.

Garlic (*Allium sativa*)

The German Commission E approves the use of garlic for elevated blood lipids and prevention of age-related vascular changes.[36] Herbalists also use garlic for hypertension. The intact garlic bulb contains alliin. When garlic bulbs are crushed, alliin is converted to allicin, the pharmacologically active moiety, and the one to which products are standardized. Garlic affects CAD by modestly reducing serum cholesterol, blood pressure, and thrombus formation.

In numerous animal studies, garlic prevents the formation of atherosclerotic plaques and reverses existing lesions. Two meta-analyses have shown that, overall, garlic lowered cholesterol by about 9% to 12%.[37, 38] In one study, trigycerides were also significantly decreased and high-density lipoprotein (HDL) cholesterol was unchanged.[38] Another meta-analysis of eight trials supported the use of garlic as an antihypertensive. All trials used the same preparation (Kwai) given over at least 4 weeks. Systolic blood pressure was lowered by 11.1 mm Hg (95% confidence interval [CI], 5.0 to 17.2) and diastolic blood pressure was lowered by 6.5 mm Hg (95% CI, 3.4 to 9.6).[39] A double-blind, randomized, controlled trial of garlic that followed 152 subjects for 4 years showed that garlic reduced the development of atherosclerosis, thus supporting the role of garlic in overall cardiovascular care.[40]

Dosage. Fresh or equivalent to 4000 mg of fresh garlic daily (one clove) or 600 to 900 mg of dried powder standardized to 1.3% allicin (Kwai). Fresh preparations are significantly more effective than dried powder preparations.

Precautions. Garlic may contribute to garlic odor, breath odor, and abdominal symptoms. A theoretical interaction of garlic with warfarin is based on the potential of garlic to decrease platelet aggregation and promote fibrinolysis.

Ginkgo biloba

See Chapter 22, Peripheral Vascular Disease, for a discussion of evidence associated with *Ginkgo biloba*.

Ginseng, American or Oriental (*Panax Species*)

The saponins in *Panax* species act as selective calcium antagonists and enhance release of NO from endothelial cells, thus providing protection during ischemia or reperfusion.[41]

Dosage. 1 to 2 g root (20 to 30 mg ginsenosides).

Precautions. Ginseng may cause nervousness, excitation, and estrogenic and hypoglycemic effects. A case report indicated that *Panax ginseng* decreases the pharmacologic effect of loop diuretics.

Ginseng, Siberian (*Eleutherococcus senticosus*)

Animal studies have shown that Siberian ginseng inhibits platelet aggregation. In human studies, it has been found to increase blood pressure in hypotensive children and promote lipid lowering in combination with other herbs.[36]

Dosage. 2 to 3 g/day for up to 3 months.

Precautions. Ginseng may produce drowsiness or nervousness.

Contraindications. Persons with hypertension or post MI should avoid this product.[41]

Interactions. Case-based data have suggested that Siberian ginseng (*Eleutherococcus*) can elevate digoxin levels, possibly by interfering with the laboratory test.[42]

Grapes (Wine, Juice, Skins, Seeds, Resveratrol)

The French Paradox—that a people could eat a diet high in saturated fats and still have low rates of heart disease—brought to light the beneficial effects of a daily intake of red wine. Many studies have shown the primary preventive benefits of consuming one to two glasses of wine.[43–45] However, wine consumption does not seem to reduce mortality in those who already have cardiovascular disease,[46] and alcohol has many untoward effects, including many drug interactions and adverse events.

Studies on grape skin extracts have illuminated the possible mechanisms by which particular molecules may be responsible for the salutary effects of wine. Red wine and red grape skins contain numerous polyphenolic compounds, including *trans*-resveratrol, proanthocyanidins, and flavonoids such as quercetin, kaempferol, and catechins that act primarily as antioxidants. Resveratrol is also found in purple grape juice, in mulberries, and in smaller amounts in peanuts. In vitro and animal studies have shown that resveratrol, in addition to being an antioxidant, is anti-inflammatory, inhibits platelet aggregation, and can cause blood vessel dilatation.[47, 48] A single small study (*n* = 24) in humans showed that resveratrol inhibits platelet aggregation.[49]

Grape seed extract has also proved useful in ways similar to those of other grape products. The mode of action appears to be the antioxidant effect of the proanthocyanidins, as demonstrated in both animal studies[50, 51] and a small human study.[52]

Dosage. Resveratrol (grape skin extract), 200 to 600 µg/day, divided twice daily. One glass of red wine contains 640 µg; a handful of peanuts, 70 µg.

Precautions. Resveratrol has estrogenic effects that may agonize or antagonize estrogen receptors; therefore, it is best to avoid use in persons with hormone-sensitive conditions.

Gugulipid (*Commiphora mukul*)

In animals, gugulipid increases binding sites for LDL, thus preventing cholesterol and triglyceride elevation.[41] In humans, two studies have reported decreased LDL, total cholesterol, and triglycerides, and one study reported increased HDL.[53]

Dosage. 100 to 500 mg daily.

Precautions. Gugulipid may produce gastrointestinal upset, headache, mild nausea, belching and hiccups, decreased propranolol, and Cardizem bioavailability. It also has thyroid-stimulating activity.

Hawthorn (*Crataegus oxycantha*)

Hawthorn leaves, flowers, and berries contain pharmacologically active proanthocyanidins, bioflavonoids, and cardiotonic amines. In vitro and experimental animal studies have suggested the following modes of action of standardized *Crataegus* extracts: (1) cyclic adenosine monophosphate–independent positive inotropy; (2) peripheral and coronary vasodilatation; (3) protection against ischemia-induced ventricular arrhythmias; (4) antioxidative properties; and (5) anti-inflammatory effects.

Hawthorn has been traditionally used to treat CAD indirectly through its hypotensive, anti-inflammatory, and antiarrhythmic actions. Herbalists have used hawthorn as a nutritive for the myocardium, especially for patients with CAD or those at high risk for CAD. Hawthorn would be given in moderate doses over many months to improve the function and structure of the heart. Animal and in vitro studies give one explanation of how hawthorn may work as a heart "nutritive." These studies have reported that hawthorn supports and prevents the destruction of the collagen matrix in the walls of blood vessels and presumably the fibrous cap of atherosclerotic lesions.[54–56] Furthermore, in one clinical trial, hawthorn was reported to improve exercise tolerance and decrease the incidence of angina.[57]

Dosage. 160 to 900 mg extract of flowers and leaves standardized to either procyanidins or flavonoids. Recommend 900 mg daily in divided doses. Do not expect this herb to act quickly. Both recent research and traditional usage suggest hawthorn takes at least 8 weeks for beneficial effects to start.

Precautions. Hawthorn may cause abdominal discomfort, fatigue, and occasional allergic rash.

Red Yeast Rice Extracts (*Monascus purpureus*)

Two human studies have documented lower LDL, total cholesterol, and triglycerides in the red yeast rice group.[58, 59] A single study found red yeast to be as effective as its analog, simvastatin (Zocor).[60]

Dosage. 1.2 to 2.4 mg proprietary red yeast product (Cholestin).

Precautions. Red yeast rice extracts may cause anaphylaxis after inhalation, gastritis, abdominal discomfort, elevated liver enzymes, heartburn, flatulence, and dizziness. Theoretically, it may produce reactions similar to those of 3-hydroxy-3-methylglutaryl coenzyme A (HMG-CoA) reductase inhibitor (statin) drugs.

NOTE

Interactions: *Grapefruit juice can increase the plasma levels of 3-hydroxy-3-methyl-glutaryl-coenzyme A (HMG-CoA) reductase inhibitors, and pectins included in antidiarrheal products appear to decrease the effectiveness of HMG-CoA reductase inhibitors.*

HERBS TO AVOID IN CORONARY ARTERY DISEASE

Ephedra

Significant problems have been associated with the use of *Ephedra* products for weight loss. *Ephedra* use may be attractive because of conventional admonishments to lose weight coupled with a paucity of effective recommendations on how to safely accomplish weight loss. *Ephedra* acts as a sympathomimetic, leading to increased arterial blood pressure, increased heart rate, increased oxygen consumption in heart muscle, and vasoconstriction.

Precautions. *Ephedra* may produce anxiety, numbness, gastroesophageal reflux, high fever, constipation, difficulty urinating, elevated liver enzymes, Bell's palsy, heart palpitations, severe hypertension, infarction of the tips of the toes, chest pain, dizziness, transient ischemic attacks, brain hemorrhage, stroke, and death.[61]

Licorice Root (*Glycyrrhiza glabra*)

Powdered or finely cut licorice root is made into an infusion and used primarily for respiratory and gastrointestinal problems. In addition to its anti-inflammatory actions, licorice has mineralocorticoid activity and, when used over long periods and at high doses, can cause hypokalemia, hypernatremia, edema, and hypertension. This can exacerbate cardiac disorders and cause pseudoaldosteronism. In addition, deleterious herb-drug interactions are possible with pharmaceuticals commonly used for cardiovascular disease, including potassium-sparing diuretics, thiazide diuretics, and digitalis.[36, 41]

PHARMACEUTICALS

Aspirin

Aspirin is clearly beneficial in secondary prevention of the vascular consequences of overt CAD. The role of aspirin in primary prevention is less clear because the risk of bleeding events is approximately equal to the protection afforded for heart attack, vascular events, and stroke combined.[1]

Dosage. 75 to 325 mg daily.

Precautions. Aspirin may cause intracranial bleeding, which, although rare, is life threatening. Gastrointestinal bleeding is more common and uses excess health care resources, but does not generally result in long-term sequelae.

NOTE

Over forty different herbs have anticoagulant effects of their own and thus could increase the risk of adverse bleeding events (Table 21–1). Other popular herbs are associated with decreased activity of warfarin that may also apply to aspirin (Table 21–2). With all persons taking aspirin or warfarin, it is imperative to inquire about the use of plant-based medicines.

Beta Blockers

As a secondary preventive in those who have had a first MI, beta blockers reduce all-cause mortality, coronary mortality, recurrent nonfatal MI, and sudden death. The greatest benefit is seen in those with the highest risk of death after MI—patients older than 50 years or those with previous MI, angina, hypertension, congestive heart failure, or a higher heart rate at baseline.[1]

Dosage. Depends on proprietary product. There is no evidence that cardioselective beta blockers are more effective.

Precautions. Beta blockers may produce shortness of breath, bronchospasm, bradycardia, hypotension, heart block, cold hands and feet, diarrhea, fatigue, reduced libido, depression, nightmares, faintness, insomnia, blacking out, and hallucinations.

Angiotensin-Converting Enzyme Inhibitors

In persons who have sustained an MI, ACE inhibitors reduce rates of death, recurrent nonfatal MI, and hospitalization for congestive heart failure.[1]

Dosage. Depends on proprietary product.

Precautions. ACE inhibitors may cause cough,

Table 21–1. Herbs That May Potentiate the Effects of Aspirin and Warfarin

Herbal Product	Effect	Evidence
Aspirin		
Ginkgo biloba	Increased risk of bleeding	Case report
Feverfew Red clover	Possible increased risk of bleeding	Theoretical
Warfarin		
Vitamin E–containing herbs (e.g., sunflower seeds)	Increased risk of bleeding owing to vitamine E interference with vitamin K–dependent clotting factors	Case reports and controlled study
Danshen Devil's claw Dong Quai Ginkgo biloba Papain Quinine	Increased risk of bleeding	Case reports
Angelica root Anise Arnica flower Asafoetida Borage seed oil Bromelain Celery Chamomile Clove Fenugreek Feverfew Garlic Ginger Horse chestnut Licorice (glycyrrhizin) Meadowsweet Onion Parsley Passion flower Quassia Red clover Reishi mushroom Rue Sweet clover Turmeric	Possible increased risk of bleeding	Theoretical

From Warber SL, Zick SM: Biologically based complementary medicine for cardiovascular disease: Help or harm? Clin Family Pract (in press); adapted from DerMarderosian.[41]

Table 21–2. Herbs That May Decrease the Effects of Warfarin

Herbal Product	Effect	Evidence
Vitamin K–containing herbs (e.g. alfalfa, green tea)	Decreased anticoagulant activity owing to potentiation of vitamin K-dependent clotting factors	Case reports
Ginseng St. John's wort Ubiquinone (coenzyme Q10)	Decreased anticoagulant activity	Case reports

From Warber SL, Zick SM: Biologically based complementary medicine for cardiovascular disease: Help or harm? Clin Family Pract (in press); adapted from DerMarderosian.[41]

dizziness, hypotension, renal failure, hyperkalemia, angina, syncope, and diarrhea.

Interactions. Topical capsaicin (cayenne pepper), used for neuritic pain, can increase the risk of cough when combined with an ACE inhibitor.

Calcium Channel Blockers

Calcium channel blockers do not reduce mortality in people after MI or with chronic CAD. If individuals do not have heart failure, diltiazem and verapamil may reduce the rates of reinfarction and refractory angina.[1]

Dosage. Depends on proprietary product.

Precautions. Calcium channel blockers may produce atrioventricular block, atrial bradycardia, heart failure, hypotension, dizziness, edema, rash, constipation, and pruritus.

Intravenous Ethylenediaminetetra-acetic Acid Chelation Therapy

The exact mode of action of ethylenediaminetetraacetic acid (EDTA) chelation therapy has yet to be determined. Hypotheses include chelation of calcium directly from atherosclerotic plaques, chelation of transitional metals with consequent reduction in free radical formation leading to less likelihood of lipid peroxidation, and inhibition of platelet aggregation in the presence of thrombin.[62]

Numerous case reports and case series have indicated that patients with CAD who are treated with EDTA chelation therapy have improved quality of life, decreased incidence of angina, increased exercise capacity, and positive electrocardiographic changes such as improved ST segments with exercise. However, in two patients who received angiography after receiving extensive EDTA chelation treatments, severe blockage of the coronary arteries was observed. There have been no large, randomized, controlled trials of chelation therapy for CAD.[62]

Dosage. Chelation therapy is administered in two treatments each week for a minimum of 20 treatments with 50 mg/kg (maximum 5 g, normally 3 g) Na$_2$EDTA in 500 to 1000 mL of normal saline solution. Heparin (1000 to 2000 units) to keep the vein patent, 2% lidocaine (1 to 10 mL) to decrease the pain of the infusion, and sodium bicarbonate (10 mEq) to maintain adequate pH during infusion are usually added to the solution. Further, the following vitamins and minerals are added to the IV solution for their proposed therapeutic qualities: 4 to 29 g sodium ascorbate (vitamin C), 200 mg elemental magnesium, and 50 to 300 mEq pyridoxine (vitamin B$_6$). Physicians also have the option of adding other B vitamins to the IV solution.

Precautions. The following reactions may be experienced: common—pain and burning at the site of the infusions; infrequent—headaches, fatigue, histamine-like reaction, nausea, vomiting, diarrhea, dermatitis, anemia, hypotension, hypocalcemia, thrombophlebitis, systemic emboli, cardiac arrhythmias, and bone marrow depression.

INVASIVE INTERVENTIONS

Percutaneous Transluminal Coronary Angioplasty with and without Stent

PTCA is more effective than medical treatment for alleviating chest pain and improving exercise tolerance. However, it does not reduce mortality, risk of MI, or the need for a later angioplasty. Placement of intracoronary stents gives superior acute and long-term clinical results. Procedural death and MI, as well as repeat procedures, are the main risks of PTCA.[1]

Coronary Artery Bypass Grafting

The greatest benefits occur for people with more severe disease, such as multivessel disease, left ventricular dysfunction, or history of MI. When compared with medical treatment, CABG may be associated with a slightly increased risk of death or MI in the first year after CABG, but at 5, 7, and 10 years there is clear survival benefit from CABG. When compared with PTCA, overall outcomes were similar, but PTCA carries a higher risk for subsequent procedures.[1]

OTHER THERAPIES TO CONSIDER

Useful alternative therapies would include the systematic approaches of Ayurvedic or traditional Chinese medicine.

THERAPEUTIC REVIEW

A summary of therapeutic options for CAD follows. Patients who present with more advanced disease or are experiencing severe symptoms require a more aggressive approach. For these patients, it is recommended that treatment begin with procedural and/or pharmaceutical intervention along with lifestyle changes. It may be possible to phase out medications after lifestyle modifications make a clinically significant impact. For individuals with a strong family history of CAD or other risk factors, primary prevention can be approached through nutrition, lifestyle modification, mind-body therapies, and the selected use of supplements.

Nutrition
- Encourage a diet high in fiber and antioxidant-rich foods, especially fruits and vegetables with intense colors such as melons, berries, and squashes.
- Encourage foods high in omega-3 fatty acids such as cold water fish (e.g., salmon, herring, sardines), nuts, and flaxseeds (3 tbsp finely ground/day) or flaxseed oil (1 tbsp or 1 to 2 500-mg capsules twice daily).
- Encourage the consumption of raw or very lightly cooked garlic (one to three medium cloves) every day. Putting garlic into soups, stir-fry dishes, or sauces at the very end of cooking (in the last 5 minutes) retains the majority of garlic's beneficial effects.
- Encourage a low-fat (especially saturated and polyunsaturated), cholesterol-free diet. Have your patient investigate programs that either encourage a Mediterranean-based diet or use the Dean Ornish diet or Dean Ornish–"like" diets.
- Encourage the consumption of water not in the form of tea, coffee, sodas, or juice. Six to eight glasses per day depending on the person's weight and physical activity level are sufficient to keep an individual well hydrated.

Lifestyle Modifications
- Have patients stop smoking. Keep telling them at every visit that smoking cessation is one of the most important things a person can do to improve the quality of life.
- Help patients to develop an exercise program that will be flexible and enjoyable enough that he or she will continue to exercise for the rest of his or her life. Having resource lists of a variety of classes (yoga, tai chi, swimming, local gymnasiums) offered in the patients geographic area is extremely helpful (see Chapter 86, Writing an Exercise Prescription).

Mind-Body
- Encourage patients to start a mind-body technique that works for them. Easily taught is a simple meditation technique in which the patient takes a comfortable position, closes the eyes, and repeats the number "1" for every expiration (10 to 15 minutes daily). This technique, combined with listening to a relaxation tape (have them available in your office for rental or sale) and instruction in "belly breathing," is often all that is needed (see Chapter 88, Breathing Exercises).
- Belly breathing: Have the patient place one hand over the chest and the other hand over the stomach. Instruct the patient to breathe in deeply and observe which hand rises first. Inform the patient that the hand over the stomach should rise first, followed by the hand over the chest. This sequence ensures that the lungs are optimally oxygenated and creates a state of deep relaxation.

Hydrotherapy
- Have patient start by doing alternating hot and cold (three cycles) over their torso and back. If this proves too difficult, the patient can either do alternating hot and cold, also three cycles, over their torso or end their showers with an alternating hot/cold application.

Botanicals
- Consider using one of the lipid-lowering herbs reported here or in the chapter on that subject. Please refer to other chapters for additional botanicals for hypertension (see Chapter 19, Hypertension), peripheral vascular disease (see Chapter 22, Peripheral Vascular Disease), and congestive heart failure (see Chapter 20, Congestive Heart Failure).
- If your patient is unable or unwilling to consume raw garlic, then advise her or him to take a garlic supplement (600 to 900 mg of dried powder standardized to 1.3%

allicin). However, many garlic supplements are ineffective because of the short shelf life (only several hours) of garlic's active constituent, allicin.
- *For patients with arrhythmias, atherosclerosis, and angina, use hawthorn, 900 mg daily in divided doses.*

Supplements
- *Start with the addition of antioxidants and a high-quality multivitamin/mineral. For example, CoQ10, 100 to 300 mg daily in divided doses, would be appropriate in individuals with angina, those taking vitamin E, or before CABG. If a patient's diet is poor and/or has little hope for improvement, recommend the addition of vitamin C, 500 mg daily, and vitamin E, 400 to 800 IU daily. In addition, a high-quality multivitamin/mineral appropriately supplies vitamin B_6 (50 to 100 mg/day in divided doses), vitamin B_{12} (2000 μg/day), and folic acid (400 μg/day) to a patient's diet, helping to reduce any risk associated with elevated homocysteine levels. Remember, giving B vitamins together causes better absorption of any B vitamin.*
- *If diet, exercise, and an appropriate mind-body technique prove insufficient, add several amino acids. We generally add L-carnitine (1000 to 3000 mg/day in divided doses) for patients with angina, arrhythmias, or post-MI, and give L-arginine (6 to 8 g) to patients after PTCA or at a high risk of developing or redeveloping atherosclerotic lesions. If L-carnitine appears inadequate, we also supplement with L-arginine for patients with angina or post-MI.*

Pharmaceuticals
- *As improvements occur with lifestyle, botanicals, supplements, and relaxation therapy, it may be possible to reduce the need for aspirin, beta blockers, and ACE inhibitors in those patients with previous overt CAD. There is no benefit in these medications for primary prevention of CAD.*
- *Combination therapy: The combination of the previously mentioned pharmaceuticals with botanicals and supplements has not been well studied. Be sure to check herbs for their interaction with aspirin or warfarin (see Tables 21–1 and 21–2).*

Chelation Therapy
- *Currently, evidence for chelation is equivocal or lacking. However, if symptoms persist or worsen despite the previous measures, chelation therapy is a less invasive approach than surgery. Chelation requires multiple clinic visits over several weeks and can be quite expensive. Physicians who practice chelation indicate that there are two populations of patients that are motivated to use this modality: those who want to avoid cardiac surgery at all costs and those who have already tried everything that conventional medicine has to offer for their heart disease.*

Surgical Therapy
- *Many patients with an acute cardiac event will receive CABG or PTCA in a relatively emergent fashion. For individuals with stable disease who begin to develop worsening symptoms despite the conservative interventions previously discussed and optimal pharmaceutical therapy, refer for evaluation and treatment with PTCA or CABG as appropriate.*

References

1. Barton S (ed): Clinical Evidence 5. London, BMJ Publishing Group, 2001, pp 63–98.
2. Keaney JF Jr: Atherosclerosis: From lesion formation to plaque activation and endothelial dysfunction. Mol Aspects Med 21(4–5):99–166, 2000.
3. Ornish DM, Brown SE, Scherwitz LW, et al: Can lifestyle changes reverse coronary atherosclerosis? The Lifestyle Heart Trial. Lancet 336:129–133, 1990.
4. Ornish D, Scherwitz LW, Billings JH, et al: Long-term lifestyle changes increase regression of coronary heart disease. JAMA 280:2001–2007, 1998.
5. Ornish D: Avoiding revascularization with lifestyle changes: The Multicenter Lifestyle Demonstration Project. Am J Cardiol 82:72T–76T, 1998.
6. Ornish D: Dietary treatment of hyperlipidemia. J Cardiovasc Risk 1:283–286, 1994.
7. Ornish D: Very-low-fat diets. Circulation 100:1013–1015, 1999.
8. Scheidt S: The current status of heart-mind relationships. J Psychosom Res 48:317–320, 2000.
9. Institute of Heart Math: Research Overview: Exploring the Role of the Heart in Human Performance. Boulder Creek, Calif, Heart Math Research Center, 1997, p 10.
10. MacLean CRK, Walton KG, Wenneberg SR, et al: Effects of the Transcendental Meditation program on adaptive mechanisms:

Changes in hormone levels and responses to stress after 4 months of practice. Psychoneuroendocrinology 22:227–295, 1995.

11. Castillo-Richmond A, Schneider RH, Alexander CN, et al: Effects of stress reduction on carotid atherosclerosis in hypertensive African Americans. Stroke 31:568–573, 2000.

12. Pandya DP, Vyas VH, Vyas SH: Mind-body therapy in the management and prevention of coronary disease. Complement Ther 25:283–293, 1999.

13. Luskin FM, Newell KA, Griffith M, et al: A review of mind-body therapies in the treatment of cardiovascular disease. Part 1: Implications for the elderly. Altern Ther Health Med 4(3):46–61, 1998.

14. Lim RF, Lin KM: Cultural formulation of psychiatric diagnosis. Case no. 03. Psychosis following Qi-gong in a Chinese immigrant. Cult Med Psychiatry 20:369–378, 1996.

15. Ives JC, Sosnoff J: Beyond the mind-body exercise hype. Physician Sportsmedicine 28(3):67–81, 2000.

16. Stampfer M, Hennekens CH, Manson JE, et al: Vitamin E consumption and the risk of coronary disease in women. N Engl J Med 328:1444, 1993.

17. Stephens NG, Parsons A, Schofield PM, et al: Randomised controlled trial of vitamin E in patients with coronary disease: Cambridge Heart Antioxidant Study (CHAOS). Lancet 347:781, 1996.

18. The α-Tocopherol, β-Carotene Cancer Prevention Study Group: The effect of vitamin E and β-carotene on the incidence of lung cancer and other cancers in male smokers. N Engl J Med 330:1029, 1994.

19. Hennekens CH, Buring JE, Manson JE: Lack of effect of long-term supplementation with β-carotene on the incidence of malignant neoplasms and cardiovascular disease. N Engl J Med 334:1145, 1996.

20. Tardif JC, Cote B, Lesperance J, et al: Probucol and multivitamins in the prevention of restenosis after coronary angioplasty. Multivitamins and Probucol Study Group. N Engl J Med 337:365, 1997.

21. Lerman A, Suwaidi JAI, Velianou JL: L-Arginine: A novel therapy for coronary artery disease? Expert Opin Investig Drugs 8:1785–1793, 1999.

22. Lerman A, Burnett JC Jr, Higano ST, et al: Long-term L-arginine supplementation improves small-vessel coronary endothelial function in humans. Circulation 97:2123–2128, 1998.

23. Sydow K, Boger RH: Homocysteine, endothelial dysfunction and cardiovascular risk: Pathomechanisms and therapeutic options. Z Kardiol 90:1–11, 2001.

24. Wald NJ, Watt H, Law M, et al: Homocysteine and ischemic heart disease: Results of a prospective study with implications regarding prevention. Arch Intern Med 158:862–867, 1998.

25. Whincup PH, Refsum H, Perry IJ, et al: Serum total homocysteine and coronary heart disease: Prospective study in middle-aged men. Heart 82:448–454, 1999.

26. Kamikawa T, Kobayashi A, Yamashita T, et al: Effects of coenzyme Q10 on exercise tolerance in chronic stable angina pectoris. Am J Cardiol 56:247–251, 1985.

27. Schardt F, Welzel D, Schiess W, Toda K: Effect of coenzyme Q10 on ischaemia-induced ST-segment depression: A double-blind, placebo-controlled crossover study. In Folkers K, Yamagami T, Littarru GP (eds): Biomedical and Clinical Aspects of Coenzyme Q, vol 6. Amsterdam, Elsevier, 1986, pp 385–403.

28. Kuklinski B, Weissenbacher E, Fahnrich A: Coenzyme Q10 and antioxidants in acute myocardial infarction. Mol Aspects Med 15(Suppl):S143–S147, 1994.

29. Chello M, Mastroroberto P, Romano R, et al: Protection by coenzyme Q10 from myocardial reperfusion injury during coronary artery bypass grafting. Ann Thorac Surg 58:1427–1432, 1994.

30. Chello M, Mastroroberto P, Romano R, et al: Protection by coenzyme Q10 of tissue reperfusion injury during abdominal aortic cross-clamping. J Cardiovasc Surg (Torino) 37:229–235, 1996.

31. Chen YF, Lin YT, Wu SC: Effectiveness of coenzyme Q10 on myocardial preservation during hypothermic cardioplegic arrest. J Thorac Cardiovasc Surg 107:242–247, 1994.

32. Englisch W, Beckers C, Unkauf M, et al: Efficacy of artichoke dry extract in patients with hyperlipoproteinemia. Arzneimittelforschung 50:260–265, 2000.

33. Shah BH, Nawaz Z, Pertani SA, et al: Inhibitory effect of curcumin, a food spice from turmeric, on platelet-activating factor– and arachidonic acid–mediated platelet aggregation through inhibition of thromboxane formation and Ca^{2+} signaling. Biochem Pharmacol 58:1167–1172, 1999.

34. Ramirez-Tortosa MC, Mesa MD, Aguilera MC, et al: Oral administration of a turmeric extract inhibits LDL oxidation and has hypocholesterolemic effects in rabbits with experimental atherosclerosis. Atherosclerosis 147:371–378, 1999.

35. Soni KB, Kuttan R: Effect of oral curcumin administration on serum peroxides and cholesterol levels in human volunteers. Indian J Physiol Pharmacol 36:273–275, 1992.

36. Blumenthal M (ed): Herbal Medicine: Expanded Commission E Monographs. Newton, Mass, Integrative Medicine Communications, 2000.

37. Warshafsky S, Kamer RS, Sivak SL: Effect of garlic on total serum cholesterol: A meta-analysis. Ann Intern Med 119:599–605, 1993.

38. Silagy C, Neil A: Garlic as a lipid lowering agent—a meta-analysis. J R Coll Physicians Lond 28:39–45, 1994.

39. Silagy CA, Neil HAW: A meta-analysis of the effect of garlic on blood pressure. J Hypertens 12:463–468, 1994.

40. Koscielny J, Klussendorf D, Latza R, et al: The antiatherosclerotic effect of *Allium sativum*. Atherosclerosis 144:237–249, 1999.

41. DerMarderosian A (ed): The Review of Natural Products. Facts and Comparisons. Philadelphia, Lippincott Williams & Wilkins, 2001.

42. McRae S: Elevated serum digoxin levels in a patient taking digoxin and Siberian ginseng. CMAJ 155:293, 1996.

43. Renaud SC, Gueguen R, Siest G, Salamon R: Wine, beer, and mortality in middle-aged men from eastern France. Arch Intern Med 159:1865–1870, 1999.

44. Kiechl S, Willeit J, Rungger G, et al: Alcohol consumption and atherosclerosis: What is the relation? Prospective results from the Bruneck Study. Stroke 29:900–907, 1998.

45. Klatsky AL, Armstrong MA, Friedman GD: Red wine, white wine, liquor, beer, and risk for coronary artery disease hospitalization. Am J Cardiol 80:416–420, 1997.

46. Shaper AG, Wannamethee SG: Alcohol intake and mortality in middle-aged men with diagnosed coronary heart disease. Heart 83:394–399, 2000.

47. RESVERATROL. Available at http://www.naturaldatabase.com/

48. Fremont L: Biological effects of resveratrol. Life Sci 66:663–673, 2000.

49. Pace-Asciak CR, Rounova O, Hahn SE, D et al: Wines and grape juices as modulators of platelet aggregation in healthy human subjects. Clin Chim Acta 246(1–2):163–182, 1996.

50. Bagchi D, Bagchi M, Stohs SJ, et al: Free radicals and grape seed proanthocyanidin extract: Importance in human health and disease prevention. Toxicology 148(2–3):187–197, 2000.

51. Bagchi D, Garg A, Krohn RL, et al: Oxygen free radical scavenging abilities of vitamins C and E, and a grape seed proanthocyanidin extract in vitro. Res Commun Mol Pathol Pharmacol 95:179–189, 1997.

52. Nuttall SL, Kendall MJ, Bombardelli E, Morazzoni P: An evaluation of the antioxidant activity of a standardized grape seed extract, Leucoselect. J Clin Pharm Ther 23:385–389, 1998.

53. Nityanand S, Srivastava JS, Asthana OP: Clinical trials with gugulipid. A new hypolipidaemic agent. J Assoc Physicians India 37:323–328, 1989.

54. Masquelier J: Pycnogenols: Recent advances in the therapeutical activity of procyanidins. Nat Prod Med Agents 1:243–256, 1981.

55. Masquelier J, Dumon MC, Dumas J: Stabilization of collagen by procyanidolic oligomers. Acta Ther 7:101–105, 1981.

56. Tixier JM, Godeau G, Robert AM, Hornebeck W: Evidence by in vivo and in vitro studies that binding of pycnogenols to elastin affects its rate of degradation by elastases. Biochem Pharmacol 33:3933–3939, 1984.

57. Weng WL, Zhang WQ, Liu FZ, et al: Therapeutic effects of *Crataegus pinnatifida* on 46 cases of angina pectoris—a double-blind study. J Tradit Chin Med 4:293–294, 1984.

58. Heber D, Yip I, Ashley JM, et al: Cholesterol-lowering effects of a proprietary Chinese red-yeast-rice dietary supplement. Am J Clin Nutr 69:231–236, 1999.

59. Wang J, Lu A, Chi J: Multicenter clinical trial of the serum lipid-lowering effects of a *Monascus purpureus* (red yeast) rice preparation from traditional Chinese medicine. Curr Ther Res 58:964–978, 1997.

60. Kou W, Lu Z, Guo J: Effect of xuezhikang on the treatment of primary hyperlipidemia. Chung Hua Nei Ko Tsa Chih 36:529–531, 1997.

61. U.S. Food and Drug Administration, Center for Feed Safety and Applied Nutrition, Office of Special Nutritionals. Search results for Metabolife. Available at http://vm.cfsan.fda.gov/

62. Zick SM, Warber SL: A review of chelation therapy for coronary artery disease. (manuscript in preparation.)

CHAPTER 22

Peripheral Vascular Disease

Sara L. Warber, M.D., and Suzanna M. Zick, N.D., M.P.H.

PATHOPHYSIOLOGY

Peripheral vascular disease (PVD) includes disease of both the arterial and venous systems. Disease of the arterial system predominantly includes peripheral vascular occlusive disease (PVOD) and its clinical manifestation, intermittent claudication. Arterial disease can also manifest as slow-healing ulcers and is the causative disorder in about 15% to 20% of lower limb ulcers. These clinical sequelae are local manifestations of the systemic disease of atherosclerosis, which also has effects on the brain, heart, and aorta. The pathophysiology of atherosclerotic arterial disease is reviewed in the chapter on coronary artery disease (CAD). In this chapter we briefly review a few well-studied interventions for intermittent claudication. Interventions included in the chapters on CAD (Chapter 21), prevention of stroke (Chapter 71), hypertension (Chapter 19), and hyperlipidemia (Chapter 31) are also likely to be useful for PVOD.

The venous system may be afflicted by chronic venous insufficiency (CVI), deep vein thrombosis, or varicose veins, with a propensity to edema, cellulitis, and venous stasis ulcers. This cascade of problems is thought to begin from valvular malfunction in the veins, increased venous compliance, and venous occlusions from atherosclerosis. The column of blood returning toward the heart is no longer moved upward but rather is pulled down by gravity, and peripheral pooling occurs. When intravessel hydrostatic pressure is greater than the surrounding tissue oncotic pressure, edema ensues. The overall slowing of venous blood flow through the area increases the risk for intravascular thrombosis, tissue cellulitis, and skin ulceration. Because the pathophysiology is thought to be primarily mechanical, the conventional treatments have been exclusively mechanical or have focused on treating the complications.

Another important source of peripheral vascular disease is the vasculitides. This chapter does not cover these disorders specifically. The clinical manifestations of the peripheral vasculitides may overlap with those of PVOD and CVI, so appropriate diagnostic workup should precede or accompany institution of the following approaches to integrative care.

INTEGRATIVE THERAPY

Lifestyle Interventions

Exercise

Large-cohort observational studies show that lack of exercise is a risk factor in arterial disease and that moderate to high levels of physical activity reduce coronary heart disease and stroke. Frequently, exercise is difficult or painful for people with PVOD, so that other interventions discussed later, such as *Ginkgo biloba* and EDTA (ethylenediamine tetraacetic acid) chelation, which potentially increase pain-free walking distance, exert an additive effect by allowing greater exercise. In the case of venous disease, it is thought that the action of the leg muscles aids the return of blood toward the heart. Therefore, exercise can be a primary treatment.[1] This potential benefit must be balanced with the fact that upright posture for exercise may exacerbate peripheral pooling. Supine bicycle exercise, rowing machines, and yoga, which use many postures, may be good choices for people with CVI.

Smoking Cessation

As has been noted for lack of exercise, observational studies have shown that smoking is a risk factor for arterial disease. It is also well known from large-cohort studies that smoking cessation is one of the most important things that people can do to modify their risk of arterial disease. In addition, smoking exacerbates Buerger's disease (thromboangiitis obliterans) of the peripheral vasculature. Therefore, smoking cessation is an important component of a treatment program directed at peripheral vascular health. Conventional approaches to smoking cessation include counseling, nicotine replacement, and use of the antidepressant bupropion. All of these approaches have been shown through systematic review to increase the likelihood of abstinence from smoking at 1 year (odds ratio [OR] of 1.32–1.46 for counseling,[2–4] 1.63–2.27 for various forms of nicotine replacement[5] and 2.73 for bupropion[6, 6a]). The use of nicotine replacement and bupropion is associated with some risk of side effects. Acupuncture for smoking cessation has also been studied but does not result in an increase in abstinence at 1 year (OR of 1.02).[7] Two studies (published in 2000) reviewing use of hypnosis for smoking cessation concluded that there is mixed evidence of its superiority to nonintervention,[8, 9] with evidence of similar effects compared with non-hypnosis behavioral treatments.[9] For selected patients, hypnosis or acupuncture may be well worth a trial in addition to or before the use of other proven treatments.

Biomechanical Measures

Compression Stockings

Use of compression stockings has been the mainstay of treatment for CVI, for treatment and prevention of venous ulcers, and for prevention of DVT. Because of the discomfort associated with wearing compression stochings, noncompliance is a well-known barrier to the success of this treatment. Indirect evidence of their utility comes from a study showing that recurrence of venous ulcers was associated with noncompliance in wearing compression hosiery.[10] To be effective, compression needs to be in excess of 35 mm Hg.[11]

NOTE

It is important to remember that about a fifth of people with venous ulcers also have arterial disease, so that compression can cause necrosis, resulting in amputation in some cases. In persons with an ankle-brachial pressure index below 0.9, compression is contraindicated.

Hydrotherapy

Hydrotherapy is the therapeutic use of hot and cold water on the exterior surface of the body. Naturopathic practitioners use hydrotherapy for chronic diseases, including PVOD and CVI. Alternating hot and cold applications can elicit a physiologic response mimicking the effect of exercise, which may be clinically beneficial for patients who cannot exercise or can exercise for only a limited duration.

Hot applications (<5 min) bring blood and lymph fluid to the skin surface, increasing local metabolism and oxygen and nutrient delivery. Following the hot application with a short cold application causes vasoconstriction, driving both blood and lymph to the body's core. This process helps to eliminate the build-up of inflammatory products, to tone the tissue, and to remove other waste products. By alternating

hot with cold, a profound pumping action is created in the region over which the water is applied.

NOTE

Method of Administering Hydrotherapy

Make sure the patient is warm. Place a wet hot towel (approximately 100°F) on the desired area. Be careful to check the temperature of the towel on a wrist before placing it on the part to be treated. Leave the hot towel on for 3 minutes and then replace the hot towel with a cold towel (45°F). Leave the cold towel on for 1 minute. Repeat this cycle three times (hot-cold, hot-cold, hot-cold). Always end with cold.

NOTE

Hydrotherapy should not be administered over open lesions, on areas of decreased or absent sensation such as in neuropathy, or over tumors. Additionally, caution should always be taken with the elderly, children, and persons who are frail.

Supplements

Omega-3 Fatty Acids

Currently, there is limited evidence that omega-3 fatty acids are beneficial for people with PVOD. Research has begun to link inflammatory markers such as C-reactive protein with increased risk for developing PVOD.[12] A case control study determined that people with PVOD had lower serum levels of the omega-3 fatty acids eicosapentaenoic acid (EPA), docosahexaenoic acid (DHA), and docosapentaenoic acid, compared with controls.[13] Omega-3 fatty acids have the ability to inhibit platelet aggregation, to reduce fibrinogen levels, and to improve endothelial function, suggesting a beneficial effect of these supplements in persons with PVOD.[14, 15] Physiologic doses of omega-3 fatty acids (less than 5 g) have been found to possibly slow progression and to promote regression of atherosclerotic lesions.[16]

Dosage. 1 to 3 g a day in divided doses or two to four 500-mg capsules twice daily.

Precautions. Large doses of more than 4 g daily may promote free radical production and if used should be given with an antioxidant (such as vitamin E or C or selenium).

L-Carnitine

Carnitine is an amino acid made from lysine or derived from eating meat and dairy products. Carnitine is responsible for transporting long-chain fatty acids into the mitochondria. Without carnitine, the carrier molecule for fatty acids, acyl coenzyme A (acyl CoA), cannot cross the cell membrane of the mitochondria, leading to decreased concentrations of fatty acids in the mitochondria and hence decreased energy production.

In individuals with peripheral arterial disease, short-term therapy with propionyl-L-carnitine (LPC) significantly improved pain-free walking distance over that observed with use of a placebo.[17] However, LPC had no clinically significant effect on muscular and subcutaneous blood flow of the lower limbs. Therefore, L-carnitine appears to exert its beneficial effect on the walking capacity of patients with intermittent claudication via improved energy metabolism within the muscle and not via improved blood flow of the lower limbs.[18, 19] In addition, LPC administration appears to improve the healing of ulcerative lesions, and can reduce the need for analgesic medication and lessen the incidence of amputation.[20]

Dosage. 1500 to 4000 mg daily in divided doses.

Precautions. Oral use can cause transient nausea and vomiting, abdominal cramps, diarrhea, and body odor.

Antioxidants

It has been proposed that oxidative stress plays an important role in the development of vascular disease, which implies that the development and progression of PVOD can be prevented or slowed by antioxidants such as alpha-lipoic acid, vitamins C and E, and beta-carotene. Currently, the mechanisms of how antioxidants affect PVOD, or whether they are clinically beneficial, is unclear.[21] There are two proposed mechanisms of how antioxidants may inhibit atherogenesis and improve PVOD. First, lipid-soluble antioxidants present in low-density lipoproteins (LDLs), including alpha-tocopherol (vitamin E), and water-soluble antioxidants present in the extracellular fluid of the arterial wall, including ascorbic acid (vitamin C), inhibit LDL oxidation through an LDL-specific antioxidant action. Second, antioxidants present in the cells of the vascular wall decrease cellular production and release of reactive oxygen species and improve the biologic activity of endothelium-derived nitric oxide.[22, 23] Despite these proposed mechanisms, neither epidemiologic nor clinical trials have been conducted to determine if antioxidants exert any positive therapeutic or preventive effects.

Dosage. Alpha-lipoic acid 20 to 50 mg daily; vitamin E 400 to 800 international units (IU) daily; vitamin C 500 mg daily; coenzyme Q10 100 to 300 mg daily.

Herbs

Ginkgo biloba has been well studied for use in intermittent claudication, and the evidence is reviewed in the following discussion.[24–32] Many of the herbs identified in the chapter on CAD may also be effective for PVOD. Three herbal products—bilberry fruit,[27] horse chestnut seed,[33–36] and Pycnogenol[37–41]—show promise for treatment of CVI.

Ginkgo biloba

Ginkgo biloba leaf extract comes from the oldest living tree in the world, with fossil evidence dating back 200 million years. Ginkgo topped the list of best-selling herbs in the United States in 1998. It is also one of the most-studied herbs, with evidence supporting its action as an inhibitor of platelet-activating factor[24] and as a vasodilator.[25] According to the German Commission E and the World Health Organization (WHO) monographs, ginkgo is approved for PVOD and postphlebitis syndrome, as well as for dementias, tinnitus, vertigo, Raynaud's disease, and acrocyanosis.[26] Its efficacy for treatment of intermittent claudication was assessed in a meta-analysis of eight randomized, double-blind, placebo-controlled trials in humans.[27] The mean improvement in pain-free walking distance in the ginkgo treatment group over the placebo treatment group was 34 m. In a head-to-head trial of *Ginkgo biloba* extract and pentoxifylline, each product caused a similar increase in pain-free walking distance and in maximal walking distance.[28]

Dosage. 120 mg daily EGb 761 (Tebonin).

Precautions. The most frequently reported adverse effects were abdominal complaints, nausea, and dyspepsia. Other adverse effects reported in the literature include allergic reactions,[26] headache, dizziness, and palpitations.[29] There are case reports of bleeding complications including subdural hematoma,[30] subarachnoid hemorrhage,[31] and spontaneous hyphema associated with aspirin plus ginkgo use.[32]

NOTE

The cost for a daily 120-mg dose of ginkgo ranges from $0.41 to $0.84, compared with $1.83 to $4.23 for a daily dose of pentoxifylline or cilostazol, pharmaceuticals approved for use in intermittent claudication.[27]

Bilberry

In Italy, the fruit of the bilberry bush (*Vaccinium myrtillus*) has been used for treatment of varicose veins, venous insufficiency, and atherosclerosis. In vitro and animal studies indicate that bilberry fruit inhibits edema formation, platelet aggregation, and thrombus formation. Preliminary studies in humans demonstrate beneficial effects on the peripheral vasculature.[94]

Dosage. 4 to 8 g of dried fruit taken with water

several times per day, or 80 to 160 mg dry extract (25% anthocyanosides) four times daily.

Precautions. No adverse effects have been reported.[26]

Horse Chestnut Seed Extract

Horse chestnut seed extract has been studied for its use in chronic venous insufficiency. Animal studies show that aescins from horse chestnut (*Aesculus hippocastanum*) inhibit vascular permeability and edema formation.[33, 34] In a randomized trial comparing horse chestnut, compression stockings, and placebo, horse chestnut and compression stockings were equal in their ability to decrease leg volume (decreases of 46.7 mL and 43.8 mL, respectively), and both were significantly more effective than placebo (which effected a decrease of only 9.8 mL).[35] A systematic review of 13 studies concluded that horse chestnut was more effective than placebo.[36]

Dosage. 250 to 312.5 mg of dry extract twice daily in slow-release form (16% to 21% aescin), equivalent to 100 mg of aescin daily.

Precautions. No adverse effects were reported in the randomized trial.[35]

Pycnogenol

Pycnogenol, an extract of the bark of the French maritime pine (*Pinus maritima*), is currently one of the best-selling herbal products in the United States, ranked eighth in 1998. Pycnogenol, containing procyandins and phenolic acids, has high bioavailability and is used in the treatment of CVI. In vitro and animal studies show that it acts as an antioxidant and as an angiotension-converting enzyme (ACE) inhibitor.[37, 38] The beneficial mechanism of action in CVI is thought to be via stabilization of the collagenous subendothelial basal membrane or scavenging free radicals. Three small human studies on its use in CVI consistently showed decreased pain, edema, and limb heaviness in the treatment group.[39-41]

Dosage. 100 mg Pycnogenol three times daily.

Precautions. No adverse effects have been reported.[38]

Biochemical Approaches

Chelation Therapy

EDTA is a chelating agent that binds minerals and removes them from the body. The exact mode of action of EDTA chelation therapy has yet to be determined. Several hypotheses have been proposed, including chelation of calcium directly from atherosclerotic plaques; induction of parathyroid hormone production; chelation of transitional metals with consequent reduction in free radical formation, leading to less likelihood of lipid perox-

idation; and inhibition of platelet aggregation in the presence of thrombin. Some or all of these actions may in fact take place; however, at present the evidence is scanty.

Case reports and reported series of patients with PVOD who have received intravenous EDTA chelation therapy have found improvement in exercise tolerance, reduction in symptoms such as pain during walking, and improvements in ankle-brachial index (ABI) values as measured by Doppler studies.[42-47] In addition, three small to moderate-sized double-blind placebo-controlled clinical trials have examined intravenous EDTA chelation therapy for PVOD.[48-51] Patients in these trials generally experienced limited improvement of symptoms and moderate improvements in ABI, without significant improvement in maximum or pain-free walking distance, when compared with placebo. However, there are several limitations to these trials and case studies, which leave the effectiveness of chelation therapy in question.

Dosage. At least two treatments a week are given for a minimum of 20 treatments with 50 mg/kg (maximum 5 g; normally 3 g) of sodium EDTA in 500 to 1000 mL of normal saline. Additives include 1000 to 2000 units of heparin to keep the vein patent, 1 to 10 mL of 2% lidocaine to decrease the pain of the infusion, and 10 mEq of sodium bicarbonate to maintain adequate pH during infusion. Furthermore, the following vitamins and minerals are added to the intravenous solution for their proposed therapeutic qualities: 4 to 29 g of sodium ascorbate (vitamin C), 200 mg of elemental magnesium, and 50 to 300 mEq of pyridoxine (vitamin B_6). Other B vitamins may be added to the intravenous solution.

Precautions. Adverse effects may include pain and burning at the site of the infusions; infrequent adverse effects include headaches, fatigue, histamine-like reaction, nausea, vomiting, diarrhea, dermatitis, anemia, hypotension, hypocalcemia, thrombophlebitis, systemic emboli, cardiac arrhythmias, and bone marrow depression.

Pharmaceuticals

For chronic venous disease of the legs, preliminary results have shown a beneficial effect of several vasodilators and an oral micronized purified flavonoid fraction, but the evidence for the efficacy of medications on venous ulcer healing is still limited. There is no evidence to routinely administer antibiotics for ulcer healing.[11] More data are available on pharmaceutical interventions for arterial disease.

Pentoxifylline

Pentoxifylline (Trental) was for several years the only drug approved in the United States for treatment of intermittent claudication. It is a xanthine derivative with several physiologic effects, including many that are antithrombogenic and antiplatelet.

Randomized controlled trials of pentoxifylline for intermittent claudication were recently reviewed; only 2 of 18 were long-term, high-quality studies, and these showed equivocal results.[52] However, another review ranked pentoxifylline ahead of ticlopidine, which increases red blood cell deformability, in terms of efficacy, safety, patient acceptance, and cost.[53] It appears that 6 months of treatment with pentoxifylline can produce an improvement in pain-free walking distance.[54]

Precautions. This drug may cause gastrointestinal disturbance, hypotension, flulike symptoms, rash, and blurred vision. Pentoxifylline should be used with caution in persons with recent surgery or peptic ulcer disease and during pregnancy (category C) or lactation. It may potentiate antihypertensives and anticoagulants.

Caution. Pentoxifylline should not be used in patients with recent cerebral or retinal hemorrhage or with caffeine or theophylline intolerance.

Dosage. 400 mg of pentoxifylline three times daily orally with food or 1200 mg intravenously (in severe cases).

Cilostazol

Cilostazol (Pletal) is both an antiplatelet and a vasodilating drug used for treatment of claudication. It acts by inhibiting cyclic adenosine monophosphate, (cAMP) phosphodiesterase in platelets and vascular smooth muscle cells. When cilostazol was compared with placebo, walking distance was doubled on cilostazol, and quality of life was improved. One head-to-head trial found cilostazol to be more effective than pentoxifylline for relief of claudication.[55]

Precautions. Fifty percent of persons taking cilostazol experience minor side effects of headache, diarrhea, or palpitations. Other possible side effects include peripheral edema and dizziness. There are no known serious adverse effects. Use caution in patients with severe underlying heart disease or hepatic dysfunction or during pregnancy (category C) or lactation.

Interactions. Cilostazol is potentiated by drugs that inhibit the cytochrome P-450 complex; caution is necessary when it is used with anticoagulants.

Caution. Cilostazol should not be used in patients with congestive heart failure.

Dosage. 100 mg cilostazol twice daily given on an empty stomach; reduce the dose to 50 mg twice daily if used with cytochrome P-450 inhibitors; avoid grapefruit juice.

Surgery

Surgery is most useful to establish blood flow to areas with decreased arterial supply.[56] There is little utility for surgery in CVI.[57] However, patients with active venous ulcers and saphenofemoral or saphenopopliteal junction incompetence do benefit from surgical treatment.[11] Surgery may also be valuable for management of severe varicose veins.

Other Therapies to Consider

Useful alternative therapies include the systematic approaches of Ayurvedic medicine and traditional Chinese medicine.

 ── *THERAPEUTIC REVIEW* ─────────────────────────────

Following is a summary of therapeutic options for patients with peripheral vascular disease. Patients who present with more advanced disease or who are experiencing severe symptoms require a more aggressive approach. For these patients, it is recommended that treatment begin with pharmaceutical intervention along with lifestyle changes. Medications can be phased out after sufficient time has passed for lifestyle modifications to make clinically significant impacts.

Nutrition
- *Encourage a diet that is high in fiber and in antioxidant-rich foods, especially fruits and vegetables with intense colors such as melons, berries, and squashes.*
- *Encourage foods high in omega-3 fatty acids such as cold water fish (salmon, herring, sardines), nuts, and flaxseed (3 tablespoons of finely ground flaxseed daily) or flaxseed oil (1 tablespoon or 1 or 2 500-mg capsules twice daily).*
- *Encourage a low-fat (especially saturated and polyunsaturated fats), cholesterol-free diet.*
- *Encourage the consumption of water not in the form of tea, coffee, sodas, or juice. Depending on weight and physical activity level, 6 to 8 glasses per day are sufficient to keep the patient well hydrated.*

THERAPEUTIC REVIEW   *continued*

Lifestyle Modifications

- *Encourage patients to stop smoking; reminders at every office visit that smoking cessation enormously improves quality of life are important.*
- *Help patients to develop an exercise program that will be flexible and enjoyable enough that exercise will become a lifelong practice. A resource list of a variety of local classes (yoga, tai chi, swimming), including those at gymnasiums and wellness centers, is extremely helpful (see Chapter 86, Writing an Exercise Prescription).*

Hydrotherapy

- *Have the patient start by doing alternating hot and cold (three cycles) applications over the torso and back. If this proves too difficult, the patient can either do alternating hot and cold, also three cycles, over the affected limbs or end the daily shower with an alternating cold-hot application.*

Botanicals

- *Start with* Ginkgo biloba *120 mg daily if the patient is suffering from intermittent claudication, Raynaud's syndrome, or phlebitis, or start with horse chestnut 250 mg daily if chronic venous insufficiency (CVI) is the chief complaint. If the patient is still experiencing symptoms, consider adding bilberry 80 to 160 mg or Pycnogenol 100 mg three times daily.*

Supplements

- *Start with L-carnitine 1500 to 4000 mg daily in divided doses if previous therapies have not reduced symptoms in persons with intermittent claudication or low blood flow to the limbs, or in patients with ulcerative lesions. The addition of coenzyme Q10, 100 to 300 mg daily in divided doses, is appropriate in individuals with low blood flow to the limbs. If the patient's diet is poor, with little hope for improvement, the addition of antioxidants is recommended, including vitamin C 500 mg daily and vitamin E 400 to 800 IU daily.*

Biomechanical Measures

- *Start use of compression stockings in persons with CVI, especially those at risk for the development of deep vein thrombosis.*

Pharmaceuticals

- *If no improvement is obtained with lifestyle interventions, botanicals, supplements, and compression stockings, discontinue botanicals and supplements and start pentoxifylline (Trental) or cilostazol (Pletal).*
- *Combination therapy: the combination of pentoxifylline or cilostazol with botanicals and supplements has not been studied. Concomitant administration of these medications and Ginkgo biloba is not recommended.*

Chelation Therapy

- *Currently, evidence for benefits of chelation is equivocal or lacking. However, if symptoms persist or worsen despite the foregoing measures, chelation therapy may be given a trial.*

Surgical Therapy

- *If the patient's symptoms persist or worsen despite the foregoing interventions or if gangrene is imminent, refer the patient for a vascular surgery evaluation and treatment.*

References

1. Junger M, Steins A, Zuder D, Klyscz T: [Physical therapy of venous diseases.] Vasa 27:73–79 1998.
2. Lancaster T, Stead LF: Individual behavioural counselling for smoking cessation (Cochrane Review). Cochrane Database Syst Rev 2:CD001292, 2000.
3. Rice VH, Stead LF: Nursing intervention for smoking cessation (Cochrane Review). Cochrane Database Syst Rev 3:CD001188, 2001.
4. Ashenden R, Silagy C, Weller D: A systematic review of the effectiveness of promoting lifestyle change in general practice. Fam Pract 1997; 14:160–176.
5. Silagy C, Mant D, Fowler G, Lancaster T: Nicotine replacement therapy for smoking cessation (Cochrane Review). Cochrane Database Syst Rev 3:CD000146, 2001.
6a. Hughes JR, Stead LF, Lancaster T: Anxiolytics for smoking cessation (Cochrane Review). Cochrane Database Syst Rev 4:CD002849, 2000.
6. Hughes JR, Stead LF, Lancaster T: Antidepressants for smoking cessation (Cochrane Review). Cochrane Database Syst Rev 4: CD000031, 2000.
7. White AR, Rampes H, Ernst E: Acupuncture for smoking cessation (Cochrane Review). Cochrane Database Syst Rev 2:CD000009, 2000.
8. Abbot NC, Stead LF, White AR, et al: Hypnotherapy for smoking

cessation (Cochrane Review). Cochrane Database Syst Rev 2:CD001008, 2000.

9. Green JP, Lynn SJ: Hypnosis and suggestion-based approaches to smoking cessation: An examination of the evidence. Int J Clin Exp Hypn. 48:195–224, 2000.

10. Cullum N, Fletcher A, Semlyen A, et al: Compression therapy for venous leg ulcers. Qual Health Care 6:226–231, 1997.

11. Clement DL: Venous ulcer reappraisal: Insights from an international task force. Veins International Task Force. J Vasc Res 36(Suppl 1):42–47, 1999.

12. Ridker PM, Cushman M, Stampfer MJ, et al: Plasma concentration of C-reactive protein and risk of developing peripheral vascular disease. Circulation 97:425–482, 1998.

13. Leng GC, Horrobin DF, Fowkes FG, et al: Plasma essential fatty acids, cigarette smoking, and dietary antioxidants in peripheral arterial disease. A population-based case-control study. Arterioscler Thromb 14:471–478, 1994.

14. Horrobin DF: Abnormal membrane concentrations of 20- and 22-carbon essential fatty acids: A common link between risk factors and coronary and peripheral vascular disease? Prostaglandins Leukot Essent Fatty Acids 53:385–396, 1995.

15. Gazso A, Horrobin D, Sinzinger H: Influence of omega-3 fatty acids on the prostaglandin metabolism in healthy volunteers and patients suffering from PVD. Agents Actions Suppl 37:151–156, 1992.

16. Von Schacky C, Angerer P, Kothny W, et al: The effect of dietary omega-3 fatty acids on coronary atherosclerosis: A randomized, double-blind, placebo-controlled trial. Ann Intern Med 30:554–562, 1999.

17. Brevetti, G, et al. Increases in walking distance in patients with peripheral vascular disease treated with L-carnitine: A double-blind, crossover study. Circulation 77:767–773, 1988.

18. Bolognesi M, Amodio P, Merkel C, et al: Effect of 8-day therapy with propionyl-L-carnitine on muscular and subcutaneous blood flow of the lower limbs in patients with peripheral arterial disease. Clin Physiol 15:417–423, 1995.

19. Sabba C, Berardi E, Antonica G, et al: Comparison between the effect of L-propionylcarnitine, L-acetylcarnitine and nitroglycerin in chronic peripheral arterial disease: A haemodynamic double blind echo-Doppler study. Eur Heart J 15:1348–1352, 1994.

20. Persico G, Amato B, Aprea G, et al: The early effects of intravenous L-propionyl carnitine on ulcerative trophic lesions of the lower limbs in arteriopathic patients: A controlled randomized study. Drugs Exp Clin Res 21:187–198, 1995.

21. Duthie GG, Bellizzi MC: Effects of antioxidants on vascular health. Br Med Bull 55:568–577, 1999.

22. May JM: How does ascorbic acid prevent endothelial dysfunction? Free Radic Biol Med 28:1421–1429, 2000.

23. Frei B: On the role of vitamin C and other antioxidants in atherogenesis and vascular dysfunction. Proc Soc Exp Biol Med 222:196–204, 1999.

24. Reuter HD: Ginkgo biloba—botany, constituents, pharmacology and clinical trials. Br J Phytother 4:3–20, 1995/6.

25. Van Beek TA, Bombardelli D, Morazzoni F: Ginkgo biloba L. Fitoterapia. 169:195–244, 1998.

26. Blumenthal M, Goldberg A, Gruenwald J, et al (eds): The Complete German Commission E Monographs: Therapeutic Guide to Herbal Medicines. Austin, Tex, American Botanical Council, 1998.

27. Pittler MH, Ernst E: Ginkgo biloba extract for the treatment of intermittent claudication: A meta-analysis of randomized trials. Am J Med 108:276–281, 2000.

28. Bohmer D, Kalinski S, Michaelis MH, Sxogy A: Behandlung der PAVK mit Ginkgo biloba-extrakt (GBE) oder Pentoxifyllin. Herz Kreislauf 1988;20:5–8.

29. Ginkgo biloba [monograph]. In DerMarderosian A (ed): Facts and Comparisons: The Review of Natural Products. Philadelphia, Lippincott Williams & Wilkins, 1999.

30. Rowin J, Lewis SL: Spntaneous bilateral subdural hematomas with chronic Ginkgo biloba ingestion. Neurology 1996; 46:1775–1776, 1996.

31. Vale S: Subarachnoid hemorrhage associated with Ginkgo biloba. Lancet 352:36, 1998.

32. Rosenblatt M, Mindel J: Spontaneous hyphemia associated with the ingestion of Ginkgo biloba extract. N Engl J Med 336:1108, 1997.

33. Guillaume M, Padioleau F: Veinotonic effect, vascular protection, antiinflammatory and free radical scavenging properties of horse chestnut extract. Arzneimittelforschung 44:25–35, 1994.

34. Matsuda H, et al: Effects of escins Ia, Ib, IIa, and IIb from horse chestnut, the seeds of Aesculus hippocastanum L., on acute inflammation in animals. Biol Pharm Bull 20:1092–1095, 1997.

35. Diehm C, et al: Comparison of leg compression stocking and oral horse-chestnut seed extract therapy in patients with chronic venous insufficiency. Lancet 347:292–294, 1996.

36. Pittler MH, Ernst E: Horse chestnut seed extract for chronic venous insufficiency. A criteria-based systematic review. Arch Dermatol 134:1356–1360, 1998.

37. Packer L, Rimbach G, Virgili F: Antioxidant activity and biologic properties of a procyanidin rich extract from pine (Pinus maritima) bark, pycnogenol. Free Radic Biol Med 27(5-6):704–724, 1999.

38. DerMarderosian A (ed): Facts and Comparisons: The Review of Natural Products. Philadelphia, Lippincott Williams & Wilkins, 2001.

39. Sarrat L: Therapeutic approach to functional disorders of lower extremities. Bordeaux Med 14:685, 1981.

40. Arcangeli P: Pycnogenol in chronic venous insufficiency. Fitoterapia 71:236–244, 2000.

41. Petrassi C, Mastromarino A, Spartera C: Pycnogenol in chronic venous insufficiency. Phytomed 7:383–388, 2000.

42. Lamar CP: Chelation therapy of occlusive arteriosclerosis in diabetic patients. Presented at the Conference on Angiology, San Juan, Puerto Rico, February, 1964, pp 379–395.

43. Lamar CP: Chelation endarterectomy for occlusive atherosclerosis. J Am Geriat Soc 14:272–294, 1966.

44. Deycher GP: Antioxidant Therapy in the Aging Process. Basel, Berkhauser Verlag, 1992.

45. Casdorph HR, Farr CH: EDTA chelation therapy III: Treatment of peripheral arterial occlusion, an alternative to amputation. J Holist Med 5:3–15, 1983.

46. Robinson SD: Chelation therapy. N Z Med J 1982; 750.

47. Godfrey ME: EDTA chelation as a treatment of arteriosclerosis. N Z Med J 93:100, 1990.

48. Olszewer E, Sabbag FC, Carter JP: A pilot double-blind study of sodium magnesium EDTA in peripheral vascular disease. J Nat Med Assoc 82:173–177, 1989.

49. Guldager B, Jelnes R, Jorgensen SJ, et al: EDTA treatment of intermittent claudication—a double-blind, placebo-controlled study. J Intern Med 231:261–267, 1992.

50. Sloth-Nielsen J, Guldager B, Mouritzen C, et al: Arteriographic finding in EDTA chelation therapy on peripheral arteriosclerosis. Am J Surg 162:122–125, 1991.

51. Van Rij AM, Solomon C, Packer SGK, Hopkins WG: Lipids: Chelation therapy for intermittent claudication: A double-blind, randomized, controlled trial. Circulation 90:1194–1199, 1994.

52. De Backer TL, Vander Stichele RH, Warie HH, Bogaert MG: Oral vasoactive medication in intermittent claudication: Utile or futile? Eur J Clin Pharmacol 56:199–206, 2000.

53. Perez Encinas M, Fernandez MA, Martin ML, et al: Multicriteria decision analysis for determining drug therapy for intermittent claudication. Methods Find Exp Clin Pharmacol 20:425–431, 1998.

54. Frampton JE, Brogden RN: Pentoxifylline (oxpentifylline). A review of its therapeutic efficacy in the management of peripheral vascular and cerebrovascular disorders. Drugs Aging 7:480–503, 1995.

55. Reilly MP, Mohler ER, 3rd: Cilostazol: Treatment of intermittent claudication. Ann Pharmacother 35:48–56, 2001.

56. Phillips TJ: Successful methods of treating leg ulcers. The tried and true, plus the novel and new. Postgrad Med 105:159–161, 165–166, 173–174, 1999.

57. Alguire PC, Mathes BM: Chronic venous insufficiency and venous ulceration. J Gen Intern Med 12:374–383, 1997.

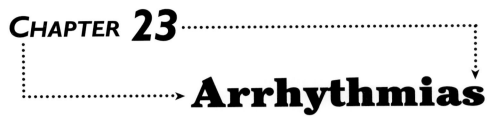

CHAPTER 23

Arrhythmias

Brian Olshansky, M.D.

Cardiac arrhythmias are slow (brady-), fast (tachy-), or irregular heart rhythm disturbances (ectopy, atrial fibrillation, and others). Arrhythmias may be a normal phenomenon related to change in autonomic tone; examples include sinus arrhythmia, sinus bradycardia, and sinus tachycardia. Interrelated reasons to evaluate and treat arrhythmias include (1) to eliminate symptoms, (2) to prevent imminent death and hemodynamic collapse, and (3) to offset long-term risk of serious symptoms and death. This chapter focuses on evaluation and treatment of arrhythmias using an integrative approach.

Common arrhythmias encountered in an office-based setting include atrial premature beats, ventricular premature beats, bradycardias, supraventricular tachycardia, nonsustained ventricular tachycardia, atrial fibrillation, and follow-up of already treated sustained ventricular tachycardia or ventricular fibrillation. Potentially symptomatic, and dangerous, arrhythmias that require evaluation for possible short- and long-term therapy include (1) sustained ventricular tachycardia in the setting of heart disease, (2) ventricular fibrillation (cardiac arrest), and (3) atrioventricular (AV) block. Junctional rhythm, atrioventricular (AV) dissociation, and ectopic beats are common, may cause concern, and may require special attention, further evaluation, and therapy. These are generally not serious enough to require long-term aggressive treatment unless associated with severe symptoms.

PATHOPHYSIOLOGY

Heart rhythm disturbances have multiple potential mechanisms and causes. The heart rhythm is a mechanical response to electrical activation of specialized fibers and atrial and ventricular myocardium. Electrical activation is generally initiated in the sinus node, which then leads to activation through various atrial conductive pathways (although this is still debated) to the AV node, the His-Purkinje system, and then the ventricles. The sinus node may be activated slowly owing to damage to this structure or because of autonomic effects. Increased vagal tone, for example, slows the sinus node rate. Abnormalities in conduction can cause disturbances throughout the normal pathways, leading to heart block and bradyarrhythmias. The autonomic nervous system can influence the

sinus node to either slow down or speed up. The autonomic nervous system can influence tissue in the heart to make it more automatic, thereby activating faster and overtaking normal sinus node rhythm. This can lead to activation by an ectopic focus. The autonomic nervous system can slow or speed conduction throughout the normal conduction pathways, and it can influence local activation of other tissue should the sinus node slow. This can cause an escape rhythm or an ectopic focus.

Heart rhythm disturbances can cause many potential problems. Abrupt change in the heart rate, especially with marked slowing or acceleration, can lead to hemodynamic compromise, syncope, and other related symptoms. Rhythm disturbances that are extraordinarily fast or that originate in the ventricles and are associated with structural heart disease can be premonitory signs of cardiac arrest. Cardiac arrest is generally due to ventricular fibrillation, which is an irregular rapid rhythm in the lower chambers of the heart; unless defibrillated, it leads to sudden death. However, most rhythm disturbances seen in clinical practice are benign.

Ectopic beats that trigger palpitations include ventricular ectopic activity (premature ventricular contractions [PVCs]), atrial ectopic activity (premature atrial contractions [PACs]), and atrial arrhythmias such as atrial fibrillation. Ventricular ectopy and atrial ectopy, when not associated with serious underlying structural heart disease, are relatively benign. Although there might be a slightly increased risk of death in any patient with PVCs (up to doubling in mortality), in someone with a normal heart, the risk remains very low; the reason to treat ectopic beats is not to prevent death but to prevent symptoms. Asymptomatic atrial and ventricular ectopy in a patient with no underlying heart disease does not require treatment.

Treatment of symptomatic atrial and ventricular ectopy, however, becomes a major problem in clinical practice for several reasons: (1) There are no good, safe, medical therapies.[1-13] Drugs used to suppress atrial ectopy frequently can be "proarrhythmic" and increase the risk for sudden death or increase the severity of the arrhythmias, and they can cause a variety of other serious complications. (2) The problem can be highly symptomatic and of concern to the patient. It can have a tremendous impact on the quality of life. (3) The severity of symptoms from benign arrhythmias varies tremendously; those who are highly symptomatic may require various therapeutic interventions, which can extend as far as drug therapy and even radiofrequency catheter ablation approaches.

Atrial fibrillation is a complex arrhythmia that has a myriad of presentations and therapeutic intervention possibilities. The general approach to treating atrial fibrillation is a triumvirate of issues: (1) ventricular rate control, (2) rhythm control, and (3) prevention of thromboembolic events. Although atrial fibrillation is associated with a doubling in mortality, this is not the reason to treat. Treatment is directed toward prevention of symptoms, yet no one has shown that treatment of the arrhythmia alone decreases mortality. Benign rhythm disturbances are extraordinarily common—atrial fibrillation occurs in 2.2 million Americans. Ectopic beats are as common but the extent of their occurrence is not completely known. Not all patients with ectopic beats are symptomatic, and the triggers for ectopic beats can be highly variable.

NOTE

Caffeinated beverages, chocolate, and even high sugar levels can trigger ectopic activity.[14, 15]

Palpitations may occur even in normal rhythm in patients with frequent ectopy or atrial fibrillation.

Symptoms

Symptoms related to arrhythmias are diverse and nonspecific, but they are crucial as they often dictate the urgency for therapy and the need for evaluation. Symptoms are related to the type and rate of the arrhythmia, the nature and severity of the underlying heart disease, and the patient. Symptoms are related to the cardiac activation sequence (relationship between atrial and ventricular contraction), rate (and rate change), regularity, and persistence and to associated conditions. Common symptoms include palpitations, dizziness, lightheadedness, syncope, chest discomfort, neck discomfort, dyspnea, weakness, and anxiety. Arrhythmias can cause symptoms by precipitating other conditions such as congestive heart failure, ischemia, and thromboemboli. Symptoms can be occult or unusual and can include tinnitus, visual changes, increased urinary frequency (due to elevation in atrial natriuretic peptide levels), abdominal discomfort, and peripheral edema. Arrhythmias may modify sympathetic and vagal tone, alter hormonal levels, elevate venous pressure, and reduce cardiac output. This can lead to an even longer list of associated symptoms. The association of heart disease with

arrhythmia determines the urgency of intervention, evaluation, and therapy, as well as the prognosis.

Palpitations

Palpitations are among the most common complaints associated with arrhythmias; the differential diagnosis is extensive. Palpitations can be intermittent or sustained, regular or irregular, and even unrelated to an arrhythmia. Catecholamine excess alone can cause a sensation of palpitations without an arrhythmia even being present.[16]

Palpitations can be a somatization of a psychiatric disorder. Of 125 outpatients referred for ambulatory electrocardiographic monitoring to evaluate palpitations, 34% had an arrhythmia and 19% had a psychiatric disorder, especially major depression or a panic disorder.[17] Those with psychiatric disorders were younger and more disabled and had a greater number of hypochondriacal concerns about their health. Their palpitations were more likely to last longer than 15 minutes, were accompanied by other symptoms, were more intense, and were associated with a greater number of emergency room visits. Several reports have confirmed the high incidence of psychiatric conditions in association with palpitations.[18, 19] Nevertheless, careful evaluation of palpitations is important to rule out organic disease.

Palpitations may occur in patients with arrhythmias, yet not be related to a rhythm disturbance. In a study of 1454 elderly patients (aged 60 to 94 years), 8.3% had palpitations. Arrhythmias, predominantly conduction abnormalities and sinus bradycardia, were found in 12.6%.[20] The prevalence of palpitations was similar in those with and without arrhythmias. In another study of 518 patients who had 24-hour electrocardiographic recordings, 34% had their typical symptoms at a time when the electrocardiogram was normal.[21]

Palpitations only rarely are the result of a life-threatening process, although they can be associated with or represent manifestations of underlying ventricular dysfunction or other structural heart disease. Palpitations in a patient with heart disease, especially coronary artery disease, should raise suspicions that the palpitations are caused by an arrhythmia.

APPROACH TO THE PATIENT

Perspective

Arrhythmias may have little meaning if they (1) have no prognostic significance, (2) do not alter hemodynamics or cardiac function, and (3) are not symptomatic. Routine screening of an asymptomatic patient is not recommended. Patients typically seek medical care for palpitations, an arrhythmia associated with symptoms, a symptom thought to be caused by an arrhythmia, or nonspecific symptoms that may be due to an arrhythmia. Occasionally, an asymptomatic patient is found to have an arrhythmia by an electrocardiogram, an ambulatory monitor, an exercise test, or a hospital monitor (placed for no specific reason). Arrhythmias such as ventricular premature beats and atrial fibrillation are so common that it is impractical, and unnecessary, for clinicians to refer every arrhythmia to a specialist. Alternatively, with major advances in the management of several cardiac arrhythmias (using ablation and implantable devices), identifying the patient who requires such an intervention can markedly improve the outcome.

Initial Evaluation and Diagnosis of the Arrhythmia

The initial evaluation includes a careful, circumspect, and complete history (directed toward the symptoms and any potential relationship to an arrhythmia, as well as an assessment of potential responsible conditions), a physical examination, and a 12-lead electrocardiogram at baseline, and, if possible, during the arrhythmia. An unhurried, careful, complete history is the key to further appropriate evaluation; it prevents the urge to perform expensive, unnecessary, or potentially risky tests. Several issues should be addressed in the history (Table 23–1).

The electrocardiogram (ECG) recorded during the arrhythmia or symptoms reveals the need for further evaluation and treatment. An ambulatory monitor or an event monitor may be needed in select patients to secure a diagnosis. If the symptoms are sporadic, but occur daily, an ambulatory (Holter) monitor is the best approach.[22–25] An event recorder or transtelephonic monitor can help make the diagnosis in a patient with less frequent palpitations. Transtelephonic devices are small, lightweight, and inexpensive. The memory feature allows recording of data without the need for immediate access to telephone transmission. An implantable monitor (Reveal, Medtronic, Minneapolis, USA) is now available[26] that can automatically record events triggered by the patient or by preselected criteria. The device can record up to 42 minutes of arrhythmia data. If episodes are associated with exercise or physical or mental stress, or if an arrhythmia cannot be documented with ambulatory or transtelephonic monitoring, exercise testing may secure a diagnosis.

Risk Assessment

It is important to determine whether an arrhythmia has prognostic importance: Is it a premonitory sign of death? Conditions that are potentially life threatening include ventricular tachycardia and atrial fibrillation in the Wolff-Parkinson-White syndrome. Not all ventricular tachycardias are life threa-

tening; a patient without heart disease, for example, with idiopathic sustained ventricular tachycardia (*not* idiopathic ventricular fibrillation) has little risk of dying. In contrast, even a single episode of nonsustained ventricular tachycardia in a patient with coronary artery disease and poor left ventricular function due to prior myocardial infarction may be associated with a poor prognosis.[27]

Rarely, an asymptomatic arrhythmia must be treated urgently. Symptoms and their relationship to the arrhythmia require careful assessment. A correlation of the arrhythmia to the symptom is preferred, although it is not always possible.

Indications for Inpatient Management

Hospital admission is required if the patient has significant underlying heart disease such as cardiomyopathy with congestive heart failure, or coronary artery disease with active ischemia; if the arrhythmia is life threatening and requires rapid reversion (e.g., a fast tachyarrhythmia, polymorphic ventricular tachycardia, or prolonged QT interval in a patient with syncope); and if the arrhythmia is uncontrolled or highly symptomatic. Hospital admission is preferred for the elderly patient who may have not only underlying heart disease but also other chronic illnesses such as kidney or liver disease that may affect antiarrhythmic therapy.

Referral to a Specialist

A cardiologist is frequently needed to help manage the complex patient with an arrhythmia; for example, a temporary pacemaker may be needed for a symptomatic bradycardia (Table 23–2). An electrophysiologist may be necessary to institute aggressive acute therapy, such as intravenous amiodarone for life-threatening ventricular tachycardia, antitachycardia pacing for acute reversion of an arrhythmia, or an implantable cardioverter-defibrillator (ICD) or to reprogram a pacemaker or an ICD.

Referral for electrophysiology study or further arrhythmia evaluation is indicated when the patient has a potentially life-threatening arrhythmia requiring interventional therapy (including survivors of aborted sudden cardiac death), if a benign but symptomatic arrhythmia cannot be controlled with straightforward medical therapy, if risky or compli-

Table 23–1. Historical Features of Importance in Evaluation of the Patient

Which arrhythmia is present?
Does the arrhythmia cause symptoms?
Does the arrhythmia have prognostic significance?
Is the problem life threatening?
Does the patient require hospital admission or extensive testing?
Is specialist consultation required, and if so, how urgently?
Is treatment required?

Table 23-2. Refer to a Specialist for the Following
....

Resuscitated ventricular fibrillation
Sustained ventricular tachycardia
Atrial fibrillation that is difficult to control or refractory to
   standard therapies
Nonsustained ventricular tachycardia
Supraventricular tachycardia that is difficult to control
Sinus bradycardia (sick sinus, tachy-brady syndrome)
Second-degree atrioventricular block
Unexplained ventricular ectopy in an athlete or in a
   symptomatic patient
Syncope with a suspected arrhythmic mechanism
Patients with devices (e.g., pacemakers, implantable
   defibrillators) who are unstable
Uncontrolled rhythm problems

cated therapy is needed (e.g., radiofrequency ablation, implantable device, or antitachycardia pacing), or if initial antiarrhythmic measures are not effective or are associated with a complication.

INTEGRATIVE THERAPY

The decision to start any type of antiarrhythmic therapy depends on the severity and frequency of arrhythmia-related symptoms, the risks of the arrhythmias, and the risks associated with the therapy itself. The need for long-term therapy must be carefully individualized to each patient because the severity and importance of symptoms are highly variable. The symptoms associated with any arrhythmia can have an impact on lifestyle, occupation, driving, and other important daily activities. These issues must be considered for every patient and are evaluated as part of a diagnostic and therapeutic approach.

Nutrition

Gastric Distention

Dietary interventions in some cases can influence some arrhythmias. A large meal can distend the stomach, thereby stimulating vagal afferents, leading to vagal efferent activation. This can initiate atrial fibrillation in patients who have vagally mediated atrial fibrillation, hypotension, bradycardia, and even syncope. Bloating from excessively fatty, fried, or poorly digestible foods and other foods to which a patient is not accustomed can create a sensation of palpitations.

Food as a Trigger

Some foods act as triggers, and patients often provide some evidence for this: Alcohol is one of the major triggers for atrial fibrillation and ventricular ectopy.[28, 29] Caffeine is frequently another trigger for ectopic beats but not necessarily atrial fibrilla-

tion.[14, 15] It is important to recognize that restriction of alcohol and caffeine may have no effect on arrhythmias. If this is the case, restriction is of no benefit and may adversely influence the patient's lifestyle. Specific food allergies can trigger a reaction, causing palpitations. (See Chapter 82, The Elimination Diet.)

The effects of diet on the autonomic nervous system are complex. Several foods increase sympathetic nervous system tone. High levels of sodium can increase the effects of catecholamines. Electrolytes can influence ventricular and atrial ectopy.[30–35]

Caffeine, theophylline, or theobromine found in coffee, tea, or chocolate, respectively, may be inciting factors or may have a positive benefit.[36–38] Trial and error with these food substances is worthwhile, but there is no particular reason to try to eliminate all these foods if they do not have an effect on the arrhythmia. Patient complaints that a specific food triggers a rhythm disturbance should be taken seriously. It is possible that this is related to some type of allergic reaction or related issue.

Botanical Triggers

Specific supplements can trigger arrhythmias. Ma huang, from the Chinese ephedra plant, contains catecholamines, including ephedrine, which can initiate ectopic rhythm disturbances.[39] It has even been suggested that Ambertose, *ginkgo biloba*, and other commonly used substances may exacerbate or even cause arrhythmias.

Blood Sugar

Severe fluctuations in blood sugar levels can trigger rhythm disturbances. A diet moderate in unrefined sugar and high in roughage may alter the autonomic effects in the gastrointestinal (GI) tract and from the sugar itself to minimize the arrhythmias due to these dietary interventions.

Diet and Anticoagulation

The diet becomes very important in arrhythmia management, especially in patients who require anticoagulation for atrial fibrillation or other arrhythmias. If the diet changes markedly and if, because of this, there are significant alterations in vitamin K levels, tremendous fluctuation is noted in the prothrombin time.

NOTE

A balanced diet low in fat and high in roughage that will lead to a moderate level of blood sugar may reduce stress on the gastrointestinal tract and improve arrhythmia symptoms.

Exercise

Exercise and physical exertion can trigger a variety of arrhythmias. Maintaining excellent physical health through exercise, however, decreases effects of the sympathetic nervous system on the heart and the heart rhythm to improve outcomes. The sympathetic nervous system often has a major contributory role in the genesis of serious and benign atrial and ventricular arrhythmias. Exercise performed regularly with enhancement of aerobic capacity decreases sensitivity to catecholamines, decreases circulating catecholamine levels, decreases sympathetic nervous system tone, and enhances vagal tone. All of these increase heart rate variability, which decreases the risk for sudden death and decreases the potential for catecholamine-initiated or sympathetically initiated atrial and ventricular arrhythmias.

Exercise can also modulate other rhythm disturbances such as sinus tachycardia. Especially in young women, inappropriate sinus tachycardia and postural orthostatic tachycardia syndrome are potential problems.[40] Inappropriate sinus tachycardia is a condition in which the sinus node appears to be hyperactive; the cause for this is not completely known. It might be, in part, related to abnormal sympathetic nervous system stimulation, but it could also be an intrinsic problem with the sinus node. Increasing exercise decreases the potential for this problem. Sinus tachycardia can occur after viral syndrome. Exercise downregulates the sympathetic nervous system and lowers catecholamine levels. By several mechanisms, it can lower heart rate. Exercise appears to be beneficial in treating many arrhythmias but it must be used with caution, as it is a double-edged sword. For patients with malignant arrhythmias, use of exercise therapy must be performed by a qualified health care provider who is knowledgeable about the risks, benefits, and methods of monitoring the patient.

Lifestyle

Tobacco and Alcohol

Lifestyle has a major impact on arrhythmias.[41–43] Cigarette smoking and other forms of nicotine have no benefit and may be harmful for any individual.[42, 44] Use of tobacco can exacerbate risk of sudden death and malignant and benign arrhythmias of all types. Cigarettes also trigger a variety of rhythm disturbances, including cardiac arrest by several potential mechanisms. If possible, it is best to try to eliminate smoking under any circumstance.

Alcohol, although it may have a beneficial effect on cardiovascular mortality, myocardial infarction, and cholesterol, has no benefit for any arrhythmia. The differences between the different types of alcohol are unclear in terms of their ability to trigger rhythm disturbances. It appears that all alcohol can trigger arrhythmias, and it is not clear that a specific type of alcohol, whether wine or hard liquor, has a greater propensity to do this.

Frequently, alcohol is used in combination with caffeine and cigarettes. The combination of alcohol and nicotine is even more likely to trigger an arrhythmia.

Mind–Body Techniques

Autonomic variations can occur with a variety of different lifestyle interventions, including acupuncture, meditation, and other mind–body issues.[45, 46] The influence can be profound and may occur by several mechanisms: (1) change in autonomic funtion, (2) placebo effect, (3) direct effect on the rhythm, (4) change in perception of the importance of the arrhythmia to the patient and, (5) shifting of attention from the arrhythmia to some other issue.

Biofeedback

Biofeedback can decrease the number, frequency, and severity of palpitations related to arrhythmias. Another issue is simply one of developing an awareness that a patient can learn to identify a rhythm disturbance as not a noxious experience. The interpretation of the severity of the rhythm disturbance amplifies the severity of the effects on symptoms. Having patients face problems can actually become an issue of empowerment whereby they can improve their perception of the arrhythmia and its implications.

Meditation

Meditation has been associated with decreased risk of sudden death due to ventricular fibrillation in high-risk patients.[45, 46] It may also change the perception of the arrhythmia as a problem for those who have a benign arrhythmia. (See Chapter 94, Learning to Meditate).

Relaxation response

Relaxation appears to have a positive benefit. Physicians have used medications (benzodiazepines) for years to treat rhythm disturbances such as atrial fibrillation and supraventricular tachycardia. If a patient develops such arrhythmias and is allowed to relax, the rhythm often stops spontaneously. (See Chapter 91, Prescribing Relaxation Techniques).

Supplements

Coenzyme Q10

Coenzyme Q10 at a dose of 100 to 300 milligrams a day may decrease episodes of atrial fibrillation by an unknown mechanism. Coenzyme Q10 can also have an effect on ventricular and atrial ectopy.[47]

Dosage. 100 to 300 mg per day.

Precautions. Long-term use of greater than 300 mg/day can increase serum aminotransferases and can also result in gastritis, nausea, diarrhea, and loss of appetite.

L-Carnitine

L-Carnitine, at a dose of 3 g or more a day, can improve mitochondrial function and left ventricular function and may prevent some atrial and ventricular arrhythmias. Several small, randomized, controlled trials of carnitine have shown a reduction in risk for sudden cardiac death and total death in patients with cardiomyopathy. The mechanism is not clear, but it may be that carnitine improves mitochondrial function and myocardial function.[48–50]

Dosage. 3 g per day.

Precautions. There are no known adverse effects of carnitine.

Calcium and Magnesium

Calcium and magnesium, approximately 1 g a day each of a salt (magnesium sulfate, for example), have been associated with a decrease in arrhythmias. Magnesium can decrease triggered activity and can slow conduction in the AV node. A variety of forms of magnesium are available, including magnesium oxide, which is available in over-the-counter preparations.

Magnesium supplementation given to patients in congestive heart failure in a double-blind, placebo-controlled trial produced improvement in arrhythmias. Individuals taking 3.2 g per day of magnesium chloride equivalent to 384 mg per day of elemental magnesium have between 23% and 52% fewer occurrences of specific arrhythmias in a 6-week follow-up period.[35]

Dosage. Elemental magnesium at 300 to 1000 mg a day. Magnesium gluconate is preferred orally because it is highly souble and is less likely to cause diarrhea.

Calcium at 1000 mg a day. Calcium citrate may be better absorbed in the elderly, but the less expensive calcium carbonate is also a good source.

Precaution. Magnesium can cause diarrhea, GI upset, nausea, and vomiting. Toxicity can lead to hypotension, drowsiness, loss of tendon reflexes, muscle weakness, and respiratory depression. Calcium can cause constipation and GI upset.

Copper and Zinc

Three cases have been reported in which ventricular premature beats disappeared after copper supplementation at a dose of 4 mg per day (and decreased PVCs).[33] It turned out that zinc made the arrhythmias worse and that extra zinc can lead to copper deficiency. However, there is a potential problem with copper, as high copper levels can lead to atherosclerosis.

Selenium

A deficiency in selenium can cause heart problems, including arrhythmias. There are no good data, however, to suggest that low selenium levels, when supplemented, improve arrhythmia status.[30, 51]

Potassium

Potassium supplementation is extraordinarily important, especially if a patient is taking drugs that are lowering potassium levels. Potassium has been implicated for all types of rhythm disturbances. High potassium levels can lead to asystole, and deficiencies can lead to torsades de pointes, ventricular fibrillation, and ectopic beats. It is clear that anyone who is at risk with long QT interval syndrome and is taking specific drugs that lower potassium should in fact take potassium supplements. This can also be done through potassium in the diet, including fruits and vegetables that contain high potassium levels. (See Chapter 85, The DASH Diet).

Omega-3 Fatty Acids

Omega-3 fatty acids appear to have a direct effect on a variety of myocardial channels that can affect arrhythmias.[52–26] Specifically, omega-3 fatty acids appear to have an effect on calcium and potassium channels.[57] Omega-3 fatty acids when given as fish oil, have been found, in men with symptomatic PVCs, to decrease the risk of PVCs by approximately 70%.[58, 59]

Fish oil has also been shown in the GISSI2 Prevenzione Trial to be associated with a decreased risk for total death and sudden death. This study included 11,324 Italians who had had myocardial infarction (MI) within the preceding 3 months. They were randomized to omega-3 polyunsaturated fatty acids (2836), vitamin E (2830), or neither (2828). Those given fish oil had a 45% reduction in sudden death and a 20% decrease in mortality.[57]

The Lyon Diet Study and the Physician's Health Study have all shown a benefit derived from the use of fish oil. The Diet and Reinfarction Trial (DART) included 2033 men with acute myocardial infarction, randomized to receive or not to receive advice on diets: decreased fat intake to 30% of total energy, at least 2 weekly portions (200 to 400 g) of fatty fish (or take 1.5 g fish oil capsules if unable to eat fish), and cereal fiber to 18 g daily. Those who were given "fish advice" survived substantially and significantly better.[60]

These data have inspired the FAAT Trial. This randomized, placebo-controlled trial compares 3 g of fish oil to cod-scented olive oil. It was undertaken to look at the incidence of recurrent ventricular arrhythmias in patients who have implanted cardiac defibrillators and are at risk for sudden death. The aim of this study is to decrease the number of shocks. Omega-3 fatty acids are available in a variety of forms, not only fish oil. A variety of plant oils can be metabolized into omega-3 fatty acids, including flaxseed oil, which also has other potential benefits, including effects on mood. As omega-3 fatty acids can improve mood, they may also have an autonomic effect that can decrease the sensation of arrhythmias or decrease arrhythmias altogether.

Dosage. 1 to 4 g of eicosapentaenoic acid (EPA) and docosahexaenoic acid (DHA) fish oil daily.

Precautions. Prolonged use of 4 g per day may have pro-oxidant effects and should, if needed, be used with an antioxidant regimen, including vitamin E, vitamin C, and selenium.

Vitamin D

A long-standing case of sick sinus syndrome was reported to resolve with supplementation of 800 units per day of vitamin D.[61] However, it is not clear that Vitamin D was the cause for this change.

Vitamin C

Recent evidence indicates that vitamin C given postoperatively to patients at risk for atrial fibrillation after coronary artery bypass graft surgery causes a marked reduction in atrial fibrillation. It appears that by whatever mechanism, vitamin C has antiarrhythmic properties and can prevent atrial fibrillation, at least in some patients. The mechanism might be by clearance of free radicals or by an anti-inflammatory influence.

Botanicals

Many of the original antiarrhythmic drugs originated from herbal therapy: quinidine (a stereo-isomer of quinine from cinchona bark), lidocaine, amiodarone (from khellin, originally from the herb *Ammi visnaga*), and digoxin (from foxglove) are a few.[62] Recent data suggest that several other herbal preparations may have antiarrhythmic effects. Several drugs used in Chinese traditional medicine have been touted as suppressing palpitations.

Japanese studies on indole alkaloids from *Uncaria rhynchophylla* and *Amsoria elliptica* contain hirsutine, hirsuteine, rhynchophylline, isorhynchophylline, and dihydrocorynantheine.[63] These and beta-yohimbine isolated from *Amsohia elliptica* have shown potential benefit for aconitine-induced arrhythmias in mice and ouabain-induced arrhythmias in guinea pigs.[63] The potency of the antiarrhythmic effects was about the same as that of ajmaline, an antiarrhythmic drug (no longer available), also an indole alkaloid. Hirsutine and dihydrocorynantheine affect action potentials of the sinoatrial node, the atria, and the ventricles.

Ciwujia (*Acanthopanax senticosus harms*)

This is used for athletic performance and for weight loss and may have antiarrhythmic effects. Ciwujia was studied in isolated rat heart with transient coronary occlusion.[64] Ciwujia extract reduced reperfusion-induced ventricular fibrillation and ventricular tachycardia. Ciwujia reduced the number of cells with abnormal action potential configurations. Ciwujia may reduce the incidence of malignant arrhythmias.[64]

Licorice (*Glycyrrhiza glabra*)

Licorice root has an antiarrhythmic property.[65] Zhigancao (prepared licorice) injection can antagonize arrhythmias induced by chloroform, catecholamines, aconitine, strophanthine K, and barium chloride. It may slow the heart rate, prolong PR and QT intervals, and antagonize the positive chronotropic response induced by catecholamines. Another component of licorice, sodium 18 beta-glycyrrhetate, strongly counteracts arrhythmia induced by chloroform, lengthens the appearance time of arrhythmia induced by $CaCl_2$, slightly retards the heart rate of rats and rabbits, and partly antagonizes the acceleration effect of isoproterenol on rabbit hearts. The clinical significance of these experimental findings is unclear.[64] Owing to the potential side-effects of this product, use for arrhythmias is not recommended at this time.

Motherwort (*Leonurus cardiaca*)

Motherwort contains bufenolide, glycosides (stachydirine), and alkaloids. A dose between 4 and 5 g of motherwort can decrease palpitations owing to a presumably mild beta-blocking effect, although the exact mechanism that motherwort exerts on the heart to decrease ectopic beats is unclear. No randomized, controlled trial has been performed using motherwort.

Khella (*Ammi visnaga*)

Khella has significant antiarrhythmic effects. In the 1950s, a compound known as khella was derived from the *Ammi visnaga* plant. It was used to treat angina due to coronary heart disease with significant improvement in those patients. It has also been used over the years by naturopaths to decrease palpitations. It turns out that khella is the original substance from which a very potent antiarrhythmic drug, amiodarone, was derived. The dose of khella depends on the arrhythmia and the endpoint to be achieved.[67-69]

Siberian Ginseng (*Eleutherococcus senticosus*)

Siberian ginseng can cause an apparent increase in digoxin.[70] It is unclear whether this is a false serum elevation, if ginseng converts to digoxin in vivo, or whether ginseng alters the metabolism of digoxin.

Hawthorn Berry (*Crataegus laevigata*)

Hawthorne berry had been used to treat atrial fibrillation and it might have an effect on other rhythm disturbances as well.[70] Hawthorne berry has bathmotropic and dromotropic effects that are ascribed to the flavonoids present. Hawthorne contains hyperoside (vitexin, rhamnose), rutin, and oligomeric procyanidins. A dose of 160 to 900 mg of the water ethanol extract is recommended. It is unclear exactly where this herb works, but it might work on the sodium-potassium ATPase pump, similar to digoxin. More likely, hawthorne acts as a phosphodiesterase inhibitor.

Angelica (*Angelica archangelica*) and Ginkgo biloba

Angelica and ginkgo biloba may have a protective influence during myocardial ischemia and reperfusion.[71] In a rat model, the incidence of ventricular premature beats and the total incidence of arrhythmia were greatly reduced.[72]

Raspberry Leaf (*Rubus idaeus*)

Raspberry leaf contains magnesium and other unknown substances that may decrease the rate of palpitation.

Pharmaceuticals

The standard first-line drug therapy approach for benign PVCs and PACs, and for episodes of atrial fibrillation is often a beta-adrenergic blocking drug. Drugs of this class alter the autonomic nervous system tone of the heart. It is unclear how effective this approach is; however, there are good data to suggest that it is not effective whatsoever. Furthermore, adverse effects are common when these therapies are used for ectopic beats.

For atrial fibrillation, various antiarrhythmic drugs are available. Their use depends on the underlying heart disease, age of the patient, severity of symptoms, and difficulty in maintaining sinus rhythm. The discussion on antiarrhythmic drug use, anticoagulation, and rate-control drugs for atrial fibrillation is beyond the scope of this chapter, but several good references are available.

For ventricular ectopy and PVCs, if beta blockers do not work, a variety of antiarrhythmic drugs can be used, including, for normal hearts without any evidence of ischemic heart disease, class IC antiarrhythmic drugs such as propafenone and flecainide.[5, 6] One concern about these antiarrhythmic drugs, like any antiarrhythmic drug, is that they can triple the mortality rate if underlying heart disease is present. Their use is never completely safe because of possible "proarrhythmic" effects.[1-8]

Occasionally, a patient with ventricular bigeminy will not perfuse the PVC and therefore will not have adequate perfusion. Treatment of the PVC can eliminate this problem.

Ablation therapy is also used to treat a variety of supraventricular and ventricular tachyarrhythmias. Atrial fibrillation, especially when paroxysmal, can be treated by ablating focal ectopic beats that originate from the pulmonary veins. This emerging technology is not completely ready for general use.

Although antiarrhythmic drugs can suppress arrhythmias, two important issues must be considered: proarrhythmia and adverse effects. All antiarrhythmic drugs have the potential to increase ectopy or induce, or aggravate, monomorphic ventricular tachycardia, torsades de pointes, ventricular fibrillation, conduction disturbances, or bradycardia. This is known as *proarrhythmia*.[1-8]

The use of antiarrhythmic drugs should be reserved for clinicians who are expert in their use. A discussion of this topic is beyond the scope of this chapter.

Although the exact incidence of proarrhythmia is not certain, it is estimated to range from 1% to 15% with various antiarrhythmic drugs. The risk varies according to the type of arrhythmia treated, the presence of structural heart disease, the QT interval, preexisting conduction disturbances, sinus node dysfunction, patient age, the presence of congestive heart failure, and left and right ventricular function. Ironically, the proarrhythmic risk is highest in patients with depressed left ventricular function (i.e., ejection fraction <0.30), the group at highest risk for an arrhythmic event and sudden death; the risk is lowest in those with no organic heart disease.

Identification of proarrhythmia has resulted in the more appropriate use of antiarrhythmic drugs, resulting in a decline in the use and a change in demographics of antiarrhythmic drug therapy. Quinidine remains the most commonly prescribed antiarrhythmic drug in the United States, especially among physicians who are not cardiologists or electrophysiologists; however, there has been increasing use of amiodarone, sotalol, and the class IC drugs in the United States.

The Risk-Benefit Ratio

The goal of therapy for any arrhythmia is to eliminate symptoms or prevent a potentially serious outcome, primarily a life-threatening arrhythmia and sudden death. These goals must be balanced against the risks associated with antiarrhythmic therapy, including proarrhythmia, and the adverse effects of individual drugs. The case of treating PVCs represents an example of the importance of a risk-benefit assessment in each individual patient.

NOTE

No study has shown that asymptomatic ventricular ectopy suppression in any group of patients improves survival. The only reason to treat is to suppress symptoms from the arrhythmias as long as treatment does not worsen the arrhythmias or the prognosis.

Antiarrhythmic Drug Therapy and Dose Titration

Therapy with some antiarrhythmic drugs is best initiated in the hospital, primarily for monitoring of early proarrhythmia. The decision to hospitalize depends on the presence and severity of structural heart disease, the indication for treatment (e.g., etiology of the arrhythmia and type and severity of associated symptoms), and the drug used. If the patient has a life-threatening arrhythmia, drug initiation and dose titration should be performed in the hospital. Follow-up 24-hour ambulatory ECG monitoring is recommended on a regular basis, for example, every 6 months, to assess for continued drug efficacy and safety. An ACC/AHA task force has published guidelines for the use of ambulatory monitoring in the assessment of antiarrhythmic drug efficacy.

New approaches to manage serious and sustained arrhythmias are emerging. Therapy is moving to device-based treatment (implanted defibrillators and pacemakers) and to ablation (to cure the arrhythmias). The use of antiarrhythmic drugs has changed drastically over the years, and the complete management approach to patients with serious or life-threatening arrhythmia is beyond the scope of this chapter. If a patient has such an arrhythmia, referral to a specialist is in order.

 ── *THERAPEUTIC REVIEW* ──────────────────

The problem of arrhythmia management is complex and multifaceted. The treatment depends on the arrhythmia and its implications, symptoms, and effect on the patient. Most serious rhythm disturbances need to be referred to a specialist, especially if they are potentially life threatening. If not, an approach to improve outcomes should involve changes in lifestyle and exercise. After these have been implemented, dietary changes may be useful. If this is not enough, mind–body effects can be substantial. Consider meditation. Acupuncture can have beneficial effects as well. Several herbal preparations may influence the presence of an arrhythmia, but care must be taken with some of these, because some supplements such as ma huang can worsen an arrhythmia or even create a new, life-threatening one.

For patients with symptomatic ectopy/PVCs:

Lifestyle/Risk
- *Determine the severity of the symptoms and their relation to the arrhythmia. Assess underlying conditions.*
- *Determine the risk to the patient.*
- *For benign ectopy, discuss the risks of drug therapy and suggest alternatives first.*
- *Eliminate dietary triggers (e.g., caffeine, chocolate, alcohol, simple carbohydrates).*
- *Increase roughage and avoid simple sugars.*

Mind-Body Techniques
- *Encourage a meditation practice*
- *Provide patient with a thorough understanding of the condition and its nature. Patients who understand will be able to tolerate the arrhythmia. Reassure the patient (if this is in order).*

Exercise
- *Determine relation to exercise; suggest an exercise program.*

Supplements/Botanicals
- *Suggest omega-3 fatty acids 1 to 2 g fish oil or flaxseed daily.*
- *Magnesium and calcium supplementation (300 to 1000 mg daily).*
- *Consider herbal approaches (motherwort—4 to 5 g of dried above-ground parts daily).*
- *Consider carnitine (3 g daily), and then CoQ10 (100 to 300 mg daily with a meal).*
- *Consider hawthorn berry 160–900 mg/day.*

Pharmaceuticals
- *Drug therapy only if resistant to the above*
  - Beta blockade titrated upward. Consider an extended-release metoprolol (Torpol XL 50, 100, 200 μg daily) or propranolol (60, 80, 120, or 160 μg daily).
  - Occasionally, calcium channel blockers are effective (diltiazem or verapamil 120–360 mg/daily).
  - Antiarrhythmic drugs as a last resort (if no structural heart disease, flecainide, propafenone, sotalol first; amiodarone only in resistant, highly symptomatic cases).

Surgical
- *Ablative therapy for bigeminy, sustained or nonsustained ventricular tacchycardia in those with no structural heart disease.*

For patient with paroxysmal atrial fibrillation:

Lifestyle/Risk
- *Correlate symptoms with arrhythmia. Determine presence of underlying conditions, including hyperthyroidism.*
- *Assess risk to the patient and need for rate control, anticoagulation, and maintenance of sinus rhythm.*
- *Determine triggers, if possible. If there is relationship, eliminate caffeine, alcohol, and any potential offending drug.*
- *If at night consider changes in diet (no large meals causing gastic distention).*

Exercise
- *If fibrillation is exercise related, consider an exercise program.*

Mind-Body Techniques
- *Relaxation techniques. Counsel patient and educate about disease process.*

Supplements/Botanicals
- *Omega-3 fatty acids (1 to 2 g fish or flaxseed oil daily).*
- *Magnesium and calcium supplementation (300 to 1000 mg daily).*
- *Hawthorn berry 160 to 900 mg daily, motherwort (4 to 5 gm daily), St. John's wort.*
- *CoQ10 (100 to 300 mg daily with a meal to enhance absorption).*

Energy
- *Acupuncture (not well tested but perhaps effective).*

Pharmaceuticals
- *Drug therapy*
  - Beta blockade (to control rhythm and rate) (see earlier for dosage).
  - Calcium channel blockade (to control rate) (diltiazem and verapamil) 120 to 360 mg daily.
  - Digoxin (little effect).
  - Antiarrhythmic drugs, depending on the patient and the conditions.
  - Warfarin (coumadin), if indicated.

Surgical
- *Ablation of the pulmonary veins.*
- *Ablation of the AV node with a pacemaker (patient remains in AF).*
- *Ablation of other inciting arrhythmia.*
- *Implantable defibrillator for atrial arrhythmias.*

References

1. Slater W, et al: Clinical predictors of arrhythmia worsening by antiarrhythmic drugs. Am J Cardiol 61:349–353, 1988.
2. Podrid PJ, et al: Aggravation of arrhythmia by antiarrhythmic drugs-incidence and predictors. Am J Cardiol 59:38E-44E, 1987.
3. Levy S, Torsades de pointes. A clearly defined syndrome or an electrocardiographic curiosity? Int J Cardiol 7:421–427, 1985.
4. Roden DM, Woosley RL, Primm RK, Incidence and clinical features of the quinidine-associated long QT syndrome: Implications for patient care. Am Heart J 111:1088–1093, 1986.
5. Preliminary report: Effect of encainide and flecainide on mortality in a randomized trial of arrhythmia suppression after myocardial infarction. The Cardiac Arrhythmia Suppression Trial (CAST) Investigators. N Engl J Med 321:406–412, 1989.
6. Effect of the antiarrhythmic agent moricizine on survival after myocardial infarction. The Cardiac Arrhythmia Suppression Trial II Investigators. N Engl J Med 327(4):227–233, 1992.
7. Velebit V, et al: Aggravation and provocation of ventricular arrhythmias by antiarrhythmic drugs. Circulation 65:886–894, 1987.
8. The 'Sicilian Gambit'. A new approach to the classification of antiarrhythmic drugs based on their actions on arrhythmogenic mechanisms. The Task Force of the Working Group on Arrhythmias of the European Society of Cardiology. Eur Heart J 12:1112–1131, 1991.
9. Pratt CM, et al: Mortality in the Survival With Oral D-sotalol (SWORD) trial: Why did patients die? Am J Cardiol 81:869–876, 1998.
10. Julian DG, et al: Randomised trial of effect of amiodarone on mortality in patients with left-ventricular dysfunction after recent myocardial infarction: EMIAT. European Myocardial Infarct Amiodarone Trial Investigators. Lancet 349:667–674, 1997.
11. Cairns JA, et al: Randomised trial of outcome after myocardial infarction in patients with frequent or repetitive ventricular premature depolarisations: CAMIAT. Canadian Amiodarone Myocardial Infarction Arrhythmia Trial Investigators. Lancet 349:675–682, 1997.
12. Janse MJ, et al: Identification of post acute myocardial infarction patients with potential benefit from prophylactic treatment with amiodarone. A substudy of EMIAT (the European Myocardial Infarct Amiodarone Trial). Eur Heart J 19:85–95, 1998.
13. Boutitie F, et al: Amiodarone interaction with beta-blockers: Analysis of the merged EMIAT (European Myocardial Infarct Amiodarone Trial) and CAMIAT (Canadian Amiodarone Myocardial Infarction Trial) databases. The EMIAT and CAMIAT Investigators. Circulation 99:2268–2275, 1999.
14. Dobmeyer DJ, et al: The arrhythmogenic effects of caffeine in human beings. N Engl J Med 308:814–816, 1983.
15. Donnerstein RL, et al: Acute effects of caffeine ingestion on signal-averaged electrocardiograms. Am Heart J 136(4 pt 1):643–646, 1998.
16. Rosano GM, et al: Palpitations: What is the mechanism, and when should we treat them? Int J Fertil Womens Med 42:94–100, 1997.
17. Barsky AJ, et al: Somatized psychiatric disorder presenting as palpitations. Arch Intern Med 156:1102–1108, 1996.
18. Barsky AJ, et al: Psychiatric disorders in medical outpatients complaining of palpitations. J Gen Intern Med 9:306–113, 1994.
19. Weber BE, Kapoor WN: Evaluation and outcomes of patients with palpitations. Am J Med 100:138–148, 1996.
20. Lok NS, Lau CP: Prevalence of palpitations, cardiac arrhythmias and their associated risk factors in ambulant elderly. Int J Cardiol 54:231–236, 1996.
21. Zeldis SM, et al: Cardiovascular complaints. Correlation with cardiac arrhythmias on 24 hour electrocardiographic monitoring. Chest 78:456–461, 1980.
22. Crawford MH, et al: ACC/AHA guidelines for ambulatory electrocardiography: Executive summary and recommendations. A report of the American College of Cardiology/American Heart Association task force on practice guidelines (committee to revise the guidelines for ambulatory electrocardiography). Circulation 100:886–893, 1999.
23. Zimetbaum PJ, Josephson ME: The evolving role of ambulatory arrhythmia monitoring in general clinical practice. Ann Intern Med 130:848–856, 1999.
24. Antman EM, et al: Transtelephonic electrocardiographic transmission for management of cardiac arrhythmias. Am J Cardiol 58:1021–1024, 1986.
25. Chadda KD, et al: The impact of transtelephonic documentation of arrhythmia on morbidity and mortality rate in sudden death survivors. Am Heart J 112:1159–1165, 1986.
26. Krahn AD, et al: Randomized assessment of syncope trial: conventional diagnostic testing versus a prolonged monitoring strategy. Circulation 104:46–51, 2001.
27. Moss AJ, et al: Improved survival with an implanted defibrillator in patients with coronary disease at high risk for ventricular arrhythmia. Multicenter Automatic Defibrillator Implantation Trial Investigators. N Engl J Med 335:1933–1940, 1996.
28. Koskinen P, Kupari M, Leinonen H: Role of alcohol in recurrences of atrial fibrillation in persons less than 65 years of age. Am J Cardiol 66:954–958, 1990.
29. Rigou DG, Pichel G, Fasah L: [Ventricular arrhythmia in young university students without evidence of heart disease]. Medicina 50:47–51, 1990.
30. Lehr D: A possible beneficial effect of selenium administration in antiarrhythmic therapy. J Am Coll Nutr 13:496–498, 1994.
31. Lumme JA, Jounela AJ: The effect of potassium and potassium plus magnesium supplementation on ventricular extrasystoles in mild hypertensives treated with hydrochlorothiazide. Int J Cardiol 25:93–97, 1989.
32. Tsuji H, et al: The associations of levels of serum potassium and magnesium with ventricular premature complexes (the Framingham Heart Study). Am J Cardiol 74: 232–235, 1994.
33. Spencer JC: Direct relationship between the body's copper/zinc ratio, ventricular premature beats, and sudden coronary death. Am J Clin Nutr 32: 1184–1185, 1979.
34. Hardarson T, et al: Cod liver oil does not reduce ventricular extrasystoles after myocardial infarction. J Intern Med 266:33–37, 1989.
35. Bashir Y, et al: Effects of long-term oral magnesium chloride replacement in congestive heart failure secondary to coronary artery disease. Am J Cardiol 72:1156–1162, 1993.
36. Mehta A et al: Caffeine and cardiac arrhythmias. An experimental study in dogs with review of literature. Acta Cardiol 52:273–283, 1997.
37. Chou, T: Wake up and smell the coffee. Caffeine, coffee, and the medical consequences. West J Med 157:544–553, 1992.
38. Myers MG, Harris L: High dose caffeine and ventricular arrhythmias. Can J Cardiol 1990. 6(3):95–98, 1990.
39. Haller CA, Benowitz NL: Adverse cardiovascular and central nervous system events associated with dietary supplements containing ephedra alkaloids. N Engl J Med 343:1833–1838, 2000.
40. Shen WK, et al: Is sinus node modification appropriate for inappropriate sinus tachycardia with features of postural orthostatic tachycardia syndrome? Pacing Clin Electrophysiol 24:217–230, 2001.
41. Lochen ML: The Tromso Study: Associations between self-reported arrhythmia, psychological conditions, and lifestyle. Scand J Prim Health Care 9:265–270, 1991.
42. Hinkle LE, Jr, et al: The risk factors for arrhythmic death in a sample of men followed for 20 years. Am J Epidemiol 127: 500–515, 1988.
43. Albert CM, et al: Moderate alcohol consumption and the risk of sudden cardiac death among US male physicians. Circulation 100:944–950, 1999.
44. McCarty MF, Fish oil may be an antidote for the cardiovascular risk of smoking. Med Hypotheses 46:337–347, 1996.
45. Alexander CN, Orme-Johnson DW, Schneider RH, Walton KG: Effects of transcendental meditation compared to other methods of relaxation and meditation in reducing risk factors, morbidity, and mortality. Homeostasis 35:243–264, 1994.
46. Zamarra, JW, et al: Usefulness of the transcendental meditation program in the treatment of patients with coronary artery disease. Am J Cardiol 77:867–870, 1996.

47. Langsjoen PH, Langsjoen AM: Overview of the use of CoQ10 in cardiovascular disease. Biofactors 9:273–284, 1999.

48. Lango R, et al: Influence of L-carnitine and its derivatives on myocardial metabolism and function in ischemic heart disease and during cardiopulmonary bypass. Cardiovasc Res 51:21–79, 2001.

49. Arsenian MA: Carnitine and its derivatives in cardiovascular disease. Prog Cardiovasc Dis 1997.40:265–786, 1997.

50. Mondillo S, et al: [Therapy of arrhythmia induced by myocardial ischemia. Association of L-carnitine, propafenone and mexiletine]. Clin Ther 146:769–774, 1995.

51. Godwin KO: Abnormal electrocardiograms in rats fed a low selenium diet. Q J Exp Physiol Cogn Med Sci 50:282–788, 1965.

52. Billman GE, Hallaq H, and Leaf A: Prevention of ischemia-induced ventricular fibrillation by omega 3 fatty acids. Proc Natl Acad Sci U S A 91:4427–4430, 1994.

53. Xiao YF, et al: Blocking effects of polyunsaturated fatty acids on Na$^+$ channels of neonatal rat ventricular myocytes. Proc Natl Acad Sci U S A 92:11000–11004, 1995.

54. Kang JX, Leaf A: Prevention and termination of beta-adrenergic agonist-induced arrhythmias by free polyunsaturated fatty acids in neonatal rat cardiac myocytes. Biochem Biophys Res Commun 208:629–636, 1995.

55. Leaf A:Omega-3 fatty acids and prevention of ventricular fibrillation. Prostaglandins Leukot Essent Fatty Acids 52:197–198, 1995.

56. Hallaq H, et al: Protective effect of eicosapentaenoic acid on ouabain toxicity in neonatal rat cardiac myocytes. Proc Natl Acad Sci U S A 87:7834–7838, 1990.

57. Hallaq H Smith TW, Leaf A: Modulation of dihydropyridine-sensitive calcium channels in heart cells by fish oil fatty acids. Proc Natl Acad Sci U S A 89:1760–1764, 1992.

58. Sellmayer A, et al: Effects of dietary fish oil on ventricular premature complexes. Am J Cardiol 76:974–977, 1995.

59. Christensen JH, Jessen T, et al: n-3 Fatty acids and ventricular extrasystoles in patients with ventricular tachyarrhythmias. Nutr Res 15:1–8, 1995.

60. Burr ML, et al: Effects of changes in fat, fish, and fibre intakes on death and myocardial reinfarction: Diet and reinfarction trial (DART). Lancet 2:757–761, 1989.

61. Kessel I: Sick sinus syndrome cured by. . . Vitamin D? Geriatrics 45:83–85, 1990.

62. Benson H, McCallie DP, Jr: Angina pectoris and the placebo effect. N Engl J Med 300:1424–1429, 1979.

63. Ozaki Y: Pharmacological studies of indole alkaloids obtained from dom plants, Uncaria rhynchophylla Miq. and Amsonia elliptica Roem Schult. Nippon Yakurigaku Zasshi 94:17–26, 1989.

64. Tian BJ, Gao TL, Song ZL: [Effects of ciwujia (Acanthopanax senticosus harms) on reperfusion-induced arrhythmia and action potential alterations in the isolated rat heart]. Zhongguo Zhong Yao Za Zhi 14:493–495, 508, 512, 1989.

65. Chen R, Yuan C: [Experimental anti-arrhythmic effects of zhigancao (prepared licorice) injection]. Zhongguo Zhong Yao Za Zhi 16: 617–619, inside back cover, 1991.

66. Klepser TB, Klepser ME: Unsafe and potentially safe herbal therapies. Am J Health Syst Pharm 56:125–138; quiz 139–141, 1999.

67. Rauwald HW, Brehm O, Odenthal KP: The involvement of a Ca^{2+} channel blocking mode of action in the pharmacology of Ammi visnaga fruits. Planta Med 60:101–510, 1994.

68. Balbaa SI, Zaki AY, Abdel-Wahab SM: A micro-method for the estimation of khellin in presence of other constituents of Ammi visnaga fruits. Planta Med 16:329–334, 1968.

69. Chen M, Stohs SJ, Staba EJ: The biosynthesis of radioactive khellin and visnagin from C14-acetate by Ammi visnaga plants. Planta Med 17:319–327, 1969.

70. Miller LG: Herbal medicinals: Selected clinical considerations focusing on known or potential drug-herb interactions. Arch Intern Med 158:2200–2211, 1998.

71. Shen J, et al: Effects of EGb 761 on nitric oxide and oxygen free radicals, myocardial damage and arrhythmia in ischemia-reperfusion injury in vivo. Biochim Biophys Acta 140:228–236, 1998.

72. Zhuang XX: [Protective effect of Angelica injection on arrhythmia during myocardial ischemia reperfusion in rat]. Zhong Xi Yi Jie He Za Zhi 11:360–361, 326, 1991.

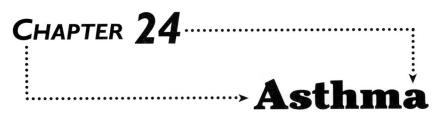

CHAPTER 24

Asthma

John Mark, M.D.

PATHOPHYSIOLOGY

Asthma was once considered a process that affected the airways with excessive mucus production, bronchial smooth muscle contraction, and swelling causing obstruction. Recently, asthma has been found to be a chronic inflammatory process with the previously mentioned findings. Airway plugs found at post-mortem examinations have mucus, serum proteins, inflammatory cells, and cellular debris. The airways are infiltrated with various inflammatory cells including eosinophils and mononuclear cells. The other findings include damage done at the epithelial cell level with cellular leakage in the microvascular space. The increased mucus production is due to increased number of goblet cells. The smooth muscle is hypertrophied and characterized by new formation of vessels and an increase of interstitial collagen. These findings are important in the theory that this chronic inflammation could ultimately lead to irreversible changes in the airway. This remodeling and fibrosis of the airway have led medical practitioners to advocate the use of anti-inflammatory medications earlier in the treatment of asthma.

Research has been aimed at determining what might trigger this response and the treatment or avoidance that might prevent this remodeling from occurring. The particular type of cellular response (mast cell, eosinophil, epithelial cells, macrophages, and activated T cells) has also been studied to determine what pharmacologic therapy would be best directed toward decreasing this inflammatory response. It has been found that these cells, along with subpopulations of T lymphocytes, may regulate this inflammation through the release of cytokines. These cytokines are thought to be important in establishing the chronicity of the asthma. The release of cytokines and chemokines from fibroblasts, endothelial cells, and epithelial cells contributes to this process. These have been important findings in researching the possible treatment for asthma.

Chronic inflammation may cause a slow and persistent cellular damage, and the repair process may in itself cause the restructuring or remodeling and eventual permanent abnormalities. This process builds on itself and amplifies the ongoing changes altering the airway physiology and architecture.

RISK FACTORS AND TRIGGERS

It is thought that asthma often begins in childhood and may be due to an interaction of several factors (Fig. 24–1). When children have atopic problems (eczema) and allergies and a genetic predisposition (chromosomes 5, 6, and 11 to 14), these may lead to a propensity for asthma. This is due to the ability to produce immunoglobulin E (IgE) to various allergens, house dust mites, and molds. The resultant IgE antibodies, mast cells, and other cells are sensitized, becoming activated when exposed to these specific allergens. Although atopy does not always lead to asthma, it is the most common predisposing factor.

Asthma symptoms can be triggered by several factors (Table 24–1).

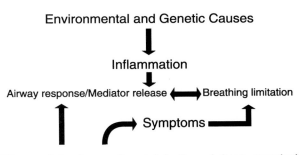

Figure 24–1. The condition of a patient's asthma may change depending on the environment, activities, and other factors. When the patient is well, monitoring and treatment are still needed to maintain control.

Table 24–1. Triggers for Symptoms of Asthma

Allergens
Viral or sinus infections
Exercise
Reflux disease (stomach acid flowing back up the esophagus)
Medications or foods
Emotional anxiety
Air pollutants such as tobacco smoke, wood smoke, chemicals, and ozone
Occupational exposure to allergens, vapors, dust, gases, or fumes
Strong odors or sprays such as perfumes, household cleaners, cooking fumes (especially from frying), paints or varnishes
Other airborne particles such as coal dust, chalk dust, or talcum powder

Viral infections such as respiratory syncytial virus have been thought to be triggers not only for their ability to cause airway swelling and obstruction but also for their influence on the cellular response of the immune system, making it more asthma prone.

MONITORING ISSUES

Peak flow monitors have been promoted by both national and international guidelines to be used to objectively measure pulmonary function in the home of patients with asthma. Often, patients may feel poorly or anxious but this may not correlate with actual pulmonary function abnormalities. Peak flow monitors (used as young as age 7 years) can be used not only to assess pulmonary function but also to dictate use of medications. If the flow is a certain value (each asthmatic patient has their own range of flows), medication could be either increased or decreased. If peak flow is significantly decreased, medical attention should be considered. The most important considerations when using peak flow meters are that the patient is motivated (effort-dependent measurement) and that the patient has guidelines (preferably written) for responding to a measured peak flow value.

INTEGRATIVE THERAPY

Environment

It is important to reduce exposure to dust mites and cockroaches that many patients with asthma are sensitive to. House dust mites are microscopic insects that live off dead skin cell flakes and are all around us, even though we cannot see them. The mites and their waste products can be allergenic. To limit exposure to dust mites, especially in the bedroom where they are most common, (1) enclose pillows and mattress in airtight polyurethane covers or use fiberfill products instead of down or foam pillows; (2) remove carpeting (hardwoods or linoleum are better) and curtains; (3) wash sheets and stuffed toys (for pediatric patients) in hot water every week; and (4) clean bedrooms frequently with a vacuum with an added high-efficiency particulate air (HEPA) filter. Cockroaches and their feces are another trigger for asthma, so cleanliness is important to decrease cockroach presence; in addition, it helps to wash floors and counters frequently to eliminate their debris.

Nutrition

Diet therapies or nutritional advice is the most common "alternative" therapy that is given by allopathic physicians for patients with asthma. It has long been thought that eliminating certain "allergenic" type foods and decreasing exposure to things such as dairy products (believed to be associated with increased mucus production) will help with chronic asthma symptoms and severity[1] (see Chapter 81, Food Allergy). The easiest way to do an elimination diet is to pick a food that the patient appears to be sensitive to, such as nuts or eggs, and then eliminate it from the diet for 2 weeks. At the end of 2 weeks, gently reintroduce the food into the diet. If there is a significant change, such as bloating or headaches, the patient may indeed be sensitive to that particular food (see Chapter 82, The Elimination Diet and Diagnosing Food Hypersensitivities). There have been few studies to support these claims, although one study did suggest that there were decreased symptoms in an adult asthmatic following a restricted diet. Some epidemiologic studies suggest that dietary habits influence lung function. The populations that have increased polyunsaturated fatty acid intake (omega-6 fatty acids) have an increased prevalence of asthma, eczema, and allergic rhinitis.

The following are the recommendations for patients with asthma:

1. **Eliminate potential allergens.**
   - Any food with a history of intolerance (gastrointestinal disturbance or eczema)
   - Sulfites (especially in dried fruits)
   - Food additives (aspartame, benzoates, and yellow dye #5)
   - Dairy products (for a trial period, as mentioned previously)
2. **Increase fruit and vegetable intake** because they are rich in antioxidants that have been shown to be low in patients with chronic lung problems such as asthma.
3. **Increase omega-3 fatty acid** intake by eating cold water fish (e.g., sardines, herring, and salmon) and decrease omega-6 fatty acids by eliminating vegetable oils, using olive oil in its place (see Chapter 84, The Anti-inflammatory Diet).

NOTE

If dairy products are decreased or eliminated (especially in children), a calcium supplement should be considered.

Exercise

Although exercise in itself can induce symptoms in patients with asthma, there have been numerous studies to show that asthma can be better controlled in patients who regularly exercise. As to what type of exercise, no study illustrates the superiority of one type of exercise over another. It had long been assumed that swimming may be beneficial because the environment is more moist and cold dry air may actually exacerbate asthma symptoms. Studies have not supported this, and it is recommended that any exercise that the patient will do on a regular basis that does not cause increased symptoms should be encouraged.

The older the patient, the better he or she does with their asthma if they follow an exercise regimen. This might, in part, have to do with a better self-image and overall improved health associated with regular exercise in adults.

Yoga

Yoga is a form of exercise that embodies many of the previously discussed therapies for improving the health of patients with asthma. It is a form of exercise, so there is a cardiovascular component; it involves using regulated breathing exercises (pranayama); and it is a mind-body method that uses relaxation and meditation, which are included in many yoga practices. It was shown in a study in adults to help decrease medication use and decrease anxiety.[2]

Botanicals

This therapeutic approach to asthma is one of the oldest and most widely used in all of asthma care worldwide. There are historical theories and treatments that have been used in breathing disorders that have persisted over thousands of years.[3] Although there is a large amount of knowledge and information regarding herbal or botanical treatment of asthma, a significant part of it is not based on any well-designed or well-performed clinical studies.[4] Many of the botanicals used are similar to pharmaceuticals in their chemical properties. There are many botanicals used traditionally, and this varies by culture.

Ginkgo (*Ginkgo biloba*)

The ginkgo tree is also known as maidenhair tree and forty-coin tree. Ginkgo products come from the leaves of a member of the ginkgo family, a living fossil more than 200 million years old. Most commercial leaf production is from plantations in South Carolina, France, and China.

Ginkgo in various forms has been used in China for hundreds of years. It is available under various brands and many have been standardized. Ginkgo's active ingredient is ginkgolide, which is thought to be a platelet-activating factor (PAF) antagonist and may decrease airway inflammation.[5] It is also thought to be a powerful antioxidant.

Studies have been done on ginkgo and its role in improving cerebral circulation and helping with memory loss. The use in degenerative dementia and for other circulatory problems has been promoted. There are few studies in asthma,[6] but improvement in pulmonary function was reported.

Dosage. The typical dose of ginkgo is 120 to 240 mg in a divided dose, two to three times per day. Allow 4 to 8 weeks to see therapeutic benefit.

Precautions. No real side effects are reported by itself, but ginkgo should be avoided if the patient is pregnant or nursing. Ginkgo has been reported to interact with warfarin, aspirin, and other anticoagulant therapy and should be avoided or monitored carefully for bleeding potential.

Coleus (*Coleus forskohlii*)

Coleus is a fairly uncommon botanical in the United States, but it has a long history of use for respiratory and asthma problems in India in Ayurvedic medicine tradition. A member of the mint family, *Coleus forskohlii* grows wild on the mountain slopes of Nepal, India, and Thailand. Traditionally, it was used for a variety of purposes, including treating skin rashes, asthma, bronchitis, insomnia, epilepsy, and angina. It is thought to act much like theophylline and has been studied as an effective bronchodilator. It has been shown to increase intracellular cyclic adenosine monophosphate levels and stabilize cells that release histamine, although its clinical value is still to be determined.[7]

Dosage. A common dosage recommendation is 50 mg two or three times a day of an extract standardized to contain 18% forskolin.

Precautions. None has been reported, but this should be used with caution with antihypertensive (beta blockers) and anticoagulant therapy.

Ma Huang (*Ephedra sinica*)

Ma huang, also known as Chinese ephedra and Chinese jointfir, has been commonly used as an asthma remedy in China for thousands of years. The pharmaceutical ephedrine (derived from *Ephedra sinica*) was used in asthma therapy until the advent of more specific beta-agonist medications. Ma huang may be in many combinations of other botanicals, including licorice and other anti-inflammatories. Botanicals and supplements containing Ephedra alkaloids have now appeared in many preparations for weight loss and increasing energy.

Dosage. Not recommended for use in the treatment of asthma.

Precautions. Ma huang botanicals and its combination products have the most serious potential for side effects. There have been reported deaths associated with its use. Central nervous system problems such as nausea, vomiting, sweating, and nervousness along with heart palpitations, tachycardia, hypertension, anxiety, and even myocardial infarction have all been recently reported.[8]

NOTE

Complications, including death, have been reported when Ma huang is taken in high doses or with caffeine-containing products. Death has been noted with only one use.

Licorice (*Glycyrrhiza glabra*)

Licorice, also known as liquorice, sweet wood, and sweet root, has been used as a cough remedy and asthma treatment. The active ingredient is glycyrrhizin, also called glycyrrhizic acid. The effect in treating asthma is in the anti-inflammatory nature of licorice and the enhancement of endogenous steroids. It is also thought to be an expectorant, aiding in the expulsion of mucus from the bronchial passages.

Dosage. Suggest using a licorice extract with the glycyrrhizin removed. A popular brand is Caved-S at 760 mg two to three times a day. If the glycyrrhizin is used, then 100 mg/day is the maximum suggested dose.

Precautions. The side effects are minimal if less than 10 mg of the glycyrrhizic acid is taken daily and prolonged use is avoided. Chronic use can cause headache, hypertension, dizziness, edema, and other signs of aldosteronism (through the binding of mineralocorticoids). It may also cause low potassium and should be avoided in those taking cardiac glycosides, blood pressure medications, corticosteroids, diuretics, or monoamine oxidase inhibitors.

NOTE

Owing to the side effects of the crude licorice, it is recommended that the deglycyrrhized licorice (DGL) be used. Most studies involving DGL deal with its role in gastroesophageal reflux and gastric ulcer disease.

Kanpo (Shinpi-To, Saiboku-To)

Combination herbs/remedies such as saiboku-to (Asian) blend black cumin, chamomile, cinnamon, cloves, rosemary, sage, spearmint, and thyme into a botanical combination that reduces asthma symptoms. It is thought to be effective through the anti-inflammatory properties of blocking 5-lipoxygenase and/or inhibiting PAF.[9] PAF is produced by several of the inflammatory cells including eosinophils, causing airway hyperreactivity, microvascular leaks, increased airway secretions, and epithelial permeability.

Dosage. This combination herbal preparation is usually prepared as a tea, taken two to four times per day, depending on the particular brand used.

Precautions. There have been no reported problems with these combination therapies.

Supplements

Vitamins and Minerals

In addition to botanical and herbal preparations for the chronic treatment of asthma, vitamins and minerals are used frequently. As with most of the treatments mentioned thus far, few studies support their use, but historically, they have been thought to help with asthma and chronic respiratory symptoms.

Vitamin C

Vitamin C has been studied, and although the results were mixed, one randomized trial did demonstrate reduced asthma symptoms. Vitamin C was also found to be protective against exercise-induced asthma.[10] It is thought that vitamin C inhibits histamine release and promotes vasodilatation by increasing prostacyclin production.

Dosage. 250 to 500 mg one to two times a day.

Vitamin B$_6$

Vitamin B$_6$ was shown in a double-blind, randomized study to improve peak flow rates in a group of adults with severe asthma.[11] In patients with low serum pyridoxine (vitamin B$_6$), supplementation helped decrease episodes of wheezing. It may be a side effect of common asthma medications to lower serum vitamin B$_6$ levels.

Dosage. 100 to 200 mg/day.

Precautions. High doses—usually over 500 mg/day—and with prolonged use have been associated with peripheral neuropathy.

Vitamin E

Intake of vitamin E is suggested in the diet or through supplementation because patients who have a high antioxidant intake have fewer pulmonary problems.

Dosage. 400 IU/day of mixed tocopherols.

Magnesium

Magnesium's role in decreasing bronchospasm has been investigated in both the conventional and the CAM communities. IV magnesium is now commonly used for serious asthma symptoms (status asthmaticus). The use of oral magnesium has been studied and, in adults, shown to decrease symptoms but not improve pulmonary function.[12]

Dosage. 200 to 400 mg/day (magnesium gluconate is the form least likely to cause diarrhea).

Precautions. A problem with using oral magnesium is the tendency of the preparations to cause diarrhea.

Selenium

Selenium is another potent antioxidant that is used in many inflammatory conditions including asthma. There are no real studies showing a deficiency or efficacy in treatment of asthma.

Dosage. 100 to 200 μg/day.

Fish Oil

The role of anti-inflammatory medication is now the standard in asthma treatment. If the diet could be altered to decrease the propensity to develop inflammatory precursors, conditions such as asthma would be less problematic. The use of omega-3 essential fatty acids in adequate amounts in the diet may limit leukotriene synthesis by blocking arachidonic acid metabolism. A rich source of omega-3 fatty acid is in fish oils. Because eating cold water oily fish (mackerel, sardines, herring, salmon, and cod) is not common in most Western diets, the use of fish oil capsules has become more standard. In populations that do eat this type of diet, it has been shown in epidemiologic studies to significantly reduce the risk of asthma and improve pulmonary function. The vegetarian sources of omega-3 fatty acids (flaxseed oil, canola oil, and soy oil) are used even less in most diets, so the study of fish oil in asthma has been investigated.[13]

Dosage. One 500-mg capsule two to three times per day. It may take several months to demonstrate benefit.

Pharmaceuticals

Bronchodilators

Bronchodilators have long been used to help alleviate the bronchospasm and difficulty breathing associated with asthma "attacks." Several different classes include the beta agonists such as albuterol (Proventil) and salmeterol (Serevent). Anticholinergic agents (ipratropium bromide [Atrovent]) are used most commonly in adults with asthma. There are also the methylxanthines (theophylline and aminophylline). The methylxanthines are used as a second- or third-line drug of choice because they have more significant side effects and need serum level monitoring.

Dosage
Albuterol (Proventil): two to four puffs of a metered-dose inhaler (MDI), one to three times per day as needed.

Salmeterol (Serevent) (long-acting beta agonist): two puffs of an MDI twice a day.
Ipratropium bromide (Atrovent): two puffs of an MDI two to four times per day.
Methylxanthines: Age- and weight-dependent.
Precautions
Beta agonists may cause rapid or irregular heartbeat, insomnia, and nervousness. The anticholinergic medications have few side effects except for occasional dry mouth or headache. The theophylline-type medications may cause tremor, shakiness, nausea, and vomiting. Overdose of methylxanthines can cause serious problems such as seizures and cardiac arrhythmias.

Anti-Inflammatory Medications

These medications are now considered the most important part of the pharmacologic approach to asthma care. There are several categories of these medications, usually listed as steroidal and nonsteroidal. The steroidal MDIs include fluticasone (Flovent) and budesonide (Pulmocort). There are also oral preparations such as prednisone, prednisolone, and methyl prednisolone. The nonsteroidal medications include cromolyn sodium (Intal) and leukotriene inhibitors (Singulair, Accolate). All of these medications act by blocking certain pathways of airway inflammation once there has been an exposure (allergic, irritant, infectious, or emotional/exercise). The oral steroids are the most potent and have the most potential for significant side effects.

Dosage. Nonsteroidal medication such as cromolyn is two puffs by MDI three to four times per day and should be used continuously. Leukotriene inhibitors differ by the specific type used. If Singulair is used, the dose is 10 mg/day for adults, 5 mg/day for children (chewable tabs). If the child is younger than 5 years, 4 mg/day is recommended (not to be used under 2 years of age).

Steroidal inhalers are usually two puffs (or one actuation) twice per day. Oral steroids are usually dosed 1 to 2 mg/kg or 20 to 40 mg/day (adults) for varying amounts of time. A short "burst" would be 4 to 5 days total.

Precautions. Nonsteroidal medications have few side effects. Cromolyn is thought to be safe with no real toxicity except for an occasional cough. Leukotriene inhibitors may cause headache and some cause hepatic dysfunction, so liver function should be monitored. The steroidal medications (especially the oral preparations) may cause problems with height and growth (in children), immune suppression, hypertension, cataracts, and hirsutism (if taken long term). The inhaled forms have rare side effects and have been followed long term in children[14] but may cause hoarseness, cough, and oral candidiasis unless a spacer is utilized and/or good mouth rinsing is done.

```
┌─────────────────────────────────────────┐
│                   NOTE                    │
│  The new anti-inflammatory steroidal     │
│  inhalers used with a spacer device have │
│  been the most innovative pharmacologic  │
│  approach to chronic asthma care.        │
└─────────────────────────────────────────┘
```

Biomechanical

Massage

Massage therapy is an ancient treatment, dating back to the second century in China. It was referred to as the "art of rubbing" and was common until the time of the large pharmaceutical use starting in the 1950s. Little material in the literature has investigated the efficacy of massage, and the studies that have been done have had problems with sampling, lack of controls, sample size, and inappropriate use of statistical analysis.[15] There have since been several studies investigating the use of massage in many areas of medicine using methodology to support the effectiveness of massage, the majority being done by the Touch Research Institute in Florida. Asthma has been studied in children, and it has been shown that daily massage improved airway caliber and control of asthma.[15] There was also a noted decrease in anxiety and improved attitude toward the subject's asthma.

Dosage. The time and duration for utilizing massage is not known for the average patient with asthma. The study that showed improvement used once a day massage for 30 days. The person doing the massage may be another family member or a friend taught massage techniques or a massage therapist.

Osteopathy

Osteopathy is another system of medical care that embraces the body as a whole and in which structure and function are closely interrelated. One main premise is that because osteopathy emphasizes that all body systems, including the musculoskeletal system, operate in unison, a disturbance in one can alter functions of the other systems. The practice of osteopathic medicine started shortly after the Civil War and included developing a form of manipulative medicine. There are several main categories of osteopathic manipulative therapies (e.g., craniosacral, strain-counterstrain, and myofascial) that have over 100 different individual treatments. Osteopathic manipulative treatments (OMT) in asthma have been used for both chronic and emergent symptoms. A report in the emergency department setting proposed that OMTs could alleviate acute symptoms.[16] There has also been a movement by the American Osteopathic Association to utilize this in the basic management of asthma.[17] No studies done in a randomized, controlled fashion have been published utilizing OMT in the treatment of asthma in children; however, there is an ongoing study in adults showing improvement (personal communication).

Dosage. The findings of the osteopathic practitioner will determine which form of OMT will be used. Again, this may affect any part of the body depending on the physical examination. Often just assisting the patient in using various parts of the chest in breathing may help.

Chiropractic

Chiropractic is the third largest regulated healthcare profession in North America and has been involved in healthcare for conditions such as asthma since the late 1800s. The theory of chiropractic care has been based around the idea that the properly adjusted body was essential for health. By using spinal manipulation therapy for the removal of subluxations, the life force is influenced and good health is attained.[18]

Some studies involving chiropractic treatments in asthma show overall improvement in lung capacity. Other findings documented abnormal spinal mechanics associated with asthma. Chiropractic adjustments may produce immediate relaxation of the neck musculature and overall may improve respiratory function. There are also chiropractic theories that various adjustments may affect respiratory symptoms by the action of treating the subluxations found and subsequent nerve function. Only one randomized clinical trial has been done and no benefit was found. The Cochrane group performed a systematic review of over 300 citations in which five randomized trials were assessed. The conclusion was that there was insufficient evidence to support the use of chiropractic manual therapies for patients with asthma, but the authors went on to suggest that more adequately sized trials be done.[19]

Dosage. Depends on the practitioner.

Precautions. Reported complications of chiropractic manual treatments have been documented but none were found in the treatment of asthma. There is often the repeated use of radiographs, making repeated radiation exposure an issue to some patients.

Mind-Body Therapy

Mind-body therapies have been used in the treatment of asthma in various ways. They are at times referred to as cognitive behavioral therapies and encompass several approaches. The ones that have been most used in asthma are discussed, and one has not been shown to be superior over another; however, depending on the patient, some therapies appear to be more acceptable. Discussing a few with the patient and the family will enhance the success of mind-body interventions. Research in this area started in the early 1960s, and approaches have included relaxation therapy, breathing exercises, biofeedback, and hypnosis/guided imagery.

The theory behind using these therapies is based on improving the inflammatory process that can be triggered by the autonomic nervous system through emotions. Numerous studies in both children and adults have shown that there is increased anxiety and even at times panic when asthma symptoms are perceived. Studies have also shown that using different types of cognitive behavioral therapies may decrease symptoms and medication use and may reduce the inflammatory response of airway cells.[20, 21]

Breathing/Relaxation

The use of breathing exercises in controlling asthma symptoms has been taught and promoted by the American Lung Association in their asthma education series. The type of breathing is often called diaphragmatic breathing or "belly breathing"(see Chapter 88, Breathing Exercises, and Chapter 91, Prescribing Relaxation Techniques, for further discussion).

Dosage. These cognitive behavioral therapies are best done when the patient feels an asthma attack coming on and also when the patient is even anxious that symptoms may be increasing. Encouraging practice of these techniques when the patient is feeling well is extremely helpful.

Hypnosis/Guided Imagery

Hypnosis has been used for achieving relaxation, relieving pain, helping with physical discomfort (even chronic pain), and altering moods. It is multidimensional and aids patients in developing a heightened concentration of an idea or image. The process may be brief or involve complex instructions, depending on the subject, the goal, and the therapist. In asthma, hypnosis has been shown to be effective in patients whose asthma is mild and if they have an emotional component to their symptoms. Studies showed that if the person was "motivated," there were decreased symptoms, decreased medication use, and improved pulmonary function.[22]

Guided imagery involves using a form of self-hypnosis in which the patient uses an image of her or his own creation after an initial relaxation period to help decrease asthma symptoms. This is especially effective in children who enjoy an active and vibrant imagination. They often can be taught this technique in less than half an hour and do well with their asthma symptoms after a few practice sessions. Guided imagery starts with initial relaxation (using diaphragmatic breathing—"belly breathing") and then progressing to an imagery session. This involves the subject developing an image and then focuses on taking control or command of the perceived airway/lung problem using this image. An

example would be of going from a closet to the outdoors where the child could once again breathe. This emotion-mediated format allows disclosure and subsequent reframing for the child and allows independence from the chronic illness.

Dosage. As with relaxation, these therapies are best when used often and especially when used when asthma symptoms are initially mild. This prepares the patient for dealing with increased symptoms during an attack.

NOTE

These cognitive therapies should not be used in place of medications, especially if symptoms are moderate or severe. If the patient is using a peak flow meter, then these therapies can be used if peak flows are in a certain range.

Disclosure/Journaling

Much like the findings in rheumatoid arthritis, some evidence has indicated that just having the patient with asthma discuss the asthma symptoms may decrease the severity and the frequency of the asthma. Journaling, in which one is writing in a journal three to five times per week for 20 to 30 minutes about asthma has been shown to decrease both symptoms and medication use. In one study, patients wrote in their journals about a stressful event that they had not discussed with others or had been unresolved; the control group just talked about daily events.[23] There was a 20% improvement in lung function vs. the control group in those who wrote about a stressful experience. (See Chapter 93, Journaling.)

Other Therapies to Consider

It is difficult to know where to put bioenergetic modalities (traditional Chinese medicine [TCM], healing touch and prayer, and homeopathy) in the stepwise approach to asthma care. These could really fit anywhere in the treatment plan from the most mild to the most severe asthma. It is important to use them in conjunction with the previously discussed therapies if the patient has moderate or severe symptoms, but they would be appropriate as first-line treatment in the interested patient with mild or intermittent asthma.

Traditional Chinese Medicine

TCM has been practiced for several thousand years and has many forms. The basis, however, is the understanding of the connections between body, mind, and spirit in health and disease. The belief in an unseen vital energy that affects the patient's health and how this energy or qi (chi) flows through the appropriate channels is the basis of this practice. The practitioner can affect this flow or intensity by manipulating the balance using acupuncture, Chinese herbs, diet, and physical therapy. It can successfully treat many medical conditions.

Acupuncture and other forms of TCM are thought to be beneficial in the treatment of asthma. Clinical observations using acupuncture and individually mixed Chinese herbs were effective, although clinical trials have not supported these observations. The National Institutes of Health 1997 Consensus Development Conference on Acupuncture did recommend acupuncture for many conditions, including asthma. One review did show modest improvement in asthma symptoms using acupuncture,[24] and another study suggested that acupuncture before exercise protected against exercise-induced asthma symptoms.[25]

Dosage. This is practitioner dependent, and the effects of TCM usually take several treatments to appear.

Precautions. Adverse side effects of acupuncture are rare but have been reported, including pneumothoraces leading to death.

Healing Touch and Prayer

Healing touch and other touch therapies such as therapeutic touch, reiki, and johrei are defined as the consciously directed process of energy exchange during which the practitioner uses touch or "nontouch" as a focus to facilitate healing. Prayer, which does not even require touch or the presence of the healer to help with symptoms and medical condition, has been used in nearly every culture for centuries. There are few studies involving this type of energy healing in the asthma patient. One small study using "hands-on" healing in adult asthmatics did show some reduction in medication.[26]

Dosage. Depends on the modality (healing touch, therapeutic touch, reiki, johrei, prayer); all have different approaches and the practitioners use various assessments.

Homeopathy

Homeopathy is thought to be an energy medicine because it is not based on the usual physical laws found in science but on the premise that using "remedies" that would cause the same symptoms (principle of like cure) and are very dilute (the more dilute, the more potent—law of dilution) have the most powerful treatment. There is a belief that the dilution in water actually imparts healing energy and that this, combined with the patient's vital force or energy, is used in healing.

There have been several studies showing efficacy of homeopathic remedies in the treatment of both asthma and allergies.[27] The study in asthma showed reduction in symptoms but no real difference in pulmonary function.

The remedies depend on the particular patient's symptom pattern and should be individually assessed by an experienced homeopath to select the correct constitutional remedy. Some of the commonly used homeopathic remedies include:

- *Arsenicum album*—used for asthma with restlessness and anxiety
- *Ipecac*—used for chest constriction and cough
- *Pulsatilla*—used for chest pressure and air hunger
- *Sambuscus*—used for asthma symptoms that wake one in the night

Dosage. Depends on the individual and the guidance of the practitioner (see Chapter 103, Therapeutic Homeopathy).

Precautions. Homeopathy is thought to be safe owing to the extreme dilution, and the treatments are inexpensive.

THERAPEUTIC REVIEW

Following is a summary of therapeutic options for treating asthma. If a patient is having persistent symptoms (daily wheezing, shortness of breath, difficulty sleeping, or difficulty exercising) or severe symptoms (even if intermittent), it would be best to prescribe more aggressive therapy such as the beta-agonist and anti-inflammatory medications. For the patient who has mild to moderate symptoms, this stepwise approach might be considered.

Lifestyle
- *As with many chronic illnesses, asthma would be best treated if prevented. Unfortunately, changing a person's lifestyle including the environment is difficult. There are cultural and regional differences just in the United States that make patient populations differ in how they approach a chronic illness and even how they use medical care.*

Environmental
- *Reducing exposure to asthma triggers can be therapeutic in itself. Such things as house dust mite reduction, frequent cleaning, use of HEPA filters, avoiding*

THERAPEUTIC REVIEW continued

secondhand smoke, and removing all pets from the home will help decrease the "irritability" of the airways.

Nutrition
- *By eliminating allergenic-type foods such as diary products (at least for a trial period), shellfish, foods with nitrites, sulfites, added food coloring, and artificial sweeteners, often asthma symptoms decrease. Patients should consider increasing organic fruits and vegetables for their antioxidant contribution as well as foods rich in omega-3 fatty acids while decreasing omega-6 fatty acid–containing ones (vegetable oils).*

Supplements
- *Increasing vitamin C (250 mg twice a day), vitamin B_6 (100 mg/day), and vitamin E (400 IU/day) may all help with chronic asthma. Magnesium (200 mg/day), selenium (100 µg/day), and fish oil capsules (1 capsule twice daily) would be additional therapy to consider.*

Mind-Body Methods
- *These techniques can be very rewarding in the treatment of asthma, and starting with breathing and relaxation is an excellent start.*
- *Guided imagery and hypnosis are readily available in most communities and will also help decrease symptoms, medication use, and physician/urgent care visits. Usually, these methods should be used regularly (one to two times daily) until familiar to the patient; they can then be used as needed for the asthma symptoms.*
- *Journaling is also recommended and patients should spend at least 20 minutes writing about their asthma or other stressors in their life three times per week.*

Exercise
- *Not only will routine exercise help with asthma (three to five periods of exercise lasting a minimum of 20 minutes per week), it will also help with self-esteem, weight loss, and cardiovascular health.*
- *Botanicals*
- *Ginkgo: 120 to 240 mg in a divided dose (two to three times/day)*
- *Coleus: 50 mg three times a day*
- *Licorice (Caved-S): 760 mg three times a day (only periodically and if no underlying cardiovascular or renal problems).*

Pharmaceuticals
- *For patients with mild to moderate symptoms that are long standing, using pharmaceuticals such as albuterol (Proventil), two puffs twice a day, and an anti-inflammatory such as fluticasone (Flovent), two puffs of the 110 MDI twice a day, may give relief much faster while the other interventions mentioned previously can be started. These medications should be considered first line if a patient has persistent or severe symptoms.*

Biomechanical
- *As adjuncts to the mentioned modalities and depending on the patient's preferences, using massage, OMT, and chiropractic therapies may be very beneficial. All three have different approaches and regimens, but finding a practitioner who is familiar with treating patients with asthma is the key.*

References

1. Ziment I: How your patients may be using herbalism to treat their asthma. J Respir Dis 19:1070–1081, 1998.
2. Vedanthan PK, Kesavalu LK, Murthy KC, et al: Clinical study of yoga techniques in university students with asthma: A controlled study. Allergy Asthma Proc 19:3–9, 1998.
3. Ziment I, Tashkin DP: Alternative medicine for allergy and asthma. J Allergy Clin Immunol 106:603–614, 2000.
4. Ernst AH: Herbal medicine for asthma: A systematic review. Thorax 55:925–929, 2000.
5. Kemper KJ, Lester MR: Alternative asthma therapies: An evidence-based review. Contemp Pediatr 16:162–195, 1999.
6. Gaby AR: Ginkgo biloba extract: A review. Altern Med Rev 1:236–242, 1996.
7. Bauer K: Pharmacodynamic effects of inhaled dry powder formulations of fenoterol and colforsin in asthma. Pharmacol Ther 53:76–83, 1993.
8. Haller CA, Benowitz NL: Adverse cardiovascular and central nervous system events associated with dietary supplements containing ephedra alkaloids. N Engl J Med 343:1833–1838, 2000.
9. Japanese Society for Allergology: Guidelines for the diagnosis and management of bronchial asthma. Allergy 50(Suppl):1–42, 1995.
10. Cohen HA, Neuman I, Nahum H: Blocking effect of vitamin C in

exercise-induced asthma. Arch Pediatr Adolesc Med 151:367–370, 1997.

11. Collipp PJ, Goldzier S, Weiss N, et al: Pyridoxine treatment of childhood bronchial asthma. Ann Allergy 35:93–97, 1975.

12. Hill J, Micklewright A, Lewis S, et al: Investigation of the effect of short-term change in dietary magnesium intake in asthma. Eur Respir J 10:2225–2228, 1997.

13. Fugh-Berman A: Alternative medicine. What works. Baltimore, Williams & Wilkins, 1997.

14. Childhood Asthma Management Program Research Group: Effect of long-term treatment with inhaled budesonide on adult height in children with asthma. N Engl J Med 343:1064–1069, 2000.

15. Field T, Henteleff T, Hernandez-Reif M, et al: Children with asthma have improved pulmonary functions after massage therapy. J Pediatr 132:854–858, 1998.

16. Paul FA, Buser BR: Osteopathic manipulative treatment applications for the emergency department patient. J Am Osteopath Assoc 96:403–409, 1996.

17. Rowane WA, Rowane MP: An osteopathic approach to asthma. J Am Osteopath Assoc 99:259–264, 1999.

18. Campbell JB, Busse JW, Injeyan HS: Chiropractors and vaccination: A historical perspective. Pediatrics 105:e43, 2000.

19. Hondras MA, Jones LK: Manual therapy for asthma. Cochrane Database of Systematic Reviews (computer file) 2:CD001002, 2000.

20. Vazquez MI, Buceta JM: Psychological treatment of asthma: Effectiveness of a self-management program with and without relaxation training. J Asthma 30:171–183, 1993.

21. Ewer TC, Stewart DE: Improvement in bronchial hyper-responsiveness in patients with moderate asthma after treatment with a hypnotic technique: A randomised controlled trial. BMJ 293:1129–1132, 1986.

22. Kohen DP, Wynne E: Applying hypnosis in a preschool family asthma education program: Uses of storytelling, imagery and relaxation. Am J Clin Hypnosis 39:169–181, 1997.

23. Smyth JM, Stone AA, Hurewitz A, et al: Effects of writing about stressful experiences on symptom reduction in patients with asthma or rheumatoid arthritis. JAMA 281:1304–1309, 1999.

24. Jobst KA: Acupuncture in asthma and pulmonary disease: An analysis of efficacy and safety. J Altern Complement Med 2:179–206, 1996.

25. Fung KP, Chow OK, So SY: Attenuation of exercise-induced asthma by acupuncture. Lancet 2:1419–1422, 1986.

26. Wacker von A: Healing in asthma. Erfahrungsheilkunde July:428, 1996.

27. Taylor MA, Reilly D, Llewellyn-Jones RH, et al: Randomised controlled trial of homeopathy versus placebo in perennial allergic rhinitis with overview of four trial series. BMJ 321:471–476, 2000.

CHAPTER 25

Allergic Rhinitis

William S. Silvers, M.D.

PATHOPHYSIOLOGY

In a patient considered to be "allergic," the mechanism of the allergic reactivity must be taken into account. By strict definition, an "allergy" is an immunoglobulin E (IgE)-mediated reaction with a complex of a specific antigen causing the release and generation of mediators of allergic inflammation.[1] However, many adverse reactions of different mechanisms may be generally regarded as "allergic," whereas the specific nature of the reaction may not be known. The "atopic" patient, however, is one with a genetic predisposition who manifests allergies following environmental exposure and sensitization.[2]

The spectrum of allergic reactivity ranges from allergic rhinitis, to asthma, to food and drug allergies and insect stings, to atopic dermatitis, to anaphylaxis. This chapter addresses the management of the "allergic patient" with upper respiratory allergies, especially allergic rhinitis. Asthma, atopic dermatitis, food "allergy," and sinusitis are covered in other chapters in this book.

The nose can be viewed as the window to the lungs, and allergic and inflammatory mechanisms studied in the lungs are often translated into treatments appropriate for study in the nose. So it is with asthma and rhinitis in evaluating the literature on integrative, complementary, and alternative medical approaches for the lower and upper respiratory tract.[3] Optimally, each approach should be studied specifically in rhinitis with standardized parameters such as with a rhinitis quality-of-life questionnaire.[4] However, the methods addressed herein are drawn from reports and reviews[5–7] believed to meet the standard of "primum non nocere" (first do no harm) and creative application of art and science for respiratory health in the context of the whole patient.

The methods described here may be employed by primary caregivers, but if the patient wishes to explore alternative practices outside the medical model, a continued relationship with the patient can be supported with timely follow-up.[8] Interest in,[9] self-treatment with,[10] practices of,[11] and demand for complementary and alternative medicine (CAM) for allergies and asthma are significant and in general are increasing.[12] Traditional allergists are also being encouraged to become more knowledgeable about alternative approaches and to meet the challenge for redefining the specialty if CAM is proved to provide improved therapies for allergy and asthma.[13, 14]

INTEGRATIVE THERAPY

Environmental Measures

Outdoor Exposure

Pollen precautions can be pursued during the pollen seasons. The sources of pollen are generally trees in the spring, grasses in the summer, and weeds in the fall in geographic regions with climate changes. Patients are advised to stay indoors with windows closed, to use air conditioning in homes and automobiles, and to purchase a HEPA (high-efficiency particulate air) filter for the home or workplace. Particulates in the air should be avoided if possible, and use of appropriate air filtration should be encouraged.[15]

Indoor Exposure

The increase in allergic reactivity as evidenced by the higher prevalence of asthma has been attributed in part to increased indoor sensitization associated with living and working in airtight buildings. House dust mite exposure in humid environments can be reduced by certain environmental precautions such as encasing the bedding and pillows with plastic and use of dehumidifiers in humid regions. During the winter, exposure to indoor allergens such as cat and dog dander is also increased. Frequent shampooing of cats is helpful to reducing ambient levels of allergens. Irritants such as tobacco smoke, wood smoke, chemical and gas fumes, and car exhaust should be specifically avoided. HEPA filters should be considered for the bedroom and main living areas of the home.

Humidification

Humidifiers can be used in dry climates to moisturize the respiratory passages. The goal should be a relative humidity of no greater than 35%, to discourage housedust mite proliferation. The humidifier can be cleaned with vinegar water.

Nasal Hygiene

One of the most helpful, inexpensive, nonpharmacologic approaches is to practice good "nasal hygiene," with frequent saline moisturization of the nasal mucosa to thin the mucus, to promote mucus evacuation, and to refresh the nasal mucosa. This concept is reviewed in detail elsewhere (see Chapter 12, Chronic Sinusitis).

The best way to clear the nasal discharge is to perform nasal washes with salt water (saline), as described in the accompanying box. Gargling with saline solution may also be beneficial.

METHOD

Nasal Moisturization and Irrigation

A saline solution is made fresh each day with 1 teaspoon of table salt and perhaps a pinch of baking soda added to a pint of warm water (preferably distilled), mixed in a clean glass or plastic bottle. At least 1 cup of the solution should be used. The patient is advised to experiment with the concentration according to preference. To make a smaller amount, $1/4$ teaspoon of salt is added to 1 cup of water.

Method 1: A small amount of saline is poured into the palm of the hand, while one nostril is held closed; then the saline is "sniffed" into the opposite nostril. This maneuver is repeated on the other side. The nasal passages are then cleared by blowing the nose well. The patient may also wish to gargle.

Method 2: A large rubber ear syringe or baby suction bulb should be purchased, and the tip of the ear syringe should be cut to enlarge the opening to about the size of the index finger. (If the opening is too big, the flow of water is too fast, causing pain.) The syringe is filled with saline; the patient leans over the sink with the head down. While the nostril is pinched closed around the tip of the syringe, the bulb is squeezed and released several times. This maneuver is repeated on the other side. The solution should run down the back of the throat and out the mouth and other nostril. The patient can be advised to use this method after showering, with the water turned off, but still standing in the steamy shower.

Method 3: Ocean Spray, Ayr Mist, Salinex, or Sinus Survival nasal solution can be used; 5 to 8 squirts are placed in each nostril. The nasal passages are then cleared by blowing the nose.

Method 4: A SinuCleanse nasal irrigation system (neti pot) can also be used. Additional information and products can be found at www.sinussurvival.com, or the manufacturer, Sinus Survival Products, can be contacted at 303-771-0033.

Method 5: Alternatively, the patient may wish to purchase an irrigation device (e.g., Waterpik) and a Grossan nasal adapter. These items may be obtained at pharmacies. With the irrigator at "low" setting, the tip of the adapter is inserted in the nostril, with the solution allowed to run down the back of the throat and out the mouth and other nostril. Although this procedure may seem arduous and somewhat unsophisticated, it is the most thorough way to wash the nasal passages.[16]

Pharmaceuticals

The medicines available today are excellent for mild to moderate allergic rhinitis.

Antihistamines and Decongestants

Over-the-counter (OTC) antihistamines and anti-histamine-decongestant combinations have been available for many years. However, the classic antihistamines, primarily the nonprescription agents diphenhydramine (Benadryl) and chlorpheniramine (Chlor-Trimeton), are associated with sedation and can influence tasks such as driving[17] and operating machinery. This caution, as well as the quality-of-life impairment with these readily available medicines, has limited their use by the public. The newer, second-generation antihistamines are nonsedating or only minimally sedating and have become widely used. Nonsedating agents include loratadine (Claritin) 10 mg once daily, fexofenadine (Allegra) 60 mg twice daily (adult dose 180 mg once daily), and decongestant combinations thereof. Cetirizine (Zyrtec) 10 mg once daily may be mildly sedating and therefore is often started with bedtime dosing.

Oral decongestants given by themselves or in combination with antihistamines may have a stimulant effect and impair sleep if taken at bedtime. These agents include pseudoephedrine and phenylephrine. Phenylpropanolamine has recently been discontinued from many medications, owing to its potential for abuse as an appetite suppressant and other potentially serious complications.

Mucolytics

The benefit of use of oral mucolytics such as guaifenesin has been poorly substantiated, but these agents are often prescribed, with doses in adults of 1200 mg twice daily needed to be effective. These drugs are safe and without side effects other than a "runny nose" in some patients. OTC guaifenesin combinations with dextromethorphan or codeine are effective for cough in age-appropriate doses (e.g., Robitussin combinations).

Topical Nasal Decongestants

Topical nasal decongestants are available over the counter (e.g., Afrin, 4-Way nasal spray) and are effective in the short term, with the potential for rebound "rhinitis medicamentosa" if overused. This condition can be treated with topical nasal steroids and discontinuation of the nasal decongestant.

Topical Nasal Anti-inflammatory Sprays

Steroids

Topical nasal steroids are available by prescription and are very effective for treatment of chronic rhinitis when inflammation is present. The main response is relief of nasal congestion. They are safe in recommended doses, although nasal dryness and bleeding are possible unless nasal saline moisturization precedes the administration of the nasal steroid and the tip is pointed toward the outside, not the septum. The available topical nasal steroids, beginning with the most recently approved, are the following: mometasone (Nasonex), 2 sprays daily, approved for use in patients as young as 3 years of age, with 0.1% systemic absorption; fluticasone (Flonase), 2 sprays daily, approved for use down to age 4 years, with 1.0% systemic absorption; budesonide (Rhinocort) aqueous or in a metered dose inhaler (MDI), effective in a dose of 1 or 2 sprays daily; and triamcinolone (Nasacort) aqueous or in an MDI, 2 sprays daily. As part of a good nasal hygiene routine, nasal spray can be used twice daily when patients brush the teeth, first irrigating with saline and, for the aesthetic-minded, inhaling of a mild eucalyptus mist, if tolerated, afterward.[18]

Antihistamines

Another topical nasal antiallergic spray available by prescription is azelastine (Astelin), which is an antihistamine with antiallergic effects. This agent is effective for treatment of seasonal and perennial allergic rhinitis and vasomotor (nonallergic) rhinitis. Dosage is 2 sprays in each nostril twice daily.

Mast Cell Stabilizer

Cromolyn sodium (NasalCrom) is an antiallergic nasal spray available over the counter. It is safe and effective for treatment of allergic rhinitis. This agent needs to be taken in a dose of 2 sprays at least 4 times daily and can be used before allergic exposure.

Anticholinergic

Ipratropium (Atrovent) is the only nasal spray effective for rhinorrhea (runny nose). It is an anticholinergic, available in concentrations of 0.03% and 0.06%; the dosage is 2 sprays 3 times daily as needed.

Immunotherapy

Allergy vaccine injection therapy (allergy immunotherapy, given as "shots") is useful when environmental exposure cannot be avoided, or if control of symptoms with medications is suboptimal, side effects are undesirable, or duration of symptomatic therapy is not appealing and the patient wants to treat the cause instead of the symptoms. In simplistic terms, allergy immunotherapy works by stimulating the production of an IgG-blocking antibody, which occupies the receptor site of the allergic IgE antibody, displacing it by competitive inhibition, thereby inhibiting the initiation and lessening the magnitude of the allergic reaction. The IgE antibody levels decline, and there is a deregulation of the immune response by a complex of mechanisms. With an increased appreciation of untreated allergic rhinitis as a disorder with systemic complications[19] (e.g., fatigue, headache, and increased asthmatic reactivity), use of allergy "shots" is now considered earlier in the treatment algorithm.

Botanicals

Bioflavonoids

Although the role of herbal medicine in allergies as effective therapy has not been studied as much as that in asthma, certain principles apply. Bioflavonoids are claimed to be active anti-inflammatory and antiallergy agents that prevent the formation of histamine and help to regulate vascular permeability and inflammation. Bioflavonoids are concentrated in onions, garlic, cayenne pepper, apples, and tea. A eucalyptus bioflavonoid preparation, Quercetin, is the most effective antihistaminic/antiallergic bioflavonoid and is taken in capsules. Other bioflavonoid-rich herbs are chamomile, feverfew, yarrow, baikal skullcap, and many mints. Other important antiallergic bioflavonoids are chlorogenic acid, caffeic acid, kaempferol, apigenin, luteolin, acacetin, and myricetin.

Essential oils of orange, tangerine, and lemon, as well as cardamom, cinnamon, and mint family plants, have antihistaminic and antiallergic effects and are believed to help to relax nasal passages and airways.[20]

Dosage. 1 or 2 1000-mg tablets of Quercetin one to three times daily.

Precautions. Quercetin is a safe supplement with no serious side effects when used orally at recommended doses.

Stinging Nettle

Stinging nettle (*Urtica dioica*) is a folk remedy for many problems. It is often used as a tonic and detoxifying remedy. The leaves are used for the relief of bronchial asthma and bronchitis. Freeze-dried stinging nettle is sometimes recommended for allergies; the rationale is that it provides a pseudohomeopathic dosage of histamine and acetylcholine. In a randomized, double-blind study of freeze-dried *Urtica dioica* in the treatment of allergic rhinitis, the stinging nettle was rated higher than placebo in the global assessments and only slightly higher in diary data comparisons.[21]

Essential oils

Dosage. 300 to 1200 mg of dried leaf two to four times daily.

Precautions. Stinging nettle should be avoided with pregnancy. It can cause diarrhea when used orally.

Butterbur (*Petasites hybridus*)

A randomized double-blind trial comparing butterbur to cetirizine (zyrtec) over 2 weeks for seasonal allergic rhinitis found butterbur was as effective as cetirizine without sedating side effects.

It is thought to work by inhibiting the biosynthesis of leukotrienes.[37]

Dosage. 8 mg (standardized to petasine content) four times daily.

Precautions. Allergic potential in those sensitive to ragweeds. Avoid using for more than 4 to 6 weeks.

Supplements

Antioxidants

A multivitamin, plus vitamin C 500 mg, once daily minimum, and vitamins A and E, is a recommended part of an antioxidant program. Grape seed extract (*Vitis vinifera*) is rich in proanthocyanidins and has been demonstrated to have antioxidant properties in some models. This botanical is a reasonable addition.[22]

Dosage. One multivitamin daily. Grape seed extract: 25 to 100 mg 1 to 3 times daily standardized to contain 40% to 80% proanthocyanidins.

Precautions. Grape seed extract may inhibit platelet aggregation and should be used with caution in patients taking anticoagulant medications.

Zinc

Zinc is described as capable of causing up to a 40% inhibition of IgE-mediated induction of histamine and leukotriene release from both basophils and mast cells, modifying the inflammatory response.[24] Owing to zinc's additional effect of promoting healing during infections, the dose can be increased during acute exacerbations of allergic rhinitis.

Dosage. 15 to 35 mg of zinc daily.

Precautions. Doses greater than 40 mg daily can lead to copper, calcium, and iron depletion. Toxic symptoms include nausea, vomiting, diarrhea, dizziness, and anemia.

Nutrition

Fluids

Hydration is of ultimate importance; with intake of at least 8 to 10 glasses of water per day recommended.

Vegetables and Fruit

Vegetables are good sources of antioxidants. Dietary modifications to include increased intake of onions, garlic, cayenne, apples, and tea can be encouraged, as well as 6 to 9 servings of fruits and vegetables daily.

Omega-3 Fatty Acids

Conventional medical practice and alternative medicine may overlap now that vitamins B and C as well as diets low in sodium and sugar and high in fish oil and magnesium intake have been reported to be beneficial in bronchospastic disorders.[27] Consumption of fish rich in omega-3 fatty acids, such as salmon and mackerel, several times a week is recommended. Other omega-3 sources include walnuts, ground flaxseed, and toasted hemp seeds.

Fats and Oils

Fats that promote inflammation should be avoided. Examples of such fats are oils rich in omega-6 fatty acids, including polyunsaturated vegetable oils (such as safflower, sunflower, sesame, and corn oils), partially hydrogenated oils (found in many snack foods), margarine, and vegetable shortening. Extra virgin olive oil, which helps fight inflammation and is high in vitamin E, should be used as the main dietary fat[28] (see Chapter 84, The Anti-Inflammatory Diet).

Chicken Soup

Chicken soup has been recommended for respiratory disorders since the time of Maimonides.[25] Its anti-inflammatory effects have recently been substantiated in the laboratory.[26]

Biomechanical Therapies

Massage

Instruction in sinus acupressure on reflexology points can be given as part of the patients's chronic sinusitis treatment program.

Chiropractic

Chiropractic has most recently been shown to have no value in asthma. By extension,[29] therefore, it is of doubtful use in rhinitis.

Traditional Chinese Medicine

Chinese herbal formulas similar to those for asthma are available for allergic rhinitis. Examples include Turtle Shell, Cistanche combination, and Jade Screen powder.[30] Although there are few well-controlled scientific studies on the efficacy, safety, and mechanisms of action of traditional Chinese medicine formulas in allergy or asthma, research is in progress, and additional data are forthcoming. Recently, the Chinese herbal medicine formula MSSM-002 was reported to suppress allergic airway hyperreactivity and to modulate T_H1/T_H2 responses in a murine model of allergic asthma.[31] Unfortunately, exotic drug preparations are likely to be unreliable in the amount of active drug content, and they may be contaminated with active drugs such as corticosteroids or with hazardous agents such as lead.[5] Practitioners need to be aware of potential and actual adverse and allergic reactions and herb-drug interactions with traditional Chinese medicines and with Chinese proprietary or patent medicines.[32]

Yoga-Type Breathing Techniques

Nasal Diaphragmatic Breathing Exercises

The patient can be instructed in nasal diaphragmatic breathing. Nasal inhalation is performed slowly, with a focus on the diaphragm; exhalation is by mouth. These exercises are preferably performed in a steam shower to humidify the nasal mucosa, with steam acting as a mucolytic and mucoevacuant. This measure also helps to remove pollen. Nasal breathing exercises can also be done over a pot of boiling water (with a towel over the head) or with use of a SteamHaler (see Chapter 88, Breathing Exercises).

Aromatic Agents

Agents such as eucalyptus, menthol, anise, fennel, tolu balsam, and camphor (with some incorporated in products such as Vicks VapoRub and Tiger Balm)[20] can soothe the inflamed nasal mucosa when inhaled as vapors.

Exercise

In the pollen season, exercise indoors should be considered, especially during peak pollen times. Membership in a health club is conducive to regular physical activity (a steam shower after the workout is also beneficial). Alternatively, brisk walking inside shopping malls is also good exercise.

Mind-Body Medicine

Laughter has been shown to produce improvement in patients experiencing the allergic diathesis of atopic dermatitis—and is always a good idea![33]

Other Therapies to Consider

Homeopathy

A randomized controlled trial of homeopathy versus placebo found significant benefit with the use of homeopathic therapy in patients with allergic rhinitis. The principal allergen was identified with skin testing in each patient, and a 30 C dilution of the appropriate homeopathic remedy was made. There was a 28% symptom reduction in the homeopathic therapy group compared with a 3% reduction in the placebo treatment group (P .0007).[34]

Constitutional homeopathy has been popularized,[35, 36] but results are highly dependent on competence of the practitioner.

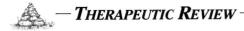 — *THERAPEUTIC REVIEW*

Environmental measures
- Use of a humidifier or dehumidifier, HEPA filter
- Dust mite precautions, dander minimization
- Nasal saline moisturization and irrigation
- Water intake of at least 8 glasses daily

Pharmaceuticals
- Oral antihistamines as needed

THERAPEUTIC REVIEW continued

- Topical nasal steroids or azelastine (Astelin) or cromolyn sodium (NasalCrom)
- Mucolytics such as guaifenesin 600 to 1200 mg twice daily
- Combination agents

Immunotherapy
- Allergy vaccine injection therapy

Botanicals
- Bioflavonoids such as eucalyptus bioflavonoids (Quercetin) 1000 mg 1 or 2 tablets 1 to 3 times daily

Supplements
- Multivitamin, vitamin C, vitamins A and E
- Grape seed extract 25 to 100 mg 1 to 3 times daily

Nutrition
- Hydration—adequate water intake cannot be over emphasized.
- Elimination of additives, processed foods, known allergens (e.g, spices, milk, nuts, eggs), yeast products
- Addition of cold water fish, such as salmon and mackerel, with omega-3 fatty acids; fruit juices and vegetables

Biomechanical therapies
- Nasal diaphragmatic breathing
- Steam shower or nasal steam inhalation
- Use of aromatics such as eucalyptus in nasal sprays or in moisturization practices may be beneficial.

References

1. Muelleman RL, Lindzon RL, Silvers WS: Allergy, hypersensitivity and anaphylaxis. In Rosen P, et al (eds). Emergency Medicine Concepts and Clinical Practice, 4th ed, vol 3, St. Louis, CV Mosby, 1998, pp 2759–2776.
2. Nelson HS: The atopic diseases. Ann Allergy 55:441, 1985.
3. Graham DM, Blaiss MS: Complementary/alternative medicine in the treatment of asthma. Ann Allergy Asthma Immunol 85:438–449, 2000.
4. Juniper EP: Measuring health-related quality of life in rhinitis. J Allergy Clin Immunol 99:S742–S749, 1997.
5. Ziment I, Tashkin DP: Alternative medicine for allergy and asthma. J Allergy Clin Immunol 106:603–614, 2000.
6. In't Veen JCCM, Sterk PJ, Bel EH: Alternative strategies in the treatment of bronchial asthma. Clin Exp Allergy 30:16–33, 2000.
7. Lewith GT, Watkins AD: Unconventional therapies in asthma: An overview. Allergy 51:761–769, 1996.
8. Eisenberg DM: Advising patients who seek alternative medical therapies. Ann Intern Med 127:61–69, 1997.
9. Silvers WS, Graham PH, Riddle JM: Alternative medicine questionnaire in a private allergy/asthma practice [abstract]. J Allergy Clin Immunol 103:308, 1999.
10. Blanc PD, Kuschner WG, Katz PP, et al: Use of herbal products, coffee or black tea, and over-the-counter medications as self-treatments among adults with asthma. J Allergy Clin Immunol 100:789–791, 1997.
11. Davis PA, Gold EB, Hackman RM, et al: The use of complementary/alternative medicine for the treatment of asthma in the United States. J Invest Allergol Clin Immunol 8:73–77, 1998.
12. Eisenberg DM, Davis RB, Ettner SL, et al: Trends in alternative medicine use in the United States, 1990-1997. JAMA 280:1569-1575, 1998.
13. Engler RJM: Alternative and complementary medicine: A source of improved therapies for asthma? A challenge for redefining the specialty? J Allergy Clin Immunol 106:627–629, 2000.
14. Bielory L: Complementary/alternative medicine: We need to become more knowledgeable. Ann Allergy Asthma Immunol 85:427–428, 2000.
15. Nelson HS, Hirsch SR, Ohman JL, et al: Recommendations for the use of residential air-cleaning devices in the treatment of allergic respiratory diseases. J Allergy Clin Immunol 82:661–669, 1988.
16. Tomooka LT, Murphy C, Davidson TM: Clinical study and literature review of nasal irrigation. Laryngoscope 110:1189–1193, 2000.
17. Weiler JM, Bloomfield JR, Woodworth GG, et al: Effects of Fexofenadine, diphenhydramine, and alcohol on driving performance: A randomized, placebo-controlled trial in the Iowa driving simulator. Ann Intern Med 132:354–363, 2000.
18. Burrow A, Eccles R, Jones AS: The effects of camphor, eucalyptus, and menthol vapour on nasal resistance to airflow and nasal sensation. Acta Otolaryngol (Stockh) 96:157–161, 1983.
19. Bousquet J, Demoly P, Michel FB: Allergen immunotherapy in the 21st century: Therapeutic vaccines for allergic diseases. Paper presented at the AAAAI Annual Meeting, Postgraduate Plenary Session, March 2001.
20. Bielory L, Lupoli K: Herbal interventions in asthma and allergy. J Asthma 36:1–65, 1999.
21. Mittman P: Randomized, double-blind study of freeze-dried Urtica dioica in the treatment of allergic rhinitis. Planta Med 56:44–77, 1990.
22. Nuttall LS, Kendall MJ, Bombardelli E, Morazzoni P: An evaluation of the antioxidant activity of a standardized grape seed extract, Leucoselect. J Clin Pharm Ther 23:385–389, 1998.
23. Scaglione F, Weiser K, Allessandria M: Effects of the standardized ginseng extract G115R in patients with chronic bronchitis: A non-blinded, randomized comparative pilot study. Clin Drug Invest 21:41–45, 2001.
24. Marone G, Columbo M, dePaulis A, et al: Physiological concentrations of zinc inhibit the release of histamine from human basophils and lung mast cells. Agents Actions 18:103–106, 1986 [erratum 18:607, 1986].
25. Cohen SG: The chicken, in history and in the soup. Allergy Proc 12:47–56, 1991.
26. Rennard BO, Ertl RF, Gossman GL, et al: Chicken soup inhibits neutrophil chemotaxis in vitro. Chest 118:1150–1157, 2000.
27. Ziment I: How your patients may be using diet to treat their asthma. J Respir Dis 19:999–1006, 1998.
28. Weil A: Managing your asthma. In Dr. Andrew Weil's Self Healing. Watertown, Mass., Thorne Communications, 2001.
29. Balon J, Aker PD, Crowther ER, et al. A comparison of active and simulated chiropractic manipulation as adjunctive treat-

ment for childhood asthma. N Engl J Med 1998;339(15):1013–1020, 1998.

30. But P, Chang C: Chinese herbal medicine in the treatment of asthma and allergies. Clin Rev Allergy Immunol 14:253–269, 1996.

31. Li X, Huang C, Zhang T, et al: The Chinese herbal medicine formula MSSM-002 suppresses allergic airway hyperactivity and modulates T_H1/T_H2 responses in a murine model of allergic asthma. J Allergy Clin Immunol 106:660–668, 2000.

32. Wong, HCG: Adverse and allergic reactions in complementary and alternative medicine [letter]. J Allergy Clin Immunol 108:149–150, 2001.

33. Kimata H: Effect of humor on allergen-induced wheal reactions. JAMA 285:738, 2001.

34. Taylor MA, Reilly D, Llewellyn-Jones RH, et al: Randomized controlled trial of homeopathy versus placebo in perennial allergic rhinitis with overview of four trial series. BMJ 321:471–476, 2000.

35. Reilly, DT, Taylor MA, McSharry C, Aitchison T: Is homeopathy a placebo response? Controlled trial of homoeopathic potency, with pollen in hayfever as model. Lancet 2:881–886, 1986.

36. Reilly DT, Taylor MA, Beattie NGM, et al: Is evidence for homoeopathy reproducible? Lancet 344:1601–1608, 1994.

37. Schapowal, A: Randomized controlled trial of butterbur and cetirizine for treating seasonal allergic rhinitis. BMJ 324:144–146, 2002.

CHAPTER 26

Insulin Resistance Syndrome

David Rakel, M.D.

PATHOPHYSIOLOGY

Identification of people with insulin resistance syndrome (IRS) can lead to therapy and lifestyle changes that may prevent progression to overt diabetes and atherosclerotic heart disease. Tissues in the body such as skeletal muscle have a reduced sensitivity to the effects of insulin-stimulated glucose uptake. Initially, the body is able to secrete more insulin to maintain euglycemia. Eventually, this adaptation is lost and the body is unable to keep up with the insulin demand, resulting in diabetes. The diagnosis of IRS and hyperinsulinemia usually precedes the diagnosis of type 2 diabetes by years to decades. Insulin resistance syndrome (also known as the metabolic syndrome, or syndrome X) is associated with hyperinsulinemia, glucose intolerance, central obesity, elevated blood pressure, dyslipidemia (↑TG, ↓HDL), and a prothrombotic state. Although the exact etiology is unclear, a genetic predisposition is likely. The condition is seen more often among inactive men with central obesity, but it can also occur in those who are of normal weight. Elevated insulin levels have been associated with atherosclerosis and with impaired fibrinolysis that results in a hypercoagulable state, leading to an increased risk for acute thrombosis (Fig. 26–1).[1] The goal of therapy should be to reduce insulin levels and enhance sensitivity, which is the focus of this chapter.

NOTE

Suspect IRS in inactive hypertensive patients (male > female) with central obesity. If fasting triglycerides are greater than 150 mg per dL, high-density lipoprotein (HDL) cholesterol is less than 40 mg per dL, and low-density lipoprotein (LDL) cholesterol is normal or elevated with an elevated uric acid, consider treatment. Fasting insulin levels may also be helpful, but order with caution owing to poor reference standards.

LIFESTYLE

Insulin resistance can be effectively treated with aggressive lifestyle changes that include exercise, weight loss, and nutritional therapy. The challenge lies in motivating the patient to do so. (See Chapter 95, Motivational Interviewing Techniques.)

Exercise

Exercise may be the single most important factor for preventing and reversing insulin resistance. Exercise improves insulin sensitivity in skeletal muscles and fat tissue, thereby reducing both insulin levels and fasting blood sugar.[2] Adding strength training (weight lifting) to endurance training maintains a high metabolic state that further improves percent body fat, insulin resistance, triglyceride levels, and systolic blood pressure.[3]

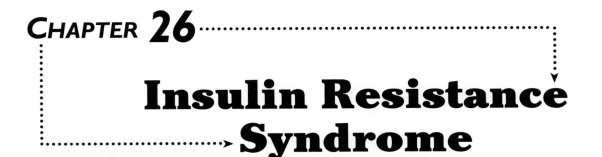

Figure 26–1. Disease path of insulin resistance syndrome. DM, diabetes mellitus.

Encourage participation in an enjoyable activity that incorporates aerobic conditioning and muscle strengthening. (See Chapter 86, Writing an Exercise Prescription.)

Weight Loss

The severity of insulin resistance is often in direct proportion to the amount of visceral body fat, despite the person's age and sex.[4] The location of the fat distribution is also a factor. Central or abdominal accumulation is associated with greater risk.[5]

Encourage a weight loss program that will result in gradual loss over time and that incorporates a regular exercise program and dietary changes. Weight loss of as little as 10 lb has been found to be beneficial.

Nicotine-Containing Products

Cigarette smoking and the use of nicotine-containing products such as the patch and chewing gum have been associated with insulin resistance, and their use should be discouraged.[6, 7]

NUTRITION

It appears that people with IRS do best with a low-carbohydrate, high-fiber, high-protein, low saturated fat, high monounsaturated fat diet. The goal is to reduce the spikes of serum glucose that result in higher insulin levels.

Low Carbohydrates

Diets with low amounts of carbohydrates have been found to improve HDL while lowering triglycerides. Carbohydrates are converted to glucose faster than are fat and protein, resulting in higher insulin levels. The more we eat foods that result in spikes in serum glucose levels, the more we expose the body to the toxic effects of high glucose and the harmful effects of insulin. One study showed a significant reduction in fasting insulin levels after 12 weeks of a 25% carbohydrate diet versus a 45% carbohydrate diet.[8]

The practitioner's goal should be to encourage foods that produce a slow and gradual insulin response. These foods can be classified as having a low glycemic index. (See Chapter 83, The Glycemic Index.) The glycemic index is a scale that tells us how fast a carbohydrate raises the level of serum glucose. The scale runs from 0 to 100, with glucose being the reference at 100. The higher the score, the higher the glucose and insulin response (Fig. 26–2). Low glycemic index foods have a score of less than 55 (e.g., oranges, peaches, and soy beans), the intermediate level is between 55 and 70 (e.g., ice cream, pineapple,

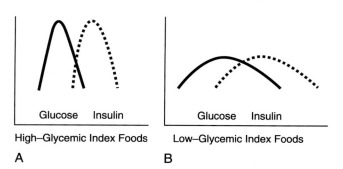

Figure 26–2. The glycemic index food (high [A], low [B]) is depicted by the *solid line*. The insulin response to the food is depicted by the *dashed line*.

and wheat bread), and high values are those greater than 70 (e.g., white bread, baked potato, and jelly beans). In one study, 2810 patients with type 1 diabetes were found to have lower glycosylated hemoglobin and higher HDL levels when they were on a low glycemic index diet.[9]

High Fiber

A high-fiber diet delays glucose absorption and binds cholesterol, thereby reducing its uptake into the body. The most benefit with respect to insulin resistance appears to come from oat fiber, guar gum, and psyllium in decreasing order. Beta-glucan, a constituent of oat bran, increases the viscosity of food in the small intestine and delays absorption that reduces postprandial plasma glucose and insulin levels.[10]

Dosage. Oat bran—3 g of soluble fiber a day. This amount is found in 75 g of dried oatmeal, which can be obtained by eating a bowl of oat bran or oatmeal for breakfast. It would be best to eat this fiber before each meal, but such a goal is unrealistic.

Guar gum—3 g in 8 oz of fluid before meals three times a day, not exceeding 15 g per day.

Psyllium (Metamucil and others)—1 tbsp in 8 oz of liquid twice a day.

Precautions. The higher the dose of these products, the greater their laxative potential and level of gastrointestinal intolerance for the patient. Be sure that the patient takes guar gum and psyllium with plenty of liquids to prevent development of an obstruction formed by these bulking agents.

High Protein

Because a low-carbohydrate diet is recommended in IRS, calories from protein need to be increased. Increasing protein results in lower serum glucose spikes because the body has to work harder to derive energy from proteins. This causes a slower release of glucose into the body. High-protein diets have been associated with greater weight loss and lower serum triglyceride levels.[11]

Encourage increased calorie consumption from protein-rich foods such as legumes, nuts, and fish.

↓Saturated Fat, ↑Monounsaturated Fat and Polyunsaturated Fats Rich in Omega-3 Fatty Acids

The key is not to reduce the total fat consumption but to create a more healthy balance of the types of fats that are consumed. A reduction in saturated fats such as those found in red meats, fried foods, and dairy products has been found to be beneficial for patients with type 2 diabetes mellitus (DM).[12]

Substituting monounsaturated fats (e.g., olive oil, canola oil) and omega-3–rich polyunsaturated fats (e.g., cold water fish, flaxseed, walnuts) improves insulin sensitivity while decreasing triglyceride and LDL levels.[13] (See Chapter 84, The Anti-inflammatory Diet.)

↑Fruits and Vegetables Rich in Carotenoids

Foods with natural yellow, orange, and red colors are generally rich in carotenoid-like pigments, which have been found to be inversely related to fasting serum insulin levels.[14] Diets rich in vitamin A (a product of the carotenoid, beta-carotene) have been associated with a reduction in insulin resistance.[15]

MIND–BODY TECHNIQUES

Studies of the fight-or-flight response have shown that stress and anxiety can result in a large release of adrenaline and cortisol from the adrenal gland. The purpose of these hormones is to provide extra energy in the form of glucose for battling the source of stress or for fleeing the scene.[16] Managing stress and anxiety reduces the number of serum glucose spikes that may help prevent or improve insulin resistance.

Lifestyle changes should be made if the amounts of stress and anxiety are out of balance for an individual. Relaxation exercises can also be recommended to provide the patient with a tool that will help in maintaining euglycemia (see Chapter 91, Prescribing Relaxation Techniques). Meditation can also be a helpful activity (see Chapter 94, Learning to Meditate).

SUPPLEMENTS

Mineral deficiencies, including calcium, magnesium, potassium, chromium, vanadium, and zinc, may promote insulin resistance. Owing to the available clinical research, the discussion here focuses on calcium, chromium, and vanadium.

Calcium

The research with regard to insulin resistance and calcium is not vast, but because calcium can also be beneficial for other conditions such as osteoporosis and hypertension, I have included it in this chapter. In one study, 20 hypertensive patients were given 1500 mg of calcium or placebo for 8 weeks. Those who received calcium had decreased fasting insulin levels and a significant increase in insulin sensitivity.[17]

Dosage. Calcium, 1500 mg a day.

Chromium

Although animal studies have shown that a deficiency of chromium can result in insulin resistance, clinical human studies are equivocal. Evidence shows that people who consume diets with the lowest amounts of chromium tend to have disruption in glucose and insulin regulation.[18]

Diet supplementation with chromium has been found to improve insulin resistance in some studies.[19] In a double-blinded, placebo-controlled study of 180 type 2 diabetics given chromium picolinate, the study group demonstrated improved glucose and fasting insulin levels, suggesting an improvement in insulin resistance.[20] In another study, 39 elderly patients with type 2 diabetes were given 200 μg chromium two times daily for 3 weeks. The patients' fasting blood glucose significantly dropped from an average of 189 to 150 mg/dL. Hemoglobin A_{1c} levels lowered from 8.15 to 7.58 g/dL, and total cholesterol fell from 225.26 to 211.42 mg/dL.[21]

Other studies have not resulted in this conclusion.

Dosage. Chromium picolinate, 200 mcg daily. Up to 500 mcg three times daily can be titrated in those with overt diabetes. Picolinate is better absorbed than the chloride or nicotinate forms.

Precautions. Toxic levels of chromium can result in cognitive, perceptual, and motor dysfunction. At elevated doses (1.5 to 2.4 mg/day), it can cause anemia, thrombocytopenia, hemolysis, hepatic dysfunction, and renal failure.

Vanadium (Vanadyl Sulfate)

Vanadium is a trace mineral that acts as a cofactor in various enzymatic reactions. It has been found to activate the insulin receptor, stimulate glucose oxidation and transport, inhibit hepatic gluconeogenesis, inhibit intestinal glucose transport, and increase glucose uptake and utilization in skeletal muscle.[22] Its ability to improve hepatic and peripheral insulin sensitivity is well documented in small clinical studies[23, 24] A study of 150 mg a day of vanadyl sulfate given to 11 type 2 diabetics resulted in significant improvement in glycemic control and cholesterol after 6 weeks of therapy. Fasting glucose levels decreased from 194 ± 16 to 155 ± 15 mg/dL, and hemoglobin A1c decreased from $8.1 \pm 0.4\%$ to $7.6 \pm 0.4\%$. It lowered plasma total cholesterol (average of 223 to 202 [$P < .05$]) and LDL cholesterol (average of 141 to 129 [$P < .05$]). Vanadyl sulfate reduced endogenous glucose production by about 20%, suggesting a greater influence on the liver than on muscle.[25] Food sources include milk, seafood, oils, cereals, and vegetables.

Dosage. 50 mg twice daily or 100 mg every day.

Precautions. Can cause green discoloration of the tongue. Elevated vanadium levels over prolonged periods of time have been associated with gastrointestinal distress, abnormal renal function tests, nervous system effects, and renal calculi. Owing to the potential toxicity and the lack of long-term studies, prolonged use of this mineral should be avoided until safety is confirmed.

α-Lipoic Acid

This is a strong antioxidant that functions as a coenzyme in the metabolism of carbohydrates and is needed to convert pyruvic acid to acetyl-coenzyme A for energy production. Studies have shown promise in its use to treat insulin resistance. Parenteral use has shown a 30% to 50% increase in insulin-stimulated glucose clearance rate.[26, 27] Orally administered α-lipoic acid has also been shown to improve insulin sensitivity in patients with diabetes. This effect was not dose dependent. A daily dose of 600 mg worked just as well as 1200 mg a day in helping to increase insulin-mediated glucose clearance by 27%.[28] A twice-daily 600-mg dose of α-lipoic acid for 4 weeks has also shown improvement in glucose metabolism in both lean and obese people with type 2 diabetes.[29]

Dosage. 600 mg a day.

Precautions. This appears to be a safe supplement with no known adverse effects. It may lead to the need to reduce insulin or diabetic pharmaceutical doses.

BOTANICALS

American Ginseng (Panax quinquefolium)

This herb should not be confused with two other forms of ginseng, Asian (*Panax*) and Siberian (*Eleutherococcus*), which can have more stimulating effects. American ginseng has been found to significantly reduce postprandial glycemia.[30] The mechanism of action remains unknown, but it may be related to a delay in carbohydrate absorption. Giving it

before meals may reduce the glycemic index of some foods. Overharvesting of this plant has placed it on the endangered species list in the United States, which may warrant other therapy choices for insulin resistance.

Dosage. 1 g before meals three times daily.

Precautions. May cause allergic reaction and gastrointestinal intolerance. May enhance the effect of some stimulating drugs and reduce the effect of warfarin, thereby reducing the protime. Use with caution in patients with hypertension.

Fenugreek (Trigonella foenum-graecum)

This herb, which comes from the pea family, affects gastrointestinal transit, slowing glucose absorption.[31] It has a high fiber content and works in the same way as psyllium, which was mentioned earlier. One unique property may be the constituent, 4-isoleucine, which appears to directly stimulate insulin.[32] If someone is unable to tolerate the previously mentioned fiber products, you may want to try giving fenugreek.

Dosage. 0.5 to 1 g of seeds two to three times daily.

Precautions. Higher doses can cause diarrhea and flatulence. Inhaling dust from ground seeds can lead to allergic reaction or asthma. The taste and odor of fenugreek resemble those of maple syrup and it may affect the urine; this should not be confused with the disease of the same name.

PHARMACEUTICALS

Avoid Sulfonylurea Drugs

These medications work by closing the adenosine triphosphate–sensitive potassium channels, which increases insulin secretion by beta cells of the pancreas. They also are associated with weight gain and vasoconstriction, both of which worsen vascular reactivity. This combination of weight gain and elevated insulin levels contradicts the goal of therapy for IRS.

Metformin Hydrochloride (Glucophage)

This medication improves insulin resistance by reducing hepatic gluconeogenesis and increasing glucose utilization in skeletal muscle and adipose tissue. It is thought to enhance the ability of insulin to bind to its receptors. It has been found to reduce very low density lipoproteins and to cause a modest reduction in triglycerides. An added benefit is mild weight loss due to anorexic effects of the drug.

Dosage. For insulin resistance, a low dose of 500 to 850 mg should be taken with a morning meal. Higher doses up to 2 g per day are used for overt diabetic therapy.

Precautions. Most common adverse effects are gastrointestinal (cramps, nausea, indigestion, and diarrhea), so take with a meal. Can cause lactic acidosis in those with renal impairment or alcoholism, metallic taste, and reduced B_{12} levels.

Thiazolidinediones (Avandia, Actos)

This class of insulin-sensitizing drugs targets the insulin receptor to make it more sensitive in the skeletal muscle, adipose tissue, and liver. It is an agonist of peroxisome proliferator–activated receptor-gamma (PPAR-gamma), which modulates a number of nuclear transcription factors that enhance the activity of the insulin-responsive glucose transport system. Although it may raise LDL by 10%, it reduces triglyceride levels and elevates HDLs, reversing the dyslipidemia seen in IRS.

Mild weight gain and edema can occur caused by fluid retention and plasma volume expansion. Estrogen levels can be lowered in those taking oral contraceptives and, most importantly, patients need to be monitored for hepatotoxicity. Research will likely show that this class of drugs can be temporarily used to enhance insulin sensitivity while lifestyle changes are made that will result in discontinuation.

Dosage. Rosiglitazone (Avandia), 2 to 4 mg each morning.

Pioglitazone (Actos), 15 mg each morning. May have a better effect on lipids.

Precautions. Hepatotoxicity—check liver function tests every 2 months for 1 year. Back pain, diarrhea, fatigue, headache, edema, weight gain, and anemia can occur.

THERAPIES TO CONSIDER

Constitutional Therapies

Traditional Chinese medicine (TCM) and Ayurvedic medicine are based on an assessment of the individual in relation to his or her environment and specific balances of energy (five elements in TCM, and the doshas [Kapha, Pitta, and Vata] in Ayurveda). Herbal treatment, diet, acupuncture, and various forms of detoxification may be used to influence health. A patient may want to work closely with a practitioner in one of these areas. Western research is lacking in studies of insulin resistance treatment from these cultural therapies, but the many years of practical experience and beneficial results should not be ignored.

L-Arginine

Although further studies are needed, a small group of patients with type 2 diabetes were given 3 g of oral L-arginine three times a day for 1 month. This resulted in improved peripheral and hepatic insulin sensitivity in a randomized, double-blind, placebo-controlled study.[33] L-Arginine an essential amino acid that is a substrate of nitric oxide synthase, increases the production of the vasodilator nitric oxide. Because of this mechanism, it is generally used for the treatment of peripheral vascular flow in those with congestive heart failure, coronary artery disease, and erectile dysfunction. Although arginine has been shown to increase insulin levels, the mechanism of action in insulin resistance is yet to be determined.

Dosage. 3 g three times daily.

Precautions. Abdominal pain, bloating, diarrhea, gout, thrombocytopenia, and elevation of BUN and creatinine can occur. L-Arginine can cause allergic reactions and may exacerbate asthma.

 THERAPEUTIC REVIEW

Laboratory evaluation:
- *Lipid panel (look for ↑TG, ↓HDL, nl or sl ↑LDL).*
- *Fasting glucose level, elevated uric acid.*
- *Consider fasting serum insulin level from reputable laboratory.*
- *Check homocysteine level as independent risk factor for heart disease (nl < 12).*

Lifestyle:
- *Encourage an exercise routine that consists of endurance and strength training.*
- *Encourage goals to achieve appropriate weight.*
- *Discourage use of nicotine-containing products.*

Nutrition:
- *Low-carbohydrate diet with focus on low glycemic index foods.*
- *High-fiber diet (add oat bran/oat cereal each day or guar gum 3g before each meal, or psyllium [Metamucil], 1 tbsp twice daily in 8 oz of water). Be sure to drink plenty of liquid with these products.*
- *High-protein diet (rich in legumes, cold water fish, and nuts)*

THERAPEUTIC REVIEW   continued

- *Low saturated fat/high monounsaturated fat. (Decrease red meat, fried foods, and dairy products. Replace vegetable oils with olive oil.)*
- *Increase yellow, orange, and red fruits and vegetables to increase intake of carotenoids.*

Mind–body:
- *Encourage lifestyle choices to reduce stress and anxiety.*
- *Recommend a relaxation technique fitted for the individual.*

NOTE

The previous recommendations highly outweigh those stated below for treating insulin resistance syndrome.

Supplements:
- *ASA, 325 mg a day due to prothrombotic state with IRS.*
- *Calcium carbonate or citrate, 1000 to 1500 mg each day.*
- *Vanadium, 100 mg each day (avoid use for longer than 2 months until long-term safety is confirmed).*
- *α-Lipoic acid, 600 mg each day.*

Some may consider adding:
- *Chromium picolinate, 200 μg each day.*

Botanicals/Pharmaceuticals:
- *If the patient is on the verge of being classified as diabetic, consider adding.*
- *American Ginseng, 1 g, before meals three times daily, or a pharmaceutical.*

If obese, consider:
- *Metformin (Glucophage), 500 to 850 mg each morning.*

If moderately overweight or of normal weight, consider:
- *Rosiglitazone (Avandia), 2 to 4 mg each morning, or*
- *Pioglitazone (Actos), 15 mg each morning.*

References

1. Meigs JB, Mittleman MA, Nathan DM, et al: Hyperinsulinemia, hyperglycemia, and impaired hemostasis: The Framingham Offspring Study. JAMA 283:221–228, 2000.
2. Horber FF, Kohler SA, Lippuner K, Jaeger P: Effect of regular physical training on age-associated alteration of body consumption in men. Eur J Clin Invest 26:279–285, 1996.
3. Wallace MB, Mills BD, Browning CL: Effects of cross-training on markers of insulin resistance/hyperinsulinemia. Med Sci Sports Exerc 29:1170–1175, 1997.
4. Belfiore F, Iannello S: Insulin resistance in obesity: Metabolic mechanisms and measurement methods. Mol Genet Metab 65:121–128, 1998.
5. Grundy SM: Hypertriglyeridemia, insulin resistance, and the metabolic syndrome. Am J Cardiol 83:25F–29F, 1999.
6. Targher G, Alberiche M, Zenere MB, et al: Cigarette smoking and insulin resistance in patients with noninsulin-dependent diabetes mellitus. J Clin Endocrinol Metab 82:3619–3624, 1997.
7. Eliasson B, Taskinen MR, Smith U: Long-term use of nicotine gum is associated with hyperinsulinemia and insulin resistance. Circulation 94:878–881, 1996.
8. Golay A, Eigenheer C, Morel Y, et al: Weight loss with low or high carbohydrate diet? Int J Obes Relat Metab Disord 20:1067–1072, 1996.
9. Buyken AE, Toeller M, Heitkamp G, et al: Glycemic index in the diet of European outpatients with type 1 diabetes: Relations to glycated hemoglobin and serum lipids. Am J Clin Nutr 73:574–581, 2001.
10. Wood PJ, Braaten JT, Scott FW, et al: Effects of dose and modification of viscous properties of oat gum on plasma glucose and insulin following an oral glucose load. Br J Nutr 72:731–743, 1993.
11. Skov AR, Toubro S, Ronn B, et al: Randomized trial on protein vs carbohydrate in ad libitum fat reduced diet for the treatment of obesity. Int J Obes Relat Metab Disord 23:528–536, 1999.
12. Knopp RH, Walden CE, Retzlaff BM, et al: Long-term cholesterol-lowering effects of 4 fat-restricted diets in hypercholesterolemic and combined hyperlipidemic men: The Dietary Alternatives Study. JAMA 278:1509–1515, 1997.
13. O'Keefe JH Jr, Nguyen T, Nelson J, et al: Potential beneficial effects of monounsaturated and polyunsaturated fats in elderly patients with or at risk of coronary artery disease. Cardiol Elder 3:5–10, 1995.
14. Ford ES, Will JC, Bowman BA, Narayan KMV: Diabetes mellitus and serum carotenoids: Findings from the third national health and nutrition examination survey. Am J Epidemiol 149:168–176, 1999.
15. Facchini F, Coulston AM, Reaven GM: Relation between dietary vitamin intake and resistance to insulin-mediated glucose disposal in healthy volunteers. Am J Clin Nutr 63:946–949, 1996.
16. Surwitt RS: Diabetes: Mind over metabolism. In Mind Body Medicine. Consumer Reports Books, 1998, pp 131–144.
17. Sanchez M, de la Sierra A, Coca A, et al: Oral calcium supplementation reduces intraplatelet free calcium concentration and insulin resistance in essential hypertensive patients. Hypertension 29:531–536, 1997.
18. Anderson RA, Polansky MM, Bryden NA, Canary JJ: Supplemental chromium effects on glucose, insulin, glucagon, and urinary chromium losses in subjects consuming controlled low-chromium diets. Am J Clin Nutr 54:909–916, 1991.
19. Railes R, Albrink MJ: Effect of chromium chloride supplemen-

tation on glucose tolerance and serum lipids including high-densitiy lipoprotein of adult men. Am J Clin Nutr 34:2670–2678, 1981.

20. Anderson RA, Cheng N, Bryden NA, et al: Elevated intakes of supplemental chromium improve glucose and insulin variables in individuals with type 2 diabetes. Diabetes 46:1786–1791, 1997.

21. Rabinovitz H, Leibovitz A, Madar Z, et al: Blood glucose and lipid levels following chromium supplementation in diabetic elderly patients on a rehabilitation program. Presented at Annual Meeting of the Gerontological Society of America, Chicago, Ill, November 18, 2000.

22. Harland BF, Harden-Williams BA: Is vanadium of human nutritional importance yet? J Am Diet Assoc 94(8):891–894, 1994.

23. Cohen N, Halberstam M, Shlimovich P, et al: Oral vanadyl sulfate improves hepatic and peripheral insulin sensitivity in patients with non-insulin-dependent diabetes mellitus. J Clin Invest 95:2501–2509, 1995.

24. Halberstam M, Cohen N, Shlimovich P, et al: Oral vanadyl sulfate improves insulin sensitivity in NIDDM but not in obese nondiabetic subjects. Diabetes 45:659–666, 1996.

25. Cusi K, DeFronzo RA, Torres M, et al: Vanadyl sulfate improves hepatic and muscle insulin sensitivity in type 2 diabetes. J Clin Endocrinol Metab 86:1410–1417, 2001.

26. Jacob S, Henriksen EJ, Tritschler HJ, et al: Enhancement of glucose disposal in patients with type 2 diabetes by alpha-lipoic acid. Arzneimittelforschung 45:872–874, 1995.

27. Jacob S, Henriksen EJ, Tritschler HJ, et al: Improvement of insulin-stimulated glucose disposal in type 2 diabetes after repeated parenteral administratioin of thioctic acid. Exp Clin Endocrinol Diabetes 104:284–288, 1996.

28. Jacob S, Ruus P, Hermann R, et al: Oral administration of RAC-alpha-lipoic acid modulates insulin sensitivity in patients with type-2 diabetes mellitus: A placebo controlled pilot trial. Free Radical Biol Med 27:309–314, 1999.

29. Konrad T, Vicini P, Kusterer K, et al: Alpha-Lipoic acid treatment decreases serum lactate and pyruvate concentrations and improves glucose effectiveness in lean and obese patients with type 2 diabetes. Diabetes Care 22:280–287, 1999.

30. Vuksan V, Sievenpiper JL, Koo VYY, et al: American Ginseng (Panax quinquefolius) reduces postprandial glycemia in nondiabetic subjects and subjects with type 2 diabetes mellitus. Arch Intern Med 160:1009–1013, 2000.

31. Sauvaire Y, Petit P, Broca C, et al: 4-Hydroxyisoleucine. A novel amino acid potentiator of insulin secretion. Diabetes 47:206–210, 1998.

32. Jellin JM, Batz F, Hitchens K: Pharmacist's Letter/Prescriber's Letter. Natural Medicines Comprehensive Database. Stockton, Calif, Therapeutic Research Faculty, 1999, pp 374–375.

33. Piatti P, Monti LD, Valsecchi G, et al: Long-term oral L-arginine administration improves peripheral and hepatic insulin sensitivity in type 2 diabetic patients. Diabetes Care 24:875–880, 2001.

CHAPTER 27

Diabetes Mellitus

Victor S. Sierpina, M.D.

PATHOPHYSIOLOGY

Diabetes mellitus (DM) lies at one end of a spectrum of diseases (Table 27–1) that includes glucose intolerance, hyperinsulinism, and insulin resistance (see Chapter 26, Insulin Resistance Syndrome). It is strongly associated with obesity and certain familial factors and is particularly prevalent in cultural or ethnic groups such as Hispanics, blacks, and Native Americans. Life style factors figure prominently in the development of DM, although type 1 (insulin-dependent) DM is thought to be due to infectious or immunologic factors. Classic clinical symptoms are polydipsia, polyphagia, and polyuria; other presenting signs and symptoms may include fatigue, diarrhea, visual symptoms, dizziness, and headache.

The pathophysiologic basis for diabetes is not merely the insufficient production of insulin but also the resistance of peripheral receptors to insulin. The main effector of glucose transport into the cell is GLUT-4; this protein is a key cellular and cytoplasmic component that controls the movement of glucose across the cellular membrane and regulates the body's response to insulin. Exercise is helpful in the management of diabetes because it promotes insulin transport across the cell membranes by stimulating GLUT-4, 90% of which is embedded in the cytoplasm, to become active by embedding in the cell membrane. Insulin also stimulates this movement, but when this mechanism is impaired by such cytokines as tumor necrosis factor-alpha (TNF-α), insulin resistance results. Another intracellular component of the insulin-signaling pathway involves peroxisome proliferator-activator receptors (PPARs), which are nuclear hormone receptor transcription factors. They induce the expression of target genes that regulate lipid homeostasis and insulin action. Defects in the insulin receptor–signaling pathway diminish insulin action, contributing to insulin resistance and, subsequently, to the development of diabetes. The resistance to insulin at the tissue level exhausts the ability of pancreatic beta cells to secrete adequate insulin output.[1]

A variety of alternative therapies are considered useful in DM (Table 27–2). However, the clinician must keep in mind the severe consequences of diabetes in the untreated state: retinopathy and blindness, coronary artery disease, renal failure, peripheral neuropathy, and vasculopathy resulting in chronic ulceration, gangrene, or amputation. As with other life-threatening conditions, the standard of care for DM requires that the practitioner adhere to proven treatments as alternative therapies are integrated. The standard of care includes pharmacologic treatment when necessary to maintain euglycemia. Several randomized controlled trials and systematic analyses have shown the benefits of improving both blood glucose levels and glycohemoglobin.[2–5] Furthermore, it was recently reported that reductions in the cost of care result from improved glycemic control.[6]

This chapter focuses primarily on type 2 non–insulin dependent diabetes; however, many of the treatments discussed are applicable to both type 1 and type 2 diabetes, although there are significant differences between the conditions (Table 27–3).

INTEGRATIVE THERAPY

Lifestyle Interventions

Diet

Because obesity is a common contributing factor in diabetes, addressing diet is essential. In addition to maintaining a low-fat diet rich in complex carbohydrates, fruits, and vegetables, a weight control and exercise program, usually involving a restriction of calories, is generally required.

The ratio and types of carbohydrates, protein, and fat constitute a crucial factor. Although most diabetic diets recommend reducing the amount of carbohydrate, Dr. James Anderson has proposed a high-carbohydrate, high-plant-fiber diet based on cereal grains, legumes, and root vegetables that restricts simple sugars and fat. This diet consists of 70% to 75% complex carbohydrates, 15% to 20% protein, and 10%

Table 27–1. The Diabetes Spectrum

Glucose intolerance $\longrightarrow$ insulin resistance $\longrightarrow$ syndrome X $\longrightarrow$ type 2 diabetes $\longrightarrow$ medical consequences

Pathologic change in:
- Heart
- Kidney
- Nerves
- Eyes
- Vascular system
- Accelerated aging

Table 27–2. Alternative Therapies for Diabetes

Therapy	Best Evidence*	Probably Useful†	Least Evidence‡
Herbals		Atremsia herba-alba Bilberry (*Vaccinium myrtillus*) for retinopathy: 80–160 mg tid Bitter melon (*Momordica charantia*) 30–60 mL of juice qd *Coccinia indica* *Gymnema sylvestre* 200 mg bid *Ginkgo biloba* for retinopathy, neuropathy, and vascular complications: 40 mg tid Gralic Green tea (*Camellia sinensis*): 2 c qd *Trigonella foenumgraecum*	Artichoke Dandelion leaves Eleutherococcus fenugreek (*Trigonella foenumgraecum*): 50 g qd defatted seed powder Ginseng: 100 mg tid Glucomannan Guar gum Horehound Juniper Lavender Myrrh Neem Primrose oil (neuropathy) Salt bush (*Atriplex halimu*) Silymarin, for cirrhosis in diabetes Spanish needles (*Bidens pilosa*) Tragacanth Yellow bells (*Tecoma stans*)

Diet and nutrition, lifestyle interventions	Regular exercise
	Weight loss
	Diet high in fiber, low in simple sugars and fats
	Pritikin diet
	Ornish diet
		Alpha-lipoic acid
		Biotin: 9 or 16 mg qd in both NIDDM and IDDM
		Chromium: 200 μg qd
		Essential fatty acids
		  Dietary: cold-water fish
		  Supplements: 480 mg qd GLA, 1 tbsp qd flaxseed oil
		Magnesium (300–500 mg qd)
		Onions
		Potassium: dietary
		Vitamin C: >2 g qd in divided doses
		Vitamin B_3, for type 1 prevention: 25 mg/kg/d
		Inositol hexaniacinate: 500–1000 mg qd for hyperlipidemia
		Vitamin B_6, 150 mg qd for neuropathy:
		Vitamin B_{12}: 1000–3000 μg qd PO
		  For neuropathy: 1000 μg/wk IM
		Vitamin E: 800–900 IU qd
		Zinc: 30 mg qd
			Flavonoids: dietary, 1–2 qd
			Manganese: 30 mg/qd

Mind-body interventions	Self-care, personal locus of control and responsibility	Biofeedback Reduction of threat of DM (adolescents) Relaxation therapy Social support Spiritual approaches Yoga	Depression, treat Qi gong
Bioelectromagnetic therapies Alternative systems of care		Therapeutic touch Acupuncture (neuropathy) Traditional Chinese medicine	Electrical stimulation Ayurveda Curanderismo Herbalism
Hands-on healing techniques			Massage

* Therapies are those that have the highest degree of scientific support for efficacy and safety.
† Therapies are often helpful, but degree of support for efficacy and safety is less.
‡ Therapies may be useful, but the practitioner needs to be aware that scientific evidence for efficacy and safety is limited.

Adapted from Sierpina VS: Integrative Health Care: Complementary and Alternative Therapies, for the Whole Person. Philadelphia, FA Davis, 2001, pp. 286–287, with permission.

DM, diabetes mellitus: GLA, gamma-linolenic acid; IDDM, insulin-dependent diabetes mellitus; NIDDM, non–insulin-dependent diabetes mellitus.

Table 27–3. Comparison of Type I and Type 2 Diabetes

Feature	Type 1	Type 2
Age at onset	Usually under 40	Usually over 40
Percentage of all diabetics	Less than 10%	Greater than 90%
Seasonal trend	Fall and winter	None
Family history	Uncommon	Common
Appearance of symptoms	Rapid	Slow
Obesity at onset	Uncommon	Common
Insulin levels	Decreased	Variable
Insulin resistance	Occasional	Often
Treatment with insulin	Always	Not required
Beta cells	Decreased	Variable
Ketoacidosis	Frequent	Rare
Complications	Frequent	Frequent

From Murray, MT, Pizzorno, JE: Diabetes mellitus. In Pizzorno JE, Murray MT (eds): Textbook of Natural Medicine. Edinburgh, Churchill Livingstone, 1999, p.1194.

to 25% fat, with a total fiber content of nearly 100 g a day.[8] This diet has many similarities to the Ornish program[9] but may be hard to follow for the average patient because it is a vegetarian diet. In general, vegetarian diets are highly beneficial to diabetics who are willing to follow them, as they are low in fat, high in fiber, and high in carotenoids and other antioxidants. Perhaps the world's most healthful diet, is the Mediterranean diet. I recommend this for my diabetic patients, especially obese ones, because of its emphasis on vegetables, grains, fish, and olive oil. Olive oil is a healthful form of monounsaturated fat that reduces the risk of atherosclerosis in diabetics, who are at very high risk for this condition as well as for resulting coronary artery disease.[10–12]

A more commonly prescribed diet that gives a proper ratio of macronutrients for diabetics is a modified high-fiber diet:

- Carbohydrates 40% to 50%
- Protein 20% to 30%
- Fat 20% to 30%

Most diabetics know not to eat "sweets." However, what they really need to understand is that eating foods with a high glycemic index—such as simple sugars, white bread and flour, other sweets, juices, sugar-containing sodas, and many processed foods (see Chapter 83, The Glycemic Index)—also creates problems. These foods are very rapidly digested, causing a surge in glucose and insulin. Low-glycemic-index foods are those high in fiber—abundant in whole grains, legumes, vegetables, and fruits—and are most likely to modulate swings in blood sugar and insulin secretion because they are absorbed more slowly. The fructose in fruit does not cause the kind of rapid rise in glucose level produced by sucrose.[13] High fiber also binds cholesterol in the gut, reducing its harmful effects of accelerating atherogenesis.

Garlic, onions, and green tea all have been shown to have beneficial effects in diabetes. Garlic (*Allium sativum*) and onion (*Allium cepa*) lower blood glucose, cholesterol, and blood pressure, suggesting their increased usefulness as a component of cooking and diet in diabetics.[14, 15] Green tea (*Camellia sinensis*) contains potent polyphenols, which have

significant antioxidant effects and immune-enhancing benefits; consumption of two cups or more per day is a rational and refreshing addition to a diabetic dietary plan.[16]

Fiber

Specific kinds of fiber such as psyllium, guar gum, pectin, and oat bran may be very useful in persons who cannot afford or are unable to chew or otherwise tolerate a high-vegetable/fruit diet, with at least five to seven servings a day. Beans and peas are the legumes with the highest protein and fiber content and are recommended in diabetes. Making breakfast a high-fiber meal instead of a high-fat one is a healthful start to the day and is best accomplished by including high-fiber cereals such as oats. All-Bran is the breakfast cereal with the highest fiber content, although adding a tablespoon or two of bulk bran (available at health food stores) to any other breakfast cereal, to low-fat yogurt, or to home-baked breads, casseroles, and other meals accomplishes much the same in enhancing fiber content.

The standard American diet (SAD) results in stools that are denser and significantly less bulky than stools produced by a high-roughage diet, as is typically consumed in Third World countries.[17] Persons indigenous to such "undeveloped countries" produce more than 2 pounds a day of bulky stool made up mostly of roughage and indigestible cellulose, whereas the SAD diet creates less than 1 pound per day of stool on average. A low-fiber diet thus not only is contributory to diabetes but is also a risk factor for the development of colon cancer, high cholesterol, hemorrhoids, and diverticulosis.

Exercise

The benefits of regular physical activity in the management of diabetes are well known:[18]

- Enhanced insulin sensitivity with a consequent diminished need for exogenous insulin

- Improved glucose tolerance
- Reduced total serum cholesterol and triglycerides with increased high-density lipoprotein levels, resulting in a more antiatherogenic state
- Improved weight loss (in obese diabetic patients)

In addition, adding muscle mass through such activities as weight lifting increases the metabolic rate and assists in weight loss, as well as stabilizing metabolic parameters, including glucose control.[19, 20]

Mind-Body Therapy

Emphasizing issues of self-care and personal responsibility for health is essential in the management of diabetes, as with any chronic disease. Because diabetic patients, particularly adolescents, often feel out of control of their bodies because of the vagaries of their disease, encouraging a personal locus of control and responsibility has clearly promoted improved glycemic control.[21] Managing stress effectively can reduce the surges in the stress hormones epinephrine and cortisol, which cause increased blood glucose levels. Such modalities as meditation, relaxation techniques, and biofeedback training all have been used to manage stress effectively and are applicable in diabetics[22] (see Chapter 91, Prescribing Relaxation Techniques).

Other stress management measures include identification or exploration of sources of social support, which improves hardiness in a stressful environment or in the case of a stressful condition such as diabetes. Prayer, yoga exercise, Qi gong, and the treatment of depression all have a place in managing diabetes. Multiple studies have shown that prayer and spiritual practice improve mental and physical health outcomes.[23, 24]

Supplements

Alpha-Lipoic Acid

Alpha-lipoic acid is a potent antioxidant. It enhances glucose uptake, prevents glycosylation, and can be useful in diabetic neuropathy. It has been used to treat pain in DM-associated neuropathy in doses of approximately 800 mg daily.[25] It is present in red meats and other mitochondria-containing foods.

Dosage. 600–800 mg daily.
Precaution. No adverse effects have been reported.

Biotin

Biotin, a water-soluble B vitamin, is a coenzyme active in the digestion of carbohydrates and also fats and protein. Dietary deficiency of biotin is rare (the recommended dietary allowance [RDA] is about 30 μg per day), as it not only is common in many foods such as oatmeal, nuts, mushrooms, and bananas but is produced in substantial quantities by gut bacteria. High doses of 8 to 16 mg per day have been reported to be helpful in regulating blood glucose and in preventing neuropathy.[26, 27]

Dosage. 8 to 16 mg daily.
Precautions. No allergies or adverse reactions have been reported.

Chromium

Chromium is widely used in non–insulin-dependent DM (NIDDM) and seems to improve glucose control in at least some patients with diabetes by facilitating uptake of glucose into the cells. Chromium in the picolinate form is also marketed as a weight loss aid, a claim for which I remain skeptical. It has been shown in a recent large study to decrease glycosylated hemoglobin, fasting and postprandial blood sugar, and insulin and cholesterol levels.[28] Some reports support its use in decreasing cholesterol and triglyceride levels as well as in enhancing glucose control.[29] In addition to the scrapings of chromium from pots and pans, it also is present in wheat germ, whole grains, brewer's yeast, and meats.

Dosage. 200 to 400 μg daily.
Precautions. Toxic levels can result in cognitive, perceptual, and motor dysfunction.

Essential Fatty Acids

Omega-3 and omega-6 fatty acids can be useful in the management of diabetes by protecting against neuropathy and atherosclerotic damage, as well as by augmenting insulin secretion and improving lipid status.[30, 31] Sources of omega-3 fatty acids include fish such as mackerel, herring, salmon, and halibut and also oils such as flaxseed oil. Sources of omega-6 fatty acids include evening primrose, borage, and black currant.

Inositol Hexaniacinate

Inositol hexaniacinate is a helpful agent for lowering cholesterol. Because it is composed of a six-sided inositol ring with six attached niacin molecules (vitamin B_3), many patients do not experience the flushing of the skin, gastrointestinal irritation, and hepatotoxicity of regular niacin. In doses of 1500 to 3000 mg per day it can significantly lower lipid levels.[32]

Dosage. Start with 500 to 1500 mg daily; increase up to 3000 mg a day for cholesterol control.
Precautions. In some patients, diabetic control may worsen with any form of niacin. In such cases, discontinuing treatment may become necessary.

Magnesium

Magnesium deficiency is common among diabetics, and supplementation may prevent diabetic complications. Magnesium is essential in glucose metabolism, and diabetics may need twice the RDA of 300 to 350 mg per day.[33] Food sources are green leafy vegetables, legumes, whole grains, molasses, nuts, seeds, and chocolate.

Dosage. 300 to 700 mg daily.

Precautions. Diarrhea and gastrointestinal intolerance are potential adverse effects.

Manganese

An important antioxidant, manganese is a cofactor in many glucose metabolic pathways. Food sources are nuts, legumes, tea, and coffee.

Dosage. At least 30 mg a day should be given as a supplementation in diabetics.[34]

Precautions. Manganese supplements can darken mucosal pigmentation and cause hypersensitivity reactions.

Vanadium

Vanadium has been shown to improve insulin sensitivity.[35] It is ubiquitous in foods but is present in only trace amounts.

Dosage. 50 to 100 mg per day.

Precautions. Vanadium supplements can cause gastrointestinal distress and green discoloration of the tongue. Long-term safety of high-dose vanadium has not been established.

Vitamin B$_6$

Because of its benefits in diabetic neuropathy, vitamin B$_6$ (pyridoxide) is an essential part of any diabetic management program. Rather than waiting for neuropathy to occur, prophylactic treatment with 50 to 100 mg a day seems the wise course.[36] Vitamin B$_6$ occurs in bananas, wheat germ, meat, fish, potatoes, brewer's yeast, and fortified breakfast cereals.

Dosage. 50 to 150 mg a day.

Precautions. Large doses in the range of 500 mg per day may actually cause neuropathy that is irreversible and indistinguishable from the neuropathy of DM.

Vitamin B$_{12}$

I use vitamin B$_{12}$ in the treatment of diabetic neuropathy in a dose of 1000 to 3000 μg per day orally or in the injectable form, with moderate success. I generally combine it with vitamin B$_6$ at 100 mg a day in established neuropathy. Vitamin B$_{12}$ deficiency may be implicated in DM retinopathy as well.[37] Vitamin B$_{12}$ comes from meat and animal products, including dairy, eggs, and fish. Patients who are vegans are more prone to vitamin B$_{12}$ deficiency and may need regular supplements.

Dosage. 1000 to 3000 μg daily a day orally or 1000 μg intramuscularly (IM) or subcutaneously (SC) each week.

Precautions. Vitamin C inactivates B$_{12}$; therefore, they should not be taken together. Oral vitamin B$_{12}$ can cause diarrhea, itching, urticaria, and a subjective feeling of generalized swelling of the body.

Vitamin C

The emperor of all vitamins, vitamin C (ascorbic acid) is essential to the treatment of diabetes. Although the RDA is now considered to be 50 to 60 mg or perhaps as high as 200 mg, much higher doses are necessary in DM to offset the marked acceleration of atherosclerosis and oxidative damage from this disease. Vitamin C is essential to collagen production, wound healing, and immunity, all of which are impaired in DM. Transport of vitamin C is facilitated by insulin; therefore, higher than normal doses are necessary to prevent a chronic, occult deficiency.[38] Natural sources are citrus fruits, melons, berries, broccoli, peppers, and many other fruits and vegetables.

Dosage. A dose of at least 1 to 2 g a day or even higher is recommended to prevent sorbitol accumulation in the red blood cells of diabetics and to inhibit protein glycosylation.[39, 40]

Vitamin E

Vitamin E is helpful in preventing the long-term complications of DM through its synergistic antioxidant effects with vitamin C, improvement of insulin action, and decrease in oxidation of LDL cholesterol.[41] Food sources include wheat germ, seeds, nuts, plant oils, and dark green leafy vegetables.

Dosage. A dose of at least 800 IU a day is recommended for every diabetic.

Zinc

Zinc is excreted in higher than normal amounts in the urine in diabetics, leading to a relative deficiency. Because of the difficulty diabetics have with wound healing, I also recommend regular zinc supplementation. Zinc is an essential factor in skin and wound healing and in immune function and also has been found to improve insulin levels in diabetics.[42, 43] Food sources are oysters, lean meats, dark meat of turkey, beans, almonds, and leavened whole-grain baked goods.

Dosage. 15 to 40 mg of zinc a day.

Precautions. Because zinc can affect copper absorption, 1 to 2 mg daily of copper, usually in a multivitamin, is recommended for anyone receiving regular zinc supplementation.

Botanicals

As seen in Table 27–2, a variety of botanical agents are used in diabetes. Others not listed here are culturally derived, such as *nopales*, or the prickly pear cactus, used as a food and hypoglycemic agent by persons of Hispanic heritage. Practitioners need to be aware that people of specific cultural or ethnic groups may use traditional herbal foods and plant agents that can significantly lower blood glucose. These medicines may interact with agents used in standard therapy.

Although I prefer the use of supplements to the use of botanicals in diabetes, the following herbal therapies are those I believe to be most useful.

Bilberry

Best known for its beneficial effects in diarrhea and eye disease, bilberry (*Vaccinium myrtillus*) contains anthocyanosides, which are beneficial in diabetics. These chemicals increase intracellular vitamin C levels, act as powerful antioxidants, stabilize capillary membranes, and improve circulation to the retina.[44]

Dosage. The usual dose is 80 to 160 mg three times daily.

Bitter Melon

Bitter melon (*Momordica charantia*), also known as balsam pear, is a gourdlike vegetable used in folk medicine for diabetes. It contains several insulin-like polypeptides, charantin, and alkaloids that lower glucose levels. It is usually available at health food stores or Asian grocery stores. A number of clinical and preclinical trials have documented its hypoglycemic effects in diabetes.[45]

Dosage. The usual dose of this bitter juice is 57 g taken on a daily basis.

Gymnema

Gymnema (*Gymnema sylvestre*) is a traditional botanical used in Ayurvedic practice as a diabetic agent. It has been found to lower glucose levels and is thought to increase insulin secretion and to enhance its action. Studies in animals and humans suggest its ability to help regenerate beta cells in the pancreas.[46] It may allow diabetics to reduce their insulin dose and has hypoglycemic effects in non–insulin-dependent diabetics as well.[47] Gurmarin and gymnemic acid block the ability of humans to taste sweets; this effect would be expected to influence dietary habits as well.

Dosage. 400 mg daily in two divided doses.

Ginkgo biloba

Ginkgo biloba is an extract from the leaves of the world's oldest species of tree. The active flavonoid glycosides and terpene lactones function as antioxidants, free radical scavengers, and membrane stabilizers and also inhibit platelet activating factor. In addition, they protect nerve cells and improve vascular function. Although ginkgo is generally recommended for cerebrovascular insufficiency, its primary application in diabetes is for intermittent claudication and peripheral vascular disease.[48] I also recommend the use of ginkgo to help protect retinal function, to prevent small vessel disease, and to protect against both central and peripheral neuronal damage.

Dosage. 40 to 80 mg of extract three times daily, standardized to 24% flavonoid glycosides and 6% terpene lactones.

Precautions. Ginkgo should be avoided in patients receiving warfarin or those who are at risk of bleeding. Despite this potential risk, there are surprisingly few case reports of bleeding complications. Ginkgo can also cause gastrointestinal distress, headache, dizziness, palpitations, and allergic skin reactions.

Pharmaceuticals

Although this chapter is devoted primarily to exploring the alternative therapies useful in diabetes, a brief summary of standard pharmacotherapy is needed to help round out the concept of integrative care. Close monitoring of blood glucose, glycohemoglobin, lipids and renal function is essential to management of diabetes whether alternative approaches, conventional medications, or both are used. Just because a patient prefers an alternative therapy, if the clinical response to that therapy is suboptimal, the pathologic implications of diabetes are severe enough to merit the inclusion of standard pharmacologic agents. In the late 1970s and early 1980s, available options for the treatment of diabetes were much fewer than today. Insulin and a limited spectrum of oral hypoglycemics in that era have been expanded dramatically in recent years. These are described in summary form below.

Alpha-Glucosidase Inhibitors

I do not use alpha-glucosidase inhibitors much because of their side effect profile. Because they block absorption of glucose from the gut, they may be useful in patients who experience postprandial hyperglycemic spikes. However, these agents have significant side effects, including diarrhea, nausea, and flatulence.

Dosage
- Acorbose (Precose): 50 to 100 mg tid
- Miglitol (Glyset): 50 mg tid

Give both with the first bite of each meal. Start with a low dose and increase as tolerated.

Sulfonylureas

Sulfonylureas are most commonly used for treatment of type 2 diabetes. These agents reduce glucose by enhancing insulin secretion. In my experience, doses higher than 10 mg per day of these agents rarely improve glucose control dramatically.

A newer agent in this class, glimepiride, does not induce hypoglycemia, as do the other sulfonylureas, and has favorable effects on the cardiovascular system.

Dosage
- Glyburide (DiaBeta, Micronase): 1.25 to 20 mg a day
- Micronized glyburide (Glynase PresTab): 0.75 to 12 mg qd or bid
- Glipizide (Glucotrol): 2.5 to 40 mg a day
- Glimepiride (Amaryl): 1 to 8 mg a day

Biguanides

One of the most useful and popular diabetic drugs to come out in the past decade, metformin has the benefit of not causing hypoglycemia. It reduces hepatic glucose production and should be considered the agent of choice in obese diabetics and in patients with dyslipidemias. It can be used as a single agent or added to sulfonylureas when these have been inadequately given as monotherapy. A newer formulation that combines both glyburide and metformin, Glucovance, is now available.

Dosage
- Metformin (Glucophage): 500 mg to 2.5 g a day in divided doses, or Glucophage XR500 mg to 2 g in a single dose or in two divided doses
- Metformin/glyburide (Glucovance): 1.25 mg of glyburide plus 250 mg of metformin; maximum of 20 mg/2000 mg of the two drugs per day in divided doses

Precautions. Metformin can be a cause of lactic acidosis and should therefore be avoided in patients with renal insufficiency or congestive heart failure.

Insulin

Standard therapy for type 1 diabetes and insulin-requiring type 2 diabetes, insulin can be used in combination with any oral agent although it is most often given in a single or twice-daily dose. The most popular and useful variety of insulin now is Humulin 70/30, which combines 70% lente and 30% regular insulin, both manufactured using human recombinant DNA methods. With this variety of insulin, two thirds of the daily dose is usually given in the morning and one third in the evening, though dosing varies widely among individuals. There are several varieties of both lente and regular insulin; the usual onset of action of lente is at 1 to 2 hours, with peak action between 6 and 12 hours, and for regular insulin, onset of action at $\frac{1}{2}$ hour and peak between 2 and 4 hours. A newer agent called Humalog is an insulin analogue with a very rapid onset of action of less than 15 minutes, so it can be taken right at mealtime, with peak action at 1 hour and duration of action of 3.5 to 4.5 hours. An extended zinc suspension, Humulin Ultralente, has a slow onset of action at 4 to 6 hours and lasts 8 to 20 hours.

All forms of insulin are given by subcutaneous injection, a step that many patients resist. However, education and reassurance are usually adequate to encourage the diabetic who needs to begin an injection regimen. Insulin pumps, which deliver a baseline coverage of insulin continuously along with mealtime boluses of insulin, have added an option to the control of brittle or hard to manage diabetes. If the use of Humulin 70/30 in divided doses fails to provide good control of the patient's diabetes, a consultation with an endocrinology colleague specializing in diabetes is recommended to optimize the patient's treatment program.

Meglitinides

Meglitinides can be used alone or with metformin, but not with sulfonylureas, and must be used carefully in patients with hepatic or renal dysfunction. These agents stimulate insulin secretion from the pancreatic cells in a different manner from that of sulfonylureas.

Dosage
- Repaglinide (Prandin): 0.5 to 5 mg before meals and two to four times a day; maximum daily dose: 16 mg
- Nateglinide (Starlix): 120 mg before meals three times a day

Thiazolidinediones

Thiazolidinediones reduce glucose levels by increasing sensitivity to glucose at the cellular level via their mechanism of binding to nuclear receptors. One drug in this class, troglitazone (Rezulin), has been taken off the market because of its potential for serious adverse effects on the liver. However, several other agents are available. All are moderately to quite expensive.

Dosage
- Pioglitazone (Actos) 15 to 30 mg a day; maximum daily dose: 45 mg
- Rosiglitazone (Avandia): 4 to 8 mg in a single or two divided doses

Standard texts go into further detail, but for an excellent summary of standard pharmacotherapy for diabetes, see the *Saunders Manual of Medical Practice*.[49] All dosing information is from the *Monthly Prescribing Reference*.[50]

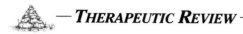 ── *THERAPEUTIC REVIEW* ──────────────

The treatment of DM calls for the highest skills of the clinician. Not only does suboptimally treated diabetes pose a risk of an acute serious complication such as diabetic ketoacidosis, nonketotic hyperosmolar coma, or other major metabolic abnormality, persistent hyperglycemia is a silent killer. It gradually damages cells, organs, and vascular systems, eventuating in severe impairment in the quality of life. The skilled clinician will therefore use a variety of conventional and alternative therapies that, combined in an integrative model, offer the best chance for the patient to lead as normal a life as possible despite a challenging disease.

Diet
- *Weight loss*
- *Complex carbohydrates; high-fiber/low-fat, Mediterranean, or other vegetarian or semivegetarian diet*
- *Green tea, onions, garlic*

Supplements
- *Vitamin C: 1 g each day*
- *Vitamin E (alpha-tocopherol): 800 IU each day*
- *Vitamin B$_6$ (pyridoxine): 50 to 150 mg each day*
- *Chromium: 200 to 400 μg a day*
- *Magnesium: 300 to 700 mg a day*
- *Zinc: 15 to 40 mg each day*

Botanicals
For retinal problems:
- *Bilberry: 80 to 160 mg 3 times daily*

For vasculopathy:
- *Ginkgo: 40 to 80 mg tid standardized to 24% flavonoid glycosides and 6% terpene lactones*

Mind-Body Medicine
- *Relaxation and stress management*
- *Encouraging personal locus of control and responsibility*
- *Yoga, tai chi, and other Asian exercise disciplines for both mental and physical conditioning*

Exercise
- *Regular daily program including an aerobic exercise such as swimming, cycling, or running*

Pharmaceuticals
- *Conventional drugs are often necessary in combination with these therapies.*

References

1. Linker L: Syndrome X. Paper presented at The Art, Science, and Practice of Holistic Medicine. Denver, December 5, 2000.
2. Herman W and the UK Prospective Diabetes Study Group: Glycaemic control in diabetes. In Clinical Evidence, issue 4. London, BMJ Publishing Group, 2000, pp 320–327.
3. UK Prospective Diabetes Study Group: Quality of life in type 2 diabetic patients is affected by complications but not by intensive policies to improve blood glucose or blood pressure control (UKPDS 37). Diabetes Care 22:1125–1136, 1999.
4. Diabetes Control and Complications Trial Research Group: The absence of a glycaemic threshold for the development of long-term complications: The perspective of the diabetes control and complications trial. Diabetes 45:1289–1298, 1996.
5. UK Prospective Diabetes Study Group: Intensive blood-glucose control with sulphonylureas or insulin compared with conventional treatment and risk of complications in patients with type 2 diabetes. Lancet 353:837–853, 1998.
6. Wagner EH, Sandhu N, Newton KM, et al: Effect of improved glycemic control of health care costs and utilization. JAMA 285:182–189, 2001.
7. Vague P: Nicotinamide may extend remission phase in insulin-dependent diabetes. Lancet 1:619–620, 1987.
8. Murray MT, Pizzorno JE: Diabetes mellitus. In Pizzorno JE, Murray MT (eds): Textbook of Natural Medicine. Edinburgh, Churchill Livingstone, 1999, pp 1203–1204.

9. Kostreski F: Ornish Program to get national test. Fam Pract News 29:1, 5, 1999.
10. De Lorgeril M: Mediterranean alpha-linolenic acid-rich diet in secondary prevention of coronary heart disease. Lancet 343:1454, 1994.
11. De Lorgeril M: Mediterranean dietary pattern in a randomized trial: Prolonged survival and possible reduced cancer rate. Arch Intern Med 158:181–187, 1998.
12. Jossa F: The Mediterranean diet in the prevention of arteriosclerosis. Recent Prog Med 87:175–181, 1996.
13. Koivisto VA, Kyki-Jarvinen H: Fructose and insulin sensitivity in patients with type 2 diabetes. J Intern Med 233:145–153, 1993.
14. Sharma KK, Gupta RK, Gupta S, et al: Antihyperglycemic effect of onion: Effect on fasting blood sugar and induced hyperglycemia in man. Indian J Med Res 65:422–429, 1977.
15. Sheela CG, Augusti KT: Antidiabetic effects of S-allyl cysteine sulphoxide isolated from garlic (*Allium sativum*). Indian J Exp Biol 30:523–526, 1992.
16. McKenna DJ, Hughes K, Jones K: Green tea [monograph]. Altern Ther 6:61–82, 2000.
17. Ardell D: Wellness promotion. Paper presented at the 34th Annual University of Texas Medical Branch Family Practice Review Course. Galveston, Tex, May 2000.
18. Murray MT, Pizzorno JE: Diabetes mellitus. In Pizzorno JE, Murray MT (eds): Textbook of Natural Medicine, Edinburgh, Churchill Livingstone, 1999, p 1215.
19. Wallace MB, Mills BD, Browning CL: Effects of cross-training on markers of insulin resistance/hyperinsulinemia. Med Sci Sports Exerc 29:1170–1175, 1997.
20. Huddleson JS: Living with heart disease and diabetes: Exercise can help. In Benson H, Stuart E (eds): The Wellness Book: The Comprehensive Guide to Maintaining Health and Treating Stress-Related Illness. New York, Simon & Schuster, 1992, pp 412–420.
21. Burroughs TE: Research on social support in adolescents with IDDM. Diabetes Educ 23:438, 1997.
22. Stuart EM, Webster A, Wells-Federman, CL: Managing stress. In Benson H, Stuart E (eds): The Wellness Book: The Comprehensive Guide to Maintaining Health and Treating Stress-Related Illness. New York, Simon & Schuster, 1992, pp 177–188.
23. Meisenhelder JB, Chandler EN: Prayer and health outcomes in church members. Altern Ther Health Med 6:56–60, 2000.
24. Matthews DA, Larson DB, Barry C: The Faith Factor, vol III: An Annotated Bibliography of Clinical Research on Spiritual Studies. NIHR, 1995.
25. Ziegler D, Ulrich H, Schatz H, et al: Effect of treatment with the anti-oxidant alpha-lipoic acid on cardiac autonomic neuropathy in patients with NIDDM. Diabetes Care 20:369–373, 1997.
26. Coggeshall JC: Biotin status and plasma glucose in diabetics. Ann N Y Acad Sci 447:389, 1985.
27. Koutsikos D, Agroyannis B, Tzanatos-Exarchou H: Biotin for diabetic peripheral neuropathy. Biomed Pharmacother 44:511–514, 1990.
28. Anderson R, Cheng N, Bryden N, et al: Beneficial effect of chromium for people with type II diabetes. Diabetes 45 (Suppl):124A, 1996.
29. Baker B: Chromium supplements tied to glucose control. Fam Pract News 15:5, 1996.
30. Keen H, Payan J, Allawi J: Treatment of diabetic neuropathy with gamma-linolenic acid. Diabetes Care 16:8–13, 1993.
31. Schmidt EB, Cyerberg J: Omega-3 fatty acids. Current status in cardiovascular medicine. Drugs 47:405–424, 1994.
32. El-Enein AMA, Hafez YS, Salem H, et al: The role of nicotinic acid and inositol hexaniacinate as anticholesterolemic and anitlipemic agents. Nutr Rep Intl 28:899–911, 1983.
33. White JR, Campbell RK: Magnesium and diabetes. A review. Ann Pharmacother 27:775–780, 1993.
34. Wimhurst JM, Manchester KL: Comparison of ability of Mg and Mn to activate the key enzymes of glycolysis. FEBS Lett 27:321–326, 1972.
35. Halberstam M: Oral vanadyl sulfate improves insulin sensitivity in NIDDM but not in obese nondiabetic subjects. Diabetes 45:659–666, 1996.
36. Jones CL, Gonzalex V: Pyridoxine deficiency: A new factor in diabetic neuropathy. J Am Podiatr Med Assoc 68:646–653, 1978.
37. Bhatt HR, Linnell JC, Matt DM: Can faulty vitamin B_{12} (cobalamin) metabolism produce diabetic retinopathy? Lancet 2:572, 1983.
38. Cunningham J: Reduced mononuclear leukocyte ascorbic acid content in adults with insulin-dependent diabetes mellitus consuming adequate dietary vitamin C. Metabolism 40:146–149, 1991.
39. Vinson JA, Staretz ME, Bose P: In vitro and in vivo reduction of erythrocyte sorbitol by ascorbic acid. Diabetes 38:1036–1041, 1998.
40. Davie SJ, Gould BJ, Yudkin JS: Effect of vitamin C on glycosylation of proteins. Diabetes 41:167–173, 1992.
41. Paolisso G, D'Amore A, Galzerano D: Daily vitamin E supplements improve metabolic control but not insulin secretion in elderly type II diabetic patients. Diabetes Care 16:1433–1437, 1993.
42. Engel ED, Erlich NE, Davis RH: Diabetes mellitus: Impaired wound healing from zinc deficiency. J Am Podiatr Med Assoc 71:536–544, 1981.
43. Hegazi SM: Effect of zinc supplementation on serum glucose, insulin, glucagon, glucose-6-phosphatase, and mineral levels in diabetics. J Clin Biochem Nutr 12:209–215, 1992.
44. Passariello N, Bisesti V, Sgambato S: Influence of anthocyanosides on the microcirculation and lipid picture in diabetic and dyslipidic subjects. Gass Med Ital 138:563–566, 1979.
45. Srivastava Y, Venkatakrishna-Bhatt H, Verma Y, et al: Antidiabetic and adaptogenic properties of *Momordica charantia* extract. An experimental and clinical evaluation. Phytother Res 7:285–289, 1993.
46. Shanmugasundaram ERB, Leela Gopinath K, Shanmugasundaram KR, et al: Possible regeneration of the islets of Langerhans in streptozotocin diabetic rats fed *Gymnema sylvestre* leaf extracts. J Ethnopharmacol 30:265–279, 1990.
47. Baskaran K, Ahamath BK, Shanmugasundaram KR, et al: Antidiabetic effect of a leaf extract from *Gymnema sylvestre* in non–insulin-dependent diabetes mellitus patients. J Ethnopharmacol 30:295–305, 1990.
48. Bauer U: 6-month double-blind clinical trial of *Ginkgo biloba* extract versus placebo in two parallel groups in patients suffering from peripheral arterial insufficiency. Arzneimittelforschung 34:716–721, 1984.
49. Wilson BE: Diabetes mellitus type II. In Rakel RE (ed): Saunders Manual of Medical Practice. Philadelphia, WB Saunders, pp 833–836, 2000.
50. Monthly Prescribing Reference. New York, Prescribing Reference, Inc, pp 108–119, Feb 2001.

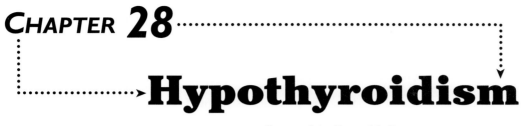

CHAPTER 28

Hypothyroidism

Susan Hadley, M.D.

PATHOPHYSIOLOGY

The thyroid gland regulates metabolism, affecting all body functions. The thyroid gland concentrates iodide (a substrate for thyroid hormone synthesis). Iodide is oxidized to iodine and undergoes organification by iodinating tyrosine residues on thyroglobulin to form monoiodothyronine (MIT) and diiodothyronine (DIT), which couple to form T_4 (thyroxine) and T_3 (triiodothyronine). T_3 and T_4 are released into the circulation. T_4 is produced solely by the thyroid gland; 20% of T_3 is produced by the thyroid gland and 80% is produced by deiodinated T_4. T_3 is considered the more metabolically active. Seventy percent of thyroid hormones circulate bound to thyroxine-binding globulin (TBG); the remainder are free. The patient's metabolic state correlates with the free component. The hypothalamic-pituitary-thyroid axis integrates thyroid metabolism control. Thyrotropin-releasing hormone (TRH), secreted by the hypothalamus, controls the secretion of thyroid-stimulating hormone (TSH), which is secreted by the pituitary gland. TSH response to TRH is regulated by the feedback inhibitory effect of the thyroid hormones.

NOTE

T_3 is considered the most metabolically active thyroid hormone.

Hypothyroidism, or insufficient synthesis of thyroid hormone, can be classified as outlined in the following sections.

Thyroid Gland

Primary

- Thyroprivic (loss of thyroid tissue): Congenital developmental defect (leading to cretinism, or juvenile hypothyroidism), primary idiopathic (usually autoimmune related), radioiodine or postradiation ablation or surgical thyroidectomy.
- Goitrous (inability to synthesize enough thyroid hormone—hypersecretion of TSH and goiter result): Heritable biosynthetic defects, maternally transmitted, iodine deficiency (intrinsic defect in the organic binding system), drug-induced (aminosalicylic acid, iodides, phenylbutazone, iodoantipyrine, lithium, antithyroid medications, amiodarone), chronic thyroiditis (Hashimoto's disease—most common cause of goitrous hypothyroidism in North America—and defective organic binding of iodide and abnormal secretion of iodoproteins are frequent), interleukin-2, and lymphokine-activated killer cells

Suprathyroid (accounts for 5%)

- Secondary: Thyroid intrinsically normal but deprived of stimulation of TSH
- Pituitary: Panhypopituitarism, isolated TSH deficiency, pituitary surgery, or postpartum pituitary necrosis
- Hypothalamic (uncommonly results from inadequate secretion of TRH): Congenital defects, infection (encephalitis), neoplasm, infiltrative type (sarcoidosis)
- Self-limited: After withdrawal of thyroid therapy, subacute thyroiditis and chronic thyroiditis with transient hypothyroidism (usually after a phase of thyrotoxicosis)[1]

CLINICAL PRESENTATION

- Children: Typically delayed growth and delayed mental development
- Adults: Cold intolerance, weight gain or difficulty losing weight, low basal body temperature, dry skin, change in menstrual cycle, constipation, fatigue, and depression

LABORATORY STUDIES IN HYPOTHYROIDISM

The single most useful test in primary hypothyroidism is an elevated TSH. Owing to suppression of TSH in secondary hypothyroidism, a TSH and free T_4 (FT_4) together are diagnostic. Decreases in serum T_4 and FT_4 are common to all varieties of hypothyroidism.

Other laboratory tests to detect hypothyroidism include increased serum cholesterol (only thyroid, not suprathyroid) and increased creatinine phosphokinase, aspartate transaminase, and lactate dehydrogenase. In subclinical hypothyroidism (most often seen with Hashimoto's), serum TSH and its response to TRH are increased, but serum T_4 and T_3 levels are normal. In more advanced thyroid failure, serum T_4 is decreased and T_3 is normal (because TSH-induced hypersecretion of T_3 relative to T_4 can lead to a more efficient conversion of T_4 to T_3).

NOTE

TSH normal—euthyroidism

TSH high—primary hypothyroidism

TSH low—TRH stimulation test:

> *Increased TSH—Primary hypothyroidism*

> *Little or no increase in TSH—pituitary hypothyroidism*

> *Increased, normal, exaggerated, peak delay in TSH—hypothalamic hypothyroidism*

Misdiagnosis of hypothyroidism is outlined in Table 28–1.[2]

SUBCLINICAL HYPOTHYROIDISM

Subclinical hypothyroidism is not uncommon. Patients who have an elevated TSH and a normal free T_4, or even a normal TSH, may still have hypothyroidism as diagnosed by their symptoms. It is reasonable to do a trial of thyroid therapy and watch these patients clinically. Confirm first that there is no risk of cardiovascular disease. Another concern of thyroid replacement is a possible link to osteoporosis (which has not yet been confirmed by studies). If osteoporosis is a concern, checking urine bone metabolites is recommended over doing bone

Table 28–1. Causes of Misdiagnosis of Hypothyroidism

Low serum T_3
Reduced serum thyroxine-binding globulin
  Genetic
  Drug effects: Androgens, glucocorticoids, danazol,
    L-asparaginase, colestipol-niacin
  Nonthyroidal illness
Displacement of T_4 from binding proteins
  Drug effects: Phenytoin, high-dose salicylates, furosemide in
    renal failure, fenclofenac, phenylbutazone
  Nonthyroidal illness
Liothyronine therapy

Elevated serum thyroid-stimulatory hormone
Recovery phase of a nonthyroidal illness
Artifactual due to interfering antimouse immunoglobulin G
  antibodies (rare)

From Rakel RE, Bope ET (eds) Conn's Current Therapy. Philadelphia, WB Saunders, 2001, p 674.

density studies. To start a patient on Armour thyroid for a "trial," the recommended dose is to start with $\frac{1}{4}$ grain (15 mg), and increase by $\frac{1}{4}$ grain (15 mg) every 2 weeks until symptoms improve.

For some patients with equivocal studies or those who do not want laboratory investigation, another useful diagnostic tool is the basal body temperature.

INTEGRATIVE THERAPY

Nutrition

Iodine deficiency in the United States is very rare—yet goiter is high in certain areas. Too much iodine can inhibit thyroid gland synthesis. The recommended daily allowance for iodine is only 150 μg per day; the average intake is typically five to six times this amount. Nature's richest sources of iodine are seaweed, clams, lobsters, oysters, sardines, and other saltwater fish. Some foods contain substances that prevent iodine utilization—for example, turnips, cabbage, mustard, soybeans, cassava root, peanuts, pine nuts, and millet; however, cooking usually inactivates these substances.[3] Although most patients with hypothyroidism will require thyroid replacement, it is important to support the thyroid gland nutritionally. It is also important that enough zinc, vitamin E, vitamin C, vitamin A, and B vitamins—riboflavin (B_2), niacin (B_3), and pyridoxine (B_6)—be consumed. These are best used when they are included in the diet.

Supplements

Zinc Picolinate

Abnormal zinc metabolism has been linked to hypothyroidism.[4]
Dosage. 30 mg each day.

Selenium

Iodothyronine 5′-deiodinase is the main enzyme responsible for peripheral T_3 production; it is a selenium-containing enzyme.[5] It has been shown that reduced peripheral conversion of T_4 to T_3 leads to hypothyroidism—selenium status influences thyroid hormones in the elderly, mainly modulating T_4 levels.[6]
Dosage. 200 to 300 μg daily.

NOTE

Selenium and vitamin C should be taken at separate times because they may interfere with each other's absorption.

Table 28-2. Commonly Prescribed Thyroid Hormone Preparations

Generic Name	Brand Name	Approximate Equivalent Dose	Preparations
Levothyroxine	Synthroid Levothyroid Eltroxin	100 μg	Tablets: 25, 50, 75, 88, 100, 112, 125, 137, 150, 175, 200, 300 μg
Liothyronine	Cytomel	25 μg	Tablets: 5, 25, 50 μg
Liotrix	Thyrolar	1 unit	1 unit=T_4 50 μg/T_3 12.5 μg $^1/_4$, $^1/_2$, 1, 2, 3 units
Thyroid USP	Armour thyroid	60–90 mg	60 mg (1 grain)=T_4 38 μg/T_3 9 μg Tablets: 15, 30, 60, 90, 120, 180, 240, 300 mg

From Rakel RE, Bope ET (eds): Conn's Current Therapy. Philadelphia, WB Saunders, 2001, p 675.

Other

Other supplement recommendations include vitamin A, 25,000 IU daily, vitamin E, 400 IU daily, riboflavin, 15 mg daily, niacin, 25 to 50 μg daily, pyridoxine, 25 to 50 μg daily, and vitamin C, 1 g daily.[3]

Botanicals

Traditional Chinese medicine botanicals may be used in the treatment of hypothyroidism (see later section, Therapies to Consider).

Pharmaceuticals

Despite the fact that only 20% of T_3 (which is considered the most biologically active) is produced by the thyroid gland, studies show that replacement therapy with T_4 and T_3 has better results, particularly regarding mood and neuropsychological function.[7]

Medical providers have been cautious about using nonsynthetic thyroid products because of the possible breakdown of the active ingredients. My experience has been that some patients using nonsynthetic thyroid have a better response. However, most providers prefer the T_4 and T_3 synthetic combination in liotrix (Thyrolar).

Armour Thyroid

Desiccated T_3 and T_4 are derived from porcine thyroid glands. T_3 is approximately four times as potent as T_4 on a microgram-for-microgram basis. One grain of Armour thyroid provides 38 μg of T_4 and 9 μg of T_3.

Thyrolar (Liotrix)

Thyrolar contains varying doses of T_4 and T_3 (five different potencies). T_3 is approximately four times as potent as T_4 on a microgram-for-microgram basis.

Liothyronine Sodium (Cytomel)

This is a synthetic T_3.

Levothyroxine Sodium (Levoxyl, Synthroid, Levothroid)

This is a synthetic L-thyroxine T_4. See Table 28-2.

THERAPIES TO CONSIDER

Traditional Chinese Medicine

Using a combination of nutrition, botanicals, and acupuncture is an extremely valuable modality for exploring the optimal treatment of hypothyroidism.

Yoga

Certain positions such as the shoulder stand combined with visualization help to stimulate the thyroid gland.

Exercise

Exercise stimulates thyroid gland secretion and increases sensitivity to thyroid hormone. Patients who are dieting may have a decreased metabolic rate, so they have a special need to exercise.

THERAPEUTIC REVIEW

In most cases of hypothyroidism, hormone supplementation will be needed. However, it is still important to support the thyroid gland nutritionally and with exercise.

Nutrition
- *Choose fresh whole foods.*
- *Avoid foods that block iodine utilization such as turnips, cabbage, mustard, cassava root, soybean, peanuts, pine nuts, and millet.*

Supplements
- *Zinc picolinate, 30 mg daily*
- *Selenium, 200 to 300 µg daily*
- *Vitamin A, 25,000 IU daily*
- *Riboflavin (vitamin B_2), 15 mg daily*
- *Niacin, 25 to 50 mg daily*
- *Pyridoxine (vitamin B_6), 25 to 50 mg daily*
- *Vitamin C, 1 g daily*

Exercise
- *15 to 20 minutes daily of aerobic exercise*

Pharmaceuticals
- *See Table 28–2 for details.*

Other
- *Traditional Chinese medicine*
- *Yoga*

Follow-up Therapy
- *Sources vary as to how often laboratory tests should be performed after therapy has been initiated. The most practical recommendation is to follow the patient clinically over 2-week periods. Additional laboratory tests may be helpful after completion of 6 weeks of therapy.*

References

1. Harrison TR, Braunwald E (eds): Harrison's Principles of Internal Medicine. 15th ed. New York, McGraw-Hill Book Co., 2001.
2. Rakel RE, Bope ET (eds): Conn's Current Therapy. Philadelphia, WB Saunders, 2001, pp 674–675.
3. Murray M, Pizzorno J: Encyclopedia of Natural Medicine. Prima Publishing, 1991, pp 389–390.
4. Nishi Y, Kawate R, Usui T: Zinc metabolism in thyroid disease. Postgrad Med J 56:833–837, 1980.
5. Olivieri O, Girelli D, Stanzial AM, et al: Selenium, zinc, and thyroid hormones in healthy subjects: Low T_3/T_4 ratio in the elderly is related to impaired selenium status. Biol Trace Elem Res 51:31–41, 1996.
6. Olivieri O, Girelli D, Azzini M, et al: Low selenium status in the elderly influences thyroid hormones. Clin Sci (Colch) 89:637–642, 1995.
7. Bunevicius R, Kazanavicius G, Zalinkevicius R, Prange AJ Jr: Effects of thyroxine as compared with thyroxine plus triiodothyronine in patients with hypothyroidism. N Engl J Med 340:469–470, 1999.

CHAPTER 29

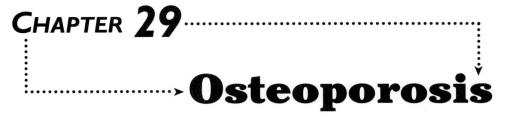

Osteoporosis

Gregory A. Plotnikoff, M.D., M.T.S., and
Sharon Norling, M.D., M.B.A.

PATHOPHYSIOLOGY

Osteoporosis is an asymptomatic bone disease resulting from an imbalance of bone formation and bone resorption. The result is low bone mass and microarchitectural deterioration of bone tissue, leading to enhanced bone fragility and a consequent increase in fracture risk.[1] Osteoporosis is the most prevalent metabolic bone disease in developed countries and is a major health problem in aging populations.[2] Currently, 13 million to 17 million American women and 8 million to 10 million American men have osteoporosis.[3] In 1995, more than $94 billion was spent on care of osteoporotic fractures.[4]

NOTE

The goal of therapy of osteoporosis is to reverse the imbalance between bone formation and bone resorption in order to prevent disabling fractures.

INTEGRATIVE THERAPY

Integrated medicine interventions for treatment of osteoporosis include (1) vitamin and mineral therapies, (2) ipriflavone and omega-3 essential fatty acid and dehydroepiandrosterone (DHEA) supplements, (3) exercise, and (4) pharmaceutical agents.

The evidence base for pharmaceutical treatment of osteoporosis is not necessarily stronger than that for nonpharmaceutical interventions. Surprisingly, there is insufficient evidence from prospective randomized controlled trials for antifracture efficacy of estrogen given for replacement therapy or of other agents such as intranasal calcitonin and the bisphosphonate etidronic acid. However, data from both observational studies and controlled trials in postmenopausal women suggest that rational mineral, vitamin, and dietary supplementation does have antifracture efficacy. Further research is needed before such interventions can be considered the standard of care.

Bisphosphonate therapy with alendronate (Fosamax) and risedronate (Actonel) is the only intervention that has been demonstrated to produce a

Table 29–1. Risk Factors for Osteoporosis

Age
Genetic
  Family history of osteoporosis
  Thin body frame or body mass index less than 20
  White or Asian ethnicity
  Women
Hormonal
  Late menarche (at older than 15 years of age)
  Premature or surgical menopause
  Prolonged amenorrhea
Life style and nutrition
  Decreased sun exposure
  High alcohol consumption
  High animal protein intake
  High caffeine consumption
  High sodium intake
  High soft drink consumption
  Immobilization
  Low calcium intake
  Low vitamin D intake
  Low vitamin K
  Practicing purdah (use of veils or the chador)
  Sedentary lifestyle
  Smoking
  Sports-induced hypothalamic amenorrhea/hypogonadism
  Use of sunscreen
  Vegetarian diet
Medical diseases
  Anorexia
  Depression
  Diabetes mellitus type 1
  Hyperparathyroidism
  Hyperprolactinemia
  Hyperthyroidism
  Hypogonadism
  Glucocorticoid excess (Cushing's syndrome)
  Liver disease
  Malabsorption
  Osteogenesis imperfecta
  Prolonged parenteral nutrition
  Rheumatoid arthritis
  Systemic mastocytosis
  Transplantation
  Turner's syndrome
Medications
  Anticonvulsants
  Chemotherapy
  Cyclosporine
  Medroxyprogesterone
  Glucocorticoids
  Gonadotropin-releasing hormone agonist or antagonist
  Heparin
  Lithium
  Methotrexate
  Phosphate-binding antacids
  Warfarin sodium

consistent reduction in the risk of multiple fractures in the elderly across trials, including a reduction in the incidence of both radiographic vertebral fractures and nonspine fractures. Therapy with the bisphosphonate raloxifene (Evista) has been demonstrated to reduce the risk of both radiographic and clinical vertebral fractures but not of nonvertebral fractures.

Nutrition

Nutritional deficits of calcium, vitamin C, vitamin D, and vitamin K play a role in the pathogenesis of osteoporosis. Nutritional deficits of boron, copper, magnesium, and manganese may also play a role. Diets rich in vegetables, fruits, and whole grains and also low in protein appear to be "bone healthy." However, such a diet may not provide adequate calcium and certainly does not provide any vitamin D.

Classic dietary recommendations for osteopenia or osteoporosis with some supporting evidence include minimizing consumption of refined foods, alcohol, caffeine, sugar, salt, phosphorus (carbonated drinks), aluminum-containing antacids, and animal proteins. These recommendations remain controversial for both scientific and cultural reasons.

Calcium

Calcium is the best known, and most controversial, of the nutritional components of the management and prevention of osteoporosis. Calcium, either from dietary sources or as a supplement, has been shown to decrease bone loss in postmenopausal women with osteoporosis. Effective sources of calcium include broccoli, kale, collard greens, mustard greens, squash, and sea vegetables. Calcium is well absorbed from vegetable sources unless they have high concentrations of oxalic acid (such as in spinach) or phytic acid (such as in wheat bran cereal).[5] Milk is often cited as an excellent source of calcium. However, the Harvard Nurses' Study of 77,761 women found that nurses who drank two or more glasses of milk daily actually suffered 1.5 times as many hip fractures and slightly more fractures of the forearm than those nurses who drank one glass per day.[6] There is thus some controversy regarding dairy products; patients can be reminded that cows get their calcium from plant sources.

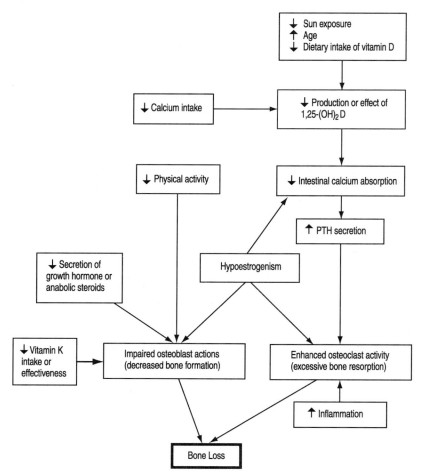

Figure 29–1. Pathophysiology of osteoporosis 1,25-(OH)$_2$D, 1,25-dihydroxyvitamin D (vitamin D component that aids calcium absorption); PTH, parathyroid hormone.

> ## NOTE
>
> *Owing to its high protein content, milk is not the best source of calcium. When the protein is broken down in the body, it causes a slight acidity of the blood, which the body compensates for by metabolizing calcium from bone to act as a buffer.*

For patients who choose to take calcium supplements, there is confusion and controversy about which form of calcium is the best. Significant amounts of lead and also aluminum have been found in bone meal, dolomite, and calcium carbonate supplements labeled "oyster shell" or "natural source."[7] Randomized crossover studies comparing the bioavailability of calcium supplements suggest that calcium citrate is better absorbed than calcium carbonate.[8–12]

Fractional calcium absorption ranges from 10% to 70% among individual patients.[13, 14] A postmenopausal woman who is not receiving estrogen therapy should take 1500 mg of calcium a day. Women receiving estrogen therapy should take 1000 mg a day.[15]

Potassium and Magnesium

Alkaline-producing dietary components such as potassium-rich and magnesium-rich fruits and vegetables have been hypothesized to contribute to maintenance of bone mineral density. Support for this theory comes from retrospective analyses of data from the original Framingham study. Dietary and supplement intakes were assessed and bone mineral density was measured. Greater intakes of each were associated with both greater bone mineral density and less decline over time in both men and women.[16] Higher intakes of magnesium and potassium in fruits and vegetables were also associated with increased bone mineral density in a cross sectional study of 62 healthy women 45 to 55 years of age.[17] No prospective trials of potassium or magnesium supplementation have been conducted.

Vitamin C

The cited studies on potassium and magnesium intake are confounded by the concomitant presence of vitamin C in fruits and vegetables. Vitamin C is an essential dietary nutrient and a necessary cofactor in the hydroxylation of lysine and proline for collagen synthesis. This collagen provides structure for the noncollagenous proteins and hence the mineral surface of bone. The importance of collagen for bones is reflected in the profound bone weakness seen in osteogenesis imperfecta (characterized by defective type I collagen) or in scurvy, a disease of failed collagen formation and secretion due to vitamin C deficiency. In the Postmenopausal Estrogen/Progestin Interventions Trial (PEPI), women with calcium intakes of greater than 500 mg per day demonstrated a positive association of vitamin C with increased bone mineral density.[18]

Vitamin D

Vitamin D is essential for growth and maintenance of healthy bones throughout life. 1,25-Dihydroxyvitamin D ($1,25[OH]_2D$) is the main regulator of intestinal calcium absorption and transport for the mineralization of the collagen matrix. Vitamin D is absorbed from the diet (sources include cod liver oil, liver, sun exposed mushrooms, fortified milk, and fortified soy milk) or is synthesized from 7-dehydrocholesterol in the skin in response to ultraviolet B light. Full synthesis requires hydroxylation in the liver and then the kidney. Therefore, vitamin D metabolism can be altered significantly by life style, aging, and gastrointestinal, renal, and hepatic disease.

Vitamin D deficiency is prevalent throughout the world, including countries in both the northern and southern latitudes. Vitamin D deficiency should be considered in anyone who drinks less than a quart of supplemented milk per day and in anyone with restricted sun exposure including the elderly and those who work indoors, wear veils, or use topical sunblock agents. The darker the skin pigmentation, the more ultraviolet B light is needed to produce vitamin D. The Institute of Medicine's Food and Nutrition Board in 1997 recommended that the daily allowance for adults younger than 50 years of age is 5 μg (200 IU), for those 50 to 70 years of age it is 10 μg (400 IU), and for those over 70, 15 μg (600 IU). For people who are sunlight-deprived, the recommendation ranges from 600 IU to 1000 IU per day to maintain a normal level of 25-hydroxyvitamin D.[19, 20]

Supplementation with 800 IU of vitamin D_3 and 1200 mg of elemental calcium has been shown prospectively to reduce the risk of hip fractures and other nonvertebral fractures among elderly women. In a population of 3270 mobile elderly women (mean age 84 ± 6 years) living in 180 nursing homes, 18 months of randomized, double-blind supplementation resulted in 43% fewer hip fractures and 32% fewer nonvertebral fractures in the treatment group.[21] In this same group, 36 months of supplementation resulted in a 29% decrease in hip fractures ($P < .01$) and a 24% decrease in all nonvertebral fractures ($P < .01$). The odds ratio for the decreased rate of hip fracture after 36 months was 0.70 (95% confidence interval [CI] of 0.62–0.78) and for all nonvertebral fractures was 0.70 (95% CI of 0.51–0.91).[22]

Although calcium alone or vitamin D alone appears to be beneficial to bone health, better results are achieved with a combination of both nutrients, as vitamin D enhances the absorption of calcium.

Vitamin K

Osteocalcin (OC) is an osteoblast-synthesized non-collagenous protein important in bone mineralization.[23, 24] Vitamin D induces its synthesis.[25] Vitamin K then helps carboxylate its glutamic acid residues to produce gamma-carboxyglutamyl residues (GLA) (not to be confused with gamma-linolenic acid). This carboxylation is crucial. These three GLA residues confer upon OC a high and relatively specific affinity for the calcium ion of the hydroxyapatite molecule.[26]

Compared with age-matched control subjects, significantly decreased serum levels of vitamin K are found in osteopenic patients with fractures.[27–29] In the Nurses' Health Study cohort of 72,327 women, higher vitamin K intake was associated with a significantly lower age-adjusted relative risk (RR) of hip fractures (RR of 0.70, 95% CI of 0.53–0.93).[30] Low dietary intake of vitamin K is associated with an elevated proportion of undercarboxylated (partially functional) OC.[31] Undercarboxylation of OC is frequently found in elderly women[32] and has been associated with increased risk of hip fracture in older women.[33–35] In one study conducted over 3 years in 183 institutionalized women 70 to 97 years of age, the age-adjusted odds ratio (OR) for hip fracture was three times higher in those with increased baseline levels of uncarboxylated OC (OR of 3.1, 99% CI of 1.7–6.0, $P < .001$).[36] Long-term warfarin therapy, which blocks gamma-carboxylation of clotting factors, is also associated with reduced bone mineral density compared with that in controls ($P < .0001$).[37]

Prospective trials of vitamin K supplementation have demonstrated corrected undercarboxylation of osteocalcin.[38–40] Few prospective clinical trials on the prevention of osteoporotic fractures with vitamin K have been published. One randomized open study conducted over 2 years in 167 osteoporotic patients in Japan demonstrated maintenance of lumbar bone mineral density with vitamin K_2 supplementation, compared with a loss of 3% in the control group. This finding translated to a significantly decreased vertebral fracture incidence (0.098 ± 0.029 event/year versus 0.212 ± 0.038 for the control group; $P < .02$).[41]

Soy

Soybeans are a low-fat, no-cholesterol food that contains high-quality protein, isoflavones (phytoestrogens), and essential fatty acids. The soy phytoestrogens bind to estrogen receptors and are believed to behave similarly to other estrogens that exhibit antiresorptive efficacy. In one trial in 66 postmenopausal women in a 6-month, parallel group, a double blind trial of soy protein at 90 mg/day with varying isoflavone content demonstrated a 2% increase in bone mineral density.[42] Isoflavone consumption in Eastern countries is on the order of 20 to 150 mg per day, compared with 2 to 5 mg per day in Western countries. Persons with osteoporosis should consume 21 servings of soy protein per week, which breaks down to about 24 to 30 g of soy protein and 48 to 60 mg of isoflavones daily.[43] No prospective treatment trials for antifracture efficacy have been conducted.

Supplements

Ipriflavone

Ipriflavone is a synthetic isoflavone derivative from soy with a long history of use in countries other than the United States. Ipriflavone has been shown to protect against bone loss in early menopause,[44] during treatment with gonadotropin-releasing hormone agonists,[45] after recent oophorectomy,[46] in postmenopausal women with low bone mass,[47] and in elderly osteoporotic women.[48] In a majority of these studies, bone mass was not increased in the ipriflavone group but was decreased in the control group, with significant between-group differences. Urinary hydroxyproline ratios indicated reduction of bone turnover.

In a large, randomized, double-blind placebo-controlled 3-year trial, published in 2001,[49] ipriflavone 200 mg 3 times a day did not prevent bone loss or affect biochemical markers of bone metabolism compared with the placebo. Some women with postmenopausal osteoporosis developed subclinical lymphocytopenia.[49] Thus far, no studies on ipriflavone have been of sufficient power to study fracture incidence in relation to ipriflavone.

From the 1980s to 1997, a total of 3132 patient-years were accumulated for study, with 2769 patients receiving ipriflavone for 6 to 96 months. The incidence of adverse reactions was not different from that of placebo, with the most common complaints being gastrointestinal.[50] The effects of overdosage in humans are unknown. Until use in cancer patients is more carefully evaluated, concentrated supplements should be taken with caution.

Dosage. 200 mg orally 3 times a day.

Precautions. Ipriflavone should be used with caution in patients with liver or kidney disease[50] and in those taking theophylline. Increased anticoagulant activity was noted when acenocoumarol was administered with ipriflavone[50]; therefore, caution is also indicated with use of this agent. For patients who choose to take ipriflavone, calcium and vitamin D supplementation may enhance the effects of the ipriflavone.

Dehydroepiandrosterone

Dehydroepiandrosterone (DHEA) and its sulfated ester dehydroepiandrosterone sulfate (DHEAS) are the most abundant circulating adrenal steroids. DHEA is a potent inhibitor of the proinflammatory and osteolytic cytokine interleukin-6 via inhibition of nuclear factor-kappa B (NF κ B). DHEAS is a precursor for the anabolic peripheral sex steroids testosterone and 17-beta-estradiol (17β-estradiol). Levels of DHEA and DHEAS correlate positively with bone mineral density at both the hip and the spine.[51] Subnormal levels of DHEAS are associated with decreased bone mineral density.[52] Women with high levels of bone resorption markers and low DHEAS levels have a markedly higher risk of fracture than that noted in postmenopausal controls (RR = 3.3, $P < .001$).[53]

NOTE

Low serum DHEAS levels have been found to be associated with 2-fold higher risk of bone fracture.

To date, no prospective trials have been conducted on DHEA supplementation for treatment of osteoporosis.

Dosage. Treatment decisions should be based on serum levels. DHEA can be started at 10 mg orally once a day and increased to bring serum levels to within normal range.

Precautions. Excessive supplementation can cause androgenic effects such as acne, hirsutism, and voice changes. No other side effects have been documented.

Omega-3 Polyunsaturated Fatty Acids

Dietary supplementation of omega-3 polyunsaturated fatty acids (PUFAs) suppresses production of the osteoclast-activating proinflammatory cytokines interleukins IL-β, IL-1α, IL-6, and TNF-α.[54] Dietary deficiencies of omega-3 fatty acids are well documented including population-wide decreased concentrations in breast milk[55] and markedly imbalanced consumption of omega-6 to omega-3 fatty acids.[56] Omega-3 fatty acids in the form of gamma-linolenic acid are found in soybean oil, canola oil, and, particularly, flaxseed oil. Additional sources include ocean-harvested cold water fish (mackerel, herring, sardines, albacore tuna, and salmon), green leafy vegetables, and walnuts (see Chapter 84, Anti-inflammatory Diet).

Excessive production of the osteoclast-activating cytokines can be indirectly measured by obtaining serum levels of C-reactive protein in persons without active infections. Unpublished data demonstrate that supplementation with omega-3 fatty acids reduces elevated C-reactive proteins. Published data in the rheumatology and gastroenterology literature demonstrate that in persons with inflammatory arthritides or bowel disease, omega-3 fatty acid supplementation markedly reduces serum levels of

specific proinflammatory cytokines such as IL-6 and TNF-α, with clinically significant benefits. Prospective data on omega-3 fatty acid supplementation for antiresorptive activity is pending.

Dosage. 2 to 4 g daily.

Precautions. When the body metabolizes these fatty acids to make energy, free radicals are produced. With high doses (greater than 4 g per day) of omega-3 fatty acids, an antioxidant such as vitamin E should be taken to reduce this accumulation.

Exercise

Bone accommodates the loads imposed on it by altering its mass and distribution of mass. When habitual loading increases, bone is gained; when loading decreases, bone is lost.[57] Some but not all intervention trials using resistance or mixed endurance-resistance exercise showed significant gains in bone mass in older men and women.[58–61] Other studies of older people, although not reporting significant gains in bone mass, indicate that exercise may lessen bone loss.[62] The modest increases in bone mineral density with strength training should not trivialize the importance of exercise for protecting older people against falls. More than 90% of hip fractures are the immediate consequence of a fall onto the hip. Among the important risk factors for falls, muscle strength is perhaps most susceptible to improvement with strength training.[63]

A complete exercise program for people with osteoporosis should include balance, postural, resistance, and weight-bearing exercises (see Chapter 86, Writing an Exercise Prescription).

- Balance exercises help patients to maintain equilibrium and can reduce the risk of falling. These exercises should be performed daily.
- Postural exercises and back extensor strengthening should be done throughout the day.
- Resistance exercises, which strengthen muscles, should be performed 2 to 3 times a week.
- Weight-bearing exercises such as walking or stair climbing should be performed at least three to five times per week. The goal is to work up to sessions that last 45 minutes.

The most important consideration is for the patient to participate safely in some activity in a frequent, regular, and sustained manner.

For osteoporotic persons, referral to a physical therapist may be necessary before an exercise program can be instituted. Severely osteoporotic patients should receive appropriate pharmaceutical therapy for 3 months before seeing a physical therapist and starting an exercise program.

Pharmaceuticals

The National Osteoporosis Foundation (NOF) recommends pharmacologic treatment of all postmenopausal women with T scores below −1.5 standard deviations (SD) below the mean and at least one other risk factor. The NOF also recommends therapy for all postmenopausal women with a T score below −2.0.

Bisphosphonates

Bisphosphonates reduce bone resorption by reducing the production of protone and lysosomal enzymes beneath the osteoclasts.[64] The result is interference with activation of osteoclastic precursors, differentiation of precursor cells into mature osteoclasts, chemotaxis, and attachment of osteoclasts to bone.[65] Bisphosphonates may also shorten the life span of osteoclasts (apoptosis).[64] However, they do not enhance bone formation.

Alendronate

Alendronate (Fosamax) is the most comprehensively studied drug currently approved for the treatment of osteoporosis. Published randomized, placebo-controlled trials of alendronate showed reduction of new vertebral fractures by 47% and reduction in the incidence of two or more vertebral fractures by 90% relative to findings in the placebo group.[67] The use of alendronate was associated with a 36% reduction in the cumulative incidence of all clinically diagnosed fractures and with a 56% reduction in the cumulative incidence of hip fractures.[66, 67]

The greatest benefit occurs in patients with the lowest bone mineral density, such as patients with T scores below 2.5 or those with preexisting vertebral fractures.[68]

Dosage. The recommended dose is 35 mg once a week for prevention and 70 mg once a week for treatment.

Precautions. Bisphosphonates must be taken with a full glass of water after fasting. Patients should maintain an upright position for 30 minutes. This increases absorption and prevents gastrointestinal ulceration.

Risedronate

Risedronate (Actonel) decreases new vertebral fractures by 36%, and the cumulative incidence of nonvertebral fractures is reduced by 39%.[69] The greatest benefit occurs in patients with T scores below 2.5 or those with preexisting vertebral fractures.[68]

Dosage. Recommended dose for risedronate is 5 mg per day.

Precautions. Same precautions as above for alendronate. Side effects include esophageal irritation, headaches, diarrhea, epigastric pain, nausea, vomiting, and arthralgias.

Estrogen Replacement Therapy

Several studies of the effects of estrogen replacement therapy (ERT), or hormone replacement therapy (HRT), alone or in combination with use of other agents, have reported data on fractures and changes in bone mineral density.[70, 71] In the randomized, placebo-controlled PEPI trial, conjugated estrogen (0.625 mg/d) increased bone mineral density by about 6% in the spine and 2.8% in the hip after 3 years. The trial did not show reduction of fractures, possibly because it was conducted in younger women, who have a low incidence of osteoporotic fractures.[68, 71] However, the antifracture efficacy data for ERT from randomized controlled trials are inconsistent and inconclusive.[72–74] Observational cohort and case-control studies have consistently reported reductions of up to 75% in the incidence of hip and wrist fractures among postmenopausal women receiving HRT, but the benefit varied widely depending on the duration of use of estrogen and time since discontinuation.[75–78] A meta-analysis of these studies estimated that estrogen use was associated with a 25% reduction in hip fracture risk.[79]

Most data suggest that at least 6 or 7 years of treatment is required to achieve a significant reduction in fracture risk, and that this benefit diminishes markedly or disappears within several years after discontinuing ERT, suggesting that estrogen should be continued indefinitely to maintain any benefit.[75, 77, 78, 80, 81]

Dosage. Conjugated equine estrogens 0.625 mg per day, oral ethinyl estradiol 0.2 mg per day, estradiol (Estrace) 1 mg orally per day, or transdermal estradiol 0.05 mg per day (1 patch twice a week) can be used. Progesterone is added for women with an intact uterus.

Precautions. ERT is associated with increased risk of endometrial cancer, breast cancer, venous thromboembolism, and gallbladder disease. Adverse effects may include endometrial bleeding, breast tenderness, fluid retention, and nausea.

Selective Estrogen Receptor Modulators: Raloxifene

Raloxifene (Evista) is a nonsteroidal benzothiophene compound that exerts tissue-specific agonist and antagonist effects as it binds to estrogen receptors. It prevents bone loss in early postmenopausal women and in one study induced a 1% to 2% gain in bone mineral density of the spine, femoral neck, and total body. The Multiple Outcomes of Raloxifene Evaluation (MORE) study showed an increase in bone mineral density in the spine of 2.5% and in the hip of 2.1% after 3 years using pooled data (doses of 60 or 120 mg per day).[69, 83] There is an estimated risk reduction of 30% for vertebral fractures, somewhat lower than that for alendronate. There are no supporting data in randomized clinical trials for a reduction in the incidence of nonvertebral fractures.

Dosage. 60 mg per day.

Precautions. Adverse effects include hot flashes, thrombophlebitis, and leg cramps.

Calcitonin

Calcitonin (Miacalcin, Calcimar) is a peptide hormone whose primary action is on bone to reduce osteoclastic bone resorption. Calcitonin is approved by the Food and Drug Administration for use in women up to 5 years post menopause. Its use is associated with slight increases in spinal bone mineral density and decreased vertebral fractures. There is no significant reduction in hip fractures. A direct comparison study found the effect of calcitonin on bone mineral density and bone resorption markers to be significantly less than that of alendronate and not significantly different from that of placebo for most sites.[83] The level of evidence for antifracture efficacy is considered marginal and insufficient for recommendations.[84] Calcitonin has an analgesic effect and has been used in osteoporosis patients who have acute or chronic pain.[68]

Dosage. 200 IU of calcitonin intranasally once daily (one spray in alternating nostrils each day), or 100 units subcutaneously or intramuscularly every other day.

Precautions. Adverse effects include nausea, vomiting, flushing, nasal ulcerations, and rhinitis.

THERAPEUTIC REVIEW

Laboratory Studies

A quantitative measurement of bone mineral density must be obtained.

Also indicated are serum measurements of vitamin D, parathyroid hormone, DHEA, C-reactive protein, alkaline phosphatase, thyroid stimulating hormone, calcium, and hemoglobin.

Nutrition

The patient should be encouraged to consume a diet rich in fruits and vegetables including the calcium-rich and vitamin K–rich cruciferous vegetables broccoli and kale.

Consumption of fortified soy milk instead of milk is recommended.

Supplements

Indications for supplementation with vitamin D depend on serum vitamin D and parathyroid hormone levels. Dosing of vitamin D is determined according to the following guidelines (normal serum vitamin D levels are 20–60 ng/ml or 50–150 nMol/L):

- *Median to high-normal vitamin D: 400 IU of vitamin D per day*
- *Low-normal vitamin D and normal PTH: 800 IU per day*
- *Below normal vitamin D and normal PTH: 1200 IU per day*
- *Markedly below normal vitamin D and symptomatic: ergocalciferol (vitamin D) 50,000 IU twice weekly for 8 weeks with follow-up serum measurements*
- *Low-normal to below normal vitamin D with elevated PTH: ergocalciferol (vitamin D) 50,000 IU twice weekly for 8 weeks with follow-up serum measurements*

DHEA supplementation is indicated to obtain at least a low normal serum level. The patient should be monitored for signs of androgenism. The dose begins at 10 mg orally once daily and is reassessed monthly.

For supplementation with refrigerated flaxseed oil and vitamin E, given the lack of prospective data, guidelines are based on anecdotal evidence and experience. Dosing may be determined by serum C-reactive protein levels according to the following guidelines (normal high sensitive C-reactive protein levels are 0–0.8 mg/dL):

- *Low-normal: 2 to 4 g of flaxseed oil per day with 400 IU of "mixed" vitamin E (D-alpha/delta/tocopherols)*
- *Median to high-normal: 8 g per day with 800 IU of "mixed" vitamin E (D-alpha/delta/gamma-tocopherols)*
- *Above normal range: 16 g per day with 1200 IU of "mixed" vitamin E (D-alpha/delta/gamma-tocopherols)*
- *Re-evaluate CRP levels in 2–3 months and adjust dosing as needed*

Consider ipriflavone therapy at 200 mg orally 3 times a day.

THERAPEUTIC REVIEW continued

Exercise

An exercise program should be initiated, if possible.

Pharmaceuticals

Consider bisphosphonate therapy:

- *Alendronate (Fosamax) 70 mg orally weekly or 10 mg orally once daily taken with 8 ounces of water on an empty stomach 30 minutes before breakfast; the patient is cautioned to remain upright for 30 minutes after taking the tablet.*
- *Risedronate (Actonel) 5 mg orally once daily taken with 8 ounces of water on an empty stomach 30 minutes before breakfast; the patient should remain upright for 30 minutes after taking the tablet.*

References

1. Consensus Development Conference V, 1993: Diagnosis, prophylaxis, and treatment of osteoporosis. Am J Med 90:646–650, 1994.
2. Bull World Health Organ 77:368–435, 1999.
3. Looker AC, Orwoll ES, Johnston CC: Prevalence of low femoral bone density in older U.S. adults from NHANES III. J Bone Miner Res 12:1761–1768, 1997.
4. Bacon WE: Secular trends in hip fracture occurrence and survival: age and sex differences. J Aging Health 8:538–553, 1996.
5. Weaver CM: Calcium bioavailability and its relation to osteoporosis. Proc Soc Exp Biol Med 200:157–160, 1992.
6. Feskanich D, Willett WC, Stampfer MJ, Colditz GA: Milk, dietary calcium, and bone fractures in women: A 12-year prospective study. Am J Public Health 87:992–997, 1997.
7. Whiting SJ: Safety of some calcium supplements questioned. Nutr Rev 52:95–97, 1994.
8. Harvey JA, et al: Superior calcium absorption from calcium citrate than calcium carbonate using external forearm counting. J Am Coll Nutr 9:583–587, 1990.
9. Harvey JA, et al: Dose dependency of calcium absorption: A comparison of calcium carbonate and calcium citrate. J Bone Miner Res 3:253–258, 1988.
10. Heller HJ, et al: Pharmacokinetic and pharmacodynamic comparison of two calcium supplements in postmenopausal women. J Clin Pharmacol 40:1237–1244, 2000.
11. Heller HJ, et al: Pharmacokinetics of calcium absorption from two commercial calcium supplements. J Clin Pharmacol 9:1151–1154, 1999.
12. Reginster JY, et al: Acute biochemical variations induced by four different calcium salts in healthy male volunteers. Osteoporos Int 3:271–275, 1993.
13. Heaney RP, Recker RR: Distribution of calcium absorption in middle-aged women. Am J Clin Nutr 43:299–305, 1986.
14. Bullamore JR, Wilkinson R, Gallagher JC, et al: Effect of age on calcium absorption. Lancet 2:535–537, 1970.
15. Consensus Conference: Osteoporosis. JAMA 252:799–802, 1984.
16. Tucker KL, Hannan MT, Chen H, et al: Potassium, magnesium, and fruit and vegetable intakes are associated with greater bone mineral density in elderly men and women. Am J Clin Nutr 69:727–736, 1999.
17. New SA, Robins SP, Campbell MK, et al: Dietary influences on bone mass and bone metabolism: Further evidence of a positive link between fruit and vegetable consumption and bone health? Am J Clin Nutr 71:142–151, 2000.
18. Hall SI, Greendale GA: The relation of dietary vitamin C intake to bone mineral density: Results from the PEPI study. Calcif Tissue Int 63:183–189, 1998.
19. Holick MF: McCollum Award Lecture, 1994: Vitamin D—new horizons for the 21st century. Am J Clin Nutr 60:619–630, 1994.
20. Glerup H, Mikkelson K, Poulsen L et al: Commonly recommended daily intake of vitamin D is not sufficient if sunlight exposure is limited. J Intern Med 247:260–268, 2000.
21. Chapuy MC, Arlot ME, Duboeuf F, et al: Vitamin D_3 and calcium to prevent hip fractures in elderly women. N Engl J Med 327:1637–1642, 1992.
22. Chapuy MC, Arlot ME, Delmas PD, Meunier PJ: Effect of calcium and cholecalciferol treatment for three years on hip fractures in elderly women. BMJ 308:1081–1082, 1994.
23. Binkley NC, Suttie JW: Vitamin K nutrition and osteoporosis. J Nutr 125:1812–1821, 1995.
24. Shearer MJ: The roles of vitamins D and K in bone health and osteoporosis prevention. Proc Nutr Soc 56:915–937, 1997.
25. Lian J, Stewart C, Puchaz E, et al: Structure of the rat osteocalcin gene and regulation of vitamin D–dependent expression. Proc Natl Acad Sci USA 86:1143–1147, 1989.
26. Hauschka PV, Lian JB, Cole DEC, Gundberg C: Osteocalcin and matrix gla protein: Vitamin K–dependent proteins in bone. Physiol Rev 69:990–1047, 1989.
27. Hart JP, Shearer MJ, Klenerman L, et al: Electrochemical detection of depressed circulating levels of vitamin K_1 in osteoporosis. J Clin Endocrinol Metab 60:1268–1269, 1985.
28. Hodges SJ, Pilkington MJ, Stamp TC, et al: Depressed levels of circulating menaquinones in patients with osteoporotic fractures of the spine and femoral neck. Bone 12:387–389, 1991.
29. Hodges SJ, Akesson K, Vergnaud P, et al: Circulating levels of vitamins K_1 and K_2 decreased in elderly women with hip fracture. J Bone Miner Res 8:1241–1245, 1993.
30. Feskanich D, Weber P, Willett WC, et al: Vitamin K intake and hip fractures in women: A prospective study. Am J Clin Nutr 69:74–79, 1999.
31. Sokoll LJ, Booth SL, O'Brien ME, et al: Changes in serum osteocalcin, plasma phylloquinone, and urinary γ-carboxyglutamic acid in response to altered intakes of phylloquinone in human subjects. Am J Clin Nutr 65:779–784, 1997.
32. Plantalech LM, Guillaumont M, Leclercq M, Delmas PD: Impaired carboxylation of serum osteocalcin in elderly women. J Bone Miner Res 6:1211–1216, 1991.
33. Szulc P, Chapuy MC, Meunier PJ, Delmas PD: Serum undercarboxylated osteocalcin is a marker of the risk of hip fracture in older women. J Clin Invest 91:1769–1774, 1993.
34. Vergnaud P, Garnero P, Meunier PJ, et al: Undercarboxylated osteocalcin measured with specific immunoassay predicts hip fracture in elderly women: The EPIDOS study. J Clin Endocrinol Metab 82:717–718, 1997.
35. Szulc P, Arlot M, Chapuy MC, et al: Serum undercarboxylated osteocalcin correlates with hip bone mineral density in elderly women. J Bone Min Res 9:1591–1595, 1994.
36. Szulc P, Chapuy MC, Meunier PJ, Delmas PD: Serum uncarboxylated osteocalcin is a marker of the risk of hip fracture: A three year follow-up study. Bone 18:487–488, 1996.
37. Sato Y, Honda Y, Kunoh H, Oizumi K: Long-term oral anticoagulation reduces bone mass in patients with previous hemispheric infarction and nonrheumatic atrial fibrillation. Stroke 28:2390–2394, 1997.
38. Douglas AS, Robin SP, Hutchison JD, et al: Carboxylation of osteocalcin in post-menopausal osteoporotic women following vitamin K and D supplementation. Bone 17:15–20, 1995.
39. Schaafsma A, Muskiet FA, Storm H, et al: Vitamin D(3) and vitamin K(1) supplementation of Dutch postmenopausal women with normal and low bone mineral densities: Effects

on serum 25-hydroxyvitamin D and carboxylated osteocalcin. Eur J Clin Nutr 54:626–631, 2000.

40. Binkley NC, Krueger DC, Engelke JA, et al: Vitamin K supplementation reduces serum concentration of under-gamma-carboxylated osteocalcin in healthy young and elderly adults. Am J Clin Nutr 72:1523–1528, 2000.

41. Shiraki M: [Vitamin K$_2$]. Nippon Rinsho 56:1525–1530, 1998.

42. Potter SM, et al: Soy protein and isoflavones: Their effects on blood lipids and bone density in postmenopausal women. Am J Clin Nutr 68(Suppl):1375S–1379S, 1998.

43. Anderson JW, Johnstone BM, Cook-Newell ME: Meta-analysis of effects of soy protein intake on serum lipids in humans. N Engl J Med 333:276–282, 1995.

44. Gennari C, Agnusdei D, Crepaldi G, et al: Effect of ipriflavone—a synthetic derivative of natural isoflavones—on bone mass loss in the early years after menopause. Menopause 5:9–15, 1998.

45. Gambacciani M, et al: Ipriflavone prevents the loss of bone mass in pharmacological menopause induced by GnRH-agonists. Calcif Tissue Int 61(Suppl 1): S15–S18, 1997.

46. Gambacciani M, Spinetti A, Cappagli B, et al: Effects of ipriflavone administration on bone mass and metabolism in ovariectomized women. J Endocrinol Invest 16:333–337, 1993.

47. Gennari C, Adami S, Agnusdei D, et al: Effect of chronic treatment with ipriflavone in postmenopoausal women with low bone mass. Calcif Tissue Int 61:(Suppl) S19–S22, 1997.

48. Agnusdei D, Bufalino L: Efficacy of ipriflavone in established osteoporosis and long-term safety. Calcif Tissue Int 61(Suppl 1):S23–S27, 1997.

49. Alexandersen P, et al: Ipriflavone in the treatment of postmenopausal osteoporosis: A randomized controlled trial. JAMA 285:1482–1488, 2001.

50. Rondelli I, et al: Steady-state pharmacokinetics of ipriflavone and its metabolites in patients with renal failure. Int J Clin Pharmacol Res 11:183–192, 1997.

51. Zofkova I, Bahbouh R, Hill M: The pathophysiologic implications of circulating androgens on bone mineral density in a normal female population. Steroids 65:857–861, 2000.

52. Fingerova H, Matlochova J: [Reduced serum dehydroepiandrosterone levels in postmenopausal osteoporosis.] Ceska Gynekol 63:110–113, 1998.

53. Garnero P, Sornay-Rendu E, Claustrat B, Delmas PD: Biochemical markers of bone turnover, endogenous hormones and the risk of fractures in postmenopausal women: The OFELY study. J Bone Miner Res 15:1526–1536, 2000.

54. Endres S, Ghorbani R, Kelley VE, et al: The effect of dietary supplementation with n-3 polyunsaturated fatty acids on the synthesis of interleukin-one and tumor necrosis factor by mononuclear cells. N Engl J Med 320:265–271, 1989.

55. Sanders TA: Polyunsaturated fatty acids in the food chain in Europe. Am J Clin Nutr 71 (1 Suppl):176S–178S, 2000.

56. Simopoulos AP: Human requirement for n-3 polyunsaturated fatty acids. Poult Sci 79:961–970, 2000.

57. Primer on the Metabolic Bone Diseases and Disorders of Mineral Metabolism. American Society for Bone and Mineral Research, 1999, p. 266.

58. Simkin A, et al: Increased trabecular bone density due to bone-loading exercises on postmenopausal osteoporotic women. Calif Tissue Int 40:59–63. 1987.

59. Dalsky G, Stocke KS, Ehsani AA, et al: Weight-bearing exercise training and lumbar bone mineral content in postmenopausal women. Ann Intern Med 108:824–828, 1988.

60. Menkes A, et al: Strength training increases regional bone mineral density and bone remodeling in middle-aged and older men. J Appl Physiol 74:2478–2484, 1993.

61. Notelovitz M, Martin D, Tesar R, et al: Estrogen therapy and variable-resistance weight training increase bone mineral in surgically menopausal women. J Bone Miner Res 6:583–590, 1991.

62. Price R, Devine A, Dick I, et al: The effects of calcium supplementation (milk powder or tablets) and exercise on bone density in postmenopausal women. J Bone Miner Res 10:1068–1075, 1995.

63. Cummings SR, Nevitt MC, Browner WS et al: Risk factors for hip fractures in white women. Study of Osteoporotic Fractures Research Group. N Engl J Med 332:767–773, 1995.

64. Rodan GA, Fleish HA: Bisphosphonates: Mechanisms of action. J Clin Invest 97:2692–2696, 1996.

65. Lowik CW, Boonekamp PM, van de Pluym G, et al: Bisphosphonates can reduce osteoclastic bone resorption by two different mechanisms. Adv Exp Med Biol 208:275–281, 1986.

66. Black DM, et al: Randomised trial of effect of alendronate on risk of fracture in women with existing vertebral fractures. Fracture Intervention Trial Research Group. Lancet 348:1535–1541, 1996.

67. Cummings SR, Black DM, Thompson DE, et al: Effect of alendronate on risk of fracture in women with low bone density but without vertebral fractures: Results from the Fracture Intervention Trial. JAMA 280:2077–2082, 1998.

68. Alkorn D, Yokes T: Treatment of postmenopausal osteoporosis. JAMA 285:1415–1418, 2001.

69. Harris ST, et al: Effects of risedronate treatment on vertebral and nonvertebral fractures in women with postmenopausal osteoporosis: A randomized controlled trial. Vertebral Efficacy with Risedronate Therapy (VERT) Study Group. JAMA 282:1344–1352, 1999.

70. O'Connell D, et al: A systematic review of the skeletal effects of estrogen therapy in postmenopausal women. II. An assessment of treatment effects. Climacteric 1:112–123, 1998.

71. Bush TL, et al: Effects of hormone therapy on bone mineral density: Results from the Postmenopausal Estrogen/Progestin Interventions (PEPI) trial. JAMA 276:1389–1396, 1996.

72. Wimalawansa SJ: A four-year randomized controlled trial of hormone replacement and bisphosphonate, alone or in combination, in women with postmenopausal osteoporosis. Am J Med 104:219–226, 1998.

73. Komulainen MH, Kroger H, Tuppurainen MT, et al: HRT and vitamin D in prevention of non-vertebral fractures in postmenopausal women: A 5 year randomized trial. Maturitas 31:45–54, 1998.

74. Lufkin EG, Wahner HW, O'Fallon WM, et al: Treatment of postmenopausal osteoporosis with transdermal estrogen. Ann Intern Med 117:1–9, 1992.

75. Kiel DP, Felson DT, Anderson JJ, et al: Hip fracture and the use of estrogens in postmenopausal women. The Framingham Study. N Engl J Med 317:1169–1174, 1987.

76. Cauley JA, Seeley DG, Ensrud K, et al: Estrogen replacement therapy and fractures in older women. Study of Osteoporotic Fractures Research Group. Ann Intern Med 122:9–16, 1995.

77. Paganini-Hill A, Chao A, Ross RK, et al: Exercise and other factors in the prevention of hip fracture: The Leisure World Study. Epidemiology 2:16–25, 1991.

78. Schneider DL, Barrett-Connor EL, Morton DJ: Timing of postmenopausal estrogen for optimal bone mineral density: The Rancho Bernardo study. JAMA 277:543–547, 1997.

79. Grady D, Rubin SM, Petitti DB, et al: Hormone therapy to prevent disease and prolong life in postmenopausal women. Ann Intern Med 117:1016–1037, 1992.

80. Michaelsson K, Baron JA, Farahmand BY, et al: Hormone replacement therapy and risk of hip fracture: Population-based case-control study The Swedish Hip Fracture Study Group. BMJ 316:1858–1863, 1998.

81. Colson F, et al: Hormonal replacement therapy (HRT): Which duration is effective to reduce the incidence of fracture in postmenopausal women? [abstract] Bone 23(Suppl):S496, 1998.

82. Ettinger B, et al for Multiple Outcomes of Raloxifene Evaluation (MORE) Investigators: Reduction of vertebral fracture risk in postmenopausal women with osteoporosis treated with raloxifene; results from a 3-year randomized clinical trial. JAMA 282:637–645, 1999.

83. Downs RW, et al: Comparison of alendronate and intranasal calcitonin for treatment of osteoporosis in postmenopausal women. J Clin Endocrinol Metab 85:1783–1788, 2000.

84. Hochberg M: Preventing fractures in postmenopausal women with osteoporosis. A review of recent controlled trials of antiresorptive agents. Drugs Aging 17:317–330, 2000.

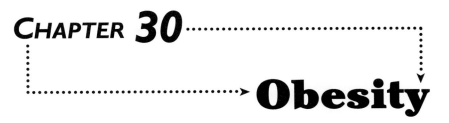

CHAPTER 30 ⋯⋯⋯⋯⋯⋯⋯⋯
Obesity

Judith Korner, M.D., Ph.D., and Louis J. Aronne, M.D.

PATHOPHYSIOLOGY

Obesity is a chronic disease that involves complex interactions among genetics, environment, and behavior. Positive energy balance is required in order for weight gain to occur; that is, energy intake must exceed energy expenditure. The pathogenesis of obesity involves a combination of various biologic factors that increase adipose tissue mass and environmental and behavioral factors that promote increased food intake and decreased physical activity (Fig. 30–1).[1] Biologic factors that modulate or partition the storage of nutrients into fat and protein include insulin and steroid, thyroid, and growth hormones, as well as hepatic and skeletal muscle metabolism and lipoprotein lipase activity.[2] Environmental and behavioral factors that may have contributed to the current epidemic of obesity are the easy availability of large portions of highly palatable foods and an increase in sedentary life style.[3]

There is also much evidence for a genetic predisposition to obesity. Except for obesity related to some rare disorders, common obesity does not exhibit typical mendelian inheritance. Recent studies suggest that the genetic contribution to obesity is about 25% to 40%.[2] Increased food intake and decreased energy expenditure may be due to imbalances or defects in substances (i.e., hormones and monoamines) produced in the brain or peripheral sites such as adipose tissue, skeletal muscle, and gastrointestinal tract (Table 30–1).[4–10]

PATIENT EVALUATION: HISTORY AND PHYSICAL EXAMINATION

The initial evaluation of an obese patient starting a weight loss regimen includes a history, physical examination, and laboratory studies. A history of eating disorders or purging is a relative contraindication to treatment, and referral to a specialist in these areas is indicated. The patient's current level of physical activity and understanding of nutrition should be assessed. Diseases associated with weight gain such as polycystic ovary disease, hypothyroidism, and Cushing's syndrome should be ruled out or treated. The physician should search for complications of obesity, such as hypertension, type 2 diabetes mellitus, hyperlipidemia, coronary heart disease, osteoarthritis of the lower extremities, gallbladder disease, gout, and certain cancers. In men, obesity is associated with colorectal and prostate cancer; in women, it is associated with endometrial, gallbladder, cervical, ovarian, and breast cancer. The patient should be questioned about symptoms and signs of sleep apnea: loud snoring, brief awakenings, sleeping in the sitting position, daytime fatigue, morning headaches, and polycythemia on laboratory evaluation. If signs of sleep apnea are present, the patient should be referred to a pulmonologist or sleep specialist.

Assessment of the patient should include the evaluation of body mass index (BMI). BMI is derived by a simple mathematical manipulation and is a useful

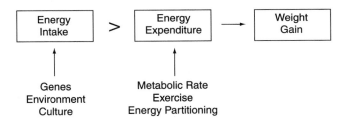

Figure 30–1. Pathogenesis of obesity.

Table 30–1. Substances That Regulate Energy Balance
⋯⋯⋯⋯⋯

Decreased Food Intake	Increased Food Intake
Leptin	Neuropeptide Y
α-Melanocyte-stimulating hormone	AGRP
Corticotropin-releasing hormone	MCH
Thyrotropin-releasing hormone	Orexin/Hypocretin
CART	Galanin
Insulin	Norepinephrine
Cholecystokinin	Ghrelin
Somatostatin	Perilipin
Glucagon-like peptide 1	
Urocortin	
Neuromedin	
Serotonin	
Dopamine	
Acrp30/apm-1/GBP28	
C75/Cerulenin	

AGRP, agouti-related protein; C75, a synthetic fatty acid synthase inhibitor; CART, cocaine- and amphetamine-regulated transcript; MCH, melanin-concentrating hormone.

$$\text{Weight (kg)/height (m)}^2$$

$$\text{or}$$

$$\text{Weight (lb)} \times 703/\text{height (in)}^2$$

Figure 30–2. Calculation of body mass index (BMI).

Table 30–2. Classification of Weight by Body Mass Index (BMI)

BMI (kg/m²)	Classification
<18.5	Underweight
18.5–24.9	Normal
25.0–29.9	Overweight
30.0–34.9	Obese class I
35.0–39.9	Obese class II
≥40	Obese class III

Adapted from Obesity: Preventing and managing the global epidemic. Report of the WHO consultation on obesity. Geneva, World Health Organization, 1997.

> ## *METHOD*
>
> *Measuring Waist Circumference: Place a measuring tape in a horizontal plane at the level of the iliac crest without compressing the skin. The value is read at the end of a normal expiration. Women with a waist circumference greater than 35 inches and men with a waist circumference greater than 40 inches should be considered to have a risk classification one level above that defined by their BMI.*

measure of fatness independent of height (Fig. 30–2). Clinical judgment is necessary in assessing a very muscular patient because BMI may overestimate the degree of fatness. The primary classification of overweight and obesity relates to BMI and the risk of developing type 2 diabetes mellitus, hypertension, and cardiovascular disease (Table 30–2).[11]

The distribution of adipose tissue is an important consideration in addition to BMI. An abdominal distribution of adipose tissue, characterized by an increase in waist circumference, is associated with an increased risk of medical complications including type 2 diabetes, dyslipidemia, hypertension, and cardiovascular disease.[12] Measurement of waist circumference should therefore be part of the evaluation of an overweight patient. A waist circumference greater than 35 inches (88 cm) in women and greater than 40 inches (102 cm) in men is considered an independent risk factor for disease even in persons of normal weight.

INTEGRATIVE THERAPY

Treatment for obesity is indicated primarily in those persons at medical risk because of their weight. These include overweight and obese patients with a BMI greater than 25 kg/m², particularly in the presence of comorbid conditions or associated with an increased waist circumference. Behavioral therapy and an exercise regimen should be an integral part of any weight loss program. A guide to the selection of the appropriate treatment based on BMI is presented in Table 30–3. Obesity treatment is usually contraindicated during pregnancy and in patients with anorexia nervosa or in the terminal stage of an illness. Medical or psychiatric illnesses should be stable before weight reduction is initiated. Patients with cholelithiasis and osteoporosis must be warned that these conditions may be aggravated by weight loss. Weight loss during lactation using a carefully monitored, mildly hypocaloric diet is possible provided that milk production is well established.

A realistic treatment goal is usually loss of 10% of initial body weight over a 6- to 12-month period. Ultimately, the goal of obesity treatment should be the lowest weight the patient can comfortably maintain. In the average patient, weight maintenance can be achieved at about a 5% to 10% reduction of total body weight. Most cardiovascular risk factors are improved even at this level of modest weight reduc-

Table 30–3. A Guide to Selecting Treatment for Obesity

Treatment	BMI Category				
	25–26.9	27–29.9	30–35	35–39.9	≥40
Diet, exercise, behavior therapy	With comorbid conditions	With comorbid conditions	+	+	+
Pharmacotherapy		With comorbid conditions	+	+	+
Surgery				With comorbid conditions	+

Prevention of weight gain with life style interventions is indicated in any patient with a BMI greater than 25 kg/m², even without comorbid conditions, but weight loss is not necessarily recommended for patients with a BMI of 25 to 29.9 kg/m² or a large waist circumference unless 2 or more comorbid conditions are present. Combined intervention with a low-calorie diet, increased physical activity, and behavior therapy provides the most successful treatment for weight loss and weight maintenance.

From: National Institutes of Health–National Heart, Lung and Blood Institute and the North American Association for the Study of Obesity: The practical guide. Identification, evaluation, and treatment of overweight and obesity in adults. NIH pub no 00–4084, 2000.

tion.[13] To prevent disappointment, the patient should be counseled that his or her body may not allow the magnitude of weight loss sought. Cosmetic goals should be discouraged.

Mind-Body Techniques

Behavioral Therapy

The goal of behavioral therapy is to overcome barriers to compliance with a diet and physical activity regimen. Behavioral therapy may consist of self-monitoring, stimulus control, reinforcement, and stress management.

Self-monitoring includes recording dietary intake (food choices, amounts, times), exercise, and changes in body weight.

Stimulus control helps the patient to identify and change cues that are associated with eating too much and exercising too little. For example, limiting exposure to food or separating eating from other activities such as reading or watching television may be helpful.

Reinforcement encourages attainment of difficult-to-achieve goals. Reinforcement may come from a social support network or getting nonfood rewards for reaching goals.

Stress management helps the patient to cope with stressful events by developing outlets besides eating for reducing stress. Evaluating setbacks and determining how to do better next time can break the chain of negative thinking and self-punishment when lapses occur.

Life Style Interventions

Exercise

Weight loss is accompanied by a reduction in total energy expenditure that counteracts the effort to lose weight and facilitates the regain of lost weight. Physical activity increases energy expenditure and is a key component of any weight maintenance program. A moderate amount of physical activity uses approximately 150 calories of energy per day. Some examples of moderate activity include walking 2 miles or pushing a stroller $1^{1}/_{2}$ miles in 30 minutes, wheeling oneself in a wheelchair for 30 to 40 minutes, bicycling 5 miles in 30 minutes, and swimming laps for 20 minutes.[12] Patients who are physically limited by obesity or arthritis may start with water exercises, bedside stretching, or seated activities. In general, the patient should build up to a 30- to 45-minute exercise regimen, daily if possible, of the greatest intensity exercise that is safe for the present level of fitness. The physician should emphasize to the patient that improvements in cardiovascular risk factors are attained through regular exercise even if

he or she remains overweight (see Chapter 86, Writing an Exercise Prescription).

Nutrition

Calorie-Restricted Diets

In order to induce weight loss, a calorie deficit must be created. General guidelines for healthy eating such as reduction in fat, sugar, and alcohol intake should be emphasized. Balanced diets should contain a minimum of 1000 to 1200 kcal per day and have adequate amounts of all essential nutrients. A diet that is individually planned to create a deficit of 500 kcal per day should produce a weight loss of about 1 pound per week. The Step I Diet, consisting of approximately 55% carbohydrate, 15% protein, and 30% fat (8% to 10% saturated fatty acids and less than 300 mg of cholesterol per day), with a total daily sodium intake of 2.4 g, will also decrease other risk factors such as high blood cholesterol and hypertension. Water intake should be at least six to eight 8-ounce glasses per day. Sample diets may be found in a set of guidelines published by the National Heart, Lung and Blood Institute (NHLBI) and may be obtained on the NHLBI website (www.nhlbi.nih.gov).[12] Supplementation with a multivitamin is also recommended. Calcium intake of 1000 to 1500 mg per day is particularly important for persons at risk for osteoporosis.

Calories consumed as fat are easier to overeat because they are "denser" (9 calories per g, versus 4 calories per g for protein and carbohydrate), are easily hidden in foods, and increase food palatability. Compared with carbohydrate, fat may have a delayed effect on satiety that makes it more likely to be overeaten. Fat-modified foods lower total fat intake but are effective in achieving weight loss only if they are also low in calories. Recent studies suggest that because people tend to consume a constant weight of food, a diet low in energy density is likely to lead to a reduction in energy intake.[14] A diet low in energy density is usually low in fat and high in water content, complex carbohydrates, and fiber. Fruits, vegetables, and grain products are low-energy-density foods. However, high-energy-density foods are not always high in fat content. For example, dry foods such as fat-free pretzels or crackers are high in energy density.

Interestingly, despite a recent reduction in fat consumption in the United States, the prevalence of overweight has continued to rise. The glycemic index (GI), defined as the area under the glucose response curve after consumption of 50 g of carbohydrate from a test food divided by the area under the curve after consumption of 50 g of carbohydrate from a control food such as white bread or glucose, may also play an important role in regulating food intake. Starchy foods such as refined grain products and potatoes generally have a high GI, whereas vegetables, legumes, and fruits are generally low-GI foods. Recent work has shown that subjects who received a low-GI diet in the morning consumed less food later in the day compared with subjects who received a high-GI diet.[15] It has been proposed that the rapid absorption of glucose from the high-GI meal results in relatively high insulin and low glucagon concentrations, which induce a "reactive hypoglycemia" that stimulates hunger and favors storage of fat[16] (see Chapter 83, The Glycemic Index). The overconsumption of low-fat but high-GI, high-energy-density foods may explain the disappointing long-term results seen with low-fat diets in some persons.

Pharmaceuticals

Medications That May Cause Weight Gain

Many commonly prescribed medications are known to cause weight gain as a side effect (Table 30–4). In considering the use of antiobesity medications, the drug history should first be reviewed for medications that may cause weight gain, and if possible the patient should be switched to others that may induce weight loss. For example, sulfonylureas and insulin tend to cause weight gain. Metformin (Glucophage) is often the best first-line drug in the obese diabetic, as it may induce weight loss, improve body composition, and optimize lipid levels. The alpha-glucosidase inhibitors acarbose (Precose) and miglitol (Glyset) may also induce weight loss. Most antidepressants and mood stabilizers cause weight gain, although bupropion (Wellbutrin, Zyban) often

Table 30–4. Drugs That May Promote Weight Gain
....

Phenothiazines	Progestational steroids
Antidepressants	Insulin
Lithium	Sulfonylureas
Neuroleptics	Thioglitazones
Antiepileptics	Antihistamines
Hormonal contraceptives	Beta-adrenergic blockers
Corticosteroids	

Adapted from Obesity: Preventing and managing the global epidemic. Report of a WHO consultation on obesity. Geneva, World Health Organization, 1997.

induces weight loss. An anticonvulsant, topiramate (Topamax), has been shown to induce weight loss, in contrast with the weight gain often seen with other agents, and there are case reports of its use to mitigate the weight gain associated with newer antipsychotic agents such as olanzipine (Zyprexa). Progesterones, corticosteroids, beta-blockers, and antihistamines, among others, all may cause weight gain.

Drugs Used for Weight Loss

The role of medication is to help patients comply with a reduced-calorie regimen. Not every patient responds to a given medicine. If a patient loses more than 4 pounds during the first month, the prognosis for losing more than 5% of body weight is good. If not, consideration should be given to changing medication after another month of treatment.

Sibutramine (Meridia) and orlistat (Xenical) (Table 30–5) are the only drugs approved for long-term use by the Food and Drug Administration. Noradrenergic agents such as phentermine (Adipex-P, Ionamin) and diethylpropion (Tenuate) have been approved for short-term use.

Sibutramine

Sibutramine (Meridia) is a serotonin and norepinephrine reuptake inhibitor (SNRI) that was originally developed as an antidepressant but has been shown to be effective in reducing body weight.[17] Although a schedule IV compound, like the other drugs in the SNRI category it has demonstrated no evidence for abuse or habituation. A 1-year-long placebo-controlled trial demonstrated that of patients receiving 15 mg of sibutramine daily, 65% lost more than 5% of body weight, compared with 29% of patients taking placebo, and 39% lost more than 10% of their body weight, compared with 8% in the placebo-treatment group (Knoll Pharmaceuticals, sibutramine package insert). Health benefits demonstrated with the use of sibutramine include reductions in triglycerides, uric acid, total cholesterol and low-density lipoprotein (LDL) cholesterol and an increase in high-density lipoprotein (HDL) cholesterol.

Table 30–5. Weight Loss Drugs Approved for Long-Term Use[*]
....

Drug/Formulation	Dose	Action	Adverse Effects
Sibutramine (Meridia) (5-, 10-, 15-mg capsules)	10 mg PO qd to start, may be increased to 15 mg or decreased to 5 mg	Norepinephrine, dopamine, and serotonin reuptake inhibitor	Increase in heart rate and blood pressure
Orlistat (Xenical) (120-mg capsules)	120 mg PO tid before meals	Inhibits pancreatic lipase, decreases fat absorption	Decrease in absorption of fat-soluble vitamins; soft stools and anal leakage

*Ephedrine and caffeine, mazindol, fluoxetine, and phentermine have also been tested for weight loss but are not approved for long-term use.

Adapted from the National Institutes of Health–National Heart, Lung and Blood Institute and the North American Association for the Study of Obesity: The practical guide. Identification, evaluation, and treatment of overweight and obesity in adults. NIH pub no 00–4084, 2000.

Dosage. 5, 10, or 15 mg once daily; 10 mg daily is the usual starting dose.

Precautions. Patients taking sibutramine may experience dry mouth, constipation, insomnia, increased appetite, dizziness, or nausea. Sibutramine is relatively contraindicated in patients with poorly controlled hypertension and atherosclerotic cardiovascular diseases including stroke and myocardial infarction. A mean increase in blood pressure of 4 mm Hg has been seen in trials. Approximately 12% of patients have an increase in systolic blood pressure of 15 mm Hg or more. Of note, a decrease in blood pressure may often be seen in patients who lose more than 5% of body weight. It is recommended that blood pressure and pulse be checked 2 to 4 weeks after the drug is started and then monthly for the first 6 months; thereafter, monitoring every 2 to 3 months is adequate or can be done more often if indicated. Some medications should not be co-administered with sibutramine, such as monoamine oxidase inhibitors, antidepressants that increase serotonin levels, pseudoephedrine, and ephedra (ma huang), a nonspecific beta agonist found in some diet products.

Orlistat

Orlistat (Xenical) is an inhibitor of pancreatic lipases that prevents the absorption of about a third of dietary fat. Analysis of patients completing a 2-year-long placebo-controlled trial demonstrated a mean weight loss of 8% after 1 year, compared with 4% in the placebo (diet-only) treatment group.[18] Orlistat slowed down the rate of weight regain in the second year, with a 6% mean weight loss maintained after 2 years of treatment compared with 2% in the placebo treatment group. Health benefits demonstrated in clinical trials of orlistat include a reduction in LDL and an increase in HDL cholesterol, reduction in blood pressure and fasting insulin levels, improvement in oral glucose tolerance test outcomes, and improved glycemic control in obese diabetics.

Dosage. 120 mg orally 3 times daily before meals. The drug is often taken once daily before dinner to start and gradually, increased to 3 times daily to minimize gastrointestinal effects.

Precautions. Gastrointestinal side effects including oily stool and fecal urgency may occur. Compliance may be enhanced with a low-fat diet. Informing the patient about these side effects and their relationship to fat intake is important, and a low-fat, high-fiber diet should be recommended. No effect on mineral balance, gallstone, or renal stone formation was seen. A reduction in the levels of vitamin D and beta-carotene was noted in some treated patients during trials and supplementation with a multivitamin taken remotely from a dose of orlistat has been recommended (orlistat package insert).

Phentermine and Diethylpropion

Noradrenergic agents such as phentermine (Ionamin, Fastin, Adipex) and diethylpropion (Tenuate) have been shown to be better than placebo in relatively small-scale, short-term studies. No large-scale, long-term studies of weight loss, health benefits, or side effects have been performed on these compounds, although they have been available since the 1960s. Accordingly, if any of these drugs are used for longer than 3 months, the patient should be informed that such use is "off-label" and has not been studied.

Dosage. For phentermine, the dose is 15 or 30 mg once daily; for diethylpropion, 75 mg long-acting once daily.

Precautions. Adverse effects include constipation, insomnia, dry mouth, tachycardia, increased blood pressure, agitation, and anxiety. These medications are relatively contraindicated in patients with poorly controlled hypertension and atherosclerotic cardiovascular diseases including stroke and myocardial infarction. These agents must not be coadministered with monoamine oxidase inhibitors, pseudoephedrine, and ephedra (ma huang). Regular monitoring of blood pressure is recommended.

Botanicals

The German Commission E monographs recognize no botanical or herbal treatments for obesity as effective.[19] Nonetheless, a bewildering variety of products is available; these are heavily promoted to the public with little evidence of their safety or efficacy. Often, anecdotal reports of success from a few individual authors are substituted for valid trials of scientific merit in evaluating these products. Unfortunately, the placebo effect of obesity treatments is substantial, and uncontrolled anecdotal trials are not adequate measures of the efficacy of any obesity treatment. Furthermore, several compounds that have proved quite effective at reducing body weight in animal trials have shown no efficacy in humans. Therefore, results obtained in animal studies cannot be generalized to humans. Although botanicals have proved effective in many areas of medicine and although several alternative therapies for obesity are promising, the promotion of ineffectual products has created increasing skepticism that these products can play a role in obesity treatment. Several recent reviews of the literature are recommended.[20–22]

Ephedrine/Caffeine/Aspirin

The combination of ephedrine and caffeine (ma huang/guarana or kola nut), with or without aspirin (white willow bark), produces significant weight loss and has been the subject of several placebo-controlled trials.[23] A recently published study documented the efficacy of a herbal version of ephedrine and caffeine.[24] This combination acts as a nonspecific beta agonist and may increase metabolic rate as well as reduce appetite. Given the risk of cardiovascular side effects including increased blood pressure, pulse, arrhthymias, anxiety, and liver function abnormalities, among others, the major issue surrounding the use of the combination is its unregulated over-the-counter status. In Denmark, for example, the combination is available as a prescription product for obesity treatment. The physician is often caught in the middle: on one hand, the Food and Drug Administration, which has not approved ephedrine as a treatment for obesity, recommends no more than 8 mg of ephedrine three times daily for only brief periods. And on the other hand, manufacturers advocate the use of as much as 100 mg of ephedrine per day for 3 months.

Precautions. Adverse effects include increased pulse, blood pressure, anxiety, agitation, and sleep disturbance.

Bladderwrack

A source of iodine, bladderwrack (*Fucus vesiculosis*) and other seaweed preparations are believed to stimulate thyroid function temporarily. Because the net result of this increased function in a patient who is euthyroid at baseline is hyperthyroidism, this product cannot be recommended. Furthermore, there is no conclusive evidence of its efficacy.

Hydroxycitric Acid

In rat studies, hydroxycitric acid—present in *Garcinia cambogia*, or brindleberry—has been shown to increase hepatic glycogen synthesis and decrease body weight gain. Human studies have not consistently documented weight loss or improvement in body composition. Although several small studies have shown modest weight loss when used alone or in conjunction with other compounds, a carefully designed, placebo-controlled trial showed no weight loss with use of 1500 mg per day of hydroxycitric acid.[26] No significant side effects were reported in clinical trials.

St. John's Wort

A plant substance with antidepressant activity related to either serotoninergic or monoamine-inhibiting properties, St. John's wort (*Hypericum perforatum*) has not been studied carefully as a weight loss agent. Early evidence from trials of serotoninergic antidepressants such as fluoxetine (Prozac) suggested weight loss as a side effect, but longer-term follow-up and clinical experience show that weight gain is more likely over time with these compounds.

Thus, St. John's wort cannot be recommended for weight loss.

Supplements

Chitosan

Chitosan is an acetylated product of chitin, a compound that makes up the exoskeleton of arthropods. Chitosan absorbs fats, and its supposed mechanism of action is mechanical binding to fat, thereby preventing its absorption from the gut. Although this mechanism is plausible, preliminary human studies suggest that no fat is found in the stool of subjects taking chitosan at recommended doses. Chitosan appears to reduce weight in animal studies, but there is conflicting evidence that it reduces body weight significantly more than placebo in humans. As a result, despite a plausible mechanism, chitosan cannot be recommended at this time as a therapeutic agent for management of obesity.

Chromium

Chromium is a trace element that functions as a cofactor in carbohydrate and lipid metabolism. Chromium deficiency leads to hallmarks of the so-called metabolic syndrome—the syndrome of insulin resistance that includes increased plasma glucose, insulin, and triglycerides and low HDL cholesterol levels. Although chromium deficiency is rare in Western nations, supplementation of chromium in deficient individuals helps to reverse the signs of insulin resistance. Evidence supporting the use of chromium for weight loss is equivocal, with some studies showing benefit and others no benefit. Cases of renal impairment and rhabdomyolysis from chronic high dosages have been reported.

Conjugated Linoleic Acid

Conjugated linoleic acid (CLA) is a fatty acid that has been found to reduce body weight and improve insulin sensitivity in Zucker rats and other animal models of obesity. In animals, CLA has slowed the gain of body fat following weight loss. Basic studies suggest that CLA inhibits lipoprotein lipase, an enzyme needed for fat deposition. Human trials in the treatment of obesity have not yet been published; thus, no recommendation can be made about its use in humans, but preliminary results were not as promising as anticipated.[25]

Pyruvate

Pyruvate is a nutritional supplement that, when used in large quantities amounting to 2% to 15% of total calories, may increase weight and fat loss in the short term when compared with placebo. A more pronounced effect may be obtained when pyruvate is combined with dihydroxyacetone. A drawback is the large quantity of pyruvate needed, between 6 and 50 g (available capsules contain 1 g of pyruvate). No study longer than 6 weeks has been reported, though one study showed greater weight loss (1.2 kg) and body fat loss (2.5 kg) in subjects taking 6 g (3 g twice daily) pyruvate per day than in persons taking a placebo.[27]

Precautions. Adverse effects include diarrhea and upset stomach.

Acupuncture

Acupuncture or acupressure behind the ear is supposed to stimulate the auricular branch of the vagal nerve and suppress appetite. For acupuncture, a permanent needle is placed behind the ear, and the patient is directed to stimulate the needle when hungry. Although patients report a short-term reduction in appetite and uncontrolled studies claim benefit, controlled trials have not shown clinically significant weight loss. There are no significant side effects.

Surgery

Obesity surgery should be considered in patients with a BMI greater than 40 or with a BMI between 35 and 40 kg/m^2 in whom other methods of treatment have failed if serious obesity-related complications are present.[13, 28] Careful screening of candidates is required if the patient is to benefit from the procedure. Surgical candidates must be motivated and well informed about the risks of the procedure, as well as the change in their lives that will occur as a result of the procedure, and its long-term effects. These changes may be relatively minor, such as the need for long-term treatment with vitamin and mineral supplements, or may include chronic vomiting or diarrhea after meals. In general, weight loss of 60% to 80% of the excess is achieved; the loss reaches its maximum at 18 months to 2 years, with some weight regain up to 5 years postoperatively and weight stability thereafter. Unfortunately, in some surgical series, up to 20% of patients ultimately regain all lost weight. Obesity surgery is best performed in specialty centers accustomed to performing procedures on high-risk obese patients. The overall mortality rate for bariatric surgery is approximately 1% but may be higher in persons with comorbid conditions.

Surgical complications such as wound dehiscence, anastomotic leak, stomal stenosis, or thrombophle-bitis occur in about 10% of patients.[29] Late complications include need for reoperation, nutritional deficiencies, dumping syndrome, cholecystitis, and failure to lose weight. Long-term follow-up is required to ensure the best results and proper nutrition in the postsurgical patient.

Vertical Banded Gastroplasty

Vertical banded gastroplasty, also known as gastric stapling or banding, is the most commonly performed procedure. A 30-mL pouch with a restricted outlet is constructed along the lesser curvature of the stomach, reducing the capacity of the stomach 100-fold. A Silastic ring or band of Marlex mesh restricts the outlet size, and four rows of staples reinforce the free wall to prevent breakdown. The amount of weight lost is correlated with the volume of the pouch and diameter of the outlet, with larger volumes and diameters yielding less weight loss but fewer side effects. Patients who undergo this procedure feel full after eating very small amounts of food and may vomit if they continue to eat. Within a few months after the procedure, up to 1 cup of food may be eaten at a time. Ingested food is digested in a normal sequence and is fully absorbed, minimizing the risk of malnutrition. In general, 70% of patients maintain a loss of 20% or more of total body weight on 5-year follow up. It is not as effective as the gastric bypass in carbohydrate cravers because of the "soft calorie syndrome," in which highly caloric liquid or meltable foods are consumed to excess, leading to weight regain.

Gastric Bypass

Gastric bypass involves constructing a small proximal gastric pouch—as with the gastroplasty—whose outlet is a limb of small bowel of varying lengths, as in a Roux-en-Y gastrojejunostomy. Increasing the length of the limb from 75 to 150 cm increases weight loss as well as the risk of long-term side effects and nutrient malabsorption. The procedure produces malabsorption of food and the dumping syndrome and is effective in patients who may not respond to the gastroplasty because of carbohydrate craving. Because of the malabsorption of vitamins and minerals, patients who have undergone gastric bypass need careful nutritional instruction and follow-up, as well as behavioral training. More weight is lost with this procedure than with gastroplasty, but the risk of complications is greater. Long-term supplementation with calcium, iron, and vitamin B_{12} is recommended. Of note, although technically challenging, laparoscopic gastric bypass surgery is now being performed on a regular basis.

—THERAPEUTIC REVIEW

Initial Examination
- *Measure the patient's weight, height, and waist circumference.*
- *Calculate BMI.*
- *Rule out or treat any medical conditions that may result in weight gain.*

Assessment for Risk Factors
- *Comorbid conditions considered important enough to warrant more aggressive therapy include type 2 diabetes mellitus, cardiovascular disease, and sleep apnea.*

Drug History
- *Discontinue medications that cause weight gain, or switch to alternatives that induce weight loss.*
- *Make sure that the patient is not using over-the-counter supplements or herbal remedies that are contraindicated with prescription medications.*

Following is a summary of the therapeutic options for weight loss stratified according to BMI, kg/m^2, and obesity-related comorbid conditions.

- *BMI 25 to 29.9*   *All patients with a BMI of greater than 25 should receive nutritional education and should begin an exercise and behavioral program.*
- *BMI ≥30, or ≥27 with ≥2 comorbid conditions*   *Pharmacotherapy should be considered if other options have not produced the desired effect.*
- *BMI ≥40, or ≥35 with ≥2 comorbid conditions*   *Bariatric surgery should be considered if other options have not produced the desired effect.*

NOTE

A realistic initial goal is to lose 10% of current weight over a 6- to 12-month period. Further weight loss can then be attempted if appropriate. Obesity is a treatable but not curable disease. When treatments are stopped, weight is usually regained.

References

1. Campfield LA, Smith FJ: The pathogenesis of obesity. Baillieres Clin Endocrinol Metab 13:13–30, 1999.
2. York D, Bouchard C: How obesity develops. Insights from the new biology. Endocrine 13:143–154, 2000.
3. Hill JO, Wyatt HR, Melanson EL: Genetic and environmental contributions to obesity. Med Clin North Am 84:333–346, 2000.
4. Fruebis J, Tsao TS, Javorschi S, et al: Proteolytic cleavage product of 30-kDa adipocyte complement-related protein increases fatty acid oxidation in muscle and causes weight loss in mice. Proc Natl Acad Sci USA 98:2005–2010, 2000.
5. Bray GA, Greenway FL: Current and potential drugs for treatment of obesity. Endocr Rev 20:805–875, 1999.
6. Wren AM, Small CJ, Ward HL, et al: The novel hypothalamic peptide ghrelin stimulates food intake and growth hormone secretion. Endocrinology 141:4325–4328, 2000.
7. Howard AD, Wang R, Pong SS, et al: Identification of receptors for neuromedin U and its role in feeding. Nature 406:70–74, 2000.
8. Bray GA, Tartaglia LA: Medicinal strategies in the treatment of obesity. Nature 404:672–677, 2000.
9. Loftus TM, Jaworsky DE, Frehywot GL, et al: Reduced food intake and body weight in mice treated with fatty acid synthase inhibitors. Science 288:2379–2381, 2000.
10. Martinez-Botas J, Anderson JB, Tessier D, et al: Absence of perilipin results in leanness and reverses obesity in Lepr *db/db* mice. Nat Genet 26:474–479, 2000.
11. World Health Organization: Obesity: Preventing and managing the global epidemic. Report of a WHO consultation on obesity. Geneva; World Health Organization, 1997.
12. National Institutes of Health–National Heart, Lung and Blood Institute and the North American Association for the Study of Obesity: The practical guide. Identification, evaluation, and treatment of overweight and obesity in adults. Bethesda, MD, 00–4084, 2000.
13. National Institutes of Health–National Heart, Lung and Blood Institute and the North American Association for the Study of Obesity: Clinical guidelines on the identification, evaluation, and treatment of overweight and obesity in adults—the evidence report. Obes Res 6 (Suppl 2):51S–209S, 1998.
14. Rolls BJ, Bell EA: Dietary approaches to the treatment of obesity. Med Clin North Am 84:401–418, 2000.
15. Spieth LE, Harnish JD, Lenders CM, et al: A low-glycemic index diet in the treatment of pediatric obesity. Arch Pediatr Adolesc Med 154:947–951, 2000.
16. Ludwig DS: Dietary glycemic index and obesity. J Nutr 130:280S–283S, 2000.
17. Bray GA, Blackburn GL, Ferguson JM, et al: Sibutramine produces dose-related weight loss. Obes Res 7:189–198, 1999.
18. Davidson MH, Hauptman J, DiGirolamo M, et al: Weight control and risk factor reduction in obese subjects treated for 2 years with orlistat: A randomized controlled trial. JAMA 281:235–242, 1999.
19. Blumenthal M (ed): The Complete German Commission E monographs: Therapeutic Guide to Herbal Medicines. Austin, Tex, American Botanical Council, 1998.
20. Allison DB, Fontaine KR, Heshka S, et al: Alternative treatments

for weight loss: A critical review. Crit Rev Food Sci Nutr 41:1–28, 2001.

21. Egger G, Cameron Smith D, Stanton R: The effectiveness of popular, non-prescription weight loss supplements. Med J Aust 171:604–608, 1999.

22. Mulhisen L, Rogers JZ: Complementary and alternative modes of therapy for the treatment of the obese patient. J Am Osteopath Assoc 99:S8–S12, 1999.

23. Astrup A, Breum L, Toubro S, et al: The effect and safety of an ephedrine/caffeine compound compared to ephedrine, caffeine and placebo in obese subjects on an energy restricted diet. A double blind trial. Int J Obes Relat Metab Disord 16:269–277, 1992.

24. Boozer CN, Nasser JA, Heymsfield SB, et al: An herbal supplement containing Ma Huang–Guarana for weight loss: A randomized, double-blind trial. Int J Obesity 25:316–324, 2001.

25. Whigham LD, Cook ME, Atkinson RL: Conjugated linoleic acid: Implications for human health. Pharmacol Res 42:503–510, 2000.

26. Heymsfield SB, Allison DB, Vasselli JR, et al: *Garcinia cambogia* (hydroxycitric acid) as a potential antiobesity agent: A randomized controlled trial. JAMA 280:1596–1600, 1998.

27. Kalman D, Colker CM, Wilets I, et al: The effects of pyruvate supplementation on body composition in overweight individuals. Nutrition 15:337–340, 1999.

28. National Institutes of Health: Gastrointestinal surgery for severe obesity. NIH Consensus Development Conference consensus statement. Bethesda, MD, National Institutes of Health, 1991.

29. Aronne LJ: Modern medical management of obesity: The role of pharmaceutical intervention. J Am Diet Assoc 98:S23–S26, 1998.

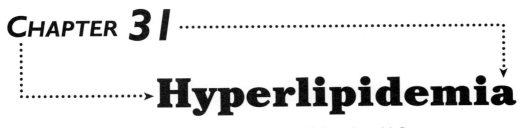

CHAPTER 31

Hyperlipidemia

Brian Olshansky, M.D.

Coronary artery disease is the most common cause of death in the United States.[1] Of all the major risk factors responsible for coronary artery disease, hypercholesterolemia has become a major concern for many Americans and has drawn the greatest attention as a risk for heart disease, even though other risk factors, such as smoking, are more potent predictors of death from heart disease.[2–6] Nevertheless, hypercholesterolemia is associated with coronary artery disease, myocardial infarction, and cardiac death. It can be due to inherent genetic defects ("primary" hypercholesterolemia), or it can be acquired as the result of obesity, physical inactivity, or a high-carbohydrate diet (>60% of energy intake) ("secondary" hypercholesterolemia). The "metabolic syndrome" is a condition involving predominantly males who have central obesity, diabetes, and hypercholesterolemia. Additional causes of secondary dyslipidemia include diabetes, hypothyroidism, obstructive liver disease, chronic renal failure, and the use of drugs that raise low-density lipoprotein (LDL) cholesterol and lower high-density lipoprotein (HDL) cholesterol (i.e., progestins, anabolic steroids, and corticosteroids). Two therapeutic approaches apply: **primary reduction** in cholesterol to prevent disease conditions and sequelae that have not yet occurred, and **secondary prevention** to modify the progression of disease in patients who already have been diagnosed with coronary heart disease.[7, 8]

Lowering the cholesterol levels in a patient who has hypercholesterolemia can reduce the long-term risk of coronary heart disease, but several caveats apply[9]: (1) Reduction of cholesterol levels does not eliminate the risk of coronary atherosclerosis and its consequences; (2) reduction of the total cholesterol level may not be enough—there may be associated elevations in other high-risk lipid markers (all of which are not defined) that require further therapy; (3) even the best pharmacologic methods to reduce cholesterol (e.g., statin therapy) can be associated with continued risk of coronary heart disease and its progression; (4) therapies can be associated with adverse effects and side effects; and (5) no therapy is always effective in lowering cholesterol.

PATHOPHYSIOLOGY

How cholesterol is related to the development of coronary artery disease is not completely understood. Cholesterol is a major building block with many important physiologic functions. For example, it creates hormones and nerve sheaths.

Cholesterol is insoluble and needs to bind to lipoproteins to be transported, and delivered, throughout the body. The mechanism for transportation of cholesterol to, and its deposition at, various sites is complex.[10] High-density lipoproteins (HDLs) transport cholesterol to the liver to eliminate it from spots where cholesterol is not needed and to metabolize it into hormones. Low-density lipoproteins (LDLs) transport cholesterol through the body to sites of action. High levels of LDLs are associated with development of coronary artery disease. Very low-density lipoproteins (VLDLs) transport triglycerides to peripheral tissue. Other lipoprotein subfractions exist; these include intermediate density lipoprotein (IDL) and lipoprotein (a) (LPa).[11]

CHOLESTEROL AND ATHEROSCLEROSIS

The oxidation-modification hypothesis states that coronary artery disease is only partly due to lipid deposition from high cholesterol and that lipid deposition occurs at least in part as the result of an inflammatory response in the endothelium.[10] It appears that cholesterol is in balance within the body. When cholesterol levels are high or when cholesterol goes into the subendothelial space (such as when there is endothelial damage), it is ingested by macrophages. These macrophages ingest only enough LDL-cholesterol, and they survive when LDL-cholesterol aggregate is not oxidized.[10] When this aggregate is oxidized, macrophages ingest through scavenger receptors that do not downregulate. These macrophages become foam cells that lyse to release toxic contents throughout the endothelial space, damaging it further. Cholesterol appears to get deposited into this space when the levels are high or when there is a need for repair of damage due to genetic endothelial structure, hypertension, smoking, or other causes. Plaque formation begins at an early age as a white plaque that progresses to an ulcerated, lipid-laden, yellow plaque, which can rupture, causing platelet aggregation and obliterating the vessel. An inflammatory response of unknown cause may further propagate the process.

Free radicals are oxidants that can bind to the LDL-cholesterol complex. Many of these are routine metabolic byproducts. Others originate from toxins such as cigarette smoke, pollutants, benzpyrene, barbecued meat, dietary factors, cellular degradation, and endothelial damage.[12] A potential oxidant, homocysteine can create oxycholesterols such as cholestane diol, which further damage the endothelium.[13–15] Reducing homocysteine levels to eliminate oxidized cholesterol is only one method of reducing all oxidized cholesterol moieties.

RISK FACTORS—CHOLESTEROL MARKERS

High levels of LDL-cholesterol (particularly) and total cholesterol are unnecessary and are associated with risk for atherosclerotic coronary artery disease. Cholesterol represents only one of many significant risk factors for coronary artery disease. The majority of coronary artery disease occurs in people with relatively normal cholesterol, even though higher levels increase the risk of coronary heart disease. Several other risk factors are now being assessed, including high-sensitivity C-reactive protein and abnormal brachial reactivity to acetylcholine.[21] These, and a host of other factors, create conditions ripe for coronary artery disease. Risk increases when the cholesterol value exceeds 200 mg/dL, but risk is continuous and increases at even higher levels. LDL-cholesterol values greater than 100 mg/dL, and perhaps even greater than 80 mg/dL, are associated with development of coronary artery disease. The HDL/total cholesterol ratio is perhaps the best cholesterol predictor of risk for coronary artery disease. When the value exceeds 1:4, risk escalates. Several types of HDL (HDL1, HDL2, and HDL3) exist. All HDL subfractions are associated with lower risk for coronary artery disease.[22, 23]

Emerging risk factors for coronary atherosclerosis include ApoB, lipoprotein (a) (LPa level >25 mg/dL is associated with coronary artery disease), fibrinogen, homocysteine, prothrombotic factors, proinflammatory factors (high-sensitivity C-reactive protein), impaired fasting glucose, subclinical atherosclerosis, even hypertriglyceridemia. ApoB may be an even better predictor than LDL-cholesterol.[22, 24]

Up to the present, no specific recommendation has been made to screen for LPa or other risk factors such as ApoB, despite the potential for increased risk.[25] Elevated triglyceride levels, perhaps, add risk but the additional risk is controversial. It is likely that high triglyceride levels add risk.[26] A long list of minor risk factors, such as chronic ingestion of soft water, has also been noted.

The absolute risk for coronary heart disease based on cholesterol levels differs by sex and racial and ethnic groups, but the relative risk is similar for all population groups (Table 31–1). Special considerations depend on the population group. Most coro-

Table 31–1. Age-Related Risk and Benefit of Therapy

Men 20 to 35 years; women 20 to 45 years: Routine cholesterol screening recommended starting at age 20. Hypercholesterolemia—LDL-lowering drugs.
Women 45 to 75 years: CHD in women delayed 10 to 15 years (compared with men).
Men >65 years; women >75 years: High LDL and low HDL still predict CHD. Benefits of LDL-lowering therapy extend to older adults.
Men 35 to 65 years: Coronary heart disease risk in men is greater than in women. High prevalence of risk factors. CHD incidence high. Strong evidence for benefit of LDL-lowering therapy.

CHD, coronary heart disease; HDL, high-density lipoprotein; LDL, low-density lipoprotein.

nary heart disease in women occurs after age 65.[35] For secondary prevention in postmenopausal women, hormone replacement therapy is of doubtful benefit and likely is harmful.[36] Benefits of statin therapy have been documented in primary and secondary prevention trials, but issues of cost effectiveness for any patient population are important.[37] Men prone to abdominal obesity who have the metabolic syndrome are at even higher risk.[39, 40] Coronary heart disease incidence is high among middle-aged men. Strong clinical trial evidence supports the benefit of LDL-lowering therapy with "statin" drugs.[41, 42]

> ## NOTE
>
> *For screening, a complete fasting lipoprotein profile is preferred (fasting total cholesterol, LDL, HDL, triglycerides). As a secondary option: Nonfasting total cholesterol and HDL can be obtained. A lipoprotein profile is recommended if total cholesterol is greater than or equal to 200 mg/dL, or if HDL is less than or equal to 40 mg/dL.*

GOALS OF THERAPY

Recent recommendations have been compiled by ATPIII[4,43](http://www.americanheart.org/Whats_News/thirdsummary.html) (Table 31–2). These have now become the standard approach to therapy. The management of cholesterol involves procedures that are more complex than simply starting a statin drug, however. Healing approaches can include use of supplements, other dietary changes, and lifestyle issues. Changes in diet and exercise and the addition of supplements can facilitate the effects of statins, can lower the incidence of hypercholesterolemia, can reduce the quantity of oxidized forms of cholesterol, and can prevent endothelial damage.[44, 45] No supplemental therapy for hypercholesterolemia should be relied on solely. Individuals may have varying desires to attempt to reduce their risks in addition to, or in lieu of, drug therapy. These desires

Table 32–2. ATP III Treatment Guidelines

LDL-Cholesterol Treatment Guidelines

Category (Risk)	Suggested LDL	Approach
Secondary prevention (CHD or its equivalent present)	100 mg/dL	Lifestyle changes, weight reduction. If elevated triglyceride or low HDL, add nicotinic or fibric acid.
2 risk factors (primary prevention) risk 10% to 20%	<130 mg/dL	Lifestyle changes. If LDL >130 @ 3mo, add drug.
2 risk factors (primary prevention) risk 10% to 20%	<130 mg/dL	Lifestyle changes. If LDL >160, add drug.
0–1 risk factor	<160 mg/dL	Lifestyle changes, if severe risk factor, emerging risks, or LDL >190, drug therapy.

ATP III Lipid and Lipoprotein Classification

LDL-Cholesterol (mg/dL)		HDL-Cholesterol (mg/dL)		Total Cholesterol (mg/dL)	
<100	Optimal	<40	Low	<200	Desirable
100–129	Near optimal/above optimal	60	High	200–239	Borderline high
130–159	Borderline high			240	High
160–189	High				
190	Very high				

New Features of ATP III Modification of Lipid and Lipoprotein Classification

LDL-cholesterol <100 mg/dL—optimal
HDL-cholesterol <40 mg/dL (Raised from <35 mg/dL)
Lower triglyceride classification cut points (<150 mg/dL fasting)
More attention to moderate elevations

CHD, coronary heart disease; HDL, high-density lipoprotein; LDL, low-density lipoprotein.

should be considered strongly as the patient is a responsible partner in the management of his or her own hypercholesterolemia. Without patient enthusiasm and compliance regarding any therapy, outcomes will not be as good as might be hoped.

LDL-cholesterol guidelines depend on risk categories and on whether the goal is primary prevention or secondary prevention.[4] The great majority of individuals will be in the primary prevention category and have the most to gain as a group.[46] The initial approach for those at risk is as follows: (1) Reduce intake of saturated fats, cholesterol, and calories; (2) increase physical activity; (3) control weight; and (4) reduce other correctable risk factors (hypertension and smoking).[47, 48] Patients who are at ideal body weight but have high LDL cholesterol or total cholesterol are at particularly high risk.

Keeping the LDL-cholesterol below 100, perhaps even less than 80 mg/dL, and the total cholesterol at less than 200 mg/dL is most desirable. Oxidized components of cholesterol are dangerous but are not generally measured and are not considered in the management of cholesterol in the recently published guidelines.

INTEGRATIVE THERAPY

Cholesterol reduction success is dependent on the attention given to the problem by the healer and the individual, and on the motivation of both to change lifestyle patterns. It is not inevitable to have a high cholesterol level or to develop heart disease at an early age, even if there are genetic factors at work. Many things alter cholesterol levels, as well as HDL and LDL levels.[5]

The patient receiving a particular therapy may benefit simply from having the intention to alter the processes that have gone on before (placebo effect), but an optimistic view motivates other important lifestyle changes that can alter the course of the disease and lower cholesterol. It is most important to try healing approaches that alter lifestyle before starting a drug therapy.[49] The greatest benefit may be in preventing heart disease by treating it early, but cholesterol reduction itself does not necessarily prevent disease, and drug therapy is very expensive over the long term.[50] The best approach is to make lifestyle changes, especially in younger patients for whom the impact can have the greatest influence.[51] Once a patient becomes older and has developed a fixed dietary and exercise regimen, altering that pattern is unlikely, or at least very difficult. Older individuals, even when motivated, may have a harder time altering lifestyle and making needed improvements. For older patients, drug therapy may be considered earlier. All individuals should be encouraged to improve lifestyle first by as many routes as possible.[52]

The problem of cholesterol elevation can be an empowering "wake-up call" to an individual. It can allow early changes in the disease process before it occurs.

It is clear that control of diet has a major impact on cholesterol, and specifically on HDL- and LDL-cholesterol levels.[53] It can also have a substantial impact on outcome. One problem is that many Americans are (apparently) unwilling to alter their lifestyle. For those who do attempt to incorporate dietary or other lifestyle changes, the longevity of these changes can be measured for the most part in months.[54] It becomes the responsibility of the patient and the healer to work diligently on making the needed changes and ensuring that these changes are permanent.[55]

NOTE

Drug therapy to keep lipid levels in control, while the diet remains laden with fat, pollutants, and oxidants, is inefficient and counterproductive.

Drug therapy is expensive and has potential risks. The cost per life-year saved in an individual taking a statin to lower total and LDL-cholesterol is in the hundreds of thousands of dollars.[56] This approach is not rational. Further, it does not address the root of the problem.

Lifestyle

Cholesterol reduction cannot be considered in a vacuum. For all potential benefits to be derived from therapy, lifestyle issues require a commitment to change behavior.[57, 58] (See Chapter 95, Motivational Interviewing Techniques.) The approach is multifaceted: Reduce stress, increase physical activity, alter diet, lower blood pressure, and stop smoking completely. Smoking decreases HDL-cholesterol and increases the chance of atherosclerosis directly by its toxic effects on the coronary vasculature.[18, 72]

Patient Adherence

Patient adherence to any therapy, especially for primary prevention, can be poor. To improve compliance, it is important that the health care provider do the following: (1) simplify medication regimens; (2) provide explicit patient instruction; (3) use good counseling techniques to teach the patient how to follow the prescribed treatment; (4) encourage the support of family and friends; (5) reward adherence; (6) increase the number of visits for patients unable to achieve treatment goal; (7) increase patient convenience and access to care; and (8) involve patients in their care through self-monitoring.[59, 60] Adherence to any therapy reduces mortality, even if that therapy is a placebo.[61]

Table 31–3. ATP III Recommended Diet

Nutrient	Recommended Intake
Saturated fat	Less than 7% of total calories
Polyunsaturated fat	Up to 10% of total calories
Monounsaturated fat	Up to 20% of total calories
Total fat	25%–35% of total calories
Carbohydrate	50%–60% of total calories
Fiber	20–30 g per day
Protein	Approximately 15% of total calories
Cholesterol	Less than 200 mg/day
Total calories (energy)	Balance energy intake and expenditure to maintain desirable body weight

Nutrition

A therapeutic diet is low in calories, oxidants, saturated fat, and cholesterol (Table 31–3). It is high in plant stanols/sterols, isoflavones such as those in soy (e.g., genestein, diadzein, and glycetein), and viscous (soluble) fiber such as apple pectin or oat bran (10 to 25 g/day).[62–64] Stanols (beta-sitosterol) bind cholesterol and fat in the gut to prevent their absorption. Soluble fiber prevents fat and cholesterol absorption and regulates blood sugar.[65] Isoflavones lower LDL-cholesterol and act as antioxidants.[10, 66]

A major emphasis must be placed on calorie reduction because a diet low in calories is associated with a better outcome. Reduction in, or elimination of, red meat, an increase in cold water fish, and reduction in both processed foods and processed cheese are recommended.[53] A total vegetarian diet is acceptable and may be optimal, but this has never been tested against other diets in carefully controlled trials.

The ATP III guidelines recommend the following: reduced intake of cholesterol-raising nutrients, saturated fats less than 7% of total calories, and dietary cholesterol less than 200 mg per day (dietary cholesterol reduction does not appear to be as rewarding as lowering the amount of saturated fat and reducing calories).[67, 68] LDL-lowering therapeutic options include plant stanols/sterols (2 g/day), viscous (soluble) fiber (10 to 25 g/day), weight reduction, and an active lifestyle (increased physical activity). This approach is appropriate for primary or secondary cholesterol prevention. Dietary changes to lower cholesterol and risk are only partially evidence-based.

Popular Diets

Several diets, including the Atkins[69] and the Ornish[57] diet, have been developed. The Atkins diet emphasizes consumption of nutrient-dense unprocessed foods and avoidance of refined carbohydrates.[70] Nutrient supplements are part of the diet. The Zone diet is a high-protein diet (30% protein, 40% carbohydrate, and 30% fat). High-fiber fruits and vegetables are allowed; a high-carbohydrate diet is thought to increase insulin levels with devastating consequence.[69] The Ornish diet is a fairly well-balanced diet that is low in calories, very low in total fat, especially saturated fat, and high in complex carbohydrates. Ornish has demonstrated that select patients can be motivated to follow both his diet and an exercise prescription.[71] This behavior improves outcomes and may be associated with regression of atherosclerosis. His diet is difficult to follow for the average patient. It is also not clear that there is an absolute requirement to maintain a very low-fat diet if overall outcome is to be affected. It is possible that a very low-fat diet can adversely affect apoprotein levels and certain forms of LDL-cholesterol, creating a greater degree of atherogenesis.[72] Many patients cannot become motivated to follow this diet.

My recommendations are less stringent about fat prescription in a low-cholesterol diet. I suggest fresh fruits and vegetables with at least six to eight servings a day. A diet high in red meat and saturated fat increases the risk for elevated cholesterol levels and atherosclerosis. It is better to switch to a diet of cold water fish (e.g., salmon, mackerel) or a vegetarian diet; these diets are high in omega-3 fatty acids and have an absence of *trans*-fatty acids (see Chapter 84, The Anti-inflammatory [Omega-3] Diet). Recent data suggest that continuous ingestion of *trans*-fatty acids, which are present in margarine and in processed foods, increases mortality among patients with coronary artery disease and hypercholesterolemia.[73, 74] The mechanisms by which this occurs are not completely clear.

Number of meals: It is likely that eating small but regular meals reduces risk.[88]

Omega-3 Fatty Acids

Omega-3 fatty acids present in fish have been associated with improved survival in patients with no coronary artery disease or hypercholesterolemia.[54] Although omega-3 fatty acids do not lower cholesterol, and they may even increase LDL-cholesterol, the oxidized forms of cholesterol are reduced; omega-3 fatty acids also have direct effects on endothelial function.[75] Triglycerides are reduced. Further, omega-3 fatty acids may have antioxidant effects. As a supplement, omega-3 fatty acids can be given as purified fish oil at between 1 and 4 g per day.[54] Other essential fatty acids in oils become metabolized in the liver to omega-3 fatty acids. Flaxseed oil, especially in the form of ground flax, is highly recommended; it avoids potential mercury toxicity from fish oils.[76, 77]

The Lyon Heart Study,[78] the GISSI 2 Prevenzione study (with 45% reduction in sudden death in the fish oil group),[79] and the Diet and Reinfarction Trial (DART) (study of 2033 man with acute myocardial infarction, randomized to receive or to not receive advice on fish)[80] demonstrate the benefits of omega-3 fatty acids in preventing the progression of coronary artery disease.

Monounsaturated fats, including olive oil, can lower LDL-cholesterol.[81] A diet low in calories and high in these fats allows weight loss to occur.

Trans-Fatty Acids

Advise patient to avoid these completely. They are polyunsaturated fats that have become saturated (hydrogenated). As opposed to *cis*-fatty acids, *trans*-fatty acids are not easily metabolized. Recent data indicate an increased mortality from heart disease and a greater risk of heart disease among those who eat this diet component.[68, 73]

Alcohol

Alcohol increases the formation of HDL3-cholesterol,[22] which has been associated with improved survival among patients with atherosclerotic heart disease; alternatively, alcohol has been used as a preventive. Tee-totaling is now considered a risk factor for heart disease. Red wine has specific bioflavonoids that act as antioxidants and are associated with a reduced risk for heart disease.[82, 83] Grape juice has similar bioflavonoids, but these appear in greater concentration in red wine. One or two drinks per day is recommended.[84] A greater amount may worsen heart disease. Alcohol can cause liver and brain damage as well; so the risks must be weighed against the benefits.

Coffee

Boiled and French pressed coffees increase cholesterol levels.[85] Although paper-filtered coffee does not increase cholesterol levels, it can increase homocysteine, a potent oxidant.[86]

Olive Oil

Olive oil (a monounsaturated oil) is recommended as data suggest that it can reduce LDL-cholesterol levels.[81]

Nuts

Eating 5 ounces of nuts each week, at least for women, reduces the risks of heart disease and of death from heart disease.[87] This was shown in a study of 86,000 women that compared those who ate nuts at this level with those who did not.[87]

Fruits and Vegetables

A diet high in fruits and vegetables is high in antioxidants, so that oxidized forms of cholesterol do not have damaging effects on the endothelium.

More than 2000 flavonoids are found in fruits and vegetables.[82, 89–91] The anthocyanins are potent antioxidants that occur in fruits such as grapes and blueberries.[92] Quercetin in onions and allyl compounds in garlic can also have strong antioxidant effects.[93] Lycopenes in tomatoes are antioxidants as well, and they may protect against the effects of hypercholesterolemia.[94] The amounts of these antioxidants vary, depending on the fruit. Antioxidants may have different effects on specific free radicals, but foods especially high in antioxidants include onions (quercetin), blueberries (anthocyanins), strawberries, watermelon, and raisins.[95] A prudent diet would be replete with fresh fruits and vegetables.

Green Tea

Green tea has several important polyphenols. It is higher in antioxidants than most fruits and vegetables. Green tea lowers cholesterol and LDL-cholesterol by about 10% to 15%, but the data are controversial.[96] Five or more cups per day is recommended. Green tea has been associated with lower LDL-cholesterol and total cholesterol and weight loss. No randomized trial has yet been performed with antioxidants in any of the foods previously mentioned, but the data are convincing enough to suggest that the use of these foods should be encouraged. No downside risk is evident. A retrospective study of tea drinkers, even black tea drinkers, indicates that, compared with coffee drinkers, tea drinkers have a substantial reduction in death from coronary artery disease.[85, 97, 98] The mechanism for this is uncertain; it may be related to other lifestyle factors. Even chocolate has potent antioxidant compounds.[99]

Likely, no one-goal, "magic bullet" antioxidant will work. It is more likely that a diet rich in antioxidant combinations neutralizes the oxidation of LDL-cholesterol and prevents damaging effects.

Rice Bran

Tocotrienols, a group of foods derived from compounds that resemble vitamin E, may lower cholesterol, but data conflict.[100, 101] The most popular product comes from rice bran. Two hundred milligrams per day has been reported to cause a 15% drop in total cholesterol and an 8% to 23% reduction in LDL-cholesterol.

Fiber

Water-soluble forms, as may occur in a diet high in pectin, may also help to lower cholesterol levels.[102] Data suggest that psyllium seed (Metamucil) can also lower cholesterol.[103] Flaxseed not only contains flax oil with its benefits, it also contains soluble fiber. Defatted flax at a dose of 20 g per day can lower LDL-

cholesterol. In one study of healthy young women, flaxseed (50 g/day) lowered LDL by 9% and total cholesterol by 6%.[104] Soluble fiber from oats, beans, psyllium seed, and fruit pectin at a dose of 20 g per day appears beneficial.[105]

Saturated Fat and Barbecued Food

Barbecuing increases benzpyrene levels; other carcinogens and free radicals that can increase oxidized LDL-cholesterol have direct toxic effects.[106] Meats to be avoided include dark meat, chicken skin, beef, pork, and veal.[107] Saturated fat from vegetable oils, particularly those with *trans*-fatty acids in hydrogenated margarine and rancid vegetable oils, should be avoided.[68, 74, 108] Palm oil and coconut oils can elevate cholesterol.

Active Cultures (Probiotics)

Yogurt, Kefir, and fermented milk may lower cholesterol.[109] These products contain beneficial bacteria such as *Lactobacillus acidophilus* and *Bifidobacteria bifidum*, among others. They work by interrupting the enterohepatic cycle by increasing bacterial bile salt hydrolase activity. As part of the "French paradox," the French eat a diet high in dairy products, but these include highly fermented cheeses, which actually may be beneficial by an unknown mechanism, despite the fact that other dairy products may be detrimental.

Soy Protein

Soy protein has been evaluated in multiple studies.[107] A meta-analysis showed that soy protein (in its water-isolated form) lowers total cholesterol and LDL-cholesterol in men and women. Soy protein, in some reports, has been shown to increase HDL-cholesterol in women. Soy protein is an antioxidant, but its direct effects on cholesterol metabolism are unclear. Soy protein contains phytoestrogens, and it may act in part in this way. Genestein is perhaps the most potent phytoestrogen in soy protein but, by itself, this isoflavone has little effect on cholesterol.[110] When the isoflavones are eliminated from water-isolated soy protein, soy protein has little effect on cholesterol. It appears that the combination of the isoflavones, along with some unknown factor in the soy protein, provides its hypocholesterolemic effect.[63] It is unclear if a specific synergistic relationship among globulins, phytates, and other compounds provides anti-atherosclerotic benefit.

Garlic

The studies regarding garlic are conflicting.[111] The s-acetyl cysteine may have a hypocholesterolemic effect but it is highly dependent on the allicin potential of the garlic.[112] Fried, cooked, and heated garlic may contain no allicin and would not be expected to be beneficial. Garlic has many other potential benefits but by itself, it cannot be relied on to alter cholesterol levels. Nevertheless, there may be a small effect on the development of atherosclerosis at the same cholesterol levels owing to the potentially beneficial effects of garlic on the endothelium.

Weight Loss

A modest (5% to 10%) weight loss has been shown to lower cholesterol (total) by more than 15% and LDL-cholesterol by more than 10%.

Exercise

Low levels of exercise have little effect on total cholesterol (one study showed an 11% reduction, but this was not significant), but moderate exercise (increasing heart rate to more than 120/min for longer than 15 minutes 3 times a week) can increase HDL-cholesterol from 4% to 22% and may have a slight effect on LPa.[67, 113, 114] One exercise that can have benefit is low-impact walking for at least 1 hour 3 to 5 times a week. Other forms of aerobic activity include running, swimming, treadmill exercise, and a long list of other activities when performed with a moderate degree of intensity. It appears that those who exercise tend to weigh less, smoke less, feel better, and have lower blood pressure.[52] Ultimately, overall outcome is improved, even if cholesterol is not reduced. All patients with high cholesterol should develop or be assisted to develop an exercise program (see Chapter 86, Writing an Exercise Prescription).

Mind–Body Approaches

Stress Reduction

No study has demonstrated that mind–body approaches alter the cholesterol profile, but mind–body approaches can modulate the risk of a patient who has high cholesterol. Meditation, for example, has been shown to lower blood pressure in hypertensive patients, and meditation has been shown to lower mortality from cardiovascular death in black patients who have multiple risk factors for cardiovascular mortality.[115, 116] Studies are under way to evaluate the mind–body connection in cholesterol lowering and in atherogenesis and its progression (Olshansky, Maharishi University: Personal communication).

Atherosclerosis is, however, associated with more anger, hostility, isolation, lack of social support, depression, and hopelessness.[27] Many of these factors lead to an alienation from self. Any method that alters and improves the mind–body connections of the individual to himself or herself will likely lower the risks.

A strong connection has been noted between depression and heart disease in men, but the impact on women has not received as much attention. A recent study at the University of Pittsburgh of 688 middle-aged women complaining of chest pain was undertaken to determine if the physical symptoms of heart disease are measures of depression and hostility correlated with physical risk factors for atherosclerosis, high blood pressure, obesity, and smoking.[27]

Women who scored in the highest range on a test for depression were three times more likely to smoke than women with the lowest depression scores. Those who showed the highest levels of hostility also had the highest levels of LDL ("bad") cholesterol.[27]

Supplements

Stanols, Sterols

A new product related to beta-sitosterol (Benecol) is now available as a special margarine; a dose of 1.7 g per day can provide a dramatic drop in cholesterol, with the LDL-cholesterol dropping by as much as 14%.[117] Several of these are available, including phytostanols, sitostanol, campestanol, stigmastanol, 5-alpha-stanols, and stanol esters. They bind to cholesterol and fat in the gut to reduce absorption. Beta-sitosterol is found in almost all plants and is found in high levels in soybeans, rice bran, wheat germ, and corn oils.

Dosage. 1.7 g per day (Benecol margarine).

Precautions. They appear effective and have been associated with no major risk to date.[118–120]

B Vitamins (B₆, B₁₂, and Folate)

These have been used to lower homocysteine, an antioxidant that may alter endothelial function and cause formation of oxidized cholesterol.[121, 122] Randomized placebo-controlled trials are under way. These vitamins lower homocysteine and may be beneficial.

Dosage. The recommended dosage of folate, until more information is available, is 1 to 3 mg per day. The dosage for vitamin B_{12} is no greater than 1 mg per day, and of vitamin B_6 is less than 30 to 60 mg per day.

Precautions. A higher dose of vitamin B_6 can cause neurologic problems.

Vitamin E

Vitamin E is available in many forms. Alpha-tocopherol may be an antioxidant, but gamma-tocopherol may be a pro-oxidant. Data conflict regarding the benefits of vitamin E.[123–125] The CHAOS trial showed a dramatic benefit with 800 units per day, but these data were not substantiated in other studies (although most studies considered a lower dose of vitamin E).[126] If there is adequate vitamin E in the diet from food sources, it is unlikely that further supplementation will be of use. Vitamin E can increase HDL-cholesterol.[127]

Omega-3 Fatty Acids

Dosage. Fish oil and other oils containing omega-3 fatty acids or converted to omega-3 fatty acids (such as flax oil) are recommended at a dose of 2 to 6 g per day.[76]

Precautions. Doses greater than 4 g per day may increase oxidation and should be used with antioxidants, vitamin E, vitamin C, and selenium.

Calcium

In some studies, it was found that calcium at supplemental levels of between 800 and 1000 mg per day may reduce cholesterol levels.[53]

L-Carnitine

L-Carnitine is required for entry of long-chain fatty acids into the mitochondria. Carnitine can improve mitochondrial function efficiency. Carnitine may have antioxidant effects by improving mitochondrial function and reducing superoxide and hydrogen peroxide formation. Carnitine can increase HDL, lower total cholesterol, and prevent oxidation of fat in the liver.

Dosage. The dose recommended is 1 to 4 g per day.[129]

Precautions. Carnitine can cause transient nausea and vomiting, abdominal cramps, diarrhea, and body odor.

Quercetin

Quercetin is present in onions, black tea, and apples. A dose as low as 35 mg may have antioxidant effects on LDL-cholesterol.[129] Vitamin C has a synergistic effect that enhances antioxidant activity.

Precautions. Nephrotoxicity can occur with doses greater than 945 mg/m^2.

Pantothine (Vitamin B$_5$)

Pantothenic acid may reduce the amount of cholesterol made in the body; it also accelerates the use of fat as an energy source. It may be most beneficial in those with elevated triglyceride levels.

Dosage. 300 mg PO up to 4 times per day may lower cholesterol and increase HDL.[129]

Precautions. Large amounts can cause diarrhea.

Chromium (Brewer's Yeast)

Chromium supplementation may reduce LDL-cholesterol and increase HDL.

Dosage. The dose is unclear but some recommend a dose as high as 200 mcg per day.[130, 131]

Precautions. Chromium can cause cognitive, perceptual, and motor dysfunction at doses of 200 to 400 mcg per day.

Botanicals

Garlic (Allium sativum)

Garlic at high, nondietetic levels can reduce cholesterol levels and have a direct beneficial effect on endothelial function, but data conflict.[132] Garlic also can inhibit platelet activation. The best form of garlic is crushed, uncooked garlic cloves. With 5000 to 6000 mcg of allicin, a drop in cholesterol of 9% to 12% can be expected. Allyl sulfur compounds inhibit cholesterol production by 40% to 60% in the liver. The compounds responsible are s-allyl cysteine, s-ethyl-cysteine, and s-propyl-cysteine. Allinin is converted to allicin when the garlic is crushed. This converts to a variety of compounds, including diallyl disulfide, ajoene, and vinyldithilins, that convert to more than 100 sulfur compounds.[133]

Dosage. Approximately 1 to 4 cloves is recommended each day, or 900 mg per day of active garlic that contains 5000 to 6000 mcg of allicin.[133]

Precautions. Body odor significantly increases at doses greater than 900 mg per day. Garlic has an antiplatelet effect, and caution should be taken among those using warfarin. Fresh crushed garlic is most effective, but if a supplement is used, it should be enteric-coated to protect constituents from destruction by stomach acid.

Fenugreek (Trigonella foenum-graecum)

Fenugreek contains steroidal saponins that inhibit cholesterol generation in the liver. Added fenugreek seeds may also raise beneficial HDL-cholesterol.

Dosage. Dose is generally 1 to 3 g three times per day with meals.[134, 135]

Precautions. Fenugreek can cause diarrhea and flatulence, as well as hypoglycemia in large doses.

Gugulipid (Commiphora mukul)

Gugulipid is an Ayurvedic herb that is the standardized extract of the Mukul myrrh tree (Commiphora mukul), which contains 5% to 10% guggulsterones. It can lower total cholesterol by 17.5% and has caused an increase of 60% in HDL-cholesterol. It is thought to work by increasing the liver's metabolism of LDL-cholesterol.

Dosage. The recommended daily dose of guggulsterones is 25 mg three times per day.

Precautions. Gugulipid also has antiplatelet properties.[136]

Red Yeast Rice

Red yeast rice is a hydroxymethyl glutaryl coenzyme A (HMG CoA) reductase inhibitor (a "statin").

Controlled clinical trials have demonstrated beneficial effects in cholesterol reduction at a dose of 2.4 g per day (equivalent to 5 to 10 mg monocolins). Lovastatin, an HMG CoA reductase inhibitor, is nearly equivalent to the monocolin in red yeast rice.[140–142]

Dosage. A product called Cholestin, produced by Pharmanex, is a 15-mg tablet that is taken once a day.

Precautions. Owing to the similar mechanism of action as lovastatin, liver enzymes should be monitored. The price of this supplement is comparable to that of statin therapy.

Green Tea

With intake of green tea, 240 to 320 mg of polyphenols may lower total and LDL-cholesterol levels substantially, but the effects are controversial and the influence on oxidized forms of LDL-cholesterol is uncertain.[143]

Psyllium (Metamucil)

Psyllium, given at 5 to 10 g per day, lowers cholesterol by 5% and LDL by 7%.[138]

Royal Jelly (Apis mellifera)

Royal jelly can prevent the cholesterol-elevating effects of nicotine and lower total cholesterol levels. The dose is 50 to 100 mg daily.[139]

Fo-ti

Some 7500 mg per day can reduce cholesterol levels substantially. A variety of other Chinese herbal preparations may help.[144, 145–149]

Many other herbs and supplements have shown effectiveness in reducing cholesterol. These include red pepper, alfalfa, turmeric, ginger, artichoke leaf, chitosan, grapeseed extract, panax ginseng (raises HDL), skullcap (raises HDL), chondroitin sulfate, copper, creatine, he shou wu, and saffron (component "crocetin" lowered cholesterol).

Pharmaceuticals

Many drug therapies have the potential to lower cholesterol.[152, 153]

HMG CoA Reductase Inhibitors (Statins)

Substantial data have been obtained from large, controlled, randomized trials that statins used for primary (West of Scotland [WOSCOPS] and Air Force/Texas Coronary Atherosclerosis Prevention Study [AFCAPS/TexCAPS]) and secondary (LIPID study, CARE trial, Scandinavian Simvastatin Study [4S]) prevention lower death risk from coronary heart disease.[46, 154, 155]

Statins reduce LDL-cholesterol by 18% to 55%, reduce triglycerides by 7% to 30%, and raise HDL-cholesterol by 5% to 15%.[156]

Statins may reduce endothelial inflammation and high-sensitivity C-reactive protein.[157] They have been shown to reduce major coronary events, coronary heart disease mortality, the need for coronary procedures (e.g., percutaneous transluminal coronary angioplasty [PTCA]/coronary artery bypass graft [CABG]), stroke, and total mortality.

Dosage

Statin Daily Dose Range
Lovastatin (Mevacor) 20–80 mg
Pravastatin (Pravachol) 20–40 mg
Simvastatin (Zocor) 20–80 mg
Fluvastatin (Lescol XL) 20–80 mg
Atorvastatin (Lipitor) 10–80 mg

Precautions. Their major side effects include myopathy and increased liver enzymes. They are unusually well tolerated. The only major contraindication is severe liver disease. A word of caution: One of these drugs (cerivastatin [Baycol]) was recently taken off the market owing to intolerable side effects (rhabdomyolysis). These drugs require long-term monitoring. Although they are a highly effective class of drugs and may have more than one beneficial effect, they are also associated with risks of adverse effects.[50, 117]

Bile Acid Sequestrants

These reduce LDL-cholesterol by 15% to 30% and raise HDL-cholesterol by 3% to 5% but may increase triglycerides. These drugs have been shown to reduce major coronary events, as well as coronary heart disease mortality.[158–160]

Dosage

Drug Dose Range
Cholestyramine (Questran) 4–16 g (start 4 g qd to bid before meals and titrate)
Colestipol (Colestid) 5–20 g (start 5 g granules qd to bid before meals; titrate by 5 g intervals)
Colesevelam (Welchol) 2.6–3.8 g (3 tablets bid with meals or 6 tablets once daily with a meal. One tablet = 625 mg)

Precautions. Side effects include gastrointestinal distress, constipation, and decreased absorption of other drugs. These drugs are contraindicated if there is an elevated triglyceride level, especially if it is over 400 mg/dL, or if there is beta-lipoproteinemia.

Nicotinic Acid

Nicotinic acid ("niacin") lowers LDL-cholesterol by 5% to 25%, lowers triglycerides by 20% to 50%, and raises HDL-cholesterol by 15% to 35%.[161, 162] Niacin can raise levels of HDL-cholesterol and lower total cholesterol. Therapy is inexpensive but it is commonly difficult to take. It causes flushing at high dosages and can cause liver toxicity. At doses as high as 3000 mg per day, niacin can lower total cholesterol by more than 10%,[163] lower LDL-cholesterol by 20%, and increase HDL-cholesterol by 30%. A slowly released form of niacin or inositol hexaniacinate can be better tolerated. It is also possible that patients can get used to the higher levels over time. Nicotinic acid reduces major coronary events and is associated with a possible reduction in total mortality.

Dosage

Immediate release (nicotinic acid) 1.5–3 g. (Start 50–100 mg PO bid–tid with meals. Increase slowly to maintenance of 1.5–3 g/day.) Comes in 25, 50, 100, and 150 mg tablets.

Extended release (Niaspan) 1–2 g. (Start 500 mg qhs with low-fat snack. Increase every 4 wk to max of 2 g.) Comes in 500, 750, and 1000 mg tablets.

Inositol hexaniacinate 1–2 g. (Start 500 mg tid with food for 2 weeks; increase to 1000 mg tid if needed.)

NOTE

Inositol hexaniacinate is a form of niacin that is popular in Europe for both cholesterol reduction and vascular claudication. It has a low incidence of both flushing and liver toxicity compared with other forms.

Precautions. Flushing, hyperglycemia, hyperuricemia, upper GI distress, and hepatotoxicity can occur. It is contraindicated with liver disease, severe gout, and peptic ulcer. Flushing may be improved by taking aspirin or ibuprofen 30 minutes before the niacin dose. The sustained-release form of niacin has more of a chance to cause liver toxicity. Monitor liver function.

Fibric Acids

Fibric acid lowers LDL-cholesterol by 5% to 20% (with normal triglycerides), may raise LDL-cholesterol (with high triglycerides), lowers triglycerides by 20% to 50%, and raises HDL-cholesterol by 10% to 20%. Fibric acids reduce progression of coronary lesions and reduce major coronary events.[35, 160]

Dosage

Gemfibrozil (Lopid) 600 mg bid. Comes in scored 600-mg tablets.

Fenofibrate (Tricor) 200 mg qd. (Start with 67 mg PO qd with meals. Increase every 4 wk to maintenance of 134–200 mg.) Comes in 67, 134, and 200 mg.

Clofibrate (Atromid-S) 1000 mg bid. Comes in 500 mg tablets.

Precautions. Side effects include dyspepsia, gallstones, and myopathy. Fibric acids are contraindicated with severe renal or hepatic disease.

Factors Favoring Drug Therapy

The HMG CoA reductase inhibitors effectively reduce total cholesterol and LDL-cholesterol.[164] They also increase HDL-cholesterol. Further, they may have other properties; these compounds may have a beneficial effect on inflammation and seem to lower the high-sensitivity C-reactive protein.

☖ — *THERAPEUTIC REVIEW* ———————————————

Death and disability from coronary atherosclerosis are not inevitable. Cholesterol reduction can improve survival and lower the risk for coronary events and the need for interventional therapy. Risk assessment is complex and involves a comprehensive view of the patient's total risk.

No simple "magic bullet" approach will succeed in all situations. Those at risk who have high cholesterol need to be given a comprehensive program of lifestyle changes, dietary recommendations, and guidelines regarding the supplements that may help. Should the cholesterol level remain high despite an aggressive attempt at lifestyle, diet, and exercise management, then drug therapy, beginning with a statin, should be provided.

Drug Therapy for Primary and Secondary Prevention

- *Initiate LDL-lowering drug therapy (after 3 months of nutrition, exercise, and mind–body therapies).*
- *Usual drug options: statin, bile acid sequestrant, nicotinic acid.*
- *Continue therapeutic lifestyle changes.*
- *Make return visit in about 6 weeks.*
- *If needed: Intensify LDL-lowering therapy (if LDL goal not achieved) by using a higher dose of statin, statin + bile acid sequestrant, or statin + nicotinic acid.*

If LDL goal is not achieved within 6 weeks, intensify drug therapy and treat other lipid risk factors (high triglycerides [200 mg/dL], low HDL-cholesterol [<40 mg/dL]). Monitor response and adherence to therapy every 4 to 6 months. Monitor liver function, particularly if combination therapy with niacin or a bile acid sequestrant is used.

References

1. AHA—Heart and Stroke Statistical Update. Dallas, American Heart Association, 2000.
2. Kannel WB, et al: Serum cholesterol, lipoproteins, and the risk of coronary heart disease. The Framingham study. Ann Intern Med 74(1):1–12, 1971.
3. Castelli WP: Epidemiology of coronary heart disease: The Framingham study. Am J Med 76(2A):4–12, 1984.
4. Wilson PW, et al: Prediction of coronary heart disease using risk factor categories. Circulation 97(18):1837–1847, 1998.
5. Kannel WB: Range of serum cholesterol values in the population developing coronary artery disease. Am J Cardiol 76(9):69C–77C, 1995.
6. Pitt B, Rubenfire M: Risk stratification for the detection of preclinical coronary artery disease. Circulation 99(20):2610–2612, 1999.
7. Pekkanen J, et al: Ten-year mortality from cardiovascular disease in relation to cholesterol level among men with and without preexisting cardiovascular disease. N Engl J Med 322(24):1700–1707, 1990.
8. Grundy SM, et al: Prevention Conference V: Beyond secondary prevention: Identifying the high-risk patient for primary prevention: Medical office assessment: Writing Group I. Circulation 101(1):E3–E11, 2000.
9. Law MR, Wald NJ, Thompson SG: By how much and how quickly does reduction in serum cholesterol concentration lower risk of ischaemic heart disease? BMJ 308(6925):367–372, 1994.
10. Diaz MN, et al: Antioxidants and atherosclerotic heart disease. N Engl J Med 337(6):408–416, 1997.
11. Nanjee MN, et al: Composition and ultrastructure of size subclasses of normal human peripheral lymph lipoproteins: Quantification of cholesterol uptake by HDL in tissue fluids. J Lipid Res 42(4):639–648, 2001.
12. Heller RF, Hartley RM, Lewis B: The effect on blood lipids of eating charcoal-grilled meat. Atherosclerosis 48(2):185–192, 1983.
13. Xu D, Neville R, Finkel T: Homocysteine accelerates endothelial cell senescence. FEBS Lett 470(1):20–24, 2000.
14. McCully KS: Vascular pathology of homocysteinemia: implications for the pathogenesis of arteriosclerosis. Am J Pathol 56(1):111–128, 1969.
15. Yan PS: Cholesterol oxidation products. Their occurrence and detection in our foodstuffs. Adv Exp Med Biol 459:79–98, 1999.
16. Patel VB, Robbins MA, Topol EJ: C-reactive protein: A "golden marker'" for inflammation and coronary artery disease. Cleve Clin J Med 68(6):521–524, 527–534, 2001.
17. Ridker PM, et al: C-reactive protein and other markers of inflammation in the prediction of cardiovascular disease in women. N Engl J Med 342(12):836–843, 2000.
18. Schachinger V, Zeiher AM: Atherosclerosis-associated endothelial dysfunction. Z Kardiol 89(suppl 9):IX/70–74, 2000.
19. Pasceri V, Willerson JT, Yeh ET: Direct proinflammatory effect of C-reactive protein on human endothelial cells. Circulation 102(18):2165–2168, 2000.
20. Fichtlscherer S, et al: Elevated C-reactive protein levels and impaired endothelial vasoreactivity in patients with coronary artery disease. Circulation 102(9):1000–1006, 2000.
21. Lieberman EH, et al: Flow-induced vasodilation of the human brachial artery is impaired in patients <40 years of age with coronary artery disease. Am J Cardiol 78(11):1210–1214, 1996.
22. Gardner CD, et al: Associations of HDL, HDL(2), and HDL(3) cholesterol and apolipoproteins A-I and B with lifestyle factors in healthy women and men: The Stanford Five City Project. Prev Med 31(4):346–356, 2000.
23. Holmer SR, et al: Lipoprotein lipase gene polymorphism, cholesterol subfractions and myocardial infarction in large samples of the general population. Cardiovasc Res 47(4):806–812, 2000.
24. Vega GL, Grundy SM: Comparison of apolipoprotein B to cholesterol in low density lipoproteins of patients with coronary heart disease. J Lipid Res 25(6):580–592, 1984.
25. Morrisett JD: The role of lipoprotein(a) in atherosclerosis. Curr Atheroscler Rep 2(3):243–250, 2000.
26. Iribarren C, et al: Relationship of lipoproteins, apolipoproteins, triglycerides and lipid ratios to plasma total cholesterol in young adults: The CARDIA Study. Coronary Artery Risk Development in Young Adults. J Cardiovasc Risk 3(4):391–396, 1996.
27. Rutledge T, et al: Psychosocial variables are associated with atherosclerosis risk factors among women with chest pain: The WISE study. Psychosom Med 63(2):282–288, 2001.
28. Reed T, et al: Family history of cancer related to cholesterol level in young adults. Genet Epidemiol 3(2):63–71, 1982.
29. Golomb BA: Cholesterol and violence: Is there a connection? Ann Intern Med 128(6):478–487, 1998.
30. Kaplan JR, Manuck SB, Shively C: The effects of fat and cholesterol on social behavior in monkeys. Psychosom Med 53(6):634–642, 1991.
31. Kaplan JR, et al: Demonstration of an association among dietary cholesterol, central serotonergic activity, and social behavior in monkeys. Psychosom Med 56(6):479–484, 1994.
32. Reisbick S, et al: Home cage behavior of rhesus monkeys with long-term deficiency of omega-3 fatty acids. Physiol Behav 55(2):231–239, 1994.
33. de Faire U, et al: Secondary preventive potential of lipid-lowering drugs. The Bezafibrate Coronary Atherosclerosis Intervention Trial (BECAIT). Eur Heart J 17(suppl F):37–42, 1996.
34. Ross SJ, et al: Body fat distribution predicts cardiac risk factors in older female coronary patients. J Cardiopulm Rehabil 17(6):419–427, 1997.
35. LaRosa JC: Triglycerides and coronary risk in women and the elderly. Arch Intern Med 157(9):961–968, 1997.
36. Mann WA, et al: Trials of the effects of drugs and hormones on lipids and lipoproteins. Curr Opin Lipidol 6(6):354–359, 1995.
37. EUROASPIRE. A European Society of Cardiology survey of secondary prevention of coronary heart disease: Principal results. EUROASPIRE Study Group. European Action on Secondary Prevention through Intervention to Reduce Events. Eur Heart J 18(10):1569–1582, 1997.
38. Price JF, Fowkes FG: Risk factors and the sex differential in coronary artery disease. Epidemiology 8(5):584–591, 1997.
39. Brochu M, et al: Coronary risk profiles in men with coronary artery disease: Effects of body composition, fat distribution, age and fitness. Coron Artery Dis 11(2):137–144, 2000.
40. Hauner H, et al: Body fat distribution in men with angiographically confirmed coronary artery disease. Atherosclerosis 85:203–210, 1990.
41. Rackley CE: Cardiovascular basis for cholesterol therapy. Cardiol Rev 8(2):124–131, 2000.
42. Rossouw JE: Lipid-lowering interventions in angiographic trials. Am J Cardiol 76(9):86C–92C, 1995.
43. Gelskey DE, Young TK, MacDonald SM: Screening with total cholesterol: Determining sensitivity and specificity of the National Cholesterol Education Program's guidelines from a population survey. J Clin Epidemiol 47(5):547–553, 1994.
44. Demke DM, et al: Effects of a fish oil concentrate in patients with hypercholesterolemia. Atherosclerosis 70:73–80, 1988.
45. Paterick TE, Fletcher GF: Endothelial function and cardiovascular prevention: Role of blood lipids, exercise, and other risk factors. Cardiol Rev 9(5):282–286, 2001.
46. Downs JR, et al: Primary prevention of acute coronary events with lovastatin in men and women with average cholesterol levels: Results of AFCAPS/TexCAPS. Air Force/Texas Coronary Atherosclerosis Prevention Study. JAMA 279(20):1615–1622, 1998.
47. Smith GD, Song F, Sheldon TA: Cholesterol lowering and mortality: The importance of considering initial level of risk. BMJ 306(6889):1367–1373, 1993.
48. Guize L, Iliou MC: (Treatment of risk factors of coronary atherosclerosis). Arch Mal Coeur Vaiss 85(11 suppl):1687–1693, 1992.
49. Boreham C, et al: Relationships between the development of biological risk factors for coronary heart disease and lifestyle parameters during adolescence: The Northern Ireland Young Hearts Project. Public Health 113(1):7–12, 1999.

50. Vogel R, Schaefer E: Should all patients with cardiovascular disease receive statin therapy? Am J Manag Care 7(5 suppl):S117–S124, 2001.

51. Hubert HB, et al: Life-style correlates of risk factor change in young adults: An eight-year study of coronary heart disease risk factors in the Framingham offspring. Am J Epidemiol 125(5):812–831, 1987.

52. Liebson PR, Amsterdam EA: Prevention of coronary heart disease. Part I. Primary prevention. Dis Mon 45(12):497–571, 1999.

53. Kromhout D: Diet and cardiovascular diseases. J Nutr Health Aging 5(3):144–149, 2001.

54. von Schacky C, et al: The effect of dietary omega-3 fatty acids on coronary atherosclerosis. A randomized, double-blind, placebo-controlled trial. Ann Intern Med 130(7):554–562, 1999.

55. Gotto AM Jr: How do we achieve optimal cardiovascular risk reduction? Clin Cardiol 24(8 suppl):III8–III12, 2001.

56. Prosser LA, et al: Cost-effectiveness of cholesterol-lowering therapies according to selected patient characteristics. Ann Intern Med 132(10):769–779, 2000.

57. Ornish D: Can lifestyle changes reverse coronary heart disease? World Rev Nutr Diet 72:38–48, 1993.

58. Ornish D, et al: Can lifestyle changes reverse coronary heart disease? The Lifestyle Heart Trial. Lancet 336(8708):129–133, 1990.

59. Braunstein JB, et al: Lipid disorders: Justification of methods and goals of treatment. Chest 120(3):979–988, 2001.

60. Van Horn L, Kavey RE: Diet and cardiovascular disease prevention: What works? Ann Behav Med 19(3):197–212, 1997.

61. Canner PFS, Prud'homme G, Berge K, Stamler J: Influence of adherence to treatment and response of cholesterol on mortality in the coronary drug project. N Engl J Med 303(18):1038–1041, 1980.

62. Lovati MR, et al: Soybean protein diet increases low density lipoprotein receptor activity in mononuclear cells from hypercholesterolemic patients. J Clin Invest 80(5):1498–1502, 1987.

63. Tovar-Palacio C, et al: Intake of soy protein and soy protein extracts influences lipid metabolism and hepatic gene expression in gerbils. J Nutr 128(5):839–842, 1998.

64. Ripsin CM, et al: Oat products and lipid lowering. A meta-analysis. JAMA 267(24):3317–3325, 1992.

65. Knopp RH, et al: Long-term blood cholesterol-lowering effects of a dietary fiber supplement. Am J Prev Med 17(1):18–23, 1999.

66. Rimm EB, et al: Vegetable, fruit, and cereal fiber intake and risk of coronary heart disease among men. JAMA 275(6):447–451, 1996.

67. Executive Summary of the Third Report of The National Cholesterol Education Program (NCEP) Expert Panel on Detection, Evaluation, and Treatment of High Blood Cholesterol in Adults (Adult Treatment Panel III). JAMA 285(19):2486–2497, 2001.

68. Kromhout D, et al: Dietary saturated and trans fatty acids and cholesterol and 25-year mortality from coronary heart disease: The Seven Countries Study. Prev Med 24(3):308–315, 1995.

69. Anderson JW, Konz EC, Jenkins DJ: Health advantages and disadvantages of weight-reducing diets: A computer analysis and critical review. J Am Coll Nutr 19(5):578–590, 2000.

70. The Atkins diet. Med Lett Drugs Ther 42(1080):52, 2000.

71. Ornish D: Reversing heart disease through diet, exercise, and stress management: An interview with Dean Ornish. Interview by Elaine R Monsen. J Am Diet Assoc 91(2):162–165, 1991.

72. Ornish D, et al: Intensive lifestyle changes for reversal of coronary heart disease. JAMA 280(23):2001–2007, 1998.

73. Oomen CM, et al: Association between trans fatty acid intake and 10-year risk of coronary heart disease in the Zutphen Elderly Study: A prospective population-based study. Lancet 357(9258):746–751, 2001.

74. Willett WC, et al: Intake of trans fatty acids and risk of coronary heart disease among women. Lancet 341(8845):581–585, 1993.

75. Heemskerk JW, Vossen RC, van Dam-Mieras MC: Polyunsaturated fatty acids and function of platelets and endothelial cells. Curr Opin Lipidol 7(1):24–29, 1996.

76. Harris WS: n-3 Fatty acids and serum lipoproteins: Human studies. Am J Clin Nutr 65(5 suppl):1645S–1654S, 1997.

77. Babu US, et al: Nutritional and hematological impact of dietary flaxseed and defatted flaxseed meal in rats. Int J Food Sci Nutr 51(2):109–117, 2000.

78. Simopoulos AP: Evolutionary aspects of omega-3 fatty acids in the food supply. Prostaglandins Leukot Essent Fatty Acids 60:421–429, 1999.

79. Dietary supplementation with n-3 polyunsaturated fatty acids and vitamin E after myocardial infarction: Results of the GISSI-Prevenzione trial. Gruppo Italiano per lo Studio della Sopravivenza nell'Infarto Miocardico. Lancet 354(9177):447–455, 1999.

80. Burr ML, et al: Diet and reinfarction trial (DART): Design, recruitment, and compliance. Eur Heart J 10(6):558–567, 1989.

81. Baggio G, et al: Olive-oil–enriched diet: Effect on serum lipoprotein levels and biliary cholesterol saturation. Am J Clin Nutr 47(6):960–964, 1988.

82. Hertog MG, et al: Dietary antioxidant flavonoids and risk of coronary heart disease: The Zutphen Elderly Study. Lancet 342(8878):1007–1011, 1993.

83. Rimm EB, et al: Review of moderate alcohol consumption and reduced risk of coronary heart disease: Is the effect due to beer, wine, or spirits? BMJ 312(7033):731–736, 1996.

84. Gronbaek M, et al: Type of alcohol consumed and mortality from all causes, coronary heart disease, and cancer. Ann Intern Med 133(6):411–419, 2000.

85. Superko HR, et al: Caffeinated and decaffeinated coffee effects on plasma lipoprotein cholesterol, apolipoproteins, and lipase activity: A controlled, randomized trial. Am J Clin Nutr 54(3):599–605, 1991.

86. Nygard O, et al: Coffee consumption and plasma total homocysteine: The Hordaland Homocysteine Study. Am J Clin Nutr 65(1):136–143, 1997.

87. Hu FB, et al: Frequent nut consumption and risk of coronary heart disease in women: Prospective cohort study. BMJ 317(7169):1341–1345, 1998.

88. Redondo MR, et al: Influence of the number of meals taken per day on cardiovascular risk factors and the energy and nutrient intakes of a group of elderly people. Int J Vitam Nutr Res 67(3):176–182, 1997.

89. Hertog MG, et al: Flavonoid intake and long-term risk of coronary heart disease and cancer in the seven countries study. Arch Intern Med 155(4):381–386, 1995.

90. Keli SO, et al: Dietary flavonoids, antioxidant vitamins, and incidence of stroke: The Zutphen study. Arch Intern Med 156(6):637–642, 1996.

91. Lairon D, Amiot MJ: Flavonoids in food and natural antioxidants in wine. Curr Opin Lipidol 10(1):23–28, 1999.

92. Prior RL, et al: Identification of procyanidins and anthocyanins in blueberries and cranberries (Vaccinium spp.) using high-performance liquid chromatography/mass spectrometry. J Agric Food Chem 49(3):1270–1276, 2001.

93. Ali M, Bordia T, Mustafa T: Effect of raw versus boiled aqueous extract of garlic and onion on platelet aggregation. Prostaglandins Leukot Essent Fatty Acids 60(1):43–47, 1999.

94. Suganuma H, Inakuma T: Protective effect of dietary tomato against endothelial dysfunction in hypercholesterolemic mice. Biosci Biotechnol Biochem 63(1):78–82, 1999.

95. Knekt P, et al: Quercetin intake and the incidence of cerebrovascular disease. Eur J Clin Nutr 54(5):415–417, 2000.

96. Weisburger JH: Tea and health: The underlying mechanisms. Proc Soc Exp Biol Med 220(4):271–275, 1999.

97. Fujiwara N, Tokudome S: Reproducibility of self-administered questionnaire in epidemiological surveys. J Epidemiol 7(2):61–69, 1997.

98. Miyake Y, et al: Relationship of coffee consumption with serum lipids and lipoproteins in Japanese men. Ann Epidemiol 9(2):121–126, 1999.

99. Hirano R, et al: Antioxidant effects of polyphenols in choco-

late on low-density lipoprotein both in vitro and ex vivo. J Nutr Sci Vitaminol (Tokyo) 46(4):199–204, 2000.

100. Qureshi AA, et al: Lowering of serum cholesterol in hypercholesterolemic humans by tocotrienols (palmvitee). Am J Clin Nutr 53(4 suppl):1021S–1026S, 1991.

101. Qureshi AA, et al: Response of hypercholesterolemic subjects to administration of tocotrienols. Lipids 30(12):1171–1177, 1995.

102. Terpstra AH, et al: Dietary pectin with high viscosity lowers plasma and liver cholesterol concentration and plasma cholesteryl ester transfer protein activity in hamsters. J Nutr 128(11):1944–1949, 1998.

103. Anderson JW, et al: Long-term cholesterol-lowering effects of psyllium as an adjunct to diet therapy in the treatment of hypercholesterolemia. Am J Clin Nutr 71(6):1433–1438, 2000.

104. Cunnane SC, et al: Nutritional attributes of traditional flaxseed in healthy young adults. Am J Clin Nutr 61(1):62–68, 1995.

105. Glore SR, et al: Soluble fiber and serum lipids: A literature review. J Am Diet Assoc 94(4):425–436, 1994.

106. Elmenhorst H, Dontenwill W: (Carcinogenic hydrocarbons in the smoke from charcoal grilling). Z Krebsforsch 70(2):157–160, 1997.

107. Anderson JW, Johnstone BM, Cook-Newell ME: Meta-analysis of the effects of soy protein intake on serum lipids. N Engl J Med 333(5):276–282, 1995.

108. Aro A, et al: Adipose tissue isomeric trans fatty acids and risk of myocardial infarction in nine countries: The EURAMIC study. Lancet 345(8945):273–278, 1995.

109. Hepner G, et al: Hypocholesterolemic effect of yogurt and milk. Am J Clin Nutr 32(1):19–24, 1979.

110. Potter SM: Soy protein and serum lipids. Curr Opin Lipidol 7(4):260–264, 1996.

111. Stevinson C, Pittler MH, Ernst E: Garlic for treating hypercholesterolemia. A meta-analysis of randomized clinical trials. Ann Intern Med 133(6):420–429, 2000.

112. Silagy C, Neil A: Garlic as a lipid lowering agent—a meta-analysis. J R Coll Physicians Lond 28(1):39–45, 1994.

113. Kokkinos PF, Fernhall B: Physical activity and high density lipoprotein cholesterol levels: What is the relationship? Sports Med 28(5):307–314, 1999.

114. Drygas W, et al: Long-term effects of different physical activity levels on coronary heart disease risk factors in middle-aged men. Int J Sports Med 21(4):235–241, 2000.

115. Patel C, et al: Trial of relaxation in reducing coronary risk: Four year follow up. BMJ (Clin Res Ed) 290(6475):1103–1106, 1985.

116. Calderon R Jr, et al: Stress, stress reduction and hypercholesterolemia in African Americans: A review. Ethn Dis 9(3):451–462, 1999.

117. Bachman DS: Cholesterol treatment with statins and/or Benecol. J Ark Med Soc 96(10):380–381, 2000.

118. Law MR: Plant sterol and stanol margarines and health. West J Med 173(1):43–47, 2000.

119. Avery JK: Making the most of cholesterol-lowering margarines. Cleve Clin J Med 68(3):194–196, 2001.

120. Plat J, Kerckhoffs DA, Mensink RP: Therapeutic potential of plant sterols and stanols. Curr Opin Lipidol 11(6):571–576, 2000.

121. Brattstrom L, Wilcken DE: Homocysteine and cardiovascular disease: Cause or effect? Am J Clin Nutr 72(2):315–323, 2000.

122. Bunout D, et al: Effects of supplementation with folic acid and antioxidant vitamins on homocysteine levels and LDL oxidation in coronary patients. Nutrition 16(2):107–110, 2000.

123. Kesaniemi YA, Grundy SM: Lack of effect of tocopherol on plasma lipids and lipoproteins in man. Am J Clin Nutr 36(2):224–228, 1982.

124. Stampfer MJ, et al: Vitamin E consumption and the risk of coronary disease in women. N Engl J Med 328(20):1444–1449, 1993.

125. Rimm EB, et al: Vitamin E consumption and the risk of coronary heart disease in men. N Engl J Med 328(20):1450–1456, 1993.

126. Ness A, Smith GD: Mortality in the CHAOS trial. Cambridge Heart Antioxidant Study. Lancet 353(9157):1017–1018, 1999.

127. Cloarec MJ, et al: Alpha-tocopherol: Effect on plasma lipoproteins in hypercholesterolemic patients. Isr J Med Sci 23(8):869–872, 1987.

128. Cara L, et al: Long-term wheat germ intake beneficially affects plasma lipids and lipoproteins in hypercholesterolemic human subjects. J Nutr 122(2):317–326, 1992.

129. Rossi CS, Siliprandi N: Effect of carnitine on serum HDL-cholesterol: Report of two cases. Johns Hopkins Med J 150(2):51–54, 1982.

130. Roeback JR Jr, et al: Effects of chromium supplementation on serum high-density lipoprotein cholesterol levels in men taking beta-blockers. A randomized, controlled trial. Ann Intern Med 115(12):917–924, 1991.

131. Newman HA, et al: Serum chromium and angiographically determined coronary artery disease. Clin Chem 24(4):541–544, 1978.

132. Borek C: Antioxidant health effects of aged garlic extract. J Nutr 131(3s):1010S–1015S, 2001.

133. Bordia A, Verma SK, Srivastava KC: Effect of garlic (*Allium sativum*) on blood lipids, blood sugar, fibrinogen and fibrinolytic activity in patients with coronary artery disease. Prostaglandins Leukot Essent Fatty Acids 58(4):257–263, 1998.

134. Bordia A, Verma SK, Srivastava KC: Effect of ginger (*Zingiber officinale* Rosc.) and fenugreek (*Trigonella foenumgraecum* L.) on blood lipids, blood sugar and platelet aggregation in patients with coronary artery disease. Prostaglandins Leukot Essent Fatty Acids 56(5):379–384, 1997.

135. Sharma RD, Raghuram TC, Rao NS: Effect of fenugreek seeds on blood glucose and serum lipids in type I diabetes. Eur J Clin Nutr 44(4):301–306, 1990.

136. Agarwal RC, et al: Clinical trial of gugulipid—a new hypolipidemic agent of plant origin in primary hyperlipidemia. Indian J Med Res 84:626–634, 1986.

137. Becker CC, et al: Effects of butter oil blends with increased concentrations of stearic, oleic and linolenic acid on blood lipids in young adults. Eur J Clin Nutr 53(7):535–541, 1999.

138. Jenkins DJ, et al: Effect of psyllium in hypercholesterolemia at two monounsaturated fatty acid intakes. Am J Clin Nutr 65(5):1524–1533, 1997.

139. Vittek J: Effect of royal jelly on serum lipids in experimental animals and humans with atherosclerosis. Experientia 51:927–935, 1995.

140. Heber D, et al: Cholesterol-lowering effects of a proprietary Chinese red-yeast-rice dietary supplement. Am J Clin Nutr 69(2):231–236, 1999.

141. Heber D, et al: An analysis of nine proprietary Chinese red yeast rice dietary supplements: Implications of variability in chemical profile and contents. J Altern Complement Med 7(2):133–139, 2001.

142. Ma J, et al: Constituents of red yeast rice, a traditional Chinese food and medicine. J Agric Food Chem 48(11):5220–5225, 2000.

143. Lou FQ, et al: A study on tea-pigment in prevention of atherosclerosis. Chin Med J (Engl) 102(8):579–583, 1989.

144. Yotsumoto H, et al: Inhibitory effects of oren-gedoku-to and its components on cholesteryl ester synthesis in cultured human hepatocyte HepG2 cells: Evidence from the cultured HepG2 cells and in vitro assay of ACAT. Planta Med 63(2):141–145, 1997.

145. Lu Y, Li JZ, Zheng X: (Effect of *Astragalus angelica* mixture on serum lipids and glomerulosclerosis in rats with nephrotic syndrome). Zhongguo Zhong Xi Yi Jie He Za Zhi 17(8):478–480, 1997.

146. Wu YJ, et al: Increase of vitamin E content in LDL and reduction of atherosclerosis in cholesterol-fed rabbits by a water-soluble antioxidant-rich fraction of *Salvia miltiorrhiza*. Arterioscler Thromb Vasc Biol 18(3):481–486, 1998.

147. Wu CZ, Inoue M, Ogihara Y: Antihypercholesterolemic action of a traditional Chinese medicine (Kampo medicine), Ogi-Keishi-Gomotsu-To-Ka-Kojin. Biol Pharm Bull 21(12):1311–1316, 1998.

148. Zhui Y, et al: Experimental study of the antiatherogenesis effect of Chinese medicine angelica and its mechanisms. Clin Hemorheol Microcirc 22(4):305–310, 2000.

149. Yamaguchi Y, et al: Antioxidant activity of the extracts from

fruiting bodies of cultured *Cordyceps sinensis*. Phytother Res 14(8):647–649, 2000.

150. Zacour AC, et al: Effect of dietary chitin on cholesterol absorption and metabolism in rats. J Nutr Sci Vitaminol (Tokyo) 38(6):609–613, 1992.

151. Yevdokimov YM, et al: Complexes between double-stranded DNA and chitosan can form cholesteric liquid-crystalline dispersions. Dokl Biophys 373–375:47–49, 2000.

152. Knopp RH: Drug treatment of lipid disorders. N Engl J Med 341(7):498–511, 1999.

153. Summary of the second report of the National Cholesterol Education Program (NCEP) Expert Panel on Detection, Evaluation, and Treatment of High Blood Cholesterol in Adults (Adult Treatment Panel II). JAMA 269(23):3015–3023, 1993.

154. Shepherd J: The West of Scotland Coronary Prevention Study: A trial of cholesterol reduction in Scottish men. Am J Cardiol 76(9):113C–117C, 1995.

155. Waters D, Pedersen TR: Review of cholesterol-lowering therapy: Coronary angiographic and events trials. Am J Med 101(4A):4A34S–4A38S, discussion 39S, 1996.

156. Wang TJ, et al: Randomized clinical trials and recent patterns in the use of statins. Am Heart J 141(6):957–963, 2001.

157. Strandberg TE, Vanhanen H, Tikkanen MJ: Effect of statins on C-reactive protein in patients with coronary artery disease. Lancet 353(9147):118–119, 1999.

158. Davidson MH, et al: Colesevelam hydrochloride (cholestagel): A new, potent bile acid sequestrant associated with a low incidence of gastrointestinal side effects. Arch Intern Med 159(16):1893–1900, 1999.

159. Beil FU, Windler E: (Goals and practical implementation of lipid therapy in coronary heart disease). Herz 22(3):134–140, 1997.

160. Farmer JA, Gotto AM Jr: Choosing the right lipid-regulating agent. A guide to selection. Drugs 52(5):649–661, 1996.

161. Brown WV: Niacin for lipid disorders. Indications, effectiveness, and safety. Postgrad Med 98(2):185–189, 192–193, 1995.

162. Inositol hexaniacinate. Altern Med Rev 3(3):222–223, 1998.

163. Lavie CJ, Mailander L, Milani RV: Marked benefit with sustained-release niacin therapy in patients with "isolated" very low levels of high-density lipoprotein cholesterol and coronary artery disease. Am J Cardiol 69(12):1083–1085, 1992.

164. Marcelino JJ, Feingold KR: Inadequate treatment with HMG-CoA reductase inhibitors by health care providers. Am J Med 100(6):605–610, 1996.

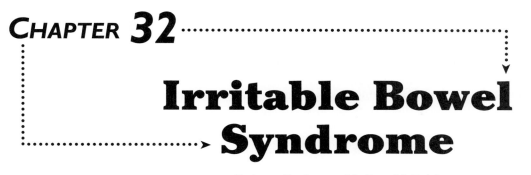

CHAPTER 32

Irritable Bowel Syndrome

Robert B. Lutz, M.D., M.P.H.

PATHOPHYSIOLOGY

Irritable bowel syndrome (IBS) is the most common gastrointestinal disease seen in clinical practice (accounting for 12% of primary care visits) and is the reason for 30% to 50% of all referrals to gastroenterologists. Symptoms compatible with IBS are reported by 10% to 22% of the American population, with a female-to-male ratio of greater than 2:1 among presenting patients. Fewer than half of adults with symptoms seek medical attention. In the United States, there appears to be no apparent relation to race, socioeconomic status, geographic location, household size, or employment status.

IBS has been characterized as a functional bowel disorder (recurrent bowel symptoms that are not readily explained by structural or biochemical abnormalities). Because there is no readily identified physiologic marker, reliance on symptomatology for diagnosis has been necessary. Various criteria are used for diagnosis; the Manning criteria have been used historically, whereas the Rome criteria (I and II), based on functional classification, are becoming the standard among gastroenterologists and clinical researchers (Table 32–1). In general, the diagnosis of IBS is suggested when the patient has abdominal pain or discomfort of at least 3 months' duration that is relieved with bowel movements or is associated with a change in frequency or consistency of stool. In addition, an irregular pattern of defecation is noted at least 25% of the time, with altered frequency (less than 3 times per week or more than 3 times per day), altered consistency, straining or urgency, or passage of mucus and bloating.

Table 32–1. Rome II Criteria for Diagnosis of Irritable Bowel Syndrome

Presence of abdominal pain or discomfort for at least 12 weeks, which Need Not be consecutive, in the preceding 12 months, with at least two of three features:
1. Relief of symptoms with defecation *and/or*
2. Onset associated with a change in frequency of stool *and/or*
3. Onset associated with a change in form (appearance) of stool

INTEGRATIVE THERAPY

Treatment is best approached from a biopsychosocial model. In this model, IBS is identified as a result of altered motility, enhanced visceral sensitivity, and brain-gut dysregulation, as modified by psychosocial influences.[1] Therefore, an integrated approach to patient care that incorporates nutrition, medications, and behavioral modalities, as well as other therapeutic options, is recommended (Table 32–2).

Table 32–2. Approach to Management of Patients with Irritable Bowel Syndrome

Establish an effective patient-physician relationship
- Acknowledge the pain
- Do not overreact
- Educate
- Reassure

Develop a treatment plan
- Set reasonable treatment goals
- Encourage the patient to take responsibility by keeping a symptom diary
- Base treatment on the severity and nature of the symptoms and the degree of disability
- Negotiate treatment
- Recognize limitations of available treatments and indications for referral

Adapted from Jones V, McLaughlan P, Shorthouse M, et al: Food intolerance: A major factor in the pathogenesis of irritable bowel syndrome. Lancet 2:1115–1117, 1982.

Nutrition Medicine/Supplements

Good basic nutritional practices are recommended, with some caveats. The majority of persons with IBS report food intolerances or exacerbation of symptoms after eating certain foodstuffs. Common offenders include wheat or wheat gluten, dairy products, corn, and citrus. Caffeine and refined sweets are also often identified. Elimination diets in which these common foodstuffs are removed for periods of 2 to 4 weeks and then slowly reintroduced may be of assistance in identifying the sensitizing agent(s) but are often very challenging to perform (see Chapter 82, The Elimination Diet). Maintenance of a food diary is strongly encouraged.[2, 3] Fiber supplementation is recommended, with caution to avoid wheat bran sources if gluten intolerance is noted. Fat may increase symptoms. Complex carbohydrate sources may increase gut bacterial fermentation, leading to gas and bloating. Therefore, some nutritionists recommend diets with simple sugars, such as monosaccharides (e.g., gluctose, fructose) and disaccharides (maltose, sucrose, lactose), for these patients. Probiotics may be beneficial in decreasing symptoms in some cases by helping to normalize the bowel flora[4] (see Chapter 97, Prescribing Probiotics).

NOTE

Rule out potential food sensitivities by having patient keep a food diary and/or a trial of an elimination diet.

Botanical Medicine

Many botanicals are currently recommended for management of IBS. Use of these agents is best directed by the nature and location of the patient's symptoms. Teas are best used for upper gastrointestinal symptoms, whereas capsules (enteric-coated) are best for lower gastrointestinal complaints.[5, 6] The classification terminology reflects herbalist groupings.

Carminatives

Carminative herbs are used to reduce flatulence and colic. They relax smooth muscle tone and reduce the incidence of spasms. They often contain volatile oils that stimulate local circulation and the secretion of gastric and gallbladder products.

Peppermint

Peppermint (*Mentha piperita*) has long been associated with promotion of digestive function. The leaves contain an oil that provides mild anesthetic properties, relieves nausea, and relaxes smooth muscle spasticity caused by histamine and cholinergic stimulation, thereby relieving spasm, while also relaxing sphincters and facilitating passage of gases of fermentation.

Dosage. One or two enteric-coated capsules (containing 0.2 ml of oil per capsule) three times daily between meals.[7–9]

Ginger

Ginger (*Zingiber officinale*) is available from health food stores. The active ingredients are gingerols, which function as 5-hydroxytryptamine (serotonin) antagonists and enhance gastrointestinal motility.

Dosage. The dose of dried ginger rhizome is 0.25 to 1 g three times per day.

Fennel

Fennel (*Foeniculum vulgare*) it is another well-known digestive.

Dosage. Fennel seeds ($^1/_2$ to 1 teaspoonful) can be consumed after meals or as needed; the recommended dose for the oil is 0.03 to 0.2 mL per day, and for the alcoholic extract, 0.5 to 2 mL per day.

German Chamomile

German chamomile (*Matricaria recutita*) has been used extensively for its anti-inflammatory (topical), antibacterial, and antispasmodic properties. The extract has also been shown to inhibit ulcer formation by serving as a mucosal restorative. It is recommended for relieving upper abdominal complaints.

Dosage. Chamomile tea is best known for its calming effect. An infusion of the flowers can be made with 1 to 2 teaspoons (2 to 3 g); for the 1:5 tincture, the dose is 1 to 4 mL three times a day between meals.

Caraway

Caraway (*Carum carvi*) is another carminative.

Dosage. Alcoholic extracts of the dried ripe fruits are used, or a tea is made by infusing 1 to 2 teaspoons of the seeds for 10 minutes.

Bitter Tonics

Bitter tonics are used to promote digestion. They are bitter-tasting herbs that increase deficient appetites and improve the acidity of stomach secretions and protein digestion, thereby increasing gastric emptying. They are recommended by herbalists for IBS, as this disorder is seen as having elements of digestive dysfunction. They are contraindicated in peptic ulcer disease and gastritis.

Gentian Root

Gentian root (*Gentiana lutea*) is one the most commonly used bitter herbs. It is most readily recognized as the active component of Angostura Bitters, the proprietary cocktail ingredient.

Dosage. Gentian root can be prepared as a decoction (by boiling the dried root for 30 minutes), taken up to four times per day, or a splash of the cocktail solution can be taken in a glass of tonic or soda water (with or without lemon), consumed before meals.

Goldenseal and Angelica

Goldenseal (*Hydrastis canadensis*) and angelica (*Angelica officinalis*) are two additional examples of bitter tonic herbs.

For persons who experience *constipation* as a major symptom of IBS, a number of botanicals are available. Two classes of botanicals are used; bulking agents and osmotic agents. The latter group should be used cautiously, as they work directly on the intestinal mucosa, often inducing a nonphysiologic bowel movement with loose stools and cramping. This effect is due to anthranoids contained within the plant. It is of note, however, that bulking agents are commonly used in persons with IBS irrespective of whether their predominant symptom is constipation or diarrhea.

Bulking Agents

Linseed

Linseed (*Linum usitatissimum*) is the dried ripened seed of flax. Linseed is high in fiber and contains mucilages, which are the key bulking constituent. This property, in addition to lubrication, helps to promote peristalsis. A few days may be needed for onset of action.

Dosage. 30 to 50 g of crushed whole seeds each day in adults.

Psyllium Seed and Husk

Psyllium (*Plantago* species) is a well-known bulking agent. The seeds contain mucilages, and the husks contain mucilages and hemicellulose. These components swell with addition of water after prolonged soaking. They promote passage of softened stool after a transit time of 6 to 12 hours.

Dosage. Dosing is based on manufacturer recommendations. A common dosage is 1 tablespoon taken with at least 8 ounces of water once or twice daily.

Wheat Bran

Wheat bran is the byproduct of the manufacture of flour from wheat (*Triticum aestivum*). Bran contains pentosans (swelling agents) as well as fiber and lignans that serve to increase stool bulk. There is also an increase in gut flora and mild irritation of the mucosa. The protein component of grain, gluten, is associated with hypersensitivity, and is therefore contraindicated in persons with this response.

Osmotic Agents

Cascara

The aged bark of cascara (*Cascara sagrada*) is used as a tincture, fluid extract, or tea (which is very bitter-tasting).

Dosage. $1/4$ to 1 tsp one to three times a day.

Precautions. Caution is indicated with concurrent use of cascara in persons receiving diuretic therapy, as excessive potassium loss may occur. With the decrease in bowel transit time, absorption of drugs may also decrease. Cascara should be used only very

infrequently and may be associated with laxative dependency.

Senna Pods and Leaves

Senna (*Cassia senna, Cassia angustifolia*) is another anthranoid-containing herb. Teas are commonly prepared from the pods and leaves, but extracts are also available. Senna is a common component of some over-the-counter laxatives.

Aloe

Aloe (*Aloe spicata* and related species) is the most powerful herbal anthranoid laxative and is widely used in Europe, but because of its drastic effects it is rarely used in the United States.

Nonspecific Antidiarrheal Agents

For persons with diarrhea-predominant IBS, herbals that have a nonspecific antidiarrheal action are sometimes used. Tannins contained in such plants serve as mild astringents, thereby decreasing inflammation. Teas made from the dried leaves of berry-containing bushes have commonly been used for this purpose. They can be consumed up to six times per day, but if symptoms persist beyond 2 to 3 days, then it is unlikely that continued usage will be beneficial.

- Blackberry (*Rubus fruticosus*)
- Blueberry (*Vaccinium* species)
- Rasberry (*Rubus idaeus*)

Demulcents

Demulcent herbs serve to coat mucosal surfaces, thereby decreasing inflammation. Marsh mallow root (*Althaea officinalis*) is an example. A common dose is 1000 mg three times per day before meals.

Physical Activity

Regular physical activity serves to enhance well-being and positively affects multiple physiologic parameters. It is recognized, for example, that physical activity may lessen feelings of depression and anxiety. This recommendation, however, should be individualized for the patient with IBS. Some activities, such as running, may enhance gastrointestinal motility and aggravate symptoms of diarrhea. Light to moderate physical activity, however, is strongly encouraged for all persons, owing to its health-related benefits.

Mind-Body Medicine

Mind-body therapies are fundamental to an integrated approach for IBS. An association of IBS with psychiatric diagnoses has been noted but is of significance only in patients who present for medical evaluation. A majority of patients with IBS report an episode of significant stress either preceding or exacerbating their symptoms.

NOTE

Persons with IBS symptoms who do not seek medical care have the same incidence of psychiatric disturbances as in the general population. Nevertheless, stress as a normal part of life may exacerbate symptoms, and identification and elimination of stress should be a key therapeutic focus.

The emphasis in these interventions is on self-understanding of factors that increase symptoms and on acquiring skills to enhance self-regulation. Many modalities have been used, both psychological and complementary and alternative medicine (CAM) techniques: cognitive-behavioral therapy, interpersonal/dynamic therapy, biofeedback, hypnotherapy and guided imagery, meditation, and stress management/relaxation (arousal reduction) training, as well as yoga and tai chi.[10-14] The practitioner should include one of these modalities that best matches the patient's lifestyle and belief structure.

Traditional Chinese Medicine

The diagnosis of IBS does not exist within traditional Chinese medicine (TCM) and other Asian treatment systems. Nonetheless, TCM has proved to be beneficial to persons suffering from characteristic symptoms of the disorder. A study demonstrated the benefits of a herbal formulation for patients with IBS; formulas that were individualized for the patient were found to be more effective than standardized herbal formulations for treating symptoms[15] (see Table 32–3).

Treatments used in TCM may include: herbal medicine, acupuncture and moxibustion, tui na (massage and acupressure), Qi gong (mind-body exercise), and dietary therapy. The individualized approach that characterizes TCM is preferred, but if a qualified TCM practitioner is not available, use of a standardized supplement that includes the herbs listed in Table 32–3 may be tried. One possibility is a product called Calm Colon (by Samra, www.samra.com/products/coloning.htm). The dose is 500 mg (1 capsule) three times daily taken with water.

In TCM, four main emotions are perceived to aggravate IBS-type symptoms: fear, anger, anxiety, and worry. Because these emotions may focus their effects in the solar plexus region, other associated symptoms may include urinary frequency, gastritis, palpitations, and dyspnea. It is helpful for persons with IBS to learn to relax deeply, and meditation linked with controlled breathing may be helpful.

Table 32–3. Standard Formulas (Capsule Ingredients) Used in Traditional Chinese Medicine for Treatment of Bowel Symptoms

Chinese Name	Pharmaceutical Name	Powdered Herb, %
Dang shen	*Codonopsis pilosulae*, radix	7
Huo xiang	*Agastaches seu pogostemi*, herba	4.5
Fang feng	*Ledebouriellae sesloidis*, radix	3
Yi yi ren	*Coicis lachryma-jobi*, semen	7
Chai hu	*Bupleurum chinense*	4.5
Yin chen	*Artemesiae capillaris*, herba	13
Bai zhu	*Atractylodis macrocephalae*, rhizoma	9
Hou po	*Magnoliae officinalis*, cortex	4.5
Chen pi	*Citri reticulatae*, pericarpium	3
Pao jiang	*Zingiberis officinalis*, rhizoma	4.5
Qin pi	*Fraxini*, cortex	4.5
Fu ling	*Poriae cocos*, sclerotium (Hoelen)	4.5
Bai zhi	*Angelicae dahuricae*, radix	2
Che qian zi	*Plantaginis*, semen	4.5
Huang bai	*Phellodendri*, cortex	4.5
Zhi gan cao	*Glycyrrhizae uralensis*, radix	4.5
Bai shao	*Paeoniae lactiflorae*, radix	3
Mu xiang	*Saussureae seu vladimirae*, radix	3
Huang lian	*Coptidis*, rhizoma	3
Wu wei zi	*Schisandrae*, fructus	7

From Bensoussan A: Treatment of irritable bowel syndrome with a Chinese herbal medicine: a randomized controlled trial. JAMA 280:1585–1589, 1998.

Pharmaceuticals

Antispasmodic Agents

Dicyclomine

Dicyclomine (Bentyl) is an anticholinergic antispasmodic agent.

Dosage. Dosage should begin with 10 to 20 mg 30 minutes before meals four times daily; the dose may be increased to 40 mg as tolerated.

Hyocyamine Sulfate

Hyoscyamine sulfate (Levsin) is another anticholinergic.

Dosage. This drug is available as 0.125-mg tablets or as an elixir containing 0.125 mg per 5 mL. The dose is 1 or 2 tablets or 5 to 10 mL of elixir every 4 hours or as needed, not to exceed 12 tablets or 60 mg per day.

Antidiarrheal Agents

Loperamide

Loperamide (Imodium) may be tried for control of symptoms of diarrhea.

Dosage. In acute cases, the dose is 2 to 4 mg every 6 to 8 hours, or 4 mg after the first loose stool and then 2 mg after each subsequent stool, not to exceed 16 mg per day; the drug should be discontinued if no improvement is obtained after 48 hours. In chromic cases, the dose is 1 to 8 mg per day as a single dose or in divided doses; the drug should be discontinued after 10 days if no improvement is obtained.

Diphenoxylate Atropine

A combination of diphenoxylate hydrochloride and atropine sulfate (Lomotil)—an opioid plus an anticholinergic—is often used to control diarrheal symptoms.

Dosage. In acute cases, the dose is 2 tablets or 10 mL 4 times a day until the diarrhea is controlled. In chronic cases, the dose is 2 tablets or 10 mL daily.

Other Therapies to Consider

Osteopathic Medicine

It is often thought that osteopathy and other related manual therapies are used only for musculoskeletal problems. However, recognition of a somatovisceral pathway amenable to manipulation has led to use of these approaches for relief of symptoms in persons with IBS.

There are many techniques in the osteopathic armamentarium. One such technique is *strain-counterstrain* (which may be combined with other direct techniques such as muscle energy or direct myofascial release).

The somatic areas that are commonly affected include the external obliques (especially the lower portion), internal obliques, and rectus abdominis;

the lower segments of the thoracic spine (T10–12); the iliocostalis thoracis/lumborum and longissimus thoracis/lumborum muscles; and the quadratus lumborum. Persons with this somatovisceral connection are often not aware of these tender points until they are discovered by careful palpation. This indirect technique seeks to release these strained somatic segments by means of initiating a reciprocal counterstrain of the antagonist muscles[16] (see Chapter 99, Strain and Counterstrain Manipulation Technique).

Homeopathy

Homeopathy is a unique healing system that makes use of very dilute remedies that best reflect a specific patient's nature. The homeopathic practitioner makes use of a *materia medica* with thousands of possible remedies.

In classic homeopathy, an extensive historical interview is performed that seeks to identify the "totality" of the patient on physical, emotional, and mental levels. To this is matched a remedy that best suits the individual patient. This remedy is administered in small and infrequent doses, and follow-up is performed to determine whether the chosen remedy should be repeated, changed, or allowed to continue its work.

 — *THERAPEUTIC REVIEW*

The treatment of IBS should be approached from the perspective that no single treatment option will work best for everyone. Accordingly, a partnership between patient and practitioner and a willingness of both to explore available options will serve to optimize management. A stepwise approach to treatment is recommended. In choosing appropriate modalities and in determining when a trial of a specific treatment is indicated, consultation with the patient to elicit his or her beliefs about healing possibilities is essential.

Nutrition

Identify any foodstuffs that may be causing symptoms. The use of a food diary is beneficial; the patient is directed to keep a close record of all foods eaten with the time of onset and nature of symptoms recorded. The food diary is typically maintained for 3 to 5 consecutive days. Trial of an elimination diet should also be considered; aggravating foods will often cause significant symptoms upon reintroduction (see Chapter 82).

A fiber supplement, especially as a source of insoluble fiber (such as methylcellulose [Citrucel], 1 scoop up to 3 times per day), should be added to the diet of all persons with IBS symptoms, irrespective of predominance.

A probiotic can also be added to the diet. Many supplement brands are available that commonly contain *Lactobacillus* species in varying concentrations; dosing is product-dependent. An easily obtainable dietary source is yogurt with active cultures, but this source may not provide an adequate concentration of live organisms (see Chapter 97).

Mind-Body Techniques

The patient's beliefs concerning the illness should be addressed. Encouragement and hope are important to assisting in managing or eliminating chronic symptoms.

THERAPEUTIC REVIEW   *continued*

Possible stressors and the patient's coping style should be identified. Possible alternatives should be provided if these coping styles are counterproductive. The patient should be made aware of the benefits of self-regulating and self-awareness practices such as meditation, guided imagery, and self-hypnosis.

Botanicals

The patient's primary symptom pattern should be determined, and botanical supplements selected on the basis of this information. This approach can begin with enteric-coated peppermint capsules, 1 or 2 taken three times a day. A bitter tonic such as gentian root may be added (if contraindications not present) and followed by other botanicals based on symptom predominance.

Traditional Chinese Medicine

Consider referral of the patient for evaluation by a TCM practitioner. A TCM treatment plan typically makes use of acupuncture, a herbal formulation, and dietary recommendations.

Osteopathy

Consider referral of the patient to an osteopathic physician who practices manual medicine. A variety of techniques are available.

Homeopathy

Consider referral of the patient to a classically trained homeopathic physician. Some modification to previously implemented treatments, such as use of botanicals, may be required.

Pharmaceuticals

The careful use of pharmaceuticals in concert with other therapeutic options as described can significantly assist in symptom management. Often, starting slowly with a simple regimen such as loperamide (Imodium) 1 to 2 mg per day, in conjunction with other modalities, can assist in demonstrating that the patient's symptoms can be managed with a multi level approach.

References

1. Drossman DA. Review article: An integrated approach to irritable bowel syndrome. Aliment Pharmacol Ther 13(Suppl 2):3–14, 1999.
2. Jones V, McLaughlan P, Shorthouse M, et al: Food intolerance: A major factor in the pathogenesis of irritable bowel syndrome. Lancet 2:1115–1117.
3. Zwetchkenbaum J: Irritable bowel syndrome and food hypersensitivity. Ann Allergy 61:47–49, 1988.
4. Nobaek S, Johansson ML, Mohn G, et al: Alteration of intestinal microflora is associated with reduction in abdominal bloating and pain in patients with irritable bowel syndrome. Am J Gastroenterol 95:1231–1238, 2000.
5. Bone K: Phytotherapy and irritable bowel syndrome. Br J Phytother 4:190–198, 1998.
6. Brown D: Irritable bowel syndrome. Q Rev Nat Med (Winter) 333–345, 1997.
7. Pittler, MH: Peppermint oil for irritable bowel syndrome: A critical review and meta-analysis. Am J Gastroenterol 93:1131–1135, 1998.
8. Rees WD, Evans BK: Treating irritable bowel syndrome with peppermint oil. BMJ 2:835–836, 1979.
9. Nash P, Gould SR, Bernardo DE: Peppermint oil does not relieve the pain of irritable bowel syndrome, Br J Clin Pract 40:292–293; 1986.
10. Bennett P, Wilkinson S: A comparison of psychological and medical treatment of the irritable bowel syndrome. Br J Clin Psychol 24:215–216, 1985.
11. Whorwell PJ, Prior A, Faragher EB, et al: Controlled trial of hypnotherapy in the treatment of severe refractory irritable bowel syndrome. Lancet 2:1232–1234, 1984.
12. Shaw G, Srivastava ED, Sadlier M et al: Stress management for irritable bowel syndrome: A controlled trial. Digestion 50:36–42, 1991.
13. Blanchard EB: Relaxation training as a treatment for IBS. Biofeedback Self-Regulation 18:125–132, 1993.
14. Haymann-Monnikes I, Arnold R: The combination of medical treatment plus multicomponent behavioral therapy is superior to medical treatment alone in the therapy of irritable bowel syndrome. Am J Gastroenterol 95:981–984, 2000.
15. Bensoussan A: Treatment of irritable bowel syndrome with a Chinese herbal medicine: A randomized controlled trial. JAMA 280:1585–1589 1998.
16. Jones LH: Jones Strain-Counterstrain. Boise, Idaho, Jones Strain Counterstrain, 1995.

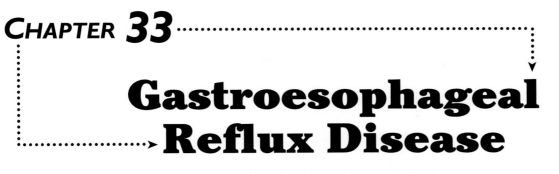

CHAPTER 33

Gastroesophageal Reflux Disease

Robert B. Lutz, M.D., M.P.H.

PATHOPHYSIOLOGY

Gastroesophageal reflux disease (GERD) is a term used to label the symptoms and/or histopathologic findings associated with reflux of stomach contents into the esophagus. Symptoms may be experienced daily or multiple times per week. This disorder is a great masquerader; with advances in understanding and improvements in diagnostic methodology, underlying GERD has been identified as the cause of such presentations as nocturnal cough, atypical chest pain, recurrent pneumonia, and persistent hoarseness. It should also be noted that the most serious complication of GERD, Barrett's esophagus, may be the initial presentation in this disorder and may be identified in persons presenting with dysphagia.

GERD is a relatively common problem in primary care, accounting for approximately 1% of all clinic visits to family practitioners.[1] It is more prevalent among the elderly and pregnant woman. From 4% to 7% of affected persons are estimated to experience daily symptoms.[2]

The mechanism for GERD is multifactorial but centers on decreased lower esophageal sphincter pressure (LES). This decrease is more often a transient phenomenon than a persistent finding. A majority of patients with GERD have a concomitant hiatal hernia. Hypersecretion of acid is not necessarily an absolute finding, although the combination of stomach acid and pepsin appears to cause the greatest degree of tissue injury. Abnormal gastric motility is the underlying disorder in GERD. Additional factors include inadequate saliva production (especially at night), with ineffective peristalsis leading to poor acid clearance; decreased esophageal tissue resistance; and exogenous substances that lower LES tone. The role of *Helicobacter pylori* is known in ulcer disease, but its role in GERD is less well defined; this organism may in some cases actually be protective.[3]

The frequency of use of complementary and alternative medicine (CAM) for chronic medical conditions has been identified as greater than 40%.[4] Frequency of use of CAM by persons with inflammatory bowel disease has been found to be approximately 34%.[5] A recent survey performed in community-based patients with GERD found the frequency of usage of CAM to be greater than 60%, but less than 4% of the patients were using CAM for their GERD symptoms. A majority of the survey participants were satisfied with use of conventional therapies and lifestyle interventions for symptom management.[6] Nevertheless, a number of therapeutic options should be considered in formulating an integrative approach to symptom management.

INTEGRATIVE THERAPY

Lifestyle Measures

Before material intervention, simple behavioral changes and lifestyle measures should be implemented. These include the following:

- Elevation of the head of the bed
- Avoidance of the recumbent position for 2 hours after meals and avoidance of eating for at least 2 hours before bedtime
- Scheduling small, frequent meals
- Weight loss, if appropriate
- Avoidance of tight, restrictive clothing
- Dietary precautions for foods that lower LES pressures and/or increase stomach acid (see Table 33-1)
- Elimination of smoking
- A review of current medications for possible side effects, e.g., oral contraceptives, theophylline, nitrates and calcium channel blockers, tricyclics, benzodiazepines, and aspirin, and other nonsteroidal anti-inflammatory drugs (NSAIDs)

Table 33–1. Substances That Lower Esophageal Sphincter Tone

Foods
Tomatoes, citrus, fat, chocolate, coffee, alcohol

Supplements
Peppermint oil

Drugs
Nitrites, theophylline, oral contraceptive pills, calcium channel blockers, benzodiazepines, tricyclic antidepressants

Botanicals

A number of herbs can be used for symptom relief, promotion of normal peristalsis, and soothing of inflamed mucosa.

Licorice Root

Licorice root (*Glycyrrhiza glabra*) has anti-inflammatory and demulcent properties. Glycyrrhizin, active ingredient of licorice, affects aldosterone metabolism, thereby increasing blood pressure; therefore, licorice root is commonly replaced with deglycyrrhizinated licorice (DGL). This preparation has been compared with H_2 blockers for treatment and maintenance therapy of peptic ulcer disease and found to be effective.[7]

NOTE

Deglycyrrhizinated licorice (DGL) is a safer form of licorice because the salt-retaining component, glycyrrhizin, is removed, resulting in less risk of hypertension, hypernatremia, and hypokalemia.

Dosage. Normal dosing of licorice root is 5 to15 g per day of cut or powdered root; or dry extracts, equivalent to 200 to 600 mg of glycyrrhizin; or 2 to 4 mL of a fluid extract in a 1:1 concentration (g/mL) taken before meals three times daily. Dosing of DGL tablets (each containing 380 mg of DGL in a 4:1 concentration) is 2 to 4 tablets chewed before each meal in acute cases (gastric or duodenal ulcers) or 1 or 2 tablets before meals in chronic cases.

Precautions. Use of licorice root is contraindicated in liver disease, renal insufficiency, and hypokalemia. It can potentiate digoxin toxicity in hypokalemia. it may increase potassium loss with concurrent thiazide usage. Its use is not recommended during pregnancy.

Marsh Mallow Root

Marsh mallow root (*Althea officinalis*) serves as a demulcent, coating and soothing inflamed mucosa. This herb is approved by the German Commission E for mild gastritis. It has no known contraindications.

Dosage. Normal dosing is 2 to 5 g of the dried root, up to three times daily or 2 to 5 mL of a fluid extract in a 1:1 concentration (g/mL), up to three times daily.

Chamomile

German chamomile (*Matricaria recutita* [syn. *Chamomilla recutita*]) has a long history of use throughout Europe. The *British Herbal Compendium* lists chamomile internally for spasms or inflammatory conditions of the gastrointestinal tract and peptic ulcer disease. It has no known contraindications.

Dosage. Teas or infusions are prepared for gastrointestinal symptoms using 3 g of the flowers in 150 mL water, to be taken three or four times daily.

Centaury

Centaury (*Centaurium erythraea*) stimulates the flow of gastric secretions and promotes digestion. Its effectiveness is seen with continued usage.

Dosage. 2 to 4 mL of a liquid extract taken before meals three times daily or steep 2 to 4 g of the flower in 150 mL of boiling water and drink the tea three times daily.

Precautions. It is contraindicated with known ulcer disease.

Mind-Body Medicine

Mind-body modalities are fundamental to an integrative approach in all medical conditions. In patients with GERD, relaxation practices and stress management techniques have been demonstrated to lessen subjective symptoms and to alleviate anxiety.[8-10] Other methods, such as self-hypnosis and imagery, can be used for relaxation, stress management, and visualization of normal gastrointestinal functioning (see Chapter 91, Prescribing Relaxation Techniques).

Traditional Chinese Medicine

As an alternative system of healing, traditional Chinese medicine (TCM) is a holistic approach to disease. For the person who is experiencing symptoms suggestive of the Western diagnosis of GERD, combination therapies are often provided that focus on herbal formulations, acupuncture, and dietetics. Therapeutic recommendations are individualized according to the patient's symptoms and other characteristics.

Physical Activity and Exercise

The health benefits of physical activity are well documented. Physiological as well as emotional and psychological components of the beneficial effect have been identified. Gastrointestinal functioning is affected by exercise (decreased splanchnic blood flow, altered peristalsis, and mass movement) and is dependent on many factors, including pre-exercise nutrition, hydration state, and exercise intensity. Results of studies in athletes have been variable, but in general, evidence suggests that exercise increases reflux. This effect is most pronounced in persons who experience symptoms at rest. Running appears to induce the highest frequency of GERD, with bicycling and weight lifting also producing symptoms. Pretreatment with H_2 blockers decreases running-related GERD.[11, 12]

Pharmaceuticals

Use of antacids and over-the-counter acid suppressants is currently recommended as appropriate initial self-directed therapy. If symptoms persist or the patient experiences dysphagia, medical attention is recommended.

Acid suppression is the mainstay of therapy for GERD. Proton pump inhibitors such as omeprazole (Prilosec), lansoprazole (Prevacid), or rabeprazole (Aciphex) provide rapid symptomatic relief and promote healing of esophagitis in the highest percentage of patients. H_2 blockers such as ranitidine (Zantac) or famotidine (Pepcid) given in divided doses may also be used and are effective in many patients with less severe GERD. Because symptoms often recur on cessation of therapy, chronic maintenance therapy to prevent symptoms and complication is often necessary. Chronic proton pump inhibitor therapy is effective and appropriate for maintenance therapy in many patients.

Other Therapies to Consider

Homeopathy has been used for management of GERD. Remedies are individualized and may consist of single or multiple ingredients. Some preparations that have been recommended include Arsenicum album, Carbo vegetabilis, Kali carbonicum, and Lycopodium. Evaluation of the patient by a trained homeopathic practitioner is recommended.

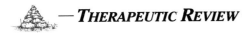 *THERAPEUTIC REVIEW*

Lifestyle Modifications

- *Elevation of the head of the bed*
- *Avoidance of the recumbent position for 2 hours after meals and avoidance of eating for at least 2 hours before bedtime*
- *Scheduling small, frequent meals*
- *Weight loss, if appropriate*
- *Avoidance of tight, restrictive clothing*
- *Dietary precautions for foods that lower LES pressures and/or increase stomach acid*
- *Elimination of smoking*
- *A review of current medications for possible side effects (oral contraceptives, theophylline, nitrates and calcium channel blockers, tricyclics, benzodiazepines, and aspirin, and other NSAIDs)*

Self-Directed Medical Interventions

- *Antacids and over-the-counter acid suppressants*

Botanical Medicine

- *Licorice root: 5 to 15 g per day of cut or powdered licorice root, or dry extracts equivalent to 200 to 600 mg of glycyrrhizin, or 2 to 4 mL of a fluid extract (1:1 [g/mL]) after meals three times daily; DGL tablets (each with 380 mg of DGL 4:1): chew 2 to 4 tablets before each meal for acute cases (gastric or duodenal ulcers) or 1 or 2 tablets before meals in chronic cases*
- *Marsh mallow root: 2 to 5 g of dried root, up to three times daily; 2 to 5 mL of fluid extract (1:1 [g/mL]) up to three times daily*

Mind-Body Medicine

Explore stress management and relaxation practices with all patients. Also consider guided imagery to promote normal gastrointestinal physiology.

Traditional Chinese Medicine

Explore the patient's interest in pursuing an alternative approach to symptom management.

Pharmaceuticals

The mainstay of GERD therapy is acid suppression. This is best accomplished with use of proton pump inhibitors, such as omeprazole (Prilosec) 20 mg twice daily for 4 weeks or lansoprazole (Prevacid) 15 mg daily for 8 weeks. H_2 receptor blockers, such as famotidine (Pepcid), 20 mg twice daily for 6 weeks or ranitidine (Zantac) 150 mg twice daily for 6 weeks, are effective in many persons with less severe symptoms. Promotility agents such as metoclopramide (Reglan) are as effective as H_2 blockers.

References

1. Centers for Disease Control and Prevention: 1995 National Ambulatory Medical Care Survey. NCHS CD-ROM series 13, No 11, 1997.
2. Sonnenberg A, El-Serag HB: Clinical epidemiology and natural history of gastroesophageal reflux disease. Yale J Biol Med 72:81–92, 2000.
3. Richter J: Do we know the cause of reflux disease? Eur J Gastroenterol Hepatol 11(Suppl 1):S3-S9, 1999.
4. Eisenberg DM, Davis RB, Ettner SL, et al: Trends in alternative medicine use in the United States, 1990-1997. JAMA 280:1569–1574, 1998.
5. Rawsthrone P, Shanahan F, Cronin NC, et al: An international survey of the use and attitudes regarding alternative medicine by patients with inflammatory bowel disease. Am J Gastroenterol 94:1298–1303, 1999 .
6. Hayden CW, Bernstein CB, Hall RA, et al: The usage of supplemental alternative medicine by community-based patients with GERD. Presented in part at the annual meeting of the American Gastroenterological Association, San Diego, Calif., 2000.
7. Morgan, AG, McAdam WA: Comparison between cimetidine and Caved-S in the treatment of gastric ulceration, and subsequent maintenance therapy. Gut 23:545–551, 1982.
8. Cuntz U, Pollman H, Enck P: [Behavior therapy in gastrointestinal functional disorders]. Z Gastroenterol 30:24–34, 1992.
9. Friedman EH: Neurobiology of relaxation training in gastroesophageal reflux disease [letter]. Gastroenterology 108:619–620, 1995.
10. McDonald-Haile J, Bradley MA, Schan CA, Richter JE: Relaxation training reduces symptom reports and acid exposure in patients with gastroesophageal reflux disease. Gastroenterology 107:61–69, 1994.
11. Kraus BB, Sinclair JW, Castell DO: Gastroesophageal reflux in runners: Characteristics and treatment. Ann Intern Med 112:429–433, 1990.
12. Van Niewenhoven MA, Bronus F, Brummer RJ: The effect of physical exercise on parameters of gastrointestinal function. Neurogastroenterol Motil 11:431–443, 1999.

CHAPTER 34

Peptic Ulcer Disease

Robert B. Lutz, M.D., M.P.H.

PATHOPHYSIOLOGY

Peptic ulcer disease (PUD) can be best understood as an imbalance between mucosal protective factors and aggressive factors. These latter include increased acid and digestive enzymes, *Helicobacter pylori,* and nonsteroidal anti-inflammatory drugs (NSAIDs). Risk factors that may increase the likelihood of PUD development include tobacco use, alcohol abuse, sleep deprivation, acid hypersecretory states (Zollinger-Ellison syndrome, possible hereditary state), localized vascular insufficiency, O blood type, and chemotherapeutic agents.

The identification and reporting of *H. pylori* by Dr. Barry J. Marshall in 1983 have served to significantly shift the focus of PUD management to identification and eradication of this bacterium. As such, the role of "stress" in PUD has been sharply downplayed. The American College of Gastroenterology, in an online patient information bulletin, states, "In the past, ulcers were incorrectly thought to be caused by stress. Doctors now know that there are two major causes of ulcers [*H. pylori* and NSAIDs]."

In spite of this stance, however, there is a strong body of evidence to support the role of stress in PUD. A recent review of the literature suggests that psychosocial factors may be estimated to contribute to 30% to 65% of PUD, in combination with either *H. pylori* infection, NSAID usage, or neither.[1] A rich body of epidemiologic evidence supports increased risks of PUD following significant traumatic events (e.g., the German *blitzkrieg* over London and the earthquake in Kobe, Japan) and with elevated levels of life and work stress.[2, 3] The increased risk of PUD in individuals of lower socioeconomic status, which has been linked to increased risk of *H. pylori* infection, may well be mediated by psychosocial factors such as deprivation and discrimination.[4]

Likewise, a focus on NSAIDs as the sole causative agent fails to answer why the majority of NSAID users never develop PUD. More than 10% of individuals who develop PUD secondary to use of NSAIDs do not have concurrent *H. pylori* infection, and more than 80% of individuals who are infected do not develop disease (however, approximately 70% of individuals with gastric ulcers and 90% of duodenal ulcer patients have *H. pylori* infection).[1, 5] Therefore, PUD is best viewed as an example of a complex model of altered physiology and increased susceptibility mediated through endogenous and exogenous factors, both physical and psychosocial. As such, it serves as a diagnosis that is highly amenable to an "integrative approach." The following provides recommendations (with research where identified) for management of PUD.

NOTE

Eighty percent of individuals infected with H. pylori *are asymptomatic. The etiology of PUD is multifactorial and warrants an integrative approach.*

LIFESTYLE CONSIDERATIONS

Tobacco

Tobacco usage causes localized vascular ischemia and inhibits the formation of protective prostaglandins. This increases the risk for development of ulcers, slows the healing of preexisting ulcers, and increases the risk of ulcer recurrence.[5] Therefore, smoking cessation is essential.

Sleep

Sleep deprivation increases physiologic stress. Therefore, appropriate restful sleep should be encouraged.

NSAIDs

All patients on NSAIDs should be warned of the potential risk of gastritis/ulcer; if symptoms develop, these should be eliminated.

Nutrition

In spite of the intuitive link between diet and peptic ulcer disease, there is currently little evidence to support a strong relationship. With the current focus on identified etiologies, nutrition has taken on a lesser role in management. Nonetheless, a few recommendations can be made. Sensible eating is encouraged, with avoidance of identified aggravating foods and possibly caffeine and alcohol. Small meals may be better than large meals. And remember that foods can affect many of the common pharmaceuticals used to conventionally treat PUD (e.g., PCN-G and citrus juice, metronidazole [Flagyl], and alcohol).

Dietary practices that emphasize fruits and vegetables are beneficial. Epidemiologic evidence has supported the relationship between fiber and vitamin A and decreased ulcer formation,[6] as well as suggesting a relationship between increased consumption of fermented dairy products and decreased ulcer prevalence. Conversely, diets high in meat and dairy, total fat, saturated and monounsaturated fatty acids, and linolenic (omega-3 fatty acids) acid demonstrate increased ulcer prevalence.[7] Bioflavonoids found in citrus fruits, berries, onions, legumes, green tea, and red wine have been demonstrated to decrease the release of histamine, thereby decreasing acid output, as well as having inhibitory effects on *H. pylori*.[8]

Vitamin C in high doses has been shown to inhibit the growth of *H. pylori* in animal studies.[9]

And of historical note, raw cabbage juice has been documented to be successful in treating PUD. In one study, 1 liter of fresh juice per day taken in divided doses provided healing in 10 days. This healing may be due to the high level of glutamine in the juice, which possibly enhances synthesis of the protective lining of the stomach.[10]

BOTANICAL MEDICINE

The roles of herbs in the treatment of PUD are to decrease inflammation and to function as demulcents. In this regard, two herbs are commonly recommended.

Licorice Root/Rhizome (*Glycyrrhiza glabra*)

Licorice has traditionally been used for the prevention and treatment of peptic ulcers. Glycyrrhizin or glycyrrhetic acid has been shown to stimulate mucus secretion by mucosal surfaces. Whereas the regular use of a high dose is potentially hazardous owing to its blockage of 5-beta-reductase and its effects on aldosterone metabolism, an extract (DGL, or deglycyrrhizinated licorice extract) has been found to be equally effective without significant adverse effects. Clinically, a comparison of cimetidine with a DGL–antacid combination found similar efficacies in ulcer healing, maintenance, and recurrence.[11]

Dosage. Normal dosing of licorice root is 5 to 15 g per day of cut or powdered root; or dry extracts equivalent to 200 to 600 mg of glycyrrhizin; or a fluidextract 1:1 (g/mL)—Take 2 to 4 mL between meals three times daily.

Dosing of DGL tablets (380 mg DGL 4:1) in acute cases (gastric or duodenal ulcers)—Chew 2 to 4 tablets before each meal; in chronic cases, chew 1 to 2 tablets before meals.

Precautions. Use of licorice root is contraindicated in patients with liver disease, renal insufficiency, and hypokalemia. It can potentiate digoxin toxicity in hypokalemia. It may increase potassium loss with concurrent thiazide usage. It is not recommended during pregnancy.

NOTE

Deglycyrrhizinated licorice (DGL) has been found to be as effective as cimetidine (Tagamet) for the treatment and prevention of peptic ulcer disease.

German Chamomile (*Matricaria recutita*)

Chamomile extract inhibits ulcer formation and promotes ulcer healing, as was documented in several clinical trials in Europe in the late 1950s.

Dosage. As its properties are affected by the mode of extraction, the hydroalcoholic extract at a dose of 1:5 strength tincture of 1 to 4 mL is desirable. Infusions, however, can work quickly to soothe irritation of gastric mucosa (1 to 2 tsp with 1 cup of water, steeped for 5 to 10 minutes and taken slowly, 3 to 4 times daily).

Marsh Mallow Root (*Althaea officinalis*)

Marsh mallow serves as a demulcent herb, coating and soothing inflamed mucosa. It is approved by the German Commission E for mild gastritis. It has no known contraindications.

Dosage. Normal dosing: Dried root 2 to 5 g, up to three times daily; fluidextract 1:1 (g/mL) 2 to 5 mL, up to three times daily.

Mind–Body Medicine

Although the current focus is on *H. pylori* and NSAID usage as etiologic factors in PUD, the role of stress has not been totally eliminated. With recognition that psychosocial factors may contribute to 30% to 65% of ulcers (whether due to *H. pylori*, NSAIDs, or neither[1]) mind–body techniques play a significant role in management. Historically, psychotherapy has been seen as beneficial[12] and psychological interventions have been recommended.[13] Likewise, techniques that facilitate stress management, address coping strategies, and promote relaxation may be beneficial. Imagery and self-hypnosis, either to promote healing or to facilitate self-regulation, can serve as useful tools for individuals.[14]

Asian Medicine

Digestion is considered of paramount importance in traditional Chinese medicine. In five-element theory, Earth is associated with digestion and the organs of stomach and spleen. The function of the stomach is to receive food, whereas the function of the spleen is to transform the food. This processed food is then sent on to the large intestine for elimination. The spleen sends the transformed "food Qi" up to the chest for further processing into usable Qi. The interruption of these functions results in subclinical or clinical symptoms.

There are at least five commonly identified TCM diagnoses for PUD. These include Liver Qi stagnation (wood attacking earth), stagnation of heat (in the stomach or liver), deficiency of Yin, Qi deficiency and cold, and blood stagnation. A differential diagnosis is required to determine which type or combination of types is present. In liver Qi stagnation, stress may play a big role; in stagnant heat or Yin deficiency, spicy foods may be involved. In Qi deficiency and cold, a weak constitution and poor diet may be causative factors. Blood stagnation is usually diagnosed when there is some bleeding involved, and it may arise from cold or heat. For liver Qi stagnation, acupuncture alone may be all that is needed, but for other diagnoses, supplemental herbs are required. Research has demonstrated the benefits of TCM therapy, either alone or in combination with conventional therapies.[15–17]

Physical Activity

The benefits of physical activity and health are well known. A recent epidemiologic study found that the risk of duodenal ulcers was decreased in men who were active (those who walked or ran 10 or more miles a week) and moderately active (those who walked or ran less than 10 miles a week or did another regular activity) compared with a reference group. These benefits were not identified in women or for gastric ulcer patients.[18]

Pharmaceuticals

All individuals with identified *H. pylori* infection and appropriate symptomatology should be treated. Treatment includes antimicrobials (e.g., metronidazole, amoxicillin, tetracycline, clarithromycin [Biaxin]) and antisecretory drugs (e.g., H_2-blocking agents such as ranitidine hydrochloride [Zantac], or proton pump inhibitors such as omeprazole [Prilosec]). There are multiple currently recommended regimens, and practitioners should familiarize themselves with a few that can be best used for particular situations. Bismuth preparations (Pepto-Bismol) have antimicrobial effects and are common components of multidrug regimens.

For those individuals in whom NSAIDs are causative, attempts should be made to eliminate or decrease usage. For chronic NSAID users, concurrent administration of misoprostol (Arthrotec, Cytotec) is recommended (decreases mucosal damage, improves ulcer healing, and reduces reactive gastritis). Omeprazole has been shown to be as effective as misoprostol for treating NSAID-related ulcers.

Individuals who have neither *H. pylori* infection nor NSAID-induced ulceration can be effectively treated with either H_2 blockers or proton pump inhibitors for 4 to 6 weeks.

THERAPIES TO CONSIDER

Mastic gum is a resin produced from the *Pistacia lentiscus* tree. It has been used for thousands of years in the Mediterranean region for gastrointestinal problems, especially dyspepsia. Interestingly, it has antimicrobial properties and has been reported to be effective in *H. pylori* eradication therapy. Normal dosing is 500 to 1000 mg twice daily for 2 weeks.

THERAPEUTIC REVIEW

Lifestyle Measures
- *Eliminate tobacco*
- *Make dietary modifications (e.g., eliminate caffeine, alcohol, identified food irritants)*
- *Get restful sleep*

Mind-Body Techniques
- *Stress management/relaxation practices*
- *Self-regulation practices (e.g., imagery, hypnosis)*

THERAPEUTIC REVIEW continued

Regular Physical Activity

Nutrition/Supplements
- *Increase intake of fruits, vegetables, and fiber*
- *Decrease meat and dairy consumption*
- *Consume antioxidants, especially sources of vitamin A (e.g., red and yellow fruits and vegetables, or mixed carotene supplements [25,000 IUs]) and vitamin C*
- *Consume bioflavonoids (sources include citrus fruits, berries, onions, legumes, and green tea)*

Botanicals
- *Licorice or DGL: Licorice root, 5 to 15 g per day of cut or powdered root, or dry extracts equivalent to 200 to 600 mg of glycyrrhizin, or a fluidextract 1:1 (g/mL): 2 to 4 mL between meals three times daily; DGL tablets (380 mg DGL 4:1)—in acute cases (gastric or duodenal ulcers), chew 2 to 4 tablets before each meal; in chronic cases, chew 1 to 2 tablets before meals.*
- *German chamomile: 1 to 4 mL of 1:5 strength tincture. Infusions, however, can work quickly to soothe irritation of gastric mucosa (1 to 2 tsp with 1 cup water, steeped for 5 to 10 minutes and taken slowly, 3 to 4 times daily).*
- *Marsh mallow root: Dried root 2 to 5 g, up to three times daily; fluidextract 1:1 (g/mL) 2 to 5 mL, up to three times daily.*
- *Mastic gum: 500 to 1000 mg bid for 2 weeks*

Pharmaceuticals
- *Multidrug regimens for elimination of* H. pylori *and acid reduction*
- *Addition of protective agents for long-term NSAID users*

Consider consultation with a practitioner of TCM.

References

1. Levenstein S: The very model of a modern etiology: A biopsychosocial view of peptic ulcer. Psychosom Med 62:176–185, 2000.
2. Levenstein S, Ackerman S, Kiecolt-Glaser J, Dubois A: Stress and peptic ulcer disease. JAMA 281:10–11, 1999.
3. Levenstein S: Peptic ulcer at the end of the 20th century: Biological and psychological risk factors [review]. Can J Gastroenterol 13:753–759, 1999.
4. Levenstein S, Kaplan GA: Socioeconomic status and ulcer. A prospective study of contributory risk factors. J Clin Gastroenterol 26:14–17, 1998.
5. Brown LF, Wilson DE: Gastroduodenal ulcers: Causes, diagnosis, prevention and treatment. Compr Ther 25:30–38, 1999.
6. Aldoori WH, Giovannucci EL, Stampfer MJ, et al: Prospective study of diet and the risk of duodenal ulcer in men. Am J Epidemiol 145:42–50, 1997.
7. Elmstahl S, Svensson U, Berglund G: Fermented milk products are associated with ulcer disease. Results from a cross-sectional population study. Eur J Clin Nutr 52:668–674, 1998.
8. Beil W, Sewing KF: Effects of flavonoids on parietal cell acid secretion, gastric mucosal prostaglandin production and *H. pylori* growth. Arzneimittelforschung 45:697–700, 1995.
9. Zhang HM, et al: Vitamin C inhibits the growth of a bacterial risk factor for gastric carcinoma, *H. pylori*. Cancer 80:1897–1903, 1997.
10. Cheney G: Rapid healing of peptic ulcers in patients receiving fresh cabbage juice. Cal Med 70:10–14, 1949.
11. Morgan AG, et al: Comparison between cimetidine and Caved-s in the treatment of gastric ulceration and subsequent maintenance therapy. Gut 23:545–551, 1982.
12. Sjoedin I, Svedlund J, Ottosson J: Controlled study of psychotherapy in chronic peptic ulcer disease. Psychosom Med 27:187–200, 1986.
13. Garrett VD: Gastrointestinal disorders. In Goreczny, Anthony J, et al (eds): Handbook of Health and Rehabilitation Psychology. Plenum Series in Rehabilitation and Health. New York, Plenum Press, 1995, pp 79–97.
14. Whorwell PJ: Use of hypnotherapy in gastrointestinal disease. Br J Hosp Med 45:27–29, 1991.
15. Ma LS, Gou TM: Combination of TCM and Western medicine in the treatment of resistant peptic ulcer. Chin Med J (Engl) 107:554–556, 1994.
16. Tougas G, Hunt RH: Relation of acupuncture and vagal gastric acid secretion [letter, comment]. Gut 36:800–801, 1995.
17. Zhou Z, Hu Y, Pi D, et al: Clinical and experimental observations on treatment of peptic ulcer with wei yang an (easing peptic ulcer) capsule. J Tradit Chin Med 11:34–39, 1991.
18. Cheng Y, Macera CA, Davis DR, Blair SN: Physical activity and peptic ulcers. Does physical activity reduce the risk of developing peptic ulcers? [see comments]. West J Med 173(2):101–107, 2000. [Comment in West J Med 173:108–109, 2000.]

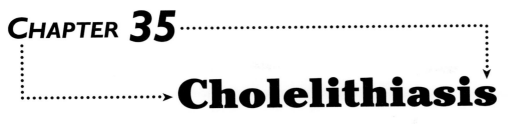

CHAPTER 35

Cholelithiasis

David Rakel, M.D.

PATHOPHYSIOLOGY

The combination of a "Western diet" high in saturated fats and a sedentary lifestyle in a population that is generally overweight creates an environment prone to gallstone formation. In fact, gallbladder disease affects about 10% of the population of the United States. There are two main types of stones—cholesterol (80%) and pigment or calcium stones (20%). It helps to remember that one of the main functions of bile is to absorb fat from the intestine, which makes it very efficient at binding cholesterol. Formation of gallstones is the result of three factors: (1) supersaturation of bile with cholesterol, (2) a decrease in bile salts that act to dissolve the cholesterol vesicles, and (3) stasis of bile flow (Fig. 35–1). Genetics may also increase risk, as can be seen in certain populations such as the Pima Indians. Although the majority of stones remain asymptomatic, conditions that influence one or more of these three factors may lead to cholelithiasis, which results in disease of the gallbladder. Table 35–1 lists conditions that may increase this risk.

LIFESTYLE

Weight Management

Slow, gradual weight loss for obese individuals reduces the amount of cholesterol in the biliary tract and decreases the risk of stone formation.

Emphasis should be placed on a slow rate of loss because drastic weight reductions have been found to increase triglycerides and biliary calcium levels, resulting in stone formation. Low-fat diets also fail to stimulate gallbladder contraction, resulting in stasis of bile and increased risk.

Exercise

A regular exercise program not only helps one to maintain a healthy weight, it also has been found to be inversely related to the risk of having a cholecystectomy. The Nurses' Health Study showed that women who spent longer than 60 hours a week sitting while working or driving were 2.32 times as likely to have a cholecystectomy. As little as 2 to 3 hours of activity a week reduced the risk by 20%.[1]

NUTRITION

Low Saturated Fat Diet

Encourage a diet low in saturated fatty foods. Reduce fried foods, dairy products, and red meat to decrease the cholesterol saturation of bile. Vegetarians are known to have a lower risk of gallstones.[2] Some evidence shows that fish oils, presumably because of their high concentration of omega-3 fatty acids, reduce the formation of gallstones owing to their ability to enhance bile flow and stabilize phospholipid-cholesterol vesicles.[3, 4] Recommend a diet low in saturated fats while increasing polyunsaturated ones rich in omega-3 fatty acids. These include cold water fish, flaxseed, and walnuts.

NOTE

Although a low saturated fat diet is beneficial, a diet low in total fat may increase the risk of gallstones because there will be less stimulation of bile flow, resulting in stasis. The goal should be to improve the types of fats consumed—that is, less of those with saturated fat and more of those rich in omega-3 essential fatty acids.

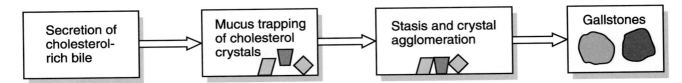

Figure 35–1. Pathophysiology of gallstones.

Table 35–1. Conditions That May Increase Risk of Cholelithiasis

↑ Cholesterol Saturation	↓ Bile Salts	↑ Stasis of Bile Flow
Estrogen = ↑ chol. secretion into bile (oral contraceptive pills, estrogen supplements, multiparous women)	Chronic loss from ileal inflammation (Crohn's disease, ileal resection)	Parenteral alimentation (no stimulation of gallbladder contraction)
Obesity	↓ Production with age	Low fat, weight-loss diets
Cholelesterol-rich diet	Low-fiber diet	Inactivity
Fibric acid– derivative drugs (gemfibrozil, clofibrate)		

High-Fiber Diet

Epidemiologic studies of vegetarians and populations who eat high-fiber diets have shown a lower rate of gallstone-related disease. One possible reason for this is that fiber reduces the absorption of deoxycholic acid. This compound is produced from bile acids by bacteria in the intestine, and it significantly reduces the solubility of cholesterol in bile promoting stone formation. Water-soluble fiber such as that found in fruits, vegetables, pectin, oat bran, and guar gum has the greatest binding capacity for this acid and may be helpful in both the prevention and reversal of gallstones.[5] Diets low in fiber and high in refined sugars and fat (Western diet) have been associated with a reduced synthesis and concentration of bile acids, leading to gallstone formation.[6]

Legumes, although rich in fiber, should be avoided because they have been found to significantly increase the cholesterol saturation of bile.

Coffee

One of the few benefits of coffee drinking does not appear to be related to its caffeine content. A prospective cohort study of 46,008 men showed that those who drank 2 to 3 cups of coffee a day over a 10-year period had a 40% lower risk of cholecystectomy or gallstone formation. This was not the case for other caffeinated drinks such as tea or soft drinks.[7] Coffee has been found to stimulate cholecystokinin release and gallbladder motility.[8]

Water

Drinking 6 to 8 cups of fluid a day ensures the water content of the bile and helps to prevent crystal agglomeration.

Food Allergy

Some research shows that food sensitivities may be a common trigger of gallbladder attacks. When 69 patients with gallstones or a postcholecystectomy syndrome were placed on a food elimination diet, all noted improvement in symptoms 3 to 5 days after treatment.[9] Foods that were found to be most likely to induce symptoms, in order of severity, were eggs, pork, onion, fowl, milk, coffee, citrus, corn, beans, and nuts. Eggs were found to result in symptoms in up to 95% of patients. For those with recurring biliary colic who want to avoid surgery, an elimination diet should be considered. (See Chapter 81, Food Allergy and Chapter 82, Recommending an Elimination Diet and Diagnosing Food Hypersensitivities.)

SUPPLEMENTS

Vitamin C

Evidence shows that a diet deficient in vitamin C results in gallstone formation.[10, 11] This may be related to its effect on reducing the amount of cholesterol in bile. A study of 2744 postmenopausal women aged 44 to 79 (HERS study) showed that ascorbic acid supplementation was associated with a significantly reduced risk of gallstones and cholecystectomy in drinkers of alcohol. The relationship between supplementation and disease in nondrinkers was not significant.[12]

Dosage. Vitamin C, 200 mg twice a day. An 8-oz glass of orange juice has about 60 mg of vitamin C.

Precautions. Dose-related effects include diarrhea, nausea, vomiting, esophagitis, heartburn, abdominal cramps, fatigue, flushing, headache, hyperoxaluria, and the predisposition to urate, oxalate, or cysteine urinary tract stones.

Vitamin E

Animal studies have shown that those who were given a vitamin E–deficient diet developed cholesterol gallstones even when they were on a cholesterol-free diet.[13] And those who were given a high-fat diet failed to develop gallstones when vitamin E was supplemented.[14] Supplementation may be beneficial in preventing gallstones, particularly in those who may not be able to eat a low-fat diet.

Dosage. Vitamin E (mixed tocopherols), 400 IU daily

Precautions. Adverse effects rarely occur but can include nausea, diarrhea, intestinal cramps, fatigue, weakness, headache, blurred vision, rash, and creatinuria.

Calcium

Similar to fiber, calcium works by binding secondary bile acids (deoxycholic acid and chenodeoxycholic acid) that reduce the solubility of cholesterol in the bile, thereby reducing the risk of cholesterol gallstones. Calcium binds these in the colon and promotes their excretion. A group of 860 middle-aged men were followed for 25 years; their risk of developing gallstones was inversely related to their calcium intake.[15]

Dosage. Calcium gluconate or citrate, 1000 to 1500 mg daily, with meals. Citrate is better absorbed in the elderly but costs more.

Precautions. Can cause gastrointestinal irritation and constipation. Decreases absorption of iron. Do not take iron supplements with calcium.

Lecithin (Phosphatidylcholine)

Lecithin is a phospholipid composed of phosphatidyl esters, one of which is phosphatidylcholine. Similar to bile salts, a low lecithin level in the body may be a causative factor in gallstone formation. Lecithin and bile salts reduce the saturation of cholesterol in the bile, which leads to stone formation. Studies have shown that oral supplementation with lecithin results in higher concentrations in the bile.[16] Unfortunately, studies have not shown that lecithin supplementation alone has a significant effect on gallstone dissolution. But it may be beneficial in prevention.

Dosage. Lecithin, 500 to 1000 mg daily.

Precautions. Diarrhea, nausea, and abdominal pain or fullness.

Liver or Gallbladder Flush

A popular remedy for gallstones among the lay population is the gallbladder flush. This may involve a number of different recipes, many of which include olive oil. A common one consists of drinking 1 cup of olive oil with the juice of two lemons each morning for 5 days. This remedy has led to stories of large gallstones being passed. However, what is thought to be gallstones is actually a soft saponified complex of minerals, olive oil, and lemon juice produced in the intestines.[17] Although the monounsaturated fat in olive oil may stimulate the gallbladder to contract and expel small stones, caution should be used in recommending a flush for someone with large stones that could become lodged in the common duct, resulting in acute cholecystitis. It would be best to avoid a gallbladder flush until an ultrasound scan is performed to document the size and severity of gallstone formation.

BOTANICALS

For treating multiple small stones or sludge within the gallbladder in someone who is asymptomatic or has mild intermittent discomfort, a combination of botanicals that both stimulate bile flow and increase bile solubility, while also working to reduce stone size, would be advantageous. Choleretic herbs help to perform the former, and peppermint oil has been found to help with gallstone dissolution.[18]

For clinical application, pick one of the choleretic herbs listed here and combine it with peppermint oil. Some herbologists mix a number of choleretics together in a tea.

Choleretic Herbs (Stimulate Bile Production and Flow)

Milk Thistle (*Silybum marianum*)

Dosage. Use a product standardized to 70% silymarin extract. Start at 150 mg twice a day, increasing to three times a day if needed.

Precautions. May have a laxative effect. Those who are allergic to plants in the Asteraceae/Compositae family (ragweed, daisies, marigolds) should be cautious about using milk thistle.

Dandelion (*Taraxacum officinale*)

Dosage. 4 to 10 g of the dried leaf, or 2 to 8 g of the dried root three times a day. Tea is prepared by steeping the same amount of the leaf or root in 150 mL of boiling water for 5 to 10 minutes and then straining. Drink 1 cup of tea three times a day. Probably the most convenient dosing is a 1:5 tincture, 5 to 10 mL three times daily.

Precautions. May lead to gastric hyperacidity. Can cause contact dermatitis topically. Like milk thistle, it can cause an allergic reaction in those with allergies to plants in the Asteraceae/Compositae family (e.g., ragweed, daisies, marigolds). Can cause hypoglycemic effects.

Artichoke (*Cynara scolymus*)

Dosage. 1 to 4 g of the leaf, stem, or root three times daily. Do not confuse with Jerusalem artichoke.

Precautions. Potential allergic reactions, including contact dermatitis if exposed topically. As with previous herb, may cause allergy in those allergic to plants in the Asteraceae/Compositae family (e.g., ragweed, daisies, marigolds).

Botanical to Enhance Gallstone Dissolution

Peppermint Oil (*Mentha piperita*)

Peppermint has a large menthol component; menthol is a volatile oil used to help dissolve gallstones.[19, 20] This effect is slow and does not work well for large stones. However, it should be considered for minimal disease with small stones.

Dosage. Enteric-coated capsules, 1 to 2 (0.2 mL/capsule) three times daily between meals

Precautions. Relaxes lower esophageal sphincter, resulting in gastroesophageal reflux and heartburn. This is the reason for the enteric-coated capsules that release the oil into the small intestine, thereby avoiding adverse effects. Peppermint can also cause allergic reaction, flushing, and headache.

PHARMACEUTICALS

Bile salt therapy reduces biliary cholesterol saturation and subsequently helps gallstones to dissolve slowly. This therapy is most successful in patients with small cholesterol stones and normally functioning gallbladders. It does not work for calcified stones. This therapy (like the botanical therapy described earlier) should be reserved for patients with mildly symptomatic gallstones who are poor surgical candidates or wish to avoid surgery. Bile acid therapy may also be warranted for those who are at high risk of forming gallstones, such as those who have rapid weight loss after surgical therapy for obesity or prolonged parenteral nutrition. Bile salt therapy may reduce gallstone formation by more than 80% in these special circumstances. If measures are not taken to reduce the risk of gallstones, a high rate of recurrence follows bile salt therapy.

Ursodiol–Ursodeoxycholic Acid (Actigall)

Dosage. 300 mg twice a day with meals. Some give a single dose at bedtime with good results.

Precautions. Dose-related elevations of hepatic enzymes (aspartate transaminase, alanine transaminase); less than 5% develop diarrhea.

> ### NOTE
> *Unless lifestyle and nutrition changes are made, all therapies except for surgical removal are associated with a high (>50%) 5-year recurrence rate of stone formation.*

SURGERY

Laparoscopic Cholecystectomy

This is the treatment of choice for symptomatic stones with gallbladder wall inflammation. The procedure can be done with a minimal hospital stay but does involve general anesthetic and is not without risk. This therapy avoids the high recurrence rate associated with other therapies.

Extracorporeal Shock Wave Lithotripsy

A successful therapy for renal stones, extracorporeal shock wave lithotripsy (ESWL) has not gained acceptance for gallstones. Although it can be effective for solitary stones, the risks of biliary colic and acute pancreatitis from fragments of pulverized stones and recurrence of stones make this therapy less appealing than laparoscopic cholecystectomy. No gallstone lithotripsy device has been approved for general use in the United States.

THERAPIES TO CONSIDER

Percutaneous Solvent Dissolution Therapy

Cholesterol gallstones can be dissolved rapidly (within hours) with organic solvents. Methyl *tert*-butyl ether or ethyl propionate can be directly instilled into the gallbladder via a percutaneous transhepatic approach. The procedure has a high success rate with few adverse effects, but it has not caught on because it is invasive and labor intensive.

THERAPEUTIC REVIEW

Therapy can be divided into two main sections—prevention and therapy.

Prevention

Lifestyle: Encourage weight management with a regular exercise regimen.
Nutrition:
- Drink 6 to 8 cups of water a day.
- Encourage a low saturated fat diet (decrease red meat, dairy, and fried foods).

THERAPEUTIC REVIEW continued

- Replace saturated fats with polyunsaturated ones rich in omega-3 fatty acids (cold water fish, flaxseed products, walnuts).
- Encourage a high-fiber diet rich in fruits and vegetables. with a goal of 6 to 8 servings a day.
- Consider supplementing with oat bran cereal each morning or psyllium (Metamucil), 1 tbsp in 8 oz water one or two times a day.
- Avoid refined sugars and legumes (beans).

Supplements:
- Vitamin C, 200 mg twice daily
- Vitamin E (mixed tocopherols), 400 IU a day. This is fat soluble, so take with meals to improve absorption.
- Calcium, 1000 to 1500 mg a day
- Lecithin, 500 to 1000 mg a day

NOTE

If the patient has severe recurring symptoms or elevation of liver enzymes, white blood cells, or amylase, immediate surgical referral is indicated.

Therapy for asymptomatic stones or mild periodic symptoms with documented small stones or sludge. Liver function (alkaline phosphatase, aspartate transaminase, alanine transaminase) normal.

Along with the above therapy, consider adding:

Nutrition: Consider an elimination diet to rule out food allergy as a possible trigger of symptoms. (See Chapter 82, The Elimination Diet and Diagnosing Food Hypersensitivities)

Botanicals: Consider one of the following choloretic herbs:
- Milk thistle *(Silybum marianum)* standardized to 70% silymarin extract. Start at 150 mg twice daily and increase to three times a day if needed.
- Dandelion *(Taraxacum officinale)* 1:5 tincture, 5 to 10 mL three times a day
- Artichoke *(Cynara scolymus),* 1 to 4 g of leaf, stem, or root three times a day
- Gallstone-dissolving herb: Peppermint oil *(Mentha piperita),* 1 to 2 enteric-coated capsules three times a day between meals

Pharmaceuticals: Ursodiol (Actigall), 300 mg twice daily with meals
- For patients with recurring symptoms, evidence of obstruction with elevated liver function tests (alkaline phosphatase, alanine transaminase, aspartate transaminase), or acute cholecystitis with thickening of the gallbladder wall on ultrasound scan, refer to surgeon for further evaluation and treatment.

Surgery: Laparoscopic cholecystectomy
- Patients with evidence of a common duct stone with obstruction (alkaline phosphatase, aspartate transaminase, alanine transaminase, amylase, bilirubin, and dilation of common duct on ultrasound) and acute right upper quadrant pain and possibly jaundice may need endoscopic retrograde cholangiopancreatography for stone removal and, if not successful, surgical exploration for retrieval.

References

1. Leitzmann MF, Rimm EB, Willett WC, et al: Recreational physical activity and the risk of cholecystectomy in women. N Engl J Med 9:341:777–784, 1999.
2. Nair P, Mayberry JF: Vegetarianism, dietary fiber and gastro-intestinal disease. Dig Dis 12:177–185, 1994.
3. Berr F, Holl J, Jungst D, et al: Dietary N-3 polyunsaturated fatty acids decrease biliary cholesterol saturation in gallstone disease. Hepatology 16:960–967, 1992.
4. Levy R, Herzberg GR: Effects of dietary fish oil and corn oil on bile flow and composition in rats. Nutr Res 15:85–98, 1995.
5. Trowell H, Burkitt D, Heaton K: Dietary Fibre, Fibre-Depleted Foods and Disease. New York, Academic Press, 1985, pp 630–632.
6. Moerman CJ, Smeets FWM, Kromhout D: Dietary risk factors for clinically diagnosed gallstones in middle-aged men. A 25-year follow-up study (The Zutphen Study). Ann Epidemiol 4:248–254, 1994.
7. Leitzmann MF, Willett WC, Rimm EB, et al: A prospective study of coffee consumption and the risk of symptomatic gallstone disease in men. JAMA 282:2212–2213, 1999.
8. Douglas BR, Jansen JB, Tham RT, et al: Coffee stimulation of

cholecystokinin release and gallbladder contraction in humans. Am J Clin Nutr 52:553–556, 1990.

9. Breneman JC: Allergy elimination diet as the most effective gallbladder diet. Ann Allergy 26:83–87, 1968.

10. Simon JA: Ascorbic acid and cholesterol gallstones. Med Hypotheses 40:81–84, 1993.

11. Jenkins SA: Biliary lipids, bile acids and gallstone formation in hypovitaminotic C guinepigs. Br J Nutr 40:317–322, 1978.

12. Simon JA, Grady D, Snabes MC, et al: Ascorbic acid supplement use and the prevalence of gallbladder disease. Heart & Estrogen-Progestin Replacement Study (HERS) Research Group. J Clin Epidemiol 51:257–265, 1998.

13. Dam H, et al: Acta Physiol Scand 36:329, 1956.

14. Christensen F, et al: Alimentary production of gallstones in hamsters. Acta Physiol Scand 27:315, 1952.

15. Moerman CJ, Smeets FWM, Kromhout D: Dietary risk factors for clinically diagnosed gallstones in middle-aged men. A 25-year follow-up study (The Zutphen Study). Ann Epidemiol 4:248–254, 1994.

16. Tuzhilin SA, Drieling DA, Narodetskaja RV, Lukash LK: The treatment of patients with gallstones by lecithin. Am J Gastroenterol 65:231, 1976.

17. Pizzorno JE, Murray MT: Gallstones. In Textbook of Natural Medicine. Edinburgh, Churchill-Livingstone, 1999, p 1245.

18. Holtz S: Nat Med 2(January):6–19, 1999.

19. Bell GD, Doran J: Gallstone dissolution in man using an essential oil preparation. BMJ 278:24, 1979.

20. Ellis WR, Bell GD: Treatment of biliary duct stones with a terpene preparation. BMJ 282:611, 1981.

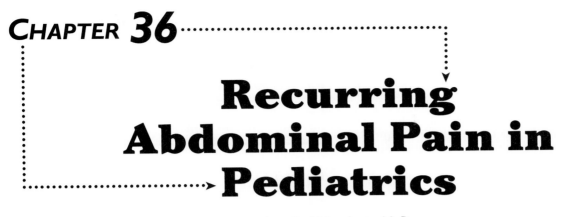

CHAPTER 36

Recurring Abdominal Pain in Pediatrics

Joy A. Weydert, M.D.

PATHOPHYSIOLOGY

Recurrent abdominal pain (RAP) in children was first defined by Apley and Naish in 1958 as at least three episodes, over a 3-month period, of pain severe enough to interfere with normal activities. RAP is one of the most common reasons for seeking medical attention.[1] It affects approximately 10% to 15% of all school-aged children and is responsible for 2% to 4% of all pediatric outpatient visits.[2] Less than 10% of those with RAP are ever found to have an organic cause for pain; however, substantial morbidity and healthcare costs are associated with this disorder. Children with RAP, on average, miss 26 days per year of school compared with only 5 days among nonpain children,[3] and RAP students have a much higher incidence of anxiety and mood disorders subsequently.[4] Parents, teachers, and physicians frequently reinforce pain behavior by providing rest periods during pain episodes, allowing absences from school, or providing medications. The etiology and pathogenesis of this disorder are unknown, but the prevailing viewpoint is that it is multidimensional, requiring a biopsychosocial approach to its understanding.

One hypothesis is that symptoms arise from changes in the "brain-gut axis," which links the neuroendocrine, immune, and enteric nervous systems with the cognitive and emotional centers of the brain. The bidirectional communications of the distal systems with the central nervous system (CNS) lead to feedback and modification by the higher cortical centers.[5] Alterations in gut wall sensory receptors, modulation of sensory transmission along the peripheral systems and the CNS, cortical perceptions, and pain memories contribute to visceral hyperalgesia.[6] Figure 36–1 presents a model for the pathogenesis of visceral hyperalgesia and the clinical expression of chronic pain.[7]

A second hypothesis states that disturbances in gastrointestinal motility, possibly triggered by physical or mental stress, may contribute to abdominal pain. Although some correlation has been seen for this, data show that patients undergoing manometry

testing have normal results despite symptoms of severe pain, or abnormal results while they are pain free.[8] Because no specific motility disturbance has been identified, studies suggest that rather than having a baseline dysmotility disorder, these

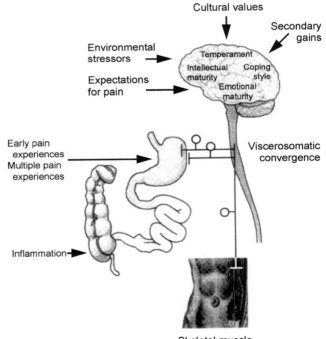

Figure 36–1. Pathogenesis of visceral hyperalgesia and clinical expression of chronic pain. Primary hyperalgesia develops when sensory neurons with cell bodies in dorsal root ganglia are recruited and sensitized after early and/or multiple pain experiences. Secondary hyperalgesia occurs when biochemical changes in pathways from the spinal cord to the cerebral cortex result in increased pain perception. Viscerosomatic convergence refers to somatic and visceral afferent nerves terminating on the same spinal interneurons, so that the affected individual is unable to define a discrete location on the body. Psychological and developmental factors (within the brain) and psychosocial factors (*arrows pointing to the brain*) alter clinical expression of pain. (From Hyams JS, Hyman PE: Recurrent abdominal pain and the biopsychosocial model of medical practice. J Pediatr 133:473–477, 1998).

patients may have an abnormal gastrointestinal motor response to a variety of stimuli such as meals, cholecystokinin, stress, or abdominal distention.

A third hypothesis is related to the behavioral profile and genetic vulnerability of the patient. Some of these children exhibit anxiety, mild depression, withdrawal, and low self-esteem. It has been postulated that this behavior pattern is frequently fostered within a family structure characterized by parental depression, enmeshment, overprotectiveness, rigidity, and lack of conflict resolution; how the disorder is experienced and addressed may be influenced by this type of environment.[9]

Children with RAP may demonstrate one of three known classical presentations, awareness of which may help guide choice of therapies.

1. Isolated paroxysmal abdominal pain (functional abdominal pain) is usually periumbilical, variable in severity and duration, and rarely associated with meals, activity, or bowel habits. There may be associated autonomic symptoms (e.g., nausea, dizziness, headache, pallor, fatigue).
2. Nonulcer dyspepsia (functional dyspepsia) is characterized by pain localized to the epigastrium or either upper abdominal quadrant. Ulcer-type pain, early satiety, nausea, vomiting, indigestion, belching, bloating, or oral regurgitation may be present. In addition, there is a temporal relationship of pain to meals.
3. Abdominal pain associated with altered bowel patterns (irritable bowel syndrome) includes pain localized to the lower abdomen that may be relieved with defecation, onset of pain associated with change in frequency of stool or form of stool, a feeling of straining or urgency, incomplete passage of stool, bloating, or abdominal distention. Diarrhea may alternate with constipation accompanied by passage of mucus.

Serious organic disease can be ruled out by a thorough history and physical examination and basic laboratory investigations. Pertinent negatives in this evaluation include the following:

1. There is no family history of inflammatory bowel disease, ulcer disease, or significant psychosocial disorder.
2. Pain does not wake the child from sleep.
3. There is no weight loss or growth delay.
4. There is no blood in the stool or bile-stained emesis.
5. The history and physical examination are entirely normal, with no fevers, rashes, joint involvement, or perianal disease.
6. The complete blood count (CBC), urinalysis, sedimentation rate, and stool test for occult blood are normal.

If a positive history is indicated, one may have to consider further testing (e.g., serology for *Helicobacter pylori*, serum transaminases, amylase, lipase, stool for pathogens, and endoscopy).

NOTE

Rather than a diagnosis of exclusion, RAP should be presented as a positive diagnosis identified as the most common cause of chronic abdominal pain in children. Parents can be further reassured that serious disease is unlikely if the history and physical examination are normal.

LIFESTYLE

Diet

If certain foods seem to exacerbate pain, they should be avoided. If symptoms are suggestive or if there is a family history of lactose intolerance, a 2- to 4-week trial of exclusion of all dairy products (e.g., milk, cheese, yogurt, ice cream) should be initiated. If there are no changes after 2 weeks, dairy products can be resumed. If some improvement is noted, dairy foods can be slowly reintroduced in small quantities as tolerated. Intake of highly processed foods should be reduced, especially of those with refined carbohydrates (e.g., snacks, candy, cookies), because the fermentation of these sugars in these foods increases gas production. Also, the elimination of caffeine in the diet and of products containing sorbitol (found in sugar-free gum or bottled fruit juices) or high-fructose corn syrup (frequently found in sweetened beverages) should be encouraged. Again, these sugars are frequently hard to digest and may lead to gas, bloating, and diarrhea.

Fiber

After 10 g of insoluble fiber is added to the diet, studies have shown a reduction of pain episodes in some children and complete resolution in others with RAP.[10] This can be accomplished by increasing the quantities of fruits, vegetables, legumes, and whole grains in the diet. Fruits and vegetables have 1 to 4 g of fiber per serving, whereas legumes have 3 to 6 g per serving. Whole wheat bread or bran muffins have approximately 2 g of fiber compared with white bread or bagels, which have less than 1 g. Breakfast cereals can also be a good source of fiber, especially those made with bran. If a child has difficulty getting adequate fiber through the diet, psyllium powder, 1 teaspoon (2 g of drug) in 8 oz of cool water or juice, may be given up to three times a day. An increase in water intake is strongly recommended, along with the increased fiber, to prevent constipation.

NOTE

Age of the child + 5 = Recommended minimum daily grams of fiber. More fiber can be added as needed.

Behavior Modification

Reinforcing pain behavior is often done unknowingly but with good intent toward the child. Families should be helped to recognize that special attention or treatment in response to pain episodes (e.g., staying home from school, dismissal from chores or responsibilities, having one-on-one attention from a parent) may foster ongoing pain behavior and diminish the child's self-reliance. School attendance should be encouraged as well as completion of personal responsibilities. Physicians can also facilitate return to a normal lifestyle by offering a thorough explanation of the diagnosis and pathophysiology, reassurance, and options for management and adaptation to the disorder.

BIOCHEMICAL THERAPY

Botanicals

Chamomile

The active ingredients in chamomile include the volatile oils alpha-bisabolol and bisabolol oxide and the flavonoids apigenin, luteolin, and quercetin. Bisabolol has effects in the gastrointestinal tract receptors, causing relaxation of the smooth muscle. Apigenin works on the CNS benzodiazepine receptors with antianxiolytic effects similar to those of Valium and Xanax but without the sedative effects.[11, 12] Chamomile can be given as a tea, as an extract, or by capsule in standardized preparations. Glyceride extracts of chamomile can be found for use in children to offset any concerns of preparations extracted with alcohol. One study done in infants with colic used an herbal tea preparation that included chamomile. This preparation was found to be effective in reducing colic episodes.[13] Currently, a research protocol is in progress at the University of Arizona to study the effects of chamomile on children with RAP.

Dosage. Adults (estimated at 150 lb), 3 g 3 to 5 times per day. Child (estimated at 75 lb), 1.5 g 3 to 5 times per day. Child (estimated at 35 lb), 0.75 g 3 to 5 times per day.

One heaping teaspoon of chamomile flowers steeped in hot water yields approximately 3 g. The extracts may come in 1-g/1 mL dilution, or 1-g/4 mL dilution. Use the following dosing as a guide:

Dosage Guideline. 1:1 Dilution/1:4 Dilution

150 lb: 15 to 30 drops three to five times/day, 2 tsp 3 to 5 times/day

75 lb: 8 to 15 drops three to five times/day, 1 tsp 3 to 5 times/day

35 lb: 4 to 8 drops three to five times/day, ½ tsp 3 to 5 times/day

Precaution. Chamomile is generally safe; however, anyone allergic to ragweed, asters, or chrysanthemums should take with caution. Chamomile is a member of the daisy family and has contributed to allergic reactions in rare cases.

Peppermint

Analysis of peppermint oil typically shows more than 40 different compounds; however, the principal components are menthol, methone, and methyl acetate. The pharmacology focuses almost entirely on its menthol component, which has carminative effects (elimination of intestinal gas), antispasmodic effects, and choleretic effects (bile flow stimulant). The mechanism of action is thought to be inhibition of smooth muscle contractions achieved through blockage of calcium channels.[14] Many studies have been conducted using peppermint oil as a treatment for irritable bowel syndrome (IBS), including one study in children.[15] Even though it did not alter the associated symptoms of IBS, such as urgency of stool, stool patterns, or belching, it did reduce the pain. Peppermint is most widely used as a tea. Because of its calcium channel blockage effects, it may cause relaxation of the lower esophageal sphincter (LES) and lead to an increase in heartburn symptoms for some. An enteric-coated capsule is available for use in the treatment of IBS. Because of its delayed release in the small intestine, there is little effect on the LES and it is less likely to cause heartburn.

Dosage. Tea—1 to 2 teaspoons of dried leaves in 8 oz of water as needed.

Capsules (187 mg)—Two capsules three times daily for adults and children who weigh more than 100 lb. One capsule three times daily for children 60 to 100 lb.

Precaution. Peppermint is generally regarded as safe; however, hypersensitivity reactions have been reported.

Ginger

Ginger contains many volatile oils (sesquesterpenes) and aromatic ketones (gingerols); the latter are thought to be more pharmacologically active. Historically, ginger has been used as far back as the 4th century BC for stomachaches, nausea, and diarrhea. It also has been used as a carminative, appetite stimulant, and choleretic. Interestingly, ginger can simultaneously improve gastric motility while exerting antispasmodic effects.[16] Studies have shown that ginger's antispasmodic effects on the visceral smooth muscle are likely due to antagonism of serotonin receptor sites. One study using a double-blind, randomized, crossover design found that the use of ginger brought about a significant reduction in nausea and vomiting among women with hyperemesis gravidarum.[17] Because of its safety profile, it is regularly used in pregnancy with no untoward fetal effects.

Dosage. Adult (estimated at 150 lb)—1 to 2 g dry powdered gingerroot per day (10 g fresh).

Children (estimated at 75 lb)—0.5 to 1 g dry powdered gingerroot per day (5 g fresh).

Children (estimated at 35 lb)—0.25 to 0.5 g dry powdered gingerroot per day (2.5 g fresh).

A one-quarter-inch slice of fresh gingerroot is approximately 10 g. This is equivalent to 1 to 2 g of a dry powder ginger that is a more concentrated form found in capsules. The fresh ginger can be brewed as a tea, sweetened with honey, or chopped and added to foods, soups, or salads. A general rule of thumb for estimating the amount of fresh ginger to use in children is to use the child's "pinky" (fifth finger) as the guide for the amount of ginger to chop.

Pharmaceuticals

Despite a lack of controlled studies with established efficacy for many drugs used in functional bowel disorders, they continue to be prescribed. For those reasons, as well as the poor adverse effect profiles (metoclopromide—irritability, dystonic reactions; cisapride—arrhythmia, adverse outcomes in prolonged QT syndrome; anticholinergics—constipation, blurred vision, tachycardia, sedation; tricyclic antidepressants—sedation, agitation, acute mental disturbance, reduction in seizure threshold), these particular drugs cannot be safely recommended for use in children.

H₂-Receptor Antagonists/Proton Pump Inhibitors

For patients with dyspepsia as their primary symptom, these drugs can be used if other strategies are unsuccessful. Few studies have been undertaken in children to support such therapy, but they may be beneficial and are relatively safe over the short term (6 to 8 wk).

Dosage. Cimetidine (Tagamet)—10 mg/kg/dose given four times daily. Comes in 100 mg OTC; 200-, 300-, 400-, 800-mg tablets and 300 mg/5-mL suspension.

Ranitidine (Zantac)—2 to 4 mg/kg/dose given twice daily. Comes in 75 mg OTC; 150 and 300 mg and 75 mg/5-mL suspension; also, 150-mg granules.

Famotidine (Pepcid)—1 to 1.2 mg/kg/day divided two or three times a day. Comes in 10 mg OTC; 20- or 40-mg tablets, and 40 mg/5-mL suspension.

*Omeprazole (Prilosec)—0.7 to 3.3 mg/kg/day daily or divided twice daily. Comes in 10-, 20-, and 40-mg capsules.

*Lansoprazole (Prevacid)—0.75 mg/kg daily. Is available in 15- and 30-mg capsules.

Adverse Effects. Headaches, diarrhea, abdominal

pain, and elevated liver function tests have been reported.

MIND–BODY THERAPY

Because of our knowledge of the brain-gut axis and associated interactions, it is only logical that mind–body therapy be used in RAP. Studies published primarily in the psychiatric journals have supported the efficacy of interventions that teach stress management, progressive muscle relaxation, or coping behaviors, or that use cognitive-behavioral therapy.[18, 19] One study showed that significant pain reduction occurred when biofeedback, cognitive-behavioral therapy, and/or parental support was added to fiber therapy as multimodal therapy for RAP.[20]

Progressive Muscle Relaxation

This technique is a way for children to learn to feel the difference between tense and relaxed muscles and to use this as a way to cope with abdominal pain. Progressive relaxation reduces the anxiety associated with pain, demonstrating the mind–body phenomenon and the patient's capacity for self-regulation. The benefit to this approach is that it is easily taught, especially to school-aged children, and can be used anywhere. Scripts can be given to parents to use, or a tape can be made or purchased for home use.

(See PMR Script in Chapter 91, Prescribing Relaxation Techniques.)

Biofeedback

This technique is a form of relaxation that uses physiologic feedback instruments to reinforce behavior. As relaxation occurs, warmth can be brought to the fingertips, increasing the distal temperature. This temperature can be monitored by sensors placed on the fingers and the positive behavior of relaxation as the temperature rises can be reinforced. Biofeedback may be beneficial for a patient who is somewhat skeptical about the ability to control body functions with the mind. Someone trained in biofeedback who has the equipment readily available can best teach this.

Hypnosis

Hypnosis is a state of focused attention whereby the mind is receptive to suggestion. The technique has been used successfully for all types of pain syndromes and is easily used in children older than 4 years of age.

(See Chapter 89, Self-Hypnosis Techniques, for

---

*The pharmacist can dissolve these capsules in an 8.4% bicarbonate suspension with good stability and bioavailability for use in children unable to swallow pills.

method on abdominal pain under teaching self-hypnosis.)

Psychotherapy

In children or families with significant psychosocial dysfunction, counseling by a child psychiatrist or clinical psychologist may be the best therapy. Cognitive-behavioral family intervention therapy, which often includes teaching specific coping skills, social skills, and relaxation techniques, has been shown to be efficacious in studies done on children with RAP.[21]

THERAPEUTIC REVIEW

Once a child has been thoroughly evaluated and organic disease has been ruled out, any of the following therapies can be used in an age-appropriate manner.

- Diet: Avoid foods that have caffeine, sorbitol, and high-fructose corn syrup, or are a source of refined carbohydrate, as these are poorly digested. Recommend a 2- to 4-week trial off all dairy products if the history is suggestive of lactose intolerance. (Refer to Chapter 82, The Elimination Diet and Diagnosing Food Hypersensitivities.)
- Fiber: Increase fiber by at least 10 g per day through addition of fruits, vegetables, legumes, and whole grains. Administer psyllium, if needed, 1 tsp in cool water, one to three times a day. Increase intake of water as well as fiber.
- Behavior: Encourage attendance at school and other usual activities. Offer strategies to overcome the reinforcement of illness behavior at school and at home.
- Botanicals: *Chamomile*, 3 g three to five times per day (150 lb); 1.5 g three to five times per day (75 lb); 0.75 g three to five times per day (35 lb). *Peppermint tea*— 1 to 2 tsp dried leaves per 8 oz hot water as required. *Enteric-coated capsules* (187 mg) 2 capsules three times daily (>100 lb); 1 capsule three times a day (60 to 99 lb). *Ginger*, 10 g fresh (or 1 to 2 g dry powdered) per day (150 lbs); 5 g fresh (or 0.5 to 1 g dry powdered) per day (75 lb); 2.5 g fresh (or 0.25 to 0.5 g dry powdered) per day (35 lb).
- Pharmaceuticals: H_2-receptor antagonists or proton pump inhibitors for a maximum of 6 to 8 weeks if dyspepsia is the primary complaint. See text for dosing.
- Mind–body therapies: Progressive muscle relaxation (refer to Chapter 91, Prescribing Relaxation Techniques). Biofeedback and hypnosis are useful (refer to Chapter 89, Self-Hypnosis Techniques). Psychotherapy may also help.

References

1. Apley J, Naish N: Recurrent abdominal pains: A field survey of 1000 school children. Arch Dis Child 33:165–170, 1958.
2. Campo JV, DiLorenzo C, Chiappetta L, et al: Adult outcomes of pediatric recurrent abdominal pain: do they just grow out of it? Pediatrics 108:E1, 2001.
3. Stone RT, Barbero GJ: Recurrent abdominal pain in childhood. Pediatrics 45:732–738, 1970.
4. Hyams JS, Burke G, Davis PM, et al: Abdominal pain and irritable bowel syndrome in adolescents: A community based study. J Pediatr 129:220–226, 1996.
5. Mayer EA, Gebhart GF: Basic and clinical aspects of visceral hyperalgesia. Gastroenterology 107:271–293, 1994.
6. Drossman DA: Chronic functional abdominal pain. Am J Gastroenterol 91:2270–2281, 1996.
7. Hyams JS, Hyman PE: Recurrent abdominal pain and the biopsychosocial model of medical practice. J Pediatr 133:473–478, 1998.
8. Youssef NN, DiLorenzo C: The role of motility in functional abdominal disorders in children. Pediatr Ann 30:24–30, 2001.
9. Boyle JT: Recurrent abdominal pain: An update. Pediatr Rev 18:310–321, 1997.
10. Feldman W, McGrath P, Hodgeson C, et al: The use of dietary fiber in the management of simple, childhood, idiopathic, recurrent abdominal pain. Am J Dis Child 9:1216–1218, 1985.
11. Forster HB, Niklas H, Lutz S: Antispasmodic effects of some medicinal plants. Planta Med 40:309–319, 1980.
12. Viola H, Wasowski C, Levi De Stein M, et al: Apigenin, a component of *Matricaria recutita* flowers, is a central benzodiazepine receptor ligand with anxiolytic effects. Planta Med 61:213–216, 1995.
13. Weizman Z, Alkrinawi S, Goldfarb D, Bitran C: Efficacy of herbal tea preparation in infantile colic. J Pediatr 122:650–652, 1993.
14. Hills JM, Aaronson PI: The mechanism of action of peppermint oil in GI smooth muscle. Gastroenterology 101:55–65, 1991.
15. Kline RM, Kline JJ, DiPalma J, Barbero G: Enteric coated, pH dependent peppermint oil capsules for the treatment of irritable bowel syndrome in children. J Pediatr 138:125–128, 2001.
16. Murray MT: Healing Power of Herbs. Rocklin, Calif, Prima Publishing, 1995.
17. Fischer-Rasmussen W: Ginger treatment of hyperemesis gravidarum. Eur J Obstet Gynecol Reprod Biol 38:19–24, 1990.
18. Finney JW, Lemanek KL, Cataldo MF, et al: Pediatric psychology in primary health care: Brief targeted therapy for recurrent abdominal pain. Behav Ther 20:283–291, 1989.
19. Edwards MC, Finney JW, Bonner M: Matching treatment with recurrent abdominal pain symptoms: An evaluation of dietary fiber and relaxation treatment. Behav Ther 22:257–267, 1991.

20. Humphreys PA, Gevirtz RN: Treatment of recurrent abdominal pain: Components analysis of four treatment protocols. J Pediatr Gastroenterol Nutr 31:(1)47–51, 2000.
21. Sanders MR, Shepherd RW, Cleghorn G, Woolford H: The treatment of recurrent abdominal pain in children: A controlled comparison of cognitive-behavior family intervention and standard pediatric care. J Consult Clin Psychol 62:306–314, 1994.

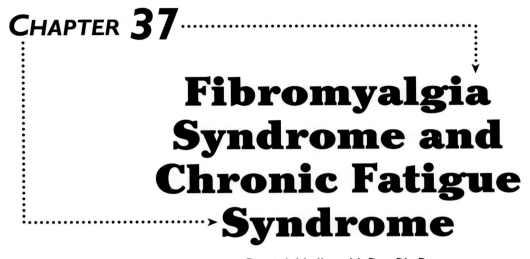

CHAPTER 37

Fibromyalgia Syndrome and Chronic Fatigue Syndrome

Daniel Muller, M.D., Ph.D.

PATHOPHYSIOLOGY

Diagnostic criteria for fibromyalgia syndrome (FMS) are twofold: (1) widespread pain and (2) tenderness in at least 11 of 18 defined points. Other characteristic signs and symptoms include nonrestorative sleep, chronic fatigue, stiffness, headache, migraine, irritable bowel syndrome, temporomandibular joint syndrome, and mood disorders.[1, 2] The degree to which psychological components contribute to pain sensitivity and symptom expression remains controversial. Some investigators have noted a high frequency of FMS patients with posttraumatic stress disorder (PTSD).[3] FMS often presents as a form of allodynia, in which normally painless stimuli are perceived as painful. Studies find little abnormality in the peripheral musculature but point to increased central nervous system (CNS) sensitivity to pain.

Chronic fatigue syndrome (CFS) is characterized by profound fatigue, often with myalgia, sleep disturbance, neurocognitive complaints, low-grade fever, nonexudative pharyngitis, and cervical or axillary adenopathy.[4] In practice there is extensive overlap of patients with the diagnosis of CFS and those with the diagnosis of FMS.[5] Minor physiologic differences between the two conditions are cited in the literature, but these differences may be due to study design and laboratory differences and may not reflect actual differences in pathophysiology. For practical purposes, however, the same approach to management is appropriate for both FMS and CFS.

FMS also can coexist with a variety of autoimmune diseases and often presents after a severe flulike syndrome, a defined infection (e.g., Lyme disease), or trauma. The increased prevalence in females may point to a hormonal influence. Cerebrospinal fluid levels of substance P are elevated, and additional abnormalities in the regulation of cortisol and in the adrenergic and serotonin systems have been noted. Antidepressant use is directed at raising CNS levels of serotonin and norepinephrine, as well as restoring sleep.

Hypothyroidism must be ruled out as a treatable cause of similar symptoms. However, a number of other, more minor alterations of the endocrine system are known to exist in FMS. Although these physiologic abnormalities, such as decreased levels of growth hormone and somatomedin, do not appear to be critical in the etiology of FMS, they may contribute to sustaining symptoms and increasing central pain sensitivity.

Alterations in the pituitary-adrenal axis in FMS appear to be quite different than are seen in clinical depression, which is somewhat surprising given the frequent concurrence of the two conditions.[6] The affinity and function of corticosteroid receptors on lymphocytes appear to be altered in FMS, which changes the cellular response when they are incubated with hormones in the laboratory.[7] There are reports of decreased numbers of T cells expressing activation markers and a deficiency of interleukin-2 release.[8] Although these immunologic changes in FMS do not meet criteria for an immunodeficiency or autoimmune disease, the lymphocyte abnormalities may reflect an altered response to hormone feedback, and altered patterns of cytokine release may contribute to fatigue and inflammatory-type symptoms.

INTEGRATIVE THERAPY

Exercise

Exercise helps to decrease the symptoms of FMS. However, overuse results in increased symptoms, often severe, and can lead to a cycle of muscle disuse. Patients may report feeling like they "ran a marathon" after only a few minutes of exercise. In one study, 9 of 16 subjects were worse or unchanged after a 14-week aerobic training intervention. However, the 3 subjects able to maintain a program of aerobic exercise no longer fulfilled criteria for FMS diagnosis 4 years later.[9] In a 21-week study of strength training, neck pain, fatigue, and depression decreased.[10] Warm water pool aerobic therapy may be helpful, particularly in severe cases.[11] The Arthritis Foundation has information on exercise programs (1-800-283-7800). Asian exercise disciplines such as tai chi and yoga can also be beneficial. A form of tai chi called the range of motion (ROM) dance is particularly suited to persons with disabilities (http://www.romdance.com; 1-800-488-4940).

Physical therapy can restore muscle balance, and local therapy with stretching, heat, and cold can be beneficial. Massage therapy has been shown to be more useful than transcutaneous nerve stimulation (TENS), but TENS was better than sham TENS and also may be helpful in some cases.[12] Treatment and exercises for all forms of soft tissue rheumatic pain are outlined in an excellent textbook.[13]

Mind–Body Therapy

Meditation

Meditation has been shown to be helpful in FMS.[14] This training increases the ability to be comfortable in the present, which can lessen the fear of future pain, and with practice can help the patient to transform the sensation of pain. Meditation is also useful for personal growth. I recommend training with a nondenominational teacher using a program such as "Mindfulness Meditation," pioneered by Dr. Jon Kabat-Zinn.[15] If no teacher is available, tapes can be helpful.

In one study, 10 of 15 subjects responded to a 14-week cognitive-behavioral and relaxation training intervention.[9] However, no patients remained improved on 4-year follow-up evaluation. Electromyographic biofeedback[16] and hypnotherapy[17] have been helpful in controlled studies. Biofeedback training can be useful in people who find difficulty with meditation.

Psychotherapeutic Interventions

Increasing disability should prompt examination of basic aspects of the patient's quality of life. A framework for such a review is the "Four Rs"[18]:

- Roles: The patient's ability to maintain self-esteem through normal roles as spouse, parent, provider, and so on may be impaired.
- Reactions: The emotional reaction to events such as the diagnosis of FMS often follows a grieving process as outlined by Kübler-Ross.[19] These stages are denial, anger, bargaining, depression, and acceptance. Patients are often stuck in anger and depression.
- Relationships: The patient may often face seemingly insurmountable problems at home or at work.

- Resources: Psychotherapy, ministers, community programs, and self-help groups may each become a key for altering this progressive decrease in ability to function; guided imagery is particularly useful.

Dr. John Sarno, a physiatrist at New York University, has written a book that some patients may find to be quite useful.[20] Dr. Sarno calls FMS and all chronic tendonitis-bursitis disorders "tension-myalgia syndromes." The short summary is that the patient may substitute physical pain for emotional pain. He believes that this simple realization can abrogate pain in certain persons. I have seen this happen in FMS, in multiple bursitis-tendinitis syndrome, and in chronic low back pain. My experience suggests that a certain level of self-awareness and acceptance of the power of the mind are required to create pain.

NOTE

Early and aggressive aerobic exercise, which can include tai chi, is an important key to decreasing the symptoms of FMS. A combination of exercise with "mindfulness meditation" affords the best chance of achieving a remission.

Nutrition

No specific diet has been shown to be effective. An anti-inflammatory diet may be helpful (see Chapter 84, Anti-Inflammatory Diet).

Chlorella

Chlorella pyrenoidosa (a fresh-water green alga) is a source of many nutrients, including protein, lipids, vitamins, and minerals. Preliminary studies in vitro and in animals have shown antitumor, immune-enhancing, and antiviral activities for chlorella. A double-blind, cross-over study has shown significant reduction in the number of FMS tender points after 3 months of supplementation.[21]

Dosage. 10 g or equivalent daily

Precautions. Chlorella contains iodine, and allergic reactions have been reported. As a significant source of vitamin K, Chlorella supplementation can antagonize the anticoagulant activity of coumadin.

Homeopathy

A placebo-controlled trial of a homeopathic treatment (R toxicodendron 6c) decreased tender points.[22] I recommend referral to a homeopathic physician for evaluation and treatment. Homeopathic remedies often will not work in the presence of pharmaceuticals.

Supplements

Calcium and magnesium

The effects of calcium and magnesium supplementation have not been studied adequately; nevertheless, in anecdotal reports, supplementation has been helpful.

Dosage. 1500 mg of calcium and 600 to 750 mg of magnesium daily; also add vitamin D 400 international units (IU) daily.

Antioxidants

Antioxidant vitamins may be helpful in FMS particularly to relieve muscle cramping. Vitamin E should be taken in a dose of 400 to 1600 (IU) daily and vitamin C in a dose of 500 mg twice per day. Selenium can be found in many foods including nuts; intake should be at least 100 μg daily but should not exceed 400 μg daily.

Other Supplements

A high-potency multivitamin with minerals and extra B vitamins is recommended.

S-Adenosylmethionine (SAMe) acts as a mild antidepressant and pain reliever and has shown moderate efficacy in FMS.[23] The recommended dose is 400 mg 2 to 3 times per day a half-hour before meals.

Omega-3 fatty acids have not been tested in FMS, but can have moderate analgesia-like activity. Omega-3 fatty acid intake can be increased by dietary means or through supplementation. Approximate doses for supplementation are eicosapentaenoic acid 30 mg/kg per day and docosahexaenoic acid 50 mg/kg per day. Gamma-linolenic acid (GLA) in a dose of 1.4 to 2.8 g per day, the equivalent of 6 to 11 g of borage oil daily, may have similar analgesic effects.

Botanicals

There are no adequate controlled trials of botanical treatments. In anecdotal reports; many treatments lead to a benefit that wanes with time, which may indicate a short-term placebo effect.

Sleep-Promoting Agents

The tricyclic antidepressants TCA are used to promote sleep, because they have been shown to be helpful in double-blind studies. Patients who would rather avoid TCAs can try St. John's wort, keeping in mind the multiple interactions with other drugs. Some patients prefer to promote sleep-using kava; they should be monitored for dermopathy and liver toxicity with chronic use. Higher doses of kava can be detrimental to driving and can potentiate the effects of alcohol and other sedating botanicals and drugs. Valerian is another possibility for promoting sleep; the patient should be warned about benzodiazepine withdrawal type symptoms after extended use. In rare cases, valerian causes hepatotoxicity. German chamomile is widely used as a tea and has mild sedative activity. Chamomile tea can be used when other botanicals are too sedating. Any of these also can be used for an anxiolytic effect.

Dosage
- St. John's wort: As extract standardized to 0.3% hypericin content, use 300 mg up to three times daily; or as tea, steep 2 to 4 g of the dried herb in 150 mL of boiling water for 5 to 10 minutes and strain; take 1 cup up to three times daily.
- Kava: As tea; simmer 2 to 4 g of root in 150 mL of boiling water for 5 to 10 minutes and strain; take 1 cup up to three times daily; or kava extract, 100 mg (70 mg of kava lactones) three times a day, or as dried root, 450 mg 1 or 2 capsules up to twice per day.
- Valerian: As tea, steep 2 to 3 g of root in 150 mL of boiling water for 5 to 10 minutes and strain; take 1 cup up to three times daily; or as a tincture, 1 to 3 mL 1 to three times daily, or as valerian extract, 400 to 900 mg 2 hours before bedtime.
- German chamomile: As tea, steep 3 g of dried flower heads in 150 mL of boiling water for 5 to 10 minutes and strain; take 1 cup up to three times daily; 2 to 8 g of dried flower heads can be taken three times daily.

Anti-inflammatory Agents

Ginger and turmeric (curcumin) have not been tested in FMS, but may exert some analgesic activity by inhibiting inflammatory prostaglandins.

Dosage
- Ginger: As dried root, 1 g two to three times per day to start: increase to up to 4 g daily; as tea, 1 g dried root steeped in 150 mL of boiling water for 5 to 10 minutes and strain; take 1 cup up to four times daily.
- Turmeric: As powdered root, 0.5 to 1 g two or three times daily.

Precautions. Ginger may stimulate increased bile flow and cause pain in the presence of cholelithiasis. Other risks include bleeding, hypertension or hypotension, and hypoglycemia. Tumeric-associated risks include bleeding, gastrointestinal intolerance, and impaired fertility.

Energy-Increasing Agents

Ginseng and gotu kola have not been tested properly in FMS or CFS but may provide some increased energy and support for the immune system. Ginseng products are used for 2 to 8 weeks and then discontinued for 2 weeks. There are three types of ginseng: Asian or panax ginseng (*Panax ginseng*), American ginseng (*Panax quinquefolius*), and Siberian ginseng (*Eleutherococcus Aconthopanax senticosus*). Asian ginseng and Siberian ginseng appear to have a more stimulating effect and may be more beneficial in treating fatigue. The German Commission E monographs state that ginseng root is helpful in counteracting weakness and fatigue, in restoring stamina, and in reversing impaired concentration. Ginseng is classified as an adaptogen, which is a term used to suggest that a substance can act to strengthen the body and increase general resistance.

Gotu kola (*Centella asiatica*) is often used in venous insufficiency and has also been used for fatigue.

Dosage
- Asian or panax ginseng (*Panax ginseng*): As powdered root, 0.6 to 3.0 g 1 to 3 times per day, A capsule extract comes in 100-, 250-, and 500-mg doses; average capsule dose: 200 to 600 mg.
- Siberian ginseng (*Eleutherococcus senticosus*): As powdered root, 0.6 to 3 g 1 to 3 times per day; As ethanolic extract, 0.5 to 6 mL 1 to 3 times per day. Note: The demand for this herb exceeds the supply, which invites products that may not have appropriate content. Recommend standardized extracts and state the content of eleutherosides, the active component. The higher the percentage the better.
- American ginseng (*Panax quinquefolius*): As powdered root, 0.6 to 3 g 1 to 3 times per day; as tea, 3 g of root steeped in 150 mL of boiling water for 5 to 10 minutes and strained; take 1 cup up to 3 times daily; as capsules, 200 to 600 mg per day.
- Gotu kola (*Centella asiatica*): As dried leaves, 600 mg 3 times per day; as tea; 600 mg of dried leaves steeped in 150 mL of boiling water for 5 to 10 minutes and strained; take 1 cup 3 times per day.

Precautions. Ginseng can cause insomnia, increase bleeding, and contribute to hypoglycemia. Gotu kola in large doses can increase cholesterol, elevate blood pressure, and cause photosensitivity, sedation, and abortion.

Pharmaceuticals

Antidepressants

Patients with a new diagnosis of FMS are usually started on treatment including a sedating TCA at night, often with an activating antidepressant in the morning, as well as low-level aerobic exercise and physical therapy. Selection and dosage of antidepressants are tailored to minimize side effects and to balance the fatigue and sleep problems for each patient. Therapeutic benefit is associated with improvements in sleep.[26, 27]

Initial drug therapy for FMS is a low dose of a sedating TCA, usually amitriptyline (Elavil) 5 to 10 mg, 1 hour before bedtime. The dose is titrated upward every 5 to 14 days as tolerated, using the minimal dose necessary to achieve restorative sleep. Excessive sedation can be an adverse effect of TCAs; therefore, an agent such as sertraline (Zoloft) 25 mg in the morning, or another of the more activating antidepressants such as fluoxetine (Prozac), can be added. Other, less sedating TCAs, such as nontriptyline, can be substituted for amitriptyline in the evening. Doxepin (Sinequan), a non-TCA antidepressant, can be particularly useful in liquid form to titrate at low doses, 2 to 5 mg, for sedation at night. Trazodone hydrochloride (Desyrel) 25 to 300 mg also can be helpful for promoting sleep. Cyclobenzaprine (Flexeril) 2.5 to 40 mg in divided doses has muscle relaxant and sedative effects. The practitioner should develop a familiarity with several different antidepressants in order to feel comfortable managing the myriad side effects.

Nonsteroidal Anti-inflammatory Drugs

Nonsteroidal anti-inflammatory drugs (NSAIDs) had a poor showing in a controlled trial testing their analgesic efficiency in fibromyalgia.[28] It may be better to try supplements or botanicals such as omega-3 fatty acids, gamma-linolenic acid (GLA), higher doses of vitamin E, ginger, or tumeric for their moderate analgesic effects.

Tramadol

One controlled trial showed a beneficial effect of tramadol (Ultram) 50 to 400 mg given in divided doses[29]; however, use of tramadol with antidepressants can cause serotonin syndrome. Tramadol can also cause excessive sedation. Tramadol may be useful in allowing a 4-week drug holiday from antidepressant therapy, to reset neural receptors, and in intermittent therapy for exacerbations. In general, I avoid the chronic use of benzodiazepines and narcotics.

NOTE

Often FMS can coexist with diagnosable autoimmune diseases such as rheumatoid arthritis or systemic lupus erthrythematosus. Identification of such disorder as the cause of pain is important to avoid treating the FMS with escalating doses of immunosuppressive medications.

Acupuncture

One high-quality trial of electroacupuncture showed almost complete remission in 20%, satisfactory benefit in 40%, and no effects in 40% of patients with FMS in a short-term study.[24] A review of several trials concluded that benefits were reduced with time.[25]

Soft Tissue Injection

The use of subcutaneous tender point injections may be helpful, particularly if they are given into palpable areas of muscle spasm. These injections are often given as 0.5 to 1 mL of 1% lidocaine per site, although dry needling or saline may work as well. The use of corticosteroids for injection should be avoided.

Surgery

There are no surgical treatments for FMS.[30] Chiari malformations and cervical stenosis can cause symptoms that can mimic FMS. However, FMS does not cause defined neurologic changes. A neurologic examination by a primary care physician can rule out neurologic abnormalities. If mild abnormalities are found, referral to a neurologist, not a neurosurgeon, is recommended.

Other Therapies to Consider

There have not been good studies on the roles of traditional Chinese medicine or Ayurvedic, homeopathic, or spiritual medicine in the management of FMS or CFS. I counsel my patients to learn about several different modalities and then record in a journal their feelings about these modalities. Then, after discussion, the patient can visit a practitioner of the selected therapy to explore the approach further. If the economic burden is not too great, addition of the therapeutic modality may be in order.

 ── *THERAPEUTIC REVIEW* ───────────────────

There is no documented "cure" for FMS. Studies have reported an improvement in 5% to 53% of patients, although 47% to 100% continue to meet criteria for FMS 2 to 5 years after diagnosis.[5, 31] Only a small minority of patients experience complete resolution of symptoms. In my practice about 75% of patients report "some" relief of symptoms with treatment. Better response to treatment is seen in patients of younger age and in those with continued employment, supportive families, and an absence of litigation and of affective disorders.[5, 32]

Lifestyle Interventions

I have observed a few remissions following complete self re-evaluation and transformation of the patient's previous life style. These changes often involved several of the following:

- *Taking up practice of an Asian discipline including movement and meditation (meditation with yoga, Qi gong, or tai chi, or an intensive aerobic exercise program).*
- *Changes in relationships at home and at work that promote taking control of the patient's life (paradoxically, part of having more control is also "letting go").*
- *Psychotherapy to investigate and change ingrained habits that maintain adverse relationships.*
- *Using treatments from complementary and alternative medicine such as acupuncture, massage, and even spiritual therapies to help the patient overcome particular problems.*
- *Spending a significant portion of time helping others perceived as more needy than the patient, usually on a voluntary basis.*

Exercise

Muscle strengthening and stretching can be invaluable to maintaining function. Physical therapy can be used initially for instruction; the "ROM dance" form of tai chi can be helpful. Warm water pool aerobics is sometimes the only tolerable exercise. As much exercise as can be tolerated should be encouraged.

THERAPEUTIC REVIEW   *continued*

Mind-Body Modalities

The practice of meditation, particularly mindfulness meditation, is highly recommended. However, a strong daily commitment of time devoted to scrutiny of body, mind, and spirit is required. Also recommended are biofeedback, relaxation exercises, and other methods to cope with stress. Tai chi and yoga training also may include a meditative component. Psychotherapy, especially guided visualization, can be helpful. I suggest that all patients read *The Mind-Body Prescription* by Dr. John Sarno.[20]

Removal of Exacerbating Factors

Eliminate consumption of coffee, smoking, and alcohol. Aggravating factors include improper body mechanics at work or play, structural features such as flat feet, and anxiety and depression. Patients, families, and appropriate personnel in the workplace must be involved in identifying goals and limitations.

Nutrition

No specific diet has been shown to be effective. An anti-inflammatory diet may be helpful (see Chapter 84). *Chlorella pyrenoidosa*, freshwater green alga, 10 g daily, can be used for a 3-month trial.

Supplements

- *Vitamin E 400 to 1600 IU daily*
- *Vitamin C 500 mg twice per day*
- *Selenium intake as nuts or supplements: at least 100 μg daily; not to exceed 400 μg daily*
- *Calcium 1.5 g daily; magnesium 600 to 750 mg daily*
- *A vitamin D supplement 400 IU per day*
- *A high-potency multivitamin with minerals and extra B vitamins*

Botanicals

Botanical sedatives can be used to promote sleep or treat anxiety.

- *St. John's wort 300 mg up to 3 times daily*
- *Kava: as dried root, 450 mg 1 or 2 capsules up to twice per day*
- *Valerian: as extract, 400 to 900 mg 2 hours before bedtime*
- *German chamomile: as tea, steep 3 g of dried flower heads in 150 ml boiling water for 5 to 10 minutes and strain; take 1 cup up to 3 times daily*

Ginger and tumeric (curcumin) may show some analgesic effects.

- *Ginger: As dried root, 1 g 2 to 3 times per day to start, increased up to 4 g daily*
- *Turmeric: As powdered root, 0.5 to 1 g 2 to 3 times daily*

Ginseng and gotu kola may provide some increased energy.

- *Siberian ginseng: As powdered root, 0.6 to 3 g 1 to 3 times per day, or ethanolic extract, 0.5 to 6 mL 1 to 3 times a day; use for 2 to 8 weeks, then abstain for 2 weeks*
- *Gotu kola: As dried leaves, 600 mg 3 times per day; as tea, 600 mg dried leaves steeped in 150 mL of boiling water for 5 to 10 minutes and strain; take 1 cup 3 times per day*

Pharmaceuticals

Therapeutic benefit is associated with improvements in sleep. Use low doses of a sedating antidepressant such as amitriptyline (Elavil) or nortriptyline 5 to 10 mg, 1 hour before bedtime, titrated upward every 5 to 14 days as tolerated. Trazodone 25 to 300 mg can also be used. For excessive sedation, add sertraline (Zoloft) 25 mg or fluoxetine (Prozac) in the morning. Cyclobenzaprine (Flexeril), 2.5 to 40 mg in divided doses, has muscle relaxant and sedative effects.

I avoid the chronic use of benzodiazapines and narcotics.

Acupuncture

A trial is worthwhile because at least short-term effects can be seen in as many as 60% of patients.

THERAPEUTIC REVIEW continued

Soft Tissue Injection

The use of subcutaneous tender point injections may be helpful, particularly if injections are given into palpable areas of muscle spasm. Use 0.5 to 1 mL of 1% lidocaine per site; steroids should be avoided.

Caution. Studies have not been done on the possible additive effects of ginger, tumeric, vitamin E, and an NSAID for increased risk of hemorrhage. Other commonly used supplements or botanicals such as ginkgo may add further risk. Particular care must be used in patients receiving other antiplatelet agents or coumadin. Mixing multiple sedating botanicals and pharmaceuticals must be avoided.

References

1. Yunus M, Masai A, Calabro J, et al: Primary fibromyalgia (fibrositis): Clinical study of 50 patients with matched normal controls. Semin Arthritis Rheum 11:151–171, 1981.
2. Wolfe F, Smythe H, Yunus M, et al: The American College of Rheumatology 1990 criteria for the classification of fibromyalgia. Arthritis Rheum 33:160–172, 1990.
3. Amir M, Kaplan Z, Neumann L, et al: Posttraumatic stress disorder, tenderness, and fibromyalgia. J Psychosomat Res 42:607–613, 1997.
4. Fukuda K, Struas SE, Hickie I, et al: The chronic fatigue syndrome: A comprehensive approach to its definition and study. Ann Intern Med 121:953, 1994.
5. Buchwald D: Fibromyalgia and chronic fatigue syndrome. Similarities and differences. Rheum Dis Clin North Am 22:219–243, 1996.
6. Hudson J, Pope H: The relationship between fibromyalgia and major depressive disorder. Rheum Dis Clin North Am 22:285–303, 1996.
7. Lentjes E, Griep E. Boersma J, et al: Glucocorticoid receptors, fibromyalgia and low back pain. Psychoneuroendocrinol 22:603–614, 1997.
8. Hader N, Rimon D, Kinarty A, Lahat N: Altered interleukin-2 secretion in patients with primary fibromyalgia syndrome. Arthritis Rheum 34:866–872, 1991.
9. Wiger SH, Stiles TC, Vogel PA: Effects of aerobic exercise versus stress management treatment in fibromyalgia. Scand J Rheum 25:77–86, 1996.
10. Hakkinen A, Hakkinen K, Hannonen P, Alen M: Strength training-induced adaptations in neuromuscular function of premenopausal women with fibromyalgia: Comparisons with healthy women. Ann Rheum Dis 60:21–26, 2001.
11. Jentoft ES, Kvalvik AG, Mengshoel AM: Effects of pool-based and land-based aerobic exercise on women with fibromyalgia/chronic widespread muscle pain. Arth Care Res 45:42–47, 2001.
12. Sunshine W, Field TM, Quintino O, et al: Fibromyalgia benefits from massage therapy and transcutaneous electrical stimulation. J Clin Rheumatol 2:18–22, 1996.
13. Sheon RP, Moskowitz RW, Goldberg VM: Soft Tissue Rheumatic Pain: Recognition, Management, and Prevention, 3rd ed. Baltimore, Williams & Wilkins, 1996.
14. Kaplan KH, Goldenberg DL, Galvin-Nadeau M: The impact of a meditation-based stress reduction program on fibromyalgia. Gen Hosp Psych 15:284–289, 1993.
15. Kabat-Zinn J: Full Catastrophe Living: Using the Wisdom of Your Body and Mind to Face Stress, Pain, Illness. New York, Bantam Doubleday Dell, 1990.
16. Ferraccioli G, Ghirelli L, Scita F, et al: EMG-biofeedback training in fibromyalgia syndrome. J Rheumatol 14:820–825, 1987.
17. Haanen HCM, Hoenderos HTW, van Romunde LKJ, et al: Controlled trial of hypnotherapy in the treatment of refractory fibromyalgia. J Rheumatol 18:72–75, 1991.
18. Neustadt DH: Commentary. Psychosocial factors in rheumatic disease. Orthop Rev 13:114–115, 1984.
19. Kübler-Ross E. On Death and Dying. New York, Macmillan Publishing, 1969.
20. Sarno JE: The Mind-Body Prescription. New York, Warner Books, 1998.
21. Merchant RE, Carmack CA, Wise CM: Nutritional supplementation with Chlorella pyrenoidosa for patients with fibromyalgia syndrome: A pilot study. Phytother Res 14:167–173, 2000.
22. Fisher P, Greenwood A, Huskisson EC, et al: Effect of homeopathic treatment on fibrositis (primary fibromyalgia). BMJ 299:365–366, 1989.
23. Jacobsen S, Danneskiold-Samose B, Anderson RB: Oral S-adenosylmethionine in primary fibromyalgia. Double-blind clinical evaluation. Scand J Rheumatol 20:294–302, 1991.
24. Deluze C, Bosia L, Zirbs A, et al: Electroacupuncture in fibromyalgia: Results of a controlled trial. BMJ 305:1249–1252, 1992.
25. Berman BM, Ezzo J, Handhazy V, Swyers JP: Is acupuncture effective in the treatment of fibromyalgia? J Fam Pract 48:213–218, 1999.
26. Simms R: Fibromyalgia syndrome: Current concepts in pathophysiology, clinical features, and management. Arthritis Care Res 9:315–328, 1996.
27. McCain G: A cost-effective approach to the diagnosis and treatment of fibromyalgia. Rheum Dis Clin North Am 22:323–349, 1996.
28. Goldenberg D, Felson D, Dinerman H: A randomized, controlled trial of amitriptyline and naproxen in the treatment of patients with fibromyalgia. Arthritis Rheum 29:655–659, 1986.
29. Russell IJ, Kamin M, Bennett RM, et al: Efficacy of tramadol in treatment of pain in fibromyalgia. J Clin Rheumatol 6:250–257, 2000.
30. Horstman J: Chiari surgery. Arthritis Today Sep-Oct: 78–82, 2000.
31. Yunus M, Bennett R, Romano, et al: Fibromyalgia consensus report: Additional comments. J Clin Rheum 3:324–349, 1997.
32. Turk DC, Okifuji A, Sinclair JD, Starz T: Pain, disability, and physical functioning in subgroups of patients with fibromyalgia. J Rheumatol 23:1255–1262, 1996.

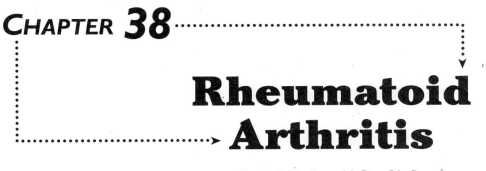

CHAPTER 38

Rheumatoid Arthritis

Daniel Muller, M.D., Ph.D.

PATHOPHYSIOLOGY

Rheumatoid arthritis (RA) is probably caused by a pathologic immune response in a genetically predisposed person to an environmental insult, typically a viral or bacterial infection.[1] Epidemiologic studies show that genes encoding the class II major histocompatibility antigens are linked to clinical features of RA. The HLADR4 and DR1 proteins present foreign and self-antigens to T cells. These molecules are presumed to play a direct role in the etiology of this autoimmune disease by presenting an "arthritogenic" viral or bacterial antigen to T cells. However, no organism has been definitively linked to the etiology of RA. The use of antibiotics is controversial, and antibiotics may have direct anti-inflammatory effects rather than acting through antibacterial activity. Other genes of the immune, endocrine, and neural systems may contribute to the pathogenesis of RA. The precise pathophysiologic cascade is not yet defined. RA is an autoimmune inflammatory disease in which immunosuppressive drugs constitute the mainstay of therapy. Certain cytokines, such as tumor necrosis factor (TNF) and interleukin-1 (IL-1), appear to play important roles, as inhibitors of these molecules decrease disease activity.[2]

Nonsteroidal anti-inflammatory drugs (NSAIDs) act to inhibit the enzymes that produce inflammatory prostaglandins, particularly thromboxanes and leukotrienes. The newer NSAIDs celecoxib (Celebrex) and rofecoxib (Vioxx) preferentially inhibit the cyclo-oxygenase-2 (COX-2) enzyme that produces these inflammatory molecules. Omega-3 fatty acids and certain botanicals such as ginger and turmeric also may act through decreasing the production or activity of inflammatory prostaglandins.

The neural, endocrine, and immune systems all share communication molecules that interact extensively. Molecules from the hypothalamic-pituitary-adrenal axis, particularly cortisol and corticotropin-releasing factor (CRF), and from the sympathetic-adrenal-medullary system are linked to disease activity in RA.[3] Corticosteroid drugs have powerful disease-suppressing activity, with equally powerful side effects such as osteoporosis. Prolactin and the estrogenic and androgenic sex hormones have been postulated to play roles as well. Other environmental factors such as nutrition, coffee, and tobacco also may contribute to the increased risk of RA.

Stress and psychological factors have been linked to the etiology of RA and to disease exacerbations.[4] In one study, psychological factors and depression accounted for at least 20% of disability in patients with RA, greater than the 14% attributable to articular signs and symptoms.[5] In another study, helplessness had a direct effect on disease activity.[6]

INTEGRATIVE THERAPY

Exercise

Joint pain can inhibit activity, leading to muscle disuse and atrophy. In turn, muscle atrophy can lead to decreased stability of joints. Light weight training can maintain or even increase muscle strength around joints, leading to increased joint stability. Stretching muscles can help to decrease flexion contractures. Aerobic exercise improves mood, decreases fatigue, and helps to control weight gain. Water exercise can be helpful as it is less stressful on joints, but weight training and walking work better to decrease bone loss (osteoporosis). The Arthritis Foundation has information on programs (1-800-283-7800). Asian exercise disciplines such as tai chi and yoga can also be beneficial. A form of tai chi called the range of motion (ROM) dance is particularly suited to persons with disabilities (http://www.romdance.com; 1-800-488-4940).

Physical Therapy and Occupational Therapy

Good physical therapy and occupational therapy programs can be invaluable in the treatment of RA. Goals are to improve range of motion and strengthen muscles. Joint protection from deformities can be aided by education and use of splints, orthotics, ambulatory aids, and other devices. Massage and local heat and cold applications can decrease inflammation, increase circulation, and relax muscles.

Mind-Body Therapy

Self-help courses given through the Arthritis Foundation provide information about diseases and medication and can help in developing coping skills. Simply writing in a journal about positive and negative emotions for 15 minutes a day can be powerful medicine, relieving symptoms by 25% or more[7] (see Chapter 95, Journaling for Health).

Meditation has been shown to be helpful for chronic pain.[8] A recent study of meditation in psoriasis, an autoimmune inflammatory skin disease, showed decreased time to clearing the skin disease.[9] There are no published studies investigating the role of meditation in RA. However, a study examining this question is underway (see Chapter 96, Recommending Meditation).

Nutrition

Food Triggers

Fasting clearly decreases symptoms in RA; however, symptoms rapidly recur with the resumption of food intake.[10] A small percentage of people with RA appear to have a food intolerance that exacerbates their disease. However, a much larger number believe that certain foods exacerbate symptoms, but this effect cannot be shown in blinded trials of food exposure. The offending foods are usually dairy products, wheat, citrus, or nuts. An elimination diet for 2 weeks with the reintroduction of the suspected food can be done with or without the supervision of a physician or a nutritionist (see Chapter 82, The Elimination Diet).

Omega-3 and Omega-9 Fatty Acids

Increased intake of omega-3 fatty acids from cold water fish, such as salmon, and from nuts, such as walnuts, flaxseed, or hempseed, can provide modest improvement in the control of RA. The role of unsaturated fatty acids in increasing symptoms is unproved; however, in view of their association with cardiovascular disease, reduction in intake is worthwhile (see Chapter 84, The Anti-inflammatory Diet).

Cooked vegetables and olive oil have been found to be independently protective for the development of RA. Omega-9 fatty acids in olive oil may confer anti-RA activity.[11]

Coffee

A high intake of coffee, 4 or more cups a day, has been linked to increased risk of RA.[12] Intake should be decreased to below this level, or the patient can switch to green tea, for the possible benefit from its antioxidant polyphenols.

Elimination of Tobacco Use

Smoking causes oxidant stress on connective tissue, as evident from the increased wrinkles seen in long-term smokers. One study has shown an association between smoking and increased risk of RA; therefore, RA patients should be counseled to avoid tobacco.[13]

Supplements

Essential Fatty Acids

Omega-3 fatty acids can be increased by dietary means or through supplementation. Approximate doses for supplementation are eicosapentaenoic acid 30 mg/kg per day and docosahexaenoic acid 50 mg/kg per day.[14]

Gamma-linolenic acid (GLA), 1.4 to 2.8 g per day, the equivalent of 6 to 11 g of borage oil daily, also has been shown to be helpful.[15] Effects may not be felt for 6 weeks or more, and continued improvement may occur after many months.

Antioxidants

Antioxidant vitamins may be helpful in RA, as they seem to be in osteoarthritis. Additionally, vitamin E has some analgesic effects.[16] Vitamin E should be taken at 1200 international units (IU) daily, and vitamin C at 500 mg twice per day. Selenium can be found in many foods including nuts; intake should be at least 100 μg daily, not to exceed 400 μg daily.

Recommended intake of calcium to prevent osteoporosis is 1500 mg daily. It is probably prudent to add magnesium at 600 to 750 mg daily and a vitamin D supplement at 400 IU per day.

Botanicals

Ginger

Ginger (*Zingiber officinale)* may have efficacy in RA by inhibiting inflammatory prostaglandins.[17]

Dosage. As the dried root, 1 g 2 to 3 times per day to start; increase up to 4 g daily. As a tea, 1 g of dried root steeped in 150 mL of boiling water for 5 to 10 minutes and strained; use 1 cup up to 4 times daily.

Precautions. The stimulation of increased bile flow can cause pain in the presence of cholelithiasis. Other risks include bleeding, hypertension or hypotension, and hypoglycemia.

Turmeric

Turmeric (curcumin) in an open trial has been shown to be similar to NSAIDs in efficacy.[18]

Dosage. As powdered root, 0.5 to 1 g 2 to 3 times daily.

Precautions. Risks include bleeding, gastrointestinal intolerance, and impaired fertility.

NOTE

Echinacea should be avoided by patients with rheumatoid arthritis, as there have been anecdotal reports of increased symptoms in persons with autoimmune disease.

Pharmaceuticals

Nonsteroidal Anti-inflammatory Drugs

NSAIDs can be used short term with minor risk of gastrointestinal toxicity. The long-term use of NSAIDs, particularly in the elderly, poses significant risks for gastrointestinal bleeding. There are many NSAIDs, and many of the newer ones are restricted on some formularies. The classic NSAIDs are ibuprofen (Motrin) used in a dose of 800 mg 3 times daily and naproxen (Naprosyn) in a dose of 500 mg twice daily. Both have antiplatelet activity. There are some advantages of using the COX-II inhibitors celecoxib and rofecoxib, as they have much less gastrointestinal toxicity. Additionally, they share a lack of antiplatelet effects with other newer NSAIDs. It should be kept in mind that these drugs also have the potential for renal toxicity and are no more effective than older NSAIDs.[19, 20] Recent data point to the possibility of increased thrombosis in patients taking COX II inhibitors who have a preexisting increased risk of thrombosis.[21] Celecoxib (Celebrex) is used in a dose of 200 mg twice daily; rofecoxib (Vioxx) is used in a dose of 25 to 50 mg once a day.

Corticosteroids

Corticosteroids can rapidly decrease RA symptoms, often within a few hours at high doses. However, both short-term and long-term toxic effects are well known. High and even moderate doses can lead to avascular necrosis of joints such as the hip, knee, or shoulder; luckily, this is a rare occurrence. With proper care and early diagnosis of avascular necrosis, disability and joint replacement may be avoided. With long-term use, osteoporosis is a significant risk with doses above 7.5 mg daily of prednisone or equivalent. Other risks include atherosclerosis, diabetes mellitus, cushingoid features, acne, and infection. Often a minor disease flare can be treated with a moderately high dose such as 30 to 40 mg of prednisone orally and a rapid taper over the course of 1 to 2 weeks. In some patients, some small dose of corticosteroids appears necessary for optional function;

prednisone 5 to 7.5 mg daily is often used for this purpose. A common method of treating a flare is to give a long-acting depot preparation such as triamcinolone acetonide (Kenalog) 80 mg intramuscularly. This approach can often control disease for 1 to 2 months, long enough for the slower acting disease-modifying antirheumatic drugs (DMARDs) to start working. For disease flares in isolated joints, once infection is ruled out, an intra-articular injection of triamcinolone (Kenalog) 2.5 to 40 mg can be given to control local disease.

NOTE

Remember: *A single joint with severely decreased range of motion and increased pain is presumed to be infected until proven otherwise. The patient should be hospitalized overnight for joint aspiration to obtain culture specimens; blood should also be drawn for cultures, followed by administration of intravenous antibiotics until results of culture are known.*

Antibiotics

Antibiotics, particularly minocycline (Minocin) in a twice-daily dose of 100 mg, may be useful in patients with less severe disease.[22] Side effects include gastrointestinal intolerance, dizziness, photosensitivity rash, vaginitis, skin and gingival discoloration, and rarely hepatic, lung, and kidney injury. The salutary effects of these agents may not be due to their antibacterial activity, because the tetracyclines also show immunomodulatory and anti-inflammatory activities.

Disease-Modifying Antirheumatic Drugs

Disease-modifying antirheumatic drugs (DMARDs) are also referred to as slow-acting antirheumatic drugs (SAARDs) because they usually take 6 weeks to 3 months to show activity.

Hydroxychloroquine and Sulfasalazine

Hydroxychloroquine (Plaquenil) and sulfasalazine (Azulfidine-EN) each are used early in disease when a diagnosis may not be clear or there is no characteristic erosive disease. Both drugs have little short-term and long-term toxicity.

Dosage. The current accepted dose of hydroxychloroquine (Plaquenil) is 200 mg twice daily, which carries little risk of toxicity; nevertheless, an ophthalmologic examination to test for retinal toxicity (see precautions) is recommended every 6 to 12 months. To reduce gastrointestinal intolerance, sulfasalazine is usually used in an enteric-coated form;

dosing is started at 500 mg a day and raised by 1 tablet every few days until a dose of 1 g twice daily is reached.

Precautions. Hydroxychloroquine when used in high doses carries a risk of retinal toxicity due to deposition of the drug into the retina. Sulfasalazine can uncommonly cause rash, hepatotoxicity, and leukopenia.

Methotrexate

Of all of the so-called DMARDs, methotrexate (Rheumatrex) has been shown to be tolerated for longer periods of treatment than any other drug.[23] Methotrexate is a folate antagonist and has a multitude of immunomodulatory activities, but its exact mechanism of action in RA is unknown. Doses of methotrexate for RA are usually between 5 and 25 mg given once a week. The dose is usually given orally in tablet form; however, the liquid form can be used orally and is sometimes less expensive. A common practice is to start with 7.5 mg orally once per week, although many practitioners recommend starting higher doses such 10 to 15 mg per week. With use of higher doses of 20 mg and above, patients are often taught to self-administer the dose subcutaneously once per week to avoid possible problems with gastrointestinal absorption. To decrease side effects, I always prescribe folic acid 1 to 2 mg to be taken each day. A decision to start methotrexate therapy or to raise or decrease the dose should be placed in the hands of a practitioner with extensive experience. Methotrexate is the standard by which all other drugs are judged, yet few patients achieve remission, and less than a majority achieve a 50% improvement on composite scores.

Contraindications to use of methotrexate include preexisting hepatic, renal, or pulmonary disease; unwillingness to discontinue alcohol; and recent malignancy. There are many side effects, the most prominent being hepatitis, bone marrow suppression, pneumonitis, mouth sores, nausea, and headache. A complete blood count, platelet count, and determination of aspartate transaminase, albumin, and creatinine levels are done initially and then every 2 weeks for 6 weeks after methotrexate therapy is begun. Thereafter, monitoring can be done every 4 to 8 weeks. A baseline hepatitis screen and chest radiography are recommended. Tuberculosis skin testing is reserved for patients with strong risk factors or abnormal appearance on chest x-ray film.

Other Immunosuppressive Drugs

Many other immunosuppressive drugs are used in RA. Leflunomide (Arava) is a newer drug that is similar in efficacy to methotrexate.[24] Leflunomide interferes with pyrimidine synthesis, whereas methotrexate interferes with purine synthesis. Leflunomide has fewer hepatotoxic effects and possibly little bone marrow toxicity but is much more likely to cause diarrhea. Azathioprine (Imuran) is metabolized to 6-mercaptopurine and interferes with inosinic acid synthesis. It is often is substituted for methotrexate; however, its use is associated with gastrointestinal and bone marrow toxicity. Other immunosuppressive drugs less commonly used are mycophenolate mofetil (CellCept), cyclosporine (Neoral), tacrolimus (Prograf), and chlorambucil (Leukeran). Cyclophosphamide (Cytoxan) is often used to treat rheumatoid vasculitis.

Recombinant Biologics

Recent advance in the therapy of RA targets cytokines, the communication molecules used in the immune system.[2] Etanercept (Enbrel) and infliximab (Remicade) are tumor necrosis factor (TNF) inhibitors. Etanercept is given subcutaneously twice per week, whereas infliximab is usually given intravenously once every 2 months. These drugs are most often used with a cytotoxic agent, usually methotrexate, to reduce the development of autoantibodies. Short-term safety is very high, with little toxicity. There are no data on long-term safety and efficacy. Use of these agents carries a risk of life-threatening exacerbations of severe infections, especially sepsis. These drugs may exacerbate demyelinating disorders; therefore, they should be avoided in patients with suspected or proven multiple sclerosis or optic neuritis. An interleukin-1 receptor antagonist, anakinra (Kineret), has recently been approved for the treatment of RA. It is given subcutaneously daily and also increases the risk of serious infection.

Acupuncture

A single small controlled trial of acupuncture in RA showed decreased knee pain for an average of 1 to 3 months.[25]

Surgery

Loss of joint function and intractable pain may be indications for surgical intervention. Synovectomy can be helpful when systemic therapy and intra-articular corticosteroids are ineffective. Joint replacement can help to restore function and to increase independent activity. Patients with RA have an increased risk of surgical and postoperative complications. Cervical spine disease can lead to spinal instability and risk of neurologic injury. Replacement of one joint can result in increased stress on other joints during recovery and rehabilitation. Long-term corticosteroid use can cause fragility of vessels and connective tissue.

Other Therapies to Consider

There have not been good studies on the role of traditional Chinese medicine or Ayurvedic, homeopathy, or spiritual therapies in the management of RA. Patients should learn about several different modalities and then record their feelings about these modalities in a journal. They may then choose to visit a practitioner of a selected modality for a trial of the techniques. If the economic burden is not too great, further exploration of that therapeutic modality may be in order.

THERAPEUTIC REVIEW

Evidence is accumulating that current allopathic treatments are successful in slowing joint destruction and in decreasing the mortality associated with RA.[23,26] In addition, the rates of extra-articular manifestations of RA, such as Felty's syndrome and rheumatoid vasculitis, seem to be decreasing. Therefore, in any but the mildest cases of RA, an integrated approach should include the so-called DMARDs, usually starting with methotrexate.

Exercise
Muscle strengthening and stretching can be invaluable for maintaining function. Physical therapy can be used initially for instruction; tai chi in the form of the ROM dance can be helpful.

Mind-Body Techniques
Meditation is highly recommended for RA patients willing to devote the daily time to looking more closely at the connection between body, mind, and spirit. Also recommended are relaxation exercises, and the development of methods to cope with stress. Tai chi and yoga also may include a meditative component to the training.
Journaling should be encouraged (see Chapter 93).

Removal of Exacerbating Factors
Use of coffee, tobacco, and alcohol should be eliminated. With suspected intolerance to dairy products, wheat, citrus, or nuts, a trial of an elimination diet for 2 weeks with the reintroduction of the suspected food can be undertaken.

Nutrition
A diet rich in omega-3 fatty acids is achieved by increasing intake of cold water fish or adding flaxseed meal or flaxseed oil. Olive oil should be increased in the diet as well. An anti-inflammatory diet is also recommended (see Chapter 84).

Supplements
Omega-3 fatty acids are recommended; doses for supplementation are eicosapentaenoic acid 30 mg/kg per day and docosahexaenoic acid 50 mg/kg per day, along with gamma-linolenic acid (GLA) 1.4 to 2.8 g per day, the equivalent of 6 to 11 g of borage oil daily.
Vitamin E should be taken in a dose of 1200 IU daily, and vitamin C in dose of 500 mg twice per day. Selenium intake as nuts or supplements should be at least 100 μg daily, not to exceed 400 μg daily. Recommended intake of calcium is 1.5 g daily; magnesium 600 to 750 mg daily and a vitamin D supplement of 400 IU per day are also recommended.

Botanicals
Start with ginger at 1 g 2 times a day to a maximum of 4 g daily. If no effect is seen after 6 to 8 weeks, turmeric 0.5 to 1 g 2 to 3 times daily can be tried.
Avoid echinacea.

Pharmaceuticals
NSAIDs are used as little as possible owing to gastrointestinal toxicity. The classic NSAIDs are ibuprofen (Motrin) 800 mg 3 times daily and naproxen (Naprosyn) 500 mg twice daily. The COX-2 inhibitors decrease but do not eliminate the risk of gastrointestinal bleeding. Celecoxib (Celebrex) is used at 200 mg twice daily; rofecoxib (Vioxx) is used at 25 to 50 mg once a day.
A majority of patients with RA are receiving combinations of drugs. Most patients are given methotrexate therapy unless there are contraindications or side effects. A common combination is methotrexate and hydroxychloroquine. Corticosteroids in moderately high doses with a rapid taper are often used for exacerbations. Commonly, a TNF inhibitor such as etanercept or infliximab is

added if methotrexate is only partially effective. Leflunomide or azathioprine is often substituted for methotrexate if there are intolerable side effects with methotrexate. Methotrexate and leflunomide can be used together with only a modest increase in risk of side effects. The DMARDs and the recombinant biologics have many varied side effects, some of which are only now being defined. The immunosuppressive pharmaceuticals should be used only with input from a subspecialist rheumatologist.

Acupuncture

Acupuncture can be tried for any patient with RA. This modality may be less effective in patients taking corticosteriods.

Surgery

Loss of joint function and intractable pain may be indications for surgical intervention. Synovectomy can be helpful when systemic therapy and intra-articular corticosteroids are ineffective. Joint replacement can help to restore function and to increase independent activity.

Caution: Studies have not been done on the possible additive effects of ginger, turmeric, vitamin E, and an NSAID for increased risk of hemorrhage. Other commonly used supplements or botanicals such as ginkgo may add further risk. Particular care must be used in patients taking other antiplatelet agents or warfarin sodium (Coumadin). In addition the interactions of supplements and botanicals on allopathic pharmaceuticals are not fully understood. All health care professionals involved in the patient's care must be aware of all therapies being used. The addition of any new treatment should prompt increased laboratory monitoring for patients receiving immunosuppressive pharmaceuticals.

References

1. Muller D: The molecular biology of autoimmunity. Immunol Allergy Clin North Am 16:659-682, 1996.
2. Choy EHS, Panayi GS: Cytokine pathways and inflammation in rheumatoid arthritis. N Engl J Med 344:907-916, 2001.
3. Straub RH, Cutolo M: Involvement of the hypothalamic-pituitary-adrenal/gonadal axis and the peripheral nervous system in rheumatoid arthritis. Arthritis Rheum 44:493-507, 2001.
4. Huyser B, Parker JC: Stress and rheumatoid arthritis: An integrated review. Arthritis Care Res 11:135-145, 1998.
5. Escalante A, Del Rincon I: How much disability in rheumatoid arthritis is explained by rheumatoid arthritis? Arthritis Rheum 42:1712-1721, 1999.
6. Parker JC, Smarr KL, Angelone EO, et al.: Psychological factors, immunologic activation, and disease activity in rheumatoid arthritis. Arthritis Care Res 5:196-201, 1992.
7. Smyth JM, Stone AA, Hurewitz A, Kaell A: Effects of writing about stressful experiences on symptom reduction in patients with asthma or rheumatoid arthritis. JAMA 281:1304-1309, 1999.
8. Kabat-Zinn J, Lipworth L, Burney R: The clinical use of mindfulness meditation for the self-regulation of chronic pain. J Behav Med 8:163-190, 1985.
9. Kabat-Zinn J, Wheeler W, Light T, et al.: Influence of a mindfulness meditation-based stress reduction intervention on rates of skin clearing in patients with moderate to severe psoriasis undergoing phototherapy (UVB) and photochemotherapy. Psychosom Med 60:625-632, 1998.
10. Henderson CJ, Panush RS: Diets, nutritional supplements, and nutritional therapies in rheumatic diseases. Rheum Dis Clin North Am 25:937-968, 1999.
11. Linos A, Kaklamani VG, Kaklamani E, et al.: Dietary factors in relation to rheumatoid arthritis: A role for olive oil and cooked vegetables? Am J Clin Nutr 70:1077-1082, 1999.
12. Heliovaara M, Aho K, Knekt P, et al.: Coffee consumption, rheumatoid factor, and the risk of rheumatoid arthritis. Ann Rheum Dis 59:631-635, 2000.
13. Hutchinson D, Shepstone L, Moots R, et al.: Heavy cigarette smoking is strongly associated with rheumatoid arthritis (RA), particularly in patients without a family history of RA. Ann Rheum Dis 60:223-227, 2001.
14. Mangge H, Herman J, Schauenstein K: Diet and rheumatoid arthritis—a review. Scand J Rheumatol 28:201-209, 1999.
15. Ernst E, Chrubasik S: Phyto-anti-inflammatories: A systemic review of randomized, placebo-controlled, double-blind trials. Rheum Dis Clin North Am 26:13-27, 2000.
16. Edmonds SE, Winyard PG, Guo R, et al.: Putative analgesic activity of repeated doses of vitamin E in the treatment of rheumatoid arthritis. Results of a placebo-controlled double-blind trial. Ann Rheum Dis 56:649-655, 1997.
17. Sirivastava KC, Mustafa T: Ginger (*Zingiber officinale*) and rheumatic disorders. Med Hypotheses 29:25-28, 1989.
18. Deodhar SD, Sethi R, Srimal RC: Preliminary studies on anti-rheumatic activity of curcumin (deferaloyl methane). Indian J Med Res 71:632-634, 1980.
19. Langman MJ, Jensen DM, Watson DJ, et al.: Adverse upper gastrointestinal effects of rofecoxib compared with NSAIDs. JAMA 282:1929-1933, 1999.
20. Silverstein FE, Faich G, Goldstein JL, et al.: Gastrointestinal toxicity with celecoxib vs. nonsteroidal anti-inflammatory drugs for osteoarthritis and rheumatoid arthritis: The CLASS study: A randomized controlled trial. JAMA 284:1247-1255, 2000.
21. Crofford LJ, Oates JC, McCune WJ, et al.: Thrombosis in patients with connective tissue diseases treated with specific cyclooxygenase 2 inhibitors; a report of four cases. Arthritis Rheum 43:1891-1896, 2000.
22. Alarcon GS: Minocycline for the treatment of rheumatoid arthritis. Rheum Dis Clin North Am 24:489-499, 1998.
23. Pincus T: Assessment of long-term outcomes of rheumatoid arthritis. Rheum Dis Clin North Am 21:619-654, 1995.
24. Breedveld FC, Dayer JM: Leflunomide: Mode of action in the treatment of rheumatoid arthritis. Ann Rheum Dis 59:841-849, 2000.
25. Man SC, Baragar FD: Preliminary clinical study of acupuncture in rheumatoid arthritis. J Rheumatol 1:126-129, 1974.
26. Krause D, Schleusser B, Herborn G, Rau R: Response to methotrexate treatment is associated with reduced mortality in patients with severe rheumatoid arthritis. Arthritis Rheum 43:14-21, 2000.

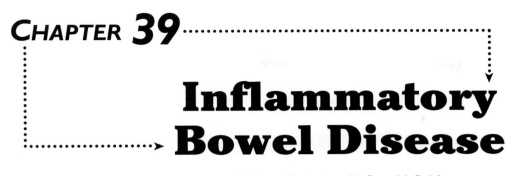

CHAPTER 39

Inflammatory Bowel Disease

Robert B. Lutz, M.D., M.P.H.

EPIDEMIOLOGY

The term *inflammatory bowel disease* (IBD) is used to describe two chronic relapsing and remitting diseases, ulcerative colitis (UC) and Crohn's disease (CD). There is growing recognition that these two conditions represent related polygenic diseases that are initiated by environmental factors.[1] Their prevalence is approximately 0.2%, with an incidence rate of 2 to 4 per 100,000.[2] They demonstrate ethnic, geographic, and socioeconomic variations, suggesting a multifactorial etiology. The peak incidence of occurrence is between the ages of 15 and 30 years, with a smaller peak noted in individuals between ages 60 and 80 years. UC demonstrates a male-to-female ratio of approximately 1:1, and CD demonstrates a female-to-male ratio of 1.1 to 1.8:1.[3]

PATHOPHYSIOLOGY

The gastrointestinal tract serves as a major barrier to antigens and exhibits a continuous level of controlled inflammation. An intact mucosal barrier and immune system, concurrent with appropriate genetic down-regulation, controls the amount of inflammation that exists. Genetic defects that prevent appropriate immune response down-regulation, in the presence of appropriate antigenic stimulation, lead to a cycle of increased inflammation, tissue damage, and tissue repair. Both arms of the immune system (cellular and humoral) are initiated by antigen exposure, possibly in differing fashion, leading to the development of UC or CD. A number of cellular products (cytokines, interleukins, and tumor necrosis factor [TNF]) interact with gut epithelium and vascular endothelium to initiate and amplify this immune response. Cell types, including macrophages, leukocytes, and lymphocytes, stimulate production of numerous nonspecific pro-inflammatory substances (eicosanoids, free radicals, and nitric oxide) that further aggravate the problem. Tissue repair may occur with quiescence of the inflammatory flare, mediated by growth factors, short-chain fatty acids, and other substances.[2, 4]

A precipitating infectious source has been sought without success. Animal models, supported by a growing body of clinical research, suggest that commensal gastrointestinal flora may, in part, be responsible for initiation and perpetuation of this inflammatory cascade. For example, treatment with antibiotics early in the course of disease may lead to improvement. This is less evident in advanced disease because prolonged inflammation may lead to bacterial resistance and a cascade of events that is perpetuated by other cross-reacting antigens.

NOTE

It is of interest that appendectomy, both in animal models and in humans, lessens the risk for colitis, suggesting a role for this lymphoid structure in modulating the immune response in genetically predisposed individuals.

INTEGRATIVE APPROACH

Nutrition

Nutritional interventions are of great significance in the management of IBD because individuals with these disorders commonly experience protein-energy malnutrition and deficiencies of vitamins, minerals, and trace elements. Malabsorption results in deficiencies of the fat-soluble vitamins (A, D, E, K), B vitamins, and calories. Malnutrition may occur from problems of absorption and exudative loss from inflamed mucosa, anorexia owing to symptoms, and the effects of conventional pharmaceuticals that may create increased demands for certain micronutrients resulting from effects on metabolism and absorption (e.g., corticosteroids and calcium and vitamin D metabolism, sulfasalazine, and folate malabsorption). Additionally, growing consideration is given to the role that certain foods may have in serving as antigens to aggravate the underlying inflammatory process.

Traditional nutritional interventions have included the replacement of micronutrients (e.g., B vitamins, protein) often through the use of parenteral and enteral formulas. Although effective in some situations (e.g., significant malnutrition, preoperative management, or when pharmaceutical intervention would be contraindicated, such as corticosteroids in growing children), the side effects, complications, and overall effectiveness make these less than optimal choices. Likewise, elemental diets (diets that contain all essential nutrients, with protein being provided only as predigested or free-form amino acids) have been noted to be effective, especially in CD, but relapse often occurs upon return to routine eating habits.

Adequate Protein Intake

General nutritional guidelines should begin with replacement of nutritional deficiencies of both micronutrients and macronutrients. Adequate caloric intake is essential, especially in individuals who weigh less than 90% of ideal body weight. Protein requirements are increased in IBD as a result of the catabolic effects of inflammation. A positive nitrogen balance can be achieved by providing 1 to 1.5 g/kg protein per day (e.g., $\frac{1}{2}$ cup firm tofu provides ~20 g protein), increasing to 2 g/kg/day in malnourished individuals.

Fiber

Regular use of dietary fiber should be encouraged. Although some fiber sources may be too "rough" for sensitive mucosa and gluten sensitivities may exist in many individuals with IBD, sources of unprocessed carbohydrate should be cautiously added to the diet. It is believed that fiber serves to normalize the intestinal microflora.

Food Irritants

An approach that has been advocated by the Functional Medicine Research Center has been referred to as the "4Rs": remove, replace, reinoculate, and repair. This framework has logical plausibility and has been reported by practitioners to be beneficial (Table 39–1) (see Chapter 104, Functional Medicine, for a functional medicine approach to IBD).

Individuals are encouraged to maintain a diary to identify potential food sensitivities or allergies.

Identification of these foodstuffs can be done by means of immunoglobulin G (IgG) and IgE food sensitivity panels or by having the individual follow an elimination diet (see Chapter 82, The Elimination Diet and Diagnosing Food Sensitivities). In addition, individuals will often have a list of aggravating foods they have identified (e.g., caffeine, refined sugar and sweets, dairy, corn, and gluten). Addressing these intolerances may be challenging because these foods

Table 39–1. The 4Rs (Remove, Replace, Reinoculate, Repair) Approach
....

1. Remove: This step emphasizes removal of pathogen microflora, allergens, and potential toxins. Pharmaceuticals (e.g. metronidazole [Flagyl] or ciprofloxacin) are used, either empirically or after appropriate identification of pathogenic microflora. Extended treatments are often called for, alternating antibiotics for up to 4 months. Elimination or oligoantigenic diets (use only foods known to have minimal allergenic potential) eliminate exposure to food irritants.
2. Replace: The focus is to provide nutritional factors that may be lacking or in insufficient quantities to promote normal digestive functioning. Gastrointestinal enzymes and hydrochloric acid are commonly supplemented. Laboratory analysis may be necessary for identification of deficiencies.
3. Reinoculate: The reintroduction of appropriate microflora into the gastrointestinal tract is achieved through the use of probiotic supplements and cultured and/or fermented foods. Recent clinical studies have documented the benefits of this step.[4]
4. Repair: The final step in this approach focuses on nutritional support of the gastrointestinal mucosa by providing materials necessary for structure and function. Antioxidants, B-vitamins, amino acids (cysteine, *N*-acetylcysteine, and glutamine), and glutathione are commonly provided. Also consider using gamma-linoleic acid (evening primrose oil; normal dosing is 500–1000 mg tid, but doses up to 4–6 g/day have been used in some situations), and sources of omega-3 fatty acids (cold water fishes, fish oil supplements as sources of EPA/DHA, or flaxseed 1 tbsp of oil or ground seed qd). Finally, butyric acid promotes growth of epithelium.

EPA/DHA, eicosapentaenoic acid/docosahexaenoic acid.

are often common in the Western diet and may not be readily apparent (e.g., corn oil in packaged goods). Difficulties also arise when eating away from home. Therefore, some advise "rotation diets" that regularly cycle families of foods, attempting to minimize the exposure to aggravating foods.

NOTE
Always consider the role of dietary practices in the cause and treatment of these disorders.

Other potential food irritants are fats and oils, and especially those with high concentrations of omega-6 fatty acids. It is thought that the development of the "Western diet," which is high in animal fats and omega-6 fatty acids and noted to be "pro-inflammatory," may contribute to the increasing rates of disease in industrialized nations. Conversely, the benefits of diets high in omega-3 fatty acids have been identified in individuals with IBD and are believed to be due to their anti-inflammatory effects. Animal models that have provided fats in the form of omega-3 fatty acids and monounsaturated fats have demonstrated decreased inflammation. Therefore, encouraging decreased consumption of pro-inflammatory fats while encouraging consumption of sources rich in this essential fatty acid (cold water fish and flaxseed) may be beneficial. In addition, dietary supplementation with a source of gamma-linoleic acid (evening primrose oil, borage oil) has been seen to decrease mucosal inflammation in animal models[5] (see Chapter 84, The Anti-Inflammatory Diet).

Supplements

Vitamins and Minerals

Supplementation with a multivitamin and multimineral complex is important. Individuals with IBD commonly experience malabsorption of many micronutrients, especially the fat-soluble and B vitamins. Supplementation with antioxidants is also recommended, although it is not readily apparent whether the low levels found in IBD are due to inadequate intake or to increased consumption by overworked antioxidant defenses. Zinc, copper, and manganese serve as cofactors for superoxide dismutase, and selenium functions as a cofactor for glutathione peroxidase. These are important elements of the antioxidant mechanism. Adequate calcium and vitamin D are necessary to prevent osteoporosis, a common finding in IBD.

Butyrate

A number of novel dietary interventions are being explored. Butyrate, a short-chain fatty acid, serves as a major source of energy for the cells of the colon. Deficiency states have been noted in patients with UC, and animal models that provide pectin (food source of butyrate) demonstrate decreased colonic inflammation. Preliminary trials with butyrate enemas have demonstrated effectiveness comparable with that of corticosteroids and mesalamine enemas in quieting active UC.

Glutamine

Glutamine (an amino acid) functions as a source of energy for the small intestine. During inflammation, demands are increased and supplementation improves functioning of the gastrointestinal mucosa. Theoretically, providing supplemental glutamine should serve to enhance the immune functioning of the gut.
Dosage. 7 g twice daily.
Precautions. No adverse effects are seen with doses up to 21 g/day.

Botanicals

Herbal treatments for IBD are directed toward modifying the inflammatory process and supporting mucosal healing. Their effects are gradual, and therefore, they may be best used for maintenance therapy.

Supportive literature is difficult to find for specific herbs in the treatment of IBD. Nonetheless, herbal therapies are reported to be among the most widely used CAM methods, with aloe and ginseng being the two most commonly cited.[6, 7] As such, the following herbs are of potential benefit, based upon their mechanism of action; research where available is noted.

A number of herbs used in traditional medical systems have anti-inflammatory properties. They are commonly viewed as being beneficial for rheumatic as well as gastrointestinal conditions. They function to inhibit the inflammatory cascade of eicosanoids and have recently been labeled *herbal COX-II inhibitors* because of their mechanism of action(s). Their actions on the gut may also be mediated by volatile oils that serve as antispasmodics.

Anti-Inflammatory Herbs

Ginger (*Zingiber officinale*). Aqueous extracts inhibit prostaglandin synthesis, including both cyclooxygenase and lipoxygenase pathways.
Dosages. Common dosing for this herb is 1 to 2 g/day of powdered ginger extract, taken in divided doses.
Turmeric (*Curcuma longa*). This herb is a common recommendation in Ayurvedic medicine. It treats inflammation as well as having hepatoprotective activity, immunostimulant properties, and antimicrobial and antiviral actions.
Dosages. Studies of inflammation have used doses of 1200 mg/day, divided three times a day.
Boswellia (*Boswellia serrata*). This herb is a relative of ginger. Preparations of the rhizome of this traditional Ayurvedic herb were given to patients with documented mild to moderate UC, in doses of 350 mg three times per day for 6 weeks. A control group received sulfasalazine (1 g three times a day). The treatment group had a somewhat greater improvement in monitored parameters and remission rates (82% vs. 75%).[8]
Dosages. 350 mg orally three times a day.

Demulcents

Some mucilaginous herbs function as demulcents (coat and soothe inflamed mucosal surfaces) and may promote mucosal healing.
Linseed (*Linum usitatissimum*). Commonly used as a bulk laxative, this herb contains fiber and mucilages.
Dosages. A common home remedy in Germany calls for soaking 30 to 50 g of crushed seeds for 30 minutes. These are combined with 10 parts water to 1 part seeds and consumed.
Marsh Mallow Root (*Althea officinalis*). This herb also has high concentrations of mucilages. It is commonly taken three times per day, as either a

capsule or a tincture. It may slow absorption of other medications.

Carminative Herbs

Carminative herbs help to relieve gas and spasm. Peppermint *(Mentha piperita)* is used for its volatile oils that relieve spasm and bloating (1 to 2 capsules containing 0.2 mL oil/capsule three times a day between meals). Chamomile *(Matricaria recutita or nobile)* has been approved by the German Commission E for gastrointestinal spasms and inflammatory diseases of the gastrointestinal tract. Teas of the flowers can be consumed three to four times per day.

Others

Aloe Vera. Aloe vera as been identified by Hilsden as one of the most common herbs used by patients with IBD.[6] This herb has traditional uses in both traditional Chinese medicine (TCM) and Ayurvedic practices, to clear constipation "due to fire" and as a general laxative. The soothing properties of the mucilaginous gel are well recognized. Animal studies have identified anti-inflammatory properties (human studies are lacking). The latex leaf lining, however, serves as a potent cathartic and is contraindicated in individuals with IBD.[10]

Robert's Formula. Naturopathic physicians have historically recommended Modified Robert's Formula for IBD, although no research exists to document its efficacy or actions. It contains a number of herbs (e.g., echinacea, goldenseal, slippery elm) that have various beneficial properties.[11] Capsules of this formulation may be obtained from Phytopharmica and dosed 2 capsules three times per day.

Mind–Body Therapy

The study of psychoneuroimmunology has led to a greater understanding of the role of the mind in modulating the effects of the immune system. Anecdotally, clinicians as well as patients have noted the association between emotional states and flare-ups of IBD. Unfortunately, to date, there are few studies demonstrating the effectiveness of mind-body techniques, such as visualization, hypnosis, relaxation, and meditation, on IBD management. Irrespective of this, the potential benefits for such therapies with minimal experienced side effects make mind-body interventions an important consideration for working with individuals.[12, 13] Normal functioning immune and gastrointestinal systems, stress release and coping skills, and relaxation and other related ideas are often used to assist individuals to gain greater understanding and insight about their disease and to help control symptoms (see Chapter 91, Relaxation Techniques).

> **NOTE**
>
> *Mind-body approaches that address identification of coping strategies for stressors are important considerations.*

Traditional Chinese Medicine

This healing system approaches individuals with IBD from a different conceptual framework than that of conventional Western medicine. Instead of focusing on the disease and its presentation, TCM looks at the whole person who is experiencing a constellation of symptoms and seeks to restore balance and harmony to the system. From this perspective, IBD is viewed as a problem of "dampness and heat" and therefore is treated by "clearing heat and transforming dampness." Herbal formulations are administered that serve to enhance digestive function (supplementing the spleen and fortifying the stomach). Specifically, the herbs used have immune modulating and anti-inflammatory properties. They may facilitate a lowering of conventional pharmaceutical dosing. Acupuncture enhances the effectiveness of herbal treatments.[14, 15]

Conventional Therapy

The goals of conventional therapy are to lessen the symptoms of active disease, lessen inflammation, support mucosal healing, and prevent recurrent inflammation. The complex nature of these disorders and their chronic nature have traditionally required coordination of efforts between gastroenterologists, primary care physicians, and surgeons. Pharmaceutical intervention and surgery are the primary available options. Surgery is necessary in more than 70% of individuals with CD within 20 years of diagnosis and in almost 25% of individuals with UC. Whereas surgical cure for UC may be experienced, this is unlikely in CD. In addition, postsurgical recurrence is exceedingly common in CD and often occurs in the original location of disease involvement.

Pharmaceuticals

A number of pharmaceutical agents are used to treat IBD, with choice based on patient characteristics (e.g., age, severity of symptoms, and responsiveness to initial therapy) and current disease status. The side effects of these agents are considerable.

The classes of medications include:

- 5-Aminosalicylates (e.g., sulfasalazine [Azulfidine], mesalamine [Pentasa])
- Antibiotics (e.g., metronidazole [Flagyl], ciprofloxacin)

- Corticosteroids (e.g., prednisone, budesonide CIR)
- Immunomodulators (e.g., 6-mercaptopurine, azathioprine [Imuran], methotrexate, cyclosporine)
- Biologic response modifiers/TNF-alpha blockers (e.g., infliximab [Remicade])

Treatment of UC often begins with oral or topical 5-aminosalicylic acid (5-ASA) derivatives (e.g., 4.8 g/day or oral dose) for proximal disease. Corticosteroids are used for moderate to severe disease or refractory situations. Azathioprine or 6-mercaptopurine (6-MP) is used if treatment is refractory to corticosteroids or steroid dependency is of concern. Maintenance therapy uses 5-ASA, 6-MP, or azathioprine.

Management of mild to moderate CD may involve treatment with a 5-ASA member, antibiotics (metronidazole or ciprofloxacin), corticosteroids, immunomodulators (azathioprine or 6-MP), or infliximab. More severe disease may require IV corticosteroids and/or infliximab with nutritional modification (e.g., parenteral nutrition). Maintenance therapy may include antibiotics, azathioprine or 6-MP, or infliximab.

A number of new agents are currently being studied, as are novel uses for pharmaceuticals used in other therapies. These include interleukin-10, interleukin-11, thalidomide, heparin, and nicotine. Clinical trials have demonstrated that the nicotine patch is effective for the treatment of patients with active UC. This treatment, however, does not demonstrate usefulness with maintenance therapy.[4]

Other Therapies to Consider

As identified by Hilsden and associates[6] and Rawsthorne and coworkers,[7] a number of additional CAM practices are being used by patients with IBD, not just for their underlying diagnosis. These include exercise, spirituality, manual medicine (massage, osteopathy, and chiropractic), and homeopathy. The effectiveness of these modalities for symptom control can be noted only anecdotally, a common complaint by critics of complementary and alternative medicine. Consistent with findings from other studies,[16] the use of CAM by patients with IBD often occurs because of side effects of medications and/or lack of effectiveness of conventional therapies. Important in these findings is a greater sense of control that occurs with CAM usage. Therefore, physicians who work with individuals who suffer from IBD should give consideration to the symptoms as well as the lived experiences of these individuals. Providing potentially nontoxic "alternatives" not only can improve symptoms but also serves to empower the individual and facilitate a path to healing.

THERAPEUTIC REVIEW

Nutrition
- *Carefully review a dietary history and encourage the maintenance of a dietary log.*
- *Address identified deficiencies with an emphasis on protein and calories, fat-soluble vitamins (especially vitamin D), and B vitamins (especially B12 and folic acid), minerals, and trace elements (iron, zinc, calcium).*
- *Explore regular use of dietary or supplemental fiber.*
- *Consider implementation of the 4Rs. Remove dietary irritants/sensitivities, possible infectious agents, and stressors. Replace identified deficiencies. Reinoculate with probiotics (see Chapter 97, Prescribing Probiotics). Promote mucosal repair with appropriate vitamin supplementation (B vitamins and antioxidants), essential fatty acids, glutamine, and butyric acid (see Table 39–1 for more details).*

Mind–Body Therapy
Living with a chronic and often debilitating disease creates great stress for individuals. Learning to live with an illness rather than fighting it is beneficial. Consider exploring one or more of the following with your patients:
- *Self-hypnosis, guided imagery, or visualization*
- *Relaxation and stress management practices*
- *Meditation or movement practices such as tai chi or yoga*

Botanical Medicine
A number of herbs in various classes can be considered for your patient. Remember that an adequate trial may take 8 to 12 weeks.
- *Inflammation: ginger (1 to 2 g three times a day), Boswellia (350 mg three times a day), and turmeric (400 mg three times a day)*
- *Bloating and intestinal spasm: peppermint (1 to 2 capsules three times a day between meals)*
- *Demulcents: marsh mallow root (2 to 5 g daily to three times a day)*

- *Consider Modified Robert's Formula because it contains many herbs that work by different mechanisms to decrease the symptoms of IBD. It can be obtained from Eclectic Institute (888-799-4372) under the brand name of Bastyr Formula B.*

Traditional Chinese Medicine

Evaluation by a licensed practitioner of TCM can serve to alleviate symptoms and lessen reliance on conventional pharmaceuticals having significant side effects.

Physical Activity

The benefits of physical activity are directed toward improvement of cardiorespiratory fitness and stress management. Encourage all individuals to achieve the Centers for Disease Control and Prevention's recommendations of 30 minutes of accumulated activity on most, preferably all, days of the week. Tailor recommendations for the individual, taking into consideration enjoyed activities, social support, and physical limitations.

Conventional Therapy

The goal of an integrated approach for management of IBD is to lessen reliance on pharmaceuticals with recognized significant side effects. Nonetheless, judicious use of these substances is often necessary. It is sometimes possible, and strongly encouraged, that individuals with early disease be initiated on a comprehensive program of alternative options before the use of some pharmaceuticals. This is more difficult with advanced disease and during flares.

Additional Considerations

Individuals with IBD use a number of other CAM options, to include manual medicine, homeopathy, energy medicine, and spiritual practices. These practices are used for disease symptoms as well as for other causes.[6, 7] Therefore, the use of CAM should be discussed with all individuals, and a partnership based on mutual understanding should be created.

References

1. Stotland BR, Stein RB, Lichtenstein GR: Advances in inflammatory bowel disease. Med Clin North Am 84:1107–1124, 2000.
2. Papadakis KA, Targan SR: Current theories on the causes of inflammatory bowel disease. Gastroenterol Clin North Am 28:283–296, 1999.
3. Andres PG, Friedman LS: Epidemiology and the natural course of inflammatory bowel disease. Gastroenterol Clin North Am 28:255–281, 1999.
4. Sands BE: Therapy of inflammatory bowel disease. Gastroenterology 118:S68–S82, 2000.
5. Bulger EM, Helton WS: General nutritional therapeutic issues: Nutrient antioxidants in gastrointestinal diseases. Gastroenterol Clin 27:403–409, 1998.
6. Hilsden RJ, Scott CM, Verhoef MJ: Complementary medicine use by patients with inflammatory bowel disease. Am J Gastroenterol 93:697–701, 1998.
7. Rawsthorne P, Shanahan F, Cronin NC, et al: An international survey of the use and attitudes regarding alternative medicine by patients with inflammatory bowel disease. Am J Gastroenterol 94:1298–1303, 1999.
8. Parihar GI, Malhotra A, Singh P, et al: Effects of *Boswellia serrata* gum resin in patients with ulcerative colitis. Eur J Med Res 2(1):37–43, 1997.
10. Kemper K, Chiou V: Aloe vera. http://www.mcp.edu/herbal. Accessed 1999.
11. Murray MT: Natural approach to inflammatory bowel disease. Am J Nat Med 4(6):8–19, 1997.
12. Anton PA: Stress and mind-body impact on the course of inflammatory bowel diseases. Semin Gastrointest Dis 10:14–19, 1999.
13. Schafer DW: Hypnosis and the treatment of ulcerative colitis and Crohn's disease. Am J Clin Hypn 40:111–117, 1997.
14. Chen Q, Zhang H: Clinical study on 118 cases of ulcerative colitis treated by integration of traditional Chinese and Western medicine. J Tradit Chin Med 19:163–165, 1999.
15. http://www.dr-zhang.com/index.htm
16. Eisenberg DM, Davis RB, Ettner SL, et al: Trends in alternative medicine use in the United States, 1990–1997. JAMA 280:1569–1574, 1998.
17. Bland JS, Costarella L, Levin B, et al: Clinical Nutrition: A Functional Approach. Gig Harbor, Wash, The Institute for Functional Medicine, 1999.
18. Fassler KL: Ulcerative colitis: An integrated clinical approach. N Engl J Homeopath 4(4):25–31, 1995.
19. Hunter JO: Nutritional factors in inflammatory bowel disease. Eur J Gastroenterol Hepatol 10(30):235–237, 1998.

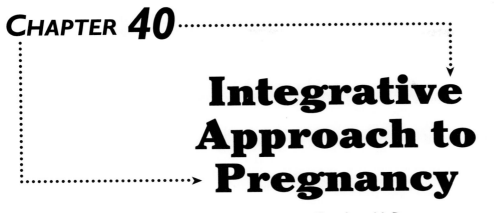

CHAPTER 40

Integrative Approach to Pregnancy

Tracy Gaudet, M.D.

Few conditions encountered in the delivery of healthcare lend themselves more perfectly to an integrative approach than pregnancy. The factors that create these circumstances are also factors that allow healthcare providers to use more integrative approaches with greater comfort when dealing with the pregnant patient. The unique aspects of pregnancy that create this "integrative-friendly" environment are:

1. Pregnancy is not a disease state.
2. Pregnancy *is* a significant life transition with little debate that all aspects of the individual are affected: mind, body, spirit, and community.
3. Pregnancy is a condition that exemplifies the power of nature and the body's capacities.
4. Pregnancy is a condition that has benefited tremendously from the advances of modern medicine.
5. Pregnancy is a condition in which the accepted goal of care is to be as minimally invasive as possible. (The same is not universally true of labor and delivery.)
6. Pregnancy is a condition in which there is general recognition of the immediate need for and benefit of optimal health.

PREGNANCY IS NOT A DISEASE STATE

Although pregnancy has certainly been managed and thought of as a disease state in the past, it is easy to recognize that it distinguishes itself from many "conditions" healthcare providers are trained to manage by the very fact that it is *not* a disease. This fact forms the basis for the argument, made by some, that physicians and hospitals should not even be in the picture when dealing with normal pregnancy. It is certainly an important distinction to both recognize and contemplate, because many of the providers who work with women and their preg-

nancies are indeed more fully trained to manage diseases than to manage normal life cycles. Optimally managing life cycles and their times of transition, such as birth and death and the processes leading up to them, requires a slightly different perspective and awareness than disease management. In fact, the management of diseases within these processes is quite distinct from the management of diseases alone. The considerations are different, and often the goals are different, when a given disease presents in the transition leading to birth (or to death.)

PREGNANCY *IS* A SIGNIFICANT LIFE TRANSITION WITH LITTLE DEBATE THAT ALL ASPECTS OF THE INDIVIDUAL ARE AFFECTED: MIND, BODY, SPIRIT, AND COMMUNITY

Very few conditions affect a person's entire being as significantly as pregnancy. A woman's anatomy, her physiology, and her psychology are all directly affected by the pregnancy. Her relationships, her spirituality, and her life in all aspects, regardless of the outcome of the pregnancy, are affected and will often be forever changed. When surveying the interplay between the healthcare delivery system and the patient, it is hard to imagine a more "holistic" one. This, of course, in no way dictates the nature of the interaction. Healthcare providers dealing with pregnancy may choose to deal with only the medical aspects of pregnancy, and do so in a very confined venue. With the possible exception of death, there does not exist a more inviting opportunity to interface with a patient in a whole person, mind-body-spirit-community level. This is true both because of the aforementioned expansive nature of pregnancy and because of the miraculous nature of this life event.

PREGNANCY IS A CONDITION THAT EXEMPLIFIES THE POWER OF NATURE AND THE BODY'S CAPACITIES

The very process of conception, pregnancy, and birth dramatically exemplifies one of the underlying principles of integrative medicine: the power of nature and of the human body, and the body's capacity to heal. Re-examining pregnancy with this awareness can be a useful tool in developing the practice of integrative medicine.

Physicians and healthcare providers are privileged to witness aspects of life and death that typically are only mysteries to general society. Contemplate the miraculous nature of pregnancy and birth, the process of creating and bringing new life into the world, the mystery that allows this to happen at all, and the fragile and yet resilient nature of the entire process. Honoring these aspects of pregnancy can create an openness not only in the patient but also in the provider. If the provider allows it, dealing with patients around pregnancy can serve as a catalyst in shifting to a practice that embraces the whole person. Intellectual barriers are softened, hearts open around births, mystery is sparked, and souls are rejuvenated. The medical profession is much in need of this dynamic, and pregnancy offers a doorway. It can certainly serve as an impetus for providing whole-person, integrative care.

PREGNANCY IS A CONDITION THAT HAS BENEFITED TREMENDOUSLY FROM THE ADVANCES OF MODERN MEDICINE

Maternal mortality and morbidity have drastically declined as the advances of modern medicine have been implemented. This factor is essential to recognize, because it underscores the imperative of *integrative* approaches to pregnancy rather than *alternative* approaches. Technology and modern interventions clearly have had a significant impact on the outcomes of pregnancy. In the United States, the number of maternal deaths per 100,000 live births has decreased from 582 to 8 in the 50 years from 1935 to 1985.[1] Failing to embrace these successful advances would be contradictory to the best practice of medicine.

PREGNANCY IS A CONDITION IN WHICH THE ACCEPTED GOAL OF CARE IS TO BE AS MINIMALLY INVASIVE AS POSSIBLE (THE SAME IS NOT UNIVERSALLY TRUE OF LABOR AND DELIVERY)

Secondary only to the care of the developing fetus, dealing with pregnancy is unique within the whole of conventional medicine. Medical interventions must be assessed based on the risk and benefit to both the mother and the fetus. This, in and of itself, makes medical decision-making more complex. Factor in that randomized controlled trials of medical interventions are virtually never conducted in pregnancy, and thus, there is a resultant paucity of data and evidence on which to base medical decisions or support the use of medical interventions. Therefore, a general principle in the conventional management of pregnancy is to avoid all medical and surgical interventions whenever possible. (This is not necessarily true of labor and delivery, however.) Consequently, pregnancy becomes the perfect condition in which to explore and integrate noninvasive alternative approaches. First, effective alternative approaches can offer relief where conventional approaches cannot be offered. Second, effective alternatives can often negate or delay the need for more invasive approaches. Third, this provides an opportunity to explore alternative approaches in a domain that, because of these unique characteristics, is less controversial both with physician colleagues and with patients.

PREGNANCY IS A CONDITION IN WHICH THERE IS GENERAL RECOGNITION OF THE IMMEDIATE NEED FOR AND BENEFIT OF OPTIMAL HEALTH

Lastly, pregnancy is a condition in which there is a greater understanding of the importance of lifestyle choices and the creation of optimal health. The dynamic of a developing fetus highlights, in a recognizable way, the significance of lifestyle choices far more dramatically than when contemplating the effects of such choices on the adult patient. The deleterious effects of substances such as tobacco, alcohol, and drugs are plainly seen on developing fetuses. The lack of appropriate nutrients clearly results in increased risk of birth defects, as is the case with folic acid and spina bifida. The overuse of supplements can increase the risk of problems as well, as is the case with high concentration of bioflavonoids and increased risk of infant and early childhood leukemia.[2, 3] The proper nutrition, exercise, and relaxation techniques can improve outcomes in pregnancy. This creates a unique opportunity to recommend behavioral changes that a woman may be hesitant to do for herself, but that she will do secondary to the new motivation provided by her pregnancy. This also allows a woman to translate the significance of these choices to her own health and to work to maintain these lifestyle changes beyond her pregnancy.

INITIATING AN INTEGRATIVE APPROACH

Conventional plus Complementary and Alternative Medicine Does Not an Integrative Approach Make

An integrative approach to pregnancy reaches far beyond incorporating complementary and alternative approaches when indicated. While there are many approaches within complementary and alternative medicine (CAM) that could be offered as adjuncts to already existing obstetric care, and although this would most likely result in improved care and is therefore very worthwhile, an integrative approach is distinct from this. It is, as the language implies, an *approach,* the framework within which the healthcare is offered, and it therefore permeates every aspect of the obstetric care. It is entirely possible to practice an integrative approach to pregnancy and have patients who never experience an "alternative" therapy. It is equally possible to have patients utilize "alternative" therapies and not have an integrative approach to their pregnancy. The integrative approach is grounded in a philosophy of care that embraces the whole person, mind-body-spirit-community, and in so doing optimizes their health and well-being.

The Significance of the "Setup"

The most important aspect of any approach is the initial encounter. It is in that "setup" that expectations are formed, by both the provider and the patient, whether spoken or not. An integrative approach to pregnancy begins with the very first visit, regardless of whether that visit is for preconceptual counseling or a first prenatal visit. No encounter is more significant. The patient presents with open inquiry and leaves with a sense of what her care will encompass and what the role of her healthcare provider will be. Whether these issues are addressed directly or not, the approach is set. Altering that at any point in the future is challenging.

It is quite possible to offer alternative therapies as appropriate throughout a woman's pregnancy, with little or no change in the setup. Indeed, it is the healthcare provider's responsibility to inform patients of all potentially beneficial therapies, regardless of their system of origin. Therefore, providers need to become educated about alternative treatments that can be safe and efficacious in preg-

nancy. This is an important objective in and of itself, and these therapies can be offered at appropriate times in a woman's pregnancy within existing obstetric care.

If, however, the healthcare provider's objective is to offer a truly integrative approach to pregnancy, then the initial encounter with the patient must be thoughtfully reconsidered.

The Initial Visit: It All Begins

The initial visit with the patient should be designed in such a way as to reflect the integrative approach. As much as possible, all aspects of your practice should invite in the whole person—mind, body, spirit, and community.
1. This approach begins with the office and nursing staff.
2. The environment matters.
3. Explain what an integrative approach to pregnancy is.
4. The questions that are asked of the patient define what is important.
5. Listening to the patient is essential.
6. Understand the patient's experience with and/or openness to alternative therapies.
7. Discuss the basis for making decisions in care during pregnancy.
8. Requests that are made of the patient reinforce the integrative approach.

This Approach Begins with the Office and Nursing Staff

The philosophy of care is often communicated long before the patient and provider meet. This can be communicated either intentionally or not, with the first call. Recruit staff at all levels who understand and are invested in an integrative philosophy. For them, it will be very rewarding to work in an environment in which they feel that their own values are supported. Support this philosophy through in-services and the interactions with the staff. An integrative approach to pregnancy begins with an integrative approach within the team itself. This will be evident to the patient from her first encounter with the medical office.

The Environment Matters

Create a space that also reflects the approach that you practice. This can be done through simple touches, with attention to such things as plants, music, color, and aromas. Make sure the space feels comfortable and inviting and speaks of health and not disease, of safety and not danger. Septic smells and cold metal send a powerful message.

Explain What an Integrative Approach to Pregnancy Is

When you first meet the patient, be certain to explain that your approach is integrative and what that means. This may have been communicated previously through your staff or through literature, but hearing it directly from the provider is crucial and allows the patient's experience and expectations to be aligned with your approach.

Three distinguishing elements of an integrative approach to pregnancy are:

1. A recognition of the whole person; mind, body, spirit, and community
2. A health orientation, rather than a disease orientation
3. The use of alternative therapies when appropriate

A Recognition of the Whole Person: Mind, Body, Spirit, and Community

An integrative approach begins by recognizing that there is likely to be no more significant event uniformly affecting all aspects of a woman's life than pregnancy. This is always complicated. Whether the pregnancy is planned or unexpected, desired or not, it is a complex event in a woman's life. A provider who begins by acknowledging this and encourages the patient to reflect on these issues in her own life has already set the stage for an integrative approach to pregnancy.

A Health Orientation, Rather Than a Disease Orientation

Often, the function of prenatal care is described as screening for the potential problems of pregnancy. Whereas this is certainly an important aspect of obstetric care, shifting the orientation to one of health rather than solely one of disease is essential to an integrative approach. One of the goals is to help the mother be as healthy as possible for the new life developing within her. This requires attention to all aspects of the mother's life—not only her habits regarding tobacco and alcohol but also her overall nutrition, her level of physical fitness, her emotional health, her spiritual health, and the strength of her community.

The Use of Alternative Therapies When Appropriate

An integrative approach also incorporates the use of safe and efficacious alternative approaches throughout pregnancy, delivery, and the postpartum period.

The Questions Asked of the Patient Define What Is Important

The initial intake for a patient communicates to the patient what you believe matters in her care. A patient history that goes beyond the conventional obstetric history initiates the approach that goes beyond the conventional obstetric care. Be certain to include questions regarding:

- Her relationship with food and a detailed nutritional history
- A detailed fitness history
- The state of her relationships, positive and negative, and how they may be affected by the pregnancy
- Her thoughts regarding sex and intimacy during pregnancy
- The degree of her social support—how does she define her community and how might this shift?
- Her greatest joys in life and how they may be affected by the pregnancy
- Her fears regarding this pregnancy
- Her greatest sorrows
- Her stressors in life and her coping strategies
- Her techniques for relaxation
- Her source of strength in difficult times
- Her darkest thoughts and feelings regarding this pregnancy
- Her brightest thoughts and feelings regarding this pregnancy

Know that unless the patient-provider relationship has been established in the context of an integrative approach, these questions are useless. The patient will respond in the socially acceptable way, so as not to be judged in a negative light. Recognizing the significance of these factors and assuring the patient that all pregnancies are complicated, although our society does not encourage this perspective, is essential. Explain that this sets the framework for her care, and it will be a valuable and significant discourse.

Listening to the Patient Is Essential

Seeking to understand the patient as fully as possible is critical to an integrative approach. This can be accomplished only by listening. Asking the right questions is just the first step. While this sounds obvious, many healthcare providers, particularly physicians, are not trained to listen well and are instead skilled at minimizing and directing conversation. Listening to your patient is key, not only in the information that you obtain but also in the relationship it begins.

Understand the Patient's Experience with and/or Openness to Alternative Therapies

When beginning to care for a woman and her pregnancy, it is important to ask what, if any, experience she has had with *alternative medicine*. Be sure to define what you mean by the term. Has she ever used any of these approaches? Is so, for what? Why did she turn to alternative medicine? What was her experience? Would she be open to your suggestions regarding uses of alternative therapies in her pregnancy? Are there certain areas she is particularly interested in or areas that she is particularly skeptical of? Make sure she knows that you are comfortable with whatever her answers are; it is simply important to know her perspective. Make certain that she also understands the significance of open communication around these issues. Many alternative therapies have the potential to affect the pregnancy and careful integration of these approaches is essential.

Discuss the Basis for Making Decisions in Care during Pregnancy

It is often useful to review with patients the way in which you will be making decisions regarding what approaches to use during her pregnancy. Obviously, the goal is the health and well-being of the mother and the fetus, but it is useful to review with the patient that, particularly in pregnancy, research is lacking on virtually all aspects of healthcare—mainstream and alternative. Given that the basic philosophy of obstetric care is to avoid anything potentially harmful, and given that the majority of things safely used outside of pregnancy have not been tested in pregnancy, our options for treating even simple things like colds or backaches are limited. This makes certain noninvasive alternative approaches particularly appealing.

A useful framework for making decisions in these often murky areas is as follows:

1. Evaluate the potential to do harm.
   a. Direct harm: The potential of the therapy itself causing harm to the mother or fetus. Sometimes there are data; at other times, it is conservative educated guesses. For example, it is certainly feasible to think that chelation therapy or ingesting megadoses of vitamins has the potential to do direct harm. It is difficult to imagine how relaxation techniques could.
   b. Indirect harm: (1) Delaying a useful therapy; (2) using the financial resources of the patient for useless therapies
2. Evaluate the potential to be of benefit.
   a. Direct evidence: What is the research on the effectiveness of this treatment? There are varying levels of research in many applicable areas, including the use of acupressure and acupuncture with hyperemesis gravidarum, moxibustion in the version of breeches, the relaxation response in pregnancy, the use of hypnosis in surgery, or the effectiveness of doulas in labor.
   b. Cultural experience: The use of certain approaches with purported success across centuries is another form of data. If there is no evidence or rationale for potential harm, a therapy may be explored on the basis of cultural experience.

   c. Personal belief: The beliefs of the patient are significant and can be a powerful therapeutic ally. In the face of no evidence of harm, a strong belief in a therapy is an important factor to consider.
3. Evaluate the "delivery system."
   a. If a provider delivers the therapy, knowing the skill of the practitioner is crucial, as in conventional medicine. If the approach involves a product, knowing the quality of the product is equally important.
4. Evaluate the integration.
   a. Some approaches and some practitioners will integrate well with you and your care plan for the patient. Others will not. Well-integrated care is essential. If the therapy is not amenable to integration, it should not be recommended.

Discuss with the patient her comfort with this approach and your commitment to her as a partner in the process. As the pregnancy progresses and as opportunities for integrating alternative therapies arise, there will be a basis of understanding around this decision-making process.

Requests That Are Made of the Patient Reinforce the Integrative Approach

Finally, the requests that you make of the patient reinforce both the nature of your integrative approach and the significance of her partnership in it. The following are some sample requests:

- Begin to journal privately about your thoughts, fears, and hopes regarding your pregnancy.
- Practice one relaxation technique daily.
- Begin a food diary.
- Do some form of physical activity three times a week.
- Pay attention to your own self care—do something nurturing for yourself at least once a week (get a massage, have a picnic by the lake, take a bubble bath).
- If you are experiencing nausea and vomiting, try candied ginger or ginger tea and an acupressure band.

In addition to standard information, be certain to include in your requests/educational information:

Avoid botanicals and megadoses of vitamins during pregnancy (their effects are not well researched).

Avoid concentrated bioflavonoids (this has been shown to be associated with an increased risk of infant and early childhood lymphomas).[2, 3]

Be certain to include oily fish in your diet (the inclusion of oily fish in the mother's diet during pregnancy has been significantly associated with the development of the visual system of the fetus).[4]

Acupuncture has been endorsed by a National

Institutes of Health consensus panel as an effective treatment for nausea in pregnancy.[5]

The use of doulas, trained laypeople who provide continuous support throughout a woman's labor, has been shown in some studies to improve obstetric outcomes, including shorter labor, decreased need for anesthesia, decreased operative deliveries, decreased cesarean sections, as well as increased breast feeding and decreased anxiety and depression postpartum.[6, 7]

THE PRACTICALITIES OF MAKING IT WORK

Just as an integrative approach to pregnancy redefines the scope of obstetric care, the method of the delivery of that care must also be redefined. It is unlikely that most practice settings could immediately accommodate this new approach. If one obstetrician, for example, is to take this expanded history with each patient, the practice would most likely not be long in existence, because it is simply not fiscally viable.

The time is right to think of new possibilities for the process by which an integrative approach to pregnancy might happen. Consider the following:

- Create an information packet that describes an integrative approach to pregnancy and get it to the patient *before* her first visit.
- Design an attractive intake form with more broad-based questions for the patient to reflect on and fill out before her visit.
- Once a month offer information sessions that all new patients attend, in which much of the general information is shared.
- Suggest that those who are interested meet monthly, on their own, as a support group.
- Ask local providers to give you descriptions of their approach and their services for your review, and place them in your office.
- Ask qualified alternative providers to offer an educational session, first for your staff, then for patients.
- Have instructive videos on topics such as relaxation techniques in your office.
- Educate the nurses, physician assistants, and nurse practitioners in these approaches.
- Enroll your patients in your commitment to create new ways to offer an integrative approach to pregnancy, and solicit their ideas and their feedback—as your partners, they will also be patient with your process.
- Be creative—the best solutions will not be found in "the same old way"—and experiment.

— *THERAPEUTIC REVIEW* —

Pregnancy offers a most unique opportunity to begin to offer integrative approaches in your practice. There is no "condition" that by its very nature is more whole person—involving mind, body, spirit, and community. There is also no "condition" that is in such need of natural, noninvasive approaches. Nor is there any other "condition" that so reminds us of the power and possibility of nature. Engaging patients in an integrative approach to their pregnancy can transform not only their experience but also the experience of the provider. Be ready to reconnect with the true meaning of healthcare and to remember the feeling that first drew you to medicine. This is an incredibly rewarding way to practice. Ultimately, as this approach is embraced, healthcare and the healthcare provider move toward greater health and wholeness, together with the patient and the yet-to-be-born.

References

1. Koonin LM, Atrash HK, Lawson HW, Smith JC: Maternal Mortality Surveillance, United States, 1979–1986. MMWR Morb Mortal Wkly Rep 40:1, 1991.
2. Strick R, Strissel PL, Borgers S, et al: Dietary bioflavonoids induce cleavage in the MLL gene and may contribute to infant leukemia. Proc Natl Acad Sci U S A 97:4790–4795, 2000.
3. Ross JA: Dietary bioflavonoids and the MLL gene: A pathway to infant leukemia? Proc Natl Acad Sci U S A 97:4411–4413, 2000.
4. Williams C, Birch EE, Emmett PM, Northstone K, and the Avon Longitudinal Study of Pregnancy and Childhood (ALSPAC) Study Team: Stereoacuity at age 3.5 y in children born full-term is associated with prenatal and postnatal dietary factors: A report from a population-based cohort study. Am J Clin Nutr 73:316–322, 2001.
5. Acupuncture. NIH Consensus Statement Online 15(5):1–34, 1997.
6. Scott KD, Berkowitz G, Klaus M: A comparison of intermittent and continuous support during labor: A meta-analysis. Am J Obstet Gynecol 180:1054–1059, 1999.
7. Klaus MH, Kennell JH: The doula: An essential ingredient of childbirth rediscovered. Acta Paediatr 86:1034–1036, 1997.

CHAPTER 41

Post-term Pregnancy

Ann L. Mattson, M.D., F.A.C.O.G., and Steffie Goodman, C.N.M., M.S.N.

PATHOPHYSIOLOGY

Post-term pregnancy is any gestation that exceeds 42 weeks (294 days) from the first day of the last menstrual period. The incidence of post-term pregnancy has been estimated from 3% to 14% of all pregnancies. It should be recognized that many cases of apparent post-term gestation actually are the result of an inaccurate assessment of gestational age.

The cause of true post-term pregnancy is not well understood. Several theories have been proposed based on observational data, including the possible roles of fetal pituitary hormones and placental enzyme functioning. In any event, initiation of labor does appear to be a hormonally mediated event in which "messengers" from the placenta or fetus may interact. Dysfunctional production or activity of one of these messengers may interfere with the timely initiation of labor.

NOTE

Verifying accurate dating of gestation should always be the first step in the management of a post-term pregnancy.

Post-term pregnancy may be associated with an increased incidence of placental abnormalities, fetal hypoxia and asphyxia, intrauterine growth restriction, macrosomia, meconium aspiration, and perinatal death. Management is based on best possible determination of gestational age (dating criteria should be reviewed) and assessment of current fetal and maternal status (antenatal surveillance). Clearly, if a medical indication exists for urgent delivery, this should be of primary concern in formulating a management approach.

INTEGRATIVE THERAPY

Behavioral/Physical Modalities

Considering Options

If maternal and fetal surveillance in the post-term gestation is reassuring, available data suggest that expectant management (i.e., no intervention) may be a reasonable option. In low-risk post-term pregnancies with a favorable cervix, no data are available suggesting that induction of labor offers an improved outcome.[1] In women with an unfavorable cervix, there may be an increased risk of cesarean birth to allay fetal distress with expectant management, but study results have been mixed.[1] Likewise, there may be an increased risk of cesarean delivery associated with induction of labor. The decision to proceed with expectant management or induction should be thoroughly discussed with the patient. If expectant management is elected, close fetal and maternal surveillance should continue and consideration given to some of the gentler potentiators of labor as described in the following sections.

Sexual Intercourse

Sexual intercourse has been commonly suggested as a means to ripen the cervix and initiate labor. Possible mechanisms include stimulation of contractions with female orgasm and a direct effect of prostaglandins from semen. Certainly, several studies have documented that intercourse causes increased contractions in women with preterm labor.[2] There have also been several studies documenting the safety of frequent intercourse in pregnancy.[2]

Nipple Stimulation

Nipple stimulation increases endogenous levels of oxytocin, a potent stimulator of uterine contractions. Historically, midwives have long used this method for initiating labor; indeed, several studies have shown it to be both safe and efficacious.[2] Of particular note, a randomized study in 1984 of 200 women at 39 weeks of gestation showed a significant reduction in post-term pregnancies (17% in control group and 5% in the intervention group).[3] Multiple regimens have been used in these studies; generally, it appears wise to advise stimulation (rolling or sucking) of one or both nipples for up to 3 hours per day (not continuous). Fetal monitoring should be considered when nipple stimulation is suggested, especially in pregnancies in which uterine hypertonus may be of concern (e.g., with placental insufficiency or oligohydramnios).

Botanicals

Red Raspberry Leaf

Red raspberry leaf (*Rubus idaeus*) is considered to be a uterine tonic. There is some evidence of stimulation and relaxation of uterine muscle in animal studies.[4] Red raspberry leaf can promote more powerful and effective uterine contractions, with more complete uterine relaxation in between.[5] This herb is reportedly useful in decreasing the likelihood of post-term gestation.[6] No data on toxicity or teratogenicity exist; the herb is generally considered safe in pregnancy on the basis of historical observation. Major components include tannins, flavonoids, and several minerals (including calcium, magnesium, and potassium).[7]

An infusion (strong tea) is preferred. Tincture or capsules may not be concentrated enough. To make an infusion, steep 1 teaspoon of dry leaf in 1 cup of boiling water for up to 20 minutes.

Dosage. Drink 1 cup up to three times per day, starting at 37 weeks of gestation.

Evening Primrose Oil

Evening primrose oil (*Oenothera biennis*) is an excellent source of essential fatty acids (CLA and gamma-linolenic acid [GLA]), which serve as precursors for prostaglandin synthesis. This herb is theoretically useful for cervical ripening, although sparse clinical data do not support this use.[8] Multiple studies have noted no toxicity.

Dosage. Evening primrose oil can be taken orally or used topically on the cervix. For oral use, the dose is 500 mg 3 times a day starting at 37 weeks of gestation. For topical use, puncture a capsule and apply the oil directly to the cervix using the fingertips or penis. Application may be repeated once or twice daily.

Precautions. Side effects are very rare but may include gastrointestinal upset and headaches.

Castor Oil

Castor oil from the castor bean (*Ricinus communis*) is a potent cathartic and taken internally is thought to cause reflex stimulation of the uterus (secondary to bowel stimulation).[9] Some authors have hypothesized that it may stimulate prostaglandin synthesis.[2] Use of castor oil was a very popular method to induce labor during the first part of the last century. Most studies trying to substantiate its clinical use in the initiation of labor have shown mixed results.[9] However, in a prospective study of 100 women at 40

to 42 weeks of gestation, half of the patients were given a single oral dose of 60 mL of castor oil. Of these patients 57.7% began labor within 24 hours, compared with 4.2% of the patients in the control group.[10] Possible toxicities include an increased incidence of meconium staining of amniotic fluid,[2] precipitous labor, and in one case report, amniotic fluid embolism 30 minutes after ingestion of castor oil (no plausible mechanism of action noted).[11]

Dosage. 2 ounces of castor oil with 2 ounces of orange juice taken orally. The dose may be repeated after 1 to 2 hours. Historically, castor oil packs covered with moist heat have been used topically to induce labor. Far fewer side effects have been noted, but efficacy data are lacking.

Precautions. Adverse effects include liquid stools and intense abdominal cramping.

Black Cohosh

Black cohosh (*Cimicifuga racemosa*) is a Native American herbal that may bind estrogen receptors and selectively inhibit luteinizing hormone. It is known to contain tannins, alkaloids, and terpenoids. Black cohosh is considered to be a uterine tonic and nerve relaxant. It may be used alone or in formula with other herbs during the last month of pregnancy to prepare for labor. Its suggested use is as an agent to ripen the cervix.[12]

NOTE

Black cohosh is more appropriately used for cervical ripening than for stimulating uterine contractions.

Dosage. 10 to 25 drops of standardized tincture of black cohosh under the tongue 4 times daily. Black cohosh may also be used as the dried herb in a size 00 capsule, 1 or 2 capsules orally 3 times a day. (Size 00 empty gelatin capsules, found at most health food stores, can be used to compound the herb at home.)

Precautions. Overdose may cause nausea, dizziness, severe headaches, central nervous system depression, visual disturbances, reduced pulse rate, and perspiration.[13]

Caution. Black cohosh must be avoided before 36 weeks of pregnancy.

Blue Cohosh

Blue cohosh (*Caulophyllum thalictoides*) is used by Native Americans to facilitate labor. It is unrelated to black cohosh. The plant contains several glycosides that have demonstrated oxytocic properties.[9] These glycosides are also potent vasoconstrictors with cardiotoxic properties. Although used historically as a potent initiator of labor, it has also been associated with serious toxicity. These toxic effects include teratogenic effects in cows, vasoconstriction of cardiac vessels, and stomach upset. Indeed, a case reported in 1998 of neonatal myocardial infarction and congestive heart failure was attributed to maternal consumption of blue cohosh.[14] Because of these concerns, blue cohosh should be used only with close maternal and fetal surveillance if at all.

Dosage. It is safest to use only very small doses of this herb. For the standardized tincture, the dose is 3 to 8 drops in water taken orally. The dose may be repeated every 30 minutes for up to 4 hours and then hourly for up to 12 hours until contractions are regular. This herb may be found in combination tinctures with black cohosh.

Precautions. See discussion above. Adverse effects may include nausea, meconium staining of amniotic fluid, uterine hyperstimulation, and hypertension. Serious toxicity has also been reported, as noted.

Caution. Blue cohosh must be avoided prior to 36 weeks of pregnancy.

Cotton Root Bark

Cotton root bark (*Gossypium*) is considered to be an oxytocin synergist. This herb has been used to both initiate and intensify uterine contractions. The seed of the plant has been shown to inhibit platelet-activating factor and leukotrienes. It may also affect levels of luteinizing hormone. No clinical data on its use as an induction agent are available. Toxicity appears to be dose-related; at high doses, adverse effects may include hypokalemia, diarrhea, hair discoloration, malnutrition, circulatory problems, and heart failure.[15]

Dosage. Not well standardized. Can be used as a tincture and taken orally.

Precautions. Cotton root is an interesting herb that seems worthy of further study. The authors' experience with it is, however, minimal, and appropriate caution should be exercised. Certainly, this herb should not be used before 36 weeks of gestation.

Concerns continue to exist about the use of many herbs in pregnancy because of the relative lack of data addressing their safety. Material in Table 41–1 may be used as an initial list (not exhaustive) of herbs that generally should not be used in pregnancy.

Mechanical Interventions

Sweeping/Stripping of Amniotic Membranes

Initially suggested in 1810 by Dr. James Hamilton, stripping of the amniotic membrane is believed to

Table 41–1. Herbals Contraindicated in Pregnancy

Angelica	Juniper
Arbor vitae	Marjoram
Barberry	Meadow saffron
Beth/birth root	Motherwort
Black cohosh	Mugwort
Blue cohosh	Pennyroyal
Cascara sagrada	Poke root
Cinchona	Rue
Cotton root bark	Squaw vine
Goldenseal	Tansy
Greater celandine	Wormwood

work by increasing cervical prostaglandin levels. Randomized controlled studies have shown that women who undergo membrane sweeping/stripping at 38 to 42 weeks of gestation deliver significantly earlier and require induction about half as often as controls.[16] This technique appears to be most successful in nulliparous women with an unfavorable cervix. Potential risks include infection, bleeding, and rupture of membranes.

Technique. During vaginal examination, a finger is placed into the cervical os and rotated so as to separate amniotic membranes from the lower uterine segment.

Precautions. The pregnant woman should always be consulted before this maneuver is attempted and warned that she may experience mild cramping or pain with the actual procedure and contractions and/or light vaginal bleeding after the procedure. It may be also helpful to use the term "cervical massage," as many women find the other terms frightening.

Foley Balloon Dilation

Foley balloon dilation is also believed to work by promoting release of cervical or amniotic prostaglandins, thereby causing cervical ripening. This technique has been studied in a few small randomized trials and found to be effective. It offers the benefit of less cost as compared with the use of prostaglandins and more timely effectiveness than with membrane stripping. [17] Potential risks are the same as for sweeping of membranes, although the risk of infection may be higher.

Technique. After sterile preparation of the cervix, an 18 French Foley catheter with a 30-mL balloon is placed through the internal os and inflated. The catheter may be left in place for up to 12 to 24 hours. Patient discomfort is usually minimal and limited to that associated with insertion of the balloon catheter. This technique is well-suited to outpatient use, as the catheter may be placed at the office and the patient sent home. The patient then returns in the morning for catheter removal and further evaluation. This technique may be used at the same time as other induction modalities directed at promoting cervical ripening (e.g., administration of prostaglandins or oxytocin).

Laminaria and Other Osmotic Dilators

Two types of dilators are recommended for use as cervical ripening agents: those made from seaweed (*Laminaria japonicum*) and a synthetic product (Dilapan). Osmotic dilators work by causing passive expansion of the cervical tissues. Dilapan dilators have been shown to be the more effective of the two types available.[18] Although there has been a suggestion of increased infectious morbidity associated with the use of osmotic dilators, the effectiveness and relative safety of these agents as compared with prostaglandins merits their consideration.[19] Use of both balloon catheters and laminaria may be indicated in the case of very unfavorable cervix.

Technique. After sterile preparation of the cervix, dilators are placed into the cervical canal using a packing or ring forceps. The number of dilators placed will vary depending on the type of dilator and status of the cervix. Vaginal packing with 4 × 4-inch gauze sponges may be used to keep the dilators in place. Dilators should generally be removed within 6 to 12 hours. Again, this method is well suited to outpatient use (see foregoing discussion on balloon catheters).

Artificial Rupture of Membranes

If the cervix is at all dilated and the presenting fetal part is firmly applied to the cervix, amniotomy may generally be accomplished easily and safely. Amniotomy has been well studied as an effective induction modality. The mode of action appears to be increased production of prostaglandins secondary to arachidonic acid release. Advantages include a greater than 80% success rate[20] and visualization of amniotic fluid. Risks include infection (with potentially increased transmission of human immunodeficiency virus and group B streptococci), bleeding, fetal injury, and cord prolapse. Of note, amniotomy should be considered only when induction and delivery can be implemented immediately, as the rate of infectious complications rises with time from amniotomy to delivery.

Pharmaceuticals

Prostaglandins

Several different types of prostaglandins are currently used for cervical ripening and induction of labor in the post-term pregnancy. They may be used orally, intravaginally, or intracervically. Several randomized controlled trials have demonstrated efficacy for prostaglandin E_2 (PGE_2), or dinoprostone (Cervidil, Prepidil) and, more recently, misoprostol (Cytotec). PGE_2 compounds have been used safely in outpatient protocols, but close maternal and fetal surveillance is indicated with the use of any of these preparations. In addition, misoprostol is not currently approved by the Food and Drug Administration for this indication, and recent case reports have indicated an increased risk of uterine rupture with its use. Risks of prostaglandin use include hyperstimulation, fetal distress, and maternal gastrointestinal upset and fever.

Dosage.

- Dinoprostone vaginal insert (Cervidil), 10 mg. Place the insert in the posterior fornix and remove after 12 hours or sooner if regular uterine contractions have developed.
- Dinoprostone gel (Prepidil), 0.5 mg intracervically. The dose may be repeated every 6 hours for up to 3 doses.
- Misoprostol (Cytotec); 25 μg in posterior fornix The dose may be repeated every 6 hours for up to 3 doses if fewer than 3 contractions occur in any 10-minute interval (the risk of uterine rupture should be kept in mind, however).

Precautions. Relative contraindications include regular or painful uterine contractions, maternal history of asthma, glaucoma, and pulmonary, cardiac, renal, or hepatic disease.

Pitocin

Pitocin has long been considered the standard agent for induction of labor. Pitocin is a synthetic analogue of endogenous oxytocin. Individual responses may vary, but it is a potent and effective stimulator of uterine contractions. Pitocin is most effective once cervical ripening has occurred and there is a favorable Bishop score. Various titration protocols have been used trying to balance efficacy, time to delivery, and side effects

Dosage. For induction, pitocin may be given in lactated Ringer's solution infused at 1 mU per minute. Generally this dosage may be increased by 1 to 2 mU every 20 minutes as long as fetal and maternal surveillance findings are normal. Dosage should not be increased once an active contraction pattern and cervical change develop. Extreme care should be taken with dosages over 20 mU per minute or duration of induction greater than 8 to 12 hours.

Precautions. Risks include uterine hyperstimulation, rupture of uterus, fetal distress, and hyponatremia. It should also be noted that use of pitocin may limit maternal mobility and increase maternal anxiety, both factors that may slow the progress of labor and prolong delivery.

Other Therapies to Consider

Hypnosis

There has been only one randomized trial to date studying the effects of hypnosis for induction of labor in post-term gestation, and that showed no effect.[21] However, the mind-body connection is a theoretically powerful factor in the initiation of labor and worth pursuing further. Certainly, this modality may be a safer intervention than the current standard of care.

Acupuncture

Use of acupuncture in the setting of post-term pregnancy can be useful as an additional mode of inducing labor. Both electrical and manual means of stimulation of relevant acupuncture points have been shown to be effective in inducing contractions or labor.[2] Use of this technique requires extensive training, however and a trained acupuncturist should be consulted if this technique is to be considered.

Homeopathy

Several remedies may be worth a try, although data are scarce. The safety of homeopathic remedies certainly cannot be disputed. Remedies of historical note include Caulophyllun, Cimicifuga, and Gelsemium. Consultation with a homeopathic practitioner is recommended.

 THERAPEUTIC REVIEW

Following is a list of therapeutic options to consider in obstetric patients to reduce the incidence of post-term pregnancy as well as its potential sequelae. Some of these recommendations are pertinent for any client who presents with an indication for induction of labor. Appropriate integrated management of post-term gestation depends on a careful balancing of fetal and maternal risks with effective and safe therapies.

Review of Pregnancy Dating Criteria
The importance of reviewing dating criteria cannot be overstated. Many apparently post-term gestations are "cured" after such careful review. This point also suggests close attention to dating criteria at each prenatal visit, particularly at the first visit.

Assessment of Maternal and Fetal Well-being
Generally accepted practice is to start routine fetal surveillance in low-risk pregnancies at 41 weeks' gestation. There is disagreement about what methods should be used and how often. An ultrasound examination at 41 weeks for evaluation of amniotic fluid levels and non-stress tests starting at 41 weeks and repeated every 2 or 3 days constitute a reasonable protocol.

Behavioral/Physical Interventions
As part of the pregnancy education program, after 36 weeks of gestation, patients may be advised to consider intercourse and gentle nipple stimulation as options for avoiding the possibility of post-term pregnancy.

Referral for Complementary Medicine Modalities
The time to consider options such as acupuncture, hypnosis, and homeopathy is generally after 40 weeks in the patient who may have some anxiety about the length of her gestation or who may be at particular risk for post-term gestation (e.g., previous pregnancy with post-term gestation).

Botanicals
Initiation of herbal combinations may be considered after 36 weeks if the pregnant woman has had a history of post-term pregnancy, large baby, or difficult previous birth or has other reasons for wanting to prevent post-term pregnancy.
Raspberry leaf may be encouraged at this time, one cup of tea up to 3 times per day.
After 40 weeks, black cohosh and cotton root may be used with or without concurrent nipple stimulation. Castor oil is another alternative.

Mechanical Techniques
The option of membrane sweeping/stripping should be discussed with the patient beginning at 38 weeks of gestation.
Once the decision has been made to induce a pregnancy, the exact methods used will depend in great part on maternal and fetal status. For induction solely for the indication of post-term gestation in a low-risk pregnancy, use of osmotic dilators or a Foley catheter is a gentle way to encourage cervical ripening. In the presence of a favorable cervix, amniotomy is a reasonable way to proceed.

THERAPEUTIC REVIEW *continued*

Pharmaceuticals

If there is an urgent indication for delivery, or the foregoing methods have been unsuccessful, pharmaceuticals should be used. If the cervix is unripe, intravaginal or cervical prostaglandins are given. If the cervix is ripe, administration of pitocin may be used as an initial step.

References

1. Management of Postterm Pregnancy. In ACOG 2001 Compendium of Selected Publications. Washington, DC, American College of Obstetricians and Gynecologists, 2000;1128.
2. Summers L: Methods of cervical ripening and labor induction. J Nurse Midwifery 42:71–85, 1997.
3. Elliot JP, Flaherty JF: The use of breast stimulation to prevent postterm pregnancy. Am J Obstet Gynecol 149:628–632, 1984.
4. Raspberry. In Facts and Comparisons: The Review of Natural Products. St. Louis, Facts and Comparisons–Wolters Kluwer, 1999.
5. Bamford DS, Percivil RC, Tothill AU: Raspberry leaf tea: A new aspect to an old problem. Br J Pharmacol 40:161–162, 1970.
6. Parsons M, Simpson M, Ponton T: Raspberry leaf and its effect on labour: Safety and efficacy. J Austral Coll Midwives 12:20–25, 1999.
7. Bergner P. The mineral content of herbal decoctions. Med Herbalism 9:6–9, 1997.
8. Dove D, Johnson P: Oral evening primrose oil: Its effect on length of pregnancy and selected intrapartum outcomes in low-risk nulliparous women. J Nurse Midwifery 44:320–324, 1999.
9. McFarlin B, Gibson M, O'Rear J, Harman P: A national survey of herbal preparation use by nurse-midwives for labor stimulation. J Nurse Midwifery 44:205–216, 1999.
10. Garry D, Figueroa R, Guillaume J, Cucco V: Use of castor oil in pregnancies at term. Altern Ther Health Med 6:77–79, 2000.
11. Steingrub JS, Lopez T, Teres D, Steingart R: Amniotic fluid embolism associated with castor oil ingestion. Crit Care Med 16:642–643, 1988.
12. Weed S: Wise Woman Herbal Childbearing Year. New York, Ash Tree Publishing, 1986, p. 59.
13. Black Cohosh. In Facts and Comparisons: The Review of Natural Products. St. Louis, Facts and Comparisons–Wolters Kluwer, 1998.
14. Jones TK, Lawson BM: Profound neonatal congestive heart failure caused by maternal consumption of blue cohosh herbal medication. J Pediatr 132: 550–552, 1998.
15. Gossypol. In Facts and Comparisons: The Review of Natural Products. St. Louis, Facts and Comparisons–Wolters Kluwer, 1994.
16. Wiriyasirivaj B, Vutyavanich T, Ruangsri RA: A randomized controlled trial of membrane stripping at term to promote labor. Obstet Gynecol 87:767–770, 1996.
17. Poma PA: Cervical ripening. A review and recommendation for clinical practice. J Reprod Med 44:657–668, 1999.
18. Blumenthal PD, Ramanauskas R: Randomized trial of Dilapan and Laminaria as cervical ripening agents before induction of labor. Obstet Gynecol 365–368, 1990.
19. Creasy R, Resnik R: Maternal-Fetal Medicine: Principles and Practice. Philadelphia, WB Saunders, 1989, p. 523.
20. Gabbe S, Niebyl J, Simpson J (eds): Obstetrics: Normal and Problem Pregnancies. New York, Churchill Livingstone, 1986, p. 372.
21. Chez R, Jonas W: Complementary and alternative medicine. Part 1: Clinical studies in obstetrics. Obstet Gynecol Surv 52:704–708, 1997.

CHAPTER **42**

Labor Pain Management

Ann Mattson, M.D., F.A.C.O.G., and Steffie Goodman, C.N.M., M.S.N.

PHYSIOLOGY

Understanding the mechanisms that cause women pain during labor is crucial to finding appropriate ways to help them. The task of managing pain in labor is sometimes complicated by concerns about how our methods of alleviating maternal pain might affect the fetus while in utero and the newborn following birth. An integrated approach to pain management is one way to address these multiple concerns.

Several mechanisms are associated with pain in labor. These can be broken down into three different categories with brief overviews as follows:

Anatomic stimuli
Hormonal balance
Emotional status

Anatomic Stimuli

During the first stage of labor, pain results from cervical dilation and uterine contractions. Pain travels via visceral afferent nerves (sympathetic) from the uterus to the spinal cord at the posterior segments of the thoracic spinal nerves 10, 11, and 12.[1] These nerves form part of the uterine and cervical plexus, the inferior hypogastric plexus, the middle hypogastric nerve, the superior hypogastric plexus or presacral nerve, and the lumbar and lower thoracic sympathetic chains.[2]

Both slow and fast nerve fibers are responsible for the transmission of pain. Fast fibers generally ensure an immediate reaction to pain, and slow fibers transmit lingering pain. At the dorsal horn of the spinal cord, nerve fiber transmissions converge before entering the brain. Here, messages to the brain are sorted and selected. According to the gate-control theory of pain, which was described in the 1960s by two researchers at McGill University, only a limited amount of information can be processed by the nervous system at one time. If too many pain signals are transmitted at once, the system becomes short-circuited. If slow nerve fibers are stimulated, and a fast fiber competes, the gate to the slow-moving fibers closes[3, 4] which explains why techniques

such as transcutaneous electrical nerve stimulation (TENS), massage, or acupuncture may help laboring women.

Adequacy of blood flow to the uterine muscle also affects the level of pain perceived throughout labor. If relaxation between contractions is insufficient to allow adequate oxygenation, the sensation of pain is worse secondary to hypoxia.[2] Thus by considering efficacy of contractions, maternal position, hemoglobin at term, and respiratory efficiency, one can promote maximum oxygenation of the uterus during labor to minimize a woman's sensation of pain.

Surrounding organs and tissues also contribute to the sensation of pain. Ligaments stretch, and traction is felt by the tubes, ovaries, and peritoneum. Pressure on the bladder, urethra, rectum, and vagina, as well as distention of the pelvic floor and perineum, contributes to pain during the second stage of labor. A ganglion of nerves located in the vagina (the pudendal or sacral nerves) are responsible for the transmission of pain from the perineum to the spinal cord.[1] Movement of pelvic bony structures also contributes to a woman's pain.

Hormonal Balance

Although one may not think of hormonal balance in association with management of painful labor, it is actually a key component of this discussion. Not much can be changed about a woman's anatomy. During labor, nerve endings will be stimulated and will transmit pain. The muscle must contract and that is going to hurt. Tissues, organs, bones, and ligaments must be stretched and moved out of the way for the baby to pass through. But a woman's hormonal status is in constant flux. It is exquisitely sensitive to both external and internal stimuli. Many women's health care issues are related to minute hormonal imbalances that can have a huge impact. It is no different in labor. Consider the hormones chiefly involved in the process of labor: prostaglandin, oxytocin, adrenocorticotropic hormone (ACTH), cortisol, catecholamines, and beta-endorphins.[1] High levels of prostaglandin, oxytocin, and beta-endorphins, along with low levels of catecholamines, cortisol, and ACTH, are optimal. A woman laboring with this combination appears quiet, inward, and immobile as she works with her contractions.

A woman's "stress" response to labor ultimately orchestrates the presence or absence of some of these hormones. If she is anxious or fearful, there will be higher levels of epinephrine, a catecholamine responsible for the fight-or-flight response, during which the hypothalamus part of the brain signals the pituitary gland to release ACTH to the adrenal glands. During early labor, this tends to slow down the labor process, decreasing the effect of oxytocin. This may work to her advantage if she is in the bush giving birth and a predator threatens early labor. The release of epinephrine would stop her labor and allow her to move to safety. The higher levels of epinephrine at the end of labor would encourage stronger contractions and would allow the birth to proceed more rapidly, which would enable her to move herself and her young to safety if needed. However, under typical labor conditions, high levels of epinephrine may not work to a woman's advantage. During early stages of labor, these levels slow labor down, which may induce exhaustion, mostly as a result of fear. A vicious cycle ensues.

Higher levels of catecholamines are also associated with decreased uterine blood flow. Again, this is part of the fight-or-flight mechanism, which may create hypoxia, more painful contractions, and fetal intolerance of labor. In addition, higher levels of catecholamines suppress the release of beta-endorphins and other endogenous pain-relieving neurotransmitters.[3] Endorphins are morphine-like substances produced in the pituitary that alleviate pain and induce a feeling of well-being. It is known that endorphin levels increase throughout labor.[1, 3] Endorphins are also found in the placenta and amniotic fluid, which suggests that they play a role for the baby as well.[3] When beta-endorphin and oxytocin levels are high, for example, during the first stage of labor, a woman gradually journeys inward, becomes quiet, and doesn't want to move much. Toward the end of labor, as physical sensations of fetal expulsion become much more powerful, catecholamine levels increase and women are much more vocal, become incredibly strong, have chills or tremble, lose control of bowels and bladder, and so forth. This is all physiologic in nature and is indicative of ideal hormonal balance in labor. As one might imagine, interruptions of any kind, such as feeling unsafe, afraid, or insecure, can ruin this delicate hormonal balance and render labor dysfunctional, thus increasing the woman's perception of pain. It is also well documented that medications used during labor, such as analgesia and regional anesthesia, decrease stress response hormones.[1] They also, however, decrease endorphin levels.[1] Practitioners must be aware of this when counseling a woman about her options for medication, or about "decreasing" an epidural during the second stage of labor.

NOTE

Women who are anxious and feel out of control of their pain during early labor have higher catecholamine levels, leading to endorphin inhibition and adrenal suppression. Greater pain and a dysfunctional labor can result.

Emotional Status

A woman's emotional status clearly may affect her perception of pain during labor. It is helpful if a woman trusts her body, the birth process, and her health care provider. The literature provides clear evidence that women who have a good support team tend to have shorter labors and better outcomes.[39, 44, 46] Women who have taken classes, have read books, and have had babies in the past are knowledgeable and confident; all of these have been shown to improve women's experiences of labor. The abilities to breathe deeply and to consciously relax affect a woman's perception of pain. Trust, confidence, support, knowledge, and the ability to relax are all elements to strive for. A woman who is afraid, anxious, alone, angry, or ignorant of the birth process tends to fight her contractions and often has a longer, more troublesome labor.

SUPPLEMENTS

Electrolytes

Two studies document an inverse relationship between the intracellular electrolytes calcium, magnesium, and potassium and labor pain. As labor progressed, it was found that serum levels of each of these electrolytes fell and pain levels increased.[5, 6] Calcium assists with muscle action and nerve function. It has been known to decrease pain, especially that associated with muscle cramps. Magnesium acts as a catalyst in the use of nutrients, including calcium and potassium. Muscular excitability, nervousness, and tremors are symptoms of magnesium deficiency. Potassium is involved in the stimulation of late nerve impulses for muscle contraction. It also functions with calcium in the regulation of neuromuscular activity. This evidence begs the question of how the use of calcium, magnesium, and potassium supplements during labor might diminish the perception of pain. Anecdotal evidence suggests that these supplements may help.

Dosage. Calcium 2000 mg combined with magnesium 1000 mg orally as a one-time dosage[7] during labor. Electrolyte replacement drinks may also be used, such as Alacer's *Emergen-C, Gatorade,* or *Recharge.*

BOTANICALS

Red Raspberry Leaf (Rubus idaeus)

This leaf is considered to be a uterine tonic. There is some evidence of stimulation and relaxation of uterine muscle in animal studies.[8] Red raspberry leaf can assist the uterus toward achieving more powerful and effective uterine contractions with more complete uterine relaxation between contractions.[9] With complete uterine relaxation between contractions, a woman's perception of pain is diminished. No data exist on toxicity or teratogenicity. Red raspberry leaf is considered safe in pregnancy based on historical observation. Major components include tannins, flavonoids, and several minerals (including calcium, magnesium, and potassium).[10]

Preparation. Infusion (strong tea) is preferred. Tincture or capsules may not be concentrated enough. To make an infusion, steep 1 teaspoon of dry leaf in 1 cup of boiling water for up to 20 minutes.

Dosage. Drink 1 cup of tea (see previous paragraph) up to three times per day, starting at 37 weeks of gestation.

Motherwort (Leonurus cadiaca)

This herb has been used to decrease pain in labor because of its ability to enhance relaxation. It is also used for its uterine stimulant property.[11-13]

Preparation and dosage. Flowering tops from fresh plants preferred. It should be taken as a tincture, using 30 to 60 drops four times daily. One source recommends 5 drops in a glass of water; effects are noticeable within 20 minutes.

NOTE

Precaution: Motherwort may cause hyperstimulation of the uterus.

Skullcap (Scutellaria lateriflora)

Skullcap is a well-known remedy for all kinds of pain, including headaches, menstrual cramps, and labor pain. It acts as a sedative. Some practitioners add St. John's wort (*Hypericum perforatum*) or valerian (*Valeriana officinalis*) to complement skullcap's properties. There is no evidence of toxicity when skullcap is ingested in "normal" doses.[14] Skullcap does not interfere with uterine contractions.

Dosage. It should be taken as a tincture, using 3 to 12 drops in hot water. This may be repeated as often as desired. Other acceptable ways to ingest this herb include capsules and tea.

Precautions. Overdose may cause giddiness, stupor, confusion, twitching of the limbs, intermittent pulse, and symptoms of epilepsy.[14]

Warning. Watch for sedative effects.

BIOMECHANICAL TECHNIQUES

Massage

Massage and counterpressure techniques may help to relieve pain during labor. Studies reflect that massage during labor is associated with shorter labors, shorter hospital stays, decreased postpartum depression, and diminished anxiety and pain during labor.[15-17] Some women like to be touched or massaged or to receive counterpressure on the lower back during labor.

Different massage techniques can be used to provide pain relief to a woman. For example, effleurage is a featherlight massage of the abdomen with fingertips only. Some women prefer more pressure than just light fingertips during or between contractions. Foot massage with lotion or oil may feel wonderful to a laboring woman. Pressure points located on the foot can also enhance uterine contractions. Lower back and hip massage combined with counterpressure techniques is particularly helpful during back labor. Placing the woman on her hands and knees or in a kneeling position can enhance this type of massage. Encouraging her to do pelvic rocks helps prevent muscles from getting too tense and helps to rotate the baby. Have the woman tell her labor support person where the massage feels best. If counterpressure helps, have the woman say where pressure should be placed and how much pressure feels best.

Hydrotherapy

Showers, tubs, and Jacuzzis offer many women incredible pain relief during labor.[18, 19] Hospitals and birth centers are redesigning their labor and delivery units to include showers, Jacuzzis, or deep tubs. Businesses advertise delivery, setup, and taking down of birthing tubs, which may be used at home or in hospitals that allow them. Water birth has become increasingly popular and accepted across the country. Literature documents safe and positive outcomes for women and babies, as well as maternal satisfaction with the birth experience.[20-22] One of the benefits to a laboring woman of taking a shower or tub bath is that often these are provided in small, dark rooms, which may be helpful in balancing labor hormones and decreasing external stimulation, thereby hastening labor.

Application of Heat or Cold

Application of heat or cold is often used to alleviate pain during labor.[17] Both can reduce muscle spasms and increase a woman's pain threshold. Heat works by dilating blood vessels, thereby hastening removal of the painful metabolites of muscle work. Heat helps to relax muscles. Cold constricts blood vessels and slows the transmission of pain impulses along nerve pathways. It also causes numbness when applied to a particular area of the body.

Technique. Heat may be applied with a hot water bottle, a microwavable hot pack, a wet towel that is warmed in a microwave oven and wrapped up, a shower, or a bath. Cold may be applied as ice packs over the back or a cool washcloth on the neck, face, or chest.

Sterile Water Injections or Intradermal Water Blocks

This is a technique whereby sterile water is injected just under the woman's skin at four sites on her back. It is reported to alleviate back labor without any adverse effects.[17, 23] It is a simple, low-cost procedure that a woman's provider can easily do. Following these injections, however, massage or counterpressure over the injection sites should be avoided. The woman remains mobile. No intravenous equipment is necessary. One recent small study compared sterile water injections; transcutaneous electrical nerve stimulation (TENS); and massage, whirlpool bath, and liberal movement for alleviating the pain of back labor. Sterile water injections were found to be more effective than either of the other two therapies.[24]

Materials needed. Tuberculin syringe, 25-gauge needle, alcohol wipes, vial of sterile water, and ballpoint pen.

Technique. Draw up 0.4 mL of sterile water in a syringe. Palpate the posterior aspect of the superior iliac spines. Mark these two sites with a pen. Measure 3 cm down from, and 1 to 2 cm medial to, each of the first two sites and mark these sites. Swab sites with alcohol. Inject 0.05 to 0.1 mL of sterile water intradermally into each of the marked sites. This forms a bleb at the site.

NOTE

Warn the woman that the injections sting for about 20 seconds or less if the injections are given with a contraction. Good relief of back pain usually occurs in approximately 2 minutes and lasts 45 to 60 minutes for about 90% of women. These injections may be repeated as needed every 1 to 2 hours.

BIOENERGETICS

Transcutaneous Electrical Nerve Stimulation

TENS is the application of electrical current to the skin using flexible silicone electrodes placed on the skin in pairs at strategic sites. Small wires connect the electrodes to a stimulator that emits a continuous series of electrical pulses. The amplitude, frequency, and duration may be controlled. The sensation is described as "tingling, tickling, or buzzing, but pleasant." It works by sending electricity to the brain along faster myelinated fibers, compared with the transmission of pain sent along unmyelinated fiber pathways. Thus the brain receives the TENS sensation and not the message of pain. It is also thought that these impulses increase the endogenous beta-endorphins. TENS is often used to treat chronic pain associated with sports-related injuries or chronic back pain. Studies report none to moderate to good pain relief with TENS units used during labor.[3, 25] TENS units are not often found on labor and delivery units, although they may be particularly useful for women with back labor. There have been no reports of poor outcomes for mothers or babies when TENS units have been used.

Technique. Place electrodes in two pairs on either side of a woman's spine. One pair goes near her waist to effect pain relief during the first stage of labor. The other pair is placed at the base of her spine for relief during the second stage of labor.

MIND-BODY THERAPY

Hypnosis/Visualization/Guided Imagery

People deal with pain in many different ways. Some find benefit in techniques such as hypnosis, visualization, or guided imagery.[26] These techniques may allow them to escape or be distracted from their pain. Imagery encourages them to imagine that they are somewhere else, more relaxed. Others may find these techniques annoying and not helpful because they want to embrace or surrender to their pain, rather than being told to pretend that they are on a beach. Visualization can be a powerful technique for some women as they visualize their cervix opening and the baby descending, with soft and bony tissues getting out of the way. Women can purchase and listen to hypnosis and visualization tapes during their pregnancy to prepare for labor and birth. These tapes can also be used during labor.

An important fact is that labor is controlled by the primitive part of a woman's brain, as it is in other mammals. This makes her extremely sensitive to stimulation, interruption, conversation, bright lights, crowded rooms, and so forth, because these functions engage her neocortex or forebrain. Stimulation of the forebrain may play a role in creating hormonal imbalance. Any time hypnosis, guided imagery, or visualization is used, particular attention should be paid to whether this is interrupting or supporting labor. Many women who maintain hormonal balance during labor appear to be in a trance-like state near the end of labor when these techniques are not used.

Music Therapy

Research on music therapy and birth indicates that music has a positive influence on metabolic rate, heart rate, blood pressure, and other bodily functions.[27] It can relax, soothe, and diminish anxiety. Studies have been done documenting the benefits to patients of listening to music with headphones during such procedures as surgeries and dental work. Listening to music during labor can be calming to a woman.[28] It may help her tune in to her breathing and her own natural rhythms. Music can also be a distraction, enabling her to tune out the rest of the world (including the laboring woman who is screaming next door). Many labor units now provide music players to laboring women.

Aromatherapy

Aromatherapy used during labor provides yet another way of stimulating a woman's central nervous system to compete with nerve impulses that transmit pain. Limited research has shown that women perceive that aromatherapy is helpful, and it decreases a woman's need for medication.[29] This can be just as useful as the stimuli of sound (music) and touch (massage, TENS, acupuncture). Documented adverse effects include nausea, itchy rash, headache, and rapid labor. None of these events is associated with adverse outcomes for mothers or babies.

Some suggested aromatherapies include rose (*Rosa centifolia*), jasmine (*Jasminum grandiflorum*), chamomile (*Chamaemelum nobile*), lemon (*Citrus limonum*), eucalyptus (*Eucalyptus globulus*), mandarin (*Citrus reticulata*), clary sage (*Salvia sclarea*), frankincense (*Boswellia carteri*), lavender (*Lavandula angustifolium*), and peppermint (*Mentha piperita*). Many other essential herbal oils can be used as well.

Aromatherapy can be applied using drops of essential oil diluted with vegetable oil as a foot massage or bath, drops in bath water, or simply oil rubbed on a washcloth or pillow and placed near the laboring woman.

Caution. Use of undiluted essential oils may cause skin irritation and is toxic if ingested.

LIFESTYLE/BEHAVIOR

Childbirth Preparation

Many types of childbirth education classes offer women and their partners important information about pregnancy, birth, postpartum events motherhood, newborn care, and breastfeeding. Some classes focus on relaxation and breathing exercises to reduce pain; others briefly discuss this and focus on giving parents much information on the entire experience, including many ways to reduce pain during labor and the risks and benefits of these methods, techniques, or medications. Some women find that being informed diminishes their anxiety and fear, and thus perceptions of pain, and makes it easier for them to think about how they would like to labor—with or without medications, for example. It is hoped that classes will encourage women to surrender to their experience, instead of having expectations that lead to a sense of failure.

Providers should encourage women to take classes and to be informed. Providing women with a list of classes or instructors may be helpful as well.

Supportive Environment/Family/ Care Providers

Many well-implemented studies document positive outcomes, that is, shorter labors, less medical intervention, and more satisfying birth experience, for women who labor with the support of a doula.[30, 31] In general, women experience less fear and anxiety if they labor in supportive environments, where they feel safe; have providers in whom they trust; and receive the active involvement and support of partners or family members. Remember that controlling fear and anxiety is key to surrendering, achieving hormonal balance, and managing pain.

Freedom of Movement and Position

All too often, women in this country are restricted to laboring in bed. Although some would elect to labor in this position, women usually say that laboring in bed is much more painful than ambulating, standing, kneeling, using a birthing ball or stool, or squatting. Changing positions helps to open the pelvis and rotate the baby.[17] Gravity in an upright position assists with fetal descent. Movement also alleviates discomforts that are associated with staying in one position for too long. Regional anesthesia can prohibit many positions.

Informed Choice/Maternal Autonomy

As with all issues of labor and birth, women and their partners should always be included in the decision-making process around issues of labor and birth pain. Remember that the mere suggestion of the need to "manage" pain may be a self-fulfilling prophecy. With great care and sensitivity, these options, risks, and benefits should be explored as part of prenatal care. At times, fetal concerns or labor progress may influence options for pain relief. This may be distressing to the woman who is in pain, or to her partner who is having a hard time witnessing her pain. Careful explanation, informed consent, and documentation remain important.

PHARMACEUTICALS

An understanding of pharmacologic options is critical to any discussion of pain during labor and birth. Optimally these conversations should take place prenatally so that women are adequately informed of the risks and benefits of, and alternatives to, drug therapies. The following discussion includes three different categories of pharmaceutical use: therapeutic rest, analgesia, and regional anesthesia.

Therapeutic Rest

A woman may experience contractions for hours or even days without being in active labor. This can happen with nulliparous and multiparous pregnant women. A woman may become emotionally and physically exhausted before active labor even begins. Rest can be encouraged in a variety of ways. A warm bath combined with some herbal teas may relax a woman enough for her to get some sleep. However, it is common practice to offer medications for therapeutic rest.

Benadryl (diphenhydramine)

This is an agent that may be useful for therapeutic rest. Women have easy access to this medication and generally experience few adverse effects. Its Pregnancy Category Rating is B, with no documented evidence of fetal toxicity in humans.
Dosage. Oral tablet/capsule, 25 to 50 mg. Take before sleep, may repeat as soon as 6 hours after first dose.

Seconal (secobarbital) and Nembutal (pentobarbital)

These are commonly used for therapeutic rest. They do cross the placenta and have a long half-life. Some women say that they are able to sleep when they take these medications. Others complain that they feel groggy and "hung over," and are unable to sleep.

Dosage. Oral tablet of either secobarbital or pentobarbital, 100 mg. Take one tablet before bedtime. May repeat once if not asleep in 30 minutes.

Morphine sulfate (MS)

Morphine is the most effective drug used for therapeutic rest. It is a narcotic and can be administered either IV or IM. It often induces several hours of sleep and a perception of decreased pain. The uterus sometimes continues to contract and a woman's cervix may dilate while she sleeps under MS. One may see decreased variability in the fetal heart rate (FHR) tracing due to fetal sleep.
Dosage. IM injection, 10 mg. Dose may be individualized based on clinical picture.
Precaution. Beware maternal respiratory depression.

Analgesia

Analgesics are medications that are given for pain relief. In labor pain management, narcotics (opiates) are most commonly used. Data indicate that these drugs do not actually reduce or relieve pain in labor but rather change a woman's perception of pain and make it more tolerable.[32, 33] All of these drugs have similar adverse effects, including dry mouth, sluggish bowels, and urinary retention. Some may cause nausea, vomiting, dizziness, and respiratory depression.

Several important facts should be considered when one is deciding whether or not to use analgesics during labor. If given too early, they can stop or slow labor. Repeated doses do not seem to work as well as initial doses. One must be aware that analgesics do cross the placenta and that the FHR tracing may show decreased variability. If there is any concern regarding an FHR tracing, narcotics may be contraindicated. In addition, narcotics given close to the time of birth (i.e., within 2 to 3 hours) may cause respiratory depression in the newborn. Finally, one must exercise caution when administering opiates that are partial opiate antagonists as they may induce acute withdrawal symptoms in women who have a history of drug abuse.

Some commonly used narcotics are discussed in the following sections.

Stadol (butorphanol)

Dosage is 0.5 to 1 mg IV or 0.5 to 2 mg IM. May be repeated every 2 to 4 hours. Stadol has opiate antagonist properties. Caution is advised when administering it to women who have a history of substance abuse.

Nubain (nalbuphine)

Dosage is 5 to 15 mg IM or IV. May be repeated every 2 to 4 hours. Maximum dose is 160 mg over 24 hours.

Sublimaze (fentanyl)

Dosage is 50 mcg IV. This dose may be repeated every 15 to 20 minutes, until a loading dose of 200 mcg is given in the first hour. This is often the drug of choice if a woman is in active labor and the birth is anticipated soon. It has a quick onset (5 minutes) and short duration (30 to 60 minutes).

Regional Anesthesia

Anesthesia is the use of various techniques designed to provide pain relief. Analgesia is one form of anesthesia (see previous section). Several other techniques can also be used during labor, including pudendal nerve blocks, continuous lumbar epidurals (CLEs), and intrathecal anesthesia (IA).

Pudendal blocks may be used for operative vaginal deliveries or with a woman for whom the very end of second stage is overwhelming. The birth attendant generally administers them. Unfortunately, the effectiveness of this nerve block varies widely.

Epidurals may provide complete regional anesthesia for the laboring mother. If a cesarean birth becomes necessary, the CLE may be adjusted to provide anesthesia for the surgery.

Few areas of the care of pregnant women are as controversial as the use of labor epidurals.[34, 35] Although it is true that CLEs often provide excellent pain relief from labor and may even be useful in the treatment of some labor complications, significant concern accompanies their use. These concerns include the following[35-37]:

Risks of catheter placement and medications
Effects on progression of labor
Limitation of maternal mobility
Effects on maternal experience of labor and birth

Maternal and fetal morbidity (urinary retention, elevated temperature, hypotension, fetal intolerance of labor)
Cascade of intervention

Remember that epidurals decrease the quantity of beta-endorphins in laboring women[1, 3] which means that turning down the CLE to assist with second-stage labor results in fewer circulating endogenous opiates; thus labor pain may be far more excruciating than in someone who has not had an epidural.

Intrathecals (IAs) are another regional anesthetic technique. Sometimes called "walking epidurals," IAs have a shorter duration than epidurals, enabling women to have increased mobility and sensation for the second stage of delivery. Fewer operative vaginal deliveries may occur with IAs for this reason.[38] An increased risk for respiratory depression during the first 24 hours after the birth has been noted.

THERAPIES TO CONSIDER

Acupuncture

Good evidence is found in the literature to suggest that acupuncture alleviates pain during labor.[17, 39, 40] Acupuncture may work to relieve pain during labor by activating the body's own painkillers, such as endorphins, enkephalins, serotonin, and other neurotransmitters associated with pain relief.[17] It has been used as anesthesia during surgery. Many more hospitals are developing and instituting integrated therapy programs, including acupuncturists who are available to women during labor and delivery. Some hospitals allow a woman to bring an acupuncturist into the hospital to assist her during labor and birth.

Homeopathy

Homeopathic remedies have been used historically during labor, but there is little clinical data to support their efficacy.[41, 42] Consultation with a homeopath is encouraged for those who wish to explore this option further.

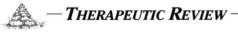 ── *THERAPEUTIC REVIEW* ─────────────────────────────

For most women, labor is an incredibly painful process characterized by a power and force that completely takes over her body. This can be frightening and overwhelming, and incredibly satisfying for many women in the end. It is a rite of passage that involves going to a deeper place within her body than ever before. It is not for us to determine how a woman "should" get through her labor. It is up to us to be a guardian of mother and baby throughout labor, and to inform her of her options along the way. Birth attendants need to trust in the process of birth and must be willing to support each woman in the way that she needs.

| Provide information and education during pregnancy | Planning ahead: Childbirth classes, recommended books, supportive prenatal visits, and discussion and development of plan for pain management and birth. Time to build relationship based on trust. |

THERAPEUTIC REVIEW continued

Assessment of hopes and dreams for birth	Does she want to try to avoid the use of pharmaceuticals or does she fully intend to have a medicated birth? Has she considered options for an integrated approach? Nonjudgmental support is optimal.
Reassessment of her needs in labor	Is it safe and reasonable to support her "hopes and dreams" for this birth? Is it still what she wants? Does she need more information?
Be present	The presence of birth attendants improves outcomes, decreases length of labor, and minimizes interventions. Your presence is reassuring and gives her confidence.
Choosing unmedicated birth	Support. Support. Support. Hydrotherapy, freedom of movement, massage, aromatherapy, visualization, music, sterile water injections for back labor, heat, supplements, acupuncture, TENS as available, botanicals as available.
Choosing medicated birth	Consider what options are safe and when they are optimally administered. Do benefits outweigh risks? If contraindicated, consider alternatives.
After the birth	A woman's experience of birth and the associated pain may leave her with unresolved feelings and concerns. Be open. Listening to these issues is also part of "managing" her pain.

References

1. Gabbe S, Niebyl J, Simpson J (eds): Obstetrics: Normal and Problem Pregnancies. New York, Churchill Livingstone, 1991.
2. Oxorn H: Human Labor and Birth. Norwalk, Conn, Appleton-Century-Crofts, 1986.
3. Lieberman A: Easing Labor Pain: The Complete Guide to a More Comfortable and Rewarding Birth. Boston, Massachusetts, The Harvard Common Press, 1987.
4. Melzack R, Wall P: The Challenge of Pain. New York, Basic Books, 1983.
5. Weissberg N, Schwartz G, Shemesh O, et al: Serum and intracellular electrolytes in patients with and without pain. Magnes Res 4(1):49–52, 1991.
6. Weissberg N, Schwartz G, Shemesh O, et al: Serum and mononuclear cell potassium, magnesium, sodium and calcium in pregnancy and labour and their relation to uterine muscle contraction. Magnes Res 5(3):173–177, 1992.
7. Weed S: Wise Woman Herbal Childbearing Year. New York, Ash Tree Publishing, 1986.
8. Raspberry. In Facts and Comparisons. The Review of Natural Products, June 1999. St. Louis, Facts and Comparisons, a Wolters Kluwer Company, 1999.
9. Bamford DS, Percivil RC, Tothill AU: Raspberry leaf tea: A new aspect to an old problem. Br Pharmacol 40:161–162, 1970.
10. Bergner P: The mineral content of herbal decoctions. Med Herb 9(2):6–9, 1997.
11. Zhang CF, Jia YS, Wei HC, et al: Studies on actions of extract of motherwort. J Tradit Chin Med 2(4):267–270, 1982.
12. Newell CA, Anderson LA, Phillipson JD: Herbal Medicines: Guide for Health Care Professionals. London, The Pharmaceutical Press, 1996.
13. Bradley P (ed): British Herbal Compendium: A Handbook of Scientific Information on Widely Used Plant Drugs. Dorset, England, British Herbal Medicine Association, 1992.
14. Skullcap In Facts and Comparisons The Review of Natural Products, May 1998. St. Louis, Facts and Comparisons, a Wolters Kluwer Company, 1998.
15 Field T, Hernandez-Reif M, Taylor S, et al: Labor pain is reduced by massage therapy. J Psychosom Obstet Gynaecol 18(4):286–291, 1997.
16. Keenan P: Benefits of massage therapy and use of a doula during labor and childbirth. Altern Ther Health Med 6(1):66–74, 2000.
17. Simkin P: Reducing pain and enhancing progress in labor: A guide to nonpharmacologic methods for maternity caregivers. Birth 22(3):161–171, 1995.
18. Rush J, Burlock S, Lambert K, et al: The effects of whirlpool baths in labor: A randomized, controlled trial. Birth 23(3):136–143, 1996.
19. Aird IA, Luckas MJ, Buckett WM, Bousfield P: Effects of intrapartum hydrotherapy on labour related parameters. Aust N Z J Obstet Gynaecol 37(2):137–142, 1997.
20. Nikodem VC: Immersion in water in pregnancy, labour, and birth. Cochrane Database Syst Rev 2:CD000111, 2000.
21. Aird IA, Luckas ML, Buckett WM, Bousfield P: Effects of intrapartum hydrotherapy on labour related parameters. Aust N Z J Obstet Gynaecol 37(2):137–142, 1997.
22. Newman A: Perinatal mortality and morbidity among babies delivered in water: Surveillance study and postal study. J. Midwifery Women's Health 45(4):362–363, 2000.
23. Ader L, Hansson B, Wallin G: Parturition pain treated by intracutaneous injections of sterile water. Pain 41:133–138, 1990.
24. Labrecque M, Nouwen A, Bergeron M, Rancourt JF: A randomized controlled trial of nonpharmacologic approaches for relief of low back pain during labor. J Fam Pract 48(4):259–263, 1999.
25. Carroll D, Tramer M, McQuay H, et al: Transcutaneous electrical nerve stimulation in labour pain: A systematic review. Br J Obstet Gynaecol 104:169–175, 1997.
26. Oster MI: Psychological preparation for labor and delivery using hypnosis. Am J Clin Hyp 37(1):12–21, 1994.
27. Geden EA, Lower M, Beattie S, Beck N: Effects of music and imagery on physiologic and self-report of analogued labor pain. Nurs Res 38(1):37–41, 1989.
28. Clark ME, McCorkie RR, Williams SB: Music therapy-assisted labor and delivery. J Music Ther 18(2):88–100, 1981.
29. Burns EE, Blamey C, Ersser S, et al: An investigation into the use of aromatherapy in intrapartum midwifery practice. J Altern Compliment Med 6(2):141–147, 2000.
30. Kennell J, Klaus M, McGrath S: Continuous emotional support during labor in a US hospital: A randomized controlled trial. JAMA 265(17):2197–2201, 1991.
31. McNiven P, Hodnett E, O'Brien-Pallas LL: Supporting women in labor: A work sampling study of the activities of labor and delivery nurses. Birth 19(1):3–7, 1992.
32. Sullivan N: Pain relief during labor and delivery. Available at *www.midwifeinfo.com/topic/painrelief.html*, 2000.

33. Faucher MA, Brucker MC: Intrapartum Pain: Pharmacologic Management. J Obstet Gynecol Neonatal Nurs 29:169–180, 2000.
34. Enkin M, Keirse MJNC, et al: A Guide to Effective Care in Pregnancy and Childbirth, 3rd ed. Oxford, Oxford University Press, 2000.
35. England P, Horowitz R: Birthing from Within. Albuquerque, NM, Partera Press, 1998.
36. Mander R: Analgesia and anesthesia in childbirth: Obscurantism and obfuscation. J Adv Nurs 28:86–93, 1998.
37. McCrea H: Satisfaction in childbirth and perceptions of personal control in pain relief during labor. J Adv Nurs 29(4):877–884, 1999.
38. Kurokawa JS, Zilkoski MW: Use of intrathecal analgesia in a rural hospital. Nurse Midwifery 41(4):338–342, 1996.
39. Chez R, Jonas W: Complementary and alternative medicine. Part 1: Clinical studies in obstetrics. Obstet Gynecol Surv 52(11):704–708, 1997.
40. Ternov K, Nilsson M, Lofberg L, et al: Acupuncture for pain relief during childbirth. Acupunct Electrother Res 23(1):19–26, 1998.
41. Cummings B: Empowering women: Homeopathy in midwifery practice. Complement Ther Nurs Midwifery 4(1):13–16, 1998.
42. Katz T: The management of pregnancy and labour with homeopathy. Complement Ther Nurs Midwifery 1(6):159–164, 1995.

CHAPTER 43

Nausea and Vomiting in Pregnancy

Ann L. Mattson M.D., F.A.C.O.G., and Steffie Goodman, C.N.M., M.S.N.

PATHOPHYSIOLOGY

Nausea and vomiting are common symptoms in early pregnancy, especially among women of Western cultures. In the United States, 60% to 80% of pregnant women experience some nausea with or without vomiting during pregnancy. Symptoms are usually mild and self-limiting, often disappearing by the 14th week of pregnancy.

The exact physiologic mechanism of these symptoms in pregnancy is very poorly understood. Suggested etiologies include a combination of biologic and psychologic factors. Most consistently recognized is the apparent relationship between elevated levels of human chorionic gonadotropin (HCG) and increased symptoms of nausea and vomiting. Symptoms often parallel the rise in HCG and are more frequent in pregnancies with unusual elevations of HCG (e.g., molar gestation, multiple gestations). Other hormones may also play a role, including thyroid, progesterone, and adrenal hormones. Ulti-

mately, one or several of these factors appear to be altering the central emetic threshold in the chemoreceptive trigger zone of the brain.

Although little is known about nausea and vomiting specific to pregnancy, some things are known about the physiologic mechanisms of nausea and vomiting in general. Noxious stimuli to peripheral receptors for 5-hydroxytryptamine (5-HT), especially in the digestive tract, cause the release of serotonin, which in turn activates visceral afferent nerves. These nerves terminate primarily in the brainstem, which contains the chemoreceptive trigger zone (Fig. 43–1). Agents circulating in the bloodstream can also activate this area.[1, 2] Hence, both local and systemic factors probably play a role in the development of nausea and vomiting.

Psychological factors have also been associated with nausea and vomiting. It is unclear whether this may be attributed to biochemical alterations, stress responses, or other mechanisms. There does appear to be an increased incidence of nausea and vomiting

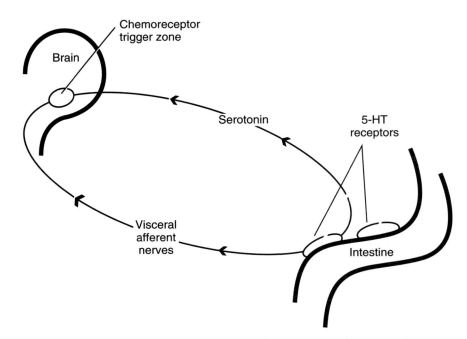

Figure 43-1. Location of visceral afferent nerves in the brainstem, which contains the chemoreceptive trigger zone. 5-HT, 5-hydroxytryptamine.

during pregnancy with certain personality disorders and adjustment disorders, but data examining these factors have been inconclusive.[3]

Hyperemesis gravidarum is the most severe form of nausea and vomiting associated with pregnancy and is seen in only about 1% to 3% of pregnant women. The diagnosis of hyperemesis is based on intractable nausea and vomiting, dehydration, weight loss, electrolyte imbalance, and ketonuria. Hyperemesis is most common in first pregnancies and white women. There also seems to be an association with certain psychological and social factors such as stress, marital status, age, and personality type. Hyperemesis may result in severe medical sequelae and, rarely, death.

LIFESTYLE

Modify the Environment

Many women find that certain odors may trigger their nausea. Avoiding strong odors such as cigarette smoke, cooking odors, and perfumes may be helpful.

Modify the Diet

These measures may seem simple but are frequently the most helpful in relieving symptoms. The underlying premise is to maintain a steady blood sugar level (avoiding hypoglycemia). At the same time, avoiding any foods that may trigger nausea and increasing intake of foods that contain helpful B vitamins may provide additional benefit.

NOTE

Specific dietary guidelines: Eliminate greasy, spicy foods. Eat small, frequent meals (at least every 2 hours). Try protein-rich snacks before bed. Always carry nutritious food/snacks. Increase intake of foods with vitamin B_6 (whole grains, wheat germ, nuts, seeds). Avoid caffeine and stay hydrated.

Rest

Fatigue may contribute to feelings of nausea and vomiting during pregnancy. Women may also need to be encouraged to get help with their daily activities and responsibilities until they feel better.

Exercise

Sometimes a simple routine of regular walking or other light to moderate exercise can be helpful in decreasing symptoms of nausea and vomiting. It can also help lessen fatigue and constipation. Eating a small snack before exercise reduces the chance of hypoglycemia.

SUPPLEMENTS

Vitamin B_6 (Pyridoxine). This supplement has been empirically recommended for the treatment of nausea and vomiting (N&V) of pregnancy for more than 45 years. The exact mechanism of this benefit is unknown, but there are now several good studies that prove its effectiveness. Most recently, Niebyl and associates showed a cessation of N&V in 74% of treated gravidas versus 46% of controls.[4] B_6 appears to be most effective in those women with moderate to severe N&V and may be more effective in reducing nausea than in decreasing the actual number of vomiting episodes. No toxicity or adverse effects are noted at recommended dosages. There were allegations in the United States in the 1970s and 1980s of possible teratogenic effects of B_6 in combination with doxylamine (Bendectin). These allegations were never substantiated, and numerous studies have failed to show any teratogenicity of either compound.[4]

Dosage. 50 mg, once or twice daily. Therapy may start as soon as symptoms of N&V develop, and it may continue as needed until they resolve.

Prenatal Vitamins. These are not directly helpful for N&V, although the B_6 present in most formulations may mitigate these symptoms for some women (please see earlier discussion). Unfortunately, for many women, prenatal vitamins may actually exacerbate symptoms of N&V. Using a different brand or route (e.g., chewable, liquid) may help. Also, varying the time of consumption may help—many women seem to find bedtime an optimal time of day for taking their prenatal vitamins. There also is a newer formulation on the market called Premesis Tx containing B_6, B_{12}, folic acid, and calcium, which may be tried in lieu of more traditional prenatal vitamin formulations.

BIOENERGETICS

Acupuncture

The treatment of N&V during pregnancy is one of the most well-documented uses of acupuncture in Western literature. Several studies have been done, including some randomized trials that demonstrate the efficacy of stimulation of the pericardium 6 (P6) Neiguan point.[5] Both acupressure and acupuncture (with or without electrical stimulation) have been shown to be efficacious in reducing nausea and actual vomiting episodes. No reports of adverse effects have been noted. (See Chapter 101, Acupuncture for Nausea and Vomiting.) Acupressure bands offer the benefits of being inexpensive and safe to use without professional referral.[6]

Technique. Apply acupressure wristbands (Sea-Band) to wrists following manufacturer's instructions as soon as symptoms of N&V develop.

MIND-BODY THERAPY

Hypnosis

Hypnotherapy has shown the capacity to affect physiologic changes that were once thought beyond voluntary control. Several studies have documented the efficacy of hypnosis for the treatment of nausea and vomiting during pregnancy.[7] Although limited by study design, these studies do show a trend toward significant clinical benefit. In one study, 88% of women with recalcitrant hyperemesis gravidarum stopped vomiting within 3 sessions of hypnotherapy.[8] Hypnosis may be considered an initial intervention, because of both its potential efficacy and its lack of adverse effects. It can also be used to address underlying psychological issues.

Technique. Refer client for consultation with an accredited hypnotherapist. The following web sites may be helpful: www.ASCH.net and www.healingmindbody.com. Training opportunities for interested providers are also noted at the ASCH site.

Counseling and Psychotherapy

Psychological associations with nausea and vomiting of pregnancy have long been recognized. This seems to be particularly evident in women with severe or protracted symptoms.[9] It may be useful to encourage women to explore this possibility through journaling or supportive counseling. For some women, psychiatric evaluation may be both necessary and therapeutic.

BOTANICALS

Red Raspberry Leaf (*Rubus idaeus*)

In addition to its uses as a uterine tonic, raspberry leaf has been widely used in early pregnancy for decreasing nausea. There are no data on toxicity or teratogenicity. It is considered safe in pregnancy based on historical observation. Major components include tannins, flavonoids, and several minerals (including calcium, magnesium, and potassium).[10]

Preparation. Infusion (strong tea) is preferred. Tincture or capsules may not be concentrated enough. To make an infusion, steep 1 teaspoon dry leaf in 1 cup of boiling water for up to 20 minutes.

Dosage. Drink 1 cup of tea (see previously) up to three times per day.

Peppermint Leaf (*Mentha piperita*)

Peppermint oil has been shown to act as an antispasmodic agent on smooth muscle.[11] Other data have indicated that this effect may be secondary to menthol's effects as a calcium antagonist.[11] Widely used historically for the treatment of morning sickness, peppermint leaf is also generally considered safe for oral ingestion in small quantities.

Dosage. Drink 1 cup of tea first thing in the morning. Tea may be prepared using fresh or dried peppermint leaves. Commercial preparations (Celestial Seasonings) may also be used. Caution would be advised regarding GI reflux and peppermint tea in pregnancy. Recommending peppermint oil in enteric-coated capsules can avoid the potential side effect and still have a beneficial effect without relaxing the lower esophageal sphincter.

Dose. 0.2 to 0.4 ml in enteric coated capsules taken three times daily between meals.

Ginger Root (*Zingiber officinale*)

Clinical trials have documented the effectiveness and safety of ginger in the treatment of motion sickness, perioperative nausea, and hyperemesis gravidarum.[12] Animal studies indicate that it may have both an effect in the gastrointestinal tract (anti-5-HT) and a direct central nervous system effect.[13] Historically, ginger has a long record of use, effectiveness, and safety in midwifery practice As compared with placebo, it is significantly more effective in reducing symptoms of hyperemesis gravidarum without notable adverse effects.[14] Although the German Commission E contraindicates ginger during pregnancy, there are no data to suggest any toxicity in pregnancy. Indeed, the Food and Drug Administration (FDA) has listed ginger as a food supplement that is generally recognized as safe (GRAS).[15]

Dosage. Make infusion using grated fresh ginger root, about 1 teaspoon ginger to 1 cup of hot water. Sip as tolerated. Drink no more than 3 cups per day. Ginger may also be consumed in other forms (including candied, pickled, snaps, tincture, and capsules). Regardless of form, the equivalent of 1 g of ginger per day is a reasonable dosage limit.

Precautions. With high levels of consumption (greater than 2 g per day), there may be an associated anticoagulant effect.

Chamomile (*Matricaria chamomilla*)

Chamomile has been used as an herbal remedy since Roman times. It has been known as both a sedative and a gastrointestinal antispasmodic agent. The primary active component appears to be bisabolol, a lipophilic compound.[16] There are no clinical trials to date on its efficacy for morning sickness. Anecdotal data would suggest that it is safe and occasionally helpful.

Dosage. Commercially prepared tea (Celestial Seasonings); sip as tolerated up to 3 to 4 cups per day.

Precautions. Beware of severe hypersensitivity reactions in those people allergic to ragweed/asters/chrysanthemums. Chamomile should not be used in persons taking anticoagulants.

PHARMACEUTICALS

Pharmaceutical treatment of nausea and vomiting in pregnancy should be reserved for those women in whom more conservative measures have been insufficient. Significant concerns also remain about fetal effects of many of these medications.

Pseudoephedrine (Sudafed)

This decongestant and smooth muscle stimulant is considered safe for use during pregnancy. Anecdotal evidence has found it useful for treating those women whose predominant symptom is ptyalism (spitting/excessive salivation). Pregnancy Category C.

Dosage. Give 30 to 60 mg orally every 4 to 6 hours as needed.

Antihistamines

Antihistamines are clinically efficacious despite an unknown mechanism of action. No evidence of teratogenicity has been found in controlled trials. The major adverse effect is drowsiness. Both of these medications are Pregnancy Category B.

Diphenhydramine (Benadryl)—25 to 50 mg orally every 8 hours.

Doxylamine (Unisom)—12.5 mg orally at bedtime and in the morning as needed. May be taken in conjunction with vitamin B_6.

Phenothiazines

Generally reserved for inpatient management of hyperemesis gravidarum, these drugs may also be useful in the short term for outpatient therapy. There have been isolated reports of fetal effects with chlorpromazine, but larger studies of promethazine and prochlorperazine have shown them to be both efficacious and free of fetal effects.[3] These latter two medications are both Pregnancy Category C. Adverse effects with these medications can be substantial and include orthostatic hypotension, sedation, tremor, extrapyramidal symptoms, dystonic reactions, and skin reactions.

Prochlorperazine (Compazine)—10-mg tablet orally every 8 hours, or 25-mg rectal suppository every 8 hours.

Promethazine (Phenergan)—25-mg tablet orally every 8 hours, or 25-mg rectal suppository every 8 hours.

Metoclopramide (Reglan)

Metoclopramide is a dopamine agonist that has been used in early pregnancy without evidence of fetal effects.[3] It increases gastrointestinal mobility and has documented efficacy as compared with placebo.[3] Adverse effects are similar to phenothiazines. Pregnancy Category B.

Dosage. 5- to 10-mg tablet orally, up to three times per day, before meals.

Ondansetron (Zofran)

A potent antiemetic that works as a 5-HT receptor antagonist. There have been no reported fetal effects, although data are limited. In efficacy trials, it has been comparable to promethazine,[3] although far better tolerated. Adverse effects include headache, fever, and gastrointestinal upset. Pregnancy Category C.

Dosage. 4-mg tablet, $\frac{1}{2}$ to 1 tablet orally every 8 hours as needed.

SURGERY

Therapeutic Abortion

There are times when the severity of nausea and vomiting/hyperemesis may be so severe that there is an actual threat of maternal disability and/or death. In these rare circumstances, it is reasonable to consider therapeutic abortion as a healing choice. Symptoms of hyperemesis resolve quickly after termination of a pregnancy. Actual techniques are beyond the scope of this publication.

THERAPIES TO CONSIDER

Homeopathy

Several remedies have been used in the treatment of morning sickness. These include *Arsenicum, Colchicum, Ipecac, Nux Vomica, Phosphorus, Pulsatilla,* and *Sepia.* Appropriate remedy selection is best done by a practitioner with extensive training in homeopathy. Homeopathic remedies may provide an excellent option for those women whose symptoms are relatively mild and who do not want to risk the use of pharmaceuticals or botanicals.

Traditional Chinese Medicine

In addition to acupuncture (see earlier discussion), traditional Chinese medicine (TCM) consultation may be useful in the treatment of nausea and vomiting. Particularly interesting are Chinese herbal approaches to these symptoms.

THERAPEUTIC REVIEW

Nausea and vomiting are symptoms commonly associated with early pregnancy. They are so common, in fact, as to be considered by many part of the normal course of pregnancy. Some have even hypothesized that this may be a mechanism for protecting the mother and embryo by causing her to avoid potentially harmful foods during the time of organogenesis.[17] In any case, the primary therapeutic goal is relief of symptoms with minimal risk to mom and baby.

Consider differential diagnosis	Although diagnosis is usually apparent, symptoms may be confused with other gastrointestinal disorders, including esophageal reflux and gastroenteritis.
Lifestyle modification	Avoid foods and odors that trigger nausea/vomiting. Get plenty of rest and try to maintain some exercise. Stay hydrated and follow dietary guidelines to avoid hypoglycemia.
Supplements	Try taking prenatal vitamin at bedtime. Vitamin B_6, 50 mg twice daily.
Acupressure	Start wearing 2 acupressure wristbands as soon as symptoms develop.
Botanicals	Try as needed for symptoms that persist despite previous therapies. Selection of tea is somewhat arbitrary, but may be based on maternal taste preferences and experienced efficacy. Ginger tea, 2 to 3 cups per day, may be most effective.
Pharmaceuticals	Start with antihistamines. The combination of doxylamine (Unisom) 12.5 mg with vitamin B_6 50 mg is often quite effective.
	If this measure is insufficient and there is evidence of worsening maternal symptoms, a trial with one of the phenothiazines may be necessary. Phenergan 25 mg given orally if possible (or rectally if not) often prevents further worsening of symptoms. For women who experience adverse effects with the phenothiazines, Reglan (5 mg every 8 hours) or Zofran (2 mg every 8 hours) should be considered.
Hospital admission	Women who develop hyperemesis gravidarum generally require hospital admission for both supportive and therapeutic treatment. Intravenous hydration is a mainstay of therapy. In addition, more intensive pharmaceutical therapy may be started. Women who require nutritional support (parenteral nutrition) may also be accommodated in the hospital setting.
	Although hyperemesis is a serious complication of pregnancy, an integrated approach as outlined previously may allow for shorter hospitalizations and a decreased need for potentially more risky interventions.

References

1. Lang IM: Noxious stimulation of emesis. Dig Dis Sci 44 (8 suppl):58S–63S, 1999.
2. Bremerkamp M: Mechanism of action of 5-HT3 receptor antagonists: Clinical overview and nursing implications. Clin J Oncol Nurs 4(5):201–207, 2000.
3. Peleg D, Jothivijayarani, Hypermesis in pregnancy. In Sciarra J., (ed): Gynecology and Obstetrics. Philadelphia, Lippincott Williams & Wilkins, 1999, pp 1–6.
4. Johnson H: Vitamin B6 can reduce nausea in pregnancy. Ob Gyn News January 1, 2001:10.
5. Chez R, Jones W: Complementary and alternative medicine. Part 1 Clinical studies in obstetrics. Obstet Gynecol Surv 52:704–708, 1997.
6. Stainton MC, Neff EJ: The efficacy of SeaBands for the control of nausea and vomiting in pregnancy. Health Care Women Int 15:563–575, 1994.
7. Simon E, Schwartz J: Medical hypnosis for hyperemesis gravidarum. Birth 26:248–254, 1999.
8. Fuchs K, Paldi E, Abramovici H, Peretz, BA: Treatment of hyperemesis gravidarum by hypnosis. Int J Clin Exp Hypn 28:312–323, 1980.
9. Murray M, Pizzorno J: Nausea and vomiting of pregnancy. In Textbook of Natural Medicine. New York, Churchill Livingstone, 1999, 1425–1427.
10. Bergner P: The mineral content of herbal decoctions. Med Herb 6–9, 1997.
11. Peppermint. In Facts and Comparisons The Review of Natural

Products, July 1990. St Louis, Facts and Comparisons, a Wolters Kluwer Company, 1990.

12. Ginger. In Facts and Comparisons The Review of Natural Products, May 2000. St Louis, Facts and Comparisons, a Wolters Kluwer Company, 2000.

13. Lumb A: Mechanism of antiemetic effect of ginger. Anesthesia 48(12):1118, 1993.

14. Fischer-Rasmussen W, Kjaer S, Dahl C, Asping U: Ginger treatment of hyperemesis gravidarum. Eur J Obstet Gynecol Reprod Biol, 38:19–24, 1990.

15. Food and Drug Administration, Department of Health and Human Services. Code of Federal Regulations, 21CFR182.10.

16. Chamomille. In Facts and Comparisons The Review of Natural Products, May 2000. St. Louis, Facts and Comparisons, a Wolters Kluwer Company, 2000.

17. Flaxmad SM, Sherman PW: Morning sickness: a mechanism for protecting mother and embryo. Q Rev Biol 75(2):113–148, 2000.

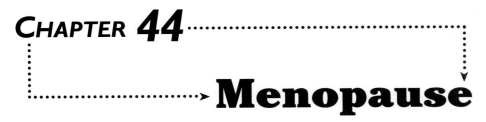

CHAPTER 44

Menopause

Monica J. Stokes, M.D., F.A.C.O.G.

PATHOPHYSIOLOGY AND DEFINITIONS

Menopause

Menopause is classically defined as the cessation of menses because of complete exhaustion of ovarian follicular function, for 6 to 12 consecutive months. The average age of onset of natural menopause is 51 years, with a range of 40 to 58 years of age. Clinically, 12 consecutive months without menses in this age range is a safer, more conservative definition that may avert undesired pregnancies in women over age 40 after the exclusion of other causes of amenorrhea. Smokers may enter menopause 2 to 3 years earlier than nonsmokers. Ovarian failure before age 40 requires significant inquiry as to the cause (e.g., autoimmune disease).

Surgical Menopause

Surgical menopause is caused by excision of all of both ovaries (bilateral oophorectomy), resulting in an abrupt withdrawal of ovarian hormones, cessation of menses, and the abrupt thrusting of the patient into a postmenopausal state. For the younger patient, other older age–related changes are not likely to occur simultaneously. Similar effects occur with induced menopause that follows the ablation of ovarian function due to chemotherapy or radiation.

Perimenopause

Perimenopause refers to the transition from regular, mostly ovulatory, menses to irregular ovulations and menses through the final months preceding complete cessation of intrinsically controlled cycling of the endometrium. This results from the progressive loss of ovarian follicular activity. Perimenopause may last from 2 to 12 years and is associated with wide fluctuations in estrogen and progesterone levels. Most commonly, the result is estrogen excess with relative progesterone deficiency, alternating with periods of hypoestrogenism. This pattern may be interrupted by intervals of regularly occurring menstrual cycles with temporary relief from symptoms.

Postmenopause

The term **postmenopause** refers to the time after complete cessation of menses (as noted previously); for clinical purposes, the ovarian reserve has been exhausted, resulting in relative estrogen and progesterone deficiencies in target tissues throughout the body. It is retrospectively dated to the final menstrual period. These changes, along with the totality of changes associated with normal aging and the woman's baseline biopsychosocial-spiritual status, may result in a variety of clinically appreciable signs and symptoms. In addition, risks begin to escalate at this age for a variety of disease or deficiency states, the type and degree of which are affected by lifelong nutrition and lifestyle habits, as well as by genetic predisposition.

After menopause, ovarian estrogen production decreases dramatically, and the circulating androgen/estrogen ratio shifts in favor of androgens. At this time, most of the circulating estrogens come from the peripheral aromatization of adrenal and ovarian androgens, making estrone the predominant circulating estrogen in postmenopausal women. Peripheral tissues capable of this hormone conversion are many, but the primary site is the stromal cell in adipose tissue. The rate of extraglandular estrone formation is directly proportional to the level of circulating androstenedione,[1] which is produced almost exclusively by the adrenal glands during this time of life. The majority of postmenopausal estradiol is derived from the (reversible) peripheral conversion of estrone to estradiol.[2]

Premenopausally, the major androgen products of the ovary are androstenedione and dehydroepiandrosterone (DHEA); postmenopausal ovarian stromal cells preferentially produce testosterone (60% of circulating testosterone in postmenopausal women comes from the ovaries; oophorectomized women do not have access to this androgen source). When menopause begins, the ovaries continue to produce testosterone at premenopausal levels for about 5 years before production begins a slow decline. Also, peripheral conversion begins of free androgens to free estrogens and of estradiol and estrone to estriol (the weakest potency of all of the endogenous estrogens; Fig. 44–1). Postmenopausal progesterone circulates in the form of 17-hydroxy-progesterone from the adrenal glands at a level similar to that noted during the follicular phase in

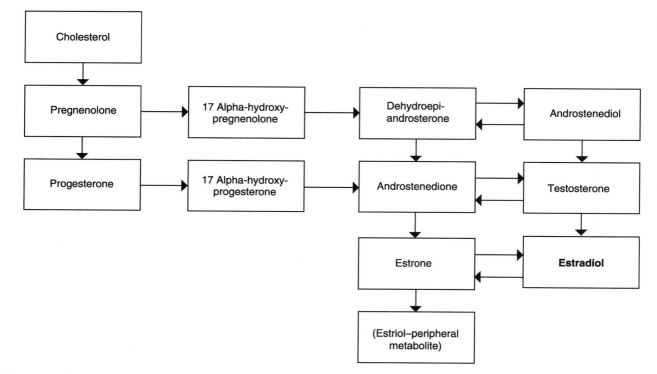

Figure 44–1. Ovarian steroidogenesis.

women of reproductive age. The principal adrenal androgen, dehydroepiandrosterone sulfate, progressively declines from between 20% to 40% of peak at menopause to 70% below lifetime peak values by age 60, whereas the secretion of other adrenal hormones remains relatively constant.

DIAGNOSIS

Women differ in how they experience symptoms of the perimenopause and menopause. Such symptoms may include irregular menses, vaginal dryness, decreased libido, night sweats, fatigue, forgetfulness, sleep disturbance, mental fogginess, palpitations, incontinence, mood swings, anxiety or depression, joint pain, weight gain, difficulty concentrating, and vasomotor symptoms. Although no symptom is life-threatening, negative experiences may affect a woman's quality of life and prompt her to seek medical advice.

DIAGNOSTIC TESTING METHODS

Follicle-Stimulating Hormone Level Testing and Monitoring

Follicle-stimulating hormone (FSH) increases gradually throughout the transitional years. A single elevated FSH level (greater than 30 to 40 mIU/mL in most laboratories) is not unequivocally positive proof that a woman is postmenopausal and incapable of reproduction.[3] In a woman who has been amenorrheic for longer than 6 months, it is more helpful, but not conclusive. FSH levels can fluctuate widely and may need to be monitored over time.

Dose-ranging estrogen studies have validated the progressive lowering of postmenopausal FSH level in response to an increased estrogen dose. However, FSH levels do not typically reach the premenopausal range to the absence of inhibin-B.

NOTE

A low (premenopausal range) FSH level in a menopausal woman receiving estrogen therapy is indicative of excessive estrogen dosing.

Selective Hormone Level Testing and Monitoring

During the perimenopausal period, spot hormone testing in blood or saliva is unreliable owing to wide fluctuations. As FSH levels steadily increase during the perimenopause, estrogen levels remain in the normal range or increase in most women. Estrogen supplementation during this period may be unnecessary and may, in fact, create or exacerbate a problem.

Generally, only free (unbound) hormone is biologically active. For estrogen, this free concentration is a function of total hormone concentration, sex hormone–binding globulin concentration (produced in the liver), albumin levels, metabolic clearance rate, and endogenous production rate (or dosage). The amount of free hormone to which any particular tissue is exposed and how it responds are highly variable.

Assessment of clinical response is all that is needed for a patient who responds easily to low-dose standard therapies. However, in several situations, testing is prudent. For example, testing may be needed when a regimen is instituted as a therapy (rather than as a preventive measure) to ensure therapeutic levels or to verify patient adherence to the regimen. A woman who remains symptomatic on adequately tailored hormone supplementation may not be absorbing the amount expected, or her sex hormone–binding globulin activity may be elevated, resulting in lower levels of bioavailable hormones. In these women, level testing is recommended, and frequently, a change in route of administration may take care of the problem. In addition, baseline assessment and follow-up spot testing are highly recommended for women who are using either customized, compounded hormones or hormones for which there are no available reputable long-term study data, yet possibly serious cosmetic and systemic effects can occur such as with androgens.

Timing

Testing related to changes in the hormone supplementation regimen should be delayed for 4 to 6 weeks (regardless of route of administration) to ensure that a steady state has been reached. For serum testing, the wait should be at least 6 to 12 hours after oral dosing or patch placement.

Salivary Testing and Monitoring

The reliability of estrogen measurements in salivary testing is inconsistent. Such testing may be helpful for noting trends in estrogen levels in patients who are not transdermally supplemented, but it appears to be most helpful for progesterone measurement. Proponents claim that there is a strong correlation between serum and salivary hormone levels, that these levels reflect only the bioavailable portion of hormones (unbound fraction), and that they are more accurate because they are atraumatic and less affected by stress hormones than are blood samples. Accuracy is further enhanced by the use of two to eleven separate measurements (number used is lab dependent). Many physicians have found salivary testing for estrogen to be less reliable than blood or urine testing and often poorly reflective of the clinical

picture (no reliable clinical study has yet been done to establish reference value ranges in the treatment of perimenopausal and menopausal women). In addition, it remains controversial whether salivary testing truly measures only the unbound (bioavailable) hormone, and low concentrations of estradiol in the saliva have increased the difficulty of measuring it accurately (more correlative data are available for progesterone).[4] Most studies using salivary analysis methods have screened only small numbers of subjects, have included only women of reproductive age, have been used to identify same-patient 24-hour and daily-cycle trends among infertile women, and have not assessed women receiving menopausal dose hormone supplementation therapy. Use of clinical acumen and 24-hour urine testing or blood testing are more highly recommended at this time. There is evidence for the reliability of salivary testing of DHEA.

Blood Testing and Monitoring

Serum levels of estradiol in a woman of reproductive age range from 30 to 40 pg/mL during the early follicular phase to approximately 250 pg/mL at midcycle. The range in postmenopausal women is 20 to 40 pg/mL (note the overlap). In perimenopausal women, this is only a snapshot during a period of widely fluctuating endogenous hormone levels. Simultaneous correlation with serum FSH level may be helpful. In supplemented patients, the therapeutic range for estradiol is 40 to 100 pg/mL. Transdermal estradiol is measured as estradiol in the circulation. The total estradiol level assayed varies with baseline endogenous estrogen production and metabolism. Oral estrogen is subjected to first-pass metabolism that converts most of it to estrone and estrone sulfate. However, the assay of estradiol alone is reflective of the dose actually prescribed and is consistent from study to study: A one-milligram oral dose of 17-beta estradiol results in a level of 60 to 80 pg/mL at 12 hours post ingestion.[5]

Urine Testing

Twenty-four-hour urine collection testing has been the gold standard for steroid hormone testing to assess baseline levels and to monitor women who are using supplementation therapy. It provides the most reliable measurements during perimenopause because most hormones are secreted in bursts within the physiology. It provides a measure of the levels of circulating hormones, but cannot specify their source (e.g., ovary or adrenal gland, peripheral conversion or exogeneous origin). Many laboratories provide a steroid hormone panel that includes metabolites of estradiol, estrone, estriol, progesterone, testosterone, and DHEA. If DHEA is being tested, its metabolites androsterone and etiocholanolone should also be measured (if these levels become too high, this indicates accelerated conversion in the body of DHEA into other steroid hormones).

INTEGRATIVE THERAPY

Preventive Healthcare

Prevention should include not only the use of early detection strategies, but the practice of health promotion behaviors as well. The perimenopause may be viewed as an opportunity for enhancement of health and well-being. Symptoms may prompt a woman to see her healthcare provider when she has not found the time for such self-care since the birth of her first (or last) child, or the last time she had a problem that brought her into the office. A plan for baseline and follow-up screening examinations (blood pressure, bone density, vision, heart disease [including fasting lipid panel], thyroid function, colonoscopy, glucose tolerance, and neoplasia or cancer [e.g., breast, gynecologic, skin, and colon]) and for vaccinations to be given now and over the next several years may be outlined. An assessment may be made of the patient's existing risk factors (both modifiable and unmodifiable), and healing and health promotion activities may be recommended that will allow her to age much more easily and gracefully. Encouragement of, and assistance with, ceasing detrimental health habits such as smoking and excessive alcohol or drug use, as well as weight management referrals, may be offered. This is also a time when a woman may be reassessing where she has been and where she would like to go in life. In the best of circumstances, the healthcare provider may serve as a supportive wellness partner and a guide to available resources and services that the patient may need or want.

Physical Activity

Exercise has repeatedly been shown to be helpful for the treatment of a wide variety of medical problems and for maintenance of good health, especially in the latter years of life. Any new activity should be advanced very slowly. Pain and injury are the primary reasons most (initially) motivated women derail from their efforts to establish a regular activity pattern. One way to encourage regular exercise is to have the patient keep an activity journal so that she can monitor her progress. Initially, the patient may agree to only 3 to 5 minutes of aerobic activity per day for 1 month. Walking is an excellent form of exercise for most women, and the journal can be used as a progress monitor and motivational tool. A well-rounded activity regimen eventually should achieve the following goals: cardiovascular endurance, strength training, flexibility, balance, and agility. Ideally, some physical activity should be performed for at least 30 minutes daily 5 to 6 days

per week (see Chapter 86, Writing an Exercise Prescription). Excessive exercise should be discouraged. Moving meditation forms such as yoga, tai chi, and qi gong may fit some women's personalities better than will more conventional forms of exercise.

Role of Sleep

Sleep disruption and insomnia are symptoms commonly reported by perimenopausal women. Sleep deprivation results in fatigue, irritability, and difficulty with concentration. The healthcare provider must first rule out the use of stimulating drugs (over the counter, prescription, or recreational) that the patient may be using. Because alcohol can increase the frequency of night flushing, it should be avoided (especially wine). Although there are many causes of sleep disturbance, the predominant one in women of this age range is vasomotor night sweats causing multiple awakenings during the night and resulting in reduced duration of rapid eye movement (REM) sleep. Estrogen is known to affect a wide range of neurotransmitters in the brain. Estrogen supplementation has been shown to improve sleep[6] and, consequently, the quality of life in these women. Progesterone supplementation has also been found to be helpful for some women. However, long-term use of the doses required to affect sleep has been anecdotally associated with fatigue and depression in some women. Education regarding sleep hygiene can be a helpful adjunct in getting the patient back into a regular sleep routine.[7, 8] Tryptophan-containing drinks such as warm milk with honey or Ovaltine taken 30 minutes before bedtime might be helpful. Chamomile (*Matricaria recutita*) and lemon balm (*Melissa officinalis*) make wonderful teas to be used at bedtime for their sedative and relaxant properties. Valerian may be used on a short-term basis while a woman is establishing these habits or is initiating hormone supplementation. Capsules of valerian root (*Valeriana officinalis*) 160 to 300 mg (standardized to 0.8% valeric acid), especially when used in combination with lemon balm extract 80 mg are effective without residual daytime sedation[9]; their effectiveness has been found in a double-blind placebo-controlled study to be comparable to that of triazolam 0.125 mg. Kava kava (*Piper methysticum*), which is usually used to treat anxiety in a dose of 45 to 70 mg of kavalactones three times per day, may be used 1 hour before bedtime in a single sedative dose of 150 to 240 mg of solid powdered kavalactone extract. Kava is best for relaxing the body, not the mind (unlike valerian), so it is not as effective in those who are unable to sleep because of racing minds. Kava has an additive effect with benzodiazepines, so if both are used in these patients, they should be given under close monitoring supervision. Pharmaceutical preparations, if used, should be prescribed for extremely short-term courses of treatment after other avenues of treatment have been exhausted.

Medical hypnotherapy training in self-hypnosis may also be helpful for treatment of willing patients.

Acupuncture has a high success rate for the treatment of insomnia. Weekly treatments are provided until a normal sleep pattern is reestablished and weekly treatments are given thereafter.

Sexuality

Loss of libido is a multifaceted problem that is increasingly reported. Active questioning on this subject should be used to elicit issues of concern. In addition to an examination with evaluation for local inflammation or infection, the diagnostic work-up should include a review of medications to identify any one (or more) known to cause sexual dysfunction in women. Evaluation continues with assessment of estrogen or androgen deficiency, prolactin excess, and issues surrounding the quality of sexual response such as dyspareunia, arousal disorders, orgasmic difficulties, and dissatisfaction, both physical and emotional. Biologic and motivational factors may overlap. Although vaginal atrophy is the most common initial cause of loss of libido in many women (may be treated with personal lubricants such as Aqua-lube and Astro-Glide or with vaginal application of progesterone or estrogen cream), anatomic and pelvic floor dysfunction also may affect physical response. Medications, use of alcohol, depression, anxiety, insomnia, and chronic stress may initiate or contribute to the problem. Finally, partner-specific physical or relational problems may need to be addressed. A sex therapist may be better qualified to deal with motivational and relational factors once the physical factors have been addressed. Excellent discussions and bibliographies on this subject have been compiled. Women who have undergone surgical menopause experience abrupt withdrawal of estrogen and testosterone and may benefit greatly from supplementation.[34]

Nutrition

Despite the supplement recommendations given later in this chapter, whole food should come first, whenever possible, to provide the natural range of vitamins, minerals, and essential fats and antioxidants. Supplements are used to augment, not substitute for, a balanced diet. Frequent small meals are preferable to large ones. Heavy foods should not be eaten after 6 or 7 pm. Avoidance of ice cold drinks is helpful for enhancing the digestive processes that occur before, during, and over several hours after each meal. The following guidelines constitute a diet aimed at symptom reduction, disease prevention, and health promotion. They also support liver metabolism and improve elimination of excess circulating hormones, while supporting the immune system and promoting anti-inflammatory prostaglandin formation. The role of inflammatory processes in a wide variety of diseases is beginning to be understood. This understanding may have wide-ranging effects on management of neurodegenerative disease and reduction in coronary vascular disease risk.

The following dietary recommendations aim to reduce symptoms of menopause, prevent disease, and promote good health:

- Increase filtered or bottled water (room temperature or warm) intake to at least 1 liter per day. Minimize fluid intake during meals.
- Eat whole, unprocessed, or minimally processed foods.
- Choose organic produce and products as often as possible to minimize exposure to xenoestrogens, pesticides, and additives.
- Maximize soluble and insoluble fiber intake, including fruits, whole grains, beans, and other legumes.
- Minimize intake of animal fats (including nonorganic dairy), sugar, caffeine, and alcohol.
- If vasomotor symptoms are an issue, avoid spicy foods (as well as other foods that seem to trigger increased hot flash intensity or frequency).
- Eat 4 to 7 vegetable servings (the more varied and deeper the colors, the better) and 3 to 5 fruits per day. Vegetables are more easily digested when taken cooked or lightly steamed. Juices and blended smoothies are a good way to take in part of this volume of fruits and vegetables.
- Use olive oil, preferentially, for cooking.
- Consider coldwater fish (omega-3 essential fatty acid source), 2 to 3 servings per week. Because of concerns about mercury and toxin accumulation in the flesh of larger, longer-lived fish, minimize intake of wild source fish to once per week.
- Ground flaxseed and flaxseed oil are excellent sources of alpha-linolenic acid (a precursor of omega-3 fatty acids). Recommended doses: 2 tablespoons of freshly ground flaxseed or 1 tablespoon of oil per day. Flax oil is heat labile, so it should be kept refrigerated and should not be used for cooking.
- Consider eating 2 to 4 servings of soy foods per day.

Supplements

The following supplements may be used in addition to, not in place of, a balanced diet:

- Calcium, 1000 to 1500 mg per day (as citrate in divided doses)
- Magnesium, 300 to 600 mg per day
- One good multivitamin per day (should contain folate [0.8 mg] and bone-supporting nutrients zinc, manganese, copper, boron, and vitamins K [1 mg][10, 11] and D [400 to 800 IU]
- B 100 complex
- Natural vitamin E with mixed tocopherols (taken with a fat-containing meal)
- Vitamin C, 200 to 500 mg twice a day

- Mixed carotenoids, 25,000 IU/day
- Selenium, 200 μg per day (taken with vitamin E).

BOTANICAL MEDICINES FOR PERIMENOPAUSAL AND MENOPAUSAL SYMPTOMATOLOGY

Remain open to alternatives to standard hormone replacement therapy, especially for the treatment of symptoms. If you are dismissive, your patients are unlikely to be open about what they are thinking about using to treat themselves. This robs you of the opportunity to learn from your patients' experiences; to identify potential hazards, given their concurrent medical and psychological issues; and to adjust your recommendations accordingly. Openness improves your credibility with patients such that they are more likely to consider your opinion about which choices may be best for them in current, unique situations. Most of the botanicals discussed here have no direct estrogen receptor action but may be effective for symptomatic relief in patients with minimal or no adverse effects. Patients should be asked to add (or remove) just one botanical to their regimen at a time (i.e., one addition per 1 to 2 weeks) to ensure that they are having no untoward effects and that any positive effect can be noted. Single botanical products should be used, from reputable companies. This rarely includes the most inexpensive commercial products. For the most part, one should discourage use of products obtained from multilevel marketing companies and products that contain more than three separate herbs, unless they are specifically prescribed Chinese or Ayurvedic remedies. Written records are helpful for patients; these should list specific products used, along with patient response to each therapy used, including botanicals and drugs. With most botanicals, full response may take 2 to 12 weeks of continuous use, depending on the specific compound. Poor-quality botanicals may never achieve an effective response. Some of the botanicals listed in the following paragraphs are extracted concentrates that provide doses outside the traditional use range. Patients must be instructed that "*natural*" does not mean "*safe at any dose.*" If patients intend to use the product outside of the range of doses recommended on the packaging, they should do so only with appropriate consultation with, and monitoring by, either a healthcare provider experienced with such issues or an experienced herbalist who has been made fully aware of the patient's concurrent medical problems and risk profile.

Phytoestrogens (Plant Estrogens)

Most foods that contain isoflavones also contain other phytochemicals. The chemical structure of the isoflavone molecule resembles those of estrogenic and antiestrogenic compounds, which have greater binding affinity for ER-beta than ER-alpha receptors.[12] Many of the possible benefits of phytoestrogens, including isoflavones, may involve systems other than estrogen receptors. Asian diets typically include 40 to 200 mg of isoflavones per day, whereas the average American diet contains 3 to 5 mg. High isoflavone intake depresses both luteinizing hormone (LH) levels and estrogen production and increases sex hormone–binding globulin levels. High fiber intake (as with beans of all types) increases gastrointestinal motility and improves the microbiologic health of the gut, which reduces enterohepatic reuptake and results in increased excretion of conjugated estrogen.

It has been suggested that increased isoflavone intake may modify endocrine function and reduce hormone-associated cancer risk (soy also contains four known anticarcinogenic non–isoflavone-related compounds). The question is whether pharmacologic dosing of isoflavones (>100 mg/d, especially in nonfood, supplement forms) may carry yet unappreciated risks (or benefits) [North American Menopause Society Consensus Opinion, March 2000]. To date, no evidence conclusively proves that a soy diet increases breast cancer risk in premenopausal or postmenopausal women, even when recurrences among women with breast cancer are considered. The major classes of phytoestrogens include isoflavones (soy, lentils, and other legumes), lignans (enterodiol and enterolactone—highest in flaxseed, but also found in most cereal grains and vegetables), and coumestans (found in addition to isoflavones in red clover, sunflower seeds, and bean sprouts).

The hormonal effects of phytoestrogens are attributed predominantly to the family of isoflavones, including genistein, diadzein, glycitein, biochanin A, and formononetin. *Whole unprocessed and minimally processed (except for fermentation) food is the safest source.* High-quality soy foods are the richest sources, although there is great variability among different soybeans and soy protein products. Processing of soy substantially lowers isoflavone content. Because processing may wholly or partially remove isoflavones from foods that originally contained them, unprocessed or minimally processed food sources (soybeans, soy flour, miso, tofu, soy milk, soy noodles, pinto beans, red lentils, and, in lesser amounts, other legumes) are recommended at this time. The estrogenic effects of soy are known to be dose dependent, and the potential negative effects of overdosing are unclear. The bioavailability of phytoestrogens is influenced by intestinal bacterial metabolism; thus, the possible biologic effects are widely variable among individuals.[13]

Currently, preliminary evidence suggests that a daily dose of 60 to 100 mg of isoflavones may benefit vasomotor symptoms, vertebral bone health and lipid profiles, low-density lipoprotein (LDL) cholesterol oxidation protection, and arterial compliance, with the resultant effect of lowering cardiovascular risk in menopausal women. It appears unlikely that doses in this range have estrogenic effects on the breast or endometrium; they also have minimal, if any, effect on prevention of vaginal atrophy. An adaptogenic effect seems to occur, with isoflavones occupying estrogenic sites in estrogen deficiency states and preventing more potent estrogens from occupying the sites in situations of estrogen excess. It is not known whether they have a neutral or weakly estrogenic effect while they occupy the sites; nor is it known how effects differ among different target tissues. Studies are ongoing, but it may be found that isoflavones are protective for the human breast at a given dosage. The problems of individual metabolism, variability of products, and optimal serum levels for treatment of specific disease states or risk factors have not yet been conclusively defined or addressed.

Black Cohosh (Cimicifuga racemosa)

This is the only botanical demonstrated in well-designed clinical studies to be effective for the treatment of vasomotor symptoms, sweating, headache, vertigo, palpitations, and sleep disturbances.[14] As with most herbs, many active compounds are known, and many have yet to be identified. The net effect may be the suppression of LH secretion in postmenopausal women.[15] Black cohosh clearly influences neuroendocrine regulatory systems but without a direct estrogen-identical mode of activity. The most recent evidence suggests that it does not stimulate proliferation of breast cancer cells.[16] It has also been demonstrated that black cohosh does not bind to estrogen receptors and does not have an estrogen effect at this level.[17, 18] It is now believed that ethanolic and isopropanolic extracts do not contain (as was previously thought) formononetin, kaempferol, or genistein.[19, 20] If this proves to be true, black cohosh could be used safely in the treatment of breast cancer survivors. The dose is based on its content of the triterpene 27-deoxyacetin, the biochemical marker of therapeutic effect.

Dosage. The dosage used in most clinical studies was 2 to 4 mg of 27-deoxyacetin twice daily.[21] Remifemin (Nature's Way) was the brand used in the majority of studies (20 to 80 mg twice daily). If the patient chooses to use a nonstandardized form, I would recommend the solid (dry powdered) extract (4:1 concentration) 250 to 600 mg three times per day.

Precautions. No toxic dose has been identified for black cohosh in animal or human studies. No adverse effects have been noted, except headache with typical therapeutic doses. Preliminary animal studies suggest that it may potentiate the effects of antihypertensive medication, but this has not yet been demonstrated in humans.[22] No mutagenic, teratogenic, or carcinogenic effects have been identified.

Black cohosh should not be confused with blue cohosh, which has a different set of indications, several contraindications, and potential adverse effects.

Dong Quai (Angelica sinensis Root)

Western herbalists have long considered dong quai a uterine tonic and antispasmodic with estrogen effects. Dong quai has been used traditionally as one component of multiherb synergistic herbal preparations in Chinese medicine for the treatment of a wide variety of symptoms and diseases, in addition to problems with menstruation and childbirth. One double-blind, placebo-controlled human trial using a low dose (4.5 g/d) showed dong quai (used in isolation) to be no more effective than placebo for the treatment of menopausal symptoms.[23] Results of in vitro studies have been conflicting in their reports of the estrogen receptor–binding capacity of dong quai. Some components stabilize blood vessels.[24]

Dosage. Forms include 1 to 4 grams of the finely chopped root as a tealike infusion in 150 mL of boiled water, steeped for 10 minutes, drink warm several times daily one half-hour before meals; a solid (dried powdered) root and rhizome preparation, 1 to 2 grams three times a day; fluidextract 1 gram: 1 to 2 mL ratio, 1.5 to 3.0 mL three times daily.[25]

Precautions. The furanocoumarins found in dong quai may cause photosensitization with the slight potential for enhancing the action of anticoagulant medications.

Chaste Tree Berry (Vitex agnus-castus)

Chaste tree berry is quite effective for the treatment of premenstrual symptoms and menstrual irregularities, both of which tend to intensify for many perimenopausal women. Another confirmed indication is for the treatment of mastalgia. It has been claimed that chaste tree berry is helpful for vasomotor symptoms as well. It is thought to work by reducing prolactin (dopaminergic effect[26]), which increases progesterone production during the luteal phase of the cycle. Postmenopausally, it is thought to normalize the hormones but the mechanism is less obvious.

Dosage. The recommended dosage of a hydroalcoholic extract preparation is the equivalent of 20 to 40 mg of fresh berries per day; a standardized preparation should contain 0.5% agnuside 175 to 225 mg per day. It may take 8 to 12 weeks for maximal effect.

Precautions. Given its probable mechanism, caution should be exercised in patients using dopamine receptor antagonists.

Evening Primrose Oil (EPO)

This oil is rich in the essential fatty acids linoleic and gamma-linolenic acid (GLA). Despite the fact that borage oil (one should use certified UPA-free products only) and black currant oil contain higher concentrations of GLA, the form in EPO is more bioavailable, reaching higher serum levels than the others with lower doses. EPO is effective for the treatment of cyclic mastalgia with comparable efficacy to bromocriptine but with fewer adverse effects (2% vs 33%).[27] It may be helpful for the treatment of nighttime hot flushes.[28] Although GLA is an omega-6 fatty acid, it is thought to preferentially contribute to the favorable series 1 prostaglandins (anti-inflammatory).

Dosage. The dose is 500 to 1000 mg three to four times per day, which can become quite expensive for the patient.

Precautions. High doses of GLA can increase the production of pro-oxidants as the body metabolizes the oil for energy. Add vitamin E 400 IU and selenium 200 μg daily for doses of >4 g GLA per day.

Licorice Root (*Glycyrrhiza glabra*)

Licorice root has been used medicinally for thousands of years for its anti-inflammatory and immunostimulatory effects (among others). It has been used as a harmonizing agent in complex herbal preparations in the treatment of premenstrual syndrome or vasomotor symptoms, its estrogen-inhibiting and progesterone-sparing effects are thought to be the modes of action. Its apparent adaptogenic effect may be attributable to glycyrrhetinic acid's antagonisms of many of estrogen's actions, as well as the estrogenic actions of isoflavones. Because of its aldosterone effect, it should be used with caution, especially in those with cardiovascular or hypertensive disease.

Dosage. A safe and effective dose for short-term (<1 month) use is 1 to 2 grams of the powdered root, or 250 to 500 mg of a solid (dry powdered) extract (4:1) three times daily.[29]

Precautions. Blood pressure and weight should be monitored because long-term use can result in sodium retention and hypokalemia. Avoid use as a single agent in those with heart disease.

Red Clover (*Trifolium ratense*)

This is a popular supplement for the treatment of both perimenopausal and menopausal symptoms. Red clover is a rich source of phytoestrogens (the isoflavones formononetin, biochanin A, genistein, and diadzein[30]) and a lesser source of coumestans. It is among the top 5% of 150 herbs assayed for both estrogen and progesterone receptor–binding capacity.[31] However, no clinical study has ever shown it to be significantly more effective than placebo or vasomotor symptoms. It may have an effect on reduction of bone resorption in premenopausal and perimenopausal women, but not in postmenopausal women. The action of bowel microorganisms on red clover produces dicoumarol, but the clinical significance of this is unknown.

Dosage. Several studies have used the brand Promensil, a 500-mg tablet that contains 40 mg per tablet per day of isoflavones, as the recommended dosing.

Precautions. Red clover can cause skin rash reactions.

Ginkgo Biloba

This herb has been shown in double-blind studies to improve memory in both elderly and college-aged women. Although no controlled studies are available of its use in menopause-related forgetfulness, a trial in any woman complaining of this symptom would be worthwhile. Ginkgo increases cerebral blood flow, is a potent antioxidant, and, in animal studies, has been found to increase the number of serotonin-binding sites in aged rats. It may also enhance the effectiveness of standard antidepressants in individuals older than 50 years of age.[32]

Dosage. Some individuals may take up to 12 weeks to respond to a 50:1 solid extract standardized to 24% ginkgo flavone glycosides and 3% to 7% terpene lactones, 40 to 80 mg three times per day.

Precautions. Mild GI complaints, headache, dizziness, palpitations, and allergic skin reactions have been reported. Avoid in patients using anticoagulant medication.

Ginseng (*Panax ginseng*)

Ginseng has a long history of use as a tonic and an adaptogen. It increases adrenocorticotropic hormone (ACTH) which stimulates adrenal cortisol and DHEA production. It produces antifatigue and antistress effects and has beneficial effects on the lipid profile in humans.

Ginsenosides exert an estrogen-like effect on the vaginal epithelium and endometrium.

Dosage. Patients should use only products from reputable, well-established companies. They should begin with use of a standardized product with a saponin content of at least 5 to 10 mg of ginsenoside Rg1 (with a ratio of Rg1 to Rb1 of 1:2) or a 5 to 8% ginsenoside product, 100 to 200 mg per day. The typical dosing schedule is two to three times daily. One should always begin at lower doses and increase gradually. Consider using ginseng cyclically (e.g., for 3 to 8 weeks followed by a ginseng-free interval of 3 weeks[33]) or adding progesterone in women who have a uterus.

Precautions. Anecdotal reports of postmenopausal bleeding have been noted in women using ginseng on a long-term basis (most likely due to the peripheral aromatization of androstenedione and DHEA to estrogens), and it is a known cause of mastalgia. The quality of marketed ginseng products in this country is widely variable, and substitutions with various other herbs or species of ginseng and ginseng-like products are more the rule than the exception. Given this situation, I recommend that ginseng products be used sparingly if they are not administered under close supervision. Avoid in those on anticoagulant medications.

St. John's Wort
(*Hypericum perforatum*)

This herb is comparable with fluoxetine (Prozac) and tricyclic antidepressants in effectiveness for the treatment of mild to moderate depression. It may concurrently increase sexual well-being as well, which is in sharp contrast with the diminution in sexual well-being associated with most antidepressants.

Dosage. The dose is 300 mg of a preparation standardized to 0.3% hypericin and 2% to 5% hyperforin (or hyperforin only) three times daily. If standardized to hyperforin, give 10 to 15 mg three times per day.

Precautions. Herb-drug interactions have been described for St. John's wort, many due to induction of cytochrome P-450 enzyme systems, resulting in lower serum levels of many drugs. It may have additive effects when given with antidepressant medications (serotonin syndrome). It also affects the levels of several neurotransmitters, including serotonin, dopamine, norepinephine, and gamma-aminobutyric acid (GABA).

BIOENERGETICS

Massage

Massage is deeply relaxing to the muscles and the mind as it raises endorphin levels and diminishes stress hormones. This helps maximize the balance within which true healing is possible.

Homeopathy

Homeopathy is a 200-year-old system of medicine (evaluation and therapy) that may be helpful for the treatment of multiple menopausal symptoms. It is based on a set of principles and "provings." The first principle is the law of similars, which indicates that "like cures like," that is, a remedy that causes a set of symptoms in a well person (a *proving*) is the remedy for an ill person who displays the same set of symptoms. As the cure progresses, different sets of self-limited symptoms may arise, which, if the correct single remedies are given in the proper sequence, occur cephalad to caudad and from inside to outside the body. Close follow-up with a homeopathic practitioner is recommended to ensure that the cure is proceeding in the proper direction, to change remedy type as necessary, and to be sure that the patient is not using something that can interfere with or resuppress portions of the process. In addition to a specific symptomatic treatment to treat, for example, hot flushes, it is helpful during this transition to have a constitutional treatment that rebalances responses of the body to hormones and provides a more long-lasting cure. Common symptomatic remedies include lachesis, sepia, sulphur, and, less commonly, kali carbonicum and calculus indicus.

Reiki, Healing Touch, Craniosacral Therapy, and Other Energy Therapies

These therapies help to rebalance the energy of the body, releasing tissue memories and allowing healing. Their use causes significant reductions in clinical symptomatology and emotional upheaval, and sometimes resolution of the presenting problem. Guided imagery techniques are often used during treatment sessions. Energy therapy may be a valuable adjunct in the treatment of menopausal women.

Ayurvedic Perspective

This system is the oldest continuous known medical tradition. Ayurvedic medicine is a prevention-oriented, consciousness-based, holistic science. It teaches that a human is a representation of, and is not separated from, the universe with its Natural Laws. Ayurveda helps the healthy person to maintain health and identify imbalances that may lead to specific diseases over months to years (if not addressed), and it enables the diseased (chronically imbalanced) person to regain health. Another concept basic to Ayurvedic science is the capability of the individual for self-healing. Ayurvedic treatment, which originated in India, is designed to promote human happiness, health, and creative growth.[35] Times of day and times of life may contribute to the manifestation of specific problems. Menopause represents a transition from one stage of life to another. It is not unusual for the body to display symptoms as it adjusts to this change. Diagnosis involves a detailed pulse evaluation and detailed questioning to determine the strength of the imbalance among body elements. Treatments rely strongly on the constitutional type of the patient, the types of disturbances present, and the specificity and intensity of the imbalance.

Chinese Medicine Perspective

In Chinese medicine, menopause is attributable to depletion of *kidney qi,* cessation of the *heavenly tenth* (*tian gui* reproductive capacity), and *vacuity* (various manifestations of deficiency) of the thoroughfare (*chong meridian*), controlling vessels (*ren channels*), and vessels of the uterus. A Chinese medicine practitioner assesses the individual constitution of the patient to determine where the imbalance lies and treats the imbalance with customized herbs that nourish the blood and yin, often in combination with acupuncture. A common pattern seen in perimenopausal/menopausal women is that of *kidney yin* deficiency (often expressed as vasomotor symptomatology) and *liver qi* stagnation (exhibited as emotional changes). Acupuncture may be used concurrently with herbs to tonify the kidney and smooth the liver qi, to instill a sense of tranquility.

MIND-BODY INTERVENTIONS

Social Support Assessment

Social support has been shown to be helpful in controlling the feelings of isolation felt by people going through illness or difficult periods in their lives. Some assessment should be made regarding the strength of a woman's friendship network and whether there is anyone she can talk with about what is going on with her. For some women, belonging to a menopause support group may be helpful. If the patient is without support, suggestions may be made regarding the availability of such support groups or women's community agencies. She can join a gym, take classes, or become involved in a special interest group activity in which she may find new and different friends.

Journaling

Keeping a written account of experiences during this passage not only is helpful for the patient, but she may choose to share it later with loved ones. Many women of this generation have no idea about what their mothers and aunts experienced; also, many of those menopause experiences were abrupt because of hysterectomies with oophorectomies before the onset of natural menopause. In addition, many women were placed immediately on hormonal therapy (there were few options then), without consideration of other interventions, because of the dominance of conventional medicine.

Cognitive-Behavioral Therapy

This is helpful for those women who would like to speak to someone outside their support network, or for those who begin this period of life with a recent history of significant problems coping with change or dealing with difficult situations. Those patients who have existing, untreated anxiety, depression, or other baseline psychiatric problems should certainly receive concurrent cognitive-behavioral therapy while appropriate medical treatment is being selected and tailored.[36] Short-term use of antidepressants or anti-anxiety herbs or pharmaceuticals may be required, but it is important that this decision be reevaluated in 3 to 6 months.

There has been considerable controversy as to whether there are increased depressive symptoms during the perimenopausal and postmenopausal periods. Depression has been associated with other times of profound hormonal change. It appears that although depressive symptoms do not universally affect women at the time of menopause, many women, especially during the perimenopause, do develop such symptoms. There is also evidence that women who have had surgical menopause,[37] previous episodes of depression, or a high degree of social or life stresses are more vulnerable to developing depressive symptoms associated with the menopausal transition.[38] Estrogen has many influences on, and interactions with, several neurotransmitter and receptor systems, and it increases the brain's excitability. Progesterone antagonizes the effects of estrogen in the brain, but the mood effect may be offset by increasing the estrogen dose while maintaining the progesterone dose at a constant level.[39] Estrogen may also potentiate the effects of some antidepressants, allowing lower doses to be used in any given patient.

Shamanic Journeying

This involves the assistance of an experienced shaman or shamanic practitioner. It is an intensive, goal-oriented method of assessing the meaning of symptoms and seeking help from other realities, in a controlled fashion, using a method of journeying. Spirit helpers and teachers from these other realms provide assistance as the subject moves toward the stated goal, or toward the true path to healing, regardless of what the subject thinks it should be. After a few sessions, the patient learns to journey on her own, and she may continue the process with guidance only as necessary.

Guided Imagery and Hypnosis

These are methods of accessing the unconscious mind in order to stimulate the innate healing processes within the individual. They are used to enlist the body's inner wisdom and resources to help alleviate problems as well as reframe current and past situations (i.e., changing internalized negative beliefs) that may be obstacles to progress toward healing. The patient may have specific goals, such as symptom amelioration, pain relief, habit resolution, or stress reduction. Individualized healing images may be formulated with the patient; these images can tap into deep, idiosyncratic meanings more potent than any the therapist can provide. A tape may be made for the patient to use regularly at home, for as long as necessary to achieve autonomy with the practice.

Meditation Training

Meditation, at the very least, relaxes the body and calms the mind. Studies have shown that it reduces stress hormone levels in the body. With practice, meditation leads to centering and consciousness expanding (feeling ill or "not right" is quite consciousness constricting) and is a way to transmit one's intentions into a greater reality. It may deepen one's spiritual life regardless of spiritual or religious convictions. Meditation also helps broaden the perspective of how one fits into the greater picture. This broadened perspective lessens the personal impact of anything that is going on. I have found that women who have a daily meditation practice are able to traverse the trials of the perimenopause and menopause with greater ease, requiring significantly less intervention. The type of meditation practiced is less important (as long as it "fits" the patient well) than the actual adherence to the recommended practice itself, daily or twice daily over a long period of time.

If one practice type is not working, encourage the patient to seek out others until she finds one that seems to "feel" right. (Examples include mindfulness, centering prayer, and transcendental and primordial sound meditation practices, as well as moving meditations such as yoga, tai chi, and qi gong.) See Chapter 94, Learning To Meditate.

Spirituality

At this time of life, many women consider connection or reconnection with spiritually centering resources. They may also consider exploring what truly brings joy and meaning to their lives. As they reassess their life path and reaffirm old goals or establish new ones, having a strong spiritual or religious anchor helps to keep them steady and provides a source of strength regardless of what events arise in their lives. If she has not done so already, this is the time the patient should give her spirit the room and freedom to breathe.

HORMONE SUPPLEMENTATION THERAPY

General

Hormone supplementation therapy as a global, systemic risk reduction strategy is in the process of being reevaluated. One prescription is no longer given "forever." Hormone regimens should be carefully tailored, reevaluated over time, and modified as the woman ages, to best meet her needs regarding comfort, adverse effect diminution, and risk reduction and to incorporate new, evidence-based information.

It has recently been suggested that the binding affinity of an estrogen (or component within an estrogen product) is not the primary predictor of biologic activity as was once thought. In addition, all types of estrogens (as well as progesterones and androgens) have direct actions between the ligand and the estrogen receptor (genomic) in various tissues, as well as nongenomic actions unrelated to this mechanism.[40] These nongenomic actions may be observed in cells with no steroid receptors; they have a variety of mediators, only some of which have been elucidated to date. These nongenomic actions may explain the apparent "estrogen" activity of many herbal preparations.

Postmenopausal hormone supplementation therapy may be thought of as a preventive healthcare decision despite the fact that menopause is a normal physiologic event in a woman's life. There is evidence to support the prevention and treatment benefits of estrogen therapy for postmenopausal women (Table 44–1).[41]

Potential major risks of estrogen supplementation can be reviewed in Table 44–2. Absolute contraindications to estrogen therapy can be found in Table 44–3.

Table 44–1. Conditions That May Be Effectively Treated or Prevented by Estrogen Therapy

Vasomotor symptoms
Sweating
Atrophic vaginitis
Genitourinary atrophy
Frequent urinary tract infections
Urge incontinence
Sexual changes related to vulvovaginal atrophy
Skin integrity
Irritability
Dizziness
Joint and muscle aches
Memory deficits
Sleep disturbances
Osteoporosis
Osteoarthritis
Periodontal disease and tooth loss
Age-related macular degeneration
Cognitive decline
Onset and progression of mild Alzheimer's disease
Symptoms of treated Parkinson's disease
Coronary heart disease
Hemoglobin A1C and insulin resistance reduction in type 2 diabetes
Colon cancer
Possibly hemorrhagic stroke and migraine headaches (if used in a continuous regimen)

Table 44-2. Risks of Estrogen Therapy

Increase in thromboembolic events
Increase in gallstone formation
Possible small increase in breast cancer risk but lower mortality risk
Endometrial (or endometriotic implant) cancer (if used by women with a uterus [or history of endometriosis] unopposed by appropriate doses of progesterone)

Table 44-3. Contraindications to Estrogen Therapy

Suspected estrogen-dependent cancer
Breast cancer
Undiagnosed genitourinary bleeding
Active thrombophlebitis or thromboembolic disorder
Active liver disease
Suspected pregnancy

Methods of Administration

Estrogen—continuous (daily)
Progesterone—continuous or sequential (13–16 days out of each month), or intravaginal micronized progesterone gel every 3 months (extended cycling with Crinone).

Routes of Administration

The route of administration of exogenous steroids can significantly affect their actions on intermediate and target organs. Several studies have compared the effects of oral estrogens vs transdermal estradiol on hepatic parameters. For example, oral conjugated estrogen increases high-density lipoprotein (HDL) cholesterol and triglyceride levels, but transdermally administered estrogen has no effect or decreases HDL or triglycerides.[42] Oral conjugated estrogens increase sex hormone–binding globulin (SHBG) levels significantly more than does transdermal estradiol (micronized estradiol falls in the middle level of effect). Issues pertinent to your patient should influence the choice of administration route based on these and other effects (Table 44–4).

Routes of administration include oral tablets (sustained-release or oil-filled capsules); continuous-release patches (two-layer, nonreservoir matrix system and the older, alcohol reservoir system); topical transdermal creams, ointments, or gels (occlusive daily application patches can be made for these); intravaginal suppositories, creams, and gels; sublingual troches (lozenges) or liquids; local estrogen release vaginal rings (Estring); intramuscular injection; subcutaneous pellet implants; and progesterone-secreting intrauterine devices (IUDs) (for those on estrogen replacement with a uterus who do not tolerate any form of systemic progesterone supplementation).

> **NOTE**
>
> **First-Pass Effect**
>
> *When hormones are given orally, they have a more direct rate of metabolism by both the flora of the gut and through the liver (first pass). This affects metabolites that have various effects on the body. For example, estrogen metabolism in the liver increases angiotensinogen (elevated blood pressure), it raises HDL and triglycerides and lowers LDL and total cholesterol (lipid effects), and increases clotting factors (thrombosis risk).*
>
> *Transdermal, transmucosal, and parenteral delivery significantly diminishes these effects.*

All of these formulations are eventually exposed to hepatic metabolism; however, only the oral forms are first partially metabolized by the gastrointestinal flora, traverse the enterohepatic circulation, and pass through the liver, being metabolized before they can begin to exert their actions. Progesterone, for example, is acted upon by gut flora, producing metabolites that have a sedating effect on the central nervous system. In the case of oral estrogen, the effects on hepatic metabolism of other substances are considerable, and this is called the first-pass effect. It explains why oral estrogen results in more beneficial lipid changes but also greater risk for thromboembolic events. Vaginal preparations of estrogen are effective for isolated treatment of vaginal atrophic changes. These are absorbed systemically and typically reach blood levels up to 25% of those attained with an equivalent oral dose, but levels may be much higher in the presence of severe atrophy and tissue erosion. This dose-related absorption cannot be relied on for consistent end-organ effects, but it is certainly adequate to cause endometrial hyperplasia (except for Estring with which there are undetectable serum estrogen levels 48 hours after placement [package insert]). Of course, any unexpected bleeding in a postmenopausal woman should be evaluated with endometrial biopsy or direct hysteroscopic visualization. A transvaginal ultrasonographic measurement of the endometrial stripe of 4 mm or less is unlikely to be associated

> **NOTE**
>
> *Generally, only free (unbound) hormone is biologically active. Anything that lowers sex hormone–binding globulin levels (e.g., obesity, hypothyroidism, androgen excess) will allow more hormone to remain free and able to act on target tissues. Conversely, SHBG-elevating circumstances (e.g., vegetarian diet, oral administration of estrogen, liver disease, hyperthyroidism) will increase binding of circulatory hormone and reduce hormone availability.[43]*

Table 44–4. Estrogen Formulations for Menopausal Women

Chemical or Generic Name/Route	Commercial or Common Name	Dose Range (per day)	Notes
17-beta Estradiol Route:			Bio-identical to human estradiol Source: Plant-soy or wild yam
Oral tablets (micronized)	Estrace, Estradiol USP	1–2 mg	1. Hepatic "first-pass effect"—increases HDL and triglycerides, clotting factors, sex hormone–binding globulin (SHBG) (as with all oral estrogens); reduces LDL 2. Peaking of serum levels within a few hours of administration, elimination within 24 hours 3. Micronized for rapid absorption but much metabolized in gastrointestinal tract before absorption, so sufficiently high doses must be used 4. Predominant metabolites reaching circulation are estrone and estrone sulfate
Transdermal patches	Climara, FemPatch Alora, Vivelle, Vivelle-Dot, Estraderm	0.025–0.1 mg delivered (25–100 μg)	1. Continuous release prevents peaking in serum 2. Recommended route for those at risk for thromboembolic disease or with hypertriglyceridemia (no "first pass") 3. Constant surface area of administration—consistent dosing 4. Adhesive may cause local skin irritation 5. Changed 2/wk (except Climara/FemPatch—once a week) 6. Press firmly on clean, dry, intact skin. Rotate application to abdomen, buttocks, lower back, lateral thorax, upper arm
Estradiol vaginal cream, ring	Estrace Estring	0.01% cream with calibrated applicator 0.5, 1, 2, 3, or 4 mg 7.5 μg release/day (2 mg per 90 days)	1. Local application and release reaching serum levels 25% of equivalent oral doses (higher if extreme atrophy) 2. Excellent for treatment of atrophic vaginal/vulvar/distal urinary symptoms 3. Creams capable of causing endometrial hyperplasia 4. Daily cream insertion until symptoms are reduced then half or full dose 2–3× wk for maintenance 5. Estring—minimal absorption into circulation and minimal effect on endometrium
Estradiol vaginal tablet	Vagifem	25-μg tablet with single-use applicator	1. Minimal systemic absorption 2. 1 tablet inserted daily for 2 wk, then 1 tablet weekly for symptom control
Estropipate (Piperazine estrone sulfate–oral)	Ogen, Ortho-Est Estropipate USP	0.625, 1.25, 2.5 mg 0.75, 1.5, 3 mg	1. Source: Plant 2. Begins bio-identical to human estrone 3. Sulfate makes formulation more soluble and protects the estrogen from rapid GI metabolism and extends time in circulation, piperazine further stabilizes 4. Vaginal cream also available (Ogen)
Esterified estrogens (oral)	Estratab, Menest	0.3 mg; 0.625 mg; 1.25 mg; 2.5 mg	1. Sources: Plant 2. Estrone sulfate (80%) and equilin sulfate (20%) 3. Approved only for symptoms, not prevention of end-organ sequelae of hypoestrogenism
Conjugated estrogens (oral)	Premarin-conjugated equine estrogens	0.3 mg, 0.625 mg, 0.9 mg, 1.25 mg, 2.5 mg	1. Source: Animal (horse)—PREgnant MAre urINe 2. Contains 10 different conjugated estrogens, including a bio-identical estrone and potent equine forms 3. Intravenous and intramuscular formulations and vaginal cream formulations available 4. The majority of studies regarding target tissue benefits have used Premarin
Synthetic (oral)	Cenestin–synthetic conjugated estrogen	0.625–1.25 mg	1. Source: Plant. Clinical data are lacking 2. Contains 9 of the 10 known conjugated estrogens found in Premarin 3. Currently approved only for vasomotor symptoms
Parenteral estrogens 1. Estradiol cypionate 2. Estradiol valerate 3. Estradiol pellets	1. Depo-Estradiol 2. Delestrogen 3. Estrapel	1. 1 mg/mL and 5 mg/mL 2. 10, 20, and 40 mg/mL 3. 25 mg pellet implant	1, 2. Administered every 3–6 weeks 3. 1–4 pellets (implanted subcutaneously with trocar in lower abdomen or gluteal region) every 6 months 4. All pellets have a cumulative effect with persistent blood levels up to 2 years after the last insertion. Monitor blood estradiol levels to remain below 100 pg/mL. 5. Mostly used in extended-care elder patients.

Table 44-4. Estrogen Formulations for Menopausal Women (Continued)

Chemical or Generic Name/Route	Commercial or Common Name	Dose Range (per day)	Notes
Combination formulations (oral) (estrogen/ progestin)			Combinations of above with synthetic progestins
17-beta estradiol+ norethindrone acetate (NETA)	Activella	1 mg 17-beta estradiol+0.5 mg NETA	
17-beta estradiol+ norgestimate (NGM)	Ortho-Prefest	1 μg 17-beta estradiol+90 mcg NGM	Estradiol on days 1–3 then estradiol + norgestimate on days 4–6. The pattern is repeated continuously
Ethinyl estradiol+NETA	Femhrt	5 mg ethinyl estradiol+1 mg NETA	Ethinyl estradiol is an extremely potent synthetic estrogen that greatly increases SHGB levels, but is not bound by SHGB; may not be the best choice for postmenopausal hormone supplementation
Conjugated equine estrogens (CEE)+ medroxyproges- sterone acetate	Prempro vs Premphase	Continuous 2.5 mg MPA vs Cyclic, sequential 5 mg MPA with 0.625 CEE (continuously) in each	Equine estrogens
Transdermal combination Preparation of norethindrone and estradiol (E^2)	CombiPatch	0.05 mg E2+0.14 mg NETA/day or 0.05 mg E2+0.25 mg NETA/day	The first approved of a series of combination patches in the pipeline for U.S. Food and Drug Administration approval
Compounded estrogen combinations (Oral or troches)	Triestrogen 80% estriol 10% estrone 10% estradiol Biestrogen 80–90% estriol 10–20% estradiol	1.25–5.0 mg/day 1.25–5.0 mg/day	1. No objective evidence to support long-term target tissue effects as yet 2. Usual dose range provides therapeutic dose of estradiol
Estriol USP (compounded oral dose, troches, or vaginal cream)	Compounded	2–5 mg/day—oral micronized Other compounded to specification	1. Weak estrogenic effect—requires higher dosing 2. In therapeutic doses, can cause endometrial hyperplasia 3. Studies in progress to evaluate potential protective effect against breast cancer in humans 4. Predominant estrogen during pregnancy (fetoplacental metabolism)
Compounding Pharmacists Estrogens and other steroids	Can produce a wide variety of dosage forms in multiple vehicles for administration (troches, creams, ointments, gels, capsules, injectables)	Wide range— Recommend communication with local or mail order pharmacy's compounding pharmacist	When using formulations and routes without clear evidence of serum level ranges with particular doses, be sure to verify with testing that the patient is getting enough but not too much estrogen, progesterone, or androgen

with neoplasia; however, it remains difficult to interpret the measurement for perimenopausal women or postmenopausal women who have used hormone supplementation for any length of time and are likely to have measurements above this level.

Definition

Synthetic Hormones

Hormones are completely designed by man and manmade; they do not exist in, and are not derived from, nature in any form (e.g., ethinyl estradiol, diethylstilbestrol).

Bio-identical Synthetic Hormones

Commonly called "natural," the plant source comes from nature, but to be formulated as drugs, these elements must be chemically modified in a laboratory from components of plants such as the Mexican yam or the soy bean (the human body does not possess the enzyme systems to make these conversions on its own). The result is a product

Table 44–5. Selected Forms of Supplemental Progesterone for Women

Chemical or Generic Name/Route	Commercial or Common Name	Dose Range (per day)	Notes
Micronized progesterone (oral capsules)	Prometrium	100 mg/capsule Cyclic: 200–300 mg/day (bid or single daily qhs administration 13–14 days per month) Continuous: 100–200 mg/day (bid or single daily qhs administration)	1. Bio-identical; plant source 2. Produces 5-alpha and 5-beta pregnenolone via gut metabolism—potential CNS-sedating effect 3. Fewer adverse effects than synthetic progestins (less thrombotic risk) 4. Adequately opposes estrogen effect on the endometrium 5. Micronized form increases GI absorption and reduces less from "first-pass" hepatic metabolism
Norethindrone acetate (oral)	Aygestin	5 mg	Synthetic—resists metabolism
Medroxy-progesterone acetate (oral)	Provera Cycrin Amen, Curretab	2.5, 5, 10 mg 5, 10 mg 10 mg	Synthetic—resists metabolism
Micronized progesterone in oil (oral capsules)	Compounded	50–300 mg/day	1. Plant source 2. Reaches higher peak serum levels at similar mg doses than Prometrium 3. First-pass effect from oral administration
Micronized progesterone in troche	Compounded	50-mg/day average dose	1. Troches dissolve between cheek and gum 2. No first-pass effect—lower doses can be used
Progesterone cream	Many companies (e.g., Pro-Gest) Prescription, over the counter, and compounded sources	20–40 mg/day	1. Choose commercial preparations that contain approx 500 mg/oz (at this concentration = 1/8–1/4 tsp/day) 2. Compounded preparations may be of higher concentrations and come with a calibrated dosing applicator 3. Check baseline levels and repeat 3 months after therapy begins (baseline <0.3 ng/mL; should increase to 3–4 ng/mL with proper use) 4. Any product that contains mineral oil prevents skin absorption even if it contains adequate amounts of progesterone 5. Improperly stabilized products deteriorate over time as they are repeatedly exposed to the air 6. Rotate application sites: upper chest, breast, inner arms, and thighs 7. Vaginal application—may use lower doses for symptom control 8. No first-pass effect
Micronized progesterone bioadhesive vaginal gel	Crinone 4% and 8%	4% (45 mg) in pre-filled applicators per vagina qod at bedtime for 12 days (6 doses) every 3 months	1. Progesterone suspended in a polycarbophil gel which adheres to vaginal mucosa—sustained release of hormone over time 2. Provides a significant local protective effect from estrogen's influence on the endometrium. Expect withdrawal bleeding flow commensurate with degree of estrogen priming and number of months between applications 3. Not yet approved by U.S. Food and Drug Administration for this indication
Progesterone in oil (Injectable)	Progesterone in oil	IM administration 100 mg q 2–3 months	1. Discomfort of injection 2. Most commonly used to induce a withdrawal bleed in an estrogen-primed endometrium

Note: In women with a uterus receiving supplemental estrogen, use of progesterone for endometrial production is necessary.

that is chemically identical to those produced by the human body (e.g., 17-beta estradiol, estrone, progesterone, and other steroids). These compounds are certainly derived from natural sources. This fact is used to describe them for marketing purposes, but there is certainly nothing "natural" about the process required for converting them into a form that the body can use. Despite this, I prefer to use these products in my practice because they are the closest available form to the native hormones our bodies produce (bio-identical).

A growing number of naturally "sourced" estrogens have been modified considerably to enhance absorption from the gut and to stabilize them so they can resist immediate metabolism by the liver. These are hybrid forms that generally achieve more potent or prolonged estrogenic effects in the body, thus allowing lower doses to be used. Examples of this are the estropipate formulations e.g., Ogen (see Table 44–4). These sulfate conjugates are cleared from the circulation at a slow rate.

Table 44–6. Testosterone Sources for Use in Women*

Chemical or Generic Name/Route	Commercial or Common Name	Dose Range (per day)	Notes
17-beta, hydroxyandrost-4-ene-3-one	Testosterone USP—used for compounding	Route dependent: 1–5 mg/day	Source: Plant **General notes regarding testosterone use (any form) in women:** 1. The long-term effects of supplemental testosterone exposure in women are unknown 2. The potential adverse effects are dose and duration of exposure dependent and include virilization (principally acne, hirsutism, and clitoromegaly), liver dysfunction, clotting factor suppression, and hypoglycemic effect. Increased low-density lipoprotein and decreased high-density lipoprotein, triglycerides, and total cholesterol 3. When used in women, close monitoring of response and for appearance of adverse effects is strongly recommended
Oral estrogen/ testosterone combinations			1. Source: Synthetic derivative 2. Most effective in women with surgical or ablative menopause (libido, energy level, mood, sense of well-being) 3. Results mixed in non-oophorectomized women; may benefit selected women.
Esterified estrogen (EstE)+ Methyltestosterone (MT)	Estratest Estratest H.S. (half-strength)	1.25 mg Est E+2.5 mg MT/day 0.625 mg EstE+1.25 mg MT/day	4. Hirsutism seen in 15%–36% of patients with long-term use 5. Combination forms approved for use in women
Conjugated equine estrogen (CEE)+ Methyltestosterone (MT)	Premarin with methyltestosterone	1. 0.625 mg CEE+5 mg MT/day 2. 1.25 mg CEE+10 mg MT	6. Oral—subject to (hepatic) first-pass effect 7. FDA approved for use in women
Methyltestosterone USP (oral tablet)	Android, testred	10 mg	1. FDA approved for use only in men 2. Subject to first-pass effect
Micronized testosterone in oil (oral capsules)	Compounded	2.5 mg–5 mg	Subject to first-pass effect
Micronized testosterone in troches	Compounded	1 mg, 2.5 mg, 5 mg	1. Troches dissolved between cheek and gum 2. No first-pass effect
Micronized testosterone in cream	Compounded	1. 2% Cream in jar 2. 2 mg/g—¼ teaspoon equals 1 g of cream	1. For libido, apply 2% cream "sparingly" (i.e., small amount on tip of finger) to perivaginal region and/or clitoris: Titrate for effect 2. If more precise dosing is required for other desired effects, choose the precisely compounded formulation
Transdermal patches (testosterone USP)	1. Androderm 2. Testoderm TTS transdermal system	Testosterone delivery/day: 1. 2.5 mg or 5 mg 2. 5 mg	1. FDA-approved use for men only 2. Daily application 3. Rotate application to back, upper buttock, and upper arm
Parenteral testosterones			FDA approval for use only in men
Testosterone cypionate	Virilon I.M. Depo-Testosterone	200 mg/mL 100 and 200 mg/mL	
Testosterone enanthate	Delatestryl	200 mg/mL	
Testosterone pellet implants	Testopel	75 mg	1. FDA approval for use only in men 2. Usually used in conjunction with estrogen pellet placement in long-term care elder patients 3. Trocar subcutaneous application 4. High supraphysiologic levels will occur initially

* The injectable forms, patches, and higher dose tablets are FDA approved only for use in men and for treatment of selected late-stage breast cancer in women. They are included here for completeness, with the realization that off-label short-term treatment situations may arise.

Natural Hormones

Despite the commercial marketing use of this term as noted previously, these are hormones that exist in nature in their original forms. Without chemical modification and with minimal processing, they are formulated as drugs (e.g., conjugated equine estrogens such as Premarin derived from the urine of pregnant mares). These formulations are similar, but not identical, to the hormones that we make in our bodies, and they are sourced from a foreign animal species.

Because conjugated equine estrogens have been studied most over the years, they have been the ones most commonly prescribed. The wisdom of the continued prescribing of these, however, has come into question for a variety of medical and political reasons.

THERAPEUTIC APPROACH FOR THE PERIMENOPAUSAL WOMAN

In perimenopausal women who present with symptoms (without other etiology), I no longer begin with hormone supplementation unless contraception is desired. In that case (in nonsmokers and those without contraindications), a low-dose oral contraceptive (20 μg estrogen dose) provides reliable contraception and predictable hormone levels, thus resolving most of the presenting problems. In women who already use a reliable form of contraception, progesterone during the last one half of their cycle will provide some symptom relief and a reliable withdrawal bleeding each month.

One of the most common presenting symptoms in perimenopausal women is menstrual irregularity, which often predates vasomotor symptoms. Although the most common cause of irregular bleeding is anovulatory cycles, any recurrence of intermenstrual bleeding or new onset of very heavy flow periods or those lasting longer than 7 days without obvious cause is reason for a screening endometrial sampling. Mild menstrual timing or flow irregularity (i.e., "a little off schedule," or "a little heavier or lighter") requires only reassurance and education, about the transition processes that may be beginning in her body, along with a reasonable estimate of what to expect. This can lead to discussion with a focus on health and well-being. Lifestyle and nutritional changes, including increased food-source phytoestrogens and botanicals used as needed, are very effective for most women. Because of the relative progesterone deficiency characteristic of many perimenopausal women, many practitioners use progesterone creams or oral progesterone. Although I use compounded progesterone creams in some women for whom my first line of treatment is ineffective, I do not employ the continuous (noncyclic) use of oral progestins or even micronized progesterone alone owing to the high incidence of fatigue and depression noted in many women with prolonged use.

THERAPEUTIC APPROACH FOR THE POSTMENOPAUSAL WOMAN

My clinical (hormonal) approach to treating the postmenopausal woman is to use the lowest dose that is effective for prevention and to control the presenting symptoms, while addressing lifestyle and nutritional issues with the patient. These recommendations, as well as mind-body approaches, may reduce the need for higher doses of hormonal interventions for symptom control. Of course, attention to the coexisting medical and risk factor issues in any given patient (as well as new study findings) must be considered in the decision-making and annual reevaluation processes. A dose of estrogen (0.3 mg) that is woefully suboptimal for treating vasomotor symptoms is quite sufficient to help maintain older women's bone density.

Twenty to thirty percent of women never fill their first prescriptions, and 20% of the women who do begin therapy discontinue use within the first year. This may be averted with appropriate counseling and supportive follow-up plans. Many women are concerned about the risk of breast cancer. Currently, the studies cumulatively reveal no risk or a slightly increased risk of breast cancer in estrogen users, and the survival rate of estrogen users diagnosed with breast cancer is considerably improved compared with that of nonusers.

After appropriate counseling regarding the risks, benefits, and expected effects and (time-limited) adverse effects of the therapy, I currently recommend beginning with a bio-identical product such as Estrace (micronized 17-beta estradiol) oral or a transdermal 17-beta estradiol and adding a micronized progesterone such as Prometrium for endometrial protection. I offer cyclic or continuous therapy to all of my patients and let them decide for themselves which regimen best fits their current lifestyle. Sequential (cyclic) therapy results in a predictably timed withdrawal bleeding, of some amount, each month. After the first few months, the volume and duration of bleeding are reduced considerably, but most women do not experience amenorrhea.

Continuous therapy causes unpredictably timed bleeding, which may last up to 6 to 12 months, after which time most women experience amenorrhea. For many women, this approach (with the eventual possibility of avoiding monthly bleeding) is acceptable and effective. If one begins with low doses and increases only as needed within the recommended dosage range with a particular product, clinical improvement over a period of 2 to 4 months is a very effective therapeutic guide. You may need to decrease or increase the dosage to minimize adverse effects and maximize symptom control. Another option is to change the route of administration or give a trial of a low-dose testosterone-containing preparation. I find that hormone testing is rarely needed for the usual patient with typical symptoms that are quickly eased (especially) with lower doses of standard therapies. For those in whom maximum standard doses are ineffective for symptom diminution after 1 to 2 months, a 24-hour urine level for estrogen and progesterone (and possibly testosterone) or serum levels may be obtained to provide a more objective measure for entry to the next steps in treatment. In these difficult cases, first change the route of administration or the type of product. Next, for these patients or for those who just would like to avoid any brand products, consider the use of custom-dosed bio-identical estrogen troches or vaginal creams; add compounded troches or vaginal progesterone gel if the patient has a uterus or a history of endometriosis. A growing school of thought holds that all women, whether they have a uterus or not, should be given some form of natural progesterone supplementation as well. Successful customization requires close communication between the patient, you, and your local compounding pharmacist. When using customized dosing of bio-identical products, consider retesting the patient after you have instituted a new combination, to ensure that she does not have extremely high hormone levels. Any patient who chooses this option should be aware that there is no evidence base to prove that these forms of administration achieve the same long-term end-organ protections (or risk profile) provided by the more traditional forms of hormone supplementation. In addition, most insurance companies do not (currently) reimburse the cost of these compounded preparations. Some mail-order pharmacies have pharmacists (see "Compounding Pharmacies," later in the chapter) who will be happy to assist you in the decision-making process.

Remember that over time each patient needs re-evaluation to be sure that (1) she is happy with her choice, (2) she is maintaining minimum effective blood levels for prevention of the target organ effects for which she is at risk, (3) no new medical issues have arisen that require regimen modifications, and (4) she is made aware of any new evidence-based supplementation type, route, dosing, or blood/saliva levels recommended for prevention of these or other risks that she may face as she grows older. If one supplement (or a combination) is ineffective and other causes for her symptoms have been ruled out, there are multiple options. It is necessary to find the right combination for your particular patient.

OTHER NONESTROGENIC TREATMENTS FOR HOT FLUSHES

1. Behavioral. Dress in layers (preferably natural fibers); do relaxation breathing exercises; carry a personal battery-operated or handheld fan; identify and avoid your triggers (e.g., spicy or very hot foods, hot rooms); lighten and simplify your make-up regimen and consider waterproof mascara and eyeliner; carry an extra undershirt or blouse to change into, if needed; participate in regular aerobic exercise. Reframe to think of it as a "power surge" rather than as something negative or disabling.
2. Progesterone cream may be very effective. Apply 20 to 40 mg/day while rotating application sites.
3. Bach Flower essences
4. Clonidine oral dosage of 0.05 to 0.1 mg once or twice per day, or a 0.1-mg patch replaced weekly, has been shown to reduce the frequency and severity of flushes in some women. Adverse effects include dizziness, fatigue, and hypotension.
5. Megestrol acetate, a synthetic progestin. Give 20 to 80 mg per day divided into two doses (titrated to clinical response [i.e., number of hot flushes/hour]).
6. Selective serotonin reuptake inhibitor. Paroxetine HCl (Paxil), 10 to 20 mg daily.

Notes About Other Hormones

Estriol

Estriol is the principal estrogen circulating during pregnancy (synthesized by the placenta). Once considered the safest of all the estrogens, estriol (although the weakest of all the estrogens in potency) in sufficient dose and duration has recently been found to exert a significant estrogen effect on the endometrium (hyperplasia), myometrium, and vagina.[44, 45] It has been found to have antiproliferative effects on breast cancer in animals. Lemon published several articles between 1966 and 1989, which claimed that estriol has anticancer effects in humans as well, but these reports have not been substantiated by other investigators as yet. High endogeneous estriol (or estradiol) levels in postmenopausal women may indicate high general endogeneous estrogen activity with its potential risk for inducing or accelerating estrogen-dependent neoplastic changes. I anxiously await more substantial data regarding the long-term end-organ protections and the cancer-protective effects of estriol in postmenopausal women, but in the interim, there appears to be no reliable justification for its sole and unopposed (by progesterone) use as a hormone supplementation therapy.

Biestrogen and Triestrogen

Triestrogen consists of 10% estradiol, 10% estrone, and 80% estriol; biestrogen consists (approximately) of estradiol (20%) and estriol (80%). It is interesting to note that a typical triestrogen preparation contains 12.5 micrograms of estradiol; the usual dosage is two tablets twice daily, resulting in a cumulative estradiol dose of 50 mcg or 0.5 mg, which may be therapeutic in the absence of the estrone and estriol. Jonathan Wright, the developer of triestrogen, states that the 2.5-mg and 5-mg dose regimens are, respectively, equivalent to 0.625 mg and 1.25 mg of conjugated estrogens. I have not been able to find reliable data on the serum levels reached with the recommended dosages, but at this dose, I have little doubt that triestrogen will achieve therapeutic serum levels. All of these estrogens undergo bio-interconversions in the body as well. The financial cost is high and most insurance companies will not cover them. Until more data are available to justify these costs, I will reserve the use of these preparations for women who insist on them and for those who cannot tolerate conventional bio-identical prescription estrogens.

Progesterone

Synthetic progestins are patentable synthetic progesterone products such as medroxyprogesterone acetate (Provera; Table 44–5). Because oral administration of unmodified progesterone results in considerable metabolism by intestinal microorganisms and digestive enzymes into inactive or less active compounds with only a small amount of biologically active compound absorbed, these compounds were synthetically modified to mimic the activity of progesterone; however, because they resist metabolism, they can be used less frequently and in lower doses. They are either C17 derivatives of progesterone (as medroxyprogesterone acetate) or C19 derivatives of testosterone (as norethindrone, norgestrel, and norgestimate). Unfortunately, these modifications were also responsible for causing many of the undesirable adverse effects that we have come to associate with synthetic progestin use, including bloating, fluid retention, weight gain, lethargy, decreased libido, and breast tenderness. Progestins also have a greater antagonistic effect on lipids than does oral micronized progesterone.[46] The central nervous system (CNS) sedating (anxiolytic) effects of oral progesterones are thought to be due to gut bacterial metabolism to 5-alpha and -beta pregnenolone metabolites that bind to brain gamma-aminobutyric acid (GABA) receptors, an effect not noted with gut-bypassing routes of administration.[47] Medroxyprogesterone acetate has the opposite brain effect, producing irritability. In addition, oral bio-identical progesterone is exposed to rapid decomposition in plasma. The bioavailability of oral progesterone is double when taken with food.

"Natural" USP progesterone is sold bulk to compounding companies and pharmacies to make oral oil-based capsules, tablets, creams, and gels. To date, just one study has showed that a large enough dose of topically applied progesterone is absorbed consistently enough to prevent proliferation of an estrogen-primed endometrium (endogeneous or exogenous source). Transdermal cream administration results in extensive metabolism in the skin (5-alpha reductase), but a recent study showed that a 60-mg dose per day of (properly applied and site rotated) topically applied progesterone cream was adequate to induce secretory transformation of the endometrium.[48] Although smaller topical doses may not protect the endometrium or bone, as little as 20 mg/day will reduce the severity and frequency of vasomotor symptoms despite poor systemic absorption.[49] *Crinone* is a newer, uterine-selective product suspended in a bioadhesive polycarbophil (adherent) vaginal gel (45 mg/day) that provides continuous local delivery of progesterone.

Despite the low plasma levels achieved, vaginal administration induces secretory transformation of the endometrium.[50]

Androgens

Well-controlled trials have shown short-term testosterone therapy to be of benefit in younger women experiencing surgical (or ablative) menopause (Table 44–6). In natural menopause, postmenopausal ovaries continue to produce testosterone and a small amount of DHEA. Few (small) clinical studies of androgen inclusion with estrogen have shown benefit (libido, energy level, mood) in older women. Some of these have used formulations that resulted in supraphysiologic doses in order to achieve the desired responses over the short term. The long-term effects of this practice are unknown at this time. Despite this, I believe that small doses of testosterone may be considered for symptomatic women in whom other treatments have been ineffective. Higher doses of androgen should be avoided owing to the potential virilizing effects (dose and duration dependent: acne, hirsutism), alterations in levels of lipids—especially HDL, hepatic function derangements, glucose levels in diabetics, and prothrombin time measurements in those on anticoagulant therapy. Response should be monitored closely with any dose used until more evidence is available on the long-term effects of exogenous androgen use in women. Commercially, methyltestosterone in combination with esterified estrogens is available, with more products on the horizon. Of course, compounding pharmacists can make daily application creams, gels, and troches to your specifications. Small amounts of the topical cream form of testosterone are well absorbed. When serum or saliva levels are checked periodically and the patient is well educated about its use, misuse, and potential adverse effects, topical dosing is quite acceptable and effective for most women.

Dehydroepiandrosterone (DHEA)

In women with known adrenal deficiency, the benefits of dehydroepiandrosterone (DHEA) have been established. Its use as a supplement in women without such deficiency and as a routine component of postmenopausal hormone supplementation is controversial. In deficient women, it appears to have a beneficial effect on sense of well-being and sexuality.[51] No study has been done to evaluate the safety of long-term DHEA supplementation in women. Animal studies suggest that DHEA may inhibit tumor-promoting substances. Biotransformation of exogenously administered DHEA results in significant increases in serum androstenedione, testosterone, and dihydrotestosterone; therefore, DHEA carries the same adverse effect profile as other androgens. In humans, unsupplemented breast cancer patients with higher circulating DHEA levels have been found to have higher survival rates than age-matched women with low circulating DHEA.[52]

Until more information is available regarding the routine, long-term use of DHEA, it seems prudent to be selective with its use, to always check a baseline level, and to closely monitor serum levels as well as clinical response or adverse reaction (virilization, hepatic function derangement); never endorse or supply more than a 50 mg/day oral dosage regimen in non–adrenal deficient patients. Over-the-counter sources of DHEA are not standardized, which may result in inconsistency with insufficient daily dosing. Lastly, one must be aware that the milligrams that are prescription-dosed by troche result in higher serum levels than do equivalent milligrams by oral dose, so lower amounts may be used.

SURGERY

Hysterectomy is the most commonly performed surgical procedure in the United States. Although most are accomplished without complication, it is not a risk-free procedure. Surgical risks include all those associated with any major abdominal or pelvic surgery. In addition, hysterectomy interrupts part of the blood supply to the ovary which may cause natural menopause to occur sooner. The practice of prophylactically removing ovaries (bilateral oophorectomy) along with the uterus in all women after age 40 to 45 should be reevaluated (if there is no pathology or specific risk factor present) owing to their significant perimenopausal and postmenopausal androgen contribution. The relative hyperestrogenism of the perimenopausal period may contribute to the incidence of menorrhagia, endometrial polyps, hyperplasia, and the growth of leiomyomata (common at these times) that are often cited as the reasons for this most common of all surgical procedures. It is important to realize that once the ovarian reserve is exhausted and the circulating estrogen levels drop, all but the polyps and atypical hyperplasia are likely to begin regressing. If the initial problems can be handled medically and the woman's hemoglobin level can be maintained with diet or modest iron replacement therapy, the reason for the surgery may be rendered moot. This may require a considerable amount of education and support of the patient to get her through this difficult time. The lure of having the problem "over and done with" is strong. If medical therapy fails in women with benign endometrial sampling results, intermediate surgical steps to treat menorrhagia might include (1) operative hysteroscopy with endometrial polyp/myoma resection, or (2) endometrial ablation done via a variety of available techniques, as well as therapeutic/diagnostic dilatation and curettage.

— THERAPEUTIC REVIEW —

Each woman in this transition is a unique individual who will have a unique menopause experience. She deserves inclusion in the decision-making process during a holistic, individual screening and management process.

Screening
- *Rule out other causes of "menopausal symptoms."*
- *Make a preventive healthcare plan with personal, population, and genetic risk factors in mind. Become a critically open-minded healthcare partner with your patient.*
- *Use testing selectively.*

Nutrition
- *Assess nutrition and supplements; make recommendations for long-term health enhancement. Discuss food first. Include whole, unprocessed, or minimally processed soy foods.*

Exercise
- *Assess activity level and make recommendations. Progress any new regimen slowly.*

Lifestyle
- *Evaluate sleep quality. Assess medication, stimulant, and alcohol use. Provide sleep hygiene advice. Intervene with herbal sleep aids if necessary, progressing to short-term pharmaceutical therapy as needed.*
- *Take a sexual history. Refer as appropriate. Surgically (or ablative) menopausal women are the most likely to benefit from existing combination estrogen/testosterone supplementation therapies. Evidence in naturally menopausal women is mixed. The long-term effects of androgens in women are unknown. Monitor closely for response if used.*
- *Encourage patient to seek social support to reduce feelings of isolation.*

THERAPEUTIC REVIEW continued

Mind-Body/Energetics/Spirituality

- *Consider behavioral, mind-body, and bioenergetic therapies for adjunctive treatment, prevention, symptom control, and health enhancement. Journaling may be very helpful. Regular meditation may be very helpful for enhancement of health and emotional and spiritual well-being.*

Botanical/Pharmaceutical

- *Consider herbal interventions in symptomatic perimenopausal women. Resist immediate initiation of estrogen as many women have normal or elevated levels (wide fluctuations). In nonsmokers who need symptom relief, menstrual cycling, and contraception, a 20-μg estrogen-containing oral contraceptive may be used in the absence of other contraindications.*
- *If hormone supplementation is agreed upon, begin with bio-identical products. Progesterone must be used in women receiving estrogen supplementation who have a uterus and may be prudent in others as well. Use the lowest doses possible to achieve the desired goals. Consider changing the route of administration before advancing to very high doses of estrogen. Reevaluate these choices periodically in the light of advancing age and the appearance of other medical or clinical issues and scientific evidence that may prompt adjustments and changes.*
- *If customized hormone supplementation is desired or necessary, educate the patient on its correct use, maintain close contact, monitor levels closely, and communicate with your local or mail-order compounding pharmacist.*

Surgery

- *Hysterectomy can often be avoided. Tailored medical therapy may be very effective. If it fails, several intermediate surgical interventions may be safer and more satisfying for your patient in the long run.*

Compounding Pharmacies

1. International Academy of Compounding Pharmacists–(800) 927–4227; Sugar Land, Texas. Provides referrals to pharmacists in your area who compound natural hormones. *www.iacprx.org*
2. Women's International Pharmacy–(800) 279–5708; Madison, Wisconsin. *www.womensinternational.com*
3. Transitions for Health–(800) 888–6814; Portland, Oregon.
4. California Pharmacy and Compounding Center–(800) 575–7776; Newport Beach, California.
5. Reed's Compounding Pharmacy–(877) REEDSRX; Tucson, Arizona. *www.treasuredesigns.com/reedsrx*

References

1. Eskine B: Menopause: Comprehensive Management, 4th ed. New York, Parthenon Publishing Group Inc, 2000.
2. Speroff L, Glass R, Kase N: Clinical Gynecologic Endocrinology and Infertility, 6th ed. Baltimore, Lippincott Williams & Wilkins, 1999, pp 31–52.
3. Stellato R, Crawford S, McKinly S, Longcope C: Can follicle-stimulating hormone be used to define menopausal status? Endocr Pract 4:137–141, 1998.
4. Lu Y, Chatterton R, Vogelsong K, May L: Direct radioimmunoassay of progesterone in saliva. J. Immunoassay 18:149–163, 1997.
5. Nachtigall L, Raju U, Banerjee S: Serum estradiol profiles in postmenopausal women undergoing three common estrogen replacement therapies: association with sex-hormone binding globulin, estradiol, and estrone levels. Menopause 7:243–250, 2000.
6. Polo-Kantola P, Erkkola R, Irjala K, et al: Effect of short-term transdermal estrogen replacement therapy on sleep: A randomized, double-blind cross-over trial in postmenopausal women. Fertil Steril 71:873–890, 1999.
7. Weil A: Getting a good night's sleep. Self Healing Newsletter. Watertown, Mass, Thorne Communications, September 1998, pp 1, 6.
8. Siegal DI: Habits worth changing. In Ourselves Growing Older: Women Aging With Knowledge and Power. New York, Touchstone Books, 1994, pp 33–34.
9. Lindahl O, Lindwall I: Double blind study of a valerian preparation. Pharmacol Biochem Behav 32:1065–1066, 1988.
10. Weber P: Management of osteoporosis: Is there a role for vitamin K? Internat J Vit Nutr Res 67:350–356, 1997.
11. Feskanich D, Weber P, Willett W, et al: Vitamin K intake and hip fractures in women: A prospective study. Am J Clin Nutr 69:74–79, 1999.
12. Kuiper G, Carlsson B, Grandien K, et al: Comparison of the ligand binding specificity and transcript tissue distribution of estrogen receptors alpha and beta. Endocrinology 138:863–870, 1997.
13. Setchell K, Cassidy A: Dietary isoflavones: Biological effects and relevance to human health. J Nutr 129(Suppl):758s–767s, 1999.
14. Lieberman SA: A review of the effectiveness of Cimicifuga racemosa for the symptoms of menopause. J Women's Health 7:525–529, 1998.
15. Duker EM, Kopanski L, Jang H, Wuttke W: Effects of extracts from C. racemosa on gonadotropin release in menopausal women and ovariectomized rats. Planta Med 57:420–424, 1991.
16. Freudenstein J, Bondinet C: Influence of isopropanolic aqueous extract of Cimicifugae racemosae rhizoma on proliferation of MCF-7 cells. In Abstract of 23rd International LOF Symposium on Phytooestrogens. Belgium, University of Gent, January 15, 1999.
17. Liske E, Therapy of climacteric complaints with Cimicifuga racemosa: Herbal medicine with clinically proven evidence. Menopause 5:250, 1998.
18. Einer-Jensen N, Zhao J, Anderson K, et al: Cimicifuga and molbrosia lack oestrogenic effects in mice and rats. Maturitas 25:149–153, 1996.
19. Liske E, Wustenberg P: Efficacy and safety of phytomedicines for gynecologic disorders with particular experience with C. racemosa and Hypericum perforatum. In Limpaphayom K, ed: 1st Asian-European Congress on the Menopause. Bangkok,

January 28–31, 1998; Bologna, Italy, Monduzzi Editore, 1998, pp 187–191.

20. Liske P: Therapeutic efficacy and safety of Cimicifuga racemosa for gynecological disorders. Adv Ther 15:45–53, 1998.

21. Blumenthal M, Goldberg A: Herbal Medicine: Expanded Commission E Monographs. Newton, Mass, Integrative Medicine Communications, American Botanical Council, 2000, pp 22–26.

22. Peppy J: Black cohosh: Cimicifuga racemosa. Am J Health Syst Pharm 56:1400–1402, 1999.

23. Hirata J, Swiersz L, Zell B, et al: Does dong quai have estrogenic effects in postmenopausal women? A double blind placebo controlled trial. Fertil Steril 68:981–986, 1997.

24. Murray M: The Healing Power of Herbs, 2nd ed. Rocklin, California, N.D. Prima Health, 1995, pp 639, 897.

25. Murray M: The Healing Power of Herbs, 2nd ed. Rocklin, California, N.D. Prima Health, 1995, pp 3, 5.

26. Frankhauser MP: Premenstrual syndrome. In Piro D, Talbert R, Yee G, eds: Pharmacotherapy: A Pathophysiologic Approach, 3rd ed. Stamford, CT, Appleton and Lange, 1997, pp 1621–1633.

27. Pye J, Mansel R, Hughes L: Clinical experience of drug treatment for mastalgia. Lancet 2:373–377, 1985.

28. Chenoy R, Hussain S, Tayob Y, et al: Effect of oral gamolenic acid from evening primrose oil on menopausal flushing. Br Med J 308:501–503, 1994.

29. Pizzorno J, Murray M: The Textbook of Natural Medicine, 2nd ed. London, Churchill Livingstone, 1999, p 772.

30. Foster S, Tyler, V: Tyler's Honest Herbal, 4th ed. Binghamton, New York, Haworth Herbal Press, 1999.

31. Zava D, Dollbaum C, Blen M, et al: Estrogen and progestin bioactivity of foods, herbs and spices. Proc Soc Exp Biol Med 217:369–378, 1998.

32. Murray M, Pizzorno J: Encyclopedia of Natural Medicine, Revised 2nd ed. Rocklin, Calif, N.D. Prima Health, 1998, p 348.

33. Liske E, Wustenberg P: The healing power of herbs. In Limpaphayom K, ed: 1st Asian-European Congress on the menopause. Bangkok, January 28–31, 1998; Bologna, Italy, Monduzzi Editore, 1998, pp 274–277.

34. Shifren L, Braunstein G, Simon J, et al: Transdermal testosterone treatment in women with impaired sexual function after oophorectomy. N Engl J Med 343:682–686, 2000.

35. Lad V: Ayurveda: The Science of Self-Healing, 2nd ed. Wilmot, Wisconsin, Lotus Light, 1984.

36. Ford D: The Dark Side of the Light Chasers. New York, Riverhead Books, 1998.

37. McKinlay J, McKinlay S, Branbilla D: The relative contribution of endocrine changes and social circumstances to depression in middle aged women. J Health Soc Behav 28:345–363, 1987.

38. Sherwin B: Impact of the changing hormonal milieu in psychological functioning. In Lobo R, ed: Treatment of the Postmenopausal Woman: Basic and Clinical Aspects. New York, Raven Press, 1994, pp 119–127.

39. Sherwin B, Gelford M: A prospective one-year study of estrogen and progestins in postmenopausal women: Effects on clinical symptoms and lipoprotein levels. Obstet Gynecol 73:759–766, 1989.

40. Revelli A, Massobrio M, Tesarik J: Nongenomic actions of steroid hormones in reproductive tissues. Endocr Rev 19:3–17, 1998.

41. Ferrava A, Kanter A, Glei D, Ackerson L: Hormone replacement therapy is associated with better glucose control in a multiethnic population with type 2 diabetes. The Northern California Kaiser Permanente Diabetes Registry. Presented at Annual Session of the ADA, Chicago, Illinois, June 1998.

42. Steinberg D, Pathosarthy S, Carew T: Beyond Cholesterol: Modifications of low density lipoproteins that increase its atherogenicity. N Engl J Med 320:915–924, 1989.

43. Siiteri P: Adipose tissue as a source of hormones. Am J Clin Nutr 45:277–282, 1987.

44. van Haaften M, Donker G, Sie-Go D, et al: Biochemical and histological effects of vaginal estriol and estradiol applications on the endometrium, myometrium and vagina of postmenopausal women. Gynecol Endocrinol 1:175–185, 1997.

45. Granberg S, Ylostald P, Wikland M, Karlsson B: Endometrial sonographic and histologic findings in women with and without hormonal replacement therapy suffering from postmenopausal bleeding. Maturitas 27:35–40, 1997.

46. The Writing Group for the PEPI Trial: Effects of estrogen/progestin regimens on heart disease risk factors in postmenopausal women. The Postmenopausal Estrogen/Progestin Interventions (PEPI) Trial. JAMA 273:199–208, 1995.

47. De Lignieres B, Dennerstein L, Backstrom T: Influence of route of administration on progesterone metabolism. Maturitas 21:251–257, 1995.

48. Burry K, Patton P, Hermsmeyer K: Percutaneous absorption of progesterone in postmenopausal women treated with transdermal estrogen. Am J Obstet Gynecol 180:1504–1511, 1999.

49. Leonetti H, Longo S, Anasti J: Transdermal progesterone cream for vasomotor symptoms and postmenopausal bone loss. Obstet Gynecol 94:225–228, 1999.

50. Miles R, Paulson R, Lobo R, et al: Pharmacokinetics and endometrial tissue levels of progesterone after administration by intramuscular and vaginal routes: A comparative study. Fertil Steril 62:485–490, 1994.

51. Wiebke A, Callies F, Van Vlijmen J, et al: Dehydroepiandrosterone replacement in women with adrenal insufficiency. N Engl J Med 341:1013–1020, 1999.

52. Mason B, Holdaway I, Skinner S, Kay R: The Relationship of urinary and plasma androgens to steroid receptors and menopausal status in breast cancer patients and their influence on survival. Breast Cancer Res Treat 32:203–212, 1994.

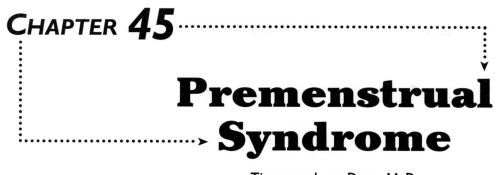

CHAPTER 45

Premenstrual Syndrome

Tieraona Low Dog, M.D.

PATHOPHYSIOLOGY

Premenstrual syndrome (PMS) is defined as a recurrent, cyclical set of physical and behavioral symptoms that occurs 7 to 14 days before the menstrual cycle and is troublesome enough to interfere with some aspects of a woman's life. PMS is estimated to affect up to 40% of menstruating women, with the most severe cases occurring in 2% to 5% of women who are between 26 and 35 years of age[1]. Although PMS has been recognized as a medical disorder for many years and most women can accurately describe the symptoms, the cause remains a mystery (Table 45–1). The complex relationships that exist among hormones may offer insight into why some women suffer more than others. Mild elevation of prolactin, a hormone that is primarily involved in regulating the development of the breast during pregnancy, has been associated with PMS,

menstrual irregularities, and breast tenderness. Low levels of thyroid hormone can contribute to depression, fatigue, and heavy menses.

Gonadal Hormones

A deficiency of progesterone or an abnormally high estrogen:progesterone ratio during the luteal phase was a popular theory for PMS for many years, although studies of hormone levels in women with PMS compared with those in women without the disorder fail to support this hypothesis.[2] Dr. Katherina Dalton first postulated this theory during the 1950s. Dr. Dalton administered natural progesterone in the form of injection, suppositories, or subcutaneous pellets, with 83% of women reporting complete relief of PMS symptoms.[3] However, because of the strict entrance criteria of the study, only 18% of

Table 45–1. Proposed Etiologies of Premenstrual Syndrome

Hormonal
Estrogen deficiency
Estrogen excess
High estrogen: progesterone ratio
Progesterone deficiency
Prolactin excess
Beta-endorphin deficiency

Fluid and Electrolyte
Aldosterone excess
Vasopressin excess
High sodium: potassium ratio
Renin/angiotensin abnormalities

Neurotransmitters
Serotonin deficiency
Cortisol excess
Hypoglycemia
Reduced glucose tolerance
Thyroid abnormalities
Adrenal insufficiency

Prostaglandins
Prostaglandin excess
Prostaglandin deficiency
Essential fatty acid deficiencies

Vitamins and Minerals
Pyridoxine deficiency
Vitamin A deficiency

Vitamin E deficiency
Magnesium deficiency
Calcium excess
Calcium deficiency
Potassium deficiency
Trace mineral deficiency
Zinc deficiency
Dopamine deficiency
Norepinephrine deficiency
Low platelet MAO activity

Hereditary
Genetic risk

Psychological factors
Beliefs around menstrual cycle
Coexisting psychiatric disorders
Poor coping skills
Poor self-esteem

Social Factors
Current marital/sexual relationships
Former marital/sexual relationships
Social stress
Psychosexual experiences
Cultural attitudes of PMS
Societal attitudes of PMS
Poor social network

PMS, Premenstrual syndrome.

women with PMS would appear to be suitable candidates for this therapy. A 1985 study using oral micronized progesterone (100 mg in the morning and 200 mg before bed time) starting 3 days after ovulation and continuing for 10 days found progesterone to be clearly superior to placebo for the symptoms of anxiety, stress, and poor concentration.[4]

Prolactin

Prolactin levels peak at ovulation and remain elevated during the luteal phase. Prolactin excess is associated with menstrual irregularities, diminished libido, depression, and hostility.[5] Some authors suggest that up to 62% of women with menstrual disorders have some degree of elevated prolactin.[6] Prolactin plays a role in breast stimulation and may be related to premenstrual breast tenderness. However, no consistent abnormalities have been found in women with PMS.[2]

Aldosterone

Aldosterone levels normally increase at ovulation and remain elevated during the luteal phase of the menstrual cycle. This elevation of aldosterone may be responsible for the congestive symptoms of PMS, such as edema, breast swelling, abdominal bloating, weight gain, and headaches. Differences in absolute levels between symptomatic and asymptomatic women are not noted in the literature.[7]

Endogenous Opiates

Some researchers have noted an increase in beta-endorpin plasma levels after ovulation. It is hypothesized that women with PMS may have a lower level of these circulating endogenous opiates or a more sudden withdrawal, causing them to experience increased sensitivity to pain and depression in the luteal phase.[8]

Vitamin B$_6$ and Magnesium

Vitamin B$_6$, (*pyridoxine*) is required for the metabolism of amino acids, carbohydrates, and lipids. The active forms of this vitamin are necessary coenzymes for the decarboxylation of 5-hydroxytryptophan to 5-HT and dopa to dopamine. Pyridoxine deficiency is associated with elevated levels of prolactin and low levels of serotonin and dopamine.[9] Pyridoxine deficiency can lead to depression, peripheral neuropathy, and mood changes.

Although serum levels of magnesium are often normal in women with PMS, researchers have noted lowered red blood cell magnesium levels in women with the disorder.[10] Calcium and dairy prod-

ucts may interfere with absorption, whereas refined sugar increases urinary excretion of magnesium. Magnesium deficiency can reduce dopamine and thyroid activity (with resultant increase in prolactin) and lead to depression, mood changes, and muscle cramping.

Hypoglycemia

The body appears to be more sensitive to insulin in the luteal phase, leading some researchers to hypothesize that transient hypoglycemia may account for some PMS symptoms.

Prostaglandins

Prostaglandins are associated with breast pain, fluid retention, abdominal cramping, headaches, irritability, and depression.[11] Physical premenstrual complaints and dysmenorrhea have been shown to respond to prostaglandin inhibitors.

Psychosocial Theory

Emotional and physical stressors have been found to influence the menstrual cycle. Travel, illness, stress, weather changes, and other environmental factors may affect ovulation, length of menstrual cycle, and severity of PMS.[12] Cultural, societal, and personal attitudes toward menstruation also appear to play a role in the presence and severity of PMS. The dynamic interplay of environment, spirit, and physiology demands an integrated biopsychosocial approach to treatment.

SYMPTOMS OF PREMENSTRUAL SYNDROME

More than 150 symptoms have been associated with premenstrual syndrome. The most common are shown in Table 45–2.

The American Psychiatric Association has defined diagnostic criteria for premenstrual dysphoric disorder, a more severe form of PMS. To be diagnosed with this disorder, a woman must have at least five of the following symptoms occurring cyclically and serious enough to interfere with her normal activities.

Table 45–2. Symptoms of Premenstrual Syndrome

Nervousness	Anxiety	Irritability
Fatigue	Lethargy	Depression
Mood swings	Water retention	Abdominal bloating
Tender breasts	Headache	Change in appetite
Back pain	Acne	Sugar cravings
Diarrhea	Low libido	Constipation
Clumsiness	Dizziness	Low self-esteem
Social isolation	Insomnia	Joint pain

1. Feeling of sadness or hopelessness, possible suicidal thoughts
2. Feelings of tension or anxiety
3. Mood swings marked by periods of teariness
4. Persistent irritability or anger
5. Disinterest in daily activities and relationships
6. Trouble concentrating
7. Fatigue or low energy
8. Food cravings or bingeing
9. Sleep disturbances
10. Feeling out of control
11. Physical symptoms such as bloating, breast tenderness, headaches, and joint or muscle pain

Although this addition to the fourth edition of the Diagnostic and Statistical Manual of Mental Disorders is useful for recognizing PMS as a valid disorder, it is somewhat disturbing that behavioral aspects are the primary focus. With the vast number of physiologic and hormonal interactions taking place in a woman's body, there would seem to be a multitude of explanations for the variety of symptoms. Thus, it is also reasonable to assume that a variety of therapies may help and that not all remedies are universally effective.

CLASSIFICATIONS OF PREMENSTRUAL SYNDROME

Dr. Guy Abraham developed a system for categorizing premenstrual syndrome into four distinct subgroups.[13] The following is a summary of these categories:

PMS-A (anxiety) is believed to be related to high levels of estrogen and deficiency of progesterone. Women experience irritability, anxiety, and emotional lability.

PMS-C (carbohydrate craving) is of unclear etiology but may be caused by enhanced intracellular binding of insulin. Women experience increased appetite, sugar and carbohydrate craving, headache, and heart palpitations.

PMS-D (depression) is most likely caused by low levels of estrogen, which leads to excessive breakdown of neurotransmitters. Low estrogen levels may be caused by enhanced adrenal androgen or progesterone secretion.

PMS-H (hyperhydration) is the result of increased water retention secondary to elevated levels of aldosterone. Elevated levels of aldosterone in the premenstrual period may be the result of excess estrogen, excessive salt intake, stress, or magnesium deficiency. Women report weight gain, breast tenderness and fullness, swelling of the hands and feet, and abdominal bloating.

Although used by many traditional and alternative practitioners, these categories should only be considered as guidelines, because the basis for these categories is not adequately confirmed by current research and most women do not neatly fall into just one of these slots.

CLINICAL EVALUATION OF PREMENSTRUAL SYNDROME

A complete physical examination, including pelvic evaluation, should be performed and laboratory tests should be done to rule out anemia or hypothyroidism. One might include a prolactin test. It is extremely useful for a woman to record her symptoms on a daily basis for at least two complete menstrual cycles to see just what her symptoms are and how they are related to her menses.

It is important to address any other underlying medical conditions that may be masked as PMS. One report found that 75% of women receiving care for PMS at specialized clinics had another diagnosis that accounted for many of their symptoms, primarily major depression and other mood disorders.[14]

INTEGRATIVE THERAPY

Once the diagnosis has been established, the first place to start is with lifestyle. One of the most effective therapies but also one of the most difficult for many women to implement is exercise.

Exercise

Exercise remains understudied in the scientific world because it does not fit well into the double-blinded, placebo-controlled study. The few studies that have been conducted on the role of exercise in PMS have clearly shown that women who engage in regular physical exercise have fewer symptoms of PMS than women who do not. Women who exercise regularly note improvement in all symptoms of PMS.[15] It is the frequency rather than the intensity of exercise that appears to decrease the negative mood and physical symptoms that occur during the premenstrual period.[16] It is postulated that exercise may reduce symptoms by decreasing estrogen levels, decreasing circulating catecholamines, improving glucose tolerance, and elevating endorphin levels.[17] Aerobic activity appears to be most beneficial; however, yoga and tai chi are probably equally effective if performed at least three times per week.

Diet and Nutrition

Many Americans eat less than an ideally healthy diet, but some researchers have found this to be even more true for women with PMS. A 1983 report noted that women with PMS consumed 275% more refined sugar, 79% more dairy products, 78% more sodium, 62% more refined carbohydrates, 77% less manganese, and 53% less iron than women without PMS.[18] These dietary excesses and deficiencies may help explain some of the symptoms women experience in the premenstrual period. Dairy products are high in sodium and interfere with magnesium absorption. Refined sugars increase the urinary excretion of magnesium.[19] Heavy intake of sugar also increases sodium and water retention due to the rapid release of insulin. Dietary salt may exacerbate swelling. Although studies give conflicting data about caffeine and premenstrual breast tenderness, many women find relief if they eliminate or reduce their consumption of caffeinated beverages and foods during the 2 weeks before their menstrual flow (Table 45–3).

Dietary Fat

Fiber-rich, low-fat diets may be beneficial for women with PMS by reducing blood levels of estrogen. Estrogen is conjugated in the liver and sent to the small intestine via bile for elimination in the feces. Intestinal bacteria can deconjugate estrogen and allow it to be reabsorbed into the body.

NOTE

Fiber-rich, low-fat diets suppress the ability of fecal bacteria to deconjugate estrogen, thereby enhancing fecal excretion.

Several studies have shown that reducing fat (< 20%) and increasing fiber for only 3 months can reduce a woman's serum estrogen level.[20] If one accepts the theory that elevated levels of estrogen can worsen PMS symptoms, consuming a diet high in fruits, vegetables, and whole grains and low in saturated fat may be wise. Four to six small meals should be consumed throughout the day to ease food cravings and ease mood swings. Alcohol consumption should be limited because it can worsen PMS symptoms.

Table 45–3. Caffeine Amounts in Common Foods and Beverages
....

Serving Size (oz)	Caffeine (mg)
Coffee, instant (6–8)	65–100
Coffee, percolated (6–8)	85–135
Coffee, filtered (6–8)	115–175
Coffee, decaffeinated (6–8)	1–5
Tea, instant (6–8)	35–70
Tea, brewed (6–8)	28–150
Tea, iced (6–8)	40–45
Chocolate, dark semisweet (1)	5–35
Chocolate, milk (1)	1–15
Cola beverage (8)	25–30

Supplements

Calcium

The data on calcium for alleviation of PMS are convincing. A large multicenter trial reported that of 497 women diagnosed with PMS, those who took 1200 mg per day of calcium carbonate had a 48% reduction in total symptoms compared with a 30% reduction in those taking placebo.[21] This effect was evident by the third month of treatment. Many women should take calcium to maintain strong bones. Recommending a trial of calcium for 3 months is certainly warranted for women with PMS.

Dosage. 1200 mg per day

Magnesium

Women with PMS have consistently been shown to have low levels of magnesium in their red blood cells. Although the evidence is less than adequate, studies have found that magnesium in doses of 200 to 400 mg per day relieves premenstrual mood fluctuations and depression. Dietary sources of magnesium include green leafy vegetables, tofu, legumes, nuts, seeds, and whole grains. Magnesium deficiency produces symptoms of fatigue, irritability, mental confusion, PMS, menstrual cramps, insomnia, muscle cramps, and heart disturbances.

Dosage. 200 to 400 mg per day

Precautions. Magnesium may cause diarrhea. Magnesium is available in many forms. The organic forms of magnesium (citrate, malate) are said to be less laxative than the inorganic salts (oxide, carbonate).

Vitamin B₆

Pyridoxine is a water soluble B vitamin that serves as a cofactor in more than 100 enzyme reactions, many of which are related to the metabolism of amino acids and proteins. Because of its involvement in the synthesis of neurotransmitters, it has been studied for numerous neurologic conditions. The use of pyridoxine (Vitamin B₆) to alleviate PMS symptoms has been evaluated in more than 28 trials since 1975. This research was inspired by the work of Adams and colleagues,[22] who first reported that vitamin B₆ successfully alleviated the depression associated with use of oral contraceptives. A systematic review was published of their work in the *British Medical Journal*.[23] Ten randomized, placebo-controlled, double-blinded, parallel or crossover studies were included. Studies of cyclical mastalgia and multivitamin preparations with at least 50 mg of vitamin B₆ were also included. Only three of these trials scored higher than 3 on the Jadad scale for methodological quality. Most trials were small (< 60 women). One of the largest studies included women who were also taking oral contraceptives, analgesics, diuretics, and psychotropic medications, which make the effects of vitamin B₆ difficult to ascertain. None of the trials included power calculations. The author of the meta-analysis, using a random effects model, found the overall odds ratio in favor of pyridoxine to be 1.57 (95% confidence interval of 1.40–1.77). When looking at the effects on depressive symptoms in five trials, the overall odds ratio in favor of pyridoxine was 2.12 (95% confidence interval of 1.80–2.48).

Current thinking postulates that pyridoxine may ease symptoms of PMS via its ability to increase the synthesis of serotonin, dopamine, norepinephrine, histamine, and taurine.[24] Serotonin is important for the regulation of sleep and appetite, and prevention of depression. Low levels of serotonin and dopamine may play a role in premenstrual symptoms.[25] Trials used doses ranging from 50 to 500 mg per day. For most women, it is probably prudent to limit single doses of B_6 to 50 mg and not to exceed 100 mg per day. Research suggests that the liver cannot process more than a 50-mg dose of pyridoxine at one time.[27] Conversion of pyridoxine to its active form is dependent on other nutrients such as magnesium and riboflavin. It may be prudent to take vitamin B_6 as part of more complete supplement.

Dosage. 50 mg a day

Precautions. Although pyridoxine is a water-soluble vitamin, it is associated with toxicity when taken in moderate to large doses over time. There are a few reports of toxicity occurring with prolonged ingestion of 150 mg per day.[26] Toxicity may occur if large doses of pyridoxine overwhelm the liver's ability to add a phosphate group to form pyridoxal-5-phosphate, the active form of vitamin B_6.

Chaste Tree (Vitex agnus-castus)

Dioscorides, the Greek physician, described the dried ripe fruits of the chaste tree some 2000 years ago. The Latin name *agnus castus* means "chaste lamb," in reference to the belief that the seeds supposedly reduced sexual desire. From this belief stemmed the other common name of the herb—monk's pepper. *Vitex agnus castus* has long been used for the alleviation of menstrual disorders. *Vitex* is a popular remedy for treating women with premenstrual syndrome in Germany, where one focused drug monitoring study found that 90% of more than 1500 women with symptoms of PMS reported improvement or resolution of symptoms while using a commercial extract of the herb (Agnolyt).[28]

Two comparative studies have been conducted with *Vitex* and pyridoxine for the treatment of PMS. One hundred seventy-five women (age range of 18–45 yr) were randomized to receive either 200 mg per day of pyridoxine or 175 mg per day of chaste tree for a 3-month trial. A reduction in total symptom score (PMTS) scale occurred in both groups. The total score decreased in the *Vitex* group from 15 to 5 and from 12 to 5 in the pyridoxine group.[29] A more recent trial also involved 175 women who were randomized to receive either one standardized *Vitex* capsule plus one placebo capsule or two 100-mg capsules of

pyridoxine. Efficacy was evaluated by use of the premenstrual tension scale (PMTS) and clinical global impression (CGI) scale. Only 127 participants were available for evaluation at the end of the 3-month trial. Overall, 77.1% of those in the *Vitex* group reported improvement compared with 60.6% in the pyridoxine group. Eighty percent of physicians rated both treatments as "adequate." No serious adverse effects were noted. Twelve women in the *Vitex* group and 5 in the pyridoxine group reported side effects including headache, gastrointestinal complaints, and skin problems.[30] These studies are difficult to interpret, because they did not use a placebo arm.

> ### NOTE
>
> *Combining chaste tree with vitamin B_6 may be a beneficial first step in the treatment of PMS.*

The proposed mechanism is increased luteinizing hormone levels that normalize the second part of the menstrual cycle. Symptoms of corpus luteum insufficiency include irregular menstrual cycles and dysfunctional uterine bleeding. Chaste tree has been found to restore progesterone concentrations and prolong the hyperthermic phase in basal body temperature curve when 40 drops of tincture are taken daily for at least 3 months.[31] *Vitex* has an inhibitory action upon prolactin due to its dopamine agonist properties. Women with hyperprolactinemia often experience menstrual dysfunction. Some researchers postulate that it is the correction of hyperprolactinemia that causes the reversal of LH suppression, resulting in full development of the corpus luteum during the luteal phase of the cycle.[32] Studies in both animals and humans have demonstrated prolactin inhibition with *Vitex*.

The German health authorities approve the use of chaste tree fruit for irregularities of the menstrual cycle, premenstrual complaints, and mastodynia.[33]

Dosage. 3 to 5 ml of the tincture (1:5) each day

Precautions. Chaste tree can rarely cause GI reactions, alopecia, headaches, tiredness, dry mouth, and increased menstrual flow.

Black Cohosh (Cimicifuga racemosa)

The eclectics used black cohosh for restlessness, nervous excitement, breast pain, and menstrual headaches.[34] Although most research has focused on black cohosh for the alleviation for menopausal complaints, a study of 135 women found a standardized extract of black cohosh to be effective in reducing the symptoms of anxiety, tension, and depression.[35] Research on an Asian species of *Cimicifuga* has indicated a possible central nervous system effect. Preliminary data suggest that the rhizome may act as a mild serotonin reuptake inhibitor.[36] If this effect occurs with *C. racemosa*, it could partially explain the positive benefits seen in women with PMS. The German health authorities have endorsed the use of black cohosh of premenstrual discomfort and dysmenorrhea.[37]

Dosage. 40 mg of the standardized extract twice daily (standardized to 2.5% triterpenes)

Precautions. The most common complaint is gastrointestinal disturbance. Other potential adverse effects include headache, heaviness of the legs, and weight gain.

Ginkgo (Ginkgo biloba)

If women primarily experience congestive symptoms in the premenstrual period (fluid retention, breast tenderness, weight gain), a trial of ginkgo may offer some relief. A double-blinded, placebo-controlled trial was conducted with 165 women complaining of premenstrual symptoms. Participants received placebo or a standardized extract of ginkgo (24% ginkgoflavones and 6% terpenes) 80 mg twice daily from day 16 of their menstrual cycle through day 5 of their next cycle. Evaluation by patient and physician found ginkgo to be effective for alleviation of breast pain and tenderness and fluid retention.[38] Ginkgo is known to augment venous tone and reduce capillary fragility.

Dosage. 80 mg of a standardized extract twice daily

Precautions. Gingko may cause gastrointestinal intolerance, headache, dizziness, palpitations, and allergic skin reactions.

Caution. Careful supervision should be maintained when gingko is used with blood thinning products.

St. John's Wort (Hypericum perforatum)

A number of herbalists recommend St. John's wort for women who complain of depression and irritability in the premenstrual period. In 1996, a meta-analysis (a review) of 23 randomized clinical trials involving 1757 patients with depression found St. John's wort to be superior to placebo and as effective as prescription medication for the treatment of mild to moderate depression.[39] The mechanism by which this herb improves mood is not completely understood.

A number of trials have been conducted using selective serotonin reuptake inhibiting (SSRI) medications. The studies have shown that approximately 60% of women with severe PMS obtain significant relief with these drugs. It would be interesting to see how St. John's wort fares in comparison with SSRIs for the alleviation of PMS.

A trial of St. John's wort is appropriate for women who have no contraindications for the herb.

Dosage. The dose is 300 mg of St. John's wort standardized to contain 4% to 5% hyperforin or 0.3% hypericin three times per day. The dose for tincture (1:5) is 2 to 3 mL three times per day.

Precautions. Those taking medications that increase photosensitivity, protease inhibitors (for HIV), cyclosporine, or other medications that are metabolized by the P450 system should avoid St. John's wort.

Kava (Piper methysticum)

Physicians sometimes prescribe alprazolam, a benzodiazepine, for the treatment of PMS. Because this drug has the potential for habituation and abuse, other anxiolytics should be tried first. This would include kava, an herb that has been used in the South Pacific for centuries as a social beverage and medicinal agent. Kava is an effective anxiolytic and is approved by the German health authorities for "conditions of nervous anxiety, stress, and restlessness."[40] I have successfully used kava in my practice for many women with PMS. It can be given from day 16 of the menstrual cycle through day 5 of the next cycle.

Dosage. The daily dose should be equal to 60 to 100 mg of kavalactones.

Precautions. Gastrointestinal distress, dizziness, headache, and pupil dilation may occur and at high doses may impair ability to drive. Chronic use at high doses can result in a pellegra-like dermopathy that results in yellow flaking of the skin and reddening of the eyes. Kava may be associated with liver toxicity in rare cases.

Other Botanicals

Numerous herbs have been used throughout history for the treatment of premenstrual complaints. Older herbals describe PMS as a type of hysteria. The word hysteria was taken from the Greek word, *hystera*, meaning uterus. The condition was so named because it was primarily noted in women. Herbs included blue cohosh (*Caulophyllum thalictroides*), false unicorn (*Chamaelirium luteum*), aletris (*Aletris farinosa*), wild yam (*Dioscorea villosa*), black haw (*Viburnum prunifolium*), and pulsatilla (*Anemone pulsatilla*). False unicorn and aletris are both under threat in the wild and so are not discussed. Neither is being successfully cultivated in quantities that would allow mass commercial sale.

Early eclectic physicians considered blue cohosh a specific remedy for "hysteria" occurring before the menstrual flow.[41] The eclectics considered wild yam to be a useful antispasmodic for dysmenorrhea and ovarian neuralgia. However, older in vitro studies of *Dioscorea villosa* extracts failed to demonstrate any antispasmodic effects on the uterus.[42] Pulsatilla, also known as pasque flower, has been shown to reduce uterine contractions in vitro,[43] and the extract exerts sedative and analgesic activity. The *British Herbal Compendium* lists as indications for pulsatilla "painful spasmodic conditions of the male and female reproductive systems; dysmenorrhea."[44] The fresh plant contains protoanemonin, a strong local irritant, but this compound is not present in the dried plant.

Society and Culture

Although many treatments discussed in this chapter have shown some degree of success, they are not universally effective and none can be touted as a true cure for PMS. The question remains as to whether premenstrual syndrome is caused by individual pathologic conditions or by cultural beliefs and societal norms. Throughout recorded history, there is documentation of menstrual taboos. Women were forbidden to sit on chairs or share eating and cooking utensils during their menses, forbidden to touch grapes on the vine for fear of causing them to rot, beaten if they bled more than 4 days in an attempt to purify them, placed in isolated huts away from other members of the group, and so forth. Would PMS exist to the extent it does if women had been elevated to a lofty position during their menses? What if women were considered sacred and powerful during the menses, asked to bless the fruits of the field and lead religious ceremonies, or seated at the head of the dining table in a place of honor? Although there is no way to adequately answer these questions, it makes sense to me that the deeply held attitudes and beliefs in many cultures and societies have either positively or negatively affected the way women feel about menstruation. A biopsychosocial model appears to be the best approach.

 THERAPEUTIC REVIEW

Lifestyle
- *Stress management*
- *Limit alcohol and drugs of abuse*
- *Regular daily exercise*

Nutrition
- *Well-balanced diet rich in fiber and low in fat*
- *Restriction of refined sugar, caffeine, and salt*
- *Calcium 1200 mg per day*
- *Vitamin B$_6$ 50 mg once or twice daily*
- *Magnesium 100 mg twice daily*
- *Chaste tree (Vitex) 3 to 5 mL tincture (1:5) or standardized extract daily*
- *Therapy for specific symptoms of PMS*

Breast Tenderness
- *Caffeine restriction*
- *Evening primrose oil 1.5 g twice daily (continuous)*
- *Ginkgo 80 mg standardized extract twice daily (ovulation through menses)*

Weight Gain
- *Ginkgo 80 mg standardized extract twice daily (ovulation through menses)*

Anxiety and Mood Swings
- *Black cohosh 40 mg standardized extract twice daily (continuous therapy)*
- *Kava 60 mg kavalactones standardized extract twice daily (ovulation through menses)*
- *Oral micronized progesterone 200 mg at bed time (ovulation through menses)*

Depression
- *St. John's wort 300 mg standardized extract three times daily (continuous therapy)*

Headache, Joint Pain, Cramps
- *Black haw or cramp bark 3 to 5 mL tincture (1:5) twice to four times daily as needed*
- *Kava 60 mg kavalactones standardized extract twice daily as needed*
- *Pulsatilla tincture (1:5) 1 mL three times daily as needed*
- *Oral micronized progesterone 200 mg at bed time (ovulation through menses)*

Insomnia
- *Kava 60 mg kavalactones standardized extract twice daily as needed*

References

1. American College of Obstetrics and Gynecology: Committee opinion. Int J Gynecol Obstet 50:80, 1995.
2. Rubinow DR, Hoban HC, Groven GN, et al: Changes in plasma hormones across the menstrual cycle in patients with menstrually related mood disorder and in control subjects. Am J Obstet Gynecol 158:5–11, 1988.
3. Keye W: Medical treatment of premenstrual syndrome. Can J Psychol 30:483–487, 1985.
4. Dennerstein L, Spencer-Gardner C, Gotts G, et al: Progesterone and the premenstrual syndrome: a double blind crossover trial. Br Med J. 290:1617–1621, 1985.
5. Kellner R, Buckman MT, Fava GA, et al: Hyperprolactinemia, distress, and hostility. Am J Psychiatry 141:759–763, 1984.
6. Bohnert KJ. Clinical study on chaste tree for menstrual disorders. Quart Rev Nat Med Spring:19–21, 1997.
7. Munday MR, Brush MG, Taylor RW: Correlations between progesterone, oestradiol, and aldosterone levels in the premenstrual syndrome. Clin Endocrinol 14:1–9, 1981.
8. Chuong CJ, Coulam CB, Kao PC, et al: Neuropeptide levels in the premenstrual syndrome. Fertil Steril 44:760–765, 1985.
9. Clare AW: Premenstrual syndrome: Single or multiple causes? Can J Psychiatry 30:474–482, 1985.
10. Sherwood RA, Rocks BF, Steward A, et al: Magnesium and premenstrual syndrome. Ann Clin Biochem 23:667–670, 1986.
11. Budoff PW: The use of prostaglandin inhibitors for the premenstrual sydrome. J Reprod Med 28:465–468, 1983.
12. Hamilton JA, Parry B, Alagna S, et al: Premenstrual mood changes: A guide to evaluation and treatment. Psychiat Ann 14:426–435, 1984.
13. Abraham GE: Nutritional factors in the etiology of premenstrual tension syndromes. J Reprod Med 28:446–464, 1983.
14. DeJong R, Rubinow DR, Roy-Byrne P, et al: Premenstrual mood disorder and psychiatric illness. Am J Psychiatry 142:1359–1361, 1985.
15. Aganoff J, Boyle G: Aerobic exercise, mood states and menstrual cycle symptoms. J Psychosom Res 38:183–192, 1994.
16. Johnson W, Carr-Nangle R, Bergeron K: Macronutrient intake, eating habits, and exercise as moderators of menstrual distress in healthy women. Psychosom Med 57:324–330, 1995.
17. Gannon L: The potential role of exercise in the alleviation of menstrual disorders and menopausal symptoms: A theoretical synthesis of current research. Women Health 14:105–127, 1988.
18. Abraham G: Nutritional factors in the etiology of the premenstrual tension syndromes. J Reprod Med 28:446–464, 1983.
19. Abraham G: Magnesium deficiency in premenstrual tension. Magnes Bull 4:68, 1982.
20. Rose D: Diet, hormones, and cancer. Ann Rev Publ Health 14:1–7, 1993.
21. Thys-Jacobs S, Starkey P, Bernstein D, Tian J: Calcium carbonate and the premenstrual syndrome: Effects on premenstrual and menstrual symptoms. Am J Obstet Gynecol 179:444–452, 1998.
22. Adams PW, Rose DP, Folkard J, et al: The effect of pyridoxine hydrochloride (vitamin B_6) upon depression associated with oral contraception. Lancet 1:897–904, 1973.
23. Wyatt KM, Dimmock PW, Jones PW et al: Efficacy of vitamin B6 in the treatment of premenstrual syndrome: Systematic review. BMJ 318:1375–1381, 1999.
24. Ebadi M, Govitrapong P: Pyridoxal phosphate and neurotransmitters in the brain. In Tryfiates G (ed): Vitamin B_6 Metabolism

and Role in Growth. Westport, CT, Food and Nutrition Press, 1980, p 223.
25. Taylor DL, Mathew RJ, Ho BT, Weinman ML, et al: Serotonin levels and platelet uptake during premenstrual tension. Neuropsychobiology 12:16–18, 1984.
26. Cohen M, Bendich A: Safety of pyridoxine—a review of human and animal studies. Toxicol Lett 34:129–139, 1986.
27. Zempleni J: Pharmacokinetics of vitamin B_6 supplements in humans. J Am Coll Nutr 14:579–586, 1995.
28. Peteres Welte C, Albrecht M: Menstrual abnormalities and PMS: *Vitex agnus-castus.* Therapiewoche Gynakol 7:49–52, 1994.
29. Schulz V, Hanself R, Tyler V: Rational Phytotherapy: A Physician's Guide to Herbal Medicine. Berlin, Springer-Verlag, 1998, pp 240–243.
30. Lauritzen C, Reuter HD, Repges R, et al: Treatment of premenstrual tension syndrome with *Vitex agnus castus*: Controlled, double-blind study versus pyridoxine. Phytomedicine 4:183–189, 1997.
31. Newall CA, et al: Herbal Medicines: A Guide for Health-Care Professionals. London, The Pharmaceutical Press, 1996, pp 19–20.
32. Bohnert KJ: Clinical study on chaste tree for menstrual disorders. Quart Rev Nat Med Spring:19–21, 1997.
33. Blumenthal M, Gruenwald J, Hall T, Rister RS (eds): The Complete German Commission E Monographs: Therapeutic Guide to Herbal Medicine. Boston, Integrative Medicine Communications, 1998, p 108.
34. Felter HW: The Eclectic Materia Medica: Pharmacology and Therapeutics. Cincinnati, OH, John K. Scudder, 1922.
35. Dittmar FW, et al: Premenstrual syndrome. Treatment with a phytopharmaceutical. Therapiewoche Gynakol 5:60–68, 1992.
36. Liao JF, Jan YM, Huang SY, et al: Evaluation with receptor binding assay on the water extracts of ten CNS-active Chinese herbal drugs. Proceedings of the National Science Council, Republic of China. Life Sci 19:151–158, 1995.
37. Blumenthal M, Gruenwald J, Hall T, Rister RS (eds): The Complete German Commission E Monographs: Therapeutic Guide to Herbal Medicine. Boston, Integrative Medicine Communications, 1998, p 90.
38. Tamborini A, Taurelle R: Value of a standardized Ginkgo biloba extract in the management of congestive symptoms of premenstrual syndrome. Rev Fr Gynecol Obstet 88:447–457, 1993.
39. Linde K, Ramirez G, Mulrow CD, et al: St. John's wort for depression—an overview and meta-analysis of randomised clinical trials. *BMJ* 313:253–258, 1996.
40. Blumenthal M, Gruenwald J, Hall T, Rister RS (eds): The Complete German Commission E Monographs: Therapeutic Guide to Herbal Medicine. Boston, Integrative Medicine Communications, 1998, p 156.
41. W.E.B: *Caulophyllum thalictroides.* Eclect Med J 57:628–630, 1987.
42. Pilcher JD: The action of certain drugs on the excised uterus of the guinea-pig. J Pharm Exp Ther 8:110–111, 1916.
43. Pilcher JD, Burman GE, Delzell WR: The action of the so-called female remedies on the excised uterus of the guinea pig. Arch Intern Med 18:557–583, 1916.
44. Bradley PR: *British Herbal Compendium:* A handbook of Scientific Information on Widely Used Plant Drugs, vol 1. British Herbal Medicine Association, Dorset, England, 1992; pp 179–180.

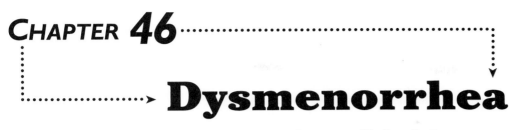

CHAPTER 46

Dysmenorrhea

Francine Rainone, Ph.D., D.O.

PATHOPHYSIOLOGY

Dysmenorrhea is painful menstruation. It is characterized by crampy lower abdominal pain and often associated with nausea, vomiting, diarrhea, headache, dizziness, and/or back pain. Primary dysmenorrhea (PD) refers to pain that occurs in the absence of pelvic pathology. It typically begins in adolescence, after ovulatory menstrual cycles are established. Symptoms usually begin a few hours before menses and persist for 1 to 3 days. Secondary dysmenorrhea refers to pain in the presence of pelvic pathology.[1] The suggestions in this chapter are restricted to the treatment of PD, assuming that secondary dysmenorrhea has been ruled out. In addition, these suggestions are not necessarily meant to apply to premenstrual syndrome (PMS). The treatment of women who suffer from both PD and PMS is not simply additive, and is beyond the scope of this chapter.

Like all chronic pain problems, the etiology of PD is multifactorial. On the biochemical level, prostaglandins (PGs) probably account for most of the symptoms.[2] Stimulation of the uterus by estrogen and progesterone increases endometrial stores of arachidonic acid (AA). During menstruation, AA is converted to $PGF_2\alpha$, the PGE_2 series, and leukotrienes (Fig. 46–1), all of which induce prolonged uterine contractions that decrease blood flow, resulting in uterine ischemia. In addition, PGF_2 and PGE_2 can cause contraction of bowel and vascular smooth muscle, resulting in nausea, vomiting, and diarrhea. In contrast the PGE_3 and PGE_1 series are primarily anti-inflammatory. The PGE_3 series is produced from eicosapentanoic acid (EPA), which competitively inhibits AA, and the PGE_1 series results from the oxidation of dihomo-gamma-linolenic acid (DGLA).[3]

Epidemiologic studies consistently find that family history in first-degree relatives, prolonged duration of menses, increased amount of bleeding, early menarche, and nulliparity are risk factors for primary dysmenorrhea.[4–6] The latter two factors suggest that prolonged exposure to estrogen contributes to PD. Family history, early menarche, and increased amount of bleeding also correlate with increased severity of pain. A simple grading scale helps to guide treatment (Table 46–1). Up to 15% of adolescent women have Grade 3 PD, the most severe type.[4]

NUTRITION

- *Arachidonic Acid* (AA): Diet is the major source of AA. Decreasing the amount of AA has been shown to decrease dysmenorrhea in adolescents.[5] Recommendations are substantial reductions in portions of red meats, poultry, and whole milk to decrease levels of AA.
- *Omega-3 fatty acids*: Increasing consumption of the precursors of the anti-inflammatory PGE_3 series has also been shown to relieve dysmenorrhea.[6] Like most practitioners, I believe the maximum effect of dietary change is experienced when increased omega-3 consumption is combined with decreased AA consumption. Three servings per week of cold-water fish, such as salmon, mackerel, and halibut (see Chapter 84, The Anti-Inflammatory Diet), are recommended; an alternative is 1 tablespoon of flaxseed oil per day. As a supplement, 2 g of EPA (fish oil) in divided doses or 3000 mg of flaxseed oil should be taken twice daily. Flaxseed has twice the amount of omega-3 fatty acids as fish oil and is much cheaper.
- DGLA: Because this acid can be metabolized to AA, compounds with high concentrations of DGLA, such as evening primrose oil, black currant oil, and borage oil, are not recommended for the treatment of PD.

BOTANICALS

- Willow bark extract (*Salix cortex*): Aspirin (acetylsalicylic acid) was originally made by hydrolysis, oxidation, and acetylation of salicin, the major active ingredient in willow bark. Willow bark inhibits cyclooxygenase but does not cause irreversible platelet aggregation. As with NSAIDs, dosing should begin the day before symptoms are expected and continue for the amount of time the symptoms usually persist.
  Dosage. 240 mg per day of salicin in divided doses
- Cramp bark (*Viburnum opulus*) and black haw (*Viburnum prunifolium*): The exact mechanism of action is not known, but these plants have a long history of use as uterine relaxants and diuretics. Black haw is known to contain tannins, oxalic acid, salicin, and salicylic acid, as well as scopoletin, which may be a uterine relaxant.[7]

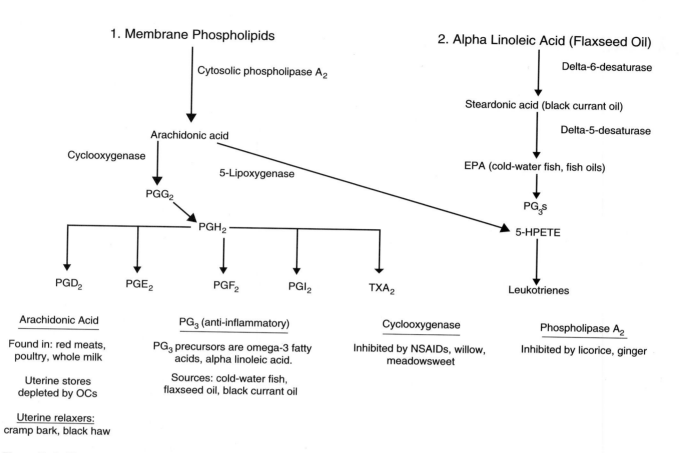

1. Membrane Phospholipids

    Cytosolic phospholipase A$_2$

Arachidonic acid

Cyclooxygenase

PGG$_2$

5-Lipoxygenase

PGH$_2$

PGD$_2$ PGE$_2$ PGF$_2$ PGI$_2$ TXA$_2$

2. Alpha Linoleic Acid (Flaxseed Oil)

    Delta-6-desaturase

Steardonic acid (black currant oil)

    Delta-5-desaturase

EPA (cold-water fish, fish oils)

PG$_3$s

5-HPETE

Leukotrienes

Arachidonic Acid

Found in: red meats, poultry, whole milk

Uterine stores depleted by OCs

Uterine relaxers: cramp bark, black haw

PG$_3$ (anti-inflammatory)

PG$_3$ precursors are omega-3 fatty acids, alpha linoleic acid.

Sources: cold-water fish, flaxseed oil, black currant oil

Cyclooxygenase

Inhibited by NSAIDs, willow, meadowsweet

Phospholipase A$_2$

Inhibited by licorice, ginger

Figure 46–1. Eicosanoid synthesis. EPA, eicosapentaenoic acid; 5-HPETE, 5-hydroperoxy eicosatetraenoic acid; NSAIDs, nonsteroidal anti-inflammatory drugs; OCs, oral contraceptives; PG, prostaglandin; TXA$_2$, thromboxane A$_2$. (Adapted from Dawood MY: Dysmenorrhea. Clin Obstet Gynecol 33:171, 1990.)

Table 46–1. Grading Scale of Dysmenorrhea

Grade	Character	Working Ability	Systemic Symptoms	Analgesics
0	Menstruation not painful: daily activity unaffected	Unaffected	None	None required
1	Menstruation mildly painful: seldom inhibits normal activity	Rarely affected	None	Rarely required
2	Moderate pain: daily activity affected, but analgesics give enough relief that absence from school/work is rare	Moderately affected	Few	Required
3	Severe pain: daily activity inhibited, analgesics give little relief	Clearly inhibited	Headache, fatigue, nausea, vomiting, diarrhea may be present	Poor effect

Adapted from Andersch B, Milsom I: An epidemiologic study of young women with dysmenorrhea. Am J Obstet Gynecol 144:655–660, 1982.

Dosage. 2 to 3 mL of a tincture made in 1:3 proportion should be taken every 2 hours or as needed. Alternatively, 4 to 8 mL of fluidextract (1:1) may be taken three or four times daily. Another alternative is to simmer 1 tablespoon of bark in 12 ounces of water for 15 minutes. One third of a cup every 2 to 3 hours should be drunk as needed.

Precautions. Black haw contains oxalates and should be avoided in people with a history of kidney stones.

Theoretically, the salicylates in black haw could trigger allergic reactions in those with aspirin allergy.

PHARMACEUTICALS

- Nonsteroidal anti-inflammatory drugs (NSAIDs): These drugs remain the first-line pharmaceutical treatment for PD. They are effective for more than 70% of patients.[8] All NSAIDs inhibit cyclooxygenase (prostaglandin synthase). The propionic acids (e.g., ibuprofen and naproxen) are generally effective for grade 2 PD. Ibuprofen, 800 mg every 6 to 8 hours, or 550 mg naproxen every 6 to 8 hours, is an appropriate dose, although lower doses can often be used. The fenamates (e.g., mefenamic acid [Ponstel]) have the advantage of both inhibiting cyclooxygenase and competing for PG binding sites, thus inhibiting the action of PGs that are already formed.[9] They should be given to women with grade 2 PD whose pain is not controlled by the propionic acids; they are the best initial choice for grade 3 PD. A loading dose of 500 mg mefenamic acid followed by 250 mg every 6 to 8 hours is often effective.

- Oral contraceptives (OCs) in monthly cycles: Combination OC pills suppress ovulation, resulting in a relatively atrophic endometrium and correspondingly lower levels of prostaglandins. After several cycles, they also decrease the amount of menstrual flow. They may be the treatment of choice for women with dysmenorrhea who desire contraception.

NOTE

Women whose pain is not relieved by any of the aforementioned methods have a high likelihood of pelvic disease. Referral for laparoscopy should be considered.

- Oral contraceptives in long cycles: Instead of prescribing 21 hormonally active pills followed by 7 placebo pills, women whose pain is unrelieved by OCs can be prescribed 3 or 5 continuously active cycles (63 and 105 consecutive active pills, respectively), followed by 7 days without medications, and perhaps followed by another 3 or 5 active cycles. This method is often effective, but many women discontinue medication because they develop breakthrough bleeding.[10]

THERAPIES TO CONSIDER

- Acupuncture: This therapy is known to increase production of endorphins, enkephalins, and dynorphins, and is widely used for PD. Numerous case series[11-13] and at least one randomized controlled trial[14] have reported acupuncture to be highly effective. This is my personal treatment of choice for those able to commit to weekly treatments for three menstrual cycles. Acupuncture is often combined with herbal and dietary treatments.
- Transcutaneous Electrical Nerve Stimulation (TENS): Women who prefer noninvasive treatments may accept TENS. Again, numerous studies have found it an effective remedy for PD.[15-17]
- Osteopathic or chiropractic manipulation: When PD is accompanied or characterized by obvious musculoskeletal disorders, such as lower back pain, increased lumbar lordosis, or leg length discrepancy, it is reasonable to suggest osteopathic or chiropractic manipulation.[18, 19] No well-designed clinical trials exist to support either approach.
- Magnesium. One controlled trial found that 4.5 mg magnesium pidolate three times daily significantly decreased pain on the first day of menses. A trend toward decrease in pain on the second and third days was found, but it did not reach significance.[20] For women whose symptoms are present primarily on the first day of menses, magnesium pidolate may be helpful.

 THERAPEUTIC REVIEW

Nutrition
- *Decrease consumption of AA. Limit servings of meat, poultry, and dairy. Increase consumption of omega-3 fatty acids. Eat three servings of salmon, mackerel, or other cold-water fish at least three times a week, and/or take one teaspoon flaxseed oil a day or 3000 mg flaxseed oil twice daily.*

Botanicals
- *240 mg salicin per day and/or 4 to 8 mL cramp bark or black haw 1:1 fluid extract three or four times a day. Other botanicals with potential benefit include meadowsweet, licorice, and ginger.*

Pharmaceuticals
- *NSAIDs. Start with propionic acid such as ibuprofen 800 mg every 6 to 8 hours for grade 2 PD. If there is no response or grade 3 PD is present, switch to mefenamic acid (Ponstel) 500 mg loading dose and then 250 mg every 6 to 8 hours. Oral contraceptives may be taken in monthly or long cycles. See earlier.*

Acupuncture/TENS:
- *Use instead of, or in combination with, any of the other therapies.*

References

1. Dawood MY: Dysmenorrhea. Clin Obstet Gynecol 33:168–178, 1990.
2. Chan WY, Dawood MY, Fuchs F: Relief of dysmenorrhea with the prostaglandin synthetase inhibitor ibuprofen: Effect on prostaglandin levels in menstrual fluid. Am J Obstet Gynecol 135:102–108, 1979.
3. Deluca P, Rothman D, Zurier RB: Marine and botanical lipids as immunomodulatory and therapeutic agents in the treatment of rheumatoid arthritis. Rheum Dis Clin North Am 21:759–777, 1995.
4. Andersch B, Milson I: An epidemiologic study of young women with dysmenorrhea. Am J Obstet Gynecol 144:655–660, 1982.
5. Harlow SD, Park M: A longitudinal study of risk factors for the occurrence, duration and severity of menstrual cramps in a cohort of college women. Br J Obstet Gynaecol 103:1134–1142, 1996.
6. Zondervan KT, Yudkin PL, Vessey MP, et al: The prevalence of chronic pelvic pain in women in the United Kingdom: A systematic review. Br J Obstet Gynaecol 105:93–99, 1998.
7. Leung AY, Foster S: Encyclopedia of Common Natural Ingredients Used in Food, Drugs and Cosmetics, 2nd ed. New York, John Wiley and Sons, 1996.
8. Owen PR: Prostaglandin synthetase inhibitors in the treatment of primary dysmenorrhea. Outcome trials reviewed. Am J Obstet Gynecol 148:96–102, 1984.
9. Budoff PW: Use of mefenamic acid in the treatment of primary dysmenorrhea. JAMA 241:2713–2716, 1979.
10. Sulak PJ, Cressman BE, Waldrop E, et al: Extending the duration of active oral contraceptive pills to manage hormone withdrawal symptoms. Obstet Gynecol 89:179–183, 1997.
11. Zhan C: Treatment of 32 cases of dysmenorrhea by puncturing hegu and sanyinjiao acupoints. J Trad Chin Med 10:33–35, 1990.
12. Wang XM: Observations of the therapeutic effects of acupuncture and moxibustion in 100 cases of dysmenorrhea. J Trad Chin Med 7:15–17, 1987.
13. Zhang YQ: A report of 49 cases of dysmenorrhea treated by acupuncture. J Trad Chin Med 4:101–102, 1984.
14. Helms JM: Acupuncture for the management of primary dysmenorrhea. Obstet Gynecol 69:51–56, 1987.
15. Milsom I, Hender N, Mannheimen CA: A comparative study of the effect of high-intensity transcutaneous nerve stimulation and oral naproxen on intrauterine pressure and menstrual pain in patients with primary dysmenorrhea. Am J Obstet Gynecol 170:123–129, 1994.
16. Kaplan B, Peled Y, Pardo J, et al: Transcutaneous electrical nerve stimulation (TENS) as a relief for dysmenorrhea. Clin Exp Obstet Gynecol 21:87–90, 1994.
17. Lundeberg T, Bondesson L, Lundstrom V: Relief of primary dysmenorrhea by transcutaneous electrical nerve stimulation. Acta Obstet Gynecol Scand 64:491–497, 1985.
18. Baker PK: Musculoskeletal origins of chronic pelvic pain. Obstet Gynecol Clin North Am 20:719–742, 1993.
19. Hitchcock ME: The manipulative approach to the management of primary dysmenorrhea. JAOA 75:909–918, 1976.
20. Benassi L, Barletta FP, Baroncini L, et al: Effectiveness of magnesium pidolate in the prophylactic treatment of primary dysmenorrhea. Clin Exp Obstet Gynecol 19:176–179, 1992.

CHAPTER 47

Uterine Fibroids (Leiomyomata)

Jean Riquelme, M.D.

PATHOPHYSIOLOGY

Uterine fibroids (leiomyomata) are monoclonal tumors of well-differentiated smooth muscle cells. They are the most commonly occurring pelvic tumor in women. Twenty percent to 25% of women aged 25 to 44 years are estimated to have uterine fibroids, although an autopsy study showed an incidence as high as 75%.[1] Incidence increases with age and is two to three times more common among African American women. The majority of women with fibroids are not bothered by them. However, some suffer symptoms that tend to fall into two major categories: abnormal uterine bleeding and pelvic discomfort.

Bleeding may be heavy and frequent, especially when the fibroid is submucosal in location. An ensuing anemia may cause the patient to present with fatigue as the major complaint. Other patients present with pelvic pressure or pain. The space-occupying effects of large fibroids include urinary frequency, dyspareunia, and even lower extremity edema. Large fibroids may interfere with a woman's fertility.

Uterine fibroids are hormone-dependent growths. They are more common among women with increased endogenous estrogen production: nulliparous women, those with early menarche, and those who are obese (body mass index [BMI] > 28 kg/m^2).[2] Fibroids involute after menopause. The effects of exogenous estrogens on fibroids is not well established. Two dietary sources of exogenous estrogens are *phytoestrogens* (endogenous plant estrogens) and *xenoestrogens* (chemicals, such as some pesticides and herbicides, that have estrogen-like effects). Even less clear is the role of progesterone in fibroid growth. Progestins that are not bioidentical to human progesterone have been shown to increase fibroid growth.[3, 4]

An integrative approach to uterine fibroids involves minimizing symptoms, removing exacerbating factors, and helping the patient to deal with a frustrating, if benign, condition.

BIOCHEMICAL

The biochemical treatment of fibroids addresses the effects of bleeding and pelvic pain and may attempt to shrink or eliminate myomata chemically.

Supplements

Iron

The abnormal bleeding caused by fibroids may cause an iron deficiency anemia. This is common when menstrual volumes exceed 60 mL/mo.

Dosage. 60 to 180 mg of elemental iron daily.

Flaxseed Oil

Flaxseed oil is a source of omega-3 fatty acids. Omega-3 fatty acids may decrease the pain of fibroids and abnormal uterine bleeding by reducing metabolism of the omega-6 fatty acids that are dominant in the Western diet and feed inflammation through the arachidonic acid pathway. Whole or ground flaxseed contains active phytoestrogens, including lignins, the effects of which on uterine fibroids is not established. For this reason, flaxseed *oil* is the recommended form of supplementation. Cost is about $7.00 for a 1-month supply.

Dosage. 1000 mg of organic flaxseed oil daily.

Precautions. For prolonged use of omega-3 supplements, consider adding vitamin E 200 to 400 IU/day to decrease the pro-oxidant effect of these oils at high doses.

NOTE

Although fish oils contain more omega-3 fatty acids per volume than flaxseed oil, it is difficult for the average consumer to find an organic source of fish oils. Organic flaxseed oil is available in most health food stores and many chain pharmacies.

Botanicals

Kuei-Chih-Fu-Ling-Wan

Kuei-chih-fu-ling-wan is a traditional Chinese remedy with five herbal components: *Cinnamomum cassia, Paeonia lactiflora, Prunus persica, Poria cocos, and Paeonia suffriticosa.* In a study of 110 premenopausal women with fibroids, this traditional medicine reduced symptoms of abnormal bleeding and dysmenorrhea in 90% of patients and shrank tumors in 60%.[5] This study was not randomized nor blinded. Kuei-chih-fu-ling-wan is available from practitioners of traditional Chinese medicine (TCM) and from some ethnic Chinese pharmacies as a patent medicine.

Dosage. Patent remedy kuei-chih-fu-ling-wan, eight pills three times daily.

Pharmaceuticals

Nonsteroidal Anti-Inflammatory Drugs

Nonsteroidal anti-inflammatory drugs (NSAIDs) reduce the pain of dysmenorrhea from fibroid tumors. Although ibuprofen, 1200 mg/day, reduces menstrual blood loss in women with primary menorrhagia, it does not diminish menorrhagia in the presence of uterine fibroids.[6] No studies support the use of one NSAID over another for pain control.

Dosage. Ibuprofen 400 to 600 mg three to four times daily for menstrual pain.

Oral Contraceptives

Opinions are mixed as to whether or not oral contraceptives help control the symptoms of fibroids. They may reduce the perceived amount of menstrual blood loss.[7] They do not relieve the space-occupying effects of fibroid tumors.

Gonadotropin-Releasing Hormone Agonists

Gonadotropin-releasing hormone (GnRH) agonists suppress both estrogen and progesterone production, causing a variable reduction in fibroid volume. Leuprolide (Lupron) is a GnRH agonist useful in reducing bleeding and normalizing blood levels in women going to fibroid surgery. It is useful for reducing the size of a myomatous uterus preoperatively, sometimes giving patients the possibility of a more conservative operation.

Dosage. Leuprolide acetate depot (Lupron) 3.75 mg IM injection, monthly for 3 months.

Precautions. Because GnRH agonists induce a menopausal state, side effects such as hot flashes, atrophic vaginitis, and decreased libido are common. Side effects and the risk of accelerated bone loss make long-term GnRH agonist therapy impractical.

BIOMECHANICAL

Biomechanical therapies include conventional treatments such as surgery and interventional radiology as well as complementary techniques such as massage, osteopathic manipulation, and chiropractic. No convincing studies of the utility of complementary techniques on reducing fibroid burden are available. Integrating massage may reduce the symptoms of pelvic pain and fatigue.

Surgery and Interventional Radiology

The Maine Women's Health Study[8] evaluated symptom and quality of life outcomes of nonsurgical management of uterine fibroids. Almost all women had reduction of symptom score and improved quality of life after conservative medical treatment. However, a certain subset of women, mainly those in whom pain rather than bleeding was the main symptom, did better with surgical management.

There are various surgical options for management of uterine fibroids. The pivotal question for the patient of childbearing potential is whether or not her fertility will be preserved.

Uterus-Preserving Techniques: Myomectomy and Uterine Artery Embolization

Myomectomy

Removal of uterine fibroids can be done either vaginally, through a hysteroscope, or abdominally (usually laparoscopically), depending on location and burden of myomata.

Depending on the operator, myomectomy improves symptoms in 80% to 90% of patients. Fifteen percent to 30% of patients experience regrowth of fibroids after 5 years. Myomectomy leaves a uterine scar that may affect future fertility.

Myolysis

Myolysis involves in situ destruction of fibroids with either heat coagulation or freezing. It is most effective in small fibroids; larger fibroids require repeated treatment. A pretreatment of GnRH agonist (see earlier) can help shrink the fibroids to a size at which myolysis is more effective. Myolysis weakens the uterine wall, so conception after myolysis is not recommended.

Uterine Artery Embolization

Uterine artery embolization is a "minimally invasive" radiology technique that has become more common recently.

Polyvinyl alcohol particles are injected intraluminally into the uterine arteries via a percutaneous catheter. Improvement in abnormal bleeding and pelvic pain develop over the next few weeks in the majority of patients. Rarely (1% to 2%), ovarian failure occurs, presumably owing to compromised circulation to the ovaries. Patients for whom preservation of fertility is a concern should be apprised of this possibility.

Removal of the Uterus: Hysterectomy

The treatment of fibroids by hysterectomy is reserved for those patients who are certain they want no further pregnancies and whose symptoms justify a more invasive procedure or when malignancy is suspected. Leiomyosarcoma is a rare tumor. In a study of 1332 women with pelvic mass, 0.23% had leiomyosarcoma or endometrial stroma carcinoma.[9] All hysterectomies render the patient infertile.

Hysterectomy may done by either a vaginal or an abdominal approach depending on fibroid burden and type of operation planned. *Supracervical hysterectomy* preserves the uterine cervix, believed to be important for orgasm in some women. *Total hysterectomy* removes the entire uterus. A *total abdominal hysterectomy* removes the entire uterus, ovaries, and fallopian tubes. In premenopausal women, total abdominal hysterectomy causes surgical menopause.

BIOENERGETICS

Bioenergetic therapies involve mobilizing the patient's energy, qi, or life force for healing. These techniques may be beneficial in alleviating the allied symptoms of fibroids, namely, pain and fatigue. With the exception of TCM, the effects of bioenergetic therapies on fibroid tumor growth has not been proven.

Traditional Chinese Medicine

TCM combines herbs, bioenergetic treatments (acupuncture and qi gong), and dietary intervention in treatment of the fibroid uterus. Chinese investigators reported a study of 100 patients with ultrasound-proven fibroids who were treated with TCM.[5] Treatment varied depending on the qi imbalance diagnosed. Nearly all patients had some benefit, with bleeding symptoms effectively reduced in 90% of patients. Half the patients experienced significant reduction in fibroid size.

LIFESTYLE

Obesity is a known risk factor for uterine fibroids. Lifestyle modification should focus on maintaining a healthy weight. It may be prudent to advise patients with fibroids to avoid ingesting xenoestrogens (see earlier). Xenoestrogens are present in the diet as herbicide and pesticide residue. They are concentrated in the fat of meat, fish, dairy products, and possibly egg yolks. Patients wishing to avoid xenoestrogens would be well advised to eat organically when possible, wash produce carefully, and minimize ingestion of fatty meat and fish.

▲ —THERAPEUTIC REVIEW

Exacerbating Factors	Work toward ideal body weight, minimize xenoestrogen exposure, and avoid artificial progesterone.
Supplements	Replace iron losses and consider an omega-3 fatty acid supplement.
Botanicals	Consider Chinese herbal medicines, in consultation with an experienced practitioner.
Pharmaceuticals	Medications may reduce symptoms of pain and bleeding. GnRH agonists are useful for reducing fibroid size on a short-term basis.
Mind-Body Therapy	Consider a program of guided imagery and relaxation to help the patient deal with symptoms or prepare for surgery.
Surgical Therapy	Surgical options are available that minimize operative risk and postoperative infertility.

References

1. Cramer SF, Patel A: The frequency of uterine leiomyomas. Am J Clin Pathol 94:435–438, 1990.
2. Marshall LM, Spiegelman D, Manson JE, et al: Risk of uterine leiomyomata among premenopausal women in relation to body size and cigarette smoking. Epidemiology 90:511–517, 1998.
3. Mixon WT, Hammond DO: Response of fibromyomas to a progestin. Am J Obstet Gynecol 82:754–760, 1961.
4. Friedman AJ, Barbieri RL, Doubilot PM, et al: A randomized, double-blind trial of a gonadotropin releasing-hormone agonist

(leuprolide) with or without medroxyprogesterone acetate in the treatment of leiomyomata uteri. Fertil Steril 49:404–409, 1988.

5. Sakamoto S, Yoshino H, Shirahata Y, et al: Pharmacotherapeutic effects of kuei-chih-fu-ling-wan (keishi-bukuryo-gan) on human uterine myomas. Am J Chin Med 20:313–317, 1992.

6. Makarainen L, Ylikorkala O: Primary and myoma-associated menorrhagia: Role of prostaglandins and effect of ibuprofen. Br J Obstet Gynaecol 93:974–978, 1986.

7. Barbieri RL: Ambulatory management of uterine leiomyomata. Clin Obstet Gynecol 42:196–205, 1999.

8. Carlson KJ, Miller BA, Fowler FJ Jr: The Maine Women's Health Study: II. Outcomes of nonsurgical management of leiomyomas, abnormal bleeding and chronic pelvic pain. Obstet Gynecol 83:566–572, 1994.

9. Parker WH, Fu YS, Berek JS: Uterine sarcoma in patients operated on for presumed leiomyoma and rapidly growing leiomyoma. Obstet Gynecol 83:414–418, 1994.

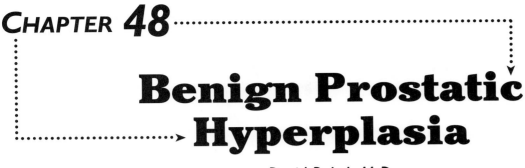

CHAPTER 48

Benign Prostatic Hyperplasia

David Rakel, M.D.

PATHOPHYSIOLOGY

Despite being one of the most common diseases of the aging male, the etiology of prostatic hyperplasia remains relatively unknown. From our current understanding, it appears to be related to age, androgens (dihydrotestosterone [DHT]), estrogens, and detrusor dysfunction of the bladder neck. There is an accumulation of DHT that inhibits prostatic cell death and promotes cell proliferation that increases the size of the gland (Fig. 48–1).

As the male passes the fifth decade of life, there is a decrease in serum testosterone levels and a rise in estrogen (as well as prolactin, luteinizing hormone, and follicle-stimulating hormone). Estrogen increases the number of androgen (DHT) receptors in the prostate and inhibits its metabolism by interfering with hydroxylation. As urinary outflow obstruction develops, the detrusor muscles of the bladder try to compensate by increasing pressure to expel urine, which leads to instability of the muscle and worsening symptoms. In summary, factors that promote the accumulation of DHT and estrogens lead to symptoms of benign prostatic hyperplasia (BPH) and obstruction of the lower urinary tract that leads to detrusor muscle dysfunction. Stimulation of the alpha adrenergic system leads to contraction of the smooth muscle fiber that leads to further flow restriction in an enlarged gland. Finally, there is reason to believe that prostaglandins and leukotrienes play a role in the inflammatory process of the prostate.

LIFESTYLE

Xenoestrogens

Xenoestrogens are foreign substances that originate outside the human body that, when incorporated into it, have hormone-like activity. This estrogen-like effect has been associated with an increased incidence of cancer and early puberty[1] and may play a role in promoting hyperplasia of the prostate. Further research is needed to better understand what long-term effect they may have.

Common xenoestrogens include dioxins (chlorinated compounds primarily from chlorine-bleached pulp and paper products), several pesticides (e.g., 2,4-D, Picloram, DDT, DDE, kelthane, and heptatochlor), nonylphenols (compounds used to soften plastics, which are also found in many paints, industrial detergents, lubricating oils, farm chemicals, toiletries, and spermicidal foams), and bisphenol-A (BPA) (plastic coating inside tin cans). BPA has been found to advance puberty and increase prostate size in animal studies.[2] It leaks into food products that are contained within tin cans that have been coated with BPA.

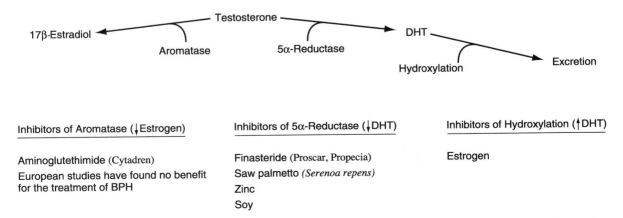

Inhibitors of Aromatase (↓Estrogen)	Inhibitors of 5α-Reductase (↓DHT)	Inhibitors of Hydroxylation (↑DHT)
Aminoglutethimide (Cytadren)	Finasteride (Proscar, Propecia)	Estrogen
European studies have found no benefit for the treatment of BPH	Saw palmetto (*Serenoa repens*)	
	Zinc	
	Soy	

Figure 48–1. Inhibitors of aramatase, 5α-reductase, and hydroxylation. BPH, benign prostatic hyperplasia; DHT, dihydrotestosterone.

Avoiding xenoestrogens completely may be futile owing to their significant presence in our daily lives. But making lifestyle choices that reduce exposure would be beneficial to our health and hormonal balance. Here are some tips we can give our patients:

- Encourage consumption of organic food.
- Wash produce thoroughly.
- Limit dairy products.
- Limit meat products, particularly from carnivorous animals at the top of the food chain.
- Avoid storing food in plastic wrap or plastic containers. Use glass.
- Avoid heating foods in the microwave that are stored in plastic.
- Filter drinking water.
- Avoid external chemical exposure including pesticides, herbicides, cleaning agents, and solvents.

NUTRITION

Soy

Soy is thought to work in two ways: as an inhibitor of 5-alpha-reductase and as a low-potency estrogen. It may block the receptor sites that the stronger estrogens use to increase the accumulation of DHT. Evidence also suggests that soy may lower serum estrone levels. A study of 35 Japanese men assigned them to either 400 mL of soy milk a day or their usual diet. After 8 weeks, those who drank the soy milk had a decrease in serum estrone levels versus the control group.[3] Epidemiologic studies in Asian men have also found that a diet rich in soy products is associated with a decreased incidence of prostate cancer.[4]

Beta-sitosterol (a major phytosterol found in soy) was found to increase urinary flow and decrease residual volume in the bladder using 20 mg daily in a double-blind, placebo-controlled study.[5] A 3.5-ounce serving of soybeans, tofu, or other soy food preparation provides approximately 90 mg of beta-sitosterol.[6] A 1-ounce preparation (which is a portion about the size of the palm of the hand) will equal approximately 25 mg.

Cholesterol

Cholesterol has been associated with not only BPH but also prostate cancer. Its metabolites (epoxycholesterols) have been found to accumulate in the hyperplastic and cancerous prostate gland. This is one reason why hypocholesterolemic drugs (3-hydroxy-3-methylglutaryl-coenzyme A [HMG-CoA] reductase inhibitors or "statins") have been associated with a lower risk of BPH and prostate cancer.[7] There is limited evidence at this time regarding the use of these drugs for this indication, but a diet low in cholesterol is beneficial not only for the prostate but also for general health.

Omega-3 Fatty Acids

A diet rich in omega-3 fatty acids will help reduce the influence of prostaglandins and leukotrienes on the inflammatory component of BPH (see Chapter 84, The Anti-Inflammatory Diet). Recommend foods rich in omega-3 fatty acids such as cold water fish (salmon, mackerel, and sardines).

SUPPLEMENTS

Zinc

Intestinal uptake of zinc is inhibited by estrogen. Because the estrogen levels increase in the aging male, zinc may be low. In fact, marginal zinc deficiency is common in the elderly, and in males, this may worsen the symptoms of BPH. In the 1970s, research showed that supplementing with zinc resulted in a reduction in the size of the gland and symptoms of BPH.[8] Further research has shown that zinc inhibits 5-alpha-reductase[9] and inhibits the binding of androgens to their receptors in the prostate.[10] This latter effect is thought to occur because of zinc's ability to inhibit prolactin that, like estrogen, increases the receptors for DHT in the prostate. So zinc not only decreases the production of DHT, it inhibits the binding to its receptors.

Coffee can decrease zinc absorption by 50%. Because caffeine stimulates the adrenergic nervous system (smooth muscle of the prostate), encourage patients with BPH to limit their intake.

Prescription drugs that can result in low serum zinc levels include thiazide diuretics, steroids, methotrexate, tetracyclines, and fluoroquinolones. Consider zinc supplementation in those patients with BPH on these medications. But do not give to those taking tetracycline or fluoroquinolone antibiotics because zinc can affect their absorption.

Dosage. 30 mg/day.

NOTE

In prescribing zinc supplementation, be aware that zinc competes with copper, calcium, and iron absorption. Make sure the patient does not take more than the recommended dose and does not take calcium and iron supplements with zinc.

BOTANICALS

Saw Palmetto (*Serenoa repens*)

The exact mechanism of action of saw palmetto remains elusive. It has been found to be a weak inhibitor of 5-alpha-reductase but may have a more active role in reducing the number of estrogen and androgen (DHT) receptors as well as having an anti-inflammatory effect on the prostate. Its principal ingredient, a sterol called beta-sitosterol, is also found in soy products (see earlier) as well as other herbs that have been used to treat diseases of the prostate including Pygeum bark, stinging nettle root, and pumpkin seed extract. Although the mechanism of action of sterols on the prostate gland remains to be found, this compound seems to be a recurring theme in the herbal treatment of this disorder.

Saw palmetto induces contraction of the inner prostatic epithelium but does not reduce the size of the gland.[11] Despite this, it has been found to improve symptom scores, nocturia, residual urine, and urinary flow in patients with BPH. It was found to be as effective as finasteride (Proscar) without the side effects.[12] Granted, finasteride has not been a great success in the treatment of BPH. It does not affect prostate-specific antigen levels.[13]

Dosage. 160 mg twice daily. Allow 8 weeks before seeing therapeutic benefit. Product lines proved to be composed of at least 85% fatty acids and 0.2% sterols include Nature's Way, CVS, Centrum, Natrol, Bayer, Quanterra, Sundown herbals, NaturPharma (Wal-Mart), and Walgreens.

NOTE

The most beneficial saw palmetto extract is composed of at least 85% fatty acids and 0.2% sterols. For example, a 160-mg pill should have a minimum of 136 mg of fatty acids and 0.32 mg of sterols.

Precautions. Mild adverse effects have included headache, nausea, diarrhea, and dizziness.

Rye Grass Pollen (*Secale cereale*)

Rye grass pollen is also known as grass pollen and grass pollen extract. Clinical studies used a form called Cernilton (flower pollen), a brand manufactured by Cernitin.

This extract has been used in Europe for BPH for longer than 35 years. Double-blind clinical studies have found it to be effective with an overall response rate near 70%.[14] Rye grass contains a substance that has been found to inhibit prostatic cell growth[15] as well as reduce inflammation of the prostate by inhibiting prostaglandins and leukotrienes.[16]

Studies have shown the greatest improvement in nocturia, urinary frequency, and residual urine volume.[17] Rye grass and flower pollen are also used for symptomatic relief of prostatitis and prostatodynia.

Dosage. Typical dose of rye grass pollen is 126 mg three times daily. Cernilton TS (TS for triple strength), a product that was used for the original studies, has 180 mg of pollen extract and is taken once or twice times a day. The cost is about $30.00 for 60 capsules. It can be ordered through www.cernitinamerica.com.

Precautions. Watch for abdominal distention, heartburn, and nausea.

Pygeum (*Prunus africana*)

Pygeum is obtained from the bark of the African plum tree. Like saw palmetto, its benefits are thought to come from fatty acids (sterols) that reduce inflammation through the inhibition of prostaglandins as well as prostatic cholesterol levels that are precursors to testosterone production. It also increases prostatic and seminal fluid secretions. Studies have shown greater improvement in nocturia and urinary flow than with residual volume.[18]

Although beneficial, Pygeum does not appear to be as effective for BPH as saw palmetto and rye grass. It is more expensive than saw palmetto and overharvesting of the bark is threatening the survival of the species.

Dosage. 100 to 200 mg/day.

Precautions. Watch for nausea and abdominal pain.

PHARMACEUTICALS

Alpha Adrenergic Blocking Agents

Alpha adrenergic blocking agents will likely give the most subjective improvement of the therapies discussed. Blocking the alpha adrenergic system results in relaxation of the smooth muscle fibers of the prostate gland causing a reduction of symptoms and improved urinary flow. The response is rapid (within hours), and studies have shown long-term efficacy.

The most commonly used drugs—terazosin (Hytrin) and doxazosin (Cardura)—require dose titration to avoid postural hypotension. The introduction of the more expensive alpha$_1$ antagonist tamsulosin (Flomax) is more specific for the prostatic tissue, reducing the incidence of hypotension and the need to titrate the dose.

Dosage

Terazosin (Hytrin): start 2 mg qhs and titrate each week to effect. Maximum, 20 mg; comes in 1, 2, 5, and 10 mg.

Doxazosin (Cardura): start 1 mg qhs and titrate each week to effect. Maximum, 8 mg; comes in 1, 2, 4, and 8 mg.

Tamsulosin (Flomax): 0.4 mg 30 minutes after a meal daily. Maximum, 0.8 mg/day; comes in 0.4 mg.

Precautions. Watch for postural hypotension, dizziness, fatigue, headache, nasal stuffiness, and retrograde ejaculation.

5-Alpha Reductase Inhibition

Finasteride (Proscar, Propecia) prevents the conversion of testosterone to DHT and lowers DHT serum levels. It can take as long as 6 months to work but does appear to halt the progression of prostatic growth. In regard to patient satisfaction and symptom reduction, it is not a great drug unless you also want to treat male pattern baldness. Finasteride may cause up to a 50% reduction of prostate-specific antigen. So monitor prostate-specific antigen levels, and if you see a rise, further evaluation of prostate cancer should be performed.

Dosage. 5 mg once a day; comes in 5-mg tablets.

Precautions. Watch for decreased ejaculatory volume (2.8%), impotence (3.7%), and decreased libido (3.3%).

SURGERY

When severe symptoms are not controlled with the therapies listed previously, consider urologic referral for minimally invasive therapy or surgical resection.

- Transurethral microwave thermotherapy uses a microwave antenna that generates heat in the transition zone, resulting in coagulation necrosis. It is performed as an outpatient therapy.
- Transurethral needle ablation involves the placement of small needles in the prostate via cystoscopy that emit radiofrequency energy resulting in necrosis of prostatic tissue.

> **NOTE**
>
> *The mimimally invasive procedures discussed previously have a decrease in morbidity compared with transurethral resection of the prostate (TURP) but are not as effective in reducing symptoms and no tissue is obtained for pathologic evaluation.*

- Transurethral resection of the prostate is the "gold standard" and will likely result in the greatest symptomatic improvement. Complications such as incontinence (1%), blood transfusion (3% to 5%), retrograde ejaculation (20% to 75%), and stricture formation (5%) are becoming less severe with the use of laser prostatectomy that results in less bleeding. Transurethral resection of the prostate is the most invasive (except for open prostatectomy) and requires a hospital stay.

OTHER THERAPIES TO CONSIDER

Homeopathy

Remedies such as *Pulsatilla, Argenticum metallicum, Baryta carbonicum,* and *Conium maculatum* have been used for enlarged prostate. Before recommending these therapies, a constitutional evaluation should be considered because each agent is prescribed based on the unique symptoms of the patient.

 — *THERAPEUTIC REVIEW*

Following is a summary of therapeutic options for BPH. If a patient presents with severe symptoms (American Urologic Association [AUA] score > 19), it would be to his benefit for you to jump ahead to a more aggressive therapy such as alpha blockers or referral to surgery. But for the patient who has mild to moderate symptoms, this ladder approach is appropriate.

Remove Exacerbating Factors
- *Avoid exposure and consumption of xenoestrogens.*
- *Stop taking over-the-counter cold remedies or diet aids (phenylpropanolamine), nasal decongestants (pseudoephedrine), herbs (ma huang, Ephedra), or caffeinated products that contain sympathomimetics that increase prostatic muscle tone.*
- *Consider stopping pharmaceutical products that have anticholinergic effects that lead to urinary retention. These include antihistamines, bowel antispasmodics, bladder antispasmodics, tricyclic antidepressants, and antipsychotics.*

Nutrition
- *Increase soy-rich foods in diet. A 1-ounce serving each day (about the size of the palm of the hand) will provide approximately 25 mg.*
- *Encourage a low-fat, cholesterol-free diet.*
- *Encourage foods rich in omega-3 fatty acids (salmon, nuts) or take 1 tbsp of fish oil twice daily or one or two 500-mg capsules of fish oil twice daily.*

THERAPEUTIC REVIEW *continued*

Supplements

- *Zinc 30 mg daily.*

Botanicals

- *Start with saw palmetto 160 mg twice daily. If there is no improvement after 8 weeks, consider adding rye grass pollen 126 mg three times daily or Pygeum 100 to 200 mg daily. Other herbal products that have potential benefit include stinging nettles and pumpkin seed extract.*

Pharmaceuticals

- *If there is no improvement with the use of botanicals, discontinue them and start an alpha adrenergic blocker (see doses given earlier).*
- *If the patient is unable to tolerate an alpha blocker, consider finasteride 5 mg daily.*
- *Combination therapy. A Veterans Administration cooperative study showed no additional benefit when finasteride was added to an alpha blocker. The combination of alpha blockers and botanicals has not been studied, but there are no contraindications to using them together.*

Surgical Therapy

- *If the patient's symptoms persist or worsen despite the measures previously discussed, refer for urologic evaluation and treatment.*

References

1. Crinnion WJ: Environmental Medicine, Part 1: The human burden of environmental toxins and their common health effects. Altern Med Rev 5:52–63, 2000.
2. Stoker TE, Robinette CL, Britt BH, et al: Prepubertal exposure to compounds that increase prolactin secretion in the male rat: Effects on the adult prostate. Biol Reprod 61:1636–1643, 1999.
3. Nagata C, Takatsuka N, Shimizu H, et al: Effect of soymilk consumption on serum estrogen and androgen concentrations in Japanese men. Cancer Epidemiol Biomarkers Prev 10(3):179–184, 2001.
4. Legumes and soybeans: Overview of their nutritional profiles and health effects [Review]. Am J Clin Nutr 70(3 Suppl):439S–450S, 1999.
5. Berges RR, Windeler J, Trampisch HJ, Senge T: Randomised, placebo-controlled, double-blind clinical trial of beta-sitosterol in patients with benign prostatic hyperplasia. Lancet 345:1529–1532, 1995.
6. Pizzorno JE, Murray MT: Benign prostatic hyperplasia. In Textbook of Natural Medicine, 2nd ed. Edinburgh, Churchill Livingstone, 1999, pp 1147–1152.
7. Padayatty SJ, Marcelli M, Shao TC, Cunningham GR: Lovastatin-induced apoptosis in prostate stromal cells. J Clin Endocrinol Metab 82:1434–1439, 1997.
8. Fahim M, Fahim Z, Der R, Harman J: Zinc treatment for the reduction of hyperplasia of the prostate. Fed Proc 35:361, 1976.
9. Leake A, Chisholm GD, Habib FK: The effect of zinc on the 5-α-reduction of testosterone by the hyperplastic human prostate gland. J Steroid Biochem 20:651–655, 1984.
10. Leake A, Chisholm GD, Busuttil A, Habib FK: Subcellular distribution of zinc in the benign and malignant human prostate: Evidence for a direct zinc androgen interaction. Acta Endocrinol 105:281–288, 1984.
11. Marks LS, Partin AW, Epstein JI, et al: Effects of a saw palmetto herbal blend in men with symptomatic benign prostatic hyperplasia. J Urol 163:1451–1456, 2000.
12. Carraro JC, Raynaud JP, Koch G, et al: Comparison of phytotherapy (Permixon) with finasteride in the treatment of benign prostate hyperplasia: A randomized international study of 1098 patients. Prostate 29:231–240, 1996.
13. Gerber GS, Zagaja GP, Bales GT, et al: Saw palmetto *(Serenoa replens)* in men with lower urinary tract symptoms: Effects on urodynamic parameters and voiding symptoms. Urology 51:1003–1007, 1998.
14. Buck AC, Cox R, Rees RW, et al: Treatment of outflow tract obstruction due to benign prostatic hyperplasia with the pollen extract, cernilton: A double-blind, placebo-controlled study. Br J Urol 66:398–404, 1990.
15. Habib FK, Ross M, Lewenstein A, et al: Identification of a prostate inhibitory substance in a pollen extract. Prostate 26:133–139, 1995.
16. Loschen G, Ebeling L: Inhibition of arachidonic acid cascade by extract of rye pollen [German]. Arzneimittelforschung 41:162–167, 1991.
17. Becker H, Ebeling L: Conservative therapy for benign prostatic hyperplasia (BPH) with cernilton. Br J Urol 66:398–404, 1988.
18. Andro MC, Riffaud JP: *Pygeum aftricanum* extract for the treatment of patients with benign prostatic hyperplasia. A review of 25 years of published experience. Curr Ther Res 56:796–817, 1995.

CHAPTER 49

Urolithiasis (Kidney and Bladder Stones)

R. W. Watkins, M.D., M.P.H.

PATHOPHYSIOLOGY

Kidney stones have plagued human beings since before recorded history. Evidence of kidney stones has been found in Egyptian mummies dating back 7000 years!

Renal calculus incidence is based on a number of genetic, nutritional, and environmental factors. More than 5% of the population of the United States will experience the pain of nephrolithiasis sometime in their lifetimes, with men being affected approximately twice as commonly as women. Renal stones tend to recur at the rate of about 75% for patients followed over 20 years.[1]

By far, the most common type of kidney stones (80%) are those composed of calcium in combination with either oxalate or phosphate.[2] The remainder are composed of either uric acid, struvite, or carbonate apatite (so-called "infection stones"), cystine, or other rare stones.

The formation of kidney stones is the result of crystallization of stone-forming salts that separate from the urine because of several possible factors. These may be environmental or metabolic in origin. More than one factor may be present in the same individual.

The major metabolic cause is hypercalciuria, which is found in roughly 50% of patients with renal calculi. Too much calcium leads to crystallization by supersaturating the urine with calcium salts. In addition, the presence of calcium inactivates negatively charged inhibitors of stone formation (citrate, magnesium, amino acids, and trace metals).

The most common cause of hypercalciuria is absorptive hypercalciuria. There is no known cause for this increased absorption from the intestinal tract. Patients with hyperparathyroidism have resorptive hypercalciuria and account for about 5% of all patients with kidney stones. Another cause is hypocitraturia, which leads to hypocitraturic calcium nephrolithiasis.

Citrate is known to slow stone formation. A major cause of low citrate in the urine is acidosis.[3] Seventy percent of patients with renal tubular acidosis eventually develop stones. Metabolic acidosis from chronic diarrhea (ileal disease, intestinal surgery), chronic urinary tract infections (enzymatic break-down of citrate by bacteria), or even lactic acidosis from strenuous exercise lowers citrate.

There are genetic and acquired forms of hyperoxaluria. Genetic or primary hyperoxaluria is quite rare. The acquired form is seen in about 10% of kidney stone patients and is the result of increased intestinal absorption of oxalate. This can be a consequence of compromised ileal function (medical or surgical). Patients with a combination of this disorder and absorptive hypercalciuria or low dietary calcium intake form stones at lower levels of oxalate because of the lack of calcium in the intestine, which is needed to bind the oxalate.[4] Uric acid stones result from a disorder in uric acid metabolism. Hyperuricosuria can produce not only uric acid stones but also calcium oxalate or phosphate or mixtures of both.[5] Roughly 15% of patients with uric acid stones have a gouty diathesis.

Cystinuria is another rare (1%) metabolic cause of kidney stones. Here, solubility of cystine is pH dependent, increasing with higher pH. When urine pH falls below 7, solubility is generally exceeded and the amino acid settles out and forms stones.

EVALUATION

A summary of recommendations from the National Institutes of Health Consensus Conference on the evaluation of stone formers is presented in Table 49–1.

INTEGRATIVE THERAPY

NUTRITION

There are a number of environmental and nutritional factors that increase risk of stone formation. In the United States, there are regional and seasonal differences in incidence, with increased risk in the summer, especially in the Southeast and Southwest. This is thought to be the result of increased dehydration and supersaturated urine. Strenuous physical exercise and excessive sweating compound the situation.

Table 49–1. Summary of Recommendations from the National Institutes of Health Consensus Conference on the Evaluation of Stone Formers[6]

Evaluation of Patient with First Stone Episode
History: medications, occupation, family history of stones or other kidney disease, inflammatory bowel disease (e.g., Crohn's disease)
Diet: intake of protein, purines, sodium, fluids, oxalate, and calcium
Laboratory tests: electrolyte, blood urea nitrogen, creatinine, calcium, phosphate and uric acid levels, urinalysis, urine culture if indicated, stone analysis if available (if not, consider qualitative cystine screening)
Radiology: plain radiographs, ultrasonography and/or intravenous pyelography (or helical computed tomography) to find more stones, radiolucent stones, or anatomic abnormalities
Consider: renal tubular acidosis, hyperparathyroidism, and sarcoidosis

Evaluation of Patient with Recurrent Stone Formation (and All Children)
Twenty-four hour urine collection: volume, pH, levels of calcium, phosphorus, sodium, uric acid, oxalate, citrate, creatinine, calcium oxalate (supersaturation), calcium phosphate, and uric acid
Repeat as necessary: 24-hour urine collection and analysis to monitor response to dietary changes and effectiveness of treatment

NIH, National Institutes of Health.
From Goldfarb DS, Coe FL: Prevention of recurrent nephrolithiasis. Am Fam Physician 60:2269–2276, 1999.

Fluid Intake

High fluid intake (to ensure a urinary output of at least 2 liters/d) has been shown to be an effective means of preventing stone recurrence. Most of this fluid should be water. In hot weather or when participating in vigorous exercise, more fluids are needed to compensate for increased loss through sweating.[7] Tap water should be tested for mineral content. "Hard" water should be treated before ingestion with a reverse osmosis filter, if possible. Caution should be used in drinking mineral water, because it may contain high levels of calcium and other minerals.

NOTE

Increased fluid intake is the cornerstone of therapy despite what other measures are taken.

Protein

A meat-rich diet and protein intake in general increase the acid content of the body and may lead to stone formation by increasing urinary uric acid and calcium and lowering citrate concentrations.[8]

Sodium

High salt intake can increase the amount of calcium in the urine. This in turn can cause increased risk of stone formation. Of course, if the patient is on a thiazide diuretic as part of therapy, it makes the medicine less effective. Higher sodium excretion also increases uric acid excretion and decreases urinary citrate concentrations.[9]

Soft Drink Consumption

A 3-year trial of 1010 men showed that those who drank at least 1.1 liters per week of soft drinks with at least one stone significantly decreased recurrence of stone formation when soft drink consumption was reduced.[10]

Grapefruit Juice

Grapefruit juice may increase the risk of kidney stone formation as evidenced in the Nurses' Health Study.[11] Other studies, however, have refuted this finding.

Oxalates

Many patients who have produced calcium oxalate stones have been encouraged to limit their intake of oxalate-containing foods. This is somewhat confusing, however, because several of the products mentioned later in the chapter have been shown to decrease incidence of kidney stones even though they contain significant amounts of oxalate! In addition, some studies have shown that eating oxalate- and calcium-containing foods together may actually decrease stone risk.[12] Studies have shown that the foods listed in Table 49–1 have the greatest influence on increasing urinary oxalate. Of course, cranberries and cranberry (or blueberry) juice are helpful in preventing urinary tract infections and thus may decrease risk of struvite stones.

Kidney stone sufferers should flatly refuse any invitation to a high tea where rhubarb pie with whole-wheat crust is served along with chocolate-covered strawberries and peanuts.

Purines

A high purine diet has been correlated with increased levels of uric acid in the urine. Thus, those with proven uric acid stones should restrict their intake of the purine-containing foods listed in Table 49–2.

Table 49-2. Foods to Avoid

Foods High in Oxalates

Spinach and other green, leafy vegetables (collards, Swiss chard), rhubarb, beets, chocolate, peanuts, tea, wheat bran, and asparagus, as well as some fruits (particularly, strawberries, cranberries, raspberries, plums, and apples)

Foods High in Purine

Alcoholic beverages, organ meats, legumes, mushrooms, asparagus, spinach, cauliflower, sardines, anchovies, and poultry all are high in purines.

SUPPLEMENTS

Calcium

In women, increased calcium from the diet may decrease risk of nephrolithiasis, whereas supplemental calcium may increase it.[13] Several large studies of both men and women have confirmed this. It is believed that calcium in the diet binds oxalate in foods and prevents both its absorption and excretion in the urine. The full story on calcium supplementation is complex. Much depends on the oxalate intake and whether the patient has any other risk factors or conditions such as absorptive hypercalciuria. Of course, the body has a number of mechanisms to maintain normal calcium levels in the serum and the urine (PTH and calcitrol), but it is prudent to restrict high calcium intake in those with absorptive hypercalciuria. High calcium intake in normal individuals poses little risk. Calcium citrate is the preferred preparation for postmenopausal women with stone disease. Although urinary calcium excretion increases with calcium citrate, urinary citrate levels also increase.[14]

Magnesium

Magnesium supplementation has been shown to lead to positive changes in lithogenic and inhibitory components. In one study, magnesium oxide (300 mg/d) was the salt used in combination with vitamin B_6 (10 mg/d). Results showed a significant decrease in calcium oxalate risk index.[15]

Dosage. Magnesium oxide 300 mg a day

Vitamin B₆

Vitamin B_6 may decrease oxalate production and thus possibly reduce the risk of kidney stone formation (at least in women). A prospective cohort study was done involving 85,557 women with no history of kidney stones. Relative risk of stone formation was .66 in those who were in the highest category of B_6 intake (≥ 40 mg/d) compared with those in the lowest category (< 3 mg/d).[16] Good food sources of B_6 are oily fish, poultry, whole grains, soybeans, avocados, baked potato with skin, bananas, nuts, and brewer's yeast.

Dosage. 50 mg per day

Vitamin C

Serum ascorbic acid levels have been shown not to correlate with kidney stone formation.[17] Thus, vitamin C need not be restricted in normal people. In fact, in the Harvard Prospective Health Professional Follow-Up study, those who had the highest vitamin C intake (> 1500 mg/d) had a lower risk of kidney stones.[18] However, since ascorbate may convert to oxalates, people with hyperoxaluria should not take vitamin C supplements.

Vitamin D

Several studies have found a positive correlation between serum vitamin D levels and urinary calcium excretion. This is thought to be the result of increased intestinal calcium absorption, which causes greater intestinal absorption of oxalate. Vitamin D may be a risk factor for kidney stone formation.[19]

BOTANICAL AND HERBAL PRODUCTS

Herbal products that have a diuretic effect have been used historically for irrigation therapy along with copious ingestion of fluids to increase urinary output in the prevention of kidney and bladder stones.

Comment. The black or green tea decoction described in the following paragraph is not a treatment guideline for urinary tract infections nor should this therapy be used as a substitute for antibiotic therapy when appropriate.

Black or Green Tea (*Camellia sinensis*)

The leaves and stems are used. Flavonoids are found in great abundance in tea, which also is a diuretic. A large cohort study of more than 85,000 women showed that those who consumed black tea had an 8% decreased risk of developing kidney stones.[11]

Dosage. For urinary stone prevention, at least one cup per day.

Precautions. Caution should be used when combining tea with other caffeine-containing supplements or supplements containing ephedra. The caffeine in tea also potentially interacts with many pharmaceuticals. It raises blood pressure, heart rate, and contractility, inhibits platelet aggregation, and increases stomach acid secretion.

Parsley Leaf and Root (*Petroselinum crispum*)[22, 24, 25]

Parsley has been used historically in several ways to affect the urologic system. It has been used as a treatment for patients with urinary tract infections, as a diuretic, and in prevention of bladder and kidney stones. Parsley has been generally recognized as safe (GRAS) by the United States Food and Drug Administration.

Parsley contains volatile oils, carotene, B vitamins, and vitamin C. It has aquaretic effects and irritates the kidney epithelium, which increases renal blood flow and glomerular filtration rate.

Dosage. A parsley tea is made by steeping 2 g of finely chopped dried root in 150 mL of boiling water for 10 to 15 minutes. The tea is then strained. One cup should be drunk two to three times a day. The maximum daily dose is 6 g. Large amounts of water should be consumed concomitantly.

Precautions. Extremely large amounts of parsley tea (200 g) can cause toxicity because of the apiole constituent (similar structure to safrole-a, which is a known hepatotoxic and carcinogenic substance). Large amounts have also been used as an abortifacient and to stimulate uterine blood flow, so it is certainly contraindicated in pregnancy. Large amounts can affect prothrombin times in patients taking coumadin because of the vitamin K content. Parsley tea is contraindicated in patients with kidney inflammation or kidney disease.

Stinging Nettle—Above-Ground Parts (*Urtica urens*)[22, 26, 27]

In the realm of urology, stinging nettle has traditionally been used for treatment of patients with inflammation and infection of the lower urinary tract, for urolithiasis, for "irrigation therapy," and as an adjunct to saw palmetto for the treatment of patients with benign prostatic hypertrophy. Active constituents are vitamins C and K, potassium, and calcium. Nettle juice increases urine output and slightly lowers systolic blood pressure. It has been shown to have diuretic activity and analgesic effects.

Dosage. A tea (decoction) is made by steeping 1.5 to 5g of the aerial portion in 150 mL of boiling water for 10 minutes. The fluid is then strained. Up to one cup three times daily may be taken with ample fluid intake for irrigation therapy. Other preparation options are fresh juice, 10 to 15 mL three times daily or dried extract (7:1) 770 mg twice daily.

Precautions. When taken orally, nettle juice may cause diarrhea. It may affect protimes in coumadin users because large amounts may have significant amounts to vitamin K. Excessive amounts may cause low blood sugar. Nettle in large doses may have depressant effects on the central nervous system.

Comment. Avoid confusion with the stinging nettle root.

PHARMACEUTICALS

Standard Drugs Used for Calcium Stones with or without Hypercalciuria

Diuretics

Thiazide diuretics in particular are often used to reduce the amount of calcium excreted by the kidneys. However, thiazides also cause increased loss of potassium and magnesium, which in turn increases citrate loss. Thus, potassium citrate or potassium-magnesium citrate should be taken along with diuretics to counter the citrate loss.

The usual starting dose of thiazide diuretics (hydrochlorothiazide or chlorthalidone) is 25 to 50 mg, with dosage increasing to 50 mg twice daily (dictated by repeat 24-urine testing if needed).

Amiloride (Midamor) is a potassium-sparing diuretic that may be used if a thiazide is not sufficient.

Potassium-Magnesium Citrate

In numerous studies, potassium citrate has been found to be effective as prophylaxis against recurrent calcium oxalate stones. One study showed an 85% drop in recurrence risk after 3 years. Citrate inhibits the crystallization of calcium oxalate and calcium phosphate and chelates calcium. Citrate reduces calcium excretion by the kidneys in individuals with distal RTA, increases intestinal loss of calcium, and restores a positive calcium balance so that bone loss is prevented.[21]

Potassium-magnesium citrate is available over the counter. The potassium citrate products mentioned here are available only by prescription but serve the same purpose as potassium-magnesium citrate, which can be given as the sole treatment for those with normal serum calcium.

Dosage. Magnesium citrate 20 to 30 mEq twice daily (OTC). Potassium citrate (Urocit-K, Polycitra-K) 20 mEq PO BID-TID (prescription). Take citrate products with food.

Precautions. Gastrointestinal intolerance

Magnesium citrate may be used in patients who develop stones secondary to impaired absorption of calcium as a result of small bowel disease.

NOTE

Any patient receiving potassium-sparing medicines, or those with urinary tract infections or kidney damage should not take citrate-containing products. Patients with a history of peptic ulcer disease should avoid these products in tablet form.

Drug for Hyperoxaluria

In addition to vitamin B_6, cholestyramine (Questran), normally used to reduce cholesterol levels, also binds oxalate in the intestine, thus reducing the oxalate load of the kidney. The powdered form is usually dissolved in water, milk, or juice. Cholestyramine may also bind many other medications; therefore, other drugs should be taken at least 1 hour before or 4 hours after cholestyramine. A daily multivitamin should be taken to prevent loss of the fat-soluble vitamins.

Dosage. 1 to 2 scoops per day
Side Effects. Bloating and constipation

Drug for Hyperuricemia

In addition to the citrates, patients may be given allopurinol (Zyloprim, Lupurin). Starting therapy with allopurinol may trigger an attack of gout. Patients may consider taking an nonsteroidal anti-inflammatory drug for 2 to 3 months after institution of allopurinol therapy. Aspirin should not be used for this purpose because it increases uric acid levels.

Dosage. 300 mg a day
Side Effects. Rash and gastrointestinal upset

Drugs for Cystine Stones[2]

First-line treatment is alkalization of the urine. If this fails, tiopronin or penicillamine decreases urinary cystine levels by forming a soluble mixed disulfide with cystine. The use of captopril is controversial but may be an option. Fluid intake of at least 4 quarts of water per day must be maintained.

Dosage. Tiopronin 200 to 500 mg twice daily or penicillamine 250 mg twice daily

Drugs for Struvite Stones

The chief way to prevent these rare stones is to prevent and treat patients with infection. If the stones cannot be removed by antibacterial methods, acetohydroxamic acid (Lithostat) may be added along with long-term antibiotic treatment. This therapy blocks the enzymes (urease) produced by the bacteria. The drug has many side effects and often causes anemia by reducing the body's iron stores. Only physicians who have experience using the drug should prescribe it.

SURGICAL AND OTHER PROCEDURES

In general, stones smaller than 6 mm should be observed for a period of time. More than 90% of stones smaller than 4 mm that are found in the distal ureter pass through the body without intervention. This number drops to 50% for stones between 4 and 6 mm. Only 20% of stones larger than 6mm pass. Of patients with these stones, 30% to 40% have a recurrence. More than 50% of patients have only one recurrence during their lives. Ten percent of recurrent stone formers have more than three recurrences.[29]

Surgery is a last resort, and surgery is performed in less than 2% of patients. Indications include stones that are too large to pass on their own and those that are damaging the kidney either through infection or obstruction (hydronephrosis). Other options are described in the following paragraphs.

Extracorporeal Shock Wave Lithotripsy[3]

Extracorporeal shock wave lithotripsy (ESWL) is the primary choice for small stones (> 1 cm) found in the upper ureter or kidney. For stones larger than 3 cm, another treatment should be employed. Success rates are usually 70% to 90%, depending on where the stone is the success rate drops to 50% when stones are located in the lower calyx, when the anatomy is unfavorable and if there are cystine stones. Occasionally, more than one treatment may be required to completely fragment all of the stones.

Recovery usually takes just a few days, but it may be complicated by discomfort as the "gravel" is passed from the body. The procedure may result in mild to moderate bruising of the skin on the back or abdomen. Transient elevation of blood pressure after lithotripsy as well as several cases of bowel perforation have been reported. Patients should be cautioned against the use of aspirin or other nonsteroidal anti-inflammatory drugs that may promote bleeding. ESWL is contraindicated in pregnancy, bleeding dyscrasias, infection, and obstruction.

Percutaneous Nephrolithotomy[31, 32]

This procedure is used when ESWL is ineffective or not readily available and for extremely large stones, cystine stones, or stones that are not accessible to ESWL. In these cases, the urologist tunnels through a small incision in the back to the kidney, inserting a nephroscope and removing the stones directly. Larger stones are usually broken up by either ultrasonography or laser lithotripsy and then removed.[33] Often, a nephrostomy tube is left in place for a short while after the procedure. Recovery usually requires less than a week in the hospital. Success rates are usually about 98% for stones found in the kidney and 88% for those in the ureter. Complications such as blood loss or fluid and electrolyte imbalance, as well as serious problems, are rare ($< 3\%$) and kidney function is usually not impaired.

Ureteroscopic Stone Removal[34]

This procedure involves passage of a ureteroscope up the urethra into the bladder and into the ureter, where the urologist uses a cagelike device to remove the stones. Overall success rates are close to 90%.

Larger stones may either be treated by laser or broken up with a pneumatic device and then removed. This procedure is used generally for stones found in the middle and lower ureter. Often, a stent is placed for a few days after removal.

— THERAPEUTIC REVIEW

There are several therapeutic options for nephrolithiasis. Increased fluid intake is the cornerstone of therapy no matter what approach is taken subsequently. Nutrition is particularly important in regard to recurrence. A number of natural and pharmaceutical therapeutic options are available, and surgery is considered only when damage to the kidney either by obstruction or infection is imminent, if the stone is too large to pass, or if it is anatomically inaccessible by other methods.

- *Remove exacerbating factors:*
  During the summer months and in warmer climates, particularly when the patient is engaging in strenuous physical activity, care must be taken to ensure that adequate fluid intake is maintained.
- *Nutrition:*
  Fluid intake should be at least 2.5 to 3 liters per day. Protein, salt, and soft drinks should be kept to a minimum. Those with stones containing oxalate should consider limiting oxalate-containing foods, and those with uric acid stones should limit their intake of foods with high purine content (see Table 49–2).
- *Supplements:*
  Calcium-containing foods seem to pose little risk, as do calcium supplements in normal individuals. Calcium citrate may be the best way to supplement calcium. Magnesium (300 mg/d) and vitamin B_6 (50 mg/d) may be helpful in prevention. Vitamin C should be restricted in those with hyperoxaluria, but high doses (> 1500 mg/d) in normal individuals may be protective.
- *Botanicals:*
  Most herbal products have traditionally been used for their mild diuretic effects in irrigation therapy. Many also contain abundant bioflavonoids that may have anti-inflammatory effects or other inhibitory attributes.
- *Pharmaceuticals:*
  Diuretics (hydrochlorothiazide or chlorthalidone) are the primary pharmaceutical option; dosages range from 25 to 50 mg. A diuretic, along with potassium citrate 20 to 30 mEq twice daily, may be the only therapy needed in most cases. Other drugs (outlined earlier) may be used to address specific metabolic or biochemical problems.
- *Surgical and other interventions:*
  The most common method of dealing with kidney stones is ESWL. For larger stones in the kidney and upper ureter or for those inaccessible to ESWL, percutaneous nephrolithotomy is used. For stones in the mid to lower ureter, ureteroscopic retrieval is the most likely method employed.

References

1. Uribarri J, Oh MS, Carroll HJ: The first kidney stone. Ann Intern Med 111:1006–1009, 1989.
2. Coe FL, Parks JH, Asplin JR: The pathogenesis and treatment of kidney stones. N Engl J Med 327:1141–1152, 1992.
3. Pak CYC: Citrate and renal calculi: An update. Miner Electr Metab 20:371–377, 1994.
4. Baggio B, Gambaro G, Marchini F, et al: An inheritable anomaly of red cell oxalate transport in primary calcium nephrolithiasis correctable with diuretics. N Engl J Med 314:599–604, 1986.
5. Coe FL: Hyperuricosuric calcium oxalate nephrolithiasis. Kidney Int 30:422–428, 1986.
6. Goldfarb DS, Coe FL: Prevention of recurrent nephrolithiasis. Am Fam Physician 60:2269–2276, 1999.
7. Borghi L, Meschi T, Amato F, et al: Urinary volume, water and recurrences in idiopathic calcium nephrolithiasis: A 5-year randomized prospective study. J Urol 155:839–843, 1996.
8. Robertson WG: Diet and kidney stones. Miner Electr Metab 13:228–234, 1987.
9. Pak CYC: Kidney stones. Lancet 351:1797–1801, 1998.
10. Shuster J, Jenkins A, Logan C, et al: Soft drink consumption and urinary stone recurrence: A randomized prevention trial. J Clin Epidemiol 45:911–916, 1992.
11. Curhan GC, Willett WC, Speizer FE, Stampfer MJ: Beverage use and risk for kidney stones in women. Arch Intern Med 128:534–540, 1998.

12. Parivar F, Low RK, Stoller ML: The influence of diet on kidney stone disease. J Urol 155:432–440, 1996.
13. Curhan GC, Willett WC, Speizer FE, Stampfer MJ. Comparison of dietary calcium with supplemental calcium and other nutrients as factors affecting the risk of kidney stones in women. Ann Intern Med 126:497–504, 1997.
14. Levine BS, Rodman JS, Wienerman S, et al: Effect of calcium citrate supplementation on urinary calcium oxalate saturation in female stone formers: Implications for prevention of osteoporosis. Am J Clin Nutr 60:592–596, 1994.
15. Rattan V, Sidhu H, Vaidyanathan S, et al: Effect of combined supplementation of magnesium oxide and pyridoxine in calcium-oxalate stone formers. Urol Res 22:161–165, 1994.
16. Curhan GC, Willett WC, Speizer FE, Stampfer MJ: Intake of vitamins B_6 and C and the risk of kidney stones in women. J Am Soc Nephrol 10:840–845, 1999.
17. Gerster H: No contribution of ascorbic acid to renal calcium oxalate stones. Ann Nutr Metab 41:269–282, 1997.
18. Simon JA, Hudes ES: Relation of serum ascorbic acid to serum vitamin B_{12}, serum ferritin, and kidney stones in US adults. Arch Intern Med, 159:619–624, 1999.
19. Giannini S, Nobile M, Castrignano R, et al: Possible link between vitamin D and hyperoxaluria in patients with renal stone disease. Clin Sci 84:51–54, 1993.
20. Ettinger B: Potassium-magnesium citrate is an effective prophylaxis against recurrent calcium oxalate nephrolithiasis. J Urol 158:2069–2073, 1997.
21. Pak CYC: Citrate and renal calculi: An update. Miner Electr Metab 20:371–377, 1994.
22. Blumenthal M, Busse WR (eds): The Complete German Commission E Monographs: Therapeutic Guide to Herbal Medicines [Trans. S. Klein]. Boston, American Botanical Council, 1998.
23. PDR for Herbal Medicines. Montvale, NJ, Medical Economics Company, 1998.
24. Robbers KE, Tyler VE: Tyler's Herbs of Choice. Binghamton, NY, Haworth Herbal Press, 1999.
25. McGuffin M: American Herbal Products Association's Botanical Safety Handbook. Boca Raton, FL, CRC Press, 1997.
26. Brinker F: Herb Contraindications and Drug Interactions, 2nd ed. Sandy, OR, Eclectic Medical Publications, 1998.
27. Newell CA, Anderson LA, Philipson JD: Herbal Medicine: A Guide for Healthcare Professionals. London, The Pharmaceutical Press, 1996.
28. Remien A, Kallistratos G, Burchardt P: Treatment of cystinuria with thiola (mercaptopropionylglycine). Eur Urol 1:227–228, 1975.
29. Strohmaier WL: Course of calcium stone disease without treatment. What can we expect? Eur Urol 37:339–344, 2000.
30. Tombolini P, Ruoppolo M, Bellorofonte C, et al: Lithotripsy in the treatment of urinary lithiasis. J Nephrol 13(Suppl 3):S71–S82, 2000.
31. Ramakumar S, Segura JW: Renal calculi. Percutaneous management. Urol Clin North Am 27:617–622, 2000.
32. Gravenstein D: Extracorporeal shock wave lithotripsy and percutaneous nephrolithotomy. Anesthesiol Clin North Am 18:953–971, 2000.
33. Sofer M, Denstedt J: Flexible ureteroscopy and lithotripsy with the Holmium:YAG. Can J Urol 7:952–956, 2000.
34. Fabrizio MD, Behari A, Bagley DH: Ureteroscopic management of intrarenal calculi. J Urol 159:1139–1143, 1998.

Bibliography

Resnick M, Persky L: Summary of the National Institutes of Arthritis, Digestive and Kidney Diseases Conference on Urolithiasis: State of the art and future research needs. J Urol 153:4–9, 1995.
National Kidney Foundation: Diet and Kidney Stones. (Call 1-800-622-9010 for a copy.)
Coe FL, Parks JH, Asplin JR: The pathogenesis and treatment of kidney stones. N Engl J Med 327:1141–1152, 1992.
Savitz G, Leslie SW: Kidney Stones Handbook: A Patient's Guide to Hope, Cure, and Prevention, 2nd ed. Roseville, CA, Four Geez Press, 1999.

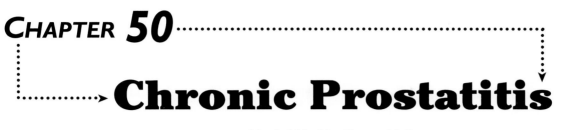

CHAPTER 50

Chronic Prostatitis

Mark W. McClure, M.D.

PATHOPHYSIOLOGY

Prostatitis is the most common reason why men younger than age fifty, and the third most common reason why men older than age fifty, see a urologist. Although the term *prostatitis* literally means "prostatic inflammation," inflammation isn't always present; neither is infection.

In an effort to standardize the terminology used to describe the different types of prostatitis, the National Institutes of Health has proposed the four categories listed in Table 50–1.[1]

NOTE

Only 5% of men with prostatitis have bacterial prostatitis.

Bacterial prostatitis is usually caused by manipulation of the urinary tract, unsafe sexual practices, and spasms of the muscular tissue in the bladder neck, prostatic urethra, and external urethral sphincter. Muscular spasms induce prostatitis by interrupting the smooth flow of urine, thereby causing reflux of urine into ducts that permeate the prostate. Chronic bacterial prostatitis, which is characterized by prostatic calculi, ductal obstruction, and chronic inflammation, is more common than acute bacterial prostatitis.

One reason why bacterial prostatitis is unusual can be traced to a substance called *antibacterial factor*. Secreted by cells that line the prostatic ducts, antibacterial factor kills bacteria on contact. Researchers have determined that zinc is the active component of antibacterial factor.[2] Although the prostate has the highest zinc concentration of any tissue in the body, men with chronic bacterial prostatitis have extremely low concentrations of zinc within their prostates, even though their blood zinc levels are usually normal.

Another reason why bacterial prostatitis is uncommon can be attributed to immune surveillance. The immune system prevents bacterial prostatitis by dispatching immune cells that either engulf bacteria (monocytes) or poison them with toxic substances such as hydrogen peroxide (lymphocytes and eosinophils).

The vast majority of men (95%) have nonbacterial prostatitis. Chronic abacterial prostatitis (also called *chronic pelvic pain syndrome*) is subdivided into two categories depending on the number of inflammatory white blood cells (WBCs) in the expressed prostatic secretions (EPS): An amount of 10 or more WBCs per high-powered field in the EPS is labeled chronic inflammatory abacterial prostatitis (category IIIa); a lesser amount is labeled chronic noninflammatory abacterial prostatitis (category IIIb).

Although controversial, the etiology of chronic inflammatory abacterial prostatitis has been linked with an occult bacterial infection, genetic factors, hormonal imbalance, aging, chemical irritants, fungal infections, and autoimmunity.[3] Researchers theorize that noninflammatory abacterial prostatitis is caused by spasms of the pelvic floor musculature, stress, and intraprostatic urinary reflux.

Although treatment guidelines can help steer physicians in the right direction, physicians in clinical practice use a process of elimination, based on the results of trial and error therapies, to diagnose and treat patients with prostatitis. For both the patient and the doctor, the hallmark of a successful treatment is the resolution of symptoms.

INTEGRATIVE THERAPIES

Physicians routinely treat prostatitis with a combination of art and science. Just the same, before instituting integrative therapies, proper medical evaluation is mandatory because other conditions, such as bladder cancer, prostate cancer, and interstitial cystitis, can mimic prostatitis symptoms. Once a proper diagnosis has been established, it is safe to proceed with the measures listed in the following paragraphs.

Table 50–1. Categories of Prostatitis

I.	Acute bacterial prostatitis
II.	Chronic bacterial prostatitis
III.	Chronic abacterial prostatitis
	IIIa. Inflammatory (>10 WBC/high-powered field [hpf] in expressed secretions)
	IIIb. Noninflammatory (<10 WBC/hpf in expressed secretions)
IV.	Asymptomatic inflammatory prostatitis

Lifestyle

Lifestyle—daily choices that are under our control—can either improve or worsen prostatitis symptoms. Healthful choices such as regular exercise, getting enough rest, eating nutritious food, and reducing stress improve the symptoms. Unhealthful choices have the opposite effect.

Nutrition

Although taken for granted, foods are a potent medicine that can either increase or decrease prostatitis symptoms.

Do's

The following measures, which can improve prostatitis symptoms, should be encouraged:

Fruits and Vegetables. Five to nine daily servings of brightly colored fruits and vegetables should be eaten. Rich in antioxidant vitamins and minerals, fruits and vegetables reduce prostatitis by neutralizing infection and inflammation-related free radical damage.

Flaxseed. Flaxseeds are a rich source of anti-inflammatory omega-3 essential fatty acids and a nutritious phytoestrogen-containing fiber called *lignan*. Flaxseeds should be ground in a coffee grinder and one teaspoon should be sprinkled over cereal or vegetables twice daily. The unused portion should be stored in the refrigerator.

Soy. Encourage two servings of soy protein daily. Soy protein reduces not only prostatic inflammation, but also the risk of prostate cancer.

Water. Drink at least sixty-four ounces of water daily. Water dilutes noxious urinary irritants.

Don'ts

The following substances can worsen prostatitis symptoms; therefore, patients should be encouraged to avoid:

Hot, spicy foods
Alcohol or caffeinated beverages
Refined sugar
Junk food or foods that are high in saturated fat.

These foods aggravate prostatitis by inducing the production of arachidonic acid and associated inflammatory prostaglandin and leukotriene molecules.

SUPPLEMENTS

Zinc

Zinc is essential for proper immune function, which may explain why men with depressed prostate zinc concentrations are more susceptible to chronic bacterial prostatitis. Unfortunately, supplemental zinc is unable to normalize prostate zinc concentration once it has become depressed.[4] On the other hand, taking oral zinc supplements can normalize seminal fluid zinc levels and reverse prostatitis-induced infertility.[5]

Dosage. 90 mg zinc gluconate (less expensive) or zinc picolinate (better absorbed) daily

Precautions. Taking more than 150 mg of zinc daily can depress serum copper levels and impair immunity.

Quercetin

A naturally occurring plant flavonoid, quercetin reduces prostatic inflammation and inhibits bacterial infection.[6] Onions, parsley, sage, tomatoes, and citrus fruits are rich natural sources of quercetin.

Dosage. Between 200 and 400 mg before meals tid. Bromelain derived from the stem of pineapple plants (*Ananas comosus*) improves the absorption of quercetin; therefore, 500 mg of bromelain tid should be taken daily along with quercetin.

Precaution. None.

Botanicals

Although effective for a variety of prostate disorders, in contrast to prescription drugs, herbs take four to six weeks to achieve maximum effect. Just the same, herbs are less expensive, cause fewer adverse effects, and often work when prescription drugs have failed. Herbs can be taken singly or in combination.

Herbs That Decrease Prostatic Inflammation

Prostatic inflammation causes pain and swelling. Referred pain radiates along the nerves that supply the prostate. The herbs discussed in the following sections can reduce prostatic inflammation.

Saw Palmetto (Serenoa repens)

Derived from the berries of the dwarf palmetto palm tree, saw palmetto inhibits two enzymes that convert arachidonic acid to prostaglandin E_2 and leukotriene molecules, thus inhibiting the inflammatory cascade.

Dosage. One capsule twice daily of a solid extract containing 160 mg of saw palmetto standardized to contain 85% to 95% fatty acids and sterols.

Precautions. Occasional upset stomach.

Rye Grass Pollen (Secale cereale)

European and Scandinavian physicians routinely use a proprietary brand of rye pollen extract (Cernilton) to successfully treat men with nonbacterial prostatitis. Rich in phytosterols, Cernilton blocks the formation of inflammatory prostaglandin and leukotriene molecules.[8]

Dosage. The typical dose of Cernilton is 126 mg three times a day.

Precautions. Although hypoallergenic, theoretically, Cernilton could cause an allergic reaction in patients with pollen allergies.

South African Star Grass (Hypoxis rooperi)

Commonly used by European physicians to treat benign prostatic hyperplasia (BPH), South African star grass is rich in phytosterols, especially beta-sitosterol. Beta-sitosterol not only reduces prostatic inflammation, it lowers serum cholesterol as well.

Dosage. Dosage depends on the formulation. Select a product that contains at least 50% beta-sitosterol. Supplement should be taken as directed.

Precautions. Occasional gastrointestinal adverse effects can occur.

Clivers (Galium aparine)

Rich in antioxidant flavonoids, clivers is a nonirritating diuretic herb that reduces prostatic inflammation.

Dosage. Drink 1 glass of water containing 30 to 40 drops of liquid extract tid.

Precautions. None.

Agrimony (Agrimonia eupatoria)

The flowering portion of agrimony is rich in antioxidants known as catechins that can put out the fire of prostatitis.

Dosage. Drink 1 glass of water containing 30 drops of liquid extract tid.

Precautions. None.

Stinging Nettle (Urtica dioica)

Nettle root is packed with polysaccharides that inhibit inflammatory prostaglandin and leukotriene molecules, thereby reducing prostatic pain and swelling.

Dosage. The normal daily dose is 3 to 6 g taken as a tablet or capsule containing 600 to 1200 mg of a 5:1 dry extract (equivalent to 3 to 6 g of dried nettle root).

Precautions. Occasional stomach upset can occur.

Herbs That Decrease Painful Urination

In addition to drinking plenty of water and avoiding urinary tract irritants, the patient seeking to alleviate dysuria can use the following herbs:

Marshmallow Root (Althaea officinalis)

Marshmallow root soothes inflamed mucous membranes.

Dosage. Available either as a tea, liquid tincture, or capsule; drink several cups of tea daily; drink 1 glass of water containing 30 to 40 drops of tincture daily; or take capsules containing an equivalent of 6 g of powdered root daily in divided doses.

Precautions. Marshmallow root can delay the absorption of drugs taken simultaneously.

Eryngo (Eryngium campestre)

The dried leaves, flowers, and roots of eryngo are used to make an herbal tincture that assuages dysuria.

Dosage. Drink 1 glass of water containing 60 drops of liquid tincture tid or qid.

Precautions. None.

Herbs That Prevent Recurrent Urinary Tract Infections

A urinary tract infection (UTI) can cause prostatitis because urine routinely refluxes into prostatic ducts during voiding.[9] Scientific research has shown that the following herbs can inhibit recurrent UTIs.

Cranberry (Vaccinium macrocarpon)

Proanthocyanidins contained in cranberries can prevent *Escherichia coli, Proteus* spp, and *Pseudomonas aeruginosa* from adhering to urothelial mucosa.[10] This is relevant because *Escherichia coli* causes 80% of the cases of bacterial prostatitis.[11]

Dosage. Drink 8 oz of *unsweetened* cranberry juice daily or take a standardized solid cranberry extract; one capsule tid for prevention, and two capsules tid if infection is present.

Precautions. None.

Uva ursi (Arctostaphylos uva-ursi)

Uva ursi leaves contain a potent urinary antiseptic called *arbutin*. Arbutin is hydrolyzed in alkaline urine to hydroquinone. Hydroquinone inhibits the following prostatitis-causing bacteria: *Proteus vulgaris, Escherichia coli, Ureaplasma urealyticum, Mycoplasma hominis, Pseudomonas aeruginosa, Staphylococcus aureus,* and *Enterococcus faecalis.*[12]

Note: Owing to its high tannin content uva ursi should not be taken for more than 1 week; it is contraindicated in pregnant women, patients with renal disease, nursing mothers, and children under the age of twelve.[13, 14]

Dosage. Uva ursi is available as a tea (add 3 g of ground herb [one heaping teaspoon] in a tea caddy to 5 oz of boiling water and drink one cup qid); a solid extract (the hydroquinone derivative, calculated as water-free arbutin, is dosed at 100 to 210 mg qid);

and as a 1:1 fluid extract (drink 1.5 to 4 mL in water tid).[15]

Precautions. Uva ursi is safe when taken as directed. Avoid medications or foods that acidify the urine (cranberries, for example) while taking uva ursi because it works best in alkaline urine.

Herbs That Prevent Muscle Spasms

Kava kava (Piper methysticum)

A drink derived from the root of this Polynesian herb has been used for centuries to reduce anxiety and relax tense muscles. The active components of kava kava, called *kavalactones*, are concentrated in the root. When compared head-to-head with a benzodiazepine, kava kava compared favorably with the prescription drug.

Dosage. Kava kava is available as a standardized liquid or solid extract (standardized for kavalactones). Depending on the preparation, one must take an equivalent amount that yields 45 to 70 mg of kavalactones tid. Products that contain this include KavaTone (Enzymatic Therapy) and Kava (Nature's Way).

Precautions. Taken as directed, kava kava is safe. However, kava kava is contraindicated in patients with endogenous depression, pregnant women, and nursing mothers. Kava kava may also cause liver damage when taken in excess and potentiate the effects of alcohol and the effectiveness of prescription antidepressant, antianxiety, and sedative medications.[16]

Petasites (Petasites officinalis)

A potent smooth muscle relaxant, petasites is useful for certain types of prostatitis.

Dosage. The typical dose of petasites is 4.5 to 7 g of root or equivalent daily. However, because unprocessed petasites root contains potentially harmful substances called *unsaturated pyrrolizidine alkaloids (UPAs)*, one should choose an alkaloid-free fluid extract instead; take 20 to 30 drops in 1 glass of water tid.[18] Limit use to a maximum of six weeks per year.[19]

Precautions. Chronic exposure to UPA can cause veno-occlusive disease. Petasites is contraindicated in pregnant women and nursing mothers.[17]

Pharmaceuticals

Anti-inflammatory Medications

Although anti-inflammatory medications can't cure prostatitis, they can reduce prostatic inflammation and pain.

Dosage. One should prescribe 200 mg of Celebrex or 50 mg Vioxx daily for two to four weeks.

Precautions. If taken on a long term basis, most nonsteroidal anti-inflammatory drugs (NSAIDs) can cause gastrointestinal bleeding and renal impairment. Selective cyclo-oxygenase 2 (COX 2) inhibitors cause fewer adverse effects.

Alpha-adrenergic Blockers

Routinely used to treat BPH, alpha-adrenergic blockers relax smooth muscle tissue in the prostatic urethra and bladder neck. Currently, the three selective alpha$_1$ blockers that are FDA approved are doxazosin (Cardura), terazosin (Hytrin), and tamsulosin (Flomax).

Dosage. Doxazosin and terazosin must be titrated to the maximum effective dosage. Tamsulosin does not require titration; take 0.4 mg 30 minutes after the same meal daily. If the medication hasn't improved prostatitis symptoms within 4 to 6 weeks, further medication is rarely helpful.

Precautions. Doxazosin and terazosin can cause postural hypotension, asthenia, and dizziness, whereas tamsulosin can cause nasal congestion and delayed or retrograde ejaculation.

Antibiotics

Ideally, antibiotics should be reserved for culture-proven bacterial infection. In clinical practice, though, antibiotics are routinely used to treat all types of prostatitis.

NOTE

Approximately one third of patients with nonbacterial prostatitis respond to antibiotics, the same proportion that respond to placebo.

Pending the results of a postprostatic massage urine culture, it is reasonable to prescribe quinolone antibiotics. If patients are allergic to quinolone antibiotics, alternate choices include sulfa, tetracycline, geocillin, or erythromycin. If the culture results are negative, the antibiotics may be stopped. On the other hand, if the patient shows clinical improvement, antibiotic therapy may be continued.

Dosage. A 1-month course of antibiotics will usually suffice; however, men with chronic bacterial prostatitis may require protracted antibiotic therapy.

Precautions. Probiotics (see Chapter 97, Prescribing Probiotics) should be taken twice daily with food in addition to antibiotics to minimize antibiotic-related gastrointestinal adverse effects.

Biomechanical Techniques

Sitz Bath

Taking a hot sitz bath for fifteen minutes twice daily increases blood flow to the prostate, reduces prostatic inflammation, and enhances immune function.

Prostatic Massage

A time-honored treatment for prostatitis, prostate massage forces secretions laden with dead bacteria and cellular debris into the prostatic urethra. According to scientific research, regular prostatic massage can improve painful prostatitis symptoms by more than 50%.[21]

Physical Therapy

According to researchers at the Cleveland Clinic, tailor-made physical therapy that targets specific muscles in the pelvis and back can alleviate prostatitis symptoms in the majority of men.[22]

Transurethral Microwave Therapy (TUMT)

Canadian researchers have shown that TUMT is an effective, safe, and durable treatment for resistant nonbacterial prostatitis.[23]

Mind-Body Interventions

Chronic prostatitis exacts a heavy emotional toll on men. According to one survey, the quality of life for these men is on par with men suffering from chronic low back pain, heart disease, or inflammatory bowel disease.[24] The following mind-body modalities can help alleviate the pain and suffering that accompany chronic prostatitis by providing men with new coping skills.

Stress reduction techniques (see Chapter 91)
Guided imagery (see Chapter 92)

Meditation (see Chapter 94)
Yoga
Psychological counseling

Stress

Although stress is a part of everyday life, heightened levels of stress worsen the symptoms of prostatitis. Mediated through the sympathetic nervous system, prolonged stress increases the incidence of urinary tract infections, depresses the immune system, and increases spasms of the bladder, urethra, and pelvic musculature.[25, 26] Although stress cannot be eliminated, it can be controlled (see Chapter 91, Prescribing Relaxation Techniques).

Biofeedback. By teaching men how to relax voluntary and involuntary muscles, biofeedback training can alleviate prostatitis symptoms.

Therapies to Consider

Homeopathy

Safe and effective homeopathic remedies for nonbacterial prostatitis such as *Pulsatilla, Kali bichromium, Causticum,* and *Chimaphilla umbellata* deserve further consideration.[27] Consult a licensed homeopathic physician.

Traditional Chinese Medicine

Chinese herbal therapies and acupuncture can improve annoying prostatitis symptoms. Consult a Traditional Chinese Medicine practitioner.

Reiki and Healing Touch

Used by millions of patients worldwide, these energetic therapies promote healing throughout the body. I have used Reiki in my practice since 1989. Consider referring receptive patients to a qualified energy worker in your area.

THERAPEUTIC REVIEW

Unless they are allergic, start symptomatic patients on a quinolone antibiotic pending culture results. If the culture is positive, further treatment should be based on the culture results. If the culture is negative, the antibiotics can be stopped. However, if there is symptomatic improvement, even though the culture results are negative, antibiotic therapy may be continued. Antibiotics should be taken for one month along with a probiotic (but not at the same time of day). Patients who fail to respond, and those who have recurrent prostatitis, should be referred to a urologist for further evaluation. Other measures that are helpful for bacterial and nonbacterial prostatitis include:

THERAPEUTIC REVIEW continued

- *Nutrition. Eat fresh fruits and vegetables; add soy to the diet; drink plenty of water; and avoid urinary irritants such as caffeinated beverages, junk food, tobacco products, alcohol, and spicy food.*
- *Mind-body. Encourage stress reduction techniques and consider meditation, counseling, and biofeedback.*
- *Supplements. Take a high-potency multivitamin daily plus additional zinc gluconate or picolinate 90 mg daily, plus quercetin 400 mg with 500 mg of bromelain tid before meals.*
- *Botanicals. Depending on the symptoms, a six-week trial of one or more of the herbs listed previously should be tried. If there is no improvement, consider trying a different herbal combination.*
- *Pharmaceuticals. Try a 2- to 4-week course of a COX-2 inhibitor to alleviate painful prostatitis symptoms. If muscle spasms are suspected, try a 4- to 6-week trial of an alpha-adrenergic blocker; if there is improvement, continue the medication; otherwise, stop.*
- *Biomechanical techniques. Recommend daily sitz baths prn and consider physical therapy and regular prostatic massage.*
- *Prostatitis symptom index. Monitor therapeutic response by asking patients to fill out a prostate symptom index before initiating therapy and monthly thereafter as long as symptoms persist (see Figure 50–1).[28]*

Pain or Discomfort

1. In the last week, have you experienced any pain or discomfort in the following areas:

	Yes	No
a. Areas between rectum and testicles (perineum)	○ 1	○ 0
b. Testicles	○ 1	○ 0
c. Tip of the penis (not related to urination)	○ 1	○ 0
d. Below your waist (in your pubic or bladder area)	○ 1	○ 0

2. In the last week, have you experienced:

	Yes	No
a. Pain or burning during urination	○ 1	○ 0
b. Pain or discomfort during or after ejaculation	○ 1	○ 0

3. How often have you had pain or discomfort in any of these areas over the last week?
- ○ 0 Never
- ○ 1 Rarely
- ○ 2 Sometimes
- ○ 3 Often
- ○ 4 Usually
- ○ 5 Always

4. Which number best describes your AVERAGE pain or discomfort on the days that you have had it over the past week?

○ 0 (No pain)　○ 1　○ 2　○ 3　○ 4　○ 5

○ 6　○ 7　○ 8　○ 9　○ 10 (Extreme pain)

Urination

5. How often have you had a sensation of not emptying your bladder completely after you finished urinating, over the last week?
- ○ 0 Not at all
- ○ 1 Less than 1 time in 5
- ○ 2 Less than half the time
- ○ 3 About half the time
- ○ 4 More than half the time
- ○ 5 Almost always

6. How often have you had to urinate less than two hours after you finished urinating, over the last week?
- ○ 0 Not at all
- ○ 1 Less than 1 time in 5
- ○ 2 Less than half the time
- ○ 3 About half the time
- ○ 4 More than half the time
- ○ 5 Almost always

Impact of symptoms

7. How much have your symptoms kept you from doing the kinds of things you would usually do, over the last week?
- ○ 0 None
- ○ 1 Only a little
- ○ 2 Some
- ○ 3 A lot

8. How much did you think about your symptoms, over the last week?
- ○ 0 None
- ○ 1 Only a little
- ○ 2 Some
- ○ 3 A lot

Quality of life

9. If you were to spend the rest of your life with your symptoms just the way they have been over the last week, how would you feel about it?
- ○ 0 Delighted
- ○ 1 Pleased
- ○ 2 Mostly satisfied
- ○ 3 Mixed (about equally satisfied and dissatisfied)
- ○ 4 Mostly dissatisfied
- ○ 5 Unhappy
- ○ 6 Terrible

Scoring the NIH-Chronic Prostatitis Symptom Index Domains

Pain: Total of items 1a, 1b, 1c, 1d, 2a, 2b, 3 and 4 _____

Urinary symptoms: Total of items 5 and 6 _____

Quality of Life Impact: Total of items 7, 8 and 9 _____

Figure 50–1. Prostatis symptom index.

References

1. Litwin MS: National Institutes of Health chronic prostatitis symptom index: Development and validation of a new outcome measure. J Urol 162:369–375, 1999.
2. Fair WR, Couch J, Wehner N: Prostatic antibacterial factor: Identity and significance. Urology 7(2):169–177, 1976.
3. Roberts RO, Lieber MM, Bostwick DG, et al: A review of clinical and pathological prostatitis syndromes. Urology 49(6):815, 1997.
4. Fair WR, Couch J, Wehner N: Prostatic antibacterial factor. Urology 7(2):169–177, 1976.
5. Marmar JL, et al: Semen zinc levels in infertile and postvasectomy patients and patients with prostatitis. Fertil Steril 26(11):1057–1063, 1975.
6. Shoskes DA, et al: Quercetin in men with category III chronic prostatitis: A preliminary prospective, double-blind, placebo-controlled trial. Urology 54(6):960–963, 1999.
7. Buck AC: Phytotherapy for the prostate. Br J Urol 78:325–336, 1996.
8. Rugendorff EW, et al: Results of treatment with pollen extract (Cernilton N) in chronic prostatitis and prostodynia. Br J Urol 71:433–438, 1993.
9. Kirby RS, et al: Intra-prostatic urinary reflux: An aetiological factor in abacterial prostatitis. Br J Urol 54:729–731, 1982.
10. Avorn J, et al: Reduction of bacteriuria and pyuria after ingestion of cranberry juice. JAMA 271(10):751–754, 1994.
11. Roberts RO, Lieber MM, Bostwick DG, et al: A review of clinical and pathological prostatitis syndromes. Urology 49(6):809, 1997.
12. Mills SY: The Essential Book of Herbal Medicine. New York, Arkana Penguin Books, 1993.
13. Fleming T (ed): PDR for Herbal Medicines. Montvale, NJ, Medical Economics Company, Inc, 1998.
14. Jellin JM, Batz F, Hitchens K: Pharmacist's Letter/Prescriber's Letter Natural Medicines Comprehensive Database. Stockton, Calif, Therapeutic Research Faculty, 1999.
15. Jellin JM: Pharmacist's Letter/Prescriber's Letter Natural Medicines Comprehensive Database, Stockton, Calif, Therapeutic Research Faculty, 1999, p 925.
16. Fleming PDR for Herbal Medicines, Montvale, NJ, Medical Economics Company, Inc, 1998, pp 1043–1044.
17. Fleming PDR for Herbal Medicines, Montvale, NJ, Medical Economics Company, Inc, 1998, pp 1020–1022.
18. Winston D: Herbal Therapeutics: Specific Indications for Herbs & Herbal Formulas, 5th ed. Broadway, NJ, Herbalist Therapeutics Research Library, 1996, p. 38.
19. Jellin JM: Pharmacist's Letter/Prescriber's Letter Natural Medicines Comprehensive Database, Stockton, Calif, Therapeutic Research Faculty, 1999, p 727.
20. Jellin JM, Batz F, Hitchens K: Pharmacist's Letter/Prescriber's Letter Natural Medicines Comprehensive Database. Stockton Calif, Therapeutic Research Faculty, 1999.
21. Talsma J: NIH-backed event formalizes approach to syndrome. Urology Times 28(4):32, 2000.
22. Talsma J: NIH-backed event formalizes approach to syndrome, Urology Times 28(4):32–33, 2000.
23. Nickel JC, Sorensen R: Transurethral microwave therapy for nonbacterial prostatitis: A randomized double-blind sham controlled study using new prostatitis specific assessment questionnaires. J Urol 155:1950–1955, 1996.
24. Wenninger K, et al: Sickness impact of chronic nonbacterial prostatitis and its correlates. J Urol 155:965–968, 1996.
25. Bakke A, Malt UF: Psychological predictors of symptoms of urinary tract infection and bacteriuria in patients treated with clean intermittent catheterization: A prospective 7-year study. Eur Urol 34:30–36, 1998.
26. Lowentritt JE, et al: Bacterial infection in prostatodynia. J Urol 154:1381, 1995.
27. Cummings S, Ullman D: Everybody's Guide To Homeopathic Medicines. New York, The Putnam Publishing Group, 1991, p 164.
28. Litwin MW, et al: The National Institutes of Health chronic prostatitis symptom index: Development and validation of a new outcome measure. J Urol 162:374, 1999.

CHAPTER 51

Osteoarthritis

Adam I. Perlman, M.D., M.P.H., and Marnee M. Spierer, M.D.

PATHOPHYSIOLOGY

Osteoarthritis (OA) is the most common form of arthritis and the second most common cause of long-term disability among adults in the United States.[1] OA is a disease of multiple etiologies and should not be considered a consequence of wear and tear, but rather a breakdown in normal physiologic pathways. OA is broadly broken down into two categories: primary OA, in which no specific risk factors, except for age, can be identified; and secondary OA, in which changes can be related to systemic and/or local factors (Fig. 51–1).

Normal Joints

Major constituents of cartilage are water, proteoglycans (which are composed of protein cores plus chondroitin sulfate and keratin sulfate side chains), and collagen, predominantly type II. Collectively, they form the extracellular matrix. Chondrocytes are metabolically active cells that are responsible for synthesis of the extracellular matrix.

Proteoglycans provide elasticity of cartilage, and collagen provides tensile strength.

Muscles and ligaments provide support and protection, and nerve endings provide proprioceptive information.

Cartilage health and function depend on compression (pumping fluid from the cartilage into the joint space and into capillaries and venules) and release (allowing cartilage to re-expand, hyperhydrate, and absorb nutrients).

Early Changes of Osteoarthritis

Increased hydration of the extracellular matrix is due to a failure of the elastic restraint of collagen.

There is increased synthesis of proteoglycans but with increased chondroitin sulfate and decreased keratin sulfate.

Progression leads to a net decrease in proteoglycans and an increase in the permeability of water.

Loss of elasticity and increased permeability of water lead to increased chondrocyte stress and increased exposure to degradative enzymes.

Late Changes of Osteoarthritis

Subchondral osteoblasts increase bone formation leading to stiffer and less compliant bones. This

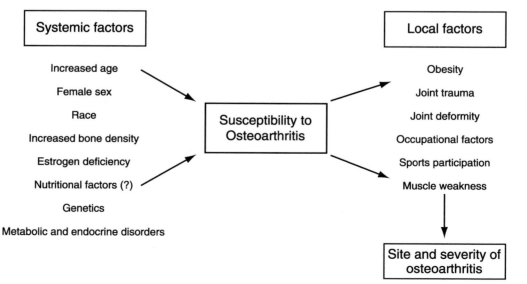

Figure 51–1. Systemic and local factors that increase susceptibility to arthritis. (Modified from Dieppe P: The classification and diagnosis of arthritis. In Kuettner K, Goldberg V (eds): Osteoarthritic Disorders. Rosemont, Ill., American Academy of Orthopaedic Surgeons, 1995, p 7.)

leads to microfractures, followed by callus formation, more stiffness, and more microfractures.

Osteophytes (outgrowths of bone) are formed and are the hallmark of OA. They ultimately cause restricted motion.

Subchondral cysts are formed in an attempt to equalize pressure.

Gross pathology includes roughening, pitting, and irregularities of the hyaline cartilage surface, proceeding to gross ulceration with focal and then diffuse areas of complete loss of cartilage.

Soft tissues around the joint are also affected. These include synovium (inflammatory infiltrates), ligaments (increased laxity), and muscles (weakened).

INTEGRATIVE THERAPY

Exercise

Three types of exercise should be incorporated into a program for OA sufferers: aerobic training, resistance training/muscle strengthening, and flexibility/range of motion.

Aerobic Exercise

The Fitness and Arthritis in Seniors Trial (FAST) looked at aerobic and resistance exercise and their effectiveness on outcomes of pain and disability and progression of disease specifically in patients with knee OA. Positive effects were found for both types of exercise.[2] In addition, aerobic training can reduce risk factors associated with disease states such as heart disease and diabetes, thereby improving overall health status. Recommended exercises include walking, biking, swimming, aerobic dance, and aerobic pool exercises.

NOTE

Two precautions should be considered before implementation of an exercise program in patients with osteroarthritis (OA): (1) exercise of an acutely inflamed or swollen joint should be deferred until the acute process subsides and (2) an exercise stress test should be performed to identify cardiac disease.[3]

Resistance Training/Muscle Strengthening

Because muscles are important shock absorbers and help stabilize the joint, periarticular muscle weakness may result in progression of structural damage to the joint in OA. In addition, insufficient loading of a joint will lead to atrophy of both articular cartilage and subchondral bone.[4] In general, strength training helps offset the loss in muscle mass and strength typically associated with normal aging.

Flexibility/Range of Motion

Flexibility is a general term that encompasses the range of motion of single or multiple joints and the ability to perform certain tasks. The range of motion of a given joint depends primarily on bone, muscle, and connective tissue structure and function. OA affects the structure of these tissues, such that range of motion and flexibility are reduced. The basis for exercise interventions to improve flexibility is that the muscle and connective tissue properties can be improved, thereby improving function.[5]

Reduction of Joint Loading

Patients with OA of the knee or hip should avoid prolonged periods of standing, kneeling, or squatting. In patients with unilateral OA of the hip or knee, a cane, when held in the contralateral hand, may reduce joint pain by reducing joint contact force. Bilateral disease may necessitate the use of crutches or a walker.[6] Although there is a paucity of literature regarding bracing and footwear, the trials that have been undertaken indicate good symptom relief using wedged insoles for patients with medial compartment knee OA.[7]

Weight Loss

Obese patients should be helped to lose weight. Studies have shown that increased weight increases the risk of developing OA.[8] Equally important, in patients who already have OA and who are symptomatic, weight loss may decrease pain and slow progression of disease.[9]

Thermal Modalities

Heat

Superficial heat penetrates the skin only a few millimeters and does not penetrate deeper joints such as the hip or knee. In contrast, a heat mitten may increase the temperature of the small joints of the hand. Application of heat can raise the pain threshold and produce muscle relaxation. Moist heat produces greater elevation of the subcutaneous temperature than does dry heat and is often preferable for relief of pain. Risk of thermal injury is increased with poor circulation or impaired sensation.[6]

Cold

Cold application is often recommended after strenuous exercise to relieve muscle aching. It may be delivered by ice packs, ice massage, or local spray. Superficial cooling can decrease muscle spasm and increase pain threshold. Cold applications should not be used in patients with Raynaud's phenomenon, cold hypersensitivity, cryoglobulinemia, or paroxysmal cold hemoglobinuria.[6]

MIND-BODY

Behavioral Interventions

Telephone Interventions

Telephone-based strategies can be an integral part of the management of chronic disease. A randomized controlled trial evaluated whether telephone-based or office-based interventions or both improved functional status of patients with OA.[10] Subjects in the intervention groups were contacted monthly by telephone and/or scheduled clinic visits by trained non-healthcare professionals. At each contact, the following items were discussed: (1) joint pain, (2) medications, (3) gastrointestinal and other medication-related symptoms, (4) date of the next scheduled outpatient visit, (5) an established mechanism by which patients could telephone a physician during weekends and evenings, and (6) barriers to keeping appointments. At 1 year, compared with the control group, persons receiving telephone calls reported less physical disability and pain and tended toward an improved psychological status.[11] The Internet may be utilized in the future to improve patient outcomes.

Group Programs

Patient education is extremely important with any disease. The Arthritis Self-Management Program (ASMP) is a community-taught, peer-led intervention in which patients gain the confidence and the necessary tools to manage their disease. A study was conducted to evaluate the effects of ASMP in patients 4 years after their participation in the program. It was found that participants in this program greatly reduced their pain, had fewer visits to their physicians, and had fewer days spent in the hospital.[12]

Acupuncture

Acupuncture is a component of traditional Chinese medicine that dates back at least 2500 years. The general theory of acupuncture is based on the premise that there are patterns of energy flow (qi) through the body that are essential for health. Disruptions of this flow are believed to be responsible for disease.

Acupuncture may correct imbalances of flow at identifiable points close to the skin. Acupuncture analgesia is believed to work through the release of opioid peptides.[13]

Numerous randomized controlled trials have been undertaken to assess the efficacy of acupuncture for treatment of pain associated with OA. In a 1975 study,[14] 40 patients were randomized to either acupuncture at standard points or acupuncture at placebo or sham points. Analysis before and after treatment showed a statistically significant improvement in tenderness and subjective report of pain in both groups.[14] In a 1982 study,[15] 32 patients with OA of the hip, knee, or humeroscapular joint were randomized either to receive weekly acupuncture or to take piroxicam (Feldene) with checkup visits at 2, 4, 6, 12, and 16 weeks. The degree of improvement in both groups at 2 weeks was equal (30%); after that, however, the acupuncture group showed greater pain relief than the piroxicam group.[15] A more recently completed pilot study[16] and a follow-up, larger, single-blind, randomized trial[17] looked at the effect of acupuncture on OA of the knee in an elderly population. The 12 patients in the pilot study showed significant improvement in pain scores and self-reported function and in performance measures of function after 8 weeks of acupuncture treatment.[16] The larger follow-up trial had 58 patients enrolled and looked at the benefit of acupuncture added to a standard non-steroidal anti-inflammatory drug (NSAID) regimen. The acupuncture-treated group had significant improvement in self-reported pain and disability scores compared with the control group.[17] A systemic review of 11 randomized controlled trials of acupuncture for OA concluded that the most rigorously conducted studies suggest acupuncture is not superior to sham needling in reducing pain from OA.[18]

Acupuncture may serve as a good adjunct to a conventional medical regimen by allowing a reduction in NSAID dosage, therefore potentially decreasing the side effects occasionally seen with long-term NSAID use.[19] Each state has its own requirements for acupuncture licensure and certification. Patients should be referred only to a licensed or a certified practitioner.

NOTE

Acupuncture often requires six or more treatments before efficacy can be truly assessed. Although it is generally safe, acupuncture may cause transient dizziness, temporary exacerbation of pain, and occasional bruising or swelling.[20]

Massage

No studies have looked at the effect of massage therapy with respect to OA specifically, but studies have been conducted on massage for the treatment of pain. A recent review looked at four randomized controlled trials to determine whether or not the use of massage in the treatment of low back pain was efficacious.[21] Each of the trials had methodological flaws, and three of the four were not designed to look at the efficacy of massage, but rather massage was the treatment used in the control group. One trial found that massage was superior to no treatment[22]; two found massage equally as effective as spinal manipulation[23, 24]; and one found massage to be less effective than spinal manipulation.[25] When massage is suggested for patients with OA, light massage, rather than deep tissue massage, is often recommended.

SUPPLEMENTS

Glucosamine Sulfate/Chondroitin Sulfate

Given degradation of cartilage in the pathogenesis of OA, cartilage-protective agents are desirable. Both glucosamine and chondroitin are important components of cartilage. Unlike traditional therapies, such as NSAIDs, that are used as symptom modifiers, these supplements are potentially structure modifying. Glucosamine's primary role is as a substrate for glycosaminoglycans and the hyaluronic acid backbone used in the formation of proteoglycans found in the structural matrix of joints.[26] Chondroitins are the main glycosaminoglycans in human joints and connective tissue, and they play a role in cartilage formation through the stimulation of chondrocyte metabolism and synthesis of collagen and proteoglycan.[27] Destructive synovial enzymes are inhibited by chondroitin.[28] Glucosamine sulfate (GS) and chondroitin sulfate (CS) are sulfate derivatives of glucosamine and chondroitin, and doubts regarding their absorption and metabolic fate have fueled skepticism about their therapeutic potential.[29] This dilemma has stimulated numerous studies.

In a recent double-blind, randomized, controlled trial,[30] 212 patients with knee OA were randomly assigned to 1500 mg of GS or placebo once daily for 3 years. Seventy-one of 106 patients on placebo completed the trial, and they showed progressive joint space narrowing on radiographs. Sixty-eight of 106 patients on GS completed the trial, and they did not show radiographic evidence of joint space narrowing. This study concluded that oral administration of GS over the long term could prevent joint structure changes in patients with OA of the knee, as well as improve symptoms.[30]

To evaluate the benefit of GS and CS for OA, a recent meta-analysis combined with systemic quality assessment was performed.[31] Fifteen double-blind, randomized, placebo-controlled trials were included in the analysis. The knee was the joint studied in all the trials, and in one study the hip was also included.

GS and/or CS was taken orally in 12 of the studies, intramuscularly in 2 of the studies, and intra-arterially in 1 of the studies. It was found that GS and/or CS demonstrated a moderate to large effect on OA symptoms. However, methodological problems may have led to exaggerated estimates of benefit. Overall, it seems that these compounds do have efficacy in treating OA symptoms, and they are safe.[31]

GS and CS are sold as dietary supplements in most health food stores as well as in many pharmacies. They are often sold in combination; however, it is unclear whether the combination is superior to either treatment alone.[20] In December 1999 and January 2000, Consumerlab.com purchased 25 brands of glucosamine, chondroitin, and combination products to test whether the products contained the amounts listed on their respective labels. Nearly one third of the products did not contain the stated amounts of the supplements.[32]

Dosage. GS 500 mg three times daily; CS 400 mg three times daily; both for a minimum of 6 weeks.

Precautions. Symptoms occurring occasionally include dyspepsia, nausea, and headache.

S-Adenosyl-L-Methionine

S-Adenyl-L-methionine (SAMe) is a physiologic molecule formed in the body from the essential amino acid methionine. It functions in a wide variety of anabolic and catabolic reactions in all living cells. Although its mechanism of action on the symptoms of OA is not fully understood, this may be related to its ability to stimulate proteoglycan synthesis in OA cartilage.[33] The U.S. Food and Drug Administration approved it for sale as a dietary supplement in 1999; however, it has been used since the mid-1970s primarily in Europe to treat depression and arthritis.[34]

A double-blind, randomized, controlled trial in 1987[35] compared 1200 mg of SAMe with 1200 mg of ibuprofen taken by 36 patients with OA of the knee, hip, or spine, or a combination, for 4 weeks. Morning stiffness, pain at rest and during motion, crepitus, swelling, and limitation of motion in the affected joints were assessed before and after treatment. The study found that both treatments were well tolerated and equally effective in lessening symptoms. It was thus concluded that SAMe exerted a beneficial effect on the symptomatology of OA.[35] Similar results were found in a trial comparing 1200 mg of SAMe and 150 mg of indomethacin; SAMe was better tolerated.[36] In a large, long-term, open trial,[34] 108 patients with OA of the knee, hip, and spine were started on 600 mg a day of SAMe for 2 weeks, followed by 400 mg daily for 2 years. Morning stiffness and pain parameters were noted to have improved after the first week of treatment, and this continued to the end of the 2-year period.[34] The Arthritis Foundation's Guide to Alternative Therapies notes that SAMe is a promising treatment worth trying for pain relief, but that more scientific evidence is needed to prove it supports cartilage repair.[37]

NOTE

To encourage SAMe production in the body, OA patients with low folic acid should consider increasing their folic acid levels through increased consumption of dark, leafy, green vegetables or supplementation.[20]

Dosage. 400 to 1600 mg daily.
Precautions. Watch for nausea and gastrointestinal distress.

Methyl Sulfonyl Methane

Methyl sulfonyl methane (MSM) is a dietary supplement commonly sold for the treatment of OA. The MSM metabolite dimethyl sulfoxide is found naturally in the human body. Because sulfur is necessary for the formation of connective tissue, MSM is thought to be useful in the treatment of OA. Animal studies have suggested that MSM may help decrease inflammatory joint disease,[38] but unfortunately, there are no published human trials. Although MSM is promoted as being nontoxic, clinical data are lacking and further scientific study is needed to define the efficacy and safety of this supplement.
Dosage. 1000 to 3000 mg three times daily.
Precautions. Watch for nausea, diarrhea, and headache.

PHARMACEUTICALS

Nonopioid Analgesics

Acetaminophen

Acetaminophen (Tylenol) acts by inhibiting prostaglandin synthesis in the central nervous system. It may relieve mild to moderate joint pain and may be used as initial therapy based on its overall cost, efficacy, and toxicity profile.[39]
Dosage. 325 to 1000 mg every 4 to 6 hours; maximum, 4 g/day.
Precautions. Reactions are infrequent with normal therapeutic doses but include nausea, rash and minor allergic reactions, transient drop in white blood cell count, liver toxicity, and prolongation of the half-life of warfarin.

Tramadol

Tramadol (Ultram) is a synthetic opioid agonist that inhibits reuptake of norepinephrine and serotonin. It should be considered for patients with moderate to severe pain in whom acetaminophen therapy has failed and who have contraindications to NSAIDs (see later).[35]
Dosage. 50 to 100 mg every 4 to 6 hours; maximum, 400 mg/day.
Precautions. Watch for nausea, constipation, drowsiness, and rarely, seizures.

Nonsteroidal Anti-Inflammatory Drugs

Nonselective NSAIDs are a group of chemically dissimilar agents that act primarily by inhibiting the cyclooxygenase (COX) enzymes, thus inhibiting the production of prostaglandins in peripheral tissues. Examples include aspirin, ibuprofen, naproxen, indomethacin, sulindac, and piroxicam. COX-2–specific inhibitors act in the same manner, but their action is confined to inflamed tissues. Examples include celecoxib (Celebrex) and rofecoxib (Vioxx). The choice between nonselective NSAIDs and COX-2–specific NSAIDs should be based on risk factors. Specifically, the risk of upper gastrointestinal bleeding should be considered. Data from epidemiologic studies demonstrate that among persons aged 65 years and older, 20% to 30% of all hospitalizations and deaths owing to peptic ulcer disease were attributable to NSAID use.[40] Risk factors include age 65 years or older, history of peptic ulcer disease, previous upper gastrointestinal bleeding, concomitant use of oral corticosteroids or anticoagulants, and possibly, smoking and alcohol consumption.[41] Patients who fall into this category may benefit from a COX-2–specific inhibitor or a nonselective NSAID with gastroprotective therapy (e.g., misoprostol, omeprazole, high-dose famotidine).

Dosage
Nonselective COX Inhibitors
Aspirin 3.6 to 5.4 g in divided doses daily.
Ibuprofen 300 to 800 mg three to four times daily; maximum, 3200 mg/day.
Naproxen 250 to 500 mg twice daily; maximum, 1500 mg/day.
Indomethacin 25 mg two to three times daily; maximum, 200 mg/day.
Sulindac 150 to 200 mg twice daily; maximum, 400 mg/day.
Piroxicam 20 mg daily or 10 mg twice daily.

COX-2 Inhibitors
Celecoxib (Celebrex) 200 mg daily or 100 mg twice daily.
Rofecoxib (Vioxx) 12.5 to 25 mg daily.
Precautions
Precautions vary with specific agent and include epigastric distress, nausea, vomiting, gastrointestinal bleeding (nonselective NSAIDs > COX-2–specific inhibitors), prolonged bleeding (aspirin), headache, dizziness, and renal toxicity.

Opioid Analgesics

Patients who have tried acetaminophen, tramadol, and NSAIDs without success may consider opiates. Opiates bind to receptors in the central nervous system to produce effects that mimic the action of endogenous peptide neurotransmitters—specifically, the relief of intense pain. They should usually be avoided for long-term use, but short-term use help in the treatment of acute exacerbations of pain.[42] Commonly used opiates include fentanyl, meperidine (Demerol), propoxyphene (Darvon), acetaminophen + propoxyphene (Darvocet), hydromorphone (Dilaudid), long-acting morphine (MS Contin), oxycodone + acetaminophen (Percocet), and acetaminophen + hydrocodone (Vicodin).

Dosage. Doses and routes vary.

Precautions. In addition to the potential for addiction of these agents, side effects include constipation, nausea, vomiting, sedation, urinary retention, and respiratory depression.

Topical Analgesics

In patients who suffer from OA of the hands or knees, topical analgesics may relieve mild to moderate pain.[43] The cream may be used alone or in combination with an oral agent. Capsaicin cream (Zostrix) is a commonly used topical agent. It exerts its pharmacologic effect by depleting local sensory nerve endings of substance P, a neuropeptide mediator of pain.

Dosage. A thin film of cream (0.025%, 0.075%) should be applied to the symptomatic joint four times a day.

Precautions. A local burning sensation is common but rarely leads to the discontinuation of therapy.

Intra-articular Steroid Injections

Injections are useful in treating a joint effusion or local inflammation that is limited to a few joints. Injections should be limited to three to four per year because of concern about the possible development of progressive cartilage damage through repeated injections in weight-bearing joints.[44]

SURGERY

Surgical treatment is usually considered only after failure of nonsurgical treatments. Two categories of surgery exist: nonbiologic and biologic.[45]

Nonbiologic Approaches

- Osteotomy: a conservative approach; may provide effective pain relief and slow disease progression; greatest benefit in those patients with only moderately advanced disease.
- Arthroscopy: removal of loose cartilage fragments can prevent locking and relieve pain; when there is substantial joint space narrowing, this type of surgery is of limited benefit.
- Arthrodesis: joint fusion; alleviates pain and is most commonly performed in the spine and in small joints of the hand and foot; in hip and knee, reserved for the very young patient with unilateral disease.
- Arthroplasty: total joint replacement; mainstay of surgical treatment of the hip, knee, and shoulder; most effective of all medical interventions; can restore patients to near-normal function; limited in durability in persons with life expectancies exceeding 20 years and those who wish to participate in high-demand activities.

Biologic Approaches

- Biologic restoration of articular cartilage using resident hyaline cartilage that is stimulated to repair its own defects.
- Biologic restoration of articular cartilage using one of three types of cartilage transplantation: osteochondral autografting, osteochondral allografting, and tissue engineering.

OTHER THERAPIES TO CONSIDER

Boswellia serrata

Boswellia serrata, also known as H15 or indish incense, Boswellia is a botanical used in traditional ayurvedic medicine, and in vitro, it decreases leukotriene synthesis.[46] A double-blind pilot study evaluated the efficacy of H15 on 37 patients with rheumatoid arthritis. Treatment with H15 showed no measurable efficacy.[46] A double-blind, randomized, controlled trial found that Boswellia improved symptoms of knee OA. The treatment included a combination of herbs rather than Boswellia alone.[47] A single-blind, randomized, controlled trial in which Boswellia was taken along with Withania, Curcuma, and a zinc complex found improvement in pain and disability in OA.[48]

Although the literature is promising, it is insufficient to support the use of *B. serrata* for OA. Taken in combination with other herbs, it may improve pain and function.

Yoga

One small, randomized, controlled trial demonstrated that weekly yoga done for 8 weeks, in addition to patient education, group discussion, and support, improved pain and tenderness in patients with hand OA.[49] Several types of yoga practices exist; it is important to begin with gentle, easy exercises.

Magnet Therapy

A popular therapy for the treatment of a variety of medical conditions is the application of a magnetic field. The biologic effects of low-level magnetic fields have been studied since the 1500s. Explanations of these effects include increased circulation and decreased inflammation.[50] Although no studies to date have looked at the effects of magnetic therapy and OA specifically, studies have looked at magnetic therapy and pain. A recent double-blind, randomized, controlled study[51] looked at bipolar magnets for the treatment of chronic low back pain. It was concluded that the application of magnets had no effect on patients' pain.[51] A 1997 study[52] compared active versus placebo magnets in a single 45-minute application to treat muscle pain in patients with postpolio syndrome. A statistically significant improvement was reported with active magnets.[52] Although magnet therapy does appear to be harmless, its therapeutic use remains questionable.

NOTE

Magnet therapy should be avoided in patients who have implanted cardiac devices (i.e., pacemakers, defibrillators).

 ── **THERAPEUTIC REVIEW** ─────────────────────

Following is a summary of therapeutic options for OA. As with other chronic diseases, it is not necessary that one therapy be used to the exclusion of others. Often, it is the combination of therapies that gives patients the most symptom relief.

Exercise	All patients should be encouraged to exercise. Flexibility, strength, and endurance are all essential components of exercise. Not only does exercise contribute to an overall healthy lifestyle, but it also helps to decrease disability and pain in patients with OA.
Joint Load Reduction	Avoid standing, kneeling, or squatting if hips and/or knees are involved. Consider using a cane, walker, or wedged insoles.
Weight Loss	Overweight patients should be encouraged to lose weight. Obesity may increase risk of developing OA, and weight loss may decrease pain and slow the progression of the disease in patients already suffering from OA.
Thermal Modalities	Heat and/or cold when applied to symptomatic joints may provide relief.
Behavioral Interventions	Both telephone-based strategies and group programs have shown positive effects on improving symptoms. These are two good options for patients who need/like more than regularly scheduled office visits to discuss their conditions.
Acupuncture	Some patients may find relief with acupuncture. It is imperative that patients be referred only to a licensed or a certified practitioner. Whereas it is generally safe, acupuncture may occasionally cause transient dizziness, pain, bruising, or swelling.
Massage	Gentle massage may improve pain, and it is often offered in conjunction with other treatments.
Supplements	Glucosamine 500 mg three times daily, chondroitin 400 mg three times daily (alone or in combination), SAMe 400 to 1600 mg once daily, and possibly, MSM 1000 to 3000 mg three times daily. As these supplements are considered structure modifying and traditional pharmaceuticals are considered symptom modifying, supplements may be taken in conjunction with traditional pharmaceuticals as well as by themselves by patients who do not require symptomatic therapy. Consumerlab.com has information regarding quality brands.

Pharmaceuticals	Begin with nonopioid analgesics such as acetaminophen or tramadol. Unless contraindicated, NSAIDs may be helpful in management of pain not treated by the nonopioids. For severe pain, opiates may be indicated for short-term use. They have potential for addiction and should be used judiciously. Topical analgesics and steroid injections have limited use but may prove helpful.
Surgery	Several options exist for patients who have failed nonsurgical treatments. Referral to an orthopedic surgeon may be warranted.

References

1. Keuttner KE, Goldberg V (eds): Osteoarthritic Disorders. Rosemont, Ill, American Academy of Orthopedic Surgeons, 1995, pp xxi–xxv.
2. Ettinger WH Jr, Burns R, Messier SP, et al: A randomized trial comparing aerobic exercise and resistance exercise to a health education program on physical disability in older people with knee osteoarthritis: The Fitness and Arthritis in Seniors Trial (FAST). JAMA 227:1:25–31, 1997.
3. Semble EL, Loeser RF, Wise CM: Therapeutic exercise for rheumatoid arthritis and osteoarthritis. Semin Arthritis Rheum 20:32–40, 1990.
4. Palmoski MJ, Colyer RA, Brandt KD: Joint motion in the absence of normal loading does not maintain normal articular cartilage. Arthritis Rheum 23:325–334, 1980.
5. American College of Sports Medicine Position Stand. Exercise and physical activity for older adults. Med Sci Sports Exerc 30:992–1008, 1998.
6. Brandt KD: The importance of nonpharmacologic approaches in management of osteoarthritis. Am J Med 105(1B):39S–44S, 1998.
7. Keating EM, Faris PM, Ritter MA, Kane J: Use of lateral heel and sole wedges in the treatment of medial osteoarthritis of the knee. Orthop Rev 22:921–924, 1993.
8. Felson DT, Zhang Y, Anthony JM, et al: Weight loss reduces the risk for symptomatic knee osteoarthritis in women. Ann Intern Med 116:535–539, 1992.
9. McGoey BV, Deitel M, Saplys RJ, Kliman ME: Effect of weight loss on musculoskeletal pain the morbidly obese. J Bone Joint Surg 72B:322–323, 1990.
10. Weinberger M: Telephone-based interventions in ambulatory care. Ann Rheum Dis 57:196–197, 1998.
11. Rene J, Weinberger M, Mazzuca SA, et al: Reduction of joint pain in patients with knee osteoarthritis who have received monthly telephone calls from lay personnel and whose medical treatment regimens have remained stable. Arthritis Rheum 35:511–515, 1992.
12. Lorig KR, Mazonson PD, Holman HR: Evidence suggesting that health education for self-management in patients with chronic arthritis has sustained health benefits while reducing health care costs. Arthritis Rheum 36:439–446, 1993.
13. Acupuncture. Natl Inst Health Consens Dev Conf Statement 15(5):1–34, 1997.
14. Gaw AC, Chang LW, Shaw LC: Efficacy of acupuncture on osteoarthritic pain: A controlled, double-blind study. N Engl J Med 293:375–378, 1975.
15. Junnila SYT: Acupuncture is superior to piroxicam for the treatment of osteoarthritis. Am J Acupunct 10:341–345, 1982.
16. Berman BM, Lao LX, Greene M, et al: Efficacy of traditional Chinese acupuncture for the treatment of symptomatic knee osteoarthritis: A pilot study. Osteoarthritis Cartilage 3:139, 1995.
17. Berman BM, Singh BB, Lao L, et al: A randomized trial of acupuncture as an adjunctive therapy in osteoarthritis of the knee. Rheumatology 38:346–354, 1999.
18. Ernst E: Acupuncture as a symptomatic treatment of osteoarthritis: A systemic review. Scand J Rheumatol 26:444–447, 1997.
19. Berman BM, Swyers JP, Ezzo J: The evidence for acupuncture as a treatment for rheumatologic conditions. Rheum Dis Clin North Am 26:103–115, 2000.
20. Perlman AI, Oza R: Evaluating alternative therapies for osteoarthritis. Women's Health Primary Care 3:365–371, 2000.
21. Ernst E: Massage therapy for low back pain: A systematic review. J Pain Symptom Manage 17:65–69, 1999.
22. Konrad K, Tatrai T, Hunka E, et al: Controlled trial of balneotherapy in treatment of low back pain. Ann Rheum Dis 51:820–822, 1992.
23. Godrey CM, Morgan PP, Schatzker J: A randomized trial of manipulation for low back pain in a medical setting. Spine 9:301–304, 1984.
24. Hoehler FK, Tobis JS, Buerger AA: Spinal manipulation for low back pain. JAMA 245:1835–1838, 1981.
25. Hseih C-YJ, Phillips RB, Adams AH, Pope MH: Functional outcomes of low back pain: Comparison of four treatment groups in a randomized controlled trial. J Manipulative Physiol Ther 15:4–9, 1992.
26. Kelly GS: The role of glucosamine sulfate and chondroitin sulfates in the treatment of degenerative joint disease. Altern Med Rev 3:27–39, 1998.
27. Fetrow CW, Avila JR: Professional's Handbook to Complementary and Alternative Medicine. Springhouse, Pa, Springhouse, 1999.
28. LaValle JB, et al: Natural Therapeutics Pocket Guide. Hudson, Ohio, Lexi-Comp, 2000.
29. Constantz RB: Hyaluronan, glucosamine and chondroitin sulfate: Roles for therapy in arthritis? In Kelley WN, Harris ED, Ruddy S, Sledge CB (eds): Textbook of Rheumatology. Philadelphia, WB Saunders, 1998.
30. Reginster JY, Deroisy R, Rovati LC, et al: Long-term effects of glucosamine sulfate on osteoarthritis progression: A randomized, placebo-controlled clinical trial. Lancet 357:251–256, 2001.
31. McAlindon TE, LaValley MP, Gulin JP, Felson DT: Glucosamine and chondroitin for treatment of osteoarthritis: A systemic quality assessment and meta-analysis. JAMA 283:1469–1475, 2000.
32. Klepser T, Nisly N: Chondroitin for the treatment of osteoarthritic pain. Am Health Consultant 38:85–96, 2000.
33. Schumacher HR Jr: Osteoarthritis: The clinical picture, pathogenesis, and management with studies on a new therapeutic agent, S-adenosylmethionine. Am J Med 83(Suppl 5A):S1–S3, 1987.
34. Konig B: A long-term (two years) clinical trial with S-adenosylmethionine for the treatment of osteoarthritis. Am J Med 83(Suppl 5A):89–94, 1987.
35. Muller-Fassbender H: Double-blind clinical trial of S-adenosylmethionine versus ibuprofen in the treatment of osteoarthritis. Am J Med 83(Suppl 5A):S81–S83, 1987.
36. Vetter G: Double-blind clinical trial with S-adenosylmethionine and indomethacin in the treatment of osteoarthritis. Am J Med 83(Suppl 5A):S78–S80, 1987.
37. Hortsman J: SAMe. In The Arthritis Foundation's Guide to

Alternative Therapies. Atlanta, Arthritis Foundation, 1999, p 224.

38. Jacob S: MSM. In The Arthritis Foundation's Guide to Alternative Therapies. Atlanta, Arthritis Foundation, 1999, p 223.

39. Holzer SS, Cuerdon T: Development of an economic model comparing acetaminophen to NSAIDs in the treatment of mild-to-moderate osteoarthritis. Am J Managed Care 2(Suppl):S15–S26, 1996.

40. Griffin MR, Piper JM, Daugherty JR, et al: Nonsteroidal anti-inflammatory drug use and increased risk for peptic ulcer disease in elderly persons. Ann Intern Med 114:257–263, 1991.

41. Simon LS, Hatoum HT, Bittman RM, et al: Risk factors for serious nonsteroidal-induced gastrointestinal complications: Regression analysis of the MUCOSA trial. Fam Med 28:204–210, 1996.

42. Hochberg MC, Altman RD, Brandt KD, et al: Guidelines for the medical management of osteoarthritis: Part I. Osteoarthritis of the hip. Arthritis Rheum 38:1535–1540, 1995.

43. Hochberg MC, McAlindon T, Felson DT: Systemic and topical treatments. In conference chair: Osteoarthritis: New insights. Part 2: Treatment approaches. Ann Intern Med 133:726–729 2000.

44. Dieppe PA, Sathapatayavongs B, Jones HE, et al: Intra-articular steroids in osteoarthritis. Rheum Rehabil 19:212–217, 1980.

45. Jacobs JJ, Goldberg V: Surgical treatment of osteoarthritis: Current and future approaches. In conference chair: Osteoar-

thritis: New insights. Part 2: Treatment approaches. Ann Intern Med 133:732–733, 2000.

46. Sander O, Herborn G, Rau R: Is H15 (resin extract of *Boswellia serrata,* "incense") a useful supplement to established drug therapy of chronic polyarthritis? Results of a double-blind pilot study [German]. Z Rheumatol 57:11–16, 1998.

47. Chopra A, Patwardhan B, Lavin P, Chitre D: A randomized placebo-controlled trial of an herbal Ayurvedic formulation in patients with active rheumatoid arthritis. Arthritis Rheum 39(Suppl):S283, 1996.

48. Kulkarni RR, Patki PS, Jog VP, et al: Treatment of osteoarthritis with a herbomineral formulation: A double-blind, placebo-controlled, cross-over study. J Ethnopharmacol 33:91–95, 1991.

49. Garfinkel MS, Schumacher HR Jr, Husain A, et al: Evaluation of a yoga based regimen for treatment of osteoarthritis of the hands. J Rheumatol 21:2341–2343, 1994.

50. Ramey DW: Magnetic and electromagnetic therapy. Sci Rev Altern Med 2:13–18, 1998.

51. Collacott EA, Zimmerman JT, White DW, Rindone JP: Bipolar permanent magnets for treatment of chronic low back pain: A pilot study. JAMA 283:1322–1325, 2000.

52. Vallbona C, Hazlewood CF, Jurida G: Response of pain to static magnetic fields in postpolio patients: A double blind pilot study. Arch Phys Med Rehabil 78:1200–1203, 1997.

CHAPTER 52

Low Back Pain

Wendy G. Kohatsu, M.D.

Low back pain is one of the most common reasons people seek medical care, yet it remains a diagnostic and a treatment challenge for both patient and physician. An estimated 70% to 80% of the population is affected by low back pain at some time in their lives, 30% to 50% of adults having low back pain per year, at a cost of approximately $60 billion dollars per year.[1] Patients suffering from chronic conditions not effectively "cured" by allopathic medicine often seek out providers of complementary and alternative medicine (CAM). Indeed, CAM therapies are used for low back pain more frequently than for any other indication, yet the evidence to date is fragmentary.[2]

An integrative approach, truly integrating the best of allopathic medicine with CAM therapies, offers a comprehensive, yet practical, way to more effectively help patients with low back pain. Physicians tend to "overmedicalize" low back pain with excessive and expensive testing; patients can often be left compartmentalizing their pain, and a whole person approach becomes lost. Successful resolution/coping with low back pain requires that the patient takes an active role in his or her own care. With the vast array of CAM therapies—ranging from acupuncture to manipulation to homeopathy—available for low back pain, it is just as easy to get lost trying to find suitable CAM therapies as it is dealing with the frustration that patients often experience with allopathic medical treatments.

Putting things in perspective, 80% of episodes of acute low back pain resolve within 6 weeks *regardless* of the approach.[3] Unfortunately, widespread acceptance of these data tends to allow a period of "benign neglect" during which function is still limited, pain is acutely felt, and pain could be more easily managed. It is sobering to note that the recurrence of low back pain is very high—up to 75% of patients have one or more relapses, and 72% continue to have pain after 1 year.[4] Many patients report persistence of activity limitations. Therefore, it is important to take action early and tailor an integrative plan to enable the patient to recover as well as prevent further episodes of low back pain.

PATHOPHYSIOLOGY

In the **integrative model,** it is important to understand that the body is a dynamic, interconnected system of which the back is a vital part. Orthopedic injuries to other parts of the body (e.g., knee, hip) can lead to muscular spasms and imbalances that trigger pain in the low back. Poor posture and gait can cause low back pain. Lifestyle factors—underexercising or overexercising, working to exhaustion, obesity—can have a profound impact on what we feel in our backs. The mind's influence on chronic, debilitating problems such as low back pain cannot be overestimated. The patient's belief in her or his ability to recover from an episode of low back pain can have a profound effect on her or his actual prognosis and can affect motivation to partake in therapy. Focusing on only the parts tends to undervalue the wholeness of the patient and limits the optimizing of health.

Several predisposing factors are considered in treating patients with low back pain (Table 52–1). It is helpful to begin to address these factors to minimize risk of recurrence.

DIAGNOSTIC CONSIDERATIONS

Part of the dilemma of diagnosing low back pain stems from the fact that the back is a complex and interconnected system that includes the spinal column and sacrum, the spinal cord and nerves, intervertebral discs, layers of muscles, and deep investing fascia (Figs. 52–1 and 52–2). Pain can arise from any of these structures.

Table 52–1. Predisposing Factors for Low Back Pain
....

Poor level of physical fitness
Prior episode(s) of low back pain
Smoking
   It is important to counsel patients on smoking cessation.
Genetics
   New studies show that there may be a genetic link for degenerative disk disease in certain populations.
Psychological stressors—depression, poor coping skills, family and marital conflicts
Psychosocial factors—job insecurity, low socioeconomic status, job dissatisfaction, worker's compensation/litigation
Occupational risk factors—whole body vibration (e.g., jackhammer use), heavy manual labor
   A recent large study showed that frequent back belt use for workers did not reduce the incidence of low back pain or claims for such.[5] It is interesting to note that, although work load may be associated with the initial complaint of low back pain, psychosocial factors strongly correlate with chronic disability.

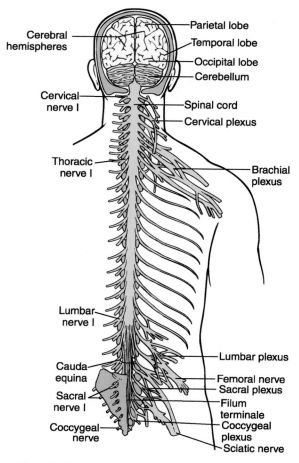

Figure 52–1. Posterior view showing the dorsal (left) and ventral (right) rami of the spinal nerves. (From Dorland's Illustrated Medical Dictionary, 29th ed. Philadelphia, WB Saunders, 2000, p. 239.)

Workup of Low Back Pain

It is, of course, necessary to conduct a thorough workup for low back pain. An integrative approach begins with history and physical examination (Table 52–2 and Fig. 52–3), with intention directed toward understanding the patient as well as the disease. It is important to simply *ASK* the patient about what he or she feels causes the back pain—daily habits, life situations/stressors. The history can reveal a chemical dependency, insomnia, occupational issues, or other factors. This inquiry often yields valuable clues that an integrative practitioner can use to better understand the disease process within the individual and to foster positive outcomes. The examination should be history focused and include a full neurologic examination. Because the psychosocial nature of low back pain can be befuddling, taking note of nonorganic clues ("Waddell signs")[6] can signal a need for greater psychological interventions such as counseling. Diagnostic categories of low back pain (Table 52–3) may be assigned after examination.

Red flags: The Agency for Health Care Policy and Research, in their Acute Low Back Pain Guideline Panel,[7] recommends being aware of the following "red flags" in the history and presentation of low back pain.

- Radiation below the knee
- History of trauma
- Atypical pain (nocturnal pain, unrelenting)
- Worse sitting (suggestive of herniation)
- Relieved with forward flexion (suggestive of spinal stenosis)
- Neurologic symptoms such as bowel or bladder incontinence, weakness, or gait impairment

Table 52–2. Physical Examination for Low Back Pain

Patient Position	Test Performed or Feature Observed	Time required (sec)	Possible Findings
All positions	Observation	Ongoing	Behavior factors, physical limitation
Standing position	Posture and gait	15	Poor postural habits, alteration owing to pain
	Toe and heel walking	10	L5 or S1 weakness
	Symmetry, asymmetry	5	Scoliosis, atrophy
	Range of motion	15	Pain response, physical limitation
Sitting position	Straight-leg raise	10	Radicular pain
	Neurologic testing	40	Neurologic deficit
Supine position	Leg length	5	Mechanical contribution
	Straight-leg raise	10	Radicular pain
	Patrick's test (fabere sign)	10	Hip involvement
Prone position	Palpation	20	Muscle dysfunction
	Hip extension, 5 to 20 degrees	10	Radicular pain (L2–L4 nerve roots)
	"Prone prop"	10	Facet joint dysfunction
Total time		2 min, 40 sec	

Fabere sign: A mnemonic for the movements required to elicit hip as etiology of pain (*f*lexion, *ab*duction, *e*xternal *r*otation, and *e*xtension). It is done by placing the lateral malleolus of the side to be tested over the top of the knee, applying gentle downward pressure on the flexed knee, causing external rotation of the hip.

"Prone prop": While prone, have the patient "prop" the body on the elbows, allowing for passive extension of the lumbar spine. This reduces compression on the anterior intervertebral disk, which may relieve pain that originates at the nerve root. But this may worsen facet joint pain owing to irritation of this joint.

From Biewen PC: A structured approach to low back pain. Postgrad Med 106(6):102–114, 1999.

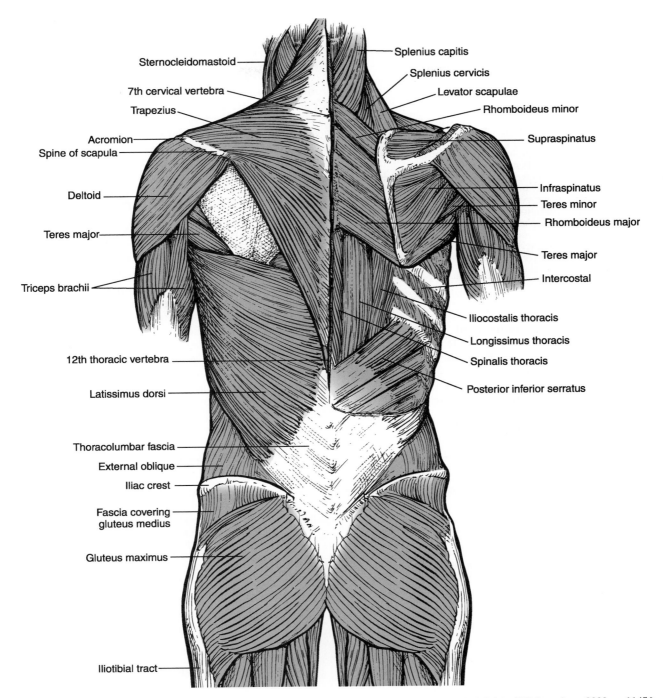

Figure 52–2. Muscles of the back. (From Dorland's Illustrated Medical Dictionary, 29th ed. Philadelphia, WB Saunders, 2000, p. 1145.)

- History of cancer, especially prostate, breast, lung, thyroid, kidney, multiple myeloma, and lymphomas

These raise suspicion for the need for further evaluation, including radiographic studies and/or surgical referral. Basic laboratory studies, if indicated, should include complete blood count, erythrocyte sedimentation rate, and urinalysis. Serious pathology such as fracture, tumor, infection, and cauda equina syndrome must be ruled out before a

diagnosis of simple, mechanical low back pain is made.

The term *low back pain* tends to be a catchall phrase that is often used but is neither precise nor clinically useful. Eighty-five percent of patients with low back pain are not given a more definitive diagnosis. Most allopathic physicians have had inadequate training in conducting a thorough physical examination of the structures (and functions) of the low back. Although most physicians may not need to distinguish between an L4 and an L3 sub-

Table 52–3. Diagnostic Categories for Low Back Pain
··········

Temporal classification
  Acute   <6 wk
  Subacute   6–12 wk
  Chronic   >12 wk
Simple versus complex low back pain[7]
  Simple—no risk factors or signs of underlying pathology
  Complex—risk factors present including: age over 50 yrs history of cancer or IV drug abuse, signs or symptoms of systemic disease (weight loss, fever, lymphadenopathy), sciatica, neurologic deficit on examination
    Only 3% of patients with low back pain present with true sciatica, and only one third of those (1% total) have acute neurologic symptomatology requiring immediate surgical consultation; note that the presence of sciatica does not automatically mean that conservative measures need to be bypassed in favor of more aggressive treatment; many patients with low back pain plus sciatica do very well with conservative treatment, including manipulation.

dysfunction may be best first approached through osteopathic manipulation, whereas muscular strain of the erector spinae may simply need to start with physical exercises at home.

Disc herniation or no? Surgery for low back pain is more prevalent in the United States than any other country, with rates increasing 55% in the 1980s. Radiographic evidence shows that 64% of people aged 45 years have silent (without pain) disc herniation on magnetic resonance imaging. Likewise, other studies show that anatomic evidence of a herniated disc is found in 20% to 30% of imaging tests of normal persons,[8] and the extent of protrusion does not often correlate with severity of symptoms. Jobs involving lifting, pulling, pushing, or carrying have *not* been associated with an increased risk for prolapsed disc,[9] contrary to popular belief.

Radiologic studies have *not* been proved to help diagnose uncomplicated low back pain. Experts conclude that "there is no firm evidence for the presence or absence of a causal relationship between radiographic findings and nonspecific low back pain" in a review of observational studies of spinal radiographic findings.[10] Likewise, patients with computed tomography scans showing spinal stenosis, disc bulging, protrusion, or extrusion compared with patients with normal findings had similar clinical examinations. Experts conclude that computed

luxation, it *is* helpful to be able to palpate differences in tissue texture, asymmetry of the lower body frame, and the like. Better education of physicians may lead to improved skill in the differentiating causes of low back pain, and, thus, to better, more informed choices for therapy. For example, back pain arising primarily from sacroiliac joint somatic

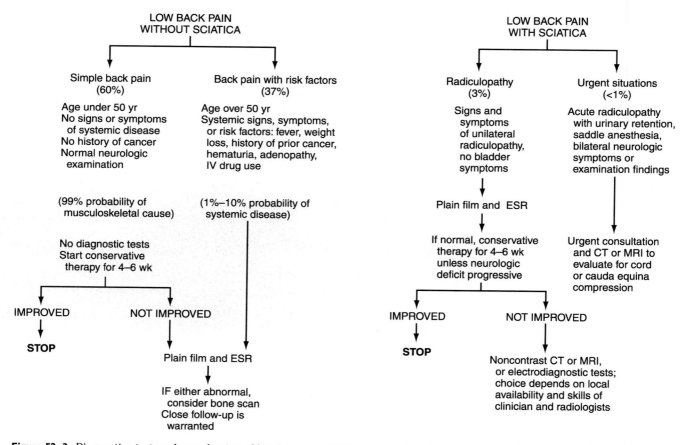

Figure 52–3. Diagnostic strategy for evaluation of low back pain. ESR, erythrocyte sedimentation rate. (Redrawn from Branch WT [ed]: Office Practice of Medicine, 3rd ed. Philadelphia, WB Saunders, 1994, p. 654.)

tomography scans of the spine to study chronic, nonprogressive back pain "do not seem to be important."[11] Therefore, radiographic studies often do not help clinicians get to the root cause of their patients' low back pain.

An excellent article by Biewen[12] outlines some of the major examination techniques that can be completed in a time-efficient manner.

INTEGRATIVE THERAPY

Given the complex anatomy of the back and lack of diagnostic consensus between physicians and alternative healthcare providers, a vast array of therapeutic options exists. Several studies have been done to scientifically assess the value of many of these therapies for low back pain, but these have been plagued by methodological flaws. Low back pain is indeed an individual's disease; no one patient exhibits back pain like another and the response to same type of treatment is highly variable. Restoration of function, not necessarily eradication of pain, is the first key goal. In the long run, the goal for patients with low back pain is to minimize dependence on any outside provider, CAM or allopathic. Self-reliance can be taught through self-care and a coordinated partnership with a primary physician.

Time and Reassurance

Reassurance to the patient of the benign nature of uncomplicated low back pain and the high rate of favorable outcomes with treatment is the essential first step in the plan of care. The second step is to work with him or her to create a therapeutic "game plan," incorporating exercise, judicious use of medications, and a defined follow-up plan if complications arise. The physician may want to include a written "prescription" that lists not only medications but also timing and amount of exercises to perform at home (see Chapter 87, Low Back Pain Exercises). Involving patients in the choice of the care plan that provides clear directions can help focus the therapy, avoid inactivity because of pain and fear, and avoid excessive treatment. With an integrative approach, it is also important to ask the patient what his or her specific goals are for the visit—for example, pain-free walking, returning to work, reducing reliance on pain medicines, so that progress may be monitored in a way that is meaningful for the patient.

Pharmacotherapy

In the most updated, evidence-based review available on the conservative treatment of low back pain,[13] common pharmaceutical agents were reviewed.

Analgesics—Analgesics (acetaminophen, opioids) were found to be as effective as nonsteroidal anti-inflammatory drugs (NSAIDs). Opioids should be considered as a third line of treatment, and limited to 1 to 3 days, for a maximum 3 weeks.[14] Patients should be informed of potential addictive properties.

NSAIDs—Strong evidence indicates that NSAIDs are not more effective than analgesics and that the various types of NSAIDs (ibuprofen, diclofenac, piroxicam, felbinac) are equally effective in comparison with each other. NSAIDs were more effective than placebo in patients with simple, acute low back pain. Optimum treatment with NSAIDs: no longer than 12 weeks. Data on the use of cyclooxygenase-2 inhibitors for low back pain are pending.

Muscle relaxants—Strong evidence demonstrates that muscle relaxants are more effective than placebo for acute low back pain, but less so for chronic low back pain. The different types of muscle relaxants were found to be equally effective. Optimum use is for 1 week, for a maximum of 4 weeks.

Antidepressants—Compared with placebo, antidepressant (amitriptyline, imipramine, trazodone) use for chronic low back pain was not found to be effective.

Botanical Medicine

Arnica—Arnica (Arnica montana) is widely known as a homeopathic medicine for acute trauma, especially of musculoskeletal origin. It is the number one ingredient in many topical homeopathic preparation (6× to 30× dilution) for bruises and muscle strain. Arnica contains sesquiterpenes and lactones that have active antioxidant properties and seem to have a different mechanism of action than NSAIDs.[15] However, there are no good studies to back up its routine use for the treatment of low back pain (see Chapter 103, Therapeutic Homeopathy).

Kava kava—Kava kava (Piper methysticum), extracted from a South Pacific root plant, has been used not only as a potent anxiolytic medication but also for its reported properties as a mild muscle relaxant. No studies have proved this effect, but observational data do support this. It is possible that all of its effects are due to its anxiolytic action.

Dosage. 100 to 250 mg by mouth three to four times daily (standardized to at least 30% kavalactones).

Precautions. The potential for significant drug-herb interactions does exist, so concomitant use of kava and benzodiazepines, barbiturates, or alcohol should be avoided. Highly concentrated extracts of kava can cause liver failure. These should only be taken under professional supervision.

Exercise Therapy

Strong evidence was found for exercise therapy for chronic low back pain, although the optimal regimen (type, frequency, duration) has yet to be determined. Exercise modalities studied include stretching, McKenzie exercises, endurance training, isometric strengthening, and intensive dynamic training. The ultimate goal of exercise therapy is to allow the patient to have greater control and ease with her or his body. Aerobic exercise has been shown to increase blood flow, mood, and pain tolerance. The optimal exercise plan is to incorporate aerobic exercise two to three times per week (20 to 30 minutes), strength training two to three times per week on alternate days, plus daily mild stretching. Small, achievable, incremental goals help the patient to gain confidence.

Robin McKenzie, a physiotherapist from New Zealand, has developed a highly evolved system of treatment that emphasizes frequent self-exercise, 2 to 3 minutes every 2 hours, slight end-range stretching, and the principle of centralization of pain.[16] He states that "the most common cause of low back pain is postural stress . . . especially poor sitting posture."[17] McKenzie exercises proved to be of significant benefit for acute low back pain as well. A randomized, controlled trial showed that these exercises were just as effective as chiropractic care provided at the same cost.[18] Responders require an average of only six or fewer visits to bring closure to their case.[16] The McKenzie Institute works directly with physicians to individualize self-treatment programs—the U.S. referral phone number is (800) 635-8380.

NOTE

Exercise is also important as a preventive measure. Lack of time is frequently cited as a reason for avoiding exercise, yet the average American watches 30 hours of television per week.

Acupuncture

Both a recent systematic review[19] and a meta-analysis[20] of acupuncture in low back pain have shown that not enough data exist to prove efficacy above placebo. This may point to the inherent methodological flaws in conducting acupuncture research. There are many different schools of classical Oriental medicine, each fostering a variation in approaches to diagnosis and treatment. Acupuncture may also not work as well when isolated from the whole system of Oriental medicine, which may also include herbs, dietary changes, and moxibustion. The skill of the acupuncturist may be highly variable; treatment outcome may depend on the particular method used as well as the skill of the practitioner.

Transcutaneous Electrical Nerve Stimulation

Transcutaneous electrical nerve stimulation (TENS) is often applied as an adjunct therapy in physical therapy. A handful of good studies have been conducted for use of TENS, with contradictory results, however. More studies may be able to provide a true therapeutic trend.[13] There is also PENS, percutaneous electrical nerve stimulation, which is essentially equivalent to electroacupuncture, in which a small current is run at various Hertz levels through needles inserted into specific points in the low back.[21]

Manipulation

Chiropractic Therapy

Spinal manipulation is of short-term benefit in some patients, particularly those with uncomplicated, acute low back pain. Meta-analyses confirm that manipulation is more effective than placebo treatment for acute low back pain, and there is also strong evidence for its use in chronic low back pain as well.[22, 23] However, there is concern that, although appropriateness of application of chiropractic manipulation is similar to allopathic medicine (46%), there is also a high rate (29%) of inappropriate use.[24] Patients should note positive effects, if any, after about four to six chiropractic treatments; if not, these should be discontinued.

Complications of spinal manipulation have been thoroughly reviewed.[25, 26] Most worrisome are the vertebrobasilar accidents that have been associated with *cervical* manipulation only. For the *lumbar area,* 62 cases were described in which spinal manipulation was associated with disc herniation or cauda equina syndrome. About half of these lumbar complications occurred during manipulation under anesthesia, now an obsolete technique. Manipulation does not appear to be contraindicated for patients with bulging discs or herniation.[27] Shekelle and coworkers[24] estimates that the rate of occurrence of cauda equina syndrome as a complication of spinal manipulation is about 1 per 100 million manipulations.

Osteopathy

Osteopathic manipulation varies from chiropractic manipulation in distinct ways. In general, osteopathy encompasses a wide variety of techniques including the familiar high-velocity, low-amplitude (HVLA) thrust, but it also includes muscle energy technique, myofascial release, counterstrain, and craniosacral treatment. In addition to the wide variety of soft tissue osteopathic manipulations, a distinct advantage to an osteopathic approach is the holistic philosophy of treating the whole person and the interrelatedness of body functions.

Two techniques commonly used by osteopathic physicians are muscle energy technique and counterstrain.

Muscle Energy

In muscle energy, the operator positions the patient so as to precisely localize a problem area—a malrotated vertebra, an overtight hamstring, and the like. The goal is to reset the length of the culprit muscle by a series of isometric contractions, thus changing Golgi tendon organ and extrafusal fiber inhibitory input to the alpha motoneuron, held for approximately 5 to 6 seconds. All of the active motion, held for 5- to 6-second intervals, is applied by the patient.

Counterstrain

Counterstrain is a passive technique in which the goal is to reset the gamma gain (intrafusal fibers) of a tightened muscle to allow it to reset to a more relaxed state. Tightness in specific muscles can cause referred pain enough to mimic neurologic back pain (see Chapter 99, Strain and Counterstrain Manipulation Technique).

Osteopathic manipulation courses are offered through continuing medical education from various osteopathic colleges and institutions for those persons seeking further training.

A recent randomized, controlled trial showed no statistical difference between a group of low back pain patients receiving osteopathic manipulative therapy compared with those receiving standard care consisting of physical therapy, TENS, ultrasound, and hot/cold packs. The osteopathic manipulative therapy group did use significantly less medication—NSAIDs, analgesics, and muscle relaxants.[28]

Greenman has compiled from his extensive work the "dirty half-dozen" osteopathic diagnoses of low back pain that have been refractory to conservative therapy or surgery[29] (Table 52–4).

Terms such as *non-neutral, pubic dysfunction,* and *posterior sacral base* are specific musculoskeletal mechanical diagnoses based on careful osteopathic evaluation. Ninety-eight percent of these "untreat-

Table 52–4. Osteopathic Diagnoses of Refractory Low Back Pain

....

Muscle imbalance—between the trunk and the thighs	100%
Non-neutral lumbar dysfunction	88%
Pubic dysfunction	76%
Short leg/pelvic tilt syndrome (>6 mm difference)	65%
Posterior sacral base (and loss of lumbar lordosis)	60%
Innominate shear	24%

able" patients fell into treatable diagnostic categories (see Table 52–4). Patients were treated 6 times over 12 weeks, with an additional 15 to 25 visits with a physical therapist. Some 75% of this population returned to work or their full prior functional status.

Massage

A recent systematic review included only four studies of sufficient quality that did not show consistent benefit for low back pain from massage. Of note, two more recent randomized controlled trials[30, 31] using massage involving *deep* tissue techniques did show short-term benefit. More studies are needed on using massage technique specifically designed for low back pain, going beyond superficial structures, and for greater length of follow-up.

Other Bodywork Therapies[32]

Trigger point therapy—Janet Travell, M.D., pioneered the practice of trigger point therapy in the United States based on the European practice in the 1930s. Originally, injections of saline and procaine were used; later an anesthetic cooling agent was employed in the "spray and stretch" technique. Bonnie Prudden developed her highly effective "pain erasure" technique by using the hands and elbows to apply pressure to the same trigger points.

Functional approaches include Feldenkrais, sensory awareness, Hanna somatics, and Alexander technique, which have in common the goal of re-educating dysfunctional movement patterns. Participants attend classes designed to enhance awareness of kinesthetic sensations in the body. The Alexander technique was founded by Frederick M. Alexander (1869 to 1955), a Shakespearean performer who solved his vocal and respiratory problems by noticing and changing his poor body posturing. This technique still remains popular with performing artists and athletes.

Rolfing—Developed by Ida Rolf in the 1960s, rolfing (also known as structural integration) is a technique working at the level of deep fascia. Rolfing is designed to reorganize the major segments of the body into proper vertical alignment.

Mind-Body Approaches

Behavior Therapy

There is limited evidence that behavior therapy (in the form of operant conditioning, cognitive treatment, or progressive muscle relaxation) is an effective treatment for chronic low back pain. Referral to a clinic specializing in the care of chronic pain may include an evaluation from a therapist specially trained to address the psychosocial issues of dealing with chronic pain.

Sarno has developed a program that has helped thousands of people overcome their back pain—expressly without drugs or surgery. He states that the primary tissue involved is muscle, and describes tension myositis syndrome (TMS) as a change of state in the muscle that is painful.[33] Sarno's approach takes a mind-body approach, with reported high rates of success: "Traditional medical diagnoses focus on the machine, the body, while the real problem seems to relate to what makes the machine work—the mind. TMS is characterized by physical pain but that acute discomfort is induced by psychologic phenomena rather than structural abnormalities or muscle deficiency."

Sarno advocates shifting attention away from physical pain to something psychological (e.g., family stress, financial concerns), talking to your brain, resuming physical activity, and *discontinuing all physical treatment*—including manipulation, heat, exercise, acupuncture, and massage. All of these work on the premise of a physical cause to low back pain and, therefore, do not belong in this setting.

Surgery

Much controversy exists as to whether surgical treatment should be attempted, and if so, which surgical approach is optimal.[34] Except for cases of acute cauda equina syndrome, surgery is considered only after failure of conservative therapies. Often, however, most patients have not fully optimized their conservative treatments. Surgical fusion of vertebrae may involve one or more levels, and although radiographic success is high (>90%), muscle stripping required to perform the surgery may lead to later weakness and fatigue. With or without an operation, more than 80% of patients with obvious surgical indications eventually recover. In patients with questionable findings, surgery benefits fewer than 40% (Agency for Health Care Policy and Research guidelines).

— *THERAPEUTIC REVIEW* —

History and Physical Examination
- *Listen for diagnostic clues in the history—including lifestyle, occupation, and patient's belief system.*
- *Conduct focused (2½-minute) physical examination.*
- *Rule out any "red flags" suggesting complications requiring further workup (see Fig. 52–3).*

Lifestyle
- *Reduce stress.*
- *Discontinue smoking.*
- *Adopt healthy eating patterns.*
- *Explore exercise habits.*
- *Weight loss, if necessary.*

Personalize Therapy Based on Function
- *The patient must take an active role in the care of his or her back.*
- *Reassure the patient of the high rate of favorable outcomes with active treatment.*
- *During the acute phase, consider physical therapy—supervised stretch, strengthening, gradual aerobic training, and/or McKenzie technique.*
- *Encourage self-care through regular exercise—aerobic exercise and strength training two to three times per week; daily mild stretching.*

Pharmaceuticals/Botanicals
- *Temporary use of analgesics and NSAIDs—NSAIDs less than 12 weeks; analgesics and muscle relaxants less than 4 weeks.*

Manual Therapy
- *Refer to physical therapy to maximize early return of function/prevention of relapse.*
- *Work with a qualified osteopathic physician or chiropractor (limit to four to six visits and check response).*
- *Consider TENS, deep tissue massage as part of manual therapy.*

Mind-Body
- *Consider intense psychosocial intervention if warranted by history and presentation.*

THERAPEUTIC REVIEW *continued*

Movement Therapy
● *Prevention of low back pain with awareness, exercise, movement therapy—consider exploring yoga, Alexander technique, Feldenkrais, and other techniques.*

Referral
● *Refer to specialists if complicated or persistent symptoms are present despite measures previously discussed—refer to specialized pain clinic; surgical referral if red flag present or neurologic symptoms develop or worsen.*

References

1. Wipf J, Deyo R: Low back pain. Med Clin North Am 79:231–245, 1995.
2. Ernst E, Pittler MH: Experts' opinion on complementary/alternative therapies for low back pain. J Manipulative Physiol Ther 22(2):87–90, 1999.
3. Cherkin DC: Primary care research on low back pain: The state of the science. Spine 23:1997–2002, 1998.
4. Van der Hoogen HJ, Koes BW, van Eijk JT, et al: On the course of low back pain in general practice: A one year follow up study. Ann Rheum Dis 57:13–19, 1998.
5. Wassell JT, Gardner LI, Landsittel DP, et al: A prospective study of back belts for prevention of back pain and injury. JAMA 284:2727–3272, 2000.
6. Waddell G, McCulloch JA, Kummel E, et al: Nonorganic physical signs in low back pain. Spine 5:117–125, 1980.
7. Clinical Practice Guideline for Acute Low Back Problems in Adults (AHCPR Pub. No. 95-0642). Rockville, Md, Agency for Health Care Policy and Research, Public Health Service, Department of Health and Human Services, 1994.
8. Boden SD, Davis DO, Dina TS, et al: Abnormal magnetic-resonance scans of the lumbar spine in asymptomatic subjects. A prospective investigation. J Bone Joint Surg 72A:403–408, 1990.
9. Kelsey JL: An epidemiological study of the relationship between occupation and acute herniated lumbar intervertebral discs. Int J Epidemiol 4:197–205, 1975.
10. van Tulder MW, Assendelft WJ, Koes BW, Bouter LM: Spinal radiographic findings and nonspecific low back pain. A systemic review of observational studies. Spine 22:427–434, 1997.
11. Elkayam O, Avrahami E, Yaron M: The lack of prognostic value of computerized tomography imaging examinations in patients with chronic non-progressive back pain. Rheumatol Int 16:19–21, 1996.
12. Biewen PC: A structured approach to low back pain. Postgrad Med 106(6):102–114, 1999.
13. Van Tulder MW, Koes BW, Bouter LM: Conservative treatment of acute and chronic nonspecific low back pain—a systematic review of randomized controlled trials of the most common interventions. Spine 22:2128–2156, 1997.
14. Wheeler AH, Hanley EN Jr: Nonoperative treatment for low back pain. Rest to restoration. Spine 20:375–378, 1995.
15. Lyss G, Schmidt TJ, Merfort I, Pahl HL: Helenalin, an anti-inflammatory sesquiterpene lacton from Arnica, selectively inhibits transcription factor NF-kappaB. Biol Chem 378:951–961, 1997.
16. Simonsen RJ: Principle-centered spine care: McKenzie principles. Occup Med 13:167–183, 1998.
17. McKenzie R: Treat Your Own Back, 7th ed. Waikanae, New Zealand, Spinal Publications, 1997.
18. Cherkin DC, Deyo RA, Battie M, et al: A comparison of physical therapy, chiropractic manipulation, and provision of an educational booklet for the treatment of patients with low back pain. N Engl J Med 339:1021–1029, 1998.
19. Van Tulder MW, Cherkin DC, Berman B, et al: The effectiveness of acupuncture in the management of acute and chronic low back pain. A systematic review within the framework of the Cochrane collaboration back review group. Spine 24:1113–1123, 1999.
20. Ernst E, White AR. Acupuncture for back pain. A meta-analysis of randomized controlled trials. Arch Int Med 1998; 158:2235–41.
21. Ghoname EA, Craig WF, White PF, et al: Percutaneous electrical nerve stimulation for low back pain—a randomized crossover study. JAMA 281:818–823, 1999.
22. Koes BW, Bouter LM, van Mameren H, et al: Randomized clinical trial of manipulative therapy and physiotherapy for persistent back and neck complaints: Results of one year follow up. BMJ 304:601–605, 1992.
23. Koes BW, Bouter LM, van Mameren H, et al: A randomized clinical trial of manual therapy and physiotherapy for persistent back and neck complaints: Subgroup analysis and relationship between outcome measures. J Manipulative Physiol Ther 1993:16:211–219.
24. Shekelle PG, Coulter I, Hurwitz EL, et al: Congruence between decisions to initiate chiropractic spinal manipulation for low back pain and appropriateness criteria in North America. Ann Intern Med 129:9–17, 1998.
25. Assendelft WJJ, Bouter LM, Knipschild PG: Complications of spinal manipulation: A comprehensive review of the literature. J Fam Pract 42:475–480, 1996.
26. Krueger BR, Okazaki H: Vertebral-basilar distribution infarction following chiropractic cervical manipulation. Mayo Clin Proc 55:322–332, 1980.
27. Haldeman S, Rubinstein SM: Cauda equina syndrome following lumbar spine manipulation. Spine 17:1469–1473, 1992.
28. Andersson GBJ, Lucente T, Davis AM, et al: A comparison of osteopathic spinal manipulation with standard care for patients with low back pain. N Engl J Med 341:1426–1431, 1999.
29. Greenman P: Clin Phys Med Rehabil Nov. 1996.
30. Cherkin DC, Eisenberg D, Sherman KJ, et al: Randomized trial comparing traditional Chinese medical, acupuncture, therapeutic massage and self-care education for chronic low back pain. Arch Intern Med 161:1081–1088, 2001.
31. Preyde M: Effectiveness of massage therapy for subacute low-back pain: A randomized controlled trial. CMAJ 162:1815–1820, 2000.
32. Knaster M: Discovering the Body's Wisdom. New York, Bantam, 1996.
33. Sarno JM: Healing Back Pain: The Mind-Body Connection. New York, Warner, 1991.
34. Nachemson A, Zdeblick TA, O'Brien JP: Controversy in spine care—lumbar disc disease with discogenic pain. What surgical treatment is most effective? Spine 21:1835–1838, 1996.

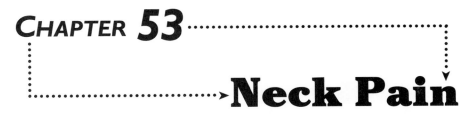

CHAPTER 53

Neck Pain

J. Adam Rindfleisch, M.D., and David Rakel, M.D.

The neck has 37 separate joints and moves an average of 600 times per hour. Understandably, it is extremely susceptible to pain. In fact, approximately 12% of women and 9% of men experience neck pain at any given time.[1] Neck pain strikes at least half of all adults at some point in their lives, and it is one of the most common complaints among patients presenting to primary care providers.[2]

PATHOPHYSIOLOGY

Neck pain can arise from multiple sources. In most cases, neck pain is due to cervical paraspinal muscle spasm or other musculoskeletal problems, and these disorders are the main focus of this chapter. However, it is important to rule out a variety of other causative disorders before a treatment regimen is initiated (Table 53–1).

In assessing musculoskeletal neck pain, it is useful to consider whether the pain is traumatic or non-traumatic in origin.[1] Traumatic neck pain is most commonly associated with hyperextension syndrome, or "whiplash." Whiplash and other traumatic injuries of the neck frequently have long-lasting

Table 53–1. Key Points in the Evaluation of Neck Pain[1]

- A tumor should be considered if the patient has pain at night or if the pain does not lessen when the body is supine.
- Neck pain with associated neurologic symptoms (e.g., dizziness, paresthesias, weakness) merits diagnostic imaging studies, most commonly computed tomography or magnetic resonance imaging study of the neck.
- Severe neck pain associated with fever is due to meningitis until proved otherwise.
- If neck pain is associated with joint pain in other areas, a systemic rheumatic disorder, such as osteoarthritis, rheumatoid arthritis, ankylosing spondylitis, or (rarely) gout, should be ruled out.
- Neck pain can arise from a source in the head or arms, such as dental disorders, temperomandibular joint disorders, and rotator cuff injuries. Of note, with cervical spine disorders, patients may describe a sensation of the eyes being pulled or pushed if there is irritation of the sympathetic nerve plexuses that surround the arteries of the neck and innervate the eyes.
- Referred neck pain can arise from nearly any organ system. Myocardial ischemia, gallbladder disease, gastrointestinal ulcers, hiatal hernias, and pancreatic inflammation are all possibilities in the differential diagnosis. Referred diaphragmatic pain and tumors of the apical lung also must be considered.
- Infrequent local sources of neck pain include the carotids, vertebral arteries, lymph nodes, and the thyroid.

sequelae if not adequately treated. It has been estimated that up to 40% of whiplash injuries result in long-term symptoms.[3]

Nontraumatic neck pain includes both soft tissue disorders and disorders that are structural/degenerative in nature. Common causes of soft tissue disorders of the neck are poor posture, repetitive activity at work, sports injuries, and pain associated with psychiatric conditions. Myofascial trigger points, which are clusters of muscle fibers locked in a contractive state, are frequently associated with soft tissue neck pain.

Mechanical/degenerative pain, in contrast, is usually related in some way to the cervical spine or spinal nerve roots. Examples of disorders causing this type of pain are cervical spondylosis and disc herniation—conditions in which imaging studies may prove useful.

The pathophysiologic basis of neck pain is complex,[3a] and our knowledge of the multitude of chemical and structural processes involved is far from complete. However, it is useful to visualize the emergence and progression of musculoskeletal neck pain according to the diagram provided in Figure 53–1.

The chain of events leading to chronic neck pain begins with irritation of the tissues by any of various mechanisms. The triggering mechanism may be infection, joint deterioration, sustained use or prolonged immobility, structural abnormality, psychological stress, or trauma. Irritation can activate nociception, resulting in pain. Eventually, muscle spasms may occur, either because of repositioning of the neck to avoid pain or because the pain stimulus directly causes involuntary muscle contraction. Inflammatory processes then ensue, leading to even more pain through a positive feedback effect. With edema formation, structural changes, and the accumulation of harmful metabolites, tissues may become ischemic. Ultimately, chronic inflammation may develop, with consequent alterations in the function of muscles, joints, and tendons. If these alterations are not interrupted or reversed in time, long-term changes in neck structure may arise, and disability can be the result.

INTEGRATIVE THERAPY

The primary goals in the treatment of neck pain are decreasing discomfort, increasing range of motion,

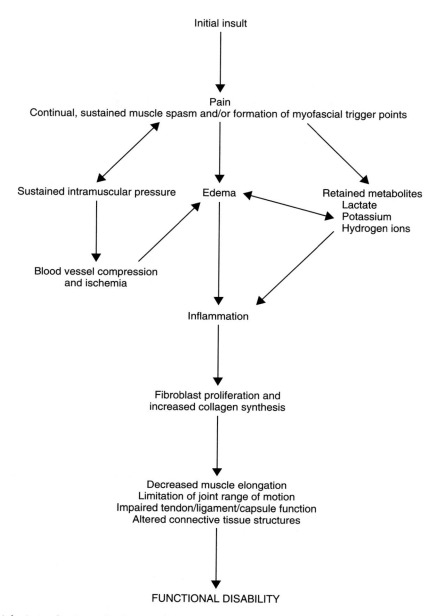

Figure 53–1. Pathophysiologic mechanisms of soft tissue cervical spine syndromes. (After Noble J, Greene HL 2nd, Levinson W, et al [eds]: Textbook of Primary Care Medicine, 3rd ed. Philadelphia, Mosby, 2001, p 1131.)

and preventing long-term disability. In order to achieve these goals, it is necessary to interrupt the process by which pain arises and is perpetuated (see Fig. 53–1). A variety of prevention and treatment methods may be helpful.

Lifestyle Interventions

Exercise

Ideally, it is preferable to prevent pain from occurring at all. Avoiding irritation of neck muscle can be accomplished in a number of ways. Regular exercise to improve posture is frequently recommended. The Alexander technique and Feldenkrais can be helpful

in retraining appropriate body posture and muscle support of the head and neck. Pilates therapy can also be helpful in building cervical muscular support.

Cervical Support

Proper neck positioning during sleep is of benefit. Prolonged flexion of the neck should be avoided; maintenance of the neck's natural lordotic curve is preferable. A number of special cervical spine pillows can prove useful, including the Cervipillow and the Wal-Pil-O.[4] The use of bifocals may lead to awkward flexion of the neck during waking hours and have the same effect as that of an improper sleeping position.

Avoidance of Repetitive Strain

Lifestyle habits can place the musculoskeletal structures of the neck under chronic stress and tension. Examples include holding a phone between the shoulder and the ear (administrative positions), carrying a heavy purse or back pack on one shoulder, leaning over a desk while reading or studying (in students), and looking back over the shoulder (in farmers). Alerting patients to these habits can lead to awareness and behavioral changes that can reduce the discomfort and bring better balance to the tone of the muscles.

A British study of 12,907 people attempted to determine whether occupational activities influenced the incidence of neck pain. The investigators concluded that there was little association between the specific occupational activities and neck pain, but that there was a significant association between perceived pain and mental stress. These workers concluded that psychosocial factors were more important than occupational activities in the incidence of neck pain.[4] Another study involving nearly 1800 workers also found no significant association between repetitive work involving the neck and arms and neck pain. Rather, they concluded that neck pain was most likely in persons who had little or no influence on their work situation.[5]

Management of Chronic Stress

Many people have a tendency to "carry" stress in the neck and trapezius muscles. A plausible explanation for the localization of stress in this manner is that the muscular tension represents the ducking reflex. Long-term stress can result in a constant readiness to duck or dodge danger, with continued tension in the muscles of the neck. It is also important to listen to metaphors that the patient may use to describe stressful lifestyle situations—for example: "My job is a pain in the neck."

Ample evidence in the literature supports an association between psychologic factors including stress, depression, anxiety, and related emotions to the severity of neck and back pain. In fact, psychologic variables have more impact on severity of pain and disability than do biomechanical and biomedical factors.[5] This knowledge and understanding should encourage the practitioner to address life style factors that may be related to these emotional states. Facilitating changes in the patient's life style to reduce stress addresses the root of the problem, allowing the body to better heal itself.

Nutrition

Essential Fatty Acids

A beneficial influence on levels of prostaglandin and leukotriene inflammatory triggers is obtained by increasing intake of omega-3 fatty acids and reducing amount of omega-6 fatty acids consumed. The traditional "Western diet" contains far higher amounts of omega-6 fatty acids in the form of partially hydrogenated vegetable oils, margarine, and processed foods. These omega-6 fatty acids are also high in trans fatty acids, which are made in the heating process when oil is partially hydrogenated. Trans fatty acids not only worsen lipid profiles but also require more energy to be broken down by the body for their metabolism. This energy breakdown creates more free radicals, which in turn mobilize arachidonic acid from cell membranes. Arachidonic acid is the main precursor in the inflammatory cascade (see Chapter 84, The Anti-Inflammatory Diet).

An interesting study showed a connection among essential fatty acids, stress, and inflammatory cytokines. The balance of omega-3 versus omega-6 fatty acids was checked in 27 college students. The researchers then measured the release of inflammatory cytokines before and after a stressful examination. They found that among those students with high blood levels of omega-6 fatty acids and low blood levels of omega-3 fatty acids, the release of inflammatory cytokines after exposure to a psychological stressor was much greater than in students with the reverse ratio.[6] Thus, the study confirmed that, as is already known, stress increases cytokines, resulting in inflammation. A second and more important finding was that the nutritional balance of essential fatty acids has an influence on the amount of inflammatory triggers the body releases under stress.

Patients should be encouraged to eat foods high in omega-3 fatty acids, such as cold water fish (salmon, mackerel, sardines, herring, and albacore tuna), flax-seed products, nuts (particularly walnuts), dark green leafy vegetables, soybeans, algae, and hemp seeds. Patients should reduce intake of foods rich in omega-6 and trans fatty acids, such as hydrogenated vegetable oils, margarine, and processed foods (anything made with fat that has a long shelf life, such as "chips," crackers, and packaged cupcakes).

NOTE

It can take months for clinical benefit to be seen after changing to an omega-3–rich, omega-6–poor diet. This therapy will probably not be of benefit in acute neck pain but will help to control chronic inflammation and will have a significant impact on general health and disease prevention.

Limiting Intake of Saturated Fats

Animal products, including red meat and dairy products, are high in saturated fat. This type of fat is a significant source of arachidonic acid. In pharmacotherapeutics, mobilization of this chemical from cell membranes is inhibited by giving steroids. In addition, a variety of anti-inflammatory agents are used to inhibit the cyclo-oxygenase (COX), leukotriene, and lipoxygenase pathways. Nonsteroidal anti-inflammatory drugs (NSAIDs) (including aspirin), leukotriene inhibitors, colchicine, and sulfasalazine prevent the metabolism of arachidonic acid into prostaglandins, thromboxanes, and leukotrienes, which promote the inflammatory process. However, little attention is paid to reducing the load of this precursor in the diet.

Patients should be encouraged to curtail intake of saturated fat (meat and dairy products) in the diet to reduce this chemical source of inflammation.

Antioxidants

Free radicals are not inherently "bad." In fact, nitric oxide—a naturally occurring free radical—is required for blood vessel dilation. The danger comes when there is an excessive number of free radicals, overwhelming the system. The imbalance can result from poor nutrition, excessive stress, toxic environmental exposure, or other factors. Large amounts of free radicals increase the mobilization of arachidonic acid, as discussed earlier.

Patients should be encouraged to consume foods rich in antioxidants such as fruits and vegetables. A helpful suggestion is to select a variety of natural food colors during food shopping. Eating green, yellow, red, purple, and orange foods ensures consumption of a range of beneficial antioxidants.

Supplements

Omega-3 Fatty Acids

As discussed previously under "Nutrition," omega-3 fatty acids have been found to reduce the amount of cytokines that stimulate the inflammatory cascade.[7] Supplementation with omega-3 fatty acids should not be done without enhancing this effect through the diet.

A leading Scandinavian treatment facility for sports injuries and rehabilitation uses a combination of essential fatty acids and antioxidants to treat inflammatory conditions in Denmark's Olympic athletes. The formula, which includes omega-3 (fish oil) and omega-6 (borage oil) fatty acids and vitamins A, B$_6$, C, and E, plus selenium and zinc, was reported to work as well as NSAIDs, but it generally required 2 to 3 weeks to take effect.[8] For patients who are unable to tolerate NSAIDs, omega-3 fatty acids may prove beneficial.

Dosage. Omega-3–rich oils: Fish oils, providing both eicosapentaenoic acid (EPA) and docosahexaenoic acid (DHA), or flaxseed oil, a source of alpha-linolenic acid (which needs to be converted into EPA/DHA): 1 to 4 g daily. Often supplied as 500-mg capsules, which can be taken with food twice daily.

Precautions. As the body metabolizes fatty acids into energy, it creates free radicals. Taking excessive doses of fatty acid supplements may be harmful because of the increased load of free radicals. The dose should not exceed 4 g a day, and if essential fatty acids are used for prolonged periods, an antioxidant regimen consisting of vitamin E 400 IU, vitamin C 200 mg, and selenium 200 μg daily is recommended.

Mind-Body Medicine

Studies show that pain perception does not correlate with the severity of injury. In a landmark study reported in the *New England Journal of Medicine*, magnetic resonance imaging examinations of 98 asymptomatic persons revealed that 52% had a bulging disc at one or more spinal levels.[9] An award-winning study conducted at Stanford University evaluated abnormal findings (high-intensity zones) on magnetic resonance images of the lumbar spine in both symptomatic and asymptomatic persons. When these areas were injected with dye (discography) to reproduce pain, the investigators found that it was not the degree of abnormality as detected by the imaging studies that best predicted pain response but the patient's underlying psychologic issues.[10] These findings are supported by the fact that many patients with debilitating pain often have normal findings on imaging studies. Pain is related to much more than what can be seen on radiographs or other imaging studies. Addressing the patient's emotions, beliefs, social support, sense of control, meaning, and purpose is necessary in order to succeed in preventing the cycle of pain and inflammation.

Addressing Emotions

In three books written for the lay reader, John E. Sarno, M.D, Professor of Clinical Rehabilitation Medicine at New York University School of Medicine, has described a syndrome that he believes is responsible for the majority of neck, back, and limb pain. The most popular of these books is entitled *Healing Back Pain*.[11] Sarno theorizes that pain is the result of mild local oxygen deprivation rather than the result of a multitude of structural abnormalities to which it is usually attributed. This altered physiology is initiated by the brain in response to noxious unconscious emotions, of which rage is the most prominent. The major source of this accumulated anger is psychological pressure, both self-imposed and derived from the outside world. The disorder is classically psychosomatic. Sarno's work describes how dealing with emotions such as anger and anxiety can release the need for the body to sympathize with pain.

```
┌──────────────────────────────────────────────┐
│                   NOTE                         │
│                                                │
│ Addressing emotions is an important therapeutic│
│ process in any patient with chronic pain. In   │
│ addi-tion, a complete workup should be done to │
│ rule out an underlying caustive physical       │
│ disorder that may be reversible.               │
└──────────────────────────────────────────────┘
```

Sarno's program is essentially one of education, in which the physical and emotional components of the disorder are explored in detail. This exploration is accomplished through lectures and in group meetings. Approximately 20% of participants also benefit from psychotherapy. He does not employ physical measures, and drugs are limited to analgesics for severe pain. A summary of Sarno's program follows:

- *Patient education is accomplished through a series of lectures.* These lectures inform the patient about how pain is related to emotional factors. Knowledge of this relationship is the "penicillin" that treats the pain.
- *When pain strikes, the patient must address underlying emotions:* When the patient becomes aware of pain, there must be a conscious switch of focus to a psychologic rather than a physical source for the pain.
- *The patient resumes physical activity:* This step involves overcoming the fear that physical activity may worsen the underlying condition. Although it is a difficult step, resuming physical activity is one of the most important tasks of the program. Sarno recommends resumption of activity after the pain has lessened and after the patient understands how emotions are involved in the process.
- *The patient discontinues all physical treatment.* Focusing on physical causes of pain distracts the mind from addressing emotions that are at the root of the condition and also reinforces the belief that the source of continued pain is physical rather than emotional.
- *Referral for counseling may be needed.* Further counseling may be required to explore emotions that have been repressed and to help the patient to understand their meaning so that a positive resolution can be reached.

This program has provided relief for many people with neck and back pain. Unfortunately, there are no well-controlled outcome studies to support its use. Nevertheless, in providing an integrative approach to management of neck pain, addressing emotions should not be overlooked. The relatively low-cost educational program outlined here has potentially few side effects and can result in significant benefit.

Journaling

Writing about stressful events can also provide an outlet for expressing emotions that may control pain and limit inflammation. A beneficial effect has been noted in people with asthma and rheumatoid arthritis who wrote for just 20 minutes on 3 consecutive days about stressful life events.[12] This technique can be used in the privacy of the patient's home, and the writing does not need to be shared with others. The therapeutic benefit comes from the organization and expression of emotional events (see Chapter 93, Journaling).

Hypnosis

One study evaluated 25 patients with head and neck pain that was treated with acupuncture. After a suitable interval ("wash out period"), the patients then received hypnotherapy for their pain. Both acupuncture and hypnosis were found to be beneficial in relieving pain. Hypnosis was slightly better, with a reduction of 4.8 points on a 10-point scale versus a 4.2-point improvement with acupuncture. Acupuncture was more appropriate for acute pain, whereas hypnosis appeared to work better for psychogenic pain. Patients who also received healing suggestions via audiotape had less pain than patients who did not[13] (see Chapter 89, Self-Hypnosis Techniques).

Interactive Guided Imagery

The technique of Interactive Guided Imagery is based on the belief that insight and knowledge are the keys to relief of symptoms. One aspect of this therapy encourages the patient to create and explore an image that represents the symptom or illness. For example, a trained guide asks the patient to allow a mental image to form that represents the neck pain. A dialogue is then begun between the patient and the image for the purpose of gaining insight into and understanding of the symptom and what the image representing the symptom may "need." The imagery acts as a bridge of communication between the conscious and unconscious mind (see Chapter 92, Guided Imagery and Interactive Guided Imagery).

Relaxation Exercises

Relaxation exercises, such as breathing techniques and progressive muscle relaxation, can be beneficial in helping to reduce sympathetic stimulation that can result in muscle tension and pain. Biofeedback from sensors placed over the trapezius muscle can help to promote relaxation. A small study of elderly patients with trapezius pain showed a 70% reduction in pain with biofeedback-assisted relaxation.[14] The limitation of relaxation is that it often provides only temporary relief. It is a beneficial tool that can empower the patient to control or eliminate neck pain or tension in the neck. It is more beneficial if one of the therapies discussed is used in conjunction with a technique that addresses underlying emotional triggers (see Chapter 91, Prescribing Relaxation Techniques).

Energy Therapies

Acupuncture

The principle that energy flows through or over the surface of the body is common to a number of healing systems used worldwide. Acupuncture and various forms of hands-on healing are frequently enlisted in the treatment of numerous disorders, including neck pain. According to these modalities, the neck is an area of significant energy flow; consequently, it can also be an area of significant pathology. In several Asian healing traditions, the throat chakra, which extends anteriorly and posteriorly relative to the neck at the level of the thyroid, is one of the seven main energy centers of the body.[15] Facilitation of healthy energy flow to the chakras is a fundamental aspect of many Eastern religious and healing traditions. In acupuncture, which is based on the idea that the body contains a number of energy channels, or meridians, needles may be inserted in more than 350 major points to improve the flow of energy (known as *qi*). Many of these points are located within, or in close proximity to, the neck.[16, 17]

At present, acupuncture is one of the best-studied forms of energy healing. Used for over 3000 years in China, it has been popular in the Western world for only a few decades. Nevertheless, more than 1 million Americans use acupuncture,[18] and greater than 5% of British general practitioners now incorporate some form of acupuncture into clinical practice.[19] Given that acupuncture is relatively safe when done by a trained practitioner,[8] it is certainly a modality worth considering if there are no contraindications[20] (Table 53–2).

One of the most thorough, evidence-based reviews of acupuncture published to date was released by the National Institutes of Health (NIH)

Table 53–2. Safety Considerations in Recommending Acupuncture

- Contraindications to acupuncture[11]
  Pregnancy
  Blood-borne viral illness
  Bleeding disorders
  Skin infections
  Pacemakers
  Cardiac arrhythmias
  Epilepsy (only electroacupuncture is contraindicated)
- Complications: Only 50 cases of severe complications were noted in the United States in a 20-year period. Most of these, such as pneumothorax and migration of broken needle fragments under the skin, can be avoided when practitioners are well trained. In the neck, the carotid arteries in particular must be carefully avoided.[8]
- Referrals should be only to board-certified or licensed acupuncturists.

in 1997.[21] The NIH Acupuncture Consensus Data Panel concluded:

"Promising results have emerged, for example, showing efficacy of acupuncture in adult postoperative and chemotherapy nausea and vomiting and in postoperative dental pain. There are other situations such as addiction, stroke rehabilitation, headache, menstrual cramps, tennis elbow, fibromyalgia, myofascial pain, osteoarthritis, low back pain, carpal tunnel syndrome, and asthma, in which acupuncture may be useful as an adjunct treatment or an acceptable alternative or be included in a comprehensive management program."[21]

A recent review of the use of acupuncture for the treatment of rheumatic conditions evaluated the results of 8 studies of osteoarthritis and 3 of fibromyalgia. It concluded that, although definitive evidence from large scale randomized controlled trials is still needed, ". . . there is moderately strong evidence from controlled trials to support the use of acupuncture as adjunctive therapy for both osteoarthritis and fibromyalgia."[22]

Evaluations of the use of acupuncture as a treatment for neck pain in general, rather than for specific disorders that may or may not cause neck pain, are somewhat less conclusive. Although several studies show some indication of benefit, there remains significant debate regarding these studies' quality, their use of adequate control groups, and what they show about acupuncture's utility relative to other neck pain treatments. Table 53–3 summarizes several recent studies that focus on acupuncture specifically for neck pain treatment.[23–29]

Although additional research would certainly be useful, it is important to bear in mind, as Mayer notes, that "[the] absence of evidence is not evidence of its absence."[53] Acupuncture is as well studied or even better studied than many of the treatments physicians most commonly use, such as rest, exercise, or pain medications, the benefits of which have also been questioned.[30] The available evidence suggests that acupuncture is worthy of consideration as an adjunct to other neck pain treatments.

Reiki and Therapeutic Touch

Other energy therapies, such as Reiki and therapeutic touch, have not yet been as thoroughly evaluated in randomized controlled trials as acupuncture has been. A 1998 study published in the *Journal of the American Medical Association* gained attention by claiming that "the claims of therapeutic touch are groundless and . . . further professional use is unjustified."[31] Evaluators made this claim after they found that a group of 21 practitioners were unable to detect the presence of the subjects' "energy fields" behind a barrier that served to obscure the healers' view. The methodology used and manner in which the experiments drew such sweeping conclusions regarding therapeutic touch are of questionable value.

Table 53–3. A Review of the Literature on Acupuncture for Neck Pain

Study	Study Characteristics	Conclusion(s)
White and Ernst[23]	Systematic literature review: 14 randomized controlled trials, 8 rated of "high quality."	"Overall, the outcomes . . . were equally balanced between positive and negative. Needle acupuncture was not superior to indistinguishable sham control in four out of five studies. Of the eight high quality trials, five were negative [not supportive of acupuncture] . . . In conclusion, the hypothesis that acupuncture is efficacious in the treatment of neck pain is not based on the available evidence from sound clinical trials. Further studies are justified."
Smith et al[24]	13 randomized controlled trials met inclusion criteria.	"With acupuncture for chronic back and neck pain, we found that the most valid trials tended to be negative. There is no convincing evidence for the analgesic efficacy of acupuncture for back or neck pain." (See the article by Cummings[25] for a response from the acupuncture literature to this article.)
Giles and Muller[26]	Australian study of 77 people comparing acupuncture, medications, and spinal manipulation for neck pain management.	"After a median intervention period of 30 days, spinal manipulation was the only intervention that achieved statistically significant improvements . . ."
Irnich et al[27]	177 patients aged 18 to 85 years; either acupuncture, massage, or sham acupuncture was used.	"Acupuncture is an effective short-term treatment for patients with chronic neck pain, but there is only limited evidence for long-term effects after five treatments." Acupuncture improved pain scores related to range of motion and cervical mobility.
David et al[28]	70 adults with pain for >6 weeks; either physical therapy or acupuncture was used.	"Both acupuncture and physiotherapy are effective forms of treatment. Since an untreated control group was not part of the study design, the magnitude of this improvement cannot be quantified."
Birch and Jamison[29]	46 patients; Japanese acupuncture, sham acupuncture, or NSAID therapy was used.	"Relevant [not sham] acupuncture with heat contributes to modest pain reduction in persons with myofascial neck pain." Difference in "real" versus "sham" acupuncture was statistically significant ($P < .05$).
Ross et al[19]	32 patients; minimal acupuncture was used.	"Minimal acupuncture may be an effective treatment for neck pain and further definitive studies are recommended." $P < .001$ for resolution of pain 3 months after treatment, according to questionnaire results.

A number of articles in the nursing literature have begun to evaluate therapeutic touch, particularly for cancer treatment. Some of the results thus far have indicated that therapeutic touch may be helpful. At this point it may only be said that, although these forms of energy healing have not been studied extensively in clinical trials, such therapies may have utility. Because they are unlikely to have adverse effects, such modalities are worthy of consideration as adjuncts to other neck pain treatment methods.

Manual Therapies

Manual therapies have been used in China for more than two millennia, and they were strongly advocated by Hippocrates in his treatise "On Joints."[32] There are four main categories of manual therapy: manipulation, mobilization, massage, and neuromuscular therapies.[33] Most manual therapy practitioners incorporate several combinations of these during treatment. *Manipulation* involves using passive maneuvers that direct force through various articulations, especially in the vertebral column. *Mobilization*, in contrast, does not involve thrust; rather, it enlists passive oscillatory movements or sustained stretching based on patient feedback.

Massage therapy focuses on manipulation of the soft tissues. *Neuromuscular therapies* take two forms: Muscle energy techniques use muscle contraction against counterforces (isometrics), whereas proprioceptive neuromuscular facilitation uses manual contact to teach the patient to improve the overall dexterity and strength of muscle movements. Most of the manual therapy research done thus far has focused on the manipulative therapies, although some studies of mobilization also exist.

Chiropractic

Chiropractic primarily involves manipulation techniques. In fact, this technique had its start with the manipulation of the cervical spine when Daniel David Palmer manipulated a janitor's neck to cure his deafness in 1895.[34] After battling with the medical community through much of the early twentieth century, chiropractic ultimately gained a widespread following. By 1975, all 50 states had licensure programs, and chiropractic was covered by Medicare and worker's compensation plans. Chiropractic holds that subluxations, or malalignments of the joints, lead to pathology. Neck pain is one of the most common complaints treated by chiropractors.

Osteopathic Manual Therapy

Like chiropractic, osteopathic medicine also involves the use of spinal manipulations. In addition, it enlists several other manual therapies as well[35] (Table 53–4).

Osteopathy was founded in 1874 by Andrew Taylor Still, M.D.[36] Concerned about the limits he observed to be associated with the allopathic medicine practiced at the time, Still developed a number of manual therapy techniques. Osteopathic practitioners commonly use these techniques as adjuncts to conventional medical treatments to aid the body in healing itself. As of 1999, there were nearly 42,000 doctors of osteopathic medicine in the United States, but only a minority practice osteopathic manual therapy (OMT).[27]

Overall, manipulative therapies have an excellent safety record in the treatment of neck pain, provided that they are performed by qualified practitioners. Bronfort and associates evaluated numerous studies involving 2600 patients who received manipulative therapies and found that no serious complications arose.[37] In 1925 to 1993, only 185 cases of adverse effects of manipulation were noted in the literature worldwide.[34] The most common adverse effects with use of high-velocity, low-amplitude manipulation were stroke (66%), disk herniation (12%), and pathologic fracture (8%). Negative outcomes can be avoided if the contraindications listed in Table 53–5 are ruled out before treatment is initiated.[38]

In general, findings regarding the utility of manual therapies for the treatment of neck pain have been quite favorable. A meta-analysis of 24 randomized controlled trials evaluating conservative treatments for adult mechanical neck disorders concluded: "Within the limits of methodologic quality, the best available evidence supports the use of manual therapies in combination with other treatments for short-term relief of neck pain."[39]

Table 53–4. Types of Manual Therapies

- High-velocity, low-amplitude (HVLA) manipulation: Similar to chiropractic but involves moving joints only within their usual physiologic ranges of motion.
- Muscle energy techniques: These enlist repeated isometric contractions with passive range of motion to increase joint mobilization or to lengthen contracted muscles. Can be used when HVLA manipulation is contraindicated.
- Strain-counterstrain: Symptomatic myofascial trigger points are identified. The muscle involved is placed in a position of shortening that inhibits the neuromuscular reflex of spasm resulting in relaxation and pain relief (see Chapter 99, Strain and Counterstrain Manipulation Technique).
- Myofascial release: Similar to deep massage but guided by areas of muscle spasm.
- Lymphatic pump techniques: These involve physical measures to facilitate lymphatic return from the extremities. Not to be used with metastatic cancer or active tuberculosis.
- Cranial osteopathy: Often practiced as a separate form of manipulative therapy by non-osteopaths (craniosacral therapy); involves sensing and adjusting the rate and amplitude of subtle oscillations of the cranial bones.

A literature review by Kjellman and coauthors[40] that focused on 27 randomized clinical trials concluded that for the 18 of the investigations that were of "high methodological quality," manipulation, active physiotherapy, and electromagnetic therapy were "effective for pain, range of motion, and activities of daily living." In contrast, a 1991 Dutch study concluded on the basis of 35 randomized trials that results were "promising" but that the efficacy of manipulation had thus far not been shown.[41] In a 1999 review, Gross and colleagues[42] also noted: "No evidence of benefit exists for manipulation or mobilization alone or over one [treatment] session. More robust design/methodology are needed." The results of some other trials[43–45] are summarized in Table 53–6.

Two techniques that primary care practitioners can incorporate into clinical practice for manual therapy of neck pain are *strain-counterstrain* and a cranial technique called *cranial base release*. Strain-counterstrain is helpful in relieving trigger points and muscle spasm of the neck (see Chapter 99, Strain and Counterstrain Manipulation Technique). The cranial base release technique (see box next page) is beneficial for patients with suboccipital neuralgia and tension headaches, which are often the result of cervical muscle tension. Identifying a beneficial effect with use of these therapies will help both diagnostically and therapeutically. These techniques constitute a small part of a very complex field of therapy of proven benefit, and appropriate referral is indicated for challenging cases.

NOTE

Chronic narcotic administration down-regulates endorphin receptors, which are partially responsible for the pain relief obtained with many mind-body therapies such as hypnosis and guided imagery. Chronic narcotic use can impede the symptom relief that comes from these therapies.

Overall, evidence-based practice appears to favor the use of manipulative manual therapies. However,

Table 53–5. Contraindications to Manipulation of the Neck[34, 37]

- Infection
- Unstable odontoid peg
- Carotid or vertebrobasilar disease
- Rheumatoid arthritis of the cervical spine
- Osteopenia
- History of pathologic fractures
- Ligament rupture and instability
- Aneurysm
- Postsurgical neck joints
- Anticoagulation therapy
- Metastatic carcinoma
- Bone tumor

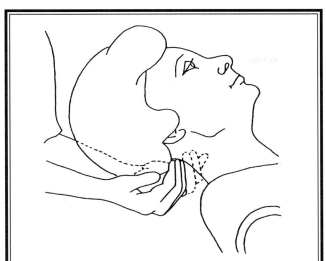

Hand positions for cranial base release. (From Chaitow L. Cranial Manipulation Theory and Practice: Osseous and Soft Tissue Approaches. New York, Churchill Livingstone, 1999, p 119.)

- *The patient is supine and the practitioner should be seated at the head of the bed with the arms resting on and supported by the table.*
- *The dorsum of the practitioner's hand rests on the table with the fingertips pointing upward at the base of the occiput into the suboccipital sulcus.*
- *The practitioner's fingertips act as a fulcrum on which the patient rests the occiput so that the back of the skull is resting on the practitioner's palms. The patient allows the head to lie heavily so that the pressure induces tissue release against the fingertips.*
- *As relaxation proceeds and the practitioner's finger pads sink deeper into the soft tissues, gentle cephalic traction is applied with the fingertips for a few minutes. This movement will allow the arch of the atlas to disengage from the occiput. Cephalic traction should be started a few minutes into the technique to allow for relaxation.*
- *This "release" of deep structures of the upper neck reduces tension and improves drainage and circulation to the head, helping to reduce intracranial congestion.[46]*

few controlled studies have concluded that such treatments should be used alone. Like acupuncture, they are useful adjuncts to a multifaceted treatment approach.

Pharmaceuticals

Antidepressants

Tricyclic antidepressants have been found to be a valuable group of agents for reducing the severity of chronic pain through modulation of descending and ascending antinociceptive pathways in the spinal cord and brain. They also help to balance the neurotransmitters serotonin and norepinephrine, which can be affected by emotions that play a role in pain severity. Therapy with a tricyclic antidepressant is the gold standard, but if a patient is unable to tolerate the characteristic anticholinergic side effects, fluoxetine (Prozac) has also been found to be beneficial.[47] Giving a tricyclic antidepressant each evening before bed for 2 to 3 weeks can of value in helping to reduce pain while the clinician also addresses the root of the condition. These sedating antidepressants will also help to improve sleep patterns and are very effective in reducing recurring tension headaches, which may be brought on by cervical muscle tension.

Dosage:
- Amitriptyline (Elavil): available as 10-, 25-, 50-, 75-, 100-, and 150-mg tablets.
- Nortriptyline (Pamelor): available as 10-, 25-, 50-, and 75-mg capsules.

Therapy can start with 10 to 25 mg in the evening; this dose can be increased by 25 mg every 3 or 4 days to 75 to 150 mg, until analgesia is obtained or side effects occur. Many patients will do well with 10 to 25 mg each day. Nortriptyline has fewer anticholinergic side effects.

- Fluoxetine (Prozac): available as 10-, 20-, and 40-mg capsules and a 20 mg/5 mL solution.

Table 53–6. Efficacy of Manual Therapies: Summary of Key Studies

Study	Description	Findings/Comments
Jordan et al[43]	119 patients with neck pain >3 months, randomized prospective study	No clinical differences among manipulative therapy, physiotherapy, or manipulation; all three resulted in meaningful improvement, but no control group was available to show that the benefit was not due just to healing over time.
McMorland and Suter[44]	119 patients at a Canadian chiropractic clinic	Significant improvements based on pain indices and visual analogue pain scales were noted in the neck pain group, but the study recognizes problems related to not having a control group.
Cassidy et al[45]	100 consecutive clinic outpatients; half treated with manipulation, half with mobilization	The study found that " . . . a single manipulation is more effective than mobilization in decreasing pain in patients with mechanical neck pain. Both treatments increase range of motion in the neck to a similar degree. Further studies are required to determine any long-term benefits of manipulation for mechanical neck pain."[45]

Therapy can start with 10 to 20 mg each morning. This dose can be increased by 10 mg weekly to no more than 60 mg if needed.

Precautions. Anticholinergic side effects of tricyclic medications include sedation, confusion, hallucinations, dry mouth, urinary retention, orthostatic hypotension, and weight gain. If doses greater than 50 mg are used for prolonged periods, serum levels should be checked. The therapeutic range for amitriptyline and nortriptyline is 150 to 300 ng/mL. With these drugs, the dose should be gradually tapered when therapy is discontinued.

Fluoxetine is more stimulating and thus should be given in the morning because it can cause insomnia. Its long half-life (7 to 9 days) warrants caution when this drug is used in the elderly.

Muscle Relaxants

Muscle relaxants have been found to be helpful for the short-term treatment of neck pain. Their chronic use should be avoided. One muscle relaxant, cyclobenzaprine (Flexeril), is pharmacologically related to tricyclic antidepressants. Although it shares the side effects of this class of medications, it can also successfully relieve pain while helping to resolve muscle spasm and tension. In treating another painful condition, fibromyalgia, a dose of 10 mg at bedtime was found to be as effective as the usual dose of 10 mg 3 times a day for pain relief while reducing side effects.[48] Using this medication each night for 2 to 3 weeks can be a useful alternative to antidepressant therapy as discussed.

Dosage. Cyclobenzaprine (Flexeril): available as 10-mg tablets. The dose is 10 mg each night at bedtime.

Precautions. Cyclobenzaprine has anticholinergic side effects including drowsiness, ataxia, dry mouth, and urinary retention. In some persons it can cause anxiety, insomnia, and restlessness. It should not be given in conjunction with amitriptyline and nortriptyline, because they are similar medications.

Nonsteroidal Anti-Inflammatory Drugs

NSAIDs constitute good example of a useful but potentially toxic class of medications. The newer COX-2 inhibitors such as celecoxib (Celebrex) and rofecoxib (Vioxx) may provide similar benefit with fewer gastrointestinal side effects. They work by blocking the production of inflammatory prostaglandins (mainly PGE_2) from arachidonic acid. NSAIDs should be used for short-term treatment of neck pain. Although side effects may differ, no one NSAID has been found to be more effective than another.[49]

Dosage:
- Ibuprofen (Motrin, Advil): available as 200-mg tablets (over the counter [OTC]) and as 400-, 600-,

and 800-mg tablets. The dose is 400 to 600 mg with food every 6 hours or as needed.
- Naproxen sodium (Aleve, Naprosyn): available as 220-mg tablets (OTC) and as 250-, 375-, and 500-mg tablets. The dose is 220 to 500 mg twice daily with food.
- COX-2 inhibitors
- Celecoxib (Celebrex): available as 100- and 200-mg capsules. The dose is 100 to 400 mg twice daily with food.
- Rofecoxib (Vioxx): available as 12.5-, 25-, and 50-mg tablets. The dose is 12.5 to 50 mg daily.

Precautions:. All COX-2 inhibitors can cause renal dysfunction, fluid retention, and central nervous system side effects. Caution is indicated when these drugs are given with warfarin. First-generation NSAIDs (ibuprofen, naproxen) can cause gastrointestinal ulceration and bleeding. These drugs should be used cautiously in patients with liver disease.

Narcotics

Short-term narcotic use is warranted for palliative treatment of severe pain. Because these drugs work by masking the severity of pain, a complete understanding of the biopsychosocial-spiritual influences of pain should be explored before the patient is placed on long-term therapy. The body expresses symptoms to ask for a change, whether in a life style habit, a repetitive strain pattern, or an emotional issue. If the symptom is simply masked with narcotics without addressing underlying factors that can result in health and resolution of symptoms, the patient is denied the opportunity to identify and implement an often much-needed change.

Dosage:
- Hydrocodone/acetaminophen (Vicodin, others): available as 5/500-mg tablets. The dose is 1 or 2 tablets every 4 to 6 hours as needed for pain.
- Codeine/acetaminophen (Tylenol No. 3 [30/300 mg], Tylenol No. 4 [60/300 mg]). The dose is 1 or 2 tablets every 4 hours as needed for pain.

Precautions. Narcotics can cause drowsiness and sedation that can be deepened by other sedating medications and alcohol. Constipation is common with prolonged use.

Botanicals

Few studies have focused specifically on the role of herbal remedies in treating musculoskeletal neck pain. However, a number of trials have evaluated the overall anti-inflammatory properties of these preparations. A review of the effects of several "phyto-anti-inflammatories" summarized the findings of 19 randomized, double-blind, placebo-controlled trials. Six botanicals in particular were found to be useful in treating inflammation associated with various rheumatic diseases.[50] Because these herbal remedies have been found to inhibit either the cyclo-oxygenase or lipoxygenase pathway, or both, a role for these remedies similar to that for pharmaceutical anti-inflammatory agents in the treatment of neck pain can be postulated. Active ingredients common to several of these herbs include gamma-linolenic acid (GLA) and alpha-linolenic acid (ALA). The review concluded:

"Herbal drugs certainly cannot compete with synthetic drugs in severe cases of pain, especially if immediate pain relief is required. For mild to moderate chronic pain, however, phyto-anti-inflammatory drugs could be tried with or even as a replacement for NSAIDs with a view to minimizing NSAID use and adverse effects."[23]

The following remedies have been found to be most useful for decreasing inflammation.

Borage Oil and Black Currant Seed Oil

Oils from borage (*Boragio officinalis*) and the seeds of the black currant (*Ribes nigrum*) are rich in GLA. They help to limit inflammation by promoting the production of less inflammatory prostaglandins (PGE$_1$). Borage oil has a higher percentage of GLA (24%) compared with black currant oil (19%), which makes it a better choice.

Dosage. For both oils: 1 g once or twice daily with meals.

Precautions. GLA can prolong bleeding time. To avoid this toxic chemical, use of products labeled "pyrrolizidine alkaloid–free" is recommended. GLA is a component of omega-6 oil and also increases arachidonic acid. A safer long-term approach may be use of an omega-3–rich product such as fish oil or flaxseed oil (see Chapter 84, The Anti-Inflammatory Diet).

Willow Bark

The bark of the willow (*Salicis cortex*) contains salicylates, flavonoids, and tannins. Its anti-inflammatory effect is largely related to its salicylate content.

Dosage. 1 to 3 g 3 or 4 times daily.

Precautions. Although limited side effects have been reported, the potential for aspirin-type side effects, including gastritis, renal irritation, and platelet inhibition, should be kept in mind.

Phytodolor

Phytodolor is a commercial mixture of the botanicals aspen (*Populus tremula*), common ash (*Fraxinus excelsior*), and goldenrod (*Solidago virgarea*). This preparation is rich in salicylates and has been found to reduce pain and NSAID dosage. Because it is a liquid, it may be useful in persons who have difficulty swallowing.

Dosage. 30 to 40 drops three times daily in water or other beverage. Phytodolor should be given for 2 to 4 weeks for full therapeutic benefit.

Stinging Nettle

Although further research is needed, stinging nettle (*Urtica dioca*) has therapeutic potential because it not only inhibits the cyclo-oxygenase and lipoxygenase pathways but also suppresses the release of inflammatory cytokines.

Dosage. The aerial parts of the plant are used. Dried extract (7:1): 770 mg twice a day; tincture (1:5 in 25% alcohol): 2 to 6 mL three times a day.

Precautions. This botanical can cause diarrhea. The root of the plant is not used, as the aboveground parts have been found to be more effective for control of inflammation.

Devil's Claw

Devil's claw (*Harpagophytum procumbens*) is another botanical that may be of benefit.

Dosage. 4.5 g of the root daily.

Precautions. This herbal may worsen gastric acidity. It also can have a hypoglycemic effect.

Surgery

Anterior diskectomy has been found to decrease pain and improve function even in patients whose chronic neck pain was not secondary to pathologic processes involving one or more nerve roots or the spinal cord.[51] However, cervical spine surgery is a therapeutic modality that should be used only when absolutely needed. There are risks of significant complications. Table 53–7 lists some of the major indications for surgery. In summary, surgery should be considered only when severe neurologic symptoms persist despite other, more conservative therapeutic efforts, or when imaging conclusively proves that no other alternative will be effective.

Table 53–7. Indications for Surgical Interventions for Neck Pain[1, 52]

- Radiculopathy: Symptoms are known to be associated with nerve root pathology.
- Myelopathy: A slowly progressive spinal cord syndrome is noted, beginning with symptoms in the legs (peripheral aspects of the spinal cord) and later progressing to the arms (more central spinal cord pathways).
- Neurologic deficits are not improved using other forms of treatment. Severe sensory deficits or muscle atrophy and weakness are present.
- Diagnostic imaging reveals an operable condition (e.g., tumor).

THERAPEUTIC REVIEW

Lifestyle adjustments
- Regular exercises, including those used in the Alexander technique, Feldenkrais, and Pilates therapy, can increase cervical muscle support.
- The normal lordotic curve of the neck should be preserved during sleep. Use of cervical spine pillows may help.
- Activities involving repetitive strain (holding the telephone on the shoulder, leaning over a desk, carrying heavy over-the-shoulder bags, looking over the shoulder) should be avoided.
- Reduction of chronic stress is indicated; psychologic causes of neck pain, such as depression and anxiety, should be identified.

Pharmaceuticals
- For chronic pain, a tricyclic antidepressant such as amitriptyline 10 to 25 mg can be given at night or an SSRI such as fluoxetine 10 to 20 mg can be given in the morning. These doses may be gradually titrated upward as needed.
- Use of a "muscle relaxant" for 2 to 3 weeks may be considered. Cyclobenzaprine 10 mg at bedtime is a reasonable choice if the patient is not already taking a tricyclic antidepressant.
- An NSAID such as ibuprofen 400 to 600 mg can be given every 6 hours with food.
- Short-term use of narcotics may be indicated for severe pain. The combination of hydrocodone and acetaminophen, 5/500 mg tablets, can be given in a dose of 1 or 2 every 4 to 6 hours as needed.

Manual therapies
- There is evidence that manipulative therapies (chiropractic and osteopathic) are of benefit.
- Cranial base release and strain-counterstrain are useful techniques that can be easily performed in the office environment.

Mind-body therapies
- Underlying emotional issues that may be causing or exacerbating pain and spasm should be addressed.
- Journaling, self-hypnosis, biofeedback-assisted relaxation, and guided imagery are all potentially useful techniques.

Energy therapies
- Acupuncture is a well-studied, potentially beneficial, and safe adjunctive treatment if performed by a trained professional.
- Therapeutic touch and other hands-on healing techniques are of potential benefit, though this is not yet clinically proved.

Nutrition
- Intake of foods high in omega-3 fatty acids (cold water fish, flaxseed products, nuts, green leafy vegetables) should be increased. Supplementation with 1 to 4 grams a day of omega-3–rich oil capsules can help to reduce inflammation.
- Foods rich in omega-6 and trans fatty acids (hydrogenated vegetable oils, margarine, processed foods) should be avoided.
- Consumption of saturated fat should be curtailed.
- Foods rich in antioxidants, including fruits and vegetables in a variety of colors, should be encouraged.

Botanicals
- If the patient is unable to tolerate NSAIDs or needs to reduce NSAID dosage, one of the following botanical products may be added:
  Borage oil, 1 g once or twice daily with meals.
  Willow bark, 1 to 3 g 3 or 4 times daily.
  Phytodolor, 30 to 40 drops in water 3 times daily.

Surgery
- Surgery is last resort, except when there is a known pathologic process involving nerve roots or the spinal cord that is surgically treatable.

References

1. Nakano KK: Neck pain. In Ruddy S, Harris ED, Sledge CB (eds): Kelley's Textbook of Rheumatology, 6th ed. Philadelphia, WB Saunders, 2001, pp 457–474.
2. Goroll: Evaluation of neck pain. In Goroll AH (ed): Primary Care Medicine. Philadelphia, Lippincott Williams & Wilkins, 2000, pp 844–847.
3. Squires B, Gargan MF, Bannister GC: Soft-tissue injuries of the cervical spine: 15 year follow-up. J Bone Joint Surg Br 78:955, 1996.
3a. Noble J, Greene HL 2nd, Levinson W, et al (eds): Textbook of Primary Care Medicine, 3rd ed. Philadelphia, Mosby, 2001.
4. Palmer KT, Walker-Bone K, Griffin MJ, et al: Prevalence and occupational associations of neck pain in the British population. Scand J Work Environ Health 27:49–56, 2001.
5. Linton SJ: A review of psychological risk factors in back and neck pain. Spine 25:1148–1156, 2000.
6. Maes M, Christophe A, Bosmans E, et al: In humans, serum polyunsaturated fatty acid levels predict the response of proinflammatory cytokines to psychologic stress. Biol Psychiatry 47:910–920, 2000.
7. James MJ, Gibson RA, Cleland LG: Dietary polyunsaturated fatty acids and inflammatory mediator production. Am J Clin Nutr 71(1 Suppl):343S–348S, 2000.
8. Fatty acids, antioxidants may help "tennis elbow." Reuters Health, April 26, 2000. Available at www.reutershealth.com
9. Jensen MC, Brant-Zawadzki MN, Obuchowski N, et al: Magnetic resonance imaging of the lumbar spine in people without back pain. N Engl J Med 331:69–73, 1994.
10. Carragee EJ, Paragioudakis SJ, Khurana S: 2000 Volvo Award winner in clinical studies: Lumbar high-intensity zone and discography in subjects without low back problems. Spine 25:2987–2992, 2000.
11. Sarno JE: Healing Back Pain: The Mind-Body Connection. New York, Warner Books, 1991.
12. Smyth JM, Stone AA, Hurewitz A, Kaell A: Effects of writing about stressful experiences on symptom reduction in patients with asthma or rheumatoid arthritis. JAMA 281:1304–1309, 1999.
13. Lu DP, Lu GP, Kleinman L: Acupuncture and clinical hypnosis for facial and head and neck pain: A single crossover comparison. Am J Clin Hypn 44:141–148, 2001.
14. Middaugh SJ, Woods SE, Kee WG, et al: Biofeedback-assisted relaxation training for the aging chronic pain patient. Biofeedback Self Regul 16:361–377, 1991.
15. Schumacher S, Woerner G (eds): The Encyclopedia of Eastern Philosophy and Religion. Boston, Shambala, 1989.
16. Kaptchuk TJ: The Web That Has No Weaver: Understanding Chinese Medicine. New York, Congdon and Weed, 1983.
17. Lyte CD: An Overview of Acupuncture. Washington, DC, U.S. Department of Health and Human Services, Health Sciences Branch, Division of Life Sciences, Office of Science and Technology, Center for Devices and Radiological Health, Food and Drug Administration, 1993.
18. Nesson R, Coan R: Safety Record of Licensed, Certified, or Registered Acupuncturists. Washington, DC, National Acupuncture Foundation, 1998.
19. Ross J, White A, Ernst E: Western, minimal acupuncture for neck pain: A cohort study. Acupunct Med 17:5–8, 1999.
20. Lewith G, Kenyon J, Lewis P: Complementary Medicine: An Integrated Approach. New York, Oxford University Press, 1996.
21. Acupuncture. NIH Consensus Statement. 15:1–34, 1997.
22. Berman BM, Swyers JP, Ezzo, J: The evidence for acupuncture as a treatment for rheumatologic conditions. Rheum Dis Clin North Am 26:103–116, 2000.
23. White AR, Ernst E: A systematic review of randomized controlled trials of acupuncture for neck pain. Rheumatology 38:143–147, 1999.
24. Smith LA, et al: Teasing apart quality and validity in systematic reviews: An example from acupuncture trials in chronic neck and back pain. Pain 86:119–132, 2000.
25. Cummings M: Teasing apart the quality and validity in systematic reviews of acupuncture. Acupunct Med, December 1, 2000.
26. Giles LG, Muller R: Chronic spinal pain syndromes: A clinical pilot trial comparing acupuncture, a nonsteroidal anti-inflammatory drug, and spinal manipulation. J Manipulative Physiol Ther 22:376–381, 1999.
27. Irnich D, et al: Randomised trial of acupuncture compared with conventional massage and "sham" laser acupuncture for treatment of chronic neck pain. BMJ 322:1574–1578, 2001.
28. David J, et al: Chronic neck pain: A comparison of acupuncture treatment and physiotherapy. Br J Rheumatol 37:1118–1122, 1998.
29. Birch S, Jamison RN: Controlled trial of Japanese acupuncture for chronic myofascial neck pain: Assessment of specific and nonspecific effects of treatment. Clin J Pain 14:248–255, 1998.
30. Aker PD, et al: Conservative management of mechanical neck pain: systematic overview and meta-analysis. BMJ 313:1291–1296, 1996.
31. Rosa L, et al: A close look at therapeutic touch. JAMA 279:1005–1010, 1998.
32. Anderson R: Spinal manipulation before chiropractic. In Haldeman S (ed): Principles and Practice of Chiropractic, 2nd ed. San Mateo, Calif, Appleton & Lange, 1992, pp 3–14.
33. Gross AR, Aker PD, Quartly C: Manual therapy in the treatment of neck pain. Rheum Dis Clin North Am, 22:579–598, 1996.
34. Hadler NM: Chiropractic. Rheum Dis Clin North Am 26:97–101, 19.
35. Lesho EP: An overview of osteopathic medicine. Arch Fam Med 8, 1999.
36. Still AT: Osteopathy: Research and Practice. Seattle, Eastland Press, 1992.
37. Bronfort G, Haas M, Bouter LM, et al: Efficacy of spinal manipulation and mobilization for low back and neck pain: A systematic review and best evidence synthesis. In Bronfort G (ed): Efficacy of Manual Therapies of the Spine. Amsterdam, EMGO Institute, 1997.
38. Vickers A, Zollman C: ABC of complementary medicine. The manipulative therapies: Osteopathy and chiropractic. BMJ 319:1176–1179, 1999.
39. Aker PD, Gross AR, Goldsmith CH, Peloso P: Conservative management of mechanical neck pain: Systematic overview and meta-analysis. BMJ 313:1291–1296, 1996.
40. Kjellman GV, Skargren EI, Oberg BE: A critical analysis of randomized clinical trials on neck pain and treatment efficacy: A review of the literature. Scand J Rehabil Med. 31:139–152, 1999.
41. Koes BW, et al: Spinal manipulation and mobilization for back and neck pain: Blinded review. BMJ 303:1298–1303, 1991.
42. Gross A, Kay T, Hondras M, Goldsmith C: Manual therapy for neck disorders. Abst Book Cochrane Colloq 7:50, 1999.
43. Jordan A, et al: Intensive training, physiotherapy, or manipulation for patients with chronic neck pain: A prospective single blinded randomized clinical trial. Spine 23:311–318, 1998.
44. McMorland G, Suter E: Chiropractic management of mechanical neck and low-back pain: A retrospective outcome-based analysis. J Manipulative Physiol Ther. 23:307–311, 2000.
45. Cassidy JD, Lopes AA, Yong-Hing K: The immediate effect of manipulation versus mobilization on pain and range of motion in the cervical spine: A randomized controlled trial. J Manipulative Physiol Ther 16:279–280, 1993.
46. Chaitow L: Cranial Manipulation Theory and Practice: Osseous and Soft Tissue Approaches. Edinburgh, Churchill Livingstone, 1999, pp 113–114.
47. Schreiber S, Vinokur S, Shavelzon V, et al: A randomized trial of fluoxetine versus amitriptyline in musculo-skeletal pain. Isr J Psychiatry Relat Sci 38:88–94, 2001.
48. Santandrea S, Montrone F, Sarzi-Puttini P, et al: A double-blind crossover study of two cyclobenzaprine regimens in primary fibromyalgia syndrome. J Int Med Res 21:74–80, 1993.
49. Tulder MW, van Scholten RJPM, Koes BW, Deyo RA: Nonsteroidal anti-inflammatory drugs for low back pain. Cochrane Back Group. Cochrane Database syst rev 3, 2001.
50. Ernst E, Chrubasik S: Phyto-anti-inflammatories: A systematic review of randomized, placebo-controlled, double-blind trials. Rheum Dis Clin North Am 26:13–27, 2000.
51. Palit M, et al: Anterior discectomy and fusion for the management of neck pain. Spine 24:2224–2228.
52. Jacchia GE, Innocenti M, Pavolini B, et al: Indications and results of surgical treatment of cervical disc disease by anterior and posterior approach. Chir Organi Mov 77:111, 1992.
53. Mayer DJ: Acupuncture: an evidence-based review of the clinical literature. Annu Rev Med 51:49-63, 2000.

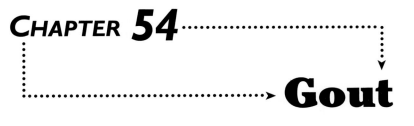

CHAPTER 54

Gout

Phillip C. DeMio, M.D.

PATHOPHYSIOLOGY

Gout is a metabolic disorder with clinical manifestations in synovial tissues (mostly joints) as well as in the kidney, with the well-known presentation of a sudden, acute, severely painful arthritis. Crystallization of uric acid in tissues is the pathophysiologic mechanism and occurs as a cumulative result of long-standing hyperuricemia, which is present in about 8% of ambulatory patients. Macroscopic crystals (tophi) slowly form during asymptomatic periods, resulting in excess tissue stores of uric acid.[1]

The joint and kidney manifestations of hyperuricemia are preventable (like other disorders such as coronary artery disease and osteoporosis). Patients should therefore be screened, when possible, for their risk of gout and urate nephropathy. In addition to prevention, accurate diagnosis at the acute presentation of gouty arthritis is of obvious importance. The needle-like microcrystals can be shed acutely from macrocrystals or may form in the nascent state to give the intense foreign body reaction with resultant acute pain and joint destruction so familiar to clinicians and patients.

Definition

Gout is here defined as an acute arthritis from uric acid crystals. Elsewhere in the literature, the term *gout* may refer to any crystalline arthropathy, whether due to urate, oxalate, pyrophosphate, or other substrates.[2]

Metabolism

Urate (uric acid) is a metabolic waste product of purine metabolism. Purines are present in about half of the genetic material, DNA and RNA (messenger, transfer, and ribosomal types); in intermediates for energy transfer, adenosine triphosphate (ATP) and guanosine triphosphate (GTP); and in second messengers such as cyclic adenosine monophosphate (cAMP). Purines also figure in one-carbon metabolism (as in *S*-adenosylmethionine) and in many other biochemical functions. Not surprisingly, metabolic pathways in humans maintain an excess of purines as a safety factor for their supply. The presence of a positive feed forward mechanism in the production

of purines further enhances their abundance and high turnover, which is another factor contributing to high levels of urate production. Furthermore, primates have no uricase (which drives one of many pathways used by other animals to dispose of uric acid.)[3] Finally, land animals do not have the continuous supply of water necessary to maintain all body urates in aqueous solution. All of these factors result in a tenuous state that always borders on urate supersaturation in both the serum and the tissues, with an ever-present tendency toward crystallization. Also, hyperuricemia is not the sole cause of crystal formation; dehydration and a lack of crystal inhibitors (mostly citrates) are also contributors.[4] Urate is produced in significant quantity only in tissues with xanthine oxidase—namely, liver and small bowel—and is excreted mainly via the kidney (about 75%), the remainder being eliminated by the small bowel. Thus, the small intestine is unique in its participation in both production and excretion of purines.

Risk Factors

The typical patient with gout is a middle-aged man. In addition to age and male gender, however, other factors are associated with an increased risk of gout.[5] Thus, gout can occur at all ages and in either gender.

> ### NOTE
>
> *Risk factors for gout and hyperuricemia include male gender, inherited metabolic or excretory deficiencies, chronic renal failure, excess dietary purines, dehydration, acid states, and certain medications and supplements. Modifying these risk factors is an excellent alternative treatment in preventing gout.*

Serum uric acid levels rise at puberty in males, whereas females experience an increase at menopause. The gender disparity seems to result from hormonal differences as well as from better excretion in females.[1] Several inherited metabolic and renal abnormalities cause overproduction or

Table 54–1. Medications and Supplements That Promote Urate Crystallization
....

Thiazide and loop diuretics
Aspirin and other salicylates
Supplemental vitamin C
Supplemental niacin

reduced clearance of urate. Many medications[6] and supplements increase the serum uric acid level and/or the tendency of urate to crystallize (see Table 54–1). Also, dehydration reduces excretion and promotes crystallization. Finally, acidemic states (as in infection, postsurgery, and ketogenic weight loss diets, or with excess alcohol consumption) heighten urate production and crystallization. Cytotoxic chemotherapy can put massive purines into the total pool.

Diagnosis

The existence of multiple non–uric acid crystalline arthropathies, as well as the possibility of septic arthritis, speaks to the importance of accurate diagnosis on the first acute arthritic episode. Thus, at clinical presentation, it is imperative to rule out infection as the cause of symptoms. This distinction is also important for long-term management of non-urate arthropathies, as no commitment to allopurinol or dietary purine avoidance is indicated in these disorders. It is therefore often recommended that arthrocentesis or bursocentesis be done for both culture and crystal analysis. This procedure allows prompt identification of infectious cases and also gives confidence regarding long-term treatment to both patient and practitioner. Neither peripheral studies (white blood cell count, other acute phase reactant assays) nor constitutional symptoms (fever, malaise) are of help in distinguishing among the various potentially causative disorders. A serum uric acid level is of no value during an acute attack, because it is the chronic purine *turnover* and the *tissue* urate saturation that lead to crystallization. In fact, the serum urate often drops acutely as urate is pulled from blood into tissues, where it causes the symptoms.[7]

INTEGRATIVE THERAPY

Prevention

Most therapies employed for prevention of gout should *not* be instituted during an acute flare of arthritis, as they worsen the pain and other inflammatory symptoms associated with the attack,[7, 8] perhaps secondary to increased shedding of microcrystals. The exception is the use of the cherry-berry

group (see later on). Preventive therapies are given to reduce or eliminate the frequency of gouty attacks, as well as to avoid damage to joints and the kidney.

NOTE

Do not initiate preventive measures during an acute gouty arthritis episode, as experience shows this worsens the attack!

Nutrition

Hydration

Water is a mainstay of treatment, is inexpensive, has virtually no untoward effects, and is available to all patients. Intake of about $2\frac{1}{2}$ liters of water, distributed throughout the day, should be encouraged (except in water-restricted patients). Adequate hydration keeps uric acid in solution and promotes its excretion. It also mobilizes other toxins and helps with many other health problems.

Purine Intake

Dietary purine intake can contribute to the formation of tophi and to the development of hyperuricemia in patients at risk.[9] In other words, in susceptible persons dietary purine can tip the metabolic "scale" toward hyperuricemia and crystallization, whereas other patients seem to tolerate unlimited purine intake with no sequelae. Therefore, patients at risk will benefit from dietary maneuvers as part of their treatment.

Basically, high-purine foods are those derived from organisms characterized by a rapid turnover of purines and high metabolism (as in organ meats and small animals), or from the floral reproductive parts of plants, with their multiple gene copies.[5] Accordingly, brain and anchovy (with high purine metabolism) and beans and mushrooms (with multiple gene copies) have high purine content. Interestingly, members of the lily family, such as asparagus, are pentaploid and therefore also are high in purines (see Table 54–2).

Dietary Recommendations

It is best to consider foods in two groups: those to be *avoided* and those to be *added*. In susceptible persons, eliminating or reducing certain foods (see Table 54–2) is very helpful. This approach can be a mainstay in management of gout in patients who do not use allopurinol owing to untoward effects or in those who prefer alternative treatments. Fatty seafoods contain significant purine, but they are also high in omega-3 fatty acids, with their own benefit

Table 54–2. Purine Content of Foods

High purine content (due to rapid turnover and metabolism): *Avoid in susceptible persons*

Organ meats (sweetbreads, brain, liver, kidney)
Young/small animals (anchovy, scallops, veal, most game meats)

Intermediate purine content: *Reduce or avoid in susceptible persons*

Floral or reproductive components of crops (high in nucleic acids)
Legumes (e.g., lentils, peas, beans, peanuts, soybeans), whole grains (especially bran)
Mushrooms, fungal fermentation products
Asparagus
Beverages (fermented or acidic, or those containing significant xanthine):
Beer
Coffee
Tea
Chocolate, cocoa
Beverages with added caffeine (e.g., some sodas)

Equivocal (see text)

Oily fish and other shellfish
Mussels
Mackerel
Herring

Low negligible purine content: *Always allowed*

Dairy
Nuts
Tubers
Eggs
Most crops not listed above

(see later on). They can be consumed in moderation. Foods always allowed are dairy products, nuts, tubers, eggs, and most crops not in the other groups.

Foods to be added include the cherry-berry group—namely, those that have a purple or red color (black cherries, purple grapes, raspberries, blueberries, and strawberries). Their action is postulated to be due to the proanthocyanidin subfraction of their bioflavonoid content; at least a half-pint a day is recommended. Alternatively, a proanthocyanidin or other bioflavonoid supplement can be employed, but those with added vitamin C (see later) should be avoided. Also, consumption of foods with significant citrates (the allowed crops in Table 54–2), should be encouraged. In addition, patients should be counseled to remain on an antiflammatory diet[10] (see chapter 84), with several modifications—specifically, avoidance of legumes, whole grains, and some seafoods (see Table 54–2). Alcohol-containing beverages contribute to acidemia and dehydration, so they should be avoided. An exception may be the darker colored wines, owing to their proanthocyanidin content as well as other antioxidant and anti-inflammatory components. Therefore, wine in moderation with proper hydration is acceptable.

Weight Loss

Weight loss diets deserve some comment here. Ketogenic-type diets cause acidemia and lead to an increase in urate production (from purine catabolism), so they contribute to hyperuricemia and gout. Such plans are often devoid of carbohydrates but are loaded with fat and high-purine foods, thus worsening ketoacidosis and hyperuricemia. In contrast, a diet based on moderate intake of carbohydrates as well as low fat intake, without excess purines, avoids acidosis and hyperuricemia. Also, dietary protein itself does not significantly contribute to urate production.[11] The available evidence thus points to a low-fat diet that minimizes purine intake.

Pharmaceuticals

Nonsteroidal Anti-inflammatory Drugs

For nonsteroidal anti-inflammatory drug (NSAID) therapy, low-dose indomethacin, 25 mg a day, can be used, but any other NSAID can be substituted except aspirin, which inhibits renal tubular urate secretion.

Dosage. Indomethacin 25 mg daily may be used.

Corticosteroids

Corticosteroids such as prednisone are also available for prophylaxis. These medications have well-known gastrointestinal side effects, and many practitioners and patients prefer to avoid them in the preventive management of gout.

Allopurinol

Allopurinol in dosages averaging 300 mg per day is also effective in reducing uric acid production and allows for greater purine excretion via urate precursors that are more soluble. It protects joints and the kidneys.[7, 12] Many patients cannot tolerate this drug owing to allergy or other effects, however, so for these patients and those who are not amenable to using prescription drugs, dietary maneuvers constitute the best approach. However, allopurinol is very helpful in patients with chronic renal failure who have difficulty in excreting urate.[7] Again, dietary maneuvers can also be used in these patients, and this approach is consistent with that indicated for the patient who needs to be on the typical "renal diet," as the two diets are low in nitrogen. Rarely, intravenous allopurinol can be used in patients with no enteral access.[13]

Dosage. Allopurinol 300 mg daily.

Supplements

Folic Acid

Folic acid is a xanthine oxidase inhibitor that decreases urate formation.

Dosage. Doses of 5000 μg daily (i.e., 5 mg) can be employed. This is about 10 times the dose for other medical purposes.

Omega-3 Fatty Acids

Omega-3 fatty acids are available in whole food and supplement forms and are of great help in controlling pain and other aspects of inflammation. Supplements such as flaxseed oil, fish oil, and evening primrose oil may be used.

For flaxseed oil preparations (e.g., Nature-Made Flaxseed Oil) one to two 1000-mg capsules three times a day is a good regimen. Fish oil can also be substituted in the same dosage. For general health purposes, I prefer fish oil for women because of its higher documented vitamin D content (beneficial in prevention of osteoporosis), whereas in men flaxseed oil is recommended because it has no cholesterol (beneficial in prevention of atherosclerosis). Either oil in bottled form can be taken in a dose of 1 teaspoon 3 times a day. Oil of evening primrose is another source. Dietary sources of omega-3 fatty acids, in increasing amount of content, include walnuts, wild seafood (especially fatty types such as salmon), and flaxseed. A 6-ounce serving of one of these foods is roughly equivalent to one dose of supplemental oil (see Chapter 85, The Anti-inflammatory Diet).

Dosage. Omega-3 oils (flaxseed oil or fish oil): 3 to 6 g divided three times daily.

Vitamin E

A vitamin E supplement can be used for prevention. Alternatively, high-vitamin-E foods include nuts and seeds with a high fat content (the best being sunflower kernels), as well as soy and peanut oil. Also, berries and pears along with grapes have a reasonable vitamin E content.

Dosage. Vitamin E 800 international units (IU) each day.

Avoidance of Excess Vitamin C and Niacin

Excess supplementation of vitamin C or niacin leads to greater production and/or crystallization of uric acid. Dietary sources of vitamin C or niacin present no problem, but supplementation in patients with a history of gout or hyperuricemia should be avoided. Hyperlipidemic patients receiving niacin for lipid control can be switched to omega-3 oils, with the added preventive benefit for gout. Also, vitamin C is said to be an obligatory supplement for the antihyperuricemic effects of folate; dietary ascorbate sources (e.g., broccoli or strawberries—which have an antiarthritic effect as well) are adequate for this purpose.

Bromelain

The bromeliad enzyme bromelain has anti-inflammatory effects; its presumed mechanism of action is lysis of inflammatory oligopeptides.

Dosage. 500 mg orally three times a day for a week, then half that dose for 2 months. Alternatively, about 6 ounces of raw pineapple can be consumed three times a day, owing to its content of similar enzymes.[14]

Botanicals

Stinging Nettle

Nettle has some inflammatory effects, presumably from antihistamine content.

Dosage. 600 mg each day, for up to 3 months. The freeze-dried preparation, *not* the alcohol tinctures, should be used.

Autumn Crocus

The Autumn crocus *(Colchicum)* is the source of colchicine, which can be very useful.

Dosage. Doses of 0.5 or 0.6 mg orally per day of the prescription medication colchicine is preferred.

Caution. Galenical (homemade or custom-made) preparations of colchicum or other sources of colchicine are dangerously toxic and should be avoided[15, 16] (see "Acute Treatment").

Acute Treatment

Caution. Institution of preventive treatment during an acute attack of gout is contraindicated, as this is known to worsen the symptoms.

Hydration

Reversal of dehydration is extremely important. However, overhydration must be avoided, as this condition seems to worsen the inflammation. Also, acidemic states must be identified and treated. Aspirin and other salicylates should be eliminated at this time, as it is very common for patients to have taken these agents in an effort to relieve the pain.

Pharmaceuticals

Nonsteroidal Anti-inflammatory Agents

NSAIDs in high doses, such as indomethacin 50 to 100 mg 3 or 4 times a day, can be used until 48 hours after the inflammatory symptoms become tolerable. Other NSAIDs except aspirin can also be employed instead.

Another choice for control of inflammation is one of the cyclo-oxygenase 2 (COX-2) inhibitors (celecoxib or rofecoxib)[7] but in general, these agents should be avoided because of the possibility that they may induce a thrombotic diathesis.[7] However, in patients who remain active and hydrated, COX-2 inhibitors may be preferred, especially to avoid the gastrointestinal effects of the other drugs. Omega-3 oils are also an excellent alternative for control of inflammation (see dosing later on).

Dosage. Indomethacin can be used in a dose of 50 to 100 mg three or four times daily.

Corticosteroids

Corticosteroids are efficacious in patients who tolerate them. They can be used by three routes of administration. Oral prednisone can be employed at 40 to 100 mg a day in divided doses (taken with food) for a week and then tapered. Parenteral doses of 40 to 125 mg of a methylprednisolone preparation given by the intravenous or intramuscular route one to three times a day can be substituted. Intra-articular injections of triamcinolone acetonide suspension at 15 to 20 mg for small joints (toe, wrist) or 40 mg for larger joints (ankle, knee, elbow) can lead to marked improvement with minimal systemic effects; they can be given every 3 weeks for 3 doses if necessary.

Colchicine

Colchicine 0.5 to 1.0 mg by mouth up to four times a day often gives prompt relief of symptoms. (Although it can be used in an intravenous form, I reserve this route of administration for corticosteroids and narcotics only.) Other preparations of colchicine include galenicals (i.e., custom made or homemade preparations made from the whole plant) derived from autumn crocus or *Gloriosa* species (i.e., the gloriosa lily)[16]. These preparations are typically liquids, such as decoctions, are heat stable, and are dangerous (see Precautions).

Precautions. Manifestations of colchicine toxicity include oral and gastrointestinal burning, as well as alopecia and ascending nephropathy. All preparations of colchicine can egress to mammalian milk, and pediatric toxicity by this route has been reported.[15] Therefore, colchicine must be avoided in lactating women. Furthermore, all colchicine preparations can cause leukopenia. Finally, I am unimpressed with the differences in efficacy between colchicine and the other medications mentioned. Therefore, use of the aforementioned alternatives should be considered first before colchicine is given.

Dosage. 0.5 to 1.0 mg of colchicine orally four times a day.

Narcotics

Narcotics can be used in oral or parenteral preparations in the usual doses given for pain, although these agents do nothing for metabolic or crystal-related problems. Therefore, other therapies need also to be used simultaneously to prevent joint destruction.

Botanicals

Glycyrrhiza (Licorice) and Boswellia

Herbal substances with biochemical effects similar to those of corticosteroids include oral *Glycyrrhiza*—licorice root extract (not deglycyrrhinated licorice [DGL])—and *Boswellia*, or Frankincense.[18, 19] The syndrome of secondary hyperaldosteronism (acute hypertension and hypokalemia) associated with intake of licorice is well documented.[19] These two substances should be expected to have steroid-like effects. I prefer the ease of control with prescription steroid medications, but in patients who are not amenable to the use of such agents, these herbal preparations can be employed. However, patients should be followed just as closely for the untoward effects mentioned. These preparations should also be taken with food to reduce any gastrointestinal side effects, although the risk of such effects seem to be less with herbals than with prescription steroids.

Stinging Nettle

Freeze-dried nettle at 600 mg once or twice a day is helpful. Only the freeze-dried preparation should be used; the alcohol tincture should be avoided.

Supplements

Folic Acid

Folic acid in doses of 10,000 to 20,000 μg per day (i.e., 10 to 20 mg) may be helpful in some patients and is worth a trial for 48 hours.

Avoidance of Excess Vitamin C and Niacin

Regarding other vitamins, supplemental vitamin C and niacin should be stopped. Furthermore, the recommendation in some urology and nutrition literature to use thousands of milligrams of high dose vitamin C supplements during an attack[20] is to be condemned, as this worsens the episode. Dietary ascorbic acid is not a problem.

Bromelain

Bromelain in a dose of 500 mg orally three times a day for a week can be used simultaneously with other treatments. A whole food alternative to bromelain is raw pineapple in the amounts recommended for prevention, earlier.

Omega-3 Fatty Acids

Omega-3 oils at 9000 to 15,000 mg per day in divided doses can also be used for acute attacks.

Vitamin E

Vitamin E supplementation at 800 IU per day orally is also a treatment that can soothe inflammation and reduce pain.

NOTE

Simultaneous administration of omega-3 fatty acids (from either food or supplement sources), vitamin E, and NSAIDs should be avoided because their anticoagulant effects are additive. One or more of these agents should be eliminated, or the dose should be moderated; patients should be instructed to report bleeding immediately.

Therapies to Consider

Nutrition

Further modifications in the anti-inflammatory diet may be of benefit. Many plants such as the cooking herbs sage, parsley, dill, and oregano, along with the floral parts of plants (plums, edible flowers), contain salicylates and other aspirin-like substances.[11] These foods should be eliminated from the diet during an attack; subsequently, the patient should be counseled to restrict intake to a minimum.

Celery seed extract or a half-pound a day of whole celery can help to relieve the acute symptoms, but because of the diuretic effect and salicylate content of the plant, in general it should be avoided in this setting. However, these preparations are highly recommended by some practitioners, and they are frequently used.

Botanicals

A myriad of other herbals have been suggested or are under investigation.[21, 22] The German Commission E, for instance, suggests everything from ash to seeds of rosehips.[23]

Traditional Chinese Medicine

Traditional chinese medicine (TCM) employs many pain-relieving and anti-inflammatory measures. Many of the medicines used are xanthine oxidase inhibitors and can be helpful for prevention and often for relief of acute symptoms.[24]

Surgery

Surgical treatment (ray amputation) has been used in extreme situations of open draining tophi and extreme pain when function has already been lost.[25]

THERAPEUTIC REVIEW

Prevention

- *Hydration*
  - Daily intake of $2\frac{1}{2}$ liters of water distributed evenly throughout the day is recommended, unless the patient is water restricted.

- *Food*
  - Avoid these foods: organ meats, young/small animals, floral or reproductive crops (legumes, mushrooms, asparagus), and the beverages beer, coffee, tea, chocolate/cocoa, or those with added caffeine.
  - Add these foods: black cherries, purple grapes, raspberries, blackberries, blueberries, and strawberries. Use a half-pound a day of raw fruit or a bioflavonoid supplement (ascorbate-free).

- *NSAIDs: Indomethacin 25 mg 1 to 3 times a day, or another NSAID (except aspirin or COX-2 inhibitors).*

- *Allopurinol: 200 to 500 mg per day orally (up to 800 mg a day if patient is undergoing concurrent cytotoxic chemotherapy).*

- *High-dose folic acid: 5000 μg per day (i.e., 5 mg); doses may be divided.*

- *Omega-3 fatty acids*
  - Flaxseed oil (e.g., Nature Made Flaxseed Oil) in a dose of three 1000 mg capsules, daily 3 times a day for females, or fish oil in the same dose for males.
  - Alternates include oil of evening primrose, and dietary omega-3 fatty acids at 6 ounces of whole food per dose of walnuts, wild seafood (especially salmon), or flaxseed.

- *Vitamin E*
  - 800 IU per day orally; doses may be divided.
  - Alternatively, foods high in vitamin E can be substituted (sunflower kernels, soy or peanut oil, berries, pears, grapes).

THERAPEUTIC REVIEW *continued*

- *Elimination of supplemental vitamin C and niacin*
  - Dietary sources are not a problem.
  - For patients with hyperlipidemias, substitute omega-3 oils at the recommended doses instead of niacin, and recheck serum lipids in 3 months.

- *Elimination of medications that cause or worsen gout—thiazide and loop diuretics, salicylates, and possibly losartan; these agents must be replaced by a suitable alternative to control the disorders for which they are prescribed.*

- *Enzyme treatment*
  - Bromelain 500 mg 3 times a day for a week to start, then half that dose for 2 months.
  - Alternatively, 6 ounces of raw pineapple can be consumed 3 times a day.

- *Autumn crocus: 0.5 or 0.6 mg orally per day of prescription colchicine (not galenicals).*

- *Stinging nettle*
  - Do not use alcohol tinctures.
  - Dried preparations at 600 mg per day for up to 3 months can be used.

Acute Treatment

- *Do not institute preventive treatment during disease flares, as this will worsen the attack, with the exception of using the cherry-berry group.*

- *Reverse the dehydration; avoid overhydration, as this can cause shedding of microcrystals with worsening pain.*

- *Nonsteroidal anti-inflammatory drugs at high dose*
  - Indomethacin 50 to 100 mg 3 to 4 times a day for at least 48 hours, or any non-aspirin NSAID.
  - COX-2 inhibitors should be avoided in the sedentary patient.

- *Corticosteroids and related herbals*
  - Prednisone in a dose of 40 to 100 mg daily for a week, then tapered.
  - Alternatively, a parenteral methylprednisolone preparation IV up to 125 mg 3 times a day or IM once a day until symptoms become tolerable.
  - Instead of these, intra-articular injections of 15 to 40 mg (depending on joint size) of triamcinolone acetonide suspension may be given every 3 weeks, for up to 3 doses.
  - Herbals with similar effects include oral *Glycyrrhiza* (licorice) and *Boswellia* (Frankincense), but they have many of the same untoward effects as for prescription steroids, and patients must be watched just as closely with these medicines.

- *High-dose folic acid: At least 10,000 µg per day (i.e., 10 mg) and up to 20,000 µg per day (i.e., 20 mg) for at least 48 hours, individed doses to lessen gastrointestinal effects.*

- *Bromelain*
  - 500 mg of bromelain orally 3 times a day for a week; then the dose is halved.
  - The whole food alternative is 6 ounces of raw pineapple 3 times a day.

- *Cherry-berry group: A half-pound or more of the whole raw fruit daily for 3 days or longer (e.g., black cherries, purple and red grapes, raspberries, blackberries, blueberries, strawberries).*

- *Colchicine*
  - Use of galencial or whole herb preparations of autumn crocus or gloriosa lily is contraindicated, as toxicity is too great. Instead, 0.5 to 1.0 mg of colchicine orally up to 4 times a day should be given until symptoms become tolerable; then other maneuvers can be instituted.
  - Colchicine should be avoided in lactating woman or those of child-bearing age.

THERAPEUTIC REVIEW continued

- *Narcotics*
  - These agents can be used in the usual routes and dosages.
  - Narcotics do nothing to prevent joint destruction, so a specific therapy must be instituted simultaneously.

References

1. Wortman RL: Gout and other disorders of purine metabolism. In Harrison TH, Fauci AS (eds): Harrison's Principles of Internal Medicine, 14th ed. New York, McGraw Hill, 1998, pp 2158–2165.
2. Reginato AJ, Hoffman GS: Arthritis due to deposition of calcium crystals. In Harrison TH, Fauci AS (eds): Harrison's Principles of Internal Medicine, 14th ed. New York, McGraw Hill, 1998, p 1941.
3. Stryer L: Biochemistry, San Francisco, WH Freeman 1975, p 548.
4. Koop CD: The Surgeon General's report on nutrition and health. US Department of Health and Human Services. Public Health Service Publication No. 88–50210. Washington, DC, US Government Printing Office, 1988, pp 383–384.
5. DeMio P: Gout: It's in the genes. Ohio Ecol Food Farm Assoc News 21:16, 2001.
6. Moser M: Clinical Management of Hypertension, Caddo, Okla, Professional Communications, 1998, pp 78–79.
7. Van Doornum S, Ryan PF: Clinical manifestations of gout and their management. Med J Aust 172:493–497, 2000.
8. McGill NW: Gout and other crystal-associated arthropathies. Baillieres Best Pract Res Clin Rheumatol 14:445–460, 2000.
9. Nelson JK, Moxness KE, Jensen MD, Gastineau CF: Mayo Clinic Diet Manual: A Handbook of Nutrition Practices, 7th ed. St. Louis, Mosby, 1994, p 345.
10. DeMio P: Anti-inflammatory diet. Ohio Ecol Food Farm Assoc News 20:17, 2000.
11. Dessein PH, et al: Beneficial effects of weight loss associated with moderate calorie/carbohydrate restriction, and increased proportional intake of protein and unsaturated fat on serum urate and lipoprotein levels in gout: A pilot study. Ann Rheum Dis; 59:539–543, 2000.
12. Brenner BM, Levy E, Hostetter T: Tubulointerstitial diseases of kidney. In Harrison TH, Fauci AS (eds): Harrison's Principles of Internal Medicine, 14th ed. New York, McGraw Hill, 1998, pp 1155–1156.
13. Smalley RV, et al: Allopurinol: Intravenous use for prevention and treatment of hyperuricemia. J Clin Oncol 18:1758–1763, 2000.
14. Dombek C: Pineapple. In The Lawrence Review of Natural Products. St. Louis, Mo, Wolters Kluwer, July 1993, pp 1–2.
15. Dombeck C: Autumn crocus. In The Lawrence Review of Natural Products. St. Louis, Mo, Wolters Kluwer, Aug 1993, pp 1–2.
16. Lampek F, McCann MA: AMA Handbook of Poisonous and Injurious Plants. Chicago, American Medical Association, 1985, pp 59–60, 85–86.
17. Abramowicz M, et al: Drugs for rheumatoid arthritis. Med Letter 42:57, 2000.
18. Hebel SK: Indian frankincense tree. In the Lawrence Review of Natural Products. St. Louis, Mo, Wolters Kluwer, June 1998, pp 1–2.
19. Hebel SK: Licorice. In The Lawrence Review of Natural Products. St. Louis, Mo, Wolters Kluwer, Feb 1998, pp 1–2.
20. Balch PA, Balch, JF: Prescription for Nutritional Healing, 3rd ed. New York Avery, 2000, p 398.
21. Badilla B, Mora G, Proveda LJ: Anti-inflammatory activity of acqueous extracts of five Costa Rican medicinal plants in Sprague-Dawley rats. Rev Biol Trop 47:723–727, 1999.
22. Deepak M, Handa SS: Antiinflammatory activity and chemical composition of extracts of *Verbena officinalis*. Phytother Res 14:463–465, 2000.
23. Blumenthal M (ed): The Complete German Commission E Monographs: Therapeutic Guide to Herbal Medicines. Boston, Integrative Medicine Communications, 1998, p 659.
24. Kong LD, et al: Inhibition of xanthine oxidase by some Chinese medical plants used to treat gout. J Ethnopharmacol 73:199–207, 2000.
25. Ertugrul Sener E, Guzel VM, Takka S: Surgical management of tophaceous gout in the hand. Arch Orthop Trauma Surg 120:482–483, 2000.

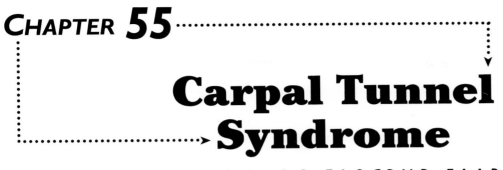

CHAPTER 55

Carpal Tunnel Syndrome

Benjamin M. Sucher, D.O., F.A.O.C.P.M.R., F.A.A.P.M.R.

INTRODUCTION, PATHO-PHYSIOLOGY, AND DIAGNOSIS

Carpal tunnel syndrome (CTS) is the most common peripheral nerve compression or entrapment disorder,[1] with a lifetime incidence of 10%.[2] It involves some type of irritation or injury to the median nerve at the wrist, with resulting symptoms of pain, numbness, tingling (paresthesias), and/or weakness. The distribution of sensory change is usually dictated by the median nerve anatomy, which typically includes the palm side of the thumb and the first two and a half fingers, with a smaller portion of the dorsal side of the same digits (near the tips). Regrettably, a diagnosis of CTS often evokes fear because many patients assume that it requires surgery for treatment.

The tunnel is relatively small, especially considering that it carries nine tendons and the median nerve. Any process that decreases space within the carpal canal causes increased pressure. Because the nerve is the softest structure within the tunnel, it usually is the most easily injured. Tendinitis, with accompanying inflammation and swelling, increases the volume of the tunnel contents and leads to elevation of pressure on the median nerve. Another process involves microtrauma. Presumably, minor insults, repeated over years, create scarring or fibrous fixation of the nerve to the walls of the tunnel, the transverse carpal ligament (TCL), or the tendons. Subsequently, movement of the tendons during normal activity can result in traction injury to the median nerve.[3]

Evaluation for CTS routinely begins with a history and physical examination, emphasizing the upper body. This includes stress tests at the wrist (phalens, tinels, carpal compression) and detailed assessment of small hand muscle strength. The electrodiagnostic examination (EDX), which includes a nerve conduction study (NCS) and needle electromyogram (EMG), is probably the most acceptable "gold standard" to confirm a diagnosis of CTS. In some cases, magnetic resonance imaging (MRI) is recommended, particularly when the clinical presentation does not match the EDX findings.[4] It is important to note that these studies evaluate different aspects of the pathology involved—electrical examinations assessing physiology and imaging techniques looking at anatomy. In effect, both may be useful, complementary, or necessary. A new and promising imaging method for assessment of CTS is diagnostic musculoskeletal ultrasound.[5] It is less costly than MRI and may provide more detailed information about the carpal tunnel and the median nerve.

Supplemental diagnosis of CTS with osteopathic palpatory assessment is very sensitive and correlates well with EDX.[6, 7] Palpatory examination is performed by lightly contacting the ventral aspect of the carpal tunnel with the thumbs while introducing gentle motion into transverse extension ("gapping" the canal), radial abduction, and lateral axial rotation of the thumb. The palpating thumbs determine whether there is any restriction to motion (0 to 5 scale, with 0 representing no restriction and 5 representing no motion). A restriction of moderate (level 2) or greater is usually present (over 90%) with CTS.[8]

It is vital to rule out other causes of upper extremity symptoms, especially before initiating any invasive or extended treatment for CTS. Key differentials include cervical radiculopathy and thoracic outlet syndrome, sometimes occurring simultaneously with CTS, the so-called double-crush syndrome.[7] Multiple other sites of compression or entrapment are possible between the wrist and the shoulder, but discussion of these areas is beyond the scope of this chapter. Osteopathic palpatory diagnosis, mechanical stress testing at other potential sites of entrapment, and EDX are all useful, if not essential, methods of confirming the diagnosis.[7]

It is important to rule out contributing causes, such as diabetes, renal or thyroid disease, a multitude of connective tissue disorders, and less often, growth hormone abnormalities such as acromegaly and amyloid disorder.[9] Other common predisposing causes or disorders include alcoholism, rheumatoid arthritis, advanced degenerative joint disease, cumulative trauma disorders (especially tendinitis), and direct or focal wrist trauma.[9] There are some unusual or rare causes such as leprosy, Lyme disease, and a variety of peripheral neuropathies.[9]

INTEGRATIVE THERAPY

Traditional treatment of CTS involves bracing and nonsteroidal anti-inflammatory drugs (NSAIDs), with less common use of diuretics and rarely oral steroids. In addition, it is prudent to consider activity modification, rest, avoiding awkward postures, and limiting repetitive movements that can challenge the structures in and about the carpal tunnel. Ergonomic modifications may also be helpful in this regard. More recent developments have demonstrated that the application of osteopathic manipulation can relieve pressure on the median nerve, alleviate symptoms of CTS, and enhance the initial treatment plan in mild and moderate cases. Manipulation is discussed in more detail in the section that follows on biomechanical principles.

Nutrition

B vitamins, in particular B_6 and B_{12}, are generally associated with proper function of peripheral nerve tissue. A well-balanced diet with traditional sources (yeast, whole grains) of these vitamins is sufficient in most cases. A diet rich in omega-3 fatty acids is also suggested, especially if tendinitis is present (see Chapter 84, The Anti-Inflammatory Diet).

Supplements

Vitamin B_6

Vitamin B_6 (pyridoxine) has been recommended by various authors as an effective treatment.[10, 11] However, most controlled studies do not support consistent results.[10, 12] There is also a concern that large doses (>200 to 500 mg daily) can cause a peripheral polyneuropathy.[10-12]

Trace Minerals

Some believe that trace mineral deficiency or imbalance plays a role in inflammation.[13] Analysis may assist in detecting such problems and guide the practitioner in selecting appropriate supplements.[13]

Botanicals

Various effects claimed for numerous botanicals[14-19] may have some application in treating CTS. Willow bark *(Salix alba)* contains salicin, which is converted to salicylic acid and may exert some helpful anti-inflammatory effect. St. John's wort *(Hypericum perforatum)*, grapeseed extract *(Vitis vinifera)*, garlic *(Allium sativum)*, and ginger *(Zingiber officinale)* also possess some anti-inflammatory activity—the latter having shown some effect in treating arthritis. As an example, some believe ginger to have cyclooxygenase 2 inhibition properties and recommend 0.5 to 1 mg of ginger root three times daily.

Precautions should be observed with all of these because dosing has not been standardized.

Pharmaceuticals

Routine use of NSAIDs has been variably effective, but poorly tolerated owing to gastrointestinal irritation and complications. The newer, selective cyclooxygenase 2 medications have been better tolerated. These drugs are particularly effective and helpful if there is concomitant tendinitis, by decreasing inflammation and thereby decreasing pressure in the tunnel and irritation on the median nerve. Dosing is recommended as suggested by the manufacturer. In addition, some compounding pharmacists are able to prepare NSAIDs in a topical or transdermal organogel base that has good penetration at superficial sites. Consider ordering ketoprofen topical gel 20% (200 mg/mL) three or four times daily, to be applied directly over the carpal tunnel. Diuretics are advocated when limb edema is present.[2] Oral steroids, such as prednisolone 20 mg daily (1 to 2 weeks, tapered), have been used effectively,[20] but carry substantial risks and are generally avoided.

BIOMECHANICAL PRINCIPLES (MANIPULATION, EXERCISE, PHYSICAL THERAPY, ORTHOSES)

Clinical research by Sucher[6-8, 21, 22] demonstrated mechanical restrictions at the level of the wrist that are significant factors contributing to CTS. Release of these restrictions using manipulation and stretching exercise has resulted in improvement of symptoms and NCS.[6, 7, 21, 22] In some cases, increased size of the carpal tunnel was documented with MRI.[22] Cadaver research by Sucher and Hinrichs[23] at Arizona State University has proved that the TCL can be elongated with sustained loads and osteopathic manipulation.

Manipulation

Manipulation may be effective after one session in some patients whereas others require multiple treatments over 2 to 4 weeks. Several techniques may be necessary to address various restrictions:

- The primary intent is to directly elongate the TCL by stretching the wrist transversely and increasing the size of the transverse carpal arch (TCA) (Fig. 55-1).[21] This increases the available space (volume) within the tunnel and reduces pressure on the nerve, thereby alleviating symptoms.
- The thenar muscles attach directly to the TCL, allowing the thumb to be used as a lever arm for

fulcrum effect, essentially applying direct traction on the TCL, which facilitates elongation (see Fig. 55–1).[21]

- Hyperextension of the wrist and digits simultaneously stretches the fascial and ligamentous structures over the carpal canal (see Fig. 55–1).[21] It also draws the flexor tendons distally, allowing the thicker musculotendinous portions to be "stuffed" into the canal, creating a bougie effect to dilate the tunnel from within. In addition, this maneuver may mobilize the median nerve by releasing adhesions between the nerve and the flexor tendons, TCL, or walls of the canal.[6]

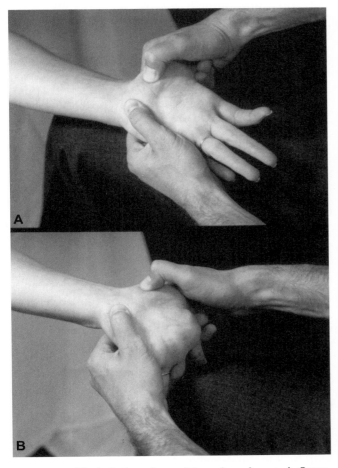

Figure 55–1 Manipulation of carpal tunnel syndrome. *A,* Operator's fingers, not visible beneath the patient's hand, press upward on the dorsal part of the wrist centrally. Operator's thumbs apply vigorous pressure along the attachment edges of the transverse carpal ligament at the medial and lateral borders of the carpal bones. In addition, the operator's right (upper) hand is pulling the patient's thumb back into radial abduction with some extension, which applies traction on the transverse carpal ligament. *B,* As in *A,* except the patient's wrist and fingers are hyperextended, further opening (extending) the canal. This also draws the thicker myotendinous portions of the flexor tendons into the tunnel, which creates a dilatory effect, and may release adhesions. The operator's thumbs have progressed away from the midline, "stripping" the ligamentous and myofascial attachments back. (*A* and *B,* From Sucher BM: Myofascial release of carpal tunnel syndrome. J Am Osteopath Assoc 93:93, 1993.)

- The base of the thumb joint, the first carpometacarpal, is a saddle joint and allows lateral axial rotation, which has been demonstrated to not only stretch the TCL but also elevate it off the median nerve at the same time. This technique, called the "opponens roll," may be better tolerated in more advanced cases of CTS.[6]
- Finally, other studies[24] have demonstrated that abduction combined with simultaneous extension of both the thumb and the little finger creates a fulcrum effect from the long flexor tendons pulling against the inside edges of the trapezium and hamate bones. The fulcrum effect creates force vectors that tend to pull the carpal bones apart and widen the TCA. This technique has been called the "guy-wire"[23] maneuver, and it is most effective when combined with transverse extension and a muscle energy technique in which the patient activates a contraction of the fingertips of digits one and five for 5 to 10 seconds. The contraction increases the forces that pull the carpal arch apart, thus enhancing the overall effect.

Stretching Exercises

Exercise, performed 5 to 10 times daily, usually works best in conjunction with the manipulation. Several self-stretching techniques have been developed, including:

- *Basic* (Fig. 55–2)[21]: This involves hyperextending the wrist and digits simultaneously as one component. The second requires taking the thumb into extension and radial abduction.
- *Advanced*: This maneuver simply combines the two basic components into one by simultaneously extending the wrist and digits while extending/abducting the thumb—use of a wall or the inside of the thigh to extend the fingers and wrist frees the other hand to apply the thumb component.[22]
- *Modified*: Several variations are available. A one-arm technique is designed to spare the patient's other hand (which may also be affected by CTS), and requires placing the involved hand (thumb and all digits) against a wall in extension.[7] A progressive enhancement of this maneuver has the fingers maintain extension and spread apart maximally, holding pressure while contracting gently with digits one and five to simulate the guy-wire effect.[7, 23] Finally, an opponens roll stretch is a development from the manipulation that elevates the TCL off the median nerve.[8]

A self-stretch exercise device, the Carpal Tunnel Stretch, is an option that eliminates the need to learn and perfect an array of stretching techniques. Individuals place their hand in the molded form and press into it with partial body weight. This forces the hand and wrist into positions similar to those achieved in the manipulation and stretching exer-

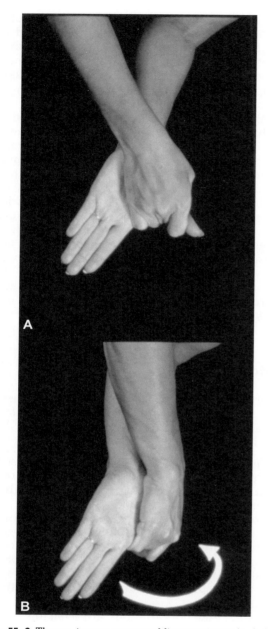

Figure 55–2 Thenar, transverse carpal ligament stretch. *A,* At the initiation of the stretch, the patient hooks the hypothenar region of the opposite hand (right hand in this illustration) into the thenar area of the hand to be stretched (left), pulling laterally while simultaneously grasping the thumb itself and extending (downward). *B,* Progressive phase of the stretch into further extension and abduction. (*A* and *B,* From Sucher BM: Myofascial release of carpal tunnel syndrome. J Am Osteopath Assoc 93:94, 1993.)

cises. The device has been studied in small numbers and has effectively treated mild to moderate cases of CTS.[6] Subsequently, it has been demonstrated to be useful in many cases as an adjunct to other treatment modalities. Caution is advised if there is significant dysfunction or pathology in the shoulder on the involved side.

Physical Therapy

Physical therapy is often useful to supplement the manipulation and stretching exercises. A typical program may require two to three sessions weekly for 2 to 4 weeks.

- *Therapeutic ultrasound* is particularly effective because it can heat the deep soft tissue structures that surround the median nerve and render them more receptive to manual techniques by increasing elasticity.[7] Caution is advised to avoid directly heating the median nerve (work on the edges of the carpal canal), because this could increase edema and compression. Exercise and/or manipulation should immediately follow ultrasound, before the patient leaves the therapy area, because the tissues will cool back to normal within 15 to 30 minutes and lose their enhanced elasticity.
- *Electrical stimulation* may have some beneficial effects by improving blood flow, reducing edema, and facilitating healing.[25] Frequencies used commonly range from 2 cycles/sec up to 100 cycles/sec or greater, and can be delivered simultaneously with the ultrasound (through the sound head) or separately with electrode pads.
- *Iontophoresis* may be indicated as an alternative, noninvasive method of delivering steroid into the carpal tunnel (as opposed to injecting it), which is safer than taking it orally. Although it has been studied in mild cases,[26] clinically it has been helpful in moderate to severe cases in which patients are unreceptive to the more invasive injection. A mild formula (4 mg/mL or 0.4% dexamethasone) is used to saturate an electrode pad that is placed directly over the median nerve. Wires are attached to the electrode from a stimulating unit that generates an external electric field that propels the ionized steroid through the skin and into the carpal tunnel.

General Precautions

Advanced or severe cases of CTS usually do not respond well to conservative treatment. Monitoring the electrophysiologic status of the median nerve with NCS is the safest and most accurate method of following the progress of the patient. However, electrical changes lag behind symptoms and mechanical or palpatory changes, and thus may not reflect improvement (or worsening) for 1 to 2 months after intervention.

Palpatory assessment will reveal changes immediately, or within days, and is a very sensitive, cost-effective method for monitoring the patient's condition from one week (or month) to the next, until electrical studies are repeated.[6–8] Arthritis or advanced degenerative changes in the hand, especially the first carpometacarpal joint, may limit the degree or extent of manipulation and stretching exercise that can be applied. Pain is also a potential limiting factor, but may be overcome to some degree with use of vapocoolant spray (i.e., ethylchloride).

Orthoses

Orthoses or wrist braces come in various types and are commonly used to treat CTS.[27]

- Prefabricated "off-the-shelf" versions are readily available, usually made of a canvas and/or elastic material with Velcro closure and a metal insert ventrally that maintains the wrist in slight extension (10 degrees to 30 degrees): the metal inserts can be removed and bent to conform to the patient for comfort and function.
- Custom-molded orthoses should be considered if the prefabricated braces are not effective or tolerated: these are routinely made of moldable plastic and Velcro. The cost is greater because they require more expensive materials and additional time to customize the fit, but they may ultimately yield better results. Referral to an occupational therapist may be indicated for fabrication and optimum fit.
- Experience has shown that braces should not be routinely or automatically prescribed. They limit motion at the wrist and may lead to excessive compensatory motion at other joints, causing new symptoms. Hyperflexion and hyperextension are both common sleep positions that can cause compression of the median nerve, and should be prevented with an orthosis if possible. In addition, an acute CTS with pronounced symptoms, or accompanied by severe tendinitis, may benefit greatly with a few days of rest in an orthosis.

Steroid Injections

- Injection of steroid into the carpal canal has been shown to be an effective CTS treatment with improvement that may persist for months.[27] It is best reserved for cases that are more severe and/or the patient refuses or needs to delay surgical treatment as long as possible (at least 2 to 3 months). Some believe steroids may impede tissue healing and prefer to avoid injection shortly before surgery.
- Because the carpal tunnel is quite small, especially when CTS is present, it does not readily accommodate large volumes of injectable material. Therefore, using the smallest amount of solution is better tolerated. A long-acting preparation, such as methylprednisolone acetate, 80 mg/mL, 0.5 to 1.0 mL, works well in most cases.
- It is critical to avoid injecting the median nerve. The palmaris longus tendon (not always present) is an excellent landmark, because the nerve is usually directly beneath it. The needle should be introduced slightly off to the medial or ulnar side

of the tunnel and can be approached either proximal or distal to the TCL.

Surgery

- The traditional surgical approach is "open," with an incision several centimeters long that completely exposes the field of operation in order to transect the TCL and relieve pressure from the median nerve.[28] Unfortunately, there is usually some accompanying weakness because of small hand muscle attachments to the TCL and loss of the tethering effect on the flexor tendons by the TCL.[29] Nonetheless, surgery is still a very effective and reasonable approach for advanced cases of CTS, or whenever nonoperative management is not working or progressive symptoms cannot be controlled.
- More recently, several surgeons are offering variations on endoscopic approach to the tunnel, involving a much smaller incision and more rapid recovery or return to work. Critics of endoscopy at the wrist suggest that because the field of view is much smaller, this leads to an increased risk of injury to some vital structures, in particular the median nerve branches.[28] When choosing this option, it is important to find a surgeon who is highly experienced and has a very low complication rate.
- Finally, a new and promising surgical technique is emerging, called *carpal tunnel balloon-plasty* (Lee Berger, M.D., email communications, July 1999). It involves a small incision and insertion of a nerve guard between the median nerve and the TCL. The guard is attached to a frame that holds it rigid to protect the nerve while a balloon is repeatedly inflated and deflated ventrally to stretch the TCL. Preliminary studies are encouraging, with rapid patient recovery. Clinical trials are continuing in several centers around the country.

Other Therapies to Consider

Acupuncture

This approach has been recognized as a viable treatment for a multitude of painful conditions. Although there is limited research to prove the efficacy, with most evidence based on case reports or studies with flawed design, the National Institutes of Health has suggested that acupuncture may be useful in CTS.[30]

Some research is supporting the claim that opioid peptide release and hypothalamic and pituitary activation may all contribute to the effects. It is generally considered as an adjunct or just one of many alternatives in a comprehensive management program.

Massage and Rolfing

Therapeutic massage and deep soft tissue release with rolfing have been observed to alleviate muscle tension from the upper extremity, with a secondary easing of mechanical strain about the carpal tunnel. The major precaution is to avoid vigorous pressure directly over the carpal canal and the median nerve, which could aggravate symptoms.

Yoga

Some promise for treating CTS has been claimed with yoga. In fact, a study by Garfinkel and colleagues[31] demonstrated that yoga was more effective than wrist splinting. They used the Iyenger approach to hatha yoga twice weekly for 8 weeks. Eleven different postures were employed that focus on the upper body, including "strengthening, stretching, and balancing," most involving hyperextension at the wrist. Some authorities on CTS commented back to the journal and challenged the conclusions (JAMA 281:2087-2089, 1999). Therefore, although yoga may be a useful adjunct to the other treatments outlined, caution is advised. In particular, it would be prudent to avoid sustaining wrist positions at the extremes of range beyond 15 to 20 seconds.

— THERAPEUTIC REVIEW

Following is a summary of therapeutic options for CTS. If a patient presents with severe symptoms, it would be reasonable to proceed with orthopedic or hand surgery referral to consider operative intervention before initiating a course of conservative treatment.

At the very least, patients should be advised of the potential risks for progressive and permanent nerve loss with residual weakness, numbness, and disability.

Avoid Stressful Postures	Institute ergonomic modifications at home and work. Use caution with yoga.
Nutrition	Eat a well-balanced diet with adequate supply of vitamins (especially B_6 and B_{12}). Consider an omega-3 fatty acid–rich diet when tendinitis is present (see Chapter 84, The Anti-Inflammatory Diet).
Supplements	Replace trace minerals if found deficient. Vitamin B_6 has not been proven effective and excess (>100 mg) could cause a diffuse neuropathy.
Botanicals	Consider white willow, grapeseed extract, ginger, St. John's wort, and garlic.
Pharmaceuticals	Use long-acting NSAIDS orally, and topical compounded preparations (ketoprofen 20%). Consider diuretics for edema; use oral steroids as a last resort.
Manipulation	Very effective in mild to moderate cases. Alleviates mechanical restrictions at the wrist (and proximally, as indicated). Works best when combined with stretching exercise, and may be enhanced by physical therapy modalities.
Exercise	Initiate stretching exercise early. Use in conjunction with manipulation, if possible. Physical therapy modalities used before exercise will enhance the response.
Physical Therapy	Facilitates exercise and manipulation. Ultrasound heats deep tissues to render them more elastic and responsive—avoid the central canal (median nerve). Electric stimulation may facilitate healing and reduce edema. Apply iontophoresis directly over the nerve in more severe cases and for inflammation.
Wrist Braces	Use these in selective cases, especially when the patient notes "bent-wrist" posturing at night and when severe tendinitis is present.

THERAPEUTIC REVIEW *continued*

Steroid Injection	Reserved for the more advanced cases in which the patient does not want surgery or may have not responded optimally to iontophoresis (if done). Use the smallest volume of medication possible, and exert great care to avoid the median nerve.
Surgery	Last resort for mild to moderate CTS, but consider as first-line treatment in severe cases or failure with conservative approaches. Many hand surgeons are avoiding endoscopic techniques in favor of better visualization with the open procedure.

Acknowledgment

Appreciation is expressed to Eugenia F. Sucher, Executive Director, Center for Carpal Tunnel Studies, for assistance with editing.

References

1. Foresti C, Quadri S, Rasella M, et al: Carpal tunnel syndrome: Which electrodiagnostic path should we follow? A prospective study of 100 consecutive patients. Electromyogr Clin Neurophysiol 36:377–384, 1996.
2. Quality Standards Subcommittee of the American Academy of Neurology: Practice parameter for carpal tunnel syndrome. Neurology 43:2406–2409, 1993.
3. Hunter JM: Recurrent carpal tunnel syndrome, epineural fibrous fixation, and traction neuropathy. Hand Clin 7:491–504, 1991.
4. Zagnoli F, Andre V, Le Dreff P, et al: Idiopathic carpal tunnel syndrome. Clinical, electrodiagnostic, and magnetic resonance imaging correlations. Rev Rheum 66:192–200, 1999.
5. Lee D, van Holsbeeck T, Janevski PK, et al: Diagnosis of carpal tunnel syndrome, ultrasound versus electromyography. Radiol Clin North Am 37:859–872, 1999.
6. Sucher BM: Palpatory diagnosis and manipulative management of carpal tunnel syndrome. J Am Osteopath Assoc 94:647–663, 1994.
7. Sucher BM: Palpatory diagnosis and manipulative management of carpal tunnel syndrome: Part 2. "Double crush" and thoracic outlet syndrome. J Am Osteopath Assoc 95:471–479, 1995.
8. Sucher BM, Glassman JH: Upper extremity syndromes. In Stanton D, Mein E (eds): Manual Medicine. Phys Med Rehabil Clin North Am 7:787–810, 1996.
9. Rosenbaum RB, Ochoa JL: Carpal Tunnel Syndrome and Other Disorders of the Median Nerve. Boston, Butterworth-Heinemann, 1993.
10. Stransky M, Rubin A, Lava NS, Reynaldo PL: Treatment of carpal tunnel syndrome with vitamin B6: A double-blind study. South Med J 82:841–842, 1989.
11. Copeland DA, Stoukides CA: Pyridoxine in carpal tunnel syndrome. Ann Pharmacother 28:1042–1044, 1994.
12. Spooner GR, Desai HB, Angel JF, et al: Using pyridoxine to treat carpal tunnel syndrome. Can Fam Physician 39:2122–2127, 1993.
13. Wilson LD: Nutritional Balancing and Hair Mineral Analysis, 2nd (revised) ed. Prescott, Ariz., LD Wilson Consultants, Inc, 1998.
14. Bisset NG (ed): Herbal Drugs and Phytopharmaceuticals. Boca Raton, Fla, CRC, 1994.
15. Covington TR (ed): The Handbook of Non-Prescription Drugs. Washington, DC, American Pharmaceutical Association, 1996.
16. Tyler VE: Herbs of Choice: The Therapeutic Use of Phytomedicinals. New York, Haworth, 1994.
17. Barnes J: Growing body of data for hypericum extract in depression. Pharma No. 1058(3–4), Oct 12, 1996.
18. Linde K, Ramirez G, Mulrow CD, et al: St. John's wort for depression—an overview and meta-analysis of randomized clinical trials. BMJ 313:253–258, 1996.
19. Tyler VE: What pharmacists should know about herbal remedies. J Am Pharm Assoc NS36(1):29–37, 1996.
20. Chang M-H, Chiang H-T, Lee SS-J, et al: Oral drug of choice in carpal tunnel syndrome. Neurology 51:390–393, 1998.
21. Sucher BM: Myofascial release of carpal tunnel syndrome. J Am Osteopath Assoc 93:92–101, 1993.
22. Sucher BM: Myofascial manipulative release of carpal tunnel syndrome: Documentation with magnetic resonance imaging. J Am Osteopath Assoc 93:1273–1278, 1993.
23. Sucher BM, Hinrichs RN: Manipulative treatment of carpal tunnel syndrome: Biomechanical and osteopathic intervention to increase the length of the transverse carpal ligament. J Am Osteopath Assoc 98:679–686, 1998.
24. Fuss FK, Wagner TF: Biomechanical alterations in the carpal arch and hand muscles after carpal tunnel release: A further approach toward understanding the function of the flexor retinaculum and the cause of postoperative grip weakness. Clin Anat 9:100–108, 1996.
25. Mysiw WJ, Jackson RD: Electrical stimulation. In Braddom RL (ed): Physical Medicine and Rehabilitation. Philadelphia, WB Saunders, 1996, pp 464–491.
26. Banta CA: A prospective, nonrandomized study of iontophoresis, wrist splinting, and antiinflammatory medication in the treatment of early-mild carpal tunnel syndrome. J Occup Med 36:166–168, 1994.
27. Burke DT: Conservative management of carpal tunnel syndrome. In Johnson EW (ed): Carpal Tunnel Syndrome. Phys Med Rehabil Clin North Am 8:513–528, 1997.
28. Einhorn N, Leddy JP: Pitfalls of endoscopic carpal tunnel release. Orthop Clin North Am 27:373–380, 1996.
29. Nancollas MP, Peimer CA, Wheeler DR, Sherwin FS: Long-term results of carpal tunnel release. J Hand Surg 20B:470–474, 1995.
30. National Institutes of Health Consensus Development Panel on Acupuncture: Acupuncture. JAMA 280;1518–1524, 1998.
31. Garfinkel MS, Singhal A, Katz WA, et al: Yoga-based intervention for carpal tunnel syndrome. JAMA 280:1601–1603, 1998.

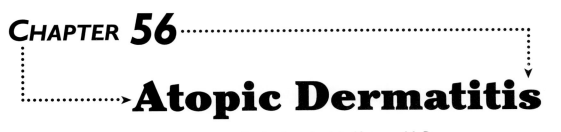

CHAPTER 56

Atopic Dermatitis

Catherine A. Hoffman, M.D.

Atopic dermatitis is a chronic inflammatory skin disease characterized by a lowered threshold of pruritus, leading to an "itch-scratch-itch" cycle.[1] Major criteria for diagnosis of atopic dermatitis as defined by Hanifin are three or more of the following: (1) pruritus; (2) typical morphology and distribution (facial and extensor surface involvement in infants and children and flexural lichenification or linearity in adults); (3) chronic or chronically relapsing dermatitis; and (4) personal or family history of atopy.[2]

An estimated 10% to 15% of the population is affected. Onset is within the first year of life in 60% of cases and within the first 5 years in 85% of cases. The condition clears spontaneously in about 40% of children and persists in some adults as hand dermatitis. Genetic inheritance is probably polygenic, with disease expression dependent on exposure to allergens. Reported concordance rate is 77% in monozygotic twins and 15% in dizygotic twins.[2]

PATHOPHYSIOLOGY OF ATOPIC DERMATITIS

The pathophysiology of atopic dermatitis is probably multifactorial. Genetic predisposition (atopy) results in immune system dysregulation, which induces and perpetuates cutaneous inflammation in response to allergens and superantigens.[1] In acute lesions of atopic dermatitis, the T_H2 response appears to be primary, whereas in chronic lesions, a switch toward a T_H1 pattern occurs, with increased levels of interferon-gamma (IFN-γ), interleukin 12 (IL-12), and granulocyte macrophage colony stimulating factor (GM-CSF) noted in the lesions in addition to the eosinophil growth factor IL-5.[1, 3–5] A decreased pruritus threshold results in scratching and release of cytokines IL-1, tumor necrosis factor alpha (TNF-α), and IL-4 from keratinocytes.[1] These cytokines induce the expression of adhesion molecules (e selectin, intercellular adhesion molecule 1 [ICAM-1], and vascular cell adhesion molecule 1 [VACM-1], which attract lymphocytes, macrophages, and eosinophils to cutaneous sites of inflammation.[1]

Peripheral blood monocytes express both high-affinity IgE receptors (FcRI) and low affinity immunoglobulin E (IgE) receptors (CD23), whereas Langerhans cells, which serve as the antigen presenting cells in the skin, express the high-affinity IgE receptor.[6, 7] By binding IgE in response to aeroallergens or food allergens, Langerhans cells serve to up regulate the IgE response in the skin.[2] Allergen-specific T_H0 cell clones expressing skin-homing receptors (cutaneous lymphocyte antigen) perpetuate the inflammatory response.[1] Specific IgE responses to *Staphylococcus aureus* superantigens are also believed to play a role in maintaining cutaneous inflammation by inhibiting monocyte apoptosis and stimulating production of cytokines GM-CSF, IL-1B, and TNF-α, which contribute to survival of monocytes.[1]

Leukotrienes derived from the lipo-oxygenase pathway may also play a role in the pathogenesis of atopic dermatitis. Increased levels of leukotriene LTB_4 are present in lesional skin.[8] LTC_4 injected intradermally has been found to result in larger wheals in atopic patients than in controls.[9]

The following section presents an overview of some basic concepts in the field of psychoneuroimmunology as a prelude to discussion of the role of stress in the pathogenesis of atopic dermatitis.

PSYCHONEUROIMMUNOLOGY

Psychoneuroimmunology is the study of behavioral, neural, endocrine, and immune system interactions.[10] Bidirectional pathways exist between the central nervous system (CNS) and the immune system.[10, 11] Links include the hypothalamic-pituitary-adrenal axis and autonomic nervous system and vagus nerve.[12] Sympathetic nerve fibers present in the spleen and lymph nodes serve as direct links between the nervous system and the immune system.[10–12] Immune cells such as lymphocytes and macrophages form close junctions with these nerves and have receptors for hormones, neuropeptides, and neurotransmitters.[10, 11] These are molecular links between the nervous system and the immune system.[12] This system may be broken down into efferent and afferent arms. The efferent arm may be thought of as pathways from the CNS to the skin, while the afferent arm consists of pathways from the skin to the CNS (Figs. 56–1 and 56–2).

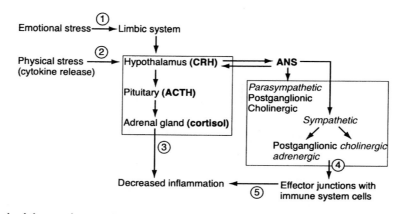

Figure 56–1. Efferent branch of the psychoneuroimmune system.
1. Emotional stress interfaces with the central nervous system via the limbic system.[13]
2. Physical stressors, such as injury, result in release of cytokines and interact via the hypothalamic-pituitary-adrenal (HPA) axis and the autonomic nervous system (ANS).[13]
3. Cortisol produced by the adrenal glands and in response to the fight or flight response downregulates inflammation.[13]
4. In the skin, the sympathetic nervous system causes vasoconstriction and sweating.
5. Thus, the HPA axis and the ANS enable us to balance our response to outside emotional and physical stressors by curtailing inflammation. Thus, self-limited responses to inflammation also may protect us from developing autoimmune disease.[13] **To summarize, the efferent arm involves stress acting on the HPA axis and the ANS to decrease inflammation.** ACTH, adrenocorticotropic hormone; CRH, corticotropin-releasing hormone. (Redrawn from Sternberg E, Chrousos G, Wilder R, Gold P: The stress response and the regulation of inflammatory disease. Ann Intern Med 117:854–866, 1992.)

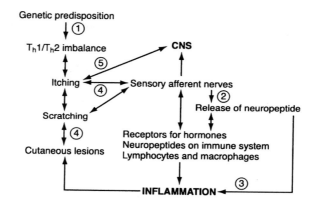

Figure 56–2. Afferent branch of the psychoneuroendocrine system.
1. If we have a genetic tendency toward atopy, resulting in a T_H1/T_H2 cell imbalance, we may develop itching.[14]
2. Sensory afferent nerves and even keratinocytes in the skin, when stimulated by scratching, release neuropeptides.[14]
3. Neuropeptides cause increased inflammation either directly or by binding to receptors on cells of the immune system.[14] They may also result in vasodilatation and wheal and flare responses.[15]
4. Stimulation of afferent sensory nerves by scratching leads to the itch-scratch-itch cycle and triggers development of cutaneous lesions.[14]
5. Note that the CNS is in the loop; thus, it is possible to disrupt the cycle using mental processes. **To summarize, the afferent branch involves stimulation of afferent nerves resulting in release of neuropeptides. This causes inflammation resulting in itching and triggers the behavior of scratching as in the itch-scratch-itch cycle.** CNS, central nervous system: T_H1, T_H2, T helper 1 and T helper 2 cells. (Redrawn from Panconesi E, Hautmann G: Psychophysiology of stress in dermatology: The psychobiologic pattern of psychosomatics. Dermatol Clin 14:399–421, 1996.)

INTEGRATIVE THERAPY IN ATOPIC DERMATITIS

Mind-Body Medicine

Stress and Atopic Dermatitis

Atopic dermatitis has long been recognized as a stress-responsive dermatosis. Retrospective reviews suggest that approximately 50% of cases are stress responsive.[16] Faulstich and coworkers found that patients with atopic dermatitis scored higher on anxiety measures than did controls.[17]

Hashiro and associates compared psychological and immunologic measures for 27 patients with moderate or severe atopic dermatitis with those for 30 normal control patients.[18] The patients with atopic dermatitis had higher self ratings on scales of depression and state of anxiety ($P < .05$ for both).

The dermatitis patients had significantly lower natural killer cell activity ($P < .01$) and IL-4 levels ($P < .05$) but tended to have higher IFN-γ levels than those in controls. These findings correlate with studies showing acute atopic dermatitis to be T_H2 mediated, whereas chronic atopic dermatitis is T_H1 driven.

Family Environment

Gil and colleagues used questionnaires and structured interviews to rate stressors, family environment, and the course of symptoms over the preceding 3 to 6 months in 44 children with severe atopic dermatitis.[19] Percentage of body surface area (BSA) involved and serum IgE levels were measured. On retrospective review it was found that major life stressors did not relate to atopic dermatitis symptoms. Children from families stressing independence and organization had fewer symptoms, whereas children from families scoring high on moral/religious ratings had more symptoms. Encouraging children to adhere to a routine and to take responsibility for their own treatment may have been the key family difference.

Koblenzer and Koblenzer reported on eight children with refractory atopic dermatitis who demonstrated whining, clinging, and demanding behavior and psychosocial delays.[20] These investigators observed that children with severe atopic dermatitis may use scratching to manipulate and to become the focus of family life.[20, 21] Feelings of anger and anxiety in family members are transmitted unconsciously to the child, exacerbating the problem.[20, 21] Helping parents to permit some scratching and to set behavioral limits and having the child sleep in his or her own bed resulted in rapid and sustained improvement.[20, 21]

Psychotherapy

In a study reported by Cole and coworkers, group psychotherapy as an adjunct to medical treatment resulted in significant improvement in 5 targeted variables in 10 adults with severe atopic dermatitis.[22] Patients served as their own controls during a 12-week baseline period, 12-week treatment period, and 1 month follow-up period.[22] The investigators found that improvement was maintained, with only slight worsening at the 1 month follow-up visit. There was a 30% decrease in the amount of topical steroids used. The investigators noted that limitations of this study were the small sample size, lack of blinding, and uncontrolled variable of increased time spent with doctors but stated that the amount of improvement noted with group therapy was clinically meaningful and worthy of additional study.

Ehlers and colleagues conducted a randomized controlled trial of one of four interventions plus standard medical care (SMC) versus SMC alone in 113 patients with atopic dermatitis.[23] They studied severity of skin lesions, amounts and types of topical steroids used, and measures of itching and scratching, distress, and psychological adjustment. Patients who received psychological treatments such as autogenic training (AT) composed of relaxation training with autosuggestions aimed at controlling scratching, cognitive-behavioral therapy (CBT), or the combination of dermatology education about atopic dermatitis and skin care plus behavioral therapy (DEBT) experienced clinical improvement that was statistically significantly greater than that obtained with SMC alone ($P < .001$ for AT and DEBT, $P < .01$ for BT). Dermatology education (DE) alone was more effective than SMC alone only after the 3 month treatment phase ($P < .01$) Psychological treatment groups, however, maintained their improvement and used lesser amounts of topical steroids during the 1-year follow-up period.

Massage Therapy

In a single blind randomized controlled trial comparing standard topical care versus standard topical care and massage therapy in 20 children with atopic dermatitis, Schachner and associates taught a specific sequence of massage strokes to follow at home.[24] After 1 month of therapy, parents had significantly lower anxiety levels ($P < .05$) and children showed significant improvement on all clinical measures: redness ($P < .001$); lichenification, scaling, and pruritus ($P < .05$); and excoriation ($P < .01$). The control group showed significant improvement only in scaling ($P < .05$). Although there were only a small number of children in this study and the follow-up period is short, the results suggest that massage therapy may be useful for both parents and children. Addition of essential oils to a massage therapy regimen did not result in additional benefit over traditional massage therapy, and such oils may provoke allergic contact dermatitis.[25]

Hypnosis

Stewart and Thomas studied the use of progressive relaxation and self hypnosis as treatment for refractory atopic dermatitis in an uncontrolled trial in 18 adult patients.[26] No objective dermatologic examination was conducted. Measurements were based on self-reporting of pruritus and amount of topical steroids used. Sixteen of the 18 patients reported decreased itching at 8 weeks, with improvement maintained for up to 2 years. There was a significant decrease in the reported amount of topical steroids used.

The same investigators treated 20 children with atopic dermatitis using a relaxation/self-hypnosis tape to be played on a nightly basis.[26] Assessments of clinical condition were based on a retrospective review of chart notes rather than by objective blinded clinical examination. Questionnaires completed up to 18 months later were used to assess response to treatment. Ten out of 12 children who completed the questionnaire reportedly experienced clinical improvement. The condition of the remaining eight children was not reported. A larger randomized controlled trial is needed to establish the benefit of hypnotherapy for treatment of atopic dermatitis.

Biofeedback

Haynes and associates studied the effect of biofeedback on atopic dermatitis in 12 patients, 8 of whom completed the study.[27] The study design consisted of a baseline phase followed by a placebo control treatment phase, in which patients were instructed to relax when they heard a tone. This phase was followed by a 4-week phase focusing on relaxation and electromyographic feedback. The investigators measured BSA involvement. Patients rated itching on a 10 point scale. There was a consistent decrease in itching during each session but not across sessions. There was a significant mean reduction in BSA involvement of approximately 50% for the duration of the program. Because of the study design, it was impossible to determine whether improvement was due to use of relaxation techniques or to biofeedback.

Phototherapy

Exacerbation of atopic dermatitis by heat and sweating complicates the use of standard ultraviolet B (UVB) phototherapy for this condition. Other phototherapy modalities such as ultraviolet A (UVA) plus UVB, narrow-band UVB (using light wavelength of 311 nm), medium- and high-dose UVA1, and cold light UVA1 therapies have been shown to be effective for treatment of atopic dermatitis.[28–34]

In one study, use of narrow-band UVB resulted in clearing skin lesions in $4^{1}/_{2}$ weeks, with remission maintained during a 2-month follow-up period.[28] In a second study, this modality was as effective as bath psoralen plus UVA (PUVA) therapy in clearing atopic dermatitis.[29] Use of air-conditioned narrow-band UVB therapy in an open trial of 21 patients was well tolerated and decreased severity of atopic dermatitis by 68%.[30]

High-dose UVA1 therapy results in longer periods of remission than those obtained with medium-dose UVA1 therapy.[31–33] Cold light UVA1 therapy was found to be more effective than both UVA-UVB therapy and conventional UVA1 therapy.[34] Skin status improved, or the lesions even cleared completely, in 3 weeks in 85.4% of patients receiving UVA1 cold light phototherapy versus 77.3% of patients receiving conventional UVA1 therapy, with improvement main-tained during a 1-month follow-up period.[34] The almost complete absence of heat load and intense sweating is a purported advantage of cold light over conventional high-dose UVA1 phototherapy.[34]

The proposed mechanism of action for high-dose UVA treatment is down-regulation of IFN γ, induction of IL-10, and apoptosis of CD$^+$ T cells in lesional skin.[31] Use of narrow-band UVB and newer UVA1 phototherapy is limited by the high cost of bulbs and equipment, lack of compatibility with preexisting light box units, and poor reimbursement by insurance companies.

Chinese Herbal Therapy

Sheehan and colleagues used a standardized decoction of 10 herbs (*Ledebouriella seseloides, Potentilla chinensis, Clematis armandii, Rehmannia glutinosa, Paeonia lactiflora, Lophatherum gracile, Dictamnus dasycarpus, Tribulus terrestris, Glycyrrhiza uralensis,* and *Schizonepeta tenuifoli*) in double blind, placebo controlled cross-over trials for the treatment of childhood and adult atopic dermatitis.[35, 36] In a study of 47 children (37 of whom completed the study), median percentage decreases in erythema scores and "surface damage" scores were 51% and 63.1% versus 6.1% and 6.2%, respectively, during the placebo phase (95% confidence interval). In a second study involving 40 adults (31 of whom completed the study), extent and severity of erythema and surface damage were significantly less for the traditional Chinese herbal therapy (TCHT) phase ($P < .0005$ for both) than for the placebo phase. There was subjective clinical improvement as determined by relief of pruritus ($P < .001$) and enhanced sleep ($P < .078$) during the TCHT treatment phase. Efficacy and safety during a 1-year follow-up period have also been established; however, monitoring of hepatic and renal function at least every 6 months during treatment is recommended.[35, 37] Armstrong and Ernst have criticized the foregoing studies on the basis of lack of intention to treat analysis, selection bias, insufficient power, and possible unblinding owing to the unpleasant taste of the TCHT decoction.[38] In addition, the placebo contained *Glycyrrhiza uralensis* (licorice) in the same quantities as were present in the active formulation.[38]

Poor palatability has limited the use of the original decoction.[39] A freeze-dried extract of the TCHT herbs used in these two trials, Zemaphyte, was formulated and found to be comparable in an open label study.[40] The dose used was four packets of Zemaphyte freeze-dried granules daily.[40] Zemaphyte therapy has been shown to block IL-4–induced expression of the low-affinity IgE receptor (CD23) on monocytes in vitro.[40, 41]

Xu and colleagues studied 10 patients with atopic dermatitis with Zemaphyte for 2 months in an uncontrolled study.[42] Erythema was decreased by 53%, and both HLA DR expression and the number of antigen presenting cells expressing CD23 were significantly reduced after treatment.[42] High-affinity IgE receptors are not affected, but levels of serum IgE complexes, soluble IL-2 receptor, and soluble VCAM were decreased following Zemaphyte treatment.[41, 42] Latchman has suggested that the success of this treatment may be in its ability to target a variety of immunologic parameters involved in the pathogenesis of atopic dermatitis: adhesion molecule expression and IL-4, IgE, and CD23 pathways.[40]

Fung and coworkers conducted a double-blind, placebo-controlled, cross-over study among 40 Chinese patients (adults and children) with recalcitrant atopic dermatitis, using Zemaphyte versus placebo for 8 consecutive weeks, each with a 4-week "wash out" period.[43] With the exception of lichenification, the median change in clinical scores for erythema, surface damage, and scaling was nonsignificant.

NOTE

Nonstandardized, unregulated Chinese herbal and proprietary medicines may be contaminated with heavy metals, substituted herbs, arsenic, Western pharmaceuticals, and other potential toxins.[44]

Pharmaceuticals

Topical Steroids

Although topical steroids have long been the mainstay of therapy for atopic dermatitis, misinformation and misuse of these medications have resulted in widespread concern regarding their use. In a questionnaire-based study of 200 dermatology outpatients with atopic dermatitis, 72.4% of patients worried about the perceived risks of skin thinning and systemic absorption effects on growth and development,[45] and 24% did not comply with treatment owing to these worries.[46] Of the patients who used hydrocortisone, 31% misclassified it as strong or very strong or did not know the potency.[46]

Precautions. Although potent and ultrapotent topical steroids may cause skin atrophy with continued or inappropriate use, careful monitoring and tapering of medications should prevent this complication. As cited by Charman and coworkers, Patel and colleagues found no discrepancies in height between adults with a history of atopic dermatitis since the age of 5 years and normal controls,[46] and most studies have failed to demonstrate clinically significant adrenal suppression from use of mild or moderate topical steroids.[46]

Tacrolimus and Pimecrolimus

Newer medications such as tacrolimus ointment (FK506), a macrolide produced by a fungus found in the soil of Mount Tsukuba, Japan, and pimecrolimus

1% cream (ascomycin; ASM 981), comprising a novel class of anti-inflammatory macrolactams, promise to revolutionize the treatment of moderate to severe atopic dermatitis and facial and eyelid dermatitis.[47, 48] Tacrolimus binds to the FK binding site on CD4+ lymphocytes.[47] This complex then binds to and competitively inhibits calcineurin, thus preventing it from activating gene promoter regions for IL-2, IL-3, IL-4, IL-5, GM-CSF, TNF-α, and IFN-γ.[49] Tacrolimus also has numerous other effects that down-regulate adhesion molecule expression, release of mast cell mediators, and high-affinity IgE receptor expression on Langerhans cells.[47] Pimecrolimus inhibits the synthesis of T_H1 and T_H2 cytokines in target cells.[48]

Double-blind, placebo-controlled, multicenter trials of tacrolimus 0.1% and 0.03% ointment versus vehicle have demonstrated 90% or greater improvement in 36.8% and 27.5% of adult patients, respectively, versus 6.6% for vehicle alone, and 50% or greater improvement in 72.7% and 61.6% versus 19.8% for vehicle alone.[45] The 0.1% strength was more effective for patients with severe disease, for those with extensive BSA involvement, and in African American patients.[45]

Tacrolimus ointment in both the 0.1% and 0.03% formulations has been demonstrated to be safe and effective in a double-blind, vehicle-controlled, multicenter study involving 351 children ages 2 to 15 with moderate to severe atopic dermatitis.[49] Significantly more children ($P < .001$) experienced improvement of 90% or greater than those receiving the vehicle.[49] In a double-blind multicenter trial involving 88 children aged 7 to 16 with moderate to severe atopic dermatitis, 69% of patients in the tacrolimus 0.03% ointment group and 67% in the 0.1% ointment group demonstrated a marked to excellent response (>75%) versus 38% in the vehicle group.[50] Use of 0.3% ointment was not markedly superior to the other two strengths, and this formulation is not currently commercially available.

Pimecrolimus 1% cream applied twice daily has been demonstrated to be effective for the treatment of moderate atopic dermatitis in a randomized, double-blind, placebo-controlled, right and left comparison study of 34 adult patients.[51] Within 3 weeks of twice daily usage, a decrease of 71.9% on the Atopic Dermatitis Severity Index was attained for treated sites, compared with a reduction of 10.3% for placebo cream–treated sites.[51]

Cyclosporine and Mycophenolate Mofetil

Cyclosporine

Cyclosporine (Neoral) has been demonstrated to be effective for the treatment of severe atopic dermatitis, but rapid rates of relapse and concerns regarding potential renal toxicity have made this agent less desirable, particularly given the efficacy of topical tacrolimus.[52]

Mycophenolate Mofetil

Oral mycophenolate mofetil at a dose of 2 g daily has also been found to be effective for the treatment of severe atopic dermatitis but staphylococcal septicemia has been reported in association with this therapy.[53, 54] The mode of action is blockade of the enzyme inosine 5′-monophosphate dehydrogenase, necessary for generating purines for DNA and RNA synthesis.[55] Detailed discussion of the use of these agents is beyond the scope of this chapter.

Antihistamines

Sedating antihistamines for bedtime use are warranted because of their soporific effect, but use for decreasing pruritus is not supported by randomized controlled trials. There is no evidence to support the use of nonsedating antihistamines[56] in atopic dermatitis.

Oral Antibiotics

Flares of atopic dermatitis are often due to secondary impetiginization, characterized by pustules, excoriations, and oozing with crusting. Treatment with oral antibiotics to cover *S. aureus* is indicated under these circumstances.

Topical Botanicals

Chamomile

Chamomile is purported to have anti-inflammatory effects when applied topically as an astringent tea to the skin, but efficacy in double-blind trials has not been established.[57] Kamillosan cream, containing chamomile extract as the active ingredient, was found to be slightly more effective than 0.5% hydrocortisone cream but was only marginally more effective than placebo in a randomized, blinded, half-side comparison trial.[58]

Glycyrrhetinic Acid

Using immunohistochemistry techniques, the enzyme ii beta-hydroxysteroid dehydrogenase, which catalyzes the conversion of cortisol to the inactive steroid cortisone in humans, was demonstrated in skin biopsy samples from healthy volunteers and from patients with psoriasis and eczema. Glycyrrhetinic acid, the major component of licorice, was found to inhibit the enzyme, thus potentiating the action of hydrocortisone.[59]

Oatmeal

Commercially available products containing oatmeal such as Aveeno are often recommended to soothe pruritus in atopic dermatitis, but data regarding efficacy and duration of relief are not available.

Diet and Dietary Supplements

Evening Primrose Oil

Normal or increased plasma levels of linoleic acid (LA) but decreased levels of its metabolites gamma linolenic acid (GLA) and arachidonic acid have been reported in patients with atopic dermatitis.[60, 61] Evening primrose oil (Epogam) is a good source of both LA and GLA and may inhibit cyclo-oxygenase; thus, its use as a supplement to treat atopic dermatitis has been studied.[61–63] However, data from clinical trials do not support the efficacy of evening primrose oil as a treatment for atopic dermatitis.[64–66]

Fish Oil

Studies of supplementation with fish oil have also failed to show consistent benefit. Treatment with evening primrose oil plus fish oil (Efamol, comprising 430 mg primrose oil and 107 mg of marine fish oil containing 17 mg of eicosapentaenoic acid and 11 mg of docosahexaenoic acid *n*-3 essential fatty acids) failed to affect clinical severity or symptom scores as compared with placebo.[7]

Food Allergies

Approximately 40% of infants and young children with moderate to severe atopic dermatitis have food allergies, but such allergies are less common in older children and adults.[68] Cow's milk, eggs, peanuts, and soy are common offending foods in infants and children. Wheat, tree nuts, fish, and shellfish are other common food allergens in children. Sicherer and Sampson have stated that although removal of the allergenic protein(s) leads to clinical improvement, a great deal of education is required because food elimination diets risk causing nutritional deficits.[68] (see Chapter 81, Food Allergy).

Skin prick testing radioallergosorbent test (RAST) techniques (in vitro testing for specific IgE antibodies), and oral food challenges are three methods of testing for food allergies. Skin prick testing is more sensitive than RAST techniques but is most useful when results are negative, as the negative predictive value is greater than 95%.[68] The positive predictive value is only 30% to 50%; thus, only about a third of positive results correlate with a positive food challenge.[68] A positive RAST result has low specificity, while a negative result is very reliable in ruling out an

IgE-mediated reaction to a particular food. Sicherer and Sampson caution that oral food challenges should be done only with medical supervision. They advise that retesting for food allergies be done on a periodic basis, as most food allergies resolve in early childhood[68] (see Chapter 82, The Elimination Diet and Diagnosing Food Hypersensitivities).

Dust Mite Allergies

Ricci and colleagues found that dust mite load and severity of atopic dermatitis decreased significantly (*P* = .022) with the use of dust mite allergen control measures during a 2-month placebo-controlled trial involving 41 children with atopic dermatitis.[69] Tan and associates found dust mite control measures such as use of Gore-Tex bed covers, benzyltannate spray, and a high-filtration vacuum cleaner to be more effective than placebo measures in decreasing atopic dermatitis severity scores (*P* = .006) and area affected (*P* = .006) in a 6-month study involving a total of 48 adults and children.[79]

— *THERAPEUTIC REVIEW* —

Mind-Body Medicine
- *The role of stress in exacerbating atopic dermatitis should be acknowledged and validated when appropriate.*
- *Discussing the role of psychological factors at the time of diagnosis can help in the patient's acceptance of this information and may be perceived as less invasive at this time.[71] If these factors are presented only later after a treatment failure, patients or family members may feel personally attacked and may feel as if they are being blamed for the failure.*
- *Patients' need to maintain control over their illness must be appreciated, as this helps them to take an active role in their treatment.*
- *Patients should be instructed in techniques such as progressive relaxation and habit-reversal techniques to provide them with an active behavioral strategy.*
- *Patients and families should be referred to support groups when appropriate.*
- *The use of massage during application of topical medications and emollients should be encouraged. Having a spouse or partner apply medications using massage techniques may be especially helpful for adult patients, who often face issues of decreased sexual attractiveness because of their skin disease.*
- *When children with atopic dermatitis do not improve as expected, the role of family dynamics in treatment failure should be explored, and the child should be encouraged to be as independent as possible in performing routine treatments.*

Phototherapy
- *Air-conditioned narrow-band UVB, medium-dose and high-dose UVA1, and cold light UVA1 therapies, although not currently widely available, are potentially promising treatments.*

Chinese Herbal Therapy
- *Treatment with standardized Zemaphyte granules (4 packets per day) has been demonstrated to be efficacious for Caucasian patients with atopic dermatitis. Complete blood count, serum creatinine, and liver enzymes should be monitored during treatment. Zemaphyte is awaiting approval from the U.S. Food and Drug Administration.*

Pharmaceuticals

Topical Steroids
- *Patient's concerns regarding the use of topical steroids should be addressed in a thoughtful manner.*
- *Appropriate strengths, vehicles, and amounts should be prescribed for the affected body area, and both strength and frequency must be tapered as improvement occurs.*
- *The use of moderate or strong topical steroids on the face or in the groin or intertriginous areas should be avoided. Even a mild topical steroid used on the face may cause perioral dermatitis and atrophy if applied frequently enough over time.*
- *Intramuscular steroids and oral steroids may be used on an occasional basis for acute flares but are contraindicated for routine or maintenance therapy in view of concerns regarding systemic side effects.*

THERAPEUTIC REVIEW   continued

Other Immunosuppressive Medications
- *Tacrolimus (FK506) ointment 0.03% or 0.1% may be used twice daily for patients with moderate to severe atopic dermatitis or facial or eyelid dermatitis.*
- *Pimecrolimus (ascomycin) 0.1% cream twice daily is indicated for moderate atopic dermatitis and may be particularly useful on the face and hands for daytime application given its cream formulation.*
- *Cyclosporine (Neoral) at 3 to 5 mg per kg per day and mycophenolate mofetil at 2 g per day should be reserved for severe refractory cases, in view of the rapid relapse rates and safety concerns. A second treatment plan should be in place before these medications are discontinued.*

Adjunct Treatments
- *Culture and treatment with appropriate oral antibiotics are indicated when secondary impetiginization manifested by pustules, erosions, and oozing is present.*
- *Sedating antihistamines are useful for their sedative rather than their antipruritic effect. Hydroxyzine (Atarax), at an adult starting dose of 10 to 25 mg orally at bedtime, and Doxepin, an antidepressant used (at low doses) for antihistamine effects, at an adult starting doses of 10 to 25 mg orally at bedtime, are choices favored by dermatologists. Both are available in suspension or syrup form for pediatric dosing. Use of nonsedating antihistamines is not supported by the literature.*

Botanicals
- *Chamomile cream is comparable in strength to 0.5% hydrocortisone cream.*
- *Topical glycyrrhetinic acid (a component of licorice) may potentiate the action of hydrocortisone, thereby serving as a steroid-sparing agent.*
- *Oatmeal baths may decrease pruritus.*

Diet
- *Testing for food allergies in young children with moderate to severe atopic dermatitis may be useful. Egg, milk, wheat, soy, and peanut are the most common culprits.*
- *Elimination diet trials should be conducted under medical supervision to prevent nutritional deficits.*

Dust Mite Precautions and Indoor Environment
- *Pillows and mattresses should be covered with Gore Tex or similar barrier fabrics.*
- *Pets should be kept out of the bedroom (and preferably outdoors).*
- *Flooring and blinds should be used instead of carpets and drapes to reduce dust accumulation.*
- *Use of hot water and high dryer temperatures (13°F or higher) in laundering is indicated to kill mites. Bedding and stuffed animals should be laundered weekly.*
- *Wet mopping and vacuuming, use of HEPA filters, and keeping ambient temperatures cool are other helpful measures.*

General Skin Care
- *Use of cooler water temperatures and gentle soaps or soap substitutes during bathing is beneficial.*
- *Moisturizers (ointments or creams rather than lotions) should be applied to moist skin rather than to dry skin.*

ACKNOWLEDGMENTS

I would like to express my appreciation to Tim Berger, M.D., for his expert advice as well as to Toby Maurer, M.D., and Rosie Chattha, M.D., for encouraging my interests in this area. I also owe special thanks to Andrew Weil, M.D., Dr. Tracy Gaudet, and the Fellows and staff at the Center for Integrative Medicine at the University of Arizona at Tucson. Thanks also to the Women's Dermatologic Society and Galderma for funding my research in this area, and to my husband, Richard, for sharing many of his weekends with this project.

References

1. Leung D: Pathogenesis of atopic dermatitis. J Allergy Clin Immunol 104:S99–S108, 1999.
2. Rudikoff D, Lebwohl M: Atopic dermatitis. Lancet 251:1715–1721, 1998.
3. Maurer D, Fiebiger E, Reininger B, et al: Expression of func-

tional high-affinity immunoglobulin E receptors (FcERI) on monocytes of atopic individuals. J Exp Med 179:745–750, 1994.

4. Stingl G, Maurer D. IgE-mediated allergen presentation via Fc epsilon RI on antigen-presenting cells. Int Arch Allergy Immunol 113:24–29, 1997.

5. Leung D: Atopic dermatitis: New insights and opportunities for therapeutic intervention. J Allergy Clin Immunol 105:860–876, 2000.

6. Hamid Q, Boguniewicz M, Leung DYM: J Clin Invest 94:870–876, 1994. (Cited in reference 5.)

7. Hamid Q, Naseer T, Minshall EM, et al: In vivo expression of IL-12 and IL-13 in atopic dermatitis. J Allergy Clin Immunol 98:225–231

8. Ruzicka, et al: Leukotrienes in skin of atopic dermatitis. Lancet 1:222–223, 1984.

9. Greaves, et al: Leukotriene B$_4$–like immunoactivity and skin disease. Lancet 2:160, 1984.

10. Ader R, Cohen N, Felten D: Psychoneuroimmunology: Interactions between the nervous and the immune system. Lancet 345:99–103, 1995.

11. Maier S, Watkins L, Fleshner M: Psychoneuroimmunology: The interface between behavior, brain and immunity. Am Psychol 49:1004–1017, 1994.

12. Pennisi E: Neuroimmunology: Tracing molecules that make the brain-body connection. Science 275:930–931, 1997.

13. Sternberg E, Chrousos G, Wilder R, Gold P: The stress response and the regulation of inflammatory disease. Ann Intern Med 117:854–866, 1992.

14. Panconesi E, Hautmann G: Psychophysiology of stress in dermatology: The psychobiologic pattern of psychosomatics Dermatol Clin 1:399–421, 1996.

15. Lotti T, Hautmann G, Panconesi E: Neuropeptides in skin. J Am Acad Dermatol 33:482–496, 1995.

16. Ruzicka T: Atopic eczema between rationality and irrationality. Arch Dermatol 1462, 1998.

17. Faulstich ME, Williamson DA, Duchmann EG, et al: Psychophysiological analysis of atopic dermatitis. J Psychosom Res 29:415–417, 1985.

18. Hashiro M, Okamura M: The relationship between the psychological and immunological state in patients with atopic dermatitis. J Dermatol Sci 16:231–235, 1998.

19. Gil KM, Keefe, FJ, Sampson HA, et al: The relation of stress and family environment to atopic dermatitis symptoms in children. J Psychosom Res 31:673–684, 1987.

20. Koblenzer CS, Koblenzer PJ: Chronic intractable atopic eczema. Arch Dermatol 124:1673–1677, 1988.

21. Hanifin JM: Parental issues in the treatment of infantile eczema. Dermatol Clin 14:423–427, 1996.

22. Cole WC, Roth HL, Sachs LB: Group psychotherapy as an aid in the medical treatment of eczema. J Am Acad Dermatol 18:286–291, 1988.

23. Ehlers A, Stangier U, Gieler U: Treatment of atopic dermatitis: A comparison of psychological and dermatologic approaches to relapse prevention. J Consult Clin Psychol 63:634–635, 1995.

24. Schachner L, Field T, Hernandez Reif M, et al: Atopic dermatitis symptoms decreased in children following massage therapy. Pediatr Dermatol 15:390–395, 1998.

25. Anderson C, Lis-Balchin M, Kirk-Smith M: Evaluation of massage with essential oils on childhood atopic eczema. Phytother Res 14:452–456, 2000.

26. Stewart A, Thomas SE: Hypnotherapy as a treatment for atopic dermatitis in adults and children Br J Dermatol 132:778–783, 1995.

27. Haynes SN, Wilson CC, Jaffe PG, Britton BT: Biofeedback treatment of atopic dermatitis. Controlled case studies of eight cases. Biofeedback and self-regulation. 4:195–209, 1979.

28. Grundmann Kollmann M, Behrens S, Podda M, et al: Phototherapy for atopic eczema with narrow band UVB. J Am Acad Dermatol 40:995–997, 1999.

29. Der Petrossian, M, Seeber A, Honigsmann H, Tanew A: Half side comparison study on the efficacy of 8-methoxypsoralen bath PUVA versus narrow band ultraviolet B phototherapy in patients with severe chronic atopic dermatitis. Br J Dermatol 142:39–43, 2000.

30. George SA, Bilsland DJ, Johnson BE, Ferguson J: Narrow band

(TL 01) UVB air conditioned phototherapy for chronic severe adult atopic dermatitis. Br J Dermatol 128:49–56, 1993.

31. Krutmann J, Diepgen T, Luger T, et al: High dose UVA1 therapy for atopic dermatitis: Results of a multicenter trial. J Am Acad Dermatol 38:589–593, 1998.

32. Abeck, D, Schmidt T, Fesq H, et al: Long term efficacy of medium dose UVA1 phototherapy in atopic dermatitis. J Am Acad Dermatol 42:254–257, 2000.

33. Schmidt T, Fesq H, Strom K, et al: Long term efficacy of medium dose UVA1 phototherapy in atopic dermatitis. J Am Acad Dermatol 42:254–257, 2000.

34. Von Kobyletzki G, Hoffmann K, Altmeyer P: Medium dose UVA1 cold-light phototherapy in the treatment of severe atopic dermatitis. J Am Acad Dermatol 41:931, 1999.

35. Sheehan MP, Atherton DJ. A controlled trial of traditional Chinese medicinal plants in widespread non-exudative atopic eczema. Br J Dermatol 126:179–184, 1992.

36. Sheehan, M, Rustin M, Atherton D, et al: Efficacy of traditional Chinese herbal therapy in adult atopic dermatitis. Lancet 340:13–17, 1992.

37. Sheehan M, Atherton D: One-year follow-up of children treated with Chinese medicinal herbs for atopic dermatitis. Br J Dermatol 130:488–493, 1994.

38. Armstrong NC, Ernst E: The treatment of eczema with Chinese herbs: A systematic review of randomized clinical trials. Br J Clin Pharmacol 48:262–264, 1999.

39. Atherton D, Sheehan M, Rustin M, et al: Treatment of atopic eczema with traditional Chinese medicinal plants. Pediat Dermatol 9:373–375, 1992.

40. Latchman Y, Banerjee P, Poulter L, et al: Association of immunological changes with clinical efficacy in atopic eczema patients treated with traditional Chinese herbal therapy (Zemaphyte). Int Arch Allergy Immunol 10:243–249, 1996.

41. Latchman Y, Bungy G, Atherton D, et al: Efficacy of traditional Chinese herbal therapy in vitro. A model system for atopic eczema: Inhibition of CD23 expression on blood monocytes. Br J Dermatol 132:592–598, 1995.

42. Xu XJ, Banerjee P, Rustin MHA, Poulter LW: Modulation by Chinese herbal therapy of immune mechanisms in the skin of patients with atopic eczema. Br J Dermatol 136:54–59, 1997.

43. Fung A, Look P, Chong LY, et al: A controlled trial of traditional Chinese herbal medicine in Chinese patients with recalcitrant atopic dermatitis. Int J Dermatol 38:387–392, 1999.

44. Chan T, Chan J, Tomlinson B, Critchley J: Chinese herbal medicines revisited: A Hong Kong perspective. Lancet 342:1532–1534, 1993.

45. Hanifin J, Ling M, Breneman D, Rafal E: Tacrolimus ointment for the treatment of atopic dermatitis in adult patients: Part 1, efficacy. J Am Acad Dermatol 44:S28–S38, 2001.

46. Charman C, Morris A, Williams H: Topical corticosteroid phobia in patient with atopic eczema. Br J Dermatol 142:931–936, 2000.

47. Fleischer A: Treatment of atopic dermatitis: Role of tacrolimus ointment as a topical noncorticosteroid therapy. J Allergy Clin Immunol 104:S126–S130, 1999.

48. Paul C, Ho V: Ascomycins in dermatology. Semin Cutan Med Surg 17:256–259, 1998.

49. Paller A, Eichenfield L, Leung D, et al: A 12-week study of tacrolimus ointment for the treatment of atopic dermatitis in pediatric patients. J Am Acad Dermatol 44:S47–S57, 2001.

50. Boguniewwicz M, Fielder V, Raimer, S et al: A randomized vehicle controlled trial of tacrolimus ointment for treatment of atopic dermatitis in children. J Allergy Clin Immunol 102:637–644, 1998.

51. Van Leent E, Graber M, Thurston M, et al: Effectiveness of the ascomycin macrolactam SDZ ASM 981 in the topical treatment of atopic dermatitis. Arch Dermatol 134:805–809, 1998.

52. Leung D, Soter N: Cellular and immunologic mechanisms in atopic dermatitis. J Am Acad Dermatol 44:S1–S12, 2001.

53. Neuber K, Schwartz I, Itschert G, Dieck AT: Treatment of atopic eczema with oral mycophenolate mofetil. Br J Dermatol 143:385–391, 2000.

54. Satchell AC, Barnetson RS: Staphylococcal septicaemia complicating treatment of atopic dermatitis with mycophenolate [letter]. Br J Dermatol 143:202–203, 2000.

55. Mehling A, Grabbe S, Voskort M, et al: Mycophenolate mofetil impairs the maturation and function of murine dendritic cells. J Immunol 165:2374–2381, 2000.

56. Klein P, Clark R: An evidence based review of the efficacy of antihistamines in relieving pruritus in atopic dermatitis. Arch Dermatol 135:1522–1525, 1999.

57. Mann C, Staba E: The chemistry, pharmacology and commercial formulations of chamomile. Part 1: Herbs, spices, and medicinal plants. In Murray M, Pizzorno J (eds): Encyclopedia of Natural Medicine, Rev 2nd ed. Prima Health, 1984, pp 235–280.

58. Patzelt Wenczler, R, Ponce-Poschl E: Proof of efficacy of Kamillosan cream in atopic eczema. Eur J Med Res 5:171–175, 2000.

59. Teelucksingh S, Mackie ADR, Burt D, et al: Potentiation of hydrocortisone activity in skin by glycyrrhetinic acid. Lancet 335:1060–1063, 1990.

60. Soyland E, Funk J, Rajka G, et al: Dietary supplementation with very long chain n-3 fatty acids in patients with atopic dermatitis. A double blind, multicentre study. Br J Dermatol 130:757–764, 1994.

61. Manku MS, Ghering D, Schlotte V, et al: Reduced levels of prostaglandin precursors in the blood of atopic patients with defective delta-6 desaturase function as a biochemical basis for atopy. Prostaglandins Leukotrienes Med 9:615–626, 1982.

62. Manku MS, Horrobin DF, Morse NL, et al: Essential fatty acids in the plasma phospholipids of patients with atopic dermatitis. Br J Dermatol 110:643–648, 1984.

63. Schaffer H: Essential fatty acids and eicosanoids in cutaneous inflammation. Int J Dermatol 281–290, 1989.

64. Bamford JTM, Gibson RW, Renier CM: Atopic eczema unresponsive to evening primrose oil (linoleic and gamma linolenic acids). J Am Acad Dermatol 13:959–965, 1985.

65. Bjornboe, A, Soyland E, Bjornboe E, et al: Effect of dietary supplementation with eicosapentaenoic acid in the treatment of atopic dermatitis. Br J Dermatol 117:463–469, 1987.

66. Fairris GM, Perkins P, Lloyd B, et al: The effect of atopic dermatitis of supplementation with selenium and vitamin E. Acta Derm Venereol (Stockh) 69:359–362, 1989.

67. Berth-Jones J, Graham-Brown RAC: Placebo controlled trial of essential fatty acid supplementation in atopic dermatitis. Lancet 341:1557–1560, 1993.

68. Sicherer S, Sampson H: Food hypersensitivity and atopic dermatitis: Pathophysiology, epidemiology, diagnosis, and management. J Allergy Clin Immunol 104:S114–S122, 1999.

69. Ricci G, Patrizi A, Specchia F, et al: Effect of house dust mite avoidance measures in children with atopic dermatitis. Br J Dermatol 143:379–384, 2000.

70. Tan BB, Weald D, Strickland I, Friedman P: Double blind controlled trial of effect of house dust mite allergen avoidance on atopic dermatitis. Lancet 347:12–18, 1996.

71. Czyzewski DI, Lopez M: Clinical psychology in the management of pediatric skin disease. Dermatol Clin 16:619–629, 1998.

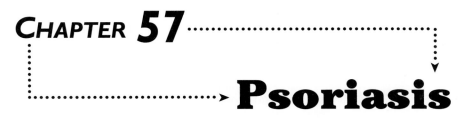

CHAPTER 57

Psoriasis

Catherine A. Hoffman, M.D.

Psoriasis is a chronic inflammatory skin disease that has been classified into following major subtypes:

- **Plaque-type psoriasis** is characterized by scaly, erythematous, variably pruritic, well-demarcated, often symmetrical plaques typically involving the scalp, elbows, knees, and lumbosacral area, but which may spread to involve a large percentage of the body surface area (BSA). Palms and soles may be affected. Dystrophic nail changes and nail pitting may occur.
- **Inverse psoriasis** affects intertriginous areas (axillae and groin).
- **Erythrodermic psoriasis** is defined as the presence of erythema and scaling involving greater than 80% of the BSA. Potential complications include high-output cardiac failure, renal failure, and sepsis.
- **Pustular psoriasis** is a life-threatening form of the disease with often confluent pustules overlying erythematous plaques and sometimes superimposed over classic psoriatic plaques. Potential complications include high-output cardiac failure, sepsis, and hypercalcemia.[1]
- **Palmar-plantar pustulosis** is a chronic, localized form involving the palms and soles.[1]
- **Guttate psoriasis** is characterized by diffuse involvement with scaly, erythematous, drop-like papules. This form may be triggered by immunogenic cross-reactivity with group A streptococci.[1]
- **Psoriatic arthritis** may accompany any of the foregoing forms of psoriasis.

PREVALENCE AND PATHOPHYSIOLOGY

Approximately 0.5% to 1.5% of the population in North America is affected by psoriasis.[2] Pathogenesis is multifactorial: Environmental and emotional stressors may trigger disease onset in a genetically predisposed person.[2] Inheritance is probably polygenic.[1] Up to 50% of affected patients have a family history of psoriasis.[1] Monozygotic twins have a 65% to 72% concordance rate, whereas dizygotic twins have a 15% to 30% concordance rate.[2] Antigens against major histocompatibility complexes (MHCs) B13, B7, Cw6, B37, DR3, Cw7, and Cw11 are associated with psoriasis.[1] Medications such as beta

blockers, lithium, and possibly nonsteroidal anti-inflammatory medications may trigger or worsen psoriasis.[1] Use of oral steroids may cause a rebound flare and may trigger a conversion to the life-threatening pustular psoriasis form.

Psoriasis is characterized by an increased rate of keratinocyte proliferation and shortening of the keratinocyte cell cycle, together with immune system dysregulation resulting in inflammation.[2] A T helper cell type 1 (T_H1) response is believed to be predominant in psoriasis, with increased levels of cytokines such as interleukin-1 (IL-1), tumor necrosis factor-alpha (TNF-α), IL-6, and IL-8.[3] CD4$^+$ T cells are present in the dermis, while CD8$^+$ cells are present in the epidermis.[2] Leukotrienes derived from the arachidonic acid and the lipo-oxygenase pathways contribute to the inflammatory response. Leukotriene B_4, known to be chemotactic for neutrophils, is elevated in psoriatic plaques, as is 5-lipo-oxygenase.[2]

Stress and Psoriasis

Epidemiologic surveys and retrospective reviews of series of patients with psoriasis indicate that stress may play a role in over a third of cases but does not correlate with severity of psoriasis.[4–8] Recall bias is an issue in these studies; nevertheless, the role of stress as a triggering factor for psoriasis in a significant proportion of patients is supported. Thus, a proportion of patients but not all patients may benefit from mind-body modalities aimed at stress reduction.

INTEGRATIVE THERAPY

Mind-Body Medicine

Psychotherapy

The effects of individual and group psychotherapy on disease course and anxiety were studied in two randomized controlled trials in 51 and 30 patients with psoriasis, respectively.[9, 10] Baseline assessments of psoriasis severity and psychological status were done in a blinded fashion, but intention-to-treat analysis was not conducted in either study.

In the study of individual psychotherapy by Zachariae and associates, medications were stopped before the study. The psoriasis area sensitivity index (PASI) score, total sign score, and laser Doppler skin blood flow measurements were obtained in a blinded fashion at baseline and at weeks 4, 8, and 12.[9] A significantly higher percentage of patients in the treatment group had decreased stress than in controls ($P < .05$). There was no difference in the PASI scale, but there was improvement in the two other measures, suggesting that psychotherapy may have a moderate beneficial effect in psoriasis ($P < .05$) There was no correlation between change in stress scores and psoriasis severity.

Price and colleagues found that patients who participated in group sessions rated them as very useful in helping them to cope with a chronic problem.[10] There was a significant decrease in anxiety scores immediately afterward and at 6-month follow-up ($P < .05$) There was no conclusive difference in clinical improvement between the two groups, but there was a trend toward improvement in the treatment group.

Meditation

In a randomized controlled trial comparing phototherapy combined with mindfulness meditation tapes played during the treatments and phototherapy alone, Kabat-Zin and associates demonstrated that use of the tapes during phototherapy resulted in an increased rate of clearing and decreased number of sessions to clear.[11] Twenty-one patients requiring ultraviolet B (UVB) therapy and 16 patients requiring psoralens plus ultraviolet A (PUVA) therapy were randomized to either a tape or a no-tape group. Intention-to-treat analysis was done. All baseline and follow-up testing was blinded. There was a 50% probability of clearing approximately 1 month earlier for patients in the UVB plus tape therapy group than in the no-tape therapy group and more than 6 weeks earlier for patients in the PUVA plus tape therapy group than in the no tape therapy group ($P = .033$).

Hypnosis

Tausk and coworkers conducted at 3-month blinded randomized controlled trial of active versus neutral hypnosis for treatment of psoriasis in 11 highly or moderately hypnotizable patients.[12] Psoriasis severity was rated using the PASI scale and visual analogue scales. There was no significant difference in PASI scores between the active and neutral hypnosis groups. Highly hypnotizable patients experienced significantly greater improvement than that seen in moderately hypnotizable patients regardless of group ($P = .01$).

Phototherapy

Ultraviolet B Therapy

Plaque-type psoriasis typically subsides during the summer and worsens during the winter.[2] UVB light treatment (with wavelengths of 290 to 320 nm) and, more recently, narrow-band UVB light treatment (with wavelengths of 311 to 312 nm) are systemic therapies for psoriasis. Mode of action is via reduction of the number of Langerhans cells and intraepidermal T cells in the skin, decreased leukocyte adhesion, and induction of the anti-inflammatory cytokine IL-10 from macrophages.[2] Narrow-band UVB therapy induces apoptosis of T cells in psoriatic plaques and reversal of regenerative epidermal hyperplasia, as demonstrated by decreased keratin 16 staining.[13, 14]

A major drawback of UVB therapy is the need for consistent thrice-weekly sessions until a maintenance phase of twice-weekly treatments can be initiated. Approximately 30 treatments are required before improvement is achieved. Risks include sunburn and potential increased risk of skin cancer. The tanning that occurs during treatment may be unacceptable to some patients. Narrow-band UVB therapy equipment is costly, and reimbursement to physicians is insufficient to cover the added expense; therefore, this treatment is less widely available. Data suggest, however, that this new treatment modality is the equivalent of PUVA with less risk of carcinogenesis, no need to wear post-treatment eye protection, and no need for psoralens.[2] Use of lasers such as the 308-nm UVB excimer laser and pulsed-dye laser may achieve more rapid onset of clearing and longer remissions.[15, 16]

Psoralens plus Ultraviolet A Therapy

Psoralens are photosensitizing compounds found in plants such as lime, lemon, parsley, celery, fig, and clove.[1] The compound 8-methoxypsoralen (8-MOP) is used either as an oral preparation or in topical lotions or bath treatments in combination with UVA phototherapy (using light wavelengths of 320 to 400 nm) on a biweekly basis. These treatments may be acceptable to patients with moderate to severe psoriasis who do not respond to UVB therapy and who do not wish to take oral medications such as acitretin (Soriatane) or methotrexate.[17] Phototoxicity, photoaging, and increased risk of cutaneous malignancies (squamous cell carcinoma, basal cell carcinomas, and melanoma) are potential adverse effects of PUVA therapy. Nausea may occur with use of oral 8-MOP.[17]

Other Phototherapeutic Regimens

Goeckerman therapy, which combines the use of

coal tar with UVB light therapy, may be considered a "natural," safe, and effective treatment for patients with extensive areas of involvement. *Ingram therapy* combines use of anthralin with UV light treatment. Both of these treatments are typically delivered at day treatment centers, as both coal tar and anthralin are messy to apply and cause staining. Use of Goeckerman therapy in the home environment has been described and may be applicable for well-informed, motivated patients who are unable or unwilling to travel to a psoriasis day treatment center.[18]

Dead Sea Climatotherapy and Balneophototherapy

Dead Sea climatotherapy combines natural UVB light exposure with soaks in the high-saline, magnesium-rich Dead Sea. Bathing in concentrated (>20%) saline combined with artificial UVB light has been used to simulate Dead Sea therapy and is known as *balneophototherapy*.[2] Retrospective and prospective studies of patients treated at the DMZ clinic at the Dead Sea indicate that the rate of clearing after 4 weeks of treatment is 75% or higher.[19] Relapse occurs in approximately 50% of patients within 1 to 3 months of returning home, but recurrences are often milder (W. Avrach [1977], as cited by Shani and coworkers[19]). In a prospective study of 100 patients with psoriasis treated for 4 weeks at the DMZ clinic, clearing of psoriatic lesions occurred in 75% of the patients, after 4 weeks of climatotherapy. Of the 100 patients, 68% were still in remission after 4 months, 43% after 6 months and 10% after 8 months (E. Knudsen, A. Worm [1996] as cited by Shani and coworkers[19]). In a recent multicenter study of 60 patients treated with narrow-band UVB plus Dead Sea salts, PASI scores significantly improved ($P < .05$), even when intention-to-treat analysis was conducted.[20] There was no control group.

Pharmaceuticals

Topical pharmaceutical products for treatment of psoriasis that may be accepted by patients searching for "natural" therapies include *calcipotriene*, a synthetic vitamin D_3 analogue; *tazarotene* (a topical retinoid related to vitamin A); and *capsaicin* (derived from the chili pepper).

Calcipotriene (Doronex)

Calcipotriene is a synthetic vitamin D_3 analogue that has been demonstrated to be effective for monotherapy for psoriasis but is often used in conjunction with a class I superpotent topical steroid in a step regimen, as the two products used together have synergistic activity.[21-23] This regimen reduces the risk of steroid atrophy and may be acceptable to

some patients who are unwilling to rely on topical steroids. Calcipotriene may also used to potentiate phototherapy and is particularly beneficial for use in difficult to treat areas such as the lower extremities.[24]

Dosage. Apply a thin layer once or twice daily for up to 8 weeks. The total maximum weekly dose is 100 g.

Precautions. Avoid the face; avoid in those with hypercalcemia or nephrolithiasis and in pregnancy.

Tazarotene Gel

The topical retinoid tazarotene (Tazorac) is typically applied once daily in conjunction with an ultrapotent topical steroid, which reduces irritation and retinoid erythema and also acts synergistically.[25] A newer cream formulation is also available. Tazarotene counteracts atrophy induced by topical steroids and has also been used in combination with phototherapy to heighten responsiveness of the skin.[26, 27]

Dosage. 0.05% or 0.1% tazarotene gel or cream applied once daily with a topical steroid cream.

Precautions. Adverse effects include photosensitivity, burning, dry skin, erythema, and pruritus (in up to 30% of patients). This drug should be avoided in pregnancy.

Capsaicin

Substance P is a neuropeptide implicated in the pathogenesis of psoriasis and itching. Because capsaicin depletes substance P from cutaneous sensory neurons, it was evaluated as an agent for potential treatment of psoriasis in a double-blind, placebo-controlled study.[28] Ninety-eight patients in the treatment group and 99 patients in the control (vehicle-only) group applied their respective products 4 times daily for 6 weeks. Patients receiving capsaicin treatment demonstrated significantly greater improvement in global evaluation (p = .024 after 4 weeks and p = .030 after 6 weeks), in pruritus relief (p = .002 and p =.060, respectively), and in reduction of combined psoriasis severity scores (p = .030 and p =.036, respectively). A transient burning sensation at application sites was the most frequently reported side effect in both treatment groups.[28]

Dosage. 0.025% or 0.075% capsaicin (Zostrix) applied three or four times daily.

Precautions. Burning often occurs initially but decreases with continued use. Careful handwashing after application is essential.

Topical Steroids

As noted, the most effective use of topical steroids is in conjunction with medications such as calcipotriene or tazarotene. Topical steroid solutions may be used on the scalp. Ointments are more efficacious than creams, but patients may prefer creams for daytime use. If topical steroids are used as monotherapy, the dosage should be tapered in frequency and the potency decreased as improvement occurs, to prevent the risk of skin atrophy. Use of oral or intramuscular steroids is contraindicated, as this may result in a rebound flare or in conversion to pustular psoriasis. Intralesional steroids may be used for treatment of refractory plaques.

Precautions. Adverse effects include skin atrophy, hyperglycemia, and adrenal suppression with prolonged use.

Cyclosporine

Cyclosporine (Neoral) is effective for the treatment of severe psoriasis. The mechanism of action is via prevention of IL-2 gene transcription.[14]

Dosage. The most effective starting dose is 5 mg per kg.[17] This dose is then tapered by 0.5 mg per kg each month until recurrence is noted.

Precautions. Careful monitoring of blood pressure, serum creatinine, electrolytes including magnesium, and lipids is necessary.[17] Plans for alternate treatment should be in place, as continuing cyclosporine therapy for longer than a 1-year period is not recommended owing to concerns about increased risk of malignancies.[17]

Specific guidelines for the use of therapies for moderate to severe psoriasis including UVB, PUVA, cyclosporine, methotrexate, and systemic retinoid therapy are beyond the scope of this chapter but have been detailed by Weinstein and Gottlieb in a text published by the National Psoriasis Foundation.[17]

New therapies for psoriasis based on T cell pathophysiology are currently undergoing clinical trials. Targets for these new medications include the following sites of interaction: CD80–CD24, CD11a–ICAM1, LFA3–CD2, and IL 8–LFA3tip. Use of TNF-α antagonists also appears promising. The National Psoriasis Foundation Web site (http://www.psoriasis.org) provides a detailed update on the current status of clinical trials and experimental therapies.

Botanicals

Aloe vera (Topical)

Significantly more patients with psoriatic plaques noted clinical improvement after treatment with *Aloe vera* extract 0.5% in a hydrophilic cream than patients whose lesions were "treated" with vehicle alone ($P < .001$)[29] in a 4-week double-blind, placebo-controlled trial. Unfortunately, the authors claim that topical aloe vera "cured" psoriasis in these patients when the clinical follow-up period was

only 12 weeks.[29] Contact dermatitis from aloe vera gel has been reported.[30]

Dosage. Aloe vera gel is available in 98% to 100% purity strengths. The gel is applied three to five times a day.

Chamomile

Although chamomile is often recommended in natural health texts as possessing anti-inflammatory activity, information based on double-blind, placebo-controlled studies is lacking.[31] Persons with a history of allergic rhinitis are advised to use caution, as this plant is a member of the ragweed family, and cross-reactivity may occur.[32]

Glycyrrhetinic Acid (Topical)

Glycyrrhetinic acid is a component of licorice with efficacy similar to or even slightly better than topically applied hydrocortisone cream (F.Q. Evans [1958], as cited by Murray and Pizzorno[31]). Glycyrrhetinic acid inhibits the enzyme ii beta-hydroxysteroid dehydrogenase, which catalyzes the conversion of cortisol to the inactive steroid. This inhibitory effect serves to potentiate the action of topically applied hydrocortisone.[33]

Milk Thistle (Oral)

Buchness has suggested that milk thistle (silymarin) may be useful to prevent hepatotoxicity in patients with psoriasis receiving methotrexate treatment. She recommends 420 mg of silymarin per day divided into three doses, with a decrease in dosage after 6 to 8 weeks to 280 mg per day.[34]

Oatmeal (Topical)

Commercially available oatmeal baths (Aveeno) may temporarily soothe pruritus associated with psoriasis. Data from randomized, controlled trials are not available.

Traditional Chinese Medicine

Chinese Herbal Medications

Both topical and systemic medications used in traditional Chinese medicine (TCM) have been employed in the treatment of psoriasis. Recent studies of topical Chinese creams have demonstrated contamination with topical steroids in many of the products.[35, 36] Contamination of herbs imported from China with heavy metals, pharmaceuticals, and toxins has also been reported.[37]

Chinese herbal medications containing furocumarins have been used topically in combination with UVA irradiation. In patients who took one such medication, Radix Angelicae dahuricae, side effects were milder than those in patients receiving 8-MOP.[38] Koo and Arain cited a study in which topical use of alkaloids with antineoplastic activity such as Camptotheca acuminata Decne (0.03% concentration) was compared with the use of 1% hydrocortisone cream; the topical alkaloids were found to be significantly more effective.[38] Contact dermatitis occurred in 9% to 15% of cases, with possible enhancement of post-inflammatory hyperpigmentation.

Tripterygium wilfordii Hook and *Tripterygium hypoglaucum Hutch* have shown modest efficacy with an acceptable side effect profile.[38] Indirubin, found in indigo naturalis, administered in doses of 100 to 300 mg per day has also been used; however, the frequency of adverse effects (primarily gastrointestinal) ranged from 26% to as high as 96%, with some toxicities rated as severe.[38] A commercially prepared version called *Pillulae indigo naturalis compositae* reportedly has fewer side effects according to Koo and Arain, although transient decreases in white blood cell counts and transient increases in liver enzymes have occurred.[38]

Injectable Radix macrotomiae seu lithospermi was shown to be more effective than an oral formulation. In an open study of 50 cases, 13 cases of psoriasis cleared and 26 greatly improved without systemic side effects.[38] Factors hampering assessment of TCM herbal therapies in the treatment of psoriasis are the differences in classification of psoriasis subtypes according to Chinese medicine and the TCM premise that herbal formulations must be tailored to individual patients, which impedes their use in standardized protocols.[38]

Acupuncture

Jerner and colleagues compared active acupuncture versus "sham" acupuncture in 56 patients with long-standing plaque-type psoriasis.[39] Patients were randomized to receive either active treatment or placebo twice weekly for 10 weeks. Severity of the skin lesions was scored (on the PASI scale) before, during, and 3 months after therapy. There were no statistically significant differences between the outcomes in the two groups during or 3 months after therapy. The PASI mean value had decreased for both groups—from 9.6 to 8.3 in the active group and from 9.2 to 6.9 in the placebo group ($P < .05$).[39]

Dietary Supplements

Fish Oil

Interest in fish oils to treat psoriasis was triggered by the observation that Eskimos, who have a diet low in arachidonic acid, have a much lower incidence of psoriasis than that in Danes.[40] Evidence from double-blind, placebo-controlled trials comparing *n*-3 fish oils and *n*-6 placebo oils has been largely unconvincing.

Bitter and coworkers reported lessening of itching ($P < .05$), erythema ($P < .05$), and scaling in patients who received 10 g of fish oil (delivered as Max-EPA capsules), compared with patients who received an equivalent amount of olive oil in placebo capsules.[41] The total number of patients enrolled in the study was 28. Bjornboe and colleagues, in a second randomized trial involving 30 patients with psoriasis, found no beneficial effect of dietary intake of 10 g per day of *n*-3 fatty acids.[42] Soyland and associates compared supplementation with 6 g of *n*-3 fatty acids (fish oil) with corn oil placebo in 145 patients with psoriasis in a double-blind randomized placebo-controlled trial. They found no significant change in PASI scores or in subjective ratings of symptoms.[43]

A possible role for fish oil supplementation may be to decrease triglyceride levels in patients with psoriasis treated with oral retinoids.[44] Lowe and coworkers studied 11 psoriatic patients with hyperlipidemia induced by etretinate therapy.[44] Fish oil supplementation with 3 g of omega-3 fatty acids daily in addition to the patient's regular diet resulted in a significant decrease in mean plasma triglyceride concentration ($P < .001$) and a significant increase in high-density-lipoprotein ("good") cholesterol ($P < .03$).[44]

Alcohol Use and Smoking

Avoiding alcohol and quitting smoking may render therapies for psoriasis more effective and may decrease the severity of psoriasis. Most studies conducted in the last decade have supported a positive association between alcohol consumption and psoriasis.[45] In addition, alcohol consumption may increase the risk of developing psoriasis. Higgins and associates reported an odds ratio of alcohol consumption as a risk factor for psoriasis of 8.01.[46] Poikalainen and colleagues conducted a case control study in 144 male patients with psoriasis and 285 unmatched controls with other skin diseases. The odds ratio for psoriasis at an alcohol intake of 100 g per day versus abstinence was 2.2 (95% confidence interval [CI] of 1.3–1.0).[47]

In a single-blind prospective study of 94 consecutive male and female inpatients with psoriasis, an average daily consumption of more than 80 g of alcohol per day was associated with a less favorable response to treatment among male but not among female patients ($P = .02$).[48] Smoking 20 cigarettes daily was associated with an odds ratio for psoriasis of 3.3, versus not smoking, in a study comparing 55 female patients and 108 unmatched controls (95% CI of 1.4–7.9).[49] The relationship between smoking and increased risk of developing palmar-plantar pustular psoriasis has been well established, with a relative risk for smokers versus nonsmokers of 7.2 in one study.[50]

Skin Care

Use of gentle skin care measures such as bathing with mild soap or soap substitutes, maintaining cooler water temperatures, and regularly applying emollients (preferably ointments or creams rather than lotions) are helpful in decreasing pruritus and subsequent "Koebnerization" of psoriatic plaques.

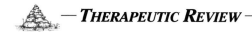 —*THERAPEUTIC REVIEW*———————————

Mind-Body Medicine

- *The role of stress in the exacerbation of the patient's symptoms should be acknowledged and validated when appropriate.*
- *The role of psychological factors should be discussed at the time of diagnosis, as this approach can help in the patient's acceptance of this information and may be perceived as less invasive at this time.[51] If such factors are presented only later after a treatment failure, patients or family member may feel personally attacked and may feel as if they are being blamed for the failure.*
- *Patients' need to maintain control over their illness should be appreciated, as this helps them to take an active role in their treatment.*
- *Patients should be instructed in techniques such as progressive relaxation and habit-reversal techniques to provide them with an active behavioral strategy.*
- *Patients should be referred to support groups when appropriate.*
- *Mindfulness meditation techniques should be incorporated during phototherapy.*
- *The use of massage during application of topical medications and emollients should be encouraged. Having a spouse or partner apply medications using massage techniques may be especially helpful for adult patients, who often face issues of decreased sexual attractiveness because of their skin disease.*

Phototherapy and Balneotherapy

- *Exposure to natural sunlight or purchase of a home UVB box should be encouraged if phototherapy is not available. Face, genitals, and uninvolved areas should be protected from exposure. Use of the new excimer UVB laser may result in prolonged remission with fewer required treatments.*
- *Calcipotriene, tazarotene, or use of hypertonic bath solutions may increase responsiveness to both conventional and narrow-band UVB therapy.*
- *Topical, bath, or traditional PUVA therapy or the Goeckerman regimen may be used for treatment of moderate to severe psoriasis.*

Pharmaceuticals, Botanicals, and Traditional Chinese Medicine

- *Use of calcipotriene (a vitamin D_3 analogue) or tazarotene (a retinoid related to vitamin A) may enable reduction in the amount of topical steroids required, may prevent atrophy from topical steroid use, and may enhance the effect of phototherapy. The use of calcipotriene should be limited to less than 100 g per week to prevent hypercalcemia.*
- *Capsaicin may decrease pruritus, but the burning sensation it causes makes it poorly tolerated.*

Topical Steroids

- *Topical steroids are most effectively used in conjunction with calcipotriene or tazarotene. Use as monotherapy may result in tachyphylaxis (decreased efficacy over time).*
- *Patients' concerns regarding the use of topical steroids should be addressed in a thoughtful manner.*
- *Appropriate strengths, vehicles, and amounts should be prescribed for the affected body area, and both strength and frequency should be tapered as improvement occurs.*
- *The use of moderate or strong topical steroids on the face or in the groin or intertriginous areas should be avoided. Even a mild topical steroid used on the face may cause perioral dermatitis and atrophy if applied frequently enough over time.*
- *The patient should be cautioned against sharing medications with others, and only enough medication should be prescribed. For adult patients, 30 g of topical steroid medication is enough to cover the entire body surface area for a single treatment, and 1 g covers a palm-sized area.*

THERAPEUTIC REVIEW *continued*

Botanicals

- *Topical* Aloe vera *cream may be effective.*
- *To decrease pruritus, topical capsaicin or oatmeal (Aveeno) baths may be used. Use of topical glycyrrhetinic acid (derived from licorice) may enable lesser amounts of topical steroids to be used.*
- *Milk thistle may be used to prevent hepatotoxicity in patients treated with medications such as acitretin (Soriatane) or methotrexate. Recommended dosing is 420 mg of silymarin per day divided into 3 doses, with a decrease in dosage after 6 to 8 weeks to 280 mg per day.*

Traditional Chinese Medicine

- *Traditional Chinese herbal therapies such as* Tripterygium wilfordii hook *and* Tripterygium hypoglaucum hutch *and commercial preparations of indigo may be helpful, but experience in the United States is lacking.*

Diet and Lifestyle Interventions

- *Use of fish oil supplements (3 g per day) or increasing intake of salmon and other fatty fish may decrease triglycerides for patients on oral retinoid therapy and may decrease pruritus but is unlikely to lessen the severity of psoriasis.*
- *Decreasing or eliminating the use of alcohol and quitting smoking not only have a positive impact on overall health but may lead to clinical improvement in patients with psoriasis.*
- *Reducing alcohol intake may also increase responsiveness to treatment.*

Skin Care

- *Use of gentle skin care (cooler water and mild soap and emollients such as creams or ointments) decreases pruritus from xerosis and may minimize "Koebnerization" from scratching.*

References

1. Arndt KA, LeBoit PE, Robinson JK, Wintroub BU: Cutaneous Medicine and Surgery. Philadelphia, WB Saunders, pp 295–317 1996.
2. Freedberg I, Eisen A, Wolff K, et al (eds): Fitzpatrick's Dermatology in General Medicine, 5th ed, Vol 1. New York, McGraw-Hill 1999.
3. Peters B, Weissman F, Gill M: Pathophysiology and treatment of psoriasis. Am J Health Syst Pharm 57:645–659, 2000.
4. Farber E: Psychoneuroimmunology and dermatology. Intl J Dermatol, 32:93–94, 1993.
5. Farber E, Nall L: Psoriasis: A stress-related disease. Cutis 51:322–326, 1993.
6. Seville RH: Psoriasis and stress. Br J Dermatol 97:297–302, 1977.
7. Massetti M, Mozzetta A, Soavi GC, et al: Psoriasis, stress and psychiatry: Psychodynamic characteristics of stressors. Acta Derm Venereol (Stockh) Suppl 186:62–64, 1994.
8. Baughman R, Sobel R. Psoriasis, stress, and strain. Arch Dermatol 103:599–605, 1971.
9. Zachariae R, Oster H, Bjerring P, Kragballe K: Effects of psychologic intervention on psoriasis: A preliminary report. J Am Acad Dermatol 34:1008–1015, 1996.
10. Price ML, Mottahedin I, Mayo PR: Can psychotherapy help patients with psoriasis? Clin Exp Dermatol 16:114–117, 1991.
11. Kabat Zinn J, Wheeler E, Light T, et al: Influence of a mindfulness meditation–based stress reduction intervention on rates of skin clearing in patients with moderate to severe psoriasis undergoing phototherapy (UVB) and photochemotherapy (PUVA). Psychosom Med 60:625–632, 1998.
12. Tausk F, Whitmore SE: A pilot study of hypnosis in the treatment of patients with psoriasis. Psychother Psychosom 68:221–225, 1999.
13. Ozawa M, Ferenczi K, Kikuchi T, et al: 312 nanometer ultraviolet B light (narrow band uVB) induces apoptosis of T cells within psoriatic lesions. J Exp Med 189:711–718, 1999.
14. Walters I, Burack L, Coven T, et al: Suberythemogenic narrow band UVB is markedly more effective than conventional UVB in treatment of psoriasis vulgaris. J Am Acad Dermatol 40:893–900, 1999.
15. Asawanonda P, Anderson R, Chang Y, Taylor C: 308 nm excimer laser for the treatment of psoriasis: A dose response study. Arch Dermatol 136:619–624, 2000.
16. Ros A, Garden J, Bakus A, Hedblad M: Psoriasis response to the pulsed dye laser. Lasers Surg Med 19:331–335, 1996.
17. Weinstein G, Gottlieb A: Therapy of Moderate to Severe Psoriasis. National Psoriasis Foundation, 1993, pp 33–55.
18. Bowman P: Take Goeckerman therapy from the office to the home. Skin Aging May 2000, pp 48–56.
19. Shani J, Harari M, Hristakieva E, et al: Dead-Sea climatotherapy versus other modalities of treatment for psoriasis: Comparative cost-effectiveness. Int J Dermatol 38:252–262, 1999.
20. Schiffner R, Schiffner-Rohe J, Wolfl G, et al: Evaluation of a multicentre study of synchronous application of narrowband ultraviolet B phototherapy (TL-01) and bathing in Dead Sea salt solution for psoriasis vulgaris. Br J Dermatol 142:740–747, 2000.
21. Ramsay C: Management of psoriasis with calcipotriol used as monotherapy. J Am Acad Dermatol 37:S53–S54, 1997.
22. Lebwohl M: Topical application of calcipotriene and corticosteroids: Combination regimens. J Am Acad Dermatol 37:S55–S58, 1997.
23. Koo J: Sequential therapy of psoriasis. Skin Aging Oct 1998.
24. Koo J: Calcipotriol/calcipotriene (Dovonex/Daivonex) in combination with phototherapy: A review. J Am Acad Dermatol 37:S59–S61, 1997.
25. Lebwohl MG, Poulin Y: Tazarotene in combination with topical corticosteroids. J Am Acad Dermatol' 39:S139–S143, 1998.
26. Koo J: Tazarotene in combination with phototherapy. J Am Acad Dermatol 39: S144–S148, 1998.
27. Behrens S, Grundmann-Kollmann M, Schiener R, et al: Combination phototherapy of psoriasis with narrow band UVB irradiation and topical tazarotene gel. J Am Acad Dermatol 42:493–495, 2000.
28. Ellis C, Berbarian B, Sulica V, et al: A double blind evaluation of topical capsaicin in pruritic psoriasis. J Am Acad Dermatol 29:438–442, 1993.

29. Syed T, Ahmad A, Holt A, et al: Management of psoriasis with *Aloe vera* extract in a hydrophilic cream: A placebo-controlled, double blind study. Trop Med Int Health 1:505–509, 1996.

30. Morrow DM, Rapaport M, Strick R: Hypersensitivity to aloe. Arch. Dermatol 116:1064–1065, 1980.

31. Murray M, Pizzorno J: Encyclopedia of Natural Medicine, rev 2nd ed. Prima Health, 1998.

32. Duke JA: The Green Pharmacy. New York, St Martin's, 1997.

33. Teelucksingh S, Mackie ADR, Burt D, et al: Potentiation of hydrocortisone activity in skin by glycyrrhetinic acid. Lancet 335:1060–1063, 1990.

34. Buchness R: Alternative medicine and dermatology. Semin Cutan Med Surg 17:284–290, 1998.

35. Chan T, Chan J, Tomlinson B, Critchley J: Chinese herbal medicines revisited: A Hong Kong perspective. Lancet 342:1532–1534, 1993.

36. Keane F, Munn S, du Vivier A, Higgins L: Analysis of Chinese herbal creams prescribed for dermatological conditions. World J Med 170:257–259, 1999.

37. Ko R, Au A, 1998. Cited by Kaltsas H: Patent poisons. AlternativeMedicine.com. Nov 12, 1999.

38. Koo J, Arain S: Traditional Chinese medicine in dermatology. Clin Dermato 17:21–27, 1999.

39. Jerner B, Skogh M, Vahlquist A: A controlled trial of acupuncture in psoriasis: No convincing effect. Acta Derm Venereol (Stockh) 77:154–156, 1997.

40. Wilkinson DI: Do dietary supplements of fish oils improve psoriasis? Cutis 46:334–336, 1990.

41. Bittiner SB, Cartwright I, Tucker WFG, Bleehan SS: A double-blind, randomised, placebo controlled trial of fish oil in psoriasis. Lancet 1:378–380, 1988.

42. Bjornboe A, Smith A, Bjornboe BE, Thuse PO, Drevon A: Effect of dietary supplementation with *n*-3 fatty acids on clinical manifestations of psoriasis. Br J Dermatol 118:77–83, 1988.

43. Soyland E, Funk J, Rajka G, et al: Effect of dietary supplementation with very long chain *n*-3 fatty acids in patients with psoriasis. N Engl J Med 328:1812–1816, 1993.

44. Lowe N, Borok M, Ashley J, Alfin-Slater R: Fish oil consumption reduces hypertriglyceridemia in psoriatic patients during etretinate therapy. Arch Dermatol 124:177, 1988.

45. Wolf R, Wof D, Ruocco V: Alcohol intake and psoriasis. Clin Dermatol 17:423–430, 1999.

46. Higgins EM, Peters, TJ, du Vivier AWP: Smoking, drinking and psoriasis. Br J Dermatol 129:749–750, 1993.

47. Poikalainen K, Reunala T, Karvonen J, et al: Alcohol intake: A risk factor for psoriasis in young and middle aged men? BMJ 300:780–783, 1990.

48. Gupta MA, Schork NJ, Gupta AK, et al: Alcohol intake and treatment responsiveness of psoriasis: A prospective study. J Am Acad Dermatol 28:730–732, 1993.

49. Poikolainen K, Reunala T, Karvonen J: Smoking, alcohol and life events related to psoriasis among women. Br J Dermatol 130:473–477, 1994.

50. O'Doherty CJ, MacIntyre C: Palmoplantar pustulosis and smoking. BMJ 291:861–864, 1985.

51. Czyzewski DI, Lopez M: Clinical psychology in the management of pediatric skin disease. Dermatol Clin 16:619–629, 1998.

CHAPTER 58

Urticaria (Acute and Chronic)

Steven Tenenbaum, M.D.

PATHOPHYSIOLOGY

Urticaria is an evanescent eruption of itching wheals (Fig. 58–1). *Acute urticaria* is defined as intermittent hives lasting from a few hours to days but no longer than 6 weeks. *Chronic urticaria* is defined as intermittent hives lasting longer than 6 weeks. Unlike acute urticaria, in which the offending agent is usually recognized and avoided, the offending agent in chronic urticaria remains elusive in up to 95% of patients. This leads to great frustration for both patient and physician, because more than 40% of patients continue to have symptoms for 1 year, and 20% have symptoms for longer than 20 years.[1] Some common triggers of chronic urticaria are listed in Table 58–1.

Even though the exact cause of chronic urticaria is usually unknown, its pathophysiology is well established. The formation of a wheal is an immunoglobulin E (IgE)–mediated allergic response. IgE binds to mast cells, effectuating the release of histamine and other mediators, which cause a localized increase in vascular permeability and transudation of fluid, resulting in a characteristic wheal. Some investiga-

tors have implicated an autoimmune phenomenon whereby autoantibodies bind to mast cells and basophils, causing the release of histamine.[2]

Treatment is based on avoiding potential triggers, blocking the effect of histamine, and treating any underlying hormonal imbalance or parasitic infection.

> ### NOTE
>
> *A thorough history and physical examination can diagnose chronic urticaria. A laboratory workup is not necessary unless the history and physical examination reveal concerns.[3] Laboratory tests to consider, when deemed necessary, are complete blood count (CBC), erythrocyte sedimentation rate (ESR), thyroid-stimulating hormone (TSH), cortisol levels, hormone levels, and stool analysis for parasites and fungi.*

INTEGRATIVE THERAPY

General Principles

The patient should be educated on the protractive nature of chronic urticaria in order to have realistic expectations of therapy. In general, botanicals and pharmaceuticals sufficiently control the symptoms, and acupuncture, homeopathy, and mind–body work can be used in an attempt to alleviate the underlying condition. One should start by trying to identify and eliminate any of the precipitating causes listed in Table 58–1.

Nutrition

Eliminate Allergenic Foods

Hyperallergenic foods such as dairy products, shellfish, red meat, wheat, eggs, beans, coffee, and nuts (see also Chapter 81, Food Allergy) should be eliminated.

An elimination diet may be tried according to the guidelines found in Chapter 82, The Elimination Diet and Diagnosing Food Hypersensitivities.

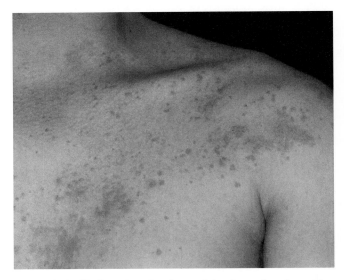

Figure 58–1. Cholinergic urticaria consists of round, red, papular wheals that occur in response to exercise, heat, or emotional stress. (From Habif T: Clinical Dermatology, 3rd ed. St. Louis, Mosby, 1996.)

Table 58–1. Triggers of Chronic Urticaria

Foods	Milk/cheese, shellfish, red meat, wheat, eggs, beans, coffee, berries, nuts
Drugs and chemicals	Nonsteroidal anti-inflammatory drugs, penicillins, sulfonamides, tartrazine dye (found in vitamins, antibiotics, and yellow #5)
Contactants	Latex, perfumes, wool
Physical stimuli	Friction resulting in dermatographism, heat (very common), cold, water, sunlight, pressure, vibration
Inhalants	Dust mite, animal dander, pollen
Infections	Viral upper respiratory infection, sinusitis, hepatitis, fungal infection, helminth infection, protozoal infection
Systemic disease	Cancer, thyroid abnormalities, collagen vascular disease

Consume an Omega-3 Fatty Acid–Rich Diet

For patients with chronic urticaria, encourage consumption of a diet rich in omega-3 fatty acids. This should be done after an elimination diet, as discussed earlier, to ensure that omega-3–rich foods such as nuts are not a potential trigger (see Chapter 84, The Anti-Inflammatory Diet).

Botanicals

Quercetin

This is a bioflavonoid (found in green vegetables, berries, onions, parsley, legumes, green tea, citrus fruit, and red grapes) whose anti-inflammatory effects are thought to be effectuated by the prevention of histamine degranulation from mast cells. Countless biochemical studies have confirmed the anti-inflammatory actions of quercetin, but no study focusing on the treatment of chronic urticaria with quercetin was found in the literature.

Dosage. 400 mg PO twice daily before meals
Precautions. None known

Stinging Nettle (*Urtica dioica*)

Stinging nettle is a perennial herb, 2 to 4 feet high, whose leaves contain medicinal properties. The leaves have been shown to be effective in the treatment of allergic rhinitis through inhibition of mast cell degranulation of histamine.[4] Stinging nettle is thought to be useful in the treatment of chronic urticaria by the same mechanism of action, but there has been no study as yet to support this notion.

Dosage. Freeze-dried, 300 mg PO three times daily. Liquid extract, $^1/_2$ to 2 tsp PO three times a day.

Precautions. Allergic skin reaction if leaves are placed on the skin.

Pot Marigold (*Calendula officinalis*)

Calendula, also known as pot marigold, is a 2-foot-tall plant whose yellow flowers contain anti-inflammatory and immune-modulating properties.[5] Calendula has been used for countless years for topical anti-inflammatory disorders but no double-blind placebo-controlled study has been undertaken to determine the effect of Calendula in the treatment of chronic urticaria. Anecdotal evidence suggests a topical soothing effect equivalent to that of calamine.

Dosage. Topical cream, ointment, or liquid extract—two to four times daily. Systemic—liquid extract, $^1/_4$ to $^1/_2$ tsp one to three times daily.

Precautions. None known

Pharmaceuticals

Antihistamines

Antihistamines are the backbone of allopathic treatment of chronic urticaria. Antihistamines compete for histamine receptors and, therefore, block the effect of histamine. Double-blind placebo-controlled studies have demonstrated the efficacy of cetirizine (Zyrtec),[6] loratadine (Claritin),[7] and fexofenadine (Allegra)[8] in the treatment of chronic idiopathic urticaria.

Dosage. Use nonsedating H_1 blocker first (cetirizine [Zyrtec] 10 mg orally [PO] daily, loratadine [Claritin] 10 mg PO daily, or fexofenadine [Allegra] 60 mg PO twice daily). Consider increasing the dose of loratadine up to 40 mg per day before adding another agent. Cetirizine can also be used at higher doses but can be more sedating than loratadine.

If there is not sufficient effect, add a sedating H_1 blocker at night (diphenhydramine [Benadryl], 25 to 50 mg PO every night, or hydroxyzine [Atarax] 25 mg PO every night).

If treatment is still inadequate, use a potent H_1 and H_2 blocker (doxepin [Sinequan] 150 mg PO every night).

Precautions. Sedation, dry mouth

Corticosteroids

Corticosteroids have potent anti-inflammatory properties. They work by inhibiting the release of leukotrienes, resulting in a marked reduction in capillary permeability. If urticarial symptoms are severe or widespread or antihistamines are ineffective, one may give a burst of corticosteroids followed by antihistamines (e.g., methylprednisolone [Medrol] Dosepack, followed by a nonsedating H_1 blocker).

Cyclosporine

If all else fails, consider referral for a 1- to 3-month trial of cyclosporine (Neoral). This immunosuppressive drug can help people to withdraw from taking high-dose steroids, but the patient should be prepared to use the agent as a short-term tool.

Dosage. 4 mg/kg per day

NOTE

Fifty percent of patients with chronic urticaria achieve resolution within 1 year. Unfortunately, 20% continue to have episodic urticaria for longer than 20 years. The mean duration of chronic urticaria in children is 16 months.[1]

Mind–Body Techniques

The therapeutic effects of hypnosis with relaxation therapy were investigated in a controlled crossover study of 15 patients with chronic urticaria. Investigators found that hypnosis with relaxation therapy significantly reduced the symptoms of chronic urticaria (pruritus) without reducing the number of hives.[9]

THERAPIES TO CONSIDER

Traditional Chinese Medicine

The symptoms of chronic urticaria are well known to traditional Chinese medicine practitioners. Most cases are secondary to fire imbalance with an excess of heat and a lack of moisture.

Nutritional recommendations include increasing the intake of cooling foods while avoiding hot foods and hot spices. The application of cool, wet compresses is also recommended.

Acupuncture has been found to be helpful in the treatment of type I allergic disease.[10] It can be used by emphasizing the following points: LI11, Sp10, Sp6, and S36.[11] The combination of ordinary acupuncture and auricular acupuncture has also been found to be highly effective in the treatment of chronic urticaria.[10] The duration of treatment may need to be 2 to 4 weeks.

Homeopathy

A complete evaluation and a constitutional remedy should be given for the treatment of chronic urticaria.

Apis mellifica

Apis is a homeopathic remedy made from the honeybee. Although there are no studies to support the efficacy of Apis in the treatment of chronic urticaria, it has long been the cornerstone of homeopathic treatment for hives. I have personally seen improvement in patients with chronic urticaria treated with Apis alone.

Dosage. 30c, take one pill once as a complete treatment; or alternatively, take 6x, one pill three times a day to prevent and control symptoms.

Precautions. None, but there may be a healing crisis with an exacerbation of symptoms before the resolution of symptoms.

Correction of Hormonal Imbalance

Restoring thyroid hormone, estrogen, progesterone, testosterone, cortisol, and DHEA levels to normal physiologic range may lead to resolution of chronic urticaria.

 THERAPEUTIC REVIEW

Below is a summary of the therapeutic options for urticaria. Remember, no laboratory investigation is needed unless something in the complete history and physical examination is alarming. Be sure to obtain a careful history of any thyroid abnormality or autoimmune disorder. Patients with chronic urticaria have a higher incidence of autoimmune thyroid disease.

- *Elimination of exacerbating factors:*
   Consider foods, drugs and chemicals, contactants, physical stimuli, inhalants, infections, and systemic disease.
- *Nutrition:*
   Consider removal of hyperallergenic foods such as dairy products, shellfish, red meat, wheat, eggs, beans, coffee, and nuts. Consider an elimination diet. Encourage a diet rich in omega-3 fatty acids (see Chapter 84, The Anti-Inflammatory Diet).
- *Botanicals:*
   Quercetin 400 mg three times daily; stinging nettle (freeze-dried) 300 mg three times daily; calendula cream, ointment, or liquid extract two times daily.

THERAPEUTIC REVIEW *continued*

- *Pharmaceuticals:*

  Start with a nonsedating antihistamine (cetirizine, 10 mg PO daily; loratadine, 10 mg PO daily; or fexofenadine, 60 mg PO twice daily). If this is not sufficiently effective, add a sedating H_1 blocker at night (diphenhydramine, 25 to 50 mg PO every night, or hydroxyzine, 25 mg PO every night). If still insufficiently effective, use a potent H_1 and H_2 blocker (doxepin, 150 mg PO daily). If the symptoms are severe, use methylprednisolone (Medrol Dosepak) followed by a nonsedating H_1 blocker or sedating H_1 blocker.

- *Mind–Body Techniques:*

  Use hypnosis and relaxation therapy.

- *Traditional Chinese Medicine:*

  Use cooling foods; eliminate hot, spicy foods. Acupuncture to LI11, Sp10, Sp6, and S36. Auricular acupuncture may be added if response is not sufficient.

- *Homeopathy:*

  Apis 30c, one pill, or Apis 6x PO, three times daily, for duration of symptoms.

- *Hormonal Balance:*

  Consider restoring levels of thyroid hormone, estrogen, progesterone, testosterone, cortisol, and DHEA to normal physiologic levels.

References

1. Volonakis M, Katsarou-Katsari A, Stratigo J: Etiologic factors in childhood chronic urticaria. Ann Allergy 69:61–65, 1992.
2. Greaves M: Chronic urticaria. J Allergy Clin Immunol 105:664–672, 2000.
3. Soter NA: The investigation of urticaria and angio-oedema. Clin Exp Dermatol 20:272, 1995.
4. Mittman P: A randomized, double-blind study of freeze dried *Urtica dioica* in the treatment of allergic rhinitis. Planta Med 56:44–47, 1990.
5. Della Loggia R, Tubaro A, Sosa S, et al: The role of terpenoids in the topical anti-inflammatory activity of *Calendula officianalis* flowers. Planta Med 60:516–20, 1994.
6. Breneman DL: Cetirizine versus hydroxyzine and placebo in chronic idiopathic urticaria. Ann Pharmacother 30:1075–1079, 1996.
7. Haria M, Fitton A, Peters DH: Loratidine. A reappraisal of its pharmacological properties and therapeutic use in allergic disorders. Drugs 48:617–637, 1994.
8. Nelson HS, Reynolds R, Mason J: Fexofenadine HCl is safe and effective for treatment of chronic idiopathic urticaria. Ann Allergy Asthma Immunol 84:517–522, 2000.
9. Schertzer CL, Lookingbill DP: Effects of relaxation therapy and hypnotizability in chronic urticaria. Arch Dermatol 123:913–916, 1987.
10. Lai X: Observation on the curative effect of acupuncture on type 1 allergic diseases. J Tradit Chin Med 13:243–248, 1993.
11. Chen CJ, Yu HS: Acupuncture treatment of urticaria. Arch Dermatol 134:1397–1399, 1998.

CHAPTER 59

Recurrent Aphthous Ulceration

Malcolm Riley, B.D.S., F.D.S., M.R.D., and David Rakel, M.D.

Recurrent aphthous ulcers (RAUs, aphthous stomatitis, canker sores) are the most common oral mucosal lesions, affecting 20% of the population in North America. They appear as recurrent ulcers with a circumscribed margin and have an erythematous halo and a gray or yellowish floor.

RAUs affect the nonkeratinized or poorly keratinized mucosa of the mouth and oropharynx. There is no specific test for RAU, and diagnosis is made from the patient's history and clinical findings (Table 59-1).

PATHOPHYSIOLOGY

RAUs appear to be multifactorial in origin, with a strong component being immune mediated. Histologically, an increase in immunoglobulin E (IgE)–bearing lymphocytes occurs, and mast cells are increased in the prodromal stages. Cytotoxic actions of lymphocytes and monocytes seem to cause the ulceration but the exact trigger is not clear.

There are three main clinical variations:

1. Minor aphthous ulcers—These are usually less than 5 mm in diameter and are the most common form (80%). Most often, one to five ulcers are present at any one time; they usually heal without scarring in 7 to 14 days.
2. Major aphthous ulcers—These are less common. The ulcers are larger and deeper, tend to have irregular edges, and are more painful. They affect the lips, soft palate, and oropharynx and can take up to 6 weeks to heal, often leaving a considerable scar. Major and minor RAUs can be associated with Behçet's syndrome and human immunodeficiency virus (HIV).
3. Herpetiform RAUs—These are 1 to 3 mm in diameter and often occur in groups of more than 100, which often coalesce to form large, irregular areas of ulceration. These are not as deep as major RAUs. They heal without scarring in 7 to 14 days; in spite of their name, they are not associated with herpesvirus, nor are they of viral origin.

Minor and major RAUs usually begin in childhood or early adolescence and have a tendency to naturally resolve later in life. Herpetiform RAUs appear later than minor and major RAUs, usually during the third decade.

INTEGRATIVE THERAPY

Nutrition

Several nutritional deficiencies have been associated with RAU. Vitamin B_{12}, iron, and folic acid have been the most studied and are commonly deficient in RAU.[1]

NOTE

Laboratory evaluation for red cell folate, serum B_{12}, and ferritin should be included in any workup of RAU.

Vitamins B_1,[2] B_2, and B_6 have also been found to be deficient in some patients with RAU.[3] There is no evidence that supplementation, in the absence of an established deficiency, has any effect on RAUs.

Table 59-1. Factors in the Etiology of Recurrent Aphthous Ulcer (RAU)

The etiology of RAU seems to be multifactorial and can include one or several of the following:

- Familial and genetic basis
- Nutritional deficiencies—B_1, B_2, B_6, B_{12}, folic acid, and Fe
- Stress
- Stopping smoking
- Menstruation
- Food allergies
- Sensitivity to toothpastes
- Medications
- Physical trauma
- Systemic conditions
  Celiac disease
  Crohn's disease
  HIV infection
  Neutropenia and other immune deficiencies
  Neumann's bipolar aphthous
  Behçet's syndrome
  MAGIC (mouth and genital ulcers with inflamed cartilage)

Diet

Gluten-Free Diet

A minority of patients with RAU have gluten-sensitive enteropathy and improve considerably on a gluten-free diet.[4] Diagnosis is usually made by means of a jejunal biopsy or with an assay of anti-gliadin antibody. There is no evidence in the literature that gluten-free diets will help patients with RAU if they do not have gluten sensitivity[5]; however, there are some anecdotal observations that some patients without gluten sensitivity may benefit from a gluten-free diet. In view of the difficulty of following a gluten-free diet, I suggest leaving this option until later.

Food Allergies

The role of food allergies in the pathogenesis of RAU is controversial. Several foods, such as milk, chocolate, coffee, nuts, strawberries, pineapple, citrus fruits, tomatoes; azo dyes; and food additives, such as monosodium glutamate (MSG), benzoic acid, tartrazine, and cinnamaldehyde have all been suggested as causes for RAU.[6, 7] Food restriction and rotation diets[8] are difficult for the patient to maintain; it is possible that RAUs triggered by food allergies are IgG mediated, and therefore, the symptoms may not be visible for up to 2 days. (See Chapter 82, The Elimination Diet and Diagnosing Food Hypersensitivities.) A reliable food allergy IgG test is available from Immunolabs at *http://www.immunolabs.com.*

Botanicals

Licorice

Licorice *(Glycyrrhiza)* has an anti-inflammatory action and has been used both as a mouthwash and as chewed tablets.[9] A licorice mouthwash, which can be made by combining $1/2$ teaspoon of licorice extract to $1/4$ cup of water, can be used four times a day. Or, one tablet of deglycyrrhizinated licorice (DGL) can be chewed into a paste and the tongue used to coat the sores with the paste; this can be done four times a day until resolution.[10] DGL does not result in the adverse effects of sodium retention and hypokalemia that can occur with straight licorice products.

Dosage. Swish, gargle, and expel mouthwash four times daily for symptomatic aphthous ulcers. Or chew one DGL tablet and apply paste to sore with the tongue four times daily.

Precautions. If the mouthwash is not swallowed, adverse effects are rare. Licorice can cause sodium retention and hypokalemia if swallowed. Care should be taken in patients with hypertension because ingestion can worsen this condition.

Other herbs such as echinacea (immune enhancing, anti-inflammatory), myrrh (antiseptic, anti-inflammatory), propolis (antiseptic, anti-inflammatory, and local anesthetic), calendula (antiseptic, anti-inflammatory) and *Rheum palmatum* (rhubarb root—antiseptic, anti-inflammatory, and astringent) have all been used traditionally to treat RAU[11] and are often found in commercial mouthwashes available through health food stores.

Homeopathy

A number of homeopathic remedies have been used historically to treat RAU; unfortunately, all evidence is anecdotal. A classical homeopath would look for a constitutional remedy that fits the whole patient. The following are symptomatic remedies that may help:

- *Mercurius solubilis* is indicated if the RAUs are associated with foul breath and increased salivation.
- Borax is indicated if the RAUs are brought on with citrus or acidic foods. The mouth usually feels dry even though some saliva may be present.
- *Arsenicum album* is indicated in patients with RAU brought on by stress and eased with hot drinks.

Dosages. All the above remedies are best given initially at a potency of 6x or 6c four times daily. (The "x" and "c" refer to the potency, which is the degree of dilution of the remedy.) They should be discontinued when the RAUs begin to improve.

Hormone Therapy

RAUs seem to follow the menstrual cycle in some women and are more common in the luteal phase. One study found significant improvement following the use of progesterone in menstrual cycle–related ulcers.[12]

Mind–Body Techniques

Stress, both emotional and physical, triggers RAU. Stress related to examinations in students commonly causes ulcers to occur. Causes of pathogenesis include known alteration of the immune response from stress and depletion of B vitamins; other causes are unknown.

Meditation and stress reduction techniques such as guided imagery and hypnosis have been shown to be useful in the management of RAU.[13, 14]

Lifestyle

Smoking

Smokers are known to have a reduced incidence of RAU. RAUs often appear when patients give up smoking, which may be related to the reduction in stress claimed by smokers. Nicotine has been used with success to treat RAU,[15] but in view of the other effects of nicotine, its use is not recommended.

Toothpaste

Sodium lauryl sulfate (SLS) is a common detergent used in toothpastes that has been shown to precipitate RAU.[16] Other ingredients may also affect RAU, so a good question to ask patients with newly developed RAU is if they have recently changed toothpastes. *Retardent* is one brand of toothpaste that does not contain SLS.

Pharmaceuticals

Anti-inflammatory Agents

Amlexanox (Aphthasol) 5% Paste

This is the only prescription medication with FDA approval for aphthous stomatitis. It accelerates healing through an unknown mechanism that inhibits inflammatory mediators (e.g., histamine, leukotrienes) from mast cells, neutrophils, and mononuclear cells. It has no direct analgesic properties.

Dosage. Apply 0.5 cm to sore with fingertip four times daily after meals and at bedtime. Start at the onset of symptoms and stop with resolution. If no resolution is noted in 7 days, reevaluate. Dispensed in a 5-g tube.

Precautions. May cause minimal burning upon application. Rash, diarrhea, nausea, and worsening stomatitis have been reported in les than 1% of cases. This medication is more expensive than the other treatments discussed here.

Triamcinolone Acetonide 0.1% in Carboxymethylcellulose Paste (Kenalog in Orabase)

Steroids such as triamcinolone and dexamethasone reduce inflammatory mediators but do not decrease frequency of occurrence.

Dosage. Apply 0.5 cm to sore, two or three times daily. Start at onset of symptoms and stop with resolution. If no resolution occurs in 7 days, reevaluate. Dispensed in a 5-g tube.

Precautions. Thrush.

Analgesic Agents

It is helpful to avoid spicy, salty, and vinegar-containing foods that may irritate and increase the pain of ulcers.

Viscous Lidocaine (Xylocaine 2% Solution)

Provides anesthetic properties that allow less pain with eating.

Dosage. Swish and expel 15 mL every 3 hr or before meals as needed for pain relief. Not to exceed 8 doses/day. Dispensed in 50-, 100-, and 450-mL bottles.

Precautions. Care should be taken not to ingest large amounts because of its potential cardiotoxicity. Benzocaine gel (10% to 20%) is a safer alternative, particularly in the pediatric population.

Cleansing Mouthwash

Chlorhexidine Gluconate 0.12% Oral Solution (Peridex or PerioGard Oral Rinse)

This is a mouthwash that has been shown to reduce the incidence, duration, and discomfort of RAUs.[17]

Dosage. 15 mL, rinse and expel for 30 seconds twice daily. Chewing sugarless gum after using can help reduce tooth discoloration.

Precautions. It can cause stinging when first used, reversible discoloration of the teeth and tongue after 1 week of use, transient taste disturbances, and burning sensation of the tongue.

Treatment for More Severe Cases

Tetracycline, Fluocinolone Acetonide, and Diphenhydramine

Tetracycline is thought to work through antimicrobial as well as anti-inflammatory mechanisms. Fluocinolone and diphenhydramine work via anti-inflammatory and anesthetic mechanisms. The authors have found this to be very helpful in severe cases that are the result of immunosuppressant therapy.

Dosage. This formula requires the help of a pharmacist for mixing. Most pharmacies are able to comply with the directions described here.

Tetracycline. At a concentration of 500 mg/5 mL (pharmacist makes the solution by dissolving a 500-mg capsule in 5 mL of water) for a total of 60 mL

Diphenhydramine syrup (Benadryl). 12.5 mg/5 mL for a total of 60 mL

Fluocinolone acetonide 0.01% solution (Synalar). Total of 30 mL

These are mixed together to make a total of 150 mL. Swish and expel 10 mL four times daily until resolution. Do not use for longer than 7 days at a time.

Precautions. Tetracycline should not be given to children younger than 9 years of age because it stains the teeth. Fluocinolone, like most steroids, can cause thrush if used for extended periods.

Systemic Pharmaceuticals

Systemic steroids (prednisone up to 40 mg/d) are indicated only in severe or persistent RAU. Thalidomide is used in severe ulceration to treat RAUs associated with HIV. H_2-receptor antagonists have been tried with limited success, as has cromolyn sodium.

THERAPIES TO CONSIDER

Traditional Chinese Medicine (TCM)

Chinese medicine views RAU as a condition caused by Heat in the Stomach, but it can also be caused by yin deficiency or toxic heat. Treatment is with topical watermelon frost and/or internally with formulas that cool stomach heat and clear toxic heat, such as dao chi pian or niu huang jie du pian. Although no reliable studies have been reported on the use of TCM in the treatment of RAU, referral to a Chinese medicine practitioner is a valid approach if other treatments are not indicated or successful.

— *THERAPEUTIC REVIEW* ————————————

The most important issue in dealing with RAU is to exclude systemic conditions, particularly Behçet's syndrome (mouth, genital, and eye ulcers). As RAUs are multifactorial in etiology, a simple list of treatments is not applicable; a good history helps in focusing on the triggers and can lead to a specific treatment plan. The following is a guide to the most common causes and treatments of RAU:

Nutrition: Fe, B$_{12}$, folate
Identification of nutritional deficiencies should be the first step in treating RAU. Ferritin, red cell folate, and serum B$_{12}$ are the most important tests, and we recommend these as the first step. It is often beneficial to give 25 mg of vitamin C with the iron to assist absorption if used.

B$_1$, B$_2$, B$_6$
Assessment of B vitamins is complex and, as these are relatively inexpensive, we suggest a trial supplementation for 3 months as the second step. There is no consensus on the doses required for these vitamins. Nutritionists suggest giving all the B vitamins together. We use a B50 complex, which contains approximately 50 mg of each taken once a day.

Diet is the third line of inquiry, unless an obvious association is found from the history.
1. If you suspect celiac disease, assess antigliadin antibody.
2. Identify any foods that trigger RAU with either an elimination diet or a food allergy test and then eliminate them for a trial period.

Botanicals
- *Licorice (Glycyrrhiza) mouthwash can be made with $^1/_2$ tsp of licorice extract to $^1/_4$ cup of water. Swish and expel four times daily. Or, chew one tablet of deglycyrrhizinated licorice (DGL) into a paste, and apply with tongue to sore four times daily.*

Homeopathy
- **Mercurius solubilis** *is indicated if the RAUs are associated with foul breath and increased salivation. Use 6x or 6c four times daily until healing begins.*
- **Borax** *is indicated if the RAUs are brought on by citrus or acidic foods. The mouth usually feels dry, although some saliva may be present. Use 6x or 6c four times daily until healing begins.*
- **Arsenicum album** *is indicated in patients whose RAUs are brought on by stress; the RAUs are eased with hot drinks. Use 6x or 6c four times daily until healing begins.*

Mind–Body Techniques
Stress is often a component of RAU; therefore, it is usually advisable to include stress reduction techniques such as meditation or guided imagery in the management approach. (See Chapter 91, Prescribing Relaxation Techniques.)

Pharmaceuticals
- *Amlexanox (Aphthasol), 5% paste, 0.5 cm to sore, four times daily.*
- *Triamcinolone acetonide 0.1% in carboxymethylcellulose paste (Kenalog in Orabase), 0.5 cm to sore two to four times daily.*

THERAPEUTIC REVIEW continued

- *Viscous lidocaine (Xylocaine 2% solution), swish 15 mL every 3 hr as needed for pain.*
- *Chlorhexidine gluconate 0.12% oral solution (Peridex or PerioGard oral rinse), 15 mL, rinse and expel twice daily.*
- *Tetracycline, 500 mg/5 mL, to make 60 mL, fluocinolone acetonide solution (Synalar), 30 mL, and diphenydramine syrup (Benadryl), 60 mL. Mix together to make 150 mL. Use 10 mL, swish, and expel four times daily.*

References

1. Wray D, Ferguson MM, Mason DK: Recurrent aphthae: Treatment with vitamin B_{12}, folic acid and iron. BMJ 2:490–493, 1975.
2. Haisraeli-Shalish M, Livneh A, Katz J: Recurrent aphthous stomatitis and thiamine deficiency. Oral Surg Oral Med Oral Pathol Oral Radiol Endod 82:634–636, 1996.
3. Nolan A, McIntosh WB, Allam BF, Lamey PJ: Recurrent aphthous ulceration: Vitamin B_1, B_2, B_6 status and the response to replacement therapy. J Oral Pathol Med 20:389–391, 1991.
4. Wray D: Gluten sensitive recurrent aphthous stomatitis. Dig Dis Sci 26:737–740, 1981.
5. Hunter IP, Ferguson MM, Scully C, et al: Effects of dietary gluten elimination in patients with recurrent minor aphthous stomatitis and no detectable gluten enteropathy. Oral Med Oral Surg Oral Pathol 75:595–597, 1993.
6. Wilson CWM: Food sensitivities, taste changes, aphthous ulcers and atopic symptoms in allergic disease. Ann Allergy 44:302–307, 1980.
7. Wright A, Ryan FP, Willingham SE, et al: Food allergy or intolerance in severe aphthous ulceration of the mouth. BMJ 292:1237–1238, 1986.
8. Hay KD, Reade PC: The use of an elimination diet in the treatment of recurrent aphthous ulceration of the oral cavity. Oral Surg Oral Med Oral Pathol 57:504–507, 1984.
9. Das SK, Gulati AK, Singh VP: Deglycyrrhizinated liquorice in apthous ulcers. J Assoc Physicians India 37:647, 1989.
10. Weil A: Self-Healing Newsletter. Watertown, Mass, Thorne Communications, March, 2001, p 5.
11. Mills S, Bone K: Principles and Practice of Phytotherapy. New York, Churchill-Livingstone, 2000.
12. Ferguson MM, McKay, Hart D, et al: Progestogen therapy for menstrually related aphthae. Int J Oral Surg 7:463–470, 1978.
13. Chalmers D, Sircus W: A trial of hypnosis in the management of recurrent mouth ulceration. Gut 5:599–600, 1964.
14. Andrews VH, Hall HR: The effects of relaxation/imagery. Training on recurrent aphthous stomatitis: A prelimary study. Psychosom Med 52:526–535, 1990.
15. Grady D, Ernster VL, Stillman L, Greenspan J: Smokeless tobacco use prevents aphthous stomatitis. Oral Surg Oral Med Oral Pathol 74:463–465, 1992.
16. Herlofson BB, Barkvoll P: The effect of two toothpaste detergents on the frequency of recurrent aphthous ulcers. Acta Odontol Scand 54:150–153, 1996.
17. Addy M, Tapper-Jones L, Seal M: Trial of astringent and antibacterial mouthwashes in the management of recurrent apthous ulceration. Br Dent J 136:452–455, 1974.

CHAPTER 60

Seborrheic Dermatitis

Alan M. Dattner, M.D.

PATHOPHYSIOLOGY

The pathophysiology of seborrheic dermatitis remains unclear. An overabundance of or inappropriate immune reaction to the common skin and follicular microflora species known as *Malassezia ovale* (formerly *Pityrosporum ovale*) has been both demonstrated and disputed in the literature.[1] Evidence both for and against an association with increased or altered sebum production has been presented. Seborrhea is aggravated by Parkinson's disease and by drugs that induce parkinsonism; clinical improvement is obtained with levo-dopa treatment of Parkinson's disease. Aggravation by emotional stress and changes associated with cases of partial denervation suggest a neurohumoral influence as well. Infantile seborrheic dermatitis, or Leiner's disease, has been reported to respond to biotin and essential fatty acids (EFAs). The observation of increased frequency and severity of seborrheic dermatitis among patients with AIDS has renewed interest in this otherwise benign disorder. These findings suggest that immune alterations may play some role in seborrheic dermatitis.

My own interpretation of the pathophysiology is that seborrheic dermatitis involves a predisposition toward a specific inflammatory desquamative reaction pattern in typically oily areas. The trigger is a specific hyperactive cross-reactive immune response to some aspect of an endotoxin or antigenic component of *M. ovale*, which begins the inflammation. The cross-reactive stimulation is a hyperactive response to the *Malassezia* organisms resulting from primary stimulation of the lymphocytes by *Candida* and other gut fungal microflora products. This phenomenon of primary stimulation and secondary response has been demonstrated in vitro[2] and in the clinical setting.[3] I believe that the immune response to the organism is biphasic, leading to both a tolerance to some components and a hyperactive response to others. Such a biphasic response would explain the mixed results in the literature showing both hyporeactivity and hyperreactivity to *Malassezia* antigens in patients with seborrheic dermatitis. The first component allows some overgrowth of *Malassezia* and related organisms (i.e., yeasts in gut and on skin). The hyperactive

response precipitates a cascade of immune-mediated activity leading to the erythema and desquamation characteristic of the disease. Resident microflora (especially *Candida*) and ingested antigens from related microflora (i.e., yeasts and molds and their by-products) provide the cross-reactive stimulus leading to both the tolerance and the hyperreactivity.

The proinflammatory response disposition comes in part from a metabolic shift toward the production of proinflammatory prostanoids, effected by the common dietary oils rich in arachidonic acid. There are insufficient anti-inflammatory precursors such as the omega-3 EFAs eicosaopentaenoic acid (EPA) and docosahexaenoic acid (DHA). Studies on psoriasis, a related skin disease, demonstrate an increased ratio of arachidonic acid to omega-3 EFAs in patients receiving fish oils, compared with that in a control group. Supplementing with fish oil reduced arachidonic acid and MDA (another inflammatory molecule) and was associated with clinical improvement.[4] Arachidonic acid is a precursor to the proinflammatory leukotriene LTB$_4$, which has been well documented to play a role in the pathogenesis of the psoriatic lesion. The mixed nature of those findings may be due in part to lack of control of other critical factors influencing both lipid metabolism—such as oxidant status of the patient and relative intake of proinflammatory lipid precursors—and biochemical influences on the delta-5 and delta-6 desaturases, which are key in the metabolism toward proinflammatory or anti-inflammatory prostanoids. An additional key factor here is that carbohydrate excess leads to excess insulin release. The excess insulin both inhibits the delta-6 desaturase and causes chronic release of proinflammatory cytokines (B. Sears, personal communication, 2001), favoring the inflammatory disease process despite the anti-inflammatory effects of ingested EFAs. Most published studies do not address this important variable, which is best done by encouraging a diet low in simple carbohydrates. It has been my experience that following such a diet leads to positive results in a significant proportion of patients with seborrheic dermatitis, as well as those with other inflammatory disorders of the skin (see Chapter 84, The Anti-Inflammatory Diet).

NOTE

In patients with seborrheic dermatitis, a diet rich in omega-3 fatty acids and low in simple sugars can lead to clinical improvement via a beneficial influence on the inflammatory cascade.

INTEGRATIVE THERAPY

Nutrition

Omega-3 Essential Fatty Acids

Omega-3 unsaturated fatty acids should be substituted for other dietary fats. Saturated, heat-altered, and partially hydrogenated fats should be eliminated from the diet because they lead to production of proinflammatory prostaglandin E_2 (PGE_2) prostanoids. Also, they block the delta-6 desaturase that catalyzes the formation of anti-inflammatory leukotriene precursors. Extra fats contribute to the unfavorable ratio of proinflammatory lipids in the cell membrane and contribute to weight gain because of their caloric content. Other indicators of a need for omega-3 oils include dry skin in winter, dryness around the nail fold area, a lack of dietary intake of such oils, depression, and a high ratio of arachidonic acid to omega-3 EFAs in the plasma or red blood cell membrane.

An excellent source of omega-3 unsaturated EFAs is EFA-enriched fish oil capsules or liquid. Cod liver oil and other cold-water fish oils are also good sources. Eating four to five portions weekly of oily cold water fish is also recommended. Flaxseed oil, which contains alpha-linolenic acid, is also a potential source, but it must undergo chain elongation involving an extra step requiring the delta-6 desaturase, and some people cannot utilize this oil effectively. Canola oil and walnut oil are lesser sources of omega-3 unsaturated EFAs.

Oils can be either taken as supplements or worked into the diet as food. For example, flaxseed oil can be used in making "smoothies" or salad dressing. These oils should not be heated because the unsaturated bonds that make them useful are unstable on heating. Because of their unsaturated nature, they should be accompanied by vitamin E in the diet. Similarly, other factors contributing to high oxidative stress in the individual patient should be corrected, or counterbalanced with additional antioxidants, to maximize the effectiveness of these oils. Omega-3 fish oil can induce glucose intolerance in diabetic patients. To counter this effect and to reduce the proinflammatory mediators from carbohydrate-stimulated insulin elevation, a proper balance of carbohydrates with protein and exercise should be achieved.

Dosage. Dosage is based on severity of presentation, a history of inadequate dietary intake of omega-3 EFAs, and low red blood cell membrane ratio of EPA to arachidonate. Whereas daily intake of 6 capsules (about 1 teaspoon) of flaxseed oil or EPA-DHA fish oils may be helpful, some patients may need as much as 20 to 40 mL (4 to 8 teaspoons) daily, worked into a "shake" to make it palatable. Vitamin E 400 to 800 IU daily should be taken to protect these unsaturated oils from oxidation.

Precautions. Fish oils have been known to prolong bleeding time via the anticoagulant effect of the PGE_3 prostaglandins for which they are precursors. Use of large doses in pregnant woman has also been associated with elevated birth weight of their infants.

Yeast Elimination

For patients who require additional measures to control their seborrhea, a yeast and mold elimination diet should be instituted. The basis of this diet is the elimination of bread, cheese, wine and beer, excessive carbohydrates (especially sugar and simple starches), and other foods containing or produced by yeast or fungus. This diet has been touted as highly effective in the popular literature, and the success of different variations is probably related to yeast reduction and also to relieving different food allergies in patients with yeast sensitivities. Probiotics such as acidophilus and bifidus should be taken before or during meals to help repopulate the normal flora of the gut (see Chapter 97, Prescribing Probiotics). Those patients who cannot give up bread should be counseled to eat true sourdough bread, for which the leavening agent is derived from limited cultures of different yeasts captured from the air.

Supplements

Vitamins

Oils, which can be used as either foods or supplements, have already been addressed. Vitamin E 400 to 800 units per day should be added as an antioxidant to protect the oils. Adequate levels of magnesium, zinc, vitamin C, and vitamin B_6 should be maintained by supplementation if any of these is insufficient in the diet, to enhance the function of the delta-6 desaturase. Vitamin B_6 cream has been used for treatment of seborrheic dermatitis of the scalp.[5, 6]

Biotin is especially useful in infantile seborrheic dermatitis,[7] and may have a role in the treatment of adult seborrhea as well. Besides contributing to the generation of anti-inflammatory prostanoids via activation of the delta-6 desaturase (as do other vitamins mentioned here), biotin is reputed to retard the formation of the mycelial form of *Candida*. Other B vitamins shown to be helpful in seborrhea are folate[8] and vitamin B_{12}.[9]

Dosage. One or two tablets of a high-potency multivitamin with mineral (even for those with a 3-

to 6-tablet-daily recommendation on the bottle label) can be used for B vitamin supplementation in most patients. If clinical improvement is not seen, extra biotin up to 7500 mg per day, folate up to 10 mg per day, and B$_6$ or pyridoxal5-phosphate 50 to 100 mg per day can be added; zinc piccolinate 50 mg and vitamin C 500 mg one to three times per day are also useful.

Probiotics

To address the yeast overgrowth, adding probiotic bacteria such as *Lactobacillus acidophilus, Bifidobacterium,* and *Saccharomyces boulardii* to the diet is nearly as important as proper diet in restoring a normal gut flora and reducing the yeast population. Caprylic acid can be added to inhibit attachment of the yeast to the intestinal wall.

Dosage. GI Flora (Allergy Research Group) is an economical, effective source of multiple probiotic strains; the dose is 1 or 2 capsules with meals. Acidophilus with Pectin (Nature's Plus) and Ultradophillus (Metagenics) are other useful sources. Dosing for caprylic acid is begun at 1 capsule 3 times daily before meals and gradually increased to 2 per meal.

Precaution. Probiotics should not be given to patients with a compromised immune system, owing to the risk of infection.

NOTE

Many companies that produce probiotics claim the absolute best species, combinations, or strains of bacteria. Clinicians are advised to start with an affordable acidophilus or bifidus preparation and then add others to their personal pharmacopoeia as evaluation of a specific product is found to be convincing and its effects are confirmed to be beneficial. Different patients will do better with different probiotic bacteria. Bifidus is thought to be more beneficial initially.

Botanicals

Grapefruit seed extract and *Artemesia annua* can also be added to reduce the yeast population. A number of new herbal preparations constituted for this purpose have emerged on the market. Pau d'arco tea is another product with reported anti-yeast activity.

Application of aloe has been shown to be useful in seborrhea.[10]

Dosage.
- The dose for Artemesia Forte (Allergy Research Group, telephone 510 639-4572) is 3 to 6 tablets daily; for Citramesia (Ecological Formulas, telephone 800 888-4585) it is 2 tablets daily. Both contain *Artemesia annua* and grapefruit seed extract.
- Another source of grapefruit seed extract is Paramicocidin (Allergy Research Group). The dose is 125 mg 2 to 6 times daily with meals.
- *Aloe vera (Aloe barbadensis)* gel may be applied directly from the cut leaf of the plant.

Mind-Body Medicine

Seborrheic dermatitis is more prevalent in patients with depression.[11] It is possible that the improvement that occurs in the summer is due either to reduced depression or to effects of increased sunlight on melatonin release.[12] Addressing depression or seasonal affective disorder with light therapy, visits to a sunnier climate, psychotherapy, Bach Flower Remedies, supplements, or medications may be considered in a patient with seborrheic dermatitis in whom disease severity varies with affective state.

Pharmaceuticals

Shampoos

The two mainstays of topical treatment of seborrheic dermatitis are tar shampoos and anti-yeast shampoos. In order of potency, the latter consist of zinc pyrithione, selenium sulfide 0.5% (over-the-counter shampoos), selenium sulfide 3%, and ketoconazole shampoos. Tar shampoos have anti-inflammatory and anti-yeast activity.

Oil Turban

Oils are applied to the scalp to loosen scale. Olive oil is particularly useful in this regard, especially in infants with thin hair. Wetting the scalp and applying a warm oil turban for an hour, with 6% salicylic acid mixed into the olive oil, may remove more adherent scale. Patients will need to remove the oil with dish washing liquid detergent before applying a therapeutic shampoo.

Topical Corticosteroids

Topical corticosteroids are another mainstay of conventional treatment of seborrheic dermatitis. Even 1% hydrocortisone cream will bring temporary improvement in seborrheic dermatitis of the face and nasolabial folds in a previously untreated patient. Liquids, gels, and even a foam vehicle are available, with a more potent fluorinated corticosteroid used to avoid the hair and reach the scalp.

Dosage. Apply sparingly once or twice daily.

Precautions. Frequent or repeated application of

corticosteroids results in tachyphylaxis (a progressively diminished response), requiring more potent steroids to obtain the same response. In addition, some patients behave as if they are addicted to the topical steroids. Repeated use on the face, especially of stronger corticosteroids, and even use of hydrocortisone on the thin tissues of the eyelids, can result in atrophy of the skin with permanent show-through of the underlying capillaries, or to problematic steroid acne.

Other Creams

Ketoconazole (Nizoral) cream applied sparingly twice daily is extremely helpful for management of seborrheic dermatitis of the face and hairline. It inhibits the *Malassezia*, gives dramatic clinical improvement, and does not cause the atrophy resulting from prolonged corticosteroid use.
Dosage. Apply twice daily to affected areas, sparingly.

Lithium Succinate

Lithium succinate 8% ointment has been reported to be helpful in seborrheic dermatitis.[13] An anti-yeast effect in vitro has been confirmed but not in vivo. The ointment is applied twice a day. It is interesting to contemplate the relationship between lithium as a drug for depression, which has been implicated as one cause of seborrhea, and direct application of lithium as a treatment for seborrhea. A common mediator pathway for both disorders may exist.

Oral Antifungals

Oral antifungals should be used only when the seborrhea is serious enough to warrant the risk of taking the drug, or when the underlying condition of overgrowth has not responded to diet and herbal treatment alone.

Nystatin

Oral nystatin is useful to reduce the *Candida* population in the gut. It has the benefit of being poorly absorbed and therefore remaining in the gut. It works by causing defective yeast cell wall formation, which results in release of intracellular contents, which has in turn been blamed for the aggravation of symptoms constituting a Herxsheimer-type reaction in some patients following a large dose.
Dosage. Dosing should begin with 1 capsule (500,000 units) per day of the powder, with addition of an extra capsule every 2 or 3 days until a total dose of a 4 capsules 3 times a day (6 million units per day total) is achieved. Dosing for the pure powder should

begin with 1/8 teaspoon per day increased to 1 teaspoon per day (6 million units per day total) in the same gradual manner.

Ketoconazole and Fluconazole

Ketoconazole (Nizoral) is well absorbed and exerts an anti-yeast effect in the gut and skin and is excreted in high concentrations in the sweat. Other oral antifungals such as fluconazole (Diflucan) have also been used for severe cases of seborrhea. An anti-yeast regimen should be instituted gradually, starting with diet, acidophilus, and supplements and botanicals before oral pharmaceuticals are used. The first reason is to avoid a rapid kill-off of a large number of organisms, which may result in a die-off effect, or Herksheimer-type reaction. The second reason is to reduce the intestinal yeast population less drastically. By altering the gut ecology to favor a more gradual reduction in yeast population, a rebound growth of yeast resistant to the most powerful agents available will not occur.

Dosage:
- Nystatin: Dosing is increased slowly from 500,000 units once a day to 2 million units 3 times daily, maintained until the patient's condition is improved and stable, and appropriate dietary changes have been effected.
- Fluconazole (Diflucan): The dose is 100 to 200 mg per day for 10 to 14 days. (Note that many drug interactions and cautions are cited in the package insert). Seborrhea is not a listed indication.
- Ketoconazole (Nizoral) 100–200 mg/day should only be used if other indications exist and liver enzymes are monitored. In general, this drug should be avoided, or the liver can be protected with silymarin (milk thistle).

Precautions. Adverse effects include elevation in liver enzymes, hepatic failure (uncommon with oral ketoconazole and less likely with fluconazole), Herxsheimer-type die-off phenomenon (especially with nystatin), and overgrowth of resistant organisms.

NOTE
Before considering an oral antifungal, reduce intestinal yeast growth with dietary measures. This will help prevent the growth of resistant strains of yeast and result in improved response from the oral antifungal.

Other Therapies to Consider

Homeopathy

A homeopathic dilution of tobacco has been reported to clear seborrheic dermatitis in a patient with tobacco sensitivity. I mention this not to recommend this specific remedy but rather to emphasize the potential benefits of choosing an appropriate homeopathic or other remedy that addresses prominent underlying imbalances in the patient. Other homeopathics including Nat mur, arsenicum alb, and bryonia may be considered, but homeopathics should be prescribed according to other characteristics of the patient besides local presentation.

Food Allergy

As in patients with atopic dermatitis, addressing food allergy by removing the offending foods from the diet may benefit some patients with recalcitrant seborrheic dermatitis.

 ## THERAPEUTIC REVIEW

Following is an outline of therapeutic options for the treatment of seborrheic dermatitis. Determining which factors lead to the disease presentation in a given patient may increase the chances of success of a given therapy. For more severe or resistant cases, a progressive, sequential approach with multiple therapeutic avenues is recommended, with either intensification of treatments or addition of systemic pharmacologic agents, as indicated by the clinical response.

- *Anti-dandruff shampoos*
  - Zinc pyrithione, selenium sulfide (Selsun), tar, or ketoconazole (Nizoral) shampoo used for 5 minutes 2 or 3 times weekly. If the patient has used one type with no clinical improvement, another can be tried.

- *Anti-yeast creams*
  - Nizoral cream, or another pharmacologic or herbal substitute, works well on the face and nonscalp areas.

- *Supplements*
  - EPA-DHA fish oils can be added at 1 to 5 mL daily or more, titrated to clinical improvement.
  - Other sources of omega-3 EFAs include oily cold-water fish such as salmon and sardines, and flaxseed oil can be used at the same dosage.
  - Vitamin E 400–800 IU daily should be given with these oils.
  - Vitamin B complex, folic acid 1 to 10 mg, vitamin B_6 500 mg, and biotin up to 8 mg a day may be beneficial in resistant cases.

- *Nutrition*
  - A low-yeast, low–simple carbohydrate diet, especially eliminating bread, cheese, wine, beer, fermented foods, and starches, is helpful in persistent cases. Some improvement may be due to removal of other food allergens.
  - Adding probiotic bacteria such as acidophilus 1 capsule per meal, or live-culture yogurt, may also help.

- *Botanicals*
  - The anti-yeast botanicals grapefruit seed extract and *Artemesia annua* may be used at 2 to 6 capsules daily.

- *Pharmaceuticals*
  - Nystatin in slowly increasing doses from 0.5 million to 6 million units daily.
  - Fluconazole (Diflucan) 100 to 200 units daily for 2 weeks or longer, for resistant cases. This agent is best used after dietary, herbal, and supplement methods have been employed to reduce the yeast flora and to attenuate the ecologic factors favoring yeast growth.
  - Triamcinolone solution or betamethasone valerate foam (Luxiq) once or twice daily can be used to relieve pruritus and inflammation.

References

1. Bergbrant IM: Seborrheic dermatitis and *Pityrosporum* yeasts. Curr Top Med Mycol 6:95-112, 1995.
2. Dattner AM, Levis WR: Clonal priming of human lymphocytes with soluble microbial antigens: High-dose paralysis, restoration, and autologous leukocyte preference. Scand J Immunol 8:403-412, 1978.
3. Albert LJ, Inman RD: Molecular mimicry and autoimmunity. N Engl J Med. 341:2068-2074, 1999.
4. Schena D, Chieregato GC, de Gironcoli M, et al: Increased erythrocyte membrane arachidonate and platelet malondialdehyde (MDA) production in psoriasis: Normalization after fish-oil. Acta Derm Venereol Suppl (Stockh) 146:42-44, 1989.
5. Schreiner AW, Rockwell E, Vilter RW: A local defect in the metabolism of pyridoxine in the skin of persons with seborrheic dermatitis of the "sicca" type. J Invest Dermatol 19:95-96, 1952.

6. Effersoe H: The effect of topical application of pyridoxine ointment on the rate of sebaceous secretion in patients with seborrheic dermatitis. Acta Derm Venereol 3:272-278, 1954.
7. Schulpis KH, Georgala S, Papakonstantinou ED, Michas T, Karikas GA: The effect of isotretinoin on biotinidase activity. Skin Pharmacol Appl Skin Physiol. 12:28-33, 1999.
8. Callaghan TJ: The effect of folic acid on seborrheic dermatitis. Cutis 3:583-588, 1967.
9. Andrews GC, Post CF, Domnkos AN: Seborrheic dermatitis: Supplemental treatment with vitamin B12. NY State Med J 50:1921-1925, 1950.
10. Vardy DA, Cohen AD, Tchetov T, et al: A double-blind, placebo-controlled trial of an *Aloe vera* (*A. barbadensis*) emulsion in the treatment of seborrheic dermatitis. J Dermatol Treat 10:7-11, 1999.
11. Maietta G, Fornaro P, Rongioletti F, Rebora A: Patients with mood depression have a high prevalence of seborrheic dermatitis. Acta Derm Venereol 70:432-434, 1990.
12. Maietta G, Rongioletti F, Rebora A: Seborrheic dermatitis and daylight. Acta Derm Venereol 71:538-539, 1991.
13. Nenoff P, Haustein UF, Munzberger C: In vitro activity of lithium succinate against *Malassezia furfur*. Dermatology 190:48-50, 1995.

CHAPTER 61

Acne Vulgaris and Acne Rosacea

Sharon K. Hull, M.D.

PATHOPHYSIOLOGY

Acne vulgaris, more commonly referred to as acne, is the most common dermatologic disease treated by physicians.[1, 2] It afflicts an estimated 17 million people in the United States, and may affect 80% to 85% of adolescents and young adults.[1, 3] A related condition, acne rosacea, more commonly affects adults between the ages of 30 and 60 years; more than 13 million people in the United States may suffer from rosacea.[4, 5] The pathophysiology of these two conditions is considerably different.

Acne Vulgaris

Acne vulgaris is a disease of the pilosebaceous unit of the skin. This structure consists of a hair follicle and its associated sebaceous (oil-producing) gland. Four separate and distinct factors are required for the development of acne vulgaris. (1) Androgens act at the sebaceous gland to increase production of sebum; this increase occurs at puberty and in hyperandrogenic states. (2) Increased sebum facilitates the growth of the gram-positive anaerobic bacterium *Propionibacterium acnes*. (3) Normal follicle desquamation is impaired, causing desquamated tissue to form a plug in the opening to the follicle. (4) *P. acnes* leads to increased conversion of sebum into free fatty acids. In susceptible persons, a hypersensitivity reaction is stimulated that may lead to inflammation of the lesion, causing severe nodular acne. Common clinical manifestations include formation of comedones (blackheads) and pustules (whiteheads). The severe, nodular form of acne occurs only in persons who have a hypersensitivity to the free fatty acids produced by *P. acnes*[3, 6] (see Fig. 61–1).

Androgen production increases at puberty, accounting for the increased occurrence of acne vulgaris around the time of sexual maturation. The skin of acne patients may exhibit higher levels of 5α-reductase, resulting in higher rates of conversion of testosterone into its more active metabolite, dihydrotestosterone. Hyperandrogenic states such as adrenal androgen excess, 21-hydroxylase deficiency, and polycystic ovary syndrome may contribute to the development of acne. Androgen-inducing medications such as steroids may also increase the likelihood of acne lesions. There is some indication that insulin resistance in skin tissue plays a role in the direct pathogenesis of this disease, consistent with the increased incidence noted in patients with polycystic ovary syndrome[7] and other hyperinsulinemic states.

Acne Rosacea

The pathophysiology of acne rosacea is a subject of significant debate, and various theories have been postulated. Of these, several possible mechanisms merit consideration.

1. The skin mite, *Demodex folliculorum*, has been noted to be present in some patients with rosacea, but it is not found consistently. This mite is known to feed on sebum and may be involved in the inflammatory response noted with this condition.[5, 8]
2. Investigators have postulated a link between the bacterium *Helicobacter pylori* and the presence of

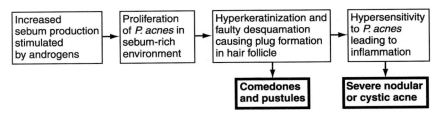

Figure 61-1. Pathophysiology of acne vulgaris. *P. acnes, Propionibacterium acnes.*

rosacea. Several studies have failed to demonstrate a clear relationship between the two, whereas others provide evidence supporting this link.[9-12]

3. There is some evidence to support an underlying connective tissue abnormality in this condition, which leads to vascular instability and chronic vasodilatation.[5]

4. Decreased levels of hydrochloric acid in gastric secretions have been noted in patients with acne rosacea, leading to the hypothesis that hypochlorhydria is a contributory factor.[13]

Clinical features of acne rosacea include the following:

- chronic vasodilatation, characterized by easy blushing and chronic erythema
- papule and pustule formation resembling that in acne vulgaris, seen most commonly over the malar eminences, nose, and cheeks, although the chest and upper arms may also be involved
- formation of telangiectasias (visible, dilated blood vessels) in affected areas of the skin
- sebaceous gland and connective tissue hypertrophy, with connective tissue overgrowth most prominent in the distal nasal area, where it causes a condition known as rhinophyma

Several "triggers" may result in symptomatic flares of this disease, including temperature extremes, hot beverages, spicy foods, and alcohol.

INTEGRATIVE THERAPY

Nutrition

A balanced diet favoring protein and low in fat over carbohydrates has been shown to be of some benefit in patients with acne, possibly owing to an improvement in insulin sensitivity that results from this nutrient balance.[7] In addition, vegetables high in vitamin A, such as sweet potatoes, carrots, and spinach and other greens, may have a beneficial effect.

A diet high in omega-3 fatty acids reduces production of inflammatory compounds such as prostaglandins and leukotrienes[14] and may alter steroid hormone metabolism in a manner to reduce androgen production; it may also improve insulin sensitivity. Consumption of oily cold-water fish such as salmon, mackerel, and sardines is recommended. Flaxseed oil is high in omega-3 fatty acids and is cheaper than fish oil supplements. Flaxseed oil, 500 mg 2 capsules twice daily, or 1 tablespoon of oil taken in food (not heated) daily, can be used. (See Chapter 84, The Anti-Inflammatory Diet.)

No clear-cut evidence exists for the direct "triggering" of acne vulgaris by specific foods such as chocolate or fats. However, such foods may contribute to the condition by impairing insulin sensitivity. Intake of foods high in exogenous hormones—particularly dairy products and some meats—should be limited.

In patient with acne rosacea, foods that tend to trigger exacerbations should be identified. Such foods typically include spicy foods, hot beverages, and alcohol. Not all patients experience the same triggers, so these foods should not be eliminated empirically.

Hygiene

Gentle cleansing with lukewarm water and use of a non–soap-based cleanser (washing with the hands and not with a washcloth or other abrasive material) are recommended. These measures prevent microabrasion of the skin, detergent irritation, and thermal injury, all of which can increase the number and severity of acne lesions.

Supplements

Several supplements may be considered in the treatment of acne vulgaris and acne rosacea.

Brewer's Yeast

Brewer's yeast (*Saccharomyces cerevisiae*) is a medicinal yeast with a high chromium content. It has been shown to improve glucose tolerance and insulin sensitivity.[7, 15] In one reported study, brewer's yeast led to clinical improvement in patients with acne.

Dosage. Dried yeast 2 g 3 times daily.

NOTE

Brewer's yeast may induce migraines in susceptible persons and may increase flatulence. This product is contraindicated in patients taking MAO inhibitors, as it may cause increased blood pressure. Use in patients with gout may precipitate disease flares.

Zinc

Zinc is an essential cofactor in wound healing, local activation of hormones, and immune function. It is essential in the production of retinal-binding protein. Use of zinc has been debated extensively, with several studies suggesting benefit and others suggesting no improvement. Zinc picolinate provides the best bioavailability among the several commercially available preparations.[7]

Dosage. Zinc picolinate 30 to 50 mg daily.

Precautions. Zinc can block copper absorption in doses greater than 50 mg per day.

Hydrochloric Acid

There is some evidence that patients with acne rosacea have concomitant hypochlorhydria on gastric analysis. These patients may benefit from hydrochloric acid supplementation.[13]

Dosage. 10 to 60 grains (1 to 6 capsules, typically 10 grains per capsule) of hydrochloric acid at each large meal. The dose should be titrated to the point at which the patient experiences a "warm" feeling in the stomach.

Vitamin A

Compounds of the class called retinols, including vitamin A, have been used extensively to treat acne. Their mechanism of action includes reduction of sebum production and reduction of follicular hyperkeratosis (implicated in plugging of follicles). The dosage required for most effective symptom reduction may lead to hypervitaminosis A (see "Precautions"). This supplement should not be used alone but should be presented in conjunction with an integrated treatment program. Vitamin A supplementation should not be used for more than 1 to 3 months.[7]

Dosage. Vitamin A 100,000 international units (IU) daily for a maximum of 1 month, then 25,000 to 50,000 IU daily.

Precautions. Hypervitaminosis A is characterized by headache, myalgia, fatigue, and elevation of liver enzymes. Prolonged use of high doses of vitamin A may result in toxicity, manifested as dry skin, anorexia, nausea and vomiting, hair loss, and hepatitis.

NOTE

Vitamin A is a teratogen when used in high dosages and is therefore contraindicated in women of childbearing age unless effective birth control methods are used for the duration of treatment and for at least 1 month after discontinuation. Vitamin A supplementation is also not recommended in children younger than 18 years of age.

Botanicals

Tea Tree Oil

The leaves of the native Australian plant *Melaleuca alternifolia* are the source of tea tree oil, widely used as a topical antimicrobial. Few clinical trials of high quality have been conducted, and the evidence regarding the benefit of this botanical is mixed.[16] One trial compared tea tree oil and a benzoyl peroxide preparation for the treatment of acne; benzoyl peroxide provided greater improvement, but tea tree oil was better tolerated by patients, with fewer side effects.[17]

Dosage. Tea tree oil 5% to 15% solution or gel, applied topically once daily.

NOTE

Tea tree oil may precipitate contact dermatitis. It should not be used in the treatment of acne rosacea, as it may worsen the associated skin problem.

Azelaic Acid

Azelaic acid is a naturally occurring dicarboxylic acid found in wheat, rye, and barley; it is reported to be both antibacterial and anticomedonal.[1] In one controlled trial, azelaic acid was found to be as effective as benzoyl peroxide and erythromycin topical preparations.[18] It appears to be both bacteriostatic and bactericidal and acts to decrease hyperkeratinization of the hair follicle.[19] Fewer side effects such as skin irritation are noted with azelaic acid then with benzoyl peroxide preparations.[3, 7]

Dosage. Azelaic acid 20% (Azelex), applied topically twice daily.

NOTE

Azelaic acid may cause hypopigmentation and should be used cautiously in patients with darker complexions.

Pharmaceuticals

Topical Pharmaceutical Preparations

Antibiotics

A number of topical antibiotic preparations are available and have been shown to be useful in treatment of acne vulgaris and acne rosacea.[3] Potential side effects are few, with the exception of skin irritation. Common preparations and dosages are listed in Table 61–1.

Retinoids

By acting as vitamin A analogues, retinoid compounds decrease desquamation, reducing formation of comedones in acne vulgaris.

Dosage.
- Tretinoin: 0.01% to 0.1% in various delivery vehicles (Retin-A) applied once daily at bedtime.
- Tazarotene: 0.05% to 0.1% (Tazorac) applied once daily at bedtime.

Table 61-1. Topical Agents for the Treatment of Acne

Preparation and Dosage	Side Effect(s)
Benzoyl peroxide 2.5%–10% (various brands), applied topically once or twice daily for acne vulgaris	Significant drying of skin, contact dermatitis in 1%–2% of users; may bleach clothing
Clindamycin (Cleocin T), applied topically once or twice daily for acne vulgaris	Drying of skin, very rare incidence of pseudomembranous colitis
Erythromycin 1.5%–2% (various brands), applied topically once or twice daily for acne vulgaris	Drying of skin
Tetracycline 2.2% (Topicycline), applied once or twice daily for acne vulgaris	Staining of skin, fluorescence under ultraviolet light
Metronidazole cream (various strengths, brands, and vehicles), applied once or twice daily for acne rosacea*	Significant skin irritation and dryness

*Data from Macsai et al.[5]

- Adapalene: 0.1% gel or solution (Differin) applied once daily at bedtime.

Precautions. Significant skin irritation may occur, depending on the concentration of the retinoid and the vehicle in which it is delivered. This irritation is worsened with sun exposure, so patients should be advised to apply it once daily at bedtime.

Systemic Pharmaceutical Preparations

Antibiotics

Oral antibiotics decrease bacterial colonization, inhibit neutrophil chemotaxis, and reduce the concentration of free fatty acids in sebaceous glands.[1] These preparations may be useful for treatment of both acne vulgaris and acne rosacea.

Dosage.
- Erythromycin: 250 to 500 mg orally twice daily.
- Tetracycline: 250 to 500 mg orally twice daily (should be taken on an empty stomach).
- Doxycycline: 50 to 100 mg orally twice daily (should be taken with food).
- Minocycline: 50 to 100 mg orally twice daily (should be taken with food).

Precautions. Adverse effects include gastrointestinal upset (nausea, diarrhea), photosensitivity, and the potential for decreased effectiveness of oral contraceptives when these agents are taken concomitantly.

Systemic Retinoids

Systemic retinoids are very effective in the treatment of severe cystic or inflammatory acne but carry with them the potential for significant side effects, including teratogenicity and depression.[20, 21]

Dosage. Isotretinoin (Accutane) 0.5 to 1 mg/kg per day in 2 divided doses.

Precautions. Only physicians experienced in managing the potential complications of their use should employ systemic retinoids. Care should be given to providing adequate contraception, monitoring patients for depression, and careful ongoing follow-up of liver enzyme level as markers for hepatic injury. Referral to a dermatologist experienced in the use and monitoring of this therapy may be indicated.

Oral Contraceptives

Oral contraceptives with low intrinsic androgenicity may be beneficial in the treatment of acne vulgaris in women, but these agents should not be used for first-line or single-agent therapy. Potential adverse effects include all side effects that accompany use of oral contraceptives.

Dosage. An oral contraceptive containing norgestimate (Ortho Tri-Cyclen, Ortho-Cyclen) or desogestrel (Desogen), 1 tablet orally daily, can be used.

Surgery

Although no surgical therapy is available to treat acne vulgaris, recent advances in laser operative techniques have proved to be beneficial in the treatment of telangiectasias associated with acne rosacea. Various surgical methods exist to treat significant rhinophyma, which may also accompany this disease. These treatment options are reserved for severe or recalcitrant disease, or for disease accompanied by significant cosmetic disfigurement.[5]

Other Therapies to Consider

Some other therapies that may be considered, but for which only limited data are available, include use of various Japanese kampo preparations[22, 23] and certain Ayurvedic therapies.[24] Homeopathic remedies may be of some benefit when selected after systematic homeopathic evaluation by a trained practitioner. At least one study suggests a potential for benefit from biofeedback-assisted relaxation and cognitive imagery.[25]

Some data exist to suggest that there is a role for vitamin E, selenium, pyridoxine, and/or pantothenic acid in the treatment of acne vulgaris.[7] Also of interest, one study suggests potential benefit from L-carnitine supplementation in managing liver and muscle side effects of isotretinoin.[26]

THERAPEUTIC REVIEW

Nutrition
- *A low-fat diet favoring proteins over carbohydrates and fats and high in foods rich in vitamin A (sweet potatoes, carrots, and spinach and other greens) should be encouraged.*
- *Intake of foods high in omega-3 fatty acids (salmon, nuts, or flaxseed) should be encouraged, or 1 tablespoon of flaxseed oil daily can be used.*
- *Potential trigger foods for acne rosacea, especially hot beverages, spicy foods, and alcohol, should be avoided.*

Hygiene
- *Use of detergent-free facial cleanser should be encouraged.*
- *Use of washcloths and hot water should be discouraged.*

Supplements
- *Brewer's yeast, 2 g 3 times daily for acne vulgaris.*
- *Zinc picolinate, 30 to 50 mg daily for acne vulgaris.*
- *Vitamin A 100,000 IU per day for a maximum of 1 month, then 25,000 to 50,000 IU per day (see with cautions about contraception and teratogenicity) for acne vulgaris.*
- *Hydrochloric acid 10 to 60 grains at each large meal (1 to 6 capsules at 10 grains per capsule), for acne rosacea; lower doses are used with smaller meals.*
- *Patients with acne rosacea should avoid use of niacin-containing products.*

Botanicals
- *Tea tree oil 5% to 15% solution or gel applied topically once daily (should not be used to treat acne rosacea).*
- *Azelaic acid 20% (Azelex) applied topically twice daily for acne vulgaris.*

Pharmaceuticals
- *Topical benzoyl peroxide, clindamycin, or erythromycin applied topically once or twice daily for acne vulgaris.*
- *Topical retinoids (tretinoin, tazarotene, or adapalene) applied once daily at bedtime for acne vulgaris.*
- *Topical metronidazole cream applied once or twice daily for acne rosacea.*
- *Oral erythromycin or tetracycline 250 to 500 mg twice daily, or oral doxycycline or minocycline 50 to 100 mg twice daily, for either acne vulgaris or acne rosacea.*
- *Oral isotretinoin (Accutane) 0.5 to 1 mg/kg per day in 2 divided doses (administered by a physician experienced in the use and monitoring of this drug) for acne vulgaris.*

Surgical Therapy
- *Laser therapy for telangiectasias, common in acne rosacea.*
- *Various scalpel and laser surgical techniques to treat rhinophyma, a severe sequela of acne rosacea.*

References

1. Krowchuk DP: Managing acne in adolescents. Pediatr Clin North Am 47:841–857, 2000.
2. Weiss JS: Current options for the topical treatment of acne vulgaris. Pediatr Dermato 14:480, 1997.
3. Russell JJ: Topical therapy for acne. Am Fam Physician 61:357–366, 2000.
4. Corr S (ed): Rosacea Awareness Month spreads public knowledge and understanding. In Drake L (ed): Rosacea Review. Boston, National Rosacea Society, 2000.
5. Acne rosacea. In Macsai MS, Mannis MJ, Huntley AC (eds): Eye and Skin Disease. Philadelphia, Lippincott-Raven, 1996, p 705.
6. Webster GF: Office dermatology. Part I: Acne and rosacea. Med Clin North Am 82:1145–1154, 1998.
7. Murray MT, Pizzorno JE: Acne vulgaris and acne conglobata. In Murray MT, Pizzorno JE (eds): Textbook of Natural Medicine, 2nd ed, vol 2. New York, Churchill Livingstone, 1999, pp 1033–1038.
8. Marks R: Concepts in the pathogenesis of rosacea. Br J Dermatol 80:170–177, 1968.
9. Herr H, You CH: Relationship between *Helicobacter pylori* and rosacea: It may be a myth. J Korean Med Sci 15:551–554, 2000.
10. Bamford JT, Tilden RL, Blankush JL, et al: Effect of treatment of *Helicobacter pylori* infection on rosacea. Arch Dermatol 135:659–663, 1999.
11. Szlachic A, Sliwowski Z, Karczewska E: *Helicobacter pylori* and its eradication in rosacea. J Physiol Pharmacol 50:777–786, 1999.
12. Wedi B, Kapp A: *Helicobacter pylori* infection and skin diseases. J Physiol Pharmacol 50:753–776, 1999.
13. Murray MT, Pizzorno JE: Rosacea. In Murray MT, Pizzorno JE (eds): Textbook of Natural Medicine, 2nd Ed, vol 2. New York, Churchill Livingstone, 1999, p. 1537-9.
14. Berbis P, Hesse S, Privat Y: Essential fatty acids and the skin. Allergy Immunol 22:225–231, 1990.
15. Blumenthal M, Goldberg A, Brinckmann J: Yeast. In Blumenthal M, Goldberg A, Brinckmann J (eds): Herbal Medicine: Expanded German Commission E Monographs. Newton,

Mass, Integrative Medicine Communications, 2000, pp 424–428.

16. Ernst E, Huntley AC: Tea tree oil: A systematic review of randomized clinical trials. Forsch Komplementarmed Klass Naturheilkd 7:17–20, 2000.

17. Bassett IB, Pannowitz DL, Barnetson RS, et al: A comparative study of tea-tree oil versus benzoyl peroxide in the treatment of acne. Med J Austr 153:455–458, 1999.

18. Nguyen QH, Bui TP: Azelaic acid: Pharmacokinetic and pharmacodynamic properties and its therapeutic role in hyperpigmentation disorders and acne. Int J Dermatol 34:75–84, 1995.

19. Azelaic acid—a well-tolerated acne treatment [web site]. Cited 2/13/2000.

20. Johnson BA, Nunley JR: Use of systemic agents in the treatment of acne vulgaris. Am Fam Physician 62:1823–1830, 1835–1836, 2000.

21. Jick SS, Kremers HM, Vasilakis-Scaramozza C: Isotretinoin use and risk of depression, psychotic symptoms, suicide and attempted suicide. Arch Dermatol 136:1231–1236, 2000.

22. Akamatsu H, Asada Y, Horio T: Effect of keigai-rengyo-to, a Japanese kampo medicine, on neutrophil functions: A possible mechanism of action of keigai-rengyo-to in acne. J Intern Med Res 1997; 25(5):255-65.

23. Higaki S, Morimatsu S, Morohashi M, et al: Susceptibility of *Propionibacterium acnes, Staphylococcus aureus* and *Staphylococcus epidermidis* to 10 kampo formulations. J Intern Med Res 25:318–324, 1997.

24. Paranjpe P, Kulkarni PH: Comparative efficacy of four Ayurvedic formulations in the treatment of acne vulbaris: A double-blind randomised placebo-controlled clinical evaluation. J Ethnopharmacol 49:127–132, 1995.

25. Hughes H, Brown BW, Lawlis GF, et al: Treatment of acne vulgaris by biofeedback relaxation and cognitive imagery. J Psychosom Res 27:185–191, 1983.

26. Georgala S, Schulpis KH, Georgala C et al: L-Carnitine supplementation in patients with cystic acne on isotretinoin therapy. J Eur Acad Dermatol Venereol 13:205–209, 1999.

CHAPTER 62

Human Papillomavirus and Warts

Sharon K. Hull, M.D.

PATHOPHYSIOLOGY

Warts represent a medical condition that has been recognized for centuries, is very common, and may occur at any age. The lesions are benign neoplasms of the epidermis caused by infection with any of a family of viruses known as human papillomavirus (HPV). Between 60 and 90 viruses are recognized within this family, and many of them are responsible for the growth of warts in various locations on the human body. The infection is transmitted by skin-to-skin contact with infected areas. Visible warts contain active, shedding virus and are probably contagious.

Warts can occur anywhere on the body, but more common locations include the following:

- the trunk, hands, feet, and fingers and toes—in these locations, warts may be associated with trauma, and periungual warts may arise after nail-biting
- the face—typically, flat warts
- the genitalia—condylomata acuminata
- the perianal area
- the undersurface of the foot—plantar warts

Perianal warts may be implicated in the development of squamous cell carcinoma of the anogenital region. Women with genital warts should be encouraged to undergo a complete gynecologic examination, including a Papanicolaou smear. DNA typing may be indicated to identify the strain of HPV involved, as certain strains are implicated in the development of cervical cancer.[1]

The functional activity of the patient's cell-mediated immunity determines the duration, size, and severity of these lesions. The virus directly infects keratinocyte cells in the skin, causing these cells to proliferate into a mass that destroys skin lines while remaining confined to the epidermis.[2]

INTEGRATIVE THERAPY

Many modes of treatment have been suggested over the centuries for this common ailment. Many of the therapies discussed here have some benefit in promotion of host defense mechanisms and cell-mediated immunity.

Nutrition and Lifestyle Interventions

A healthful diet with an abundance of fruits and vegetables, particularly those high in carotenoids such as spinach and other greens, sweet potatoes, and carrots, promotes a healthy immune system.[3] High intake of refined sugar has been implicated in decreased immunity, so reduction of sugar intake may also be advisable.[4]

Avoidance of tobacco is critical with HPV infection, especially in patients with genital warts. Cigarette smoking may be associated with a two- to threefold increase in the risk for cervical cancer in women who have certain types of HPV genital infections.[5]

Mind-Body Therapy

Guided Imagery

Interactive Guided Imagery is a mind-body approach that incorporates a wide range of therapeutic interventions, including visualization, interpretation of dreams, storytelling, and direct suggestion. Its mechanism of action is complex, calling into play all major physiologic responses known to human beings. This includes enhancement of immune function, thought to play a role in combating viral infections such as those causing warts. It is a very safe treatment, except in the case of patients who are psychotic or are prone to dissociative states (it is contraindicated in both of these situations).[6]

Several anecdotal reports indicate that this therapeutic approach may be particularly useful in the management of warts.[7] A sample visualization technique for this purpose may be found in Chapter 89, Self-Hypnosis Techniques.

Hypnotherapy

Long a subject of scorn by the medical community, hypnotherapy has been recognized as a credible medical procedure by both the American Medical Association and the American Psychological Association since 1958. Its mechanism of action involves the induction of a trance state, with suggestions to the patient of alternative ways of looking at life experiences and situations.[8, 9] Few side effects are noted, but caution is indicated in patients with certain psychiatric disorders, particularly schizophrenia and other forms of psychosis.[9]

Several case reports and data from a number of studies particularly support the use of hypnotherapy in the treatment of warts.[10–15] At least one study compared hypnosis, placebo, and salicyclic acid treatments; results indicated that only the hypnosis subjects lost more warts than the treatment controls.[16]

This therapy appears to be both safe and effective when provided by a practitioner skilled in its use.

NOTE

Caution is indicated with use of both hypnotherapy and guided imagery in patients who may be at risk for psychiatric problems, including dissociation and schizophrenia.

Supplements

Although specific supplements are not widely used to treat warts directly, several supplements may help to improve immune function and host defense mechanisms, thereby increasing the patient's ability to eradicate the HPV infection more readily.[17–19]

Vitamin C

Vitamin C (ascorbic acid) has demonstrated many positive effects on the immune system, including lymphoproliferation and lymphotrophic activity as well as increased levels of antibodies, interferon, and immunoglobulins.[19]

Dosage. Vitamin C 3000 to 8000 mg daily.[18]

NOTE

Vitamin C may induce diarrhea at higher doses. One way to deal with this side effect is to begin the dose at 1000 mg per day, increasing by 1000 mg every 2 days until the patient experiences diarrhea, and then decreasing the dose by 1000 mg daily until the diarrhea stops.

Vitamin A

Vitamin A is a fat-soluble vitamin that plays a particularly helpful role in induction of cell-mediated immunity[20] and exhibits direct viricidal activity as well. Both of these functions make it well suited for use in the treatment of HPV infections.

Dosage. Vitamin A 100,000 international units (IU) for 1 week, then 25,000 IU daily until 4 weeks after visible warts are gone.[18]

Precautions. Vitamin A is a teratogen at high dosages and is contraindicated in women of childbearing age unless effective birth control methods are used for the duration of treatment and for at least 1 month following discontinuation. It is also not recommended for use by children younger than 18 years of age. Prolonged high doses of vitamin A may result in toxicity. Signs of hypervitaminosis A include dry skin, anorexia, nausea and vomiting, hair loss, and hepatitis.

Folic Acid

Folic acid (pteroylglutamic acid) is a water-soluble vitamin that is an essential cofactor in amino acid metabolism, nucleic acid synthesis, and various enzymatic reactions. It has been suggested to be an important enhancer of immune function as well.[17]

Dosage. Folic acid 400 μg per day.

Precautions. Folic acid may impair zinc absorption. Zinc supplementation may be useful in patients taking folic acid on a regular basis. Folic acid may also impair absorption of selective serotonin reuptake inhibitors (SSRIs), so caution must be exercised in patients taking these preparations concomitantly.

Zinc

Zinc is a cofactor for many enzymatic reactions in the body; it promotes complement binding and may also have inhibitory effects on viruses.[3]

Dosage. Zinc picolinate, or zinc in an amino acid chelate, 15 to 30 mg per day.

Precautions. Zinc can inhibit copper absorption at doses greater than 50 mg a day.

Pharmaceuticals

Salicylic Acid

Salicylic acid is keratolytic and does not scar. Use of this compound requires preparation of the wart tissue by soaking in warm water and then paring of the keratinized tissue. Following this preparation, a small amount of the salicyclic acid is placed on the wart tissue and allowed to dry. Occlusive dressing with tape may enhance the effectiveness but also increases the likelihood of soreness. After 1 to 3 days, the keratin is pared again. Larger warts may be treated with 40% salicyclic acid plasters.[2]

Dosage. Salicylic acid solution 17% (DuoPlant, Occlusal, and others) applied as directed. These preparations can be obtained over the counter.

Trichloroacetic Acid and Bichloroacetic Acid

Trichloroacetic and bichloroacetic acid are strongly acidic compounds that are effective in removing wart tissue; however, they are very destructive to normal tissue and should not be applied by patients at home. A thin coating of petrolatum is applied first, in order to protect the surrounding normal skin, and then a tiny amount of the acid is used topically on the wart tissue itself. The treatment should not be repeated for 7 to 10 days. These compounds are particularly useful in treating genital warts.

Dosage. An acid solution of choice (bichloroacetic or trichloracetic acid) is applied to wart after the surrounding tissue is protected by petrolatum.

Podophyllin

Podophyllin also acts as a keratolytic; it is derived from the mayapple plant. It is highly absorbable in normal tissue, especially near mucous membranes, and can cause serious neurologic complications. A prescription form of this medication, podofilox (podophyllotoxin), is available for home application by patients who have genital or perianal warts. Caution should be used in the frequency and extent of application.

Dosage. Podofilox (Condylox) gel 0.5% is applied twice daily for 3 days and then discontinued for 4 days. This cycle may be repeated until visible wart tissue is gone. No more than 0.5 g of gel should be used per day.

Precautions. Podophyllin has significant potential for neurotoxicity if applied too liberally; limited amounts should be applied at any given treatment session. It should not be used on the cervix or vagina because of increased systemic absorption. It also has been implicated as a teratogen, so its use in pregnant and breast-feeding women is contraindicated.

Surgery

Several surgical methods are effective for treating warts:

- Paring (with a blade or scalpel) and curettage for warts on the digits, hands, and feet
- Electrocautery for warts on the trunk, digits, hands, and feet
- Liquid nitrogen for warts in any location, including the face and the cervix, with duration of freeze dependent on size and location
- Loop electrosurgical excision procedure (LEEP) and large-loop excision of the transformation zone (LLETZ), used to remove condylomata from the cervix
- Laser surgery using the carbon dioxide laser for treating large or resistant warts[21]

Other Therapies to Consider

There is a long history of use of "folk remedies" for removal of wart, including the application of a potato, onion, or fresh garlic directly to the wart. No data exist to support these therapies, but some direct irritant effect may stimulate immune response, enhancing resolution of the condition. Application of other topical irritants, including vitamin E and castor oil, has also been suggested.

Homeopathic remedies may be of some benefit when selected after systematic homeopathic evaluation by a trained practitioner.

There may also be a role for acupuncture in treating this condition. Insertion of a needle directly into the wart using a complex "open door" technique has been reported to be beneficial. Additionally, specific acupuncture points between the first and second phalanges of the thumb or toe and the TE-3, LI-4, and auricular points have been suggested.[22]

Although no studies have been found to support it, the use of echinacea as an immune system stimulant may theoretically be beneficial.

Other irritant compounds are commonly used for wart removal in allopathic medical practice. Some of these are cantharin, 5-fluorouracil, formalin, and intralesional bleomycin.[2]

Use of immune system modulators such as interferon and imiquimod is also under study at this time.

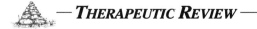 ─── *THERAPEUTIC REVIEW* ─────────────────────────

Nutrition and Lifestyle Interventions
- *High intake of vegetables, especially those high in carotenoids (spinach and other greens, sweet potatoes, carrots)*
- *Limited intake of refined sugars*
- *Avoidance of tobacco products*

Mind-Body Therapies
- *Interactive Guided Imagery approach*
- *Hypnotherapy*

THERAPEUTIC REVIEW *continued*

Supplements

- *Vitamin C 3000 to 8000 mg daily*
- *Vitamin A 100,000 IU for 1 week, then 25,000 IU daily until 4 weeks after visible warts are gone*
- *Folic acid 400 μg per day*
- *Zinc picolinate, or zinc in an amino acid chelate, 15 to 30 mg per day*

Pharmaceuticals

- *Salicylic acid 17% solution, topical*
- *Trichloroacetic or bichloroacetic acid, topical, for anogenital warts*
- *Podophyllin 25% solution of podofilox (Condylox) 0.5% gel, topical, particularly for anogenital warts*

Surgery

- *Paring and curettage*
- *Electrocautery*
- *Laser*
- *Cryosurgery*
- *Loop electrosurgical excision procedure and large loop excision of the transformation zone (LEEP/LLETZ) for cervical lesions*

References

1. Apgar BS: Changes in strategies for human papillomavirus genital disease [editorial]. Am Fam Physician 55: 1545–1546, 1548, 1997.
2. Habif TB: Clinical Dermatology, 3rd ed. St Louis, Mosby–Year Book, 1996.
3. Murray MT, Pizzorno JE: Immune support. In Murray MT, Pizzorno JE (eds): Textbook of Natural Medicine, 2nd ed, vol. 1. New York, Churchill Livingstone, 1999, pp 479–487.
4. Sanchez A: Role of sugars in human neutrophilic phagocytosis. Am J Clin Nutr 26: 1180–1184, 1973.
5. Kjellberg L, Hallmans G, Ahren A, et al: Smoking, diet, pregnancy and oral contraceptive use as risk factors for cervical intra-epithelial neoplasia in relation to huma papillomavirus infection. Br J Cancer 82: 1332–1338, 2000.
6. Rossman ML, Bresler DE: Interactive guided imagery. In Novey DW (ed): Clinician's Complete Reference to Complementary and Alternative Medicine. St Louis, Mosby, 2000, pp 64–83.
7. Grossbart TA: The skin: Matters of the flesh. In Goleman D, Gurin J (eds): Mind Body Medicine: How to Use Your Mind for Better Health. Yonkers, NY, Consumers Union of United States, 1993, pp 145–160.
8. Sierpina VS: Integrative Health Care: Complementary and Alternative Therapies for the Whole Person. Philadelphia, FA Davis, 2001.
9. Saichek KI: Hypnotherapy. In Novey DW (ed): Clinician's Complete Reference to Complementary and Alternative Medicine. St Louis, Mosby, 2000, pp 53–63.
10. Shenefelt PD: Hypnosis in dermatology. Arch Dermato 136:393–399, 2000.
11. Kohen DP, Mann-Rinehart P, Schmitz D, et al: Using hypnosis to help deaf children help themselves: Report of two cases. Am J Clin Hypn 40:288–296, 1998.
12. Noll RB: Hypnotherapy of a child with warts. J Dev Behav Pediatr 9:2, 1988.
13. Straatmeyer AJ, Rhodes NR: Condylomata acuminata: Results of treatment using hypnosis. J Am Acad Dermatol 9:434–436, 1983.
14. Spanos NP, Stenstrom RJ, Johnston JC: Hypnosis, placebo, and suggestion in the treatment of warts. Psychosom Med 50:245–260, 1988.
15. Ewin DM: Hypnotherapy for warts (verruca vulgaris): 41 consecutive cases with 33 cures. Am J Clin Hypn 35:1–10, 1992.
16. Spanos NP, Williams V, Gwynn MI: Effects of hypnotic, placebo, and salicylic acid treatments on wart regression. Psychosom Med 52:109–114, 1990.
17. Northrup C: Women's Bodies, Women's Wisdom. New York, Bantam Books, 1998.
18. Golan R: Optimal Wellness. New York, Ballantine Books, 1995.
19. Murray MT, Pizzorno JE: Recommended optimum nutrient intakes. In Murray MT, Pizzorno JE (eds): Textbook of Natural Medicine, 2nd ed, vol 1. New York, Churchill Livingstone, 1999; pp 909–937.
20. Murray MT, Pizzorno JE: Vitamin A. In Murray MT, Pizzorno JE (eds):Textbook of Natural Medicine, 2nd ed, vol 1. New York, Churchill Livingstone, 1999, pp 1007–1014.
21. Ceilley RI, Cornelison RL, Dobes WL, et al: Guidelines of care for warts: Human papillomavirus. J Am Acad Dermatol 32:98–103, 1995.
22. Filshie J, White A (eds): Medical Acupuncture: A Western Scientific Approach. Edinburgh, Churchill Livingstone, 1998.

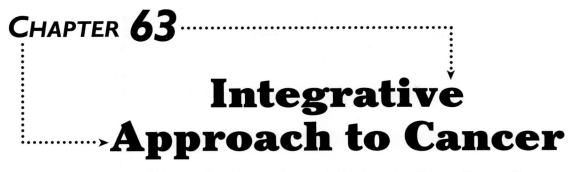

CHAPTER 63

Integrative Approach to Cancer

William Benda, M.D., and Kathryn L. Grant, Pharm.D.

At the end of the 20th century, cancer emerged as America's second leading cause of death, exceeded only by cardiovascular disease.[1] Taking into account the emotional and psychological trauma associated with an illness that strikes people of all ages, and for which the treatment is often as harsh as the disease itself, cancer may be second to none in terms of suffering experienced by those affected. In view of the enormous breadth and complexity of both biology and treatment, the scope of this chapter is limited to general philosophic and practical guidance, with more detailed investigations left to specialized references.

PATHOPHYSIOLOGY

Cancers originate as cells, normal in structure and function, that are subsequently transformed via a process called multistep carcinogenesis[1] (Fig. 63–1). Initiation of this event requires one or more alterations in cellular DNA, possibly mediated by viral, chemical, or physical events in the presence of tumor-promoting agents.[2] Subsequent genetic alterations allow these transformed cells to escape from their usual pattern of differentiation and programmed cell death (apoptosis).[3] Individual susceptibility to such transformation is influenced by additional genetic factors (e.g., abnormal DNA repair), variable expression of cellular oncogenes, or the loss of tumor suppressor genes.

PRINCIPLES OF THERAPY

Conventional cancer therapy is designed to reduce the tumor burden locally through surgical excision and irradiation, as well as by eradication of both primary and metastatic cancer cells via systemic chemotherapy. Because of the significant side effects of such invasive methods, the emotional trauma of the diagnosis is often magnified by the physical trauma of these interventions. Oncology is therefore one specialty practice in which complementary and alternative approaches may be synergistically employed in reducing both the sequelae of the disease itself and in limiting the toxicity of its manage-

ment. As more and more patients seek alternative or complementary treatments of cancer, the conventional practitioner needs to be aware of both potential benefits and risks. Fortunately, there is an

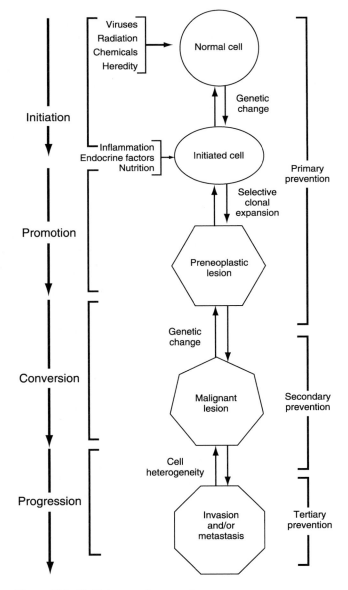

Figure 63-1. Multistep carcinogenesis.

increasing number of controlled studies to evaluate the efficacy and side effects of alternative approaches in both treatment and adjunctive support of the cancer patient (e.g., mistletoe extract [Iscador], green tea).

MANAGEMENT OF ADVERSE EFFECTS OF CANCER AND ITS TREATMENT

Each cancer patient faces significant physical, emotional, and social challenges resulting from both the disease itself and the sequelae of surgery, radiation therapy, and chemotherapy. The most common adverse events are as follows:

- Nausea and vomiting
- Weight loss and cachexia
- Pain
- Cardiac complications
- Alopecia
- Psychological distress and depression

The following discussion presents generally accepted complementary and alternative approaches to management of these problems. A review of conventional approaches is beyond the scope of this chapter, and the reader is directed to the appropriate literature.

Nausea and Vomiting

Nausea and hyperemesis are experienced by more than 75% of patients receiving combination chemotherapy.[4] Both frequency and severity are associated not only with specific chemotherapeutic agents, dosages, and schedules but also with age, gender, and prior alcohol history. Owing to the intense emotional state precipitated by the prospect and experience of chemotherapy, patients often develop anticipatory nausea and vomiting via classical behavioral conditioning.[5] Both anticipatory and delayed symptoms can be very difficult to alleviate and may lead to premature cessation of treatment, thus decreasing the potential for remission.

Management

Conventional approaches involve adjusting the chemotherapeutic agents and schedules, as well as administering antiemetic medications. The most effective regimens employ a combination of pharmaceutical agents (e.g., a serotonin type 3 receptor inhibitor, such as ondansetran [Zofran], plus dexamethasone).[4] Despite aggressive treatment, 60% of patients continue to experience protracted symptoms. Therefore, a comprehensive treatment plan may be greatly enhanced by the addition of unconventional approaches, including the following.

Ginger

This botanical has been shown to be an effective antiemetic, albeit through unknown pathways.[6]

Dosage. Patients may choose ginger root extracts (500 to 1000 mg as needed) or eat crystallized ginger (1 teaspoon or 5 g as needed).

Precautions. Ginger rarely produces adverse effects. In excessive doses it may induce a mild heartburn, and contact dermatitis has been documented after topical exposure.

Traditional Chinese Medicine

Serial acupuncture in conjunction with appropriate herbal therapy may alleviate the nausea and vomiting associated with chemotherapy and radiation therapy. The complexity of traditional Chinese medicine (TCM) requires referral to an experienced and qualified practitioner.[7] Contamination of Chinese botanical and other ingestible preparations with heavy metals, toxic chemicals, or prescription medications has been reported; therefore, the patient is advised either to use teas brewed from the fresh or dried herbs or to choose only oral products manufactured in the United States.[8] Because TCM practitioners obtain these products from various sources, quality and origin of merchandise may be of significance in choosing a practitioner for referral.

Mind-Body Techniques

Use of hypnosis to achieve physical as well as emotional states of relaxation has been shown to be of significant benefit in the prevention and management of nausea and vomiting.[9] An audiotape of the session may be created to aid the patient before or during subsequent treatments. Similar responses can be achieved by instructing the patient in appropriate guided imagery techniques, which may be self-initiated as the situation warrants.[10]

> **NOTE**
>
> *Hypnosis is beneficial, for the anticipatory nausea that is often associated with entering the facility where chemotherapy is provided.*

Marijuana

In selected patients, inhaled marijuana may be more effective than ingested synthetic tetrahydrocannabinol (THC).[11] Dosage is easily self-titrated. Although a number of states have passed legislation approving the medical use of marijuana, at present federal law claims authority in banning its use. Consideration by both the practitioner and the patient must include a full understanding of local, state, and federal statutes.[12, 13]

Weight Loss and Cachexia

Fifty percent to 80% of patients with malignancies suffer from cachexia, and the effect on survival in this patient population is seriously underestimated.[14] Significant weight loss can decrease patient tolerance of therapy and is thought to be the cause of death in as many as 20% of all cancer patients. Loss of body mass results from a number of factors, including anorexia, impaired cellular metabolism, and tumor-related increase in energy requirements. In addition, cytokines such as tumor necrosis factor-α, interleukin-1, interleukin-6, and interferon gamma may promote cachexia through induction of metabolic dysfunction.

Management

Conventional treatment of cytokine-induced abnormalities includes administration of anabolic steroids, cyproheptadine (Periactin), and megestrol (Megace). In addition, the following unconventional approaches may be considered in place of or as adjuncts to drug therapy. Unfortunately, all approaches are generally inadequate in dealing with this significant problem.

Diet and Supplementation

Nutritional requirements are optimized through patient consultation with a dietitian specifically trained in cancer management. General recommendations, however, include eating at least five to eight servings of fruits and vegetables each day, while limiting protein intake to 20% of calories and fat intake to 30% or less. Dietary supplements that may be of benefit include arginine, glutamine, and branched-chain amino acids.[14] Omega-3 fatty acids, found in freshwater fish, flaxseed, and fish oil, have been shown to inhibit cytokine production. Because flaxseed oil readily degrades without refrigeration and on exposure to heat, light, and air, the seeds should be purchased whole and ground in a coffee grinder before they are added to cereals or fruit or vegetable drinks. Whole seeds usually pass undigested through the gastrointestinal tract. Additional discussion may be found in the section on prevention of recurrences.

Marijuana

This botanical has demonstrated appetite enhancement in selected patients.[12] Legal and ethical issues are as described previously.

Pain

Perhaps the patient's greatest apprehension (aside from death) revolves around the specter of physical pain. Pain results not only from direct tumor invasion and subsequent cancer-induced syndromes but from appropriate diagnostic and therapeutic procedures as well.[15] It is estimated that in 85% of patients, cancer pain is theoretically responsive to oral opioid analgesics. However, studies have found frequent underuse of narcotics by the patient's medical team. To address this problem, several statewide, cancer pain initiatives promoted through the Joint Commission for Accreditation of Healthcare Organizations have been developed for educating healthcare professionals about pain management.[16, 17] Perhaps the most direct approach is to ask the patient about experience of pain at each follow-up visit, accept the validity of the patient's assessment, and treat accordingly.

Management

Conventional pharmacologic therapy is of great benefit. Selection of initial drugs is based on type and severity of pain. Dosages are adjusted as necessary. Although there are recommended maximums for nonopioid analgesics (owing to limiting toxic side effects), it is essential to remember that there is no analgesic ceiling for opioid dosages. Addiction occurs very rarely in cancer patients requiring these medications for pain control. Administration of meperidine (Demerol) in high dosages or over prolonged periods may result in accumulation of a toxic metabolite, producing central nervous system excitability and convulsions.[18] For this reason, meperidine is not recommended for patients with cancer.

Once the pain can no longer be controlled with oral medications, use of the intramuscular, intravenous, rectal, or topical (patches) route may be instituted. In the most severe cases, regional analgesia or neuroablative procedures may be effective. Should the patient desire or require nonpharmacologic pain control, the following alternative or adjunctive approaches should be considered.

Mind-Body Techniques

Hypnosis and guided imagery have been shown to be of significant benefit, as both psychological stress and physical tension contribute greatly to the experience of pain.[9] The therapist should be knowledgeable in issues associated with cancer and experienced in choosing the appropriate techniques.

Marijuana

As used for nausea, vomiting, and cachexia, the inhaled form of marijuana may be helpful in the control of pain in appropriate patients.[12] Again, the practitioner (and the patient) must be fully informed of all ethical and legal issues.

Support

Feelings of isolation and fear greatly amplify the subjective perception of physical pain. Emotional, psychological, and social support must be a fundamental aspect of any treatment plan and addressed by every member of the health care team who comes into contact with the patient. Discussion of support groups is found in the section on psychological distress.

Cardiac Complications

Cardiomyopathies with congestive heart failure, myocardial ischemia, and arrhythmias are not infrequent complications of chemotherapy and radiation therapy.[19]

Management

There is some evidence that use of specific antioxidant therapy before, during, and after chemotherapy or radiation therapy may limit the adverse cardiac effects of such treatments.

Coenzyme Q10

This antioxidant has demonstrated an ability to protect the myocardium from the toxic effects of anthracyclines (such as daunorubicin or idarubicin) in doses of 100 mg per day.[20, 21]

Dosage. Because coenzyme Q10 is poorly absorbed, formulations incorporating an oil base are preferred, and the dose for these gelcaps is 60 mg daily.[22] Further research is necessary to more fully delineate this antioxidant's role and optimal dose.

Vitamin E

Although animal studies have shown a protective effect of vitamin E against anthracycline-induced cardiac toxicity, studies in humans have yielded contradictory results. More research is needed to determine the appropriate dose.[23–25]

Alopecia

Alopecia is a common side effect of chemotherapy. Although regrowth of hair often occurs within 3 to 6 months, the social stigma of hair loss may lead to therapeutic noncompliance.[26]

Management

Most pharmacologic and nonmedical attempts at prevention and treatment of alopecia have proved unsuccessful and in some cases harmful. At present there are no safe and efficacious measures for prevention of alopecia or restoration of hair growth. The best approach is early determination of the patient's anticipated response, followed by continual psychological and emotional support throughout the treatment period. Mind-body techniques such as guided imagery may be of use in addressing the perceived trauma of hair loss. In some communities, hair stylists volunteer their time to assist patients with use of cosmetics, wigs, hats, and scarves.

Psychological Distress and Depression

Understandably, approximately 33% to 66% of oncology patients experience measurable levels of psychological distress.[27] The actual incidence or prevalence of major depression is unknown, although it appears to vary with the specific diagnosis and stage of disease. The highest incidence has been noted in patients with cancers of the pancreas and oropharynx, often associated with poor prognosis or surgical disfigurement. It is clear, however, that major depression has a negative impact on morbidity, length of hospitalization, disability, and mortality.

Management

Conventional approaches often utilize antidepressant medications and, in severe cases, psychostimulants such as dextroamphetamine (Dexedrine) or methylphenidate (Ritalin). Psychosocial interventions, usually incorporating referral to cancer support groups, are also employed.[28] Although a few clinical trials have shown positive patient outcomes, in actual practice, many patients quit such support groups after a short period of attendance. One explanation is that these individuals perceive themselves as more ill or less ill than the group as a whole, which adds to feelings of isolation and depression. Additionally, if the group is not appropriately facilitated, group meetings may evolve into "gripe sessions" with no evidence of positive progress. The patient's referring physician should therefore ascertain that the group and the patient are a good match in terms of diagnosis and degree of illness, as well as ensuring the presence of appropriate group leadership in providing education, problem solving, stress management, and psychosocial support. The patient's progress and level of satisfaction should be evaluated as part of all medical follow-up appointments.

Additional unconventional approaches may also prove efficacious.

Botanical Medicine

St. John's wort for depression, kava for anxiety, and valerian for insomnia may be employed in mild to moderate cases, or if the patient has an initial preference for nondrug approaches. In view of the severity of the diagnosis, pharmacologic intervention may become warranted should such botanical measures prove inadequate or symptoms intensify.

Dosage of St. John's Wort. The dose of an extract standardized to 0.3% hypericin and 6% hyperforin is 300 mg three times daily.

Precautions. Because St. John's wort has been shown to affect the cytochrome P450 enzyme system and p-glycoproteins, drug interactions have been reported with such agents as warfarin, indinavir, and cyclosporine.[29, 30] Interactions with digoxin, selective serotonin reuptake inhibitors, oral contraceptives, and theophylline are suspected but not fully documented.[31]

Dosage of Kava. The dose of the kava root standardized to 70% kavapyrones is 100 mg three times daily for anxiety and 250 to 500 mg as a hypnotic at bedtime. The gelcap form is recommended to ensure that the product is an extract of the lipophilic portions of the root.

Dosage of Valerian. The dose of valerian root standardized to 0.8% valerenic acid is 400 to 900 mg at bedtime for sleep.

Mind-Body Techniques

Along with hypnosis and guided imagery, relaxation breathing, biofeedback, and physical practices such as yoga and tai chi may be employed to achieve states of mental and emotional relaxation.[32–35]

Social Support

The importance of continuing support from family, friends, and members of the medical team cannot be emphasized strongly enough. Animal and human studies have demonstrated the severe physical and psychological trauma suffered when such contact is insufficient for the situation at hand. Patient discernment of adequate support should be confirmed at all follow-up visits.

Spiritual Practice

Here is a topic that could fill an entire book dedicated to its definition and relevance. It may be useful to consider *spirituality* as an intermediate on the continuum between *spirit*, its source, and *religion*, its social and moral expression. One thing that is clear is the beneficial effects of spiritual practice on the alleviation of the psychological depression associated with the diagnosis of cancer.[36]

In the clinical situation it may be prudent to limit discussions to a personal conceptualization of spirituality should the patient be open to such exploration. It is equally important to respect the patient who does not wish to enter into this arena. The offer may be gently made, however. Especially when considering the specter of death so often associated with the diagnosis of cancer, the practitioner is encouraged to offer an exploration of such issues, whether in the office or through appropriate referral.[37]

RECURRENCE, METASTASES, AND SECONDARY MALIGNANCIES

The frequency of both recurrences and metastatic disease is highly dependent on tumor type and treatment protocol. Secondary malignancies are less common, their frequency varying with type of original tumor, patient age, and radiotherapy or chemotherapy regimen.[38] Among patients whose original cancer was diagnosed in childhood, the frequency of a secondary cancer is 2.6% to 12.1% at 25 years after treatment. In adults, the greatest risk occurs after treatment of Hodgkin's disease; 10% to 15% of these patients develop a secondary malignancy up to 15 years after therapy.

Management

From an integrative point of view, the approach to recurrence, metastatic disease, or secondary cancer is the same as with prevention of primary malignancy. Avoidance of environmental and chemical toxins (e.g., tobacco), nutritional support, antioxidant supplementation, and employment of immunostimulating botanicals are options to be discussed with the patient. Motivation is high, as prevention of recurrence is often foremost in the mind of a patient who has already undergone the traumatic experience of the original disease and treatment.

Nutrition

Epidemiologic studies reveal that diets high in fruits and vegetables play a significant role in staving off occurrence or recurrence of cancer.[39] Although referral to a nutritionist specializing in cancer is optimal, some general recommendations apply. Patients are encouraged to choose at least five servings of fruits and vegetables per day, selecting at least one serving of fruit that is high in vitamin C (e.g., oranges, strawberries), at least one serving of vegetables that is high in vitamin A (e.g., carrots, tomatoes), and at least one serving of vegetables that is high in indole 3-carbinol (e.g., cauliflower, broccoli). A serving of fruit is roughly equivalent to one apple or $1/2$ cup of fruit juice. A serving of vegetables is roughly equivalent to 1 cup raw or $1/2$ cup cooked vegetable.

Another dietary recommendation is drinking 4 to 5 cups of green tea per day for its antioxidant value. In addition, soy in its various forms is thought to assist in prevention of hormone-dependent tumors[40, 41]; however, women with breast cancer should avoid supplementation with isoflavones and include only small amounts of soy products in the diet.[42] Although studies yield conflicting results, there is some suggestion that soy supplementation may increase the proliferation rate of breast lobular epithelium.[43] No studies have yet demonstrated that consumption of organically grown produce, rather than conventionally grown fruits and vegetables, will decrease the incidence of cancer; nevertheless, pesticides are often known carcinogens, and patients are also encouraged to select as much produce as possible that is certified organically grown.

Antioxidants

Because few people in the United States consume the recommended amount of fresh fruits and vegetables, antioxidant supplementation is often advised. Studies supporting the benefit of individual antioxidants have been disappointing[39]; therefore, some authors recommend that antioxidants be used synergistically for optimal effectiveness.[44] For example, regeneration of tocopherols (vitamin E) requires the presence of vitamin C,[47] suggesting that the two should be taken together. The recommended doses for four key antioxidants are as follows:

Vitamin C: 250 to 1000 mg daily. At this dose range, toxicities and side effects are unlikely.

Vitamin E: 400 to 800 IU mixed tocopherols daily. Because tocopherols are fat-soluble vitamins, taking amounts in excess of 800 IU daily is not recommended.

Mixed carotenes: 25,000 IU daily. Carotenes are provitamin A compounds and will not induce the toxicities of excess vitamin A ingestion. Because beta-carotene alone has not been shown to be effective and may be a pro-oxidant under certain conditions, patients should be encouraged to look for products with mixed isomers of carotenes.

Selenium: 100 μg daily. Selenium may cause toxicity in high doses, resulting in nausea, vomiting, extreme fatigue, hair loss, nail changes, and, rarely, paresthesias. The maximum recommended supplementation dose varies from country to country (e.g., 200 μg daily in the United States and 400 μg daily in China[46]).

Other antioxidants are recommended depending on the individual clinical situation. Coenzyme Q10 in doses of up to 390 mg daily slowed the rate of breast cancer metastases in one group of patients.[21] Selenium, vitamin E, and lycopene, a specific carotenoid that is not a pro-vitamin A, may play a role in preventing disease progression in patients with prostate cancer.[47]

There is significant controversy about whether patients receiving radiation therapy or chemotherapy should receive antioxidant supplementation. The theoretical concern is that these supplements may block the oxidizing effects of therapy thought to limit proliferation of cancerous cells. Research results are mixed, and given that antioxidants may protect normal cells during radiation and chemotherapy, the practitioner and the patient must weigh unknown risk versus unknown benefit before making a decision. Antioxidant therapy appears to be a concern with chemotherapeutic agents designed to damage cellular DNA (e.g., bleomycin, cisplatin, alkylating agents).[39]

Immunostimulating Botanicals

High-molecular-weight polysaccharides derived from a variety of plant and fungal sources have been shown to have a variety of biological functions, including antitumoral and immunomodulating effects.[48] Sources with the most potent polysaccharide activity are those containing beta-1,3/1,6 glucans found in mushrooms (e.g., maitake, shiitake, reishe, zhu ling). Because dietary sources for medicinal mushrooms are not readily available outside of Asia, the patient may take either an extract of at least one of the mushrooms or several in combination.

Astragalus root is another botanical with high immunostimulating polysaccharide content. The dose for a standardized astragalus preparation (70% polysaccharides) is 200 mg daily.

NOTE

Because cytokines may promote cachexia, immunostimulating botanicals should be avoided in the cachectic patient until more information regarding safety is available.

Table 63-1. Complementary and Alternative Therapies That Have Been Used for the Treatment of Cancer
....

Single Agents

714-X	Essiac tea
Aloe vera	Govallo therapy
Antineoplastons	Green Tea
Cancell/Entelev	Hydrogen peroxide
Cartilage	Immune augmentation therapy
Cat's claw	(IAT)
Chaparral	Laetrile
Coenzyme Q10	Mistletoe (Iscador)
Coley toxins	Modified citrus pectin (MCP)
Coriolus versicolor	MTH-68
	Pau d'arco
	PC-SPES

Therapeutic Systems

Chelation therapy	Hoxsey
Electromagnetic therapy	Livingston-Wheeler therapy
Fasting and juice therapies	Ozone therapy
Gerson therapy	Revici method

ALTERNATIVE TREATMENTS FOR CANCER

Over the years a vast array of alternative treatments for cancer have been offered in the United States and elsewhere. Although studies are still in progress to evaluate the efficacy and potential side effects of these therapies, patients are already using them out of desperation for a cure. Here is an area in which practice of the *art* of medicine is essential in providing guidance, information, and eventually support for whatever choice the patient makes. Discussion of even one such treatment protocol is beyond the scope of this chapter; Table 63–1 presents a list of alternative therapeutic approaches patients may be interested in using. The reader is directed to the reference section of Harwood and Pickett's online publication[49] for further inquiry into these modalities.

THERAPEUTIC REVIEW

Following is a review of the basic therapeutic options commonly recommended to the patient with cancer.

General Recommendations: Nutrition, Supplementation, and Botanicals

Nutrition
Individual nutritional consultation, ideally with an experienced registered dietitian, is essential for all patients with cancer, regardless of specific diagnosis or stage of disease. General recommendations include choosing organically grown produce, limiting protein intake to 20% of dietary calories, and increasing vegetable protein while decreasing animal protein. Fat intake should be limited to 30% or less of the dietary calories.

Antioxidant Supplementation
Patients undergoing radiation therapy or chemotherapy should consult their oncologist before making an informed decision about supplementation. The following basic antioxidants may be found in a single high-quality multivitamin taken once daily:
- *Vitamin C: 250 to 1000 mg*
- *Vitamin E: 400 to 800 IU*
- *Mixed carotenes: 25,000 IU*
- *Selenium: 100 μg*

The choice of additional antioxidants may be tailored to specific situations, such as lycopenes for prostate cancer (see Chapter 67) or coenzyme Q10 to prevent chemotherapeutic cardiotoxicity.

Immunomodulating Supplementation
All cancer patients except those who are significantly cachectic may be offered the following immunomodulating botanicals:
- *Extracts of maitake, shiitake, reishe, or zhu ling (or a combination): follow dosing on the label*
- *Astragalus: 200 mg daily*

Symptom-Specific Recommendations
- *Nausea and vomiting*
  - Ginger: 500 mg to 1000 mg of root extract or 5 g (1 teaspoonful) of candied ginger as needed
  - Traditional Chinese medicine: referral to a qualified practitioner for acupuncture and/or herbal tonics
  - Mind-body techniques: hypnosis, guided imagery
  - Marijuana: in selected patients, carefully weighing legal and ethical risks
- *Weight loss and cachexia*
  - Nutrition: consult with registered dietitian; (see under general recommendations earlier)
  - Marijuana: in selected patients, carefully weighing the legal and ethical risks
- *Pain*
  - Mind-body techniques: hypnosis, guided imagery
  - Marijuana: in selected patients, carefully weighing the legal and ethical risks
  - Support: from family, friends, and all health care practitioners associated with the patient

THERAPEUTIC REVIEW *continued*

- *Cardiac complications*
  - Coenzyme Q10: 60 mg (gelcaps) daily
  - Vitamin E: the appropriate dose has not been established
- *Alopecia*
  - Mind-body techniques: guided imagery
  - Body and appearance perception enhancement: consultation with cosmetologists educated or trained to work with patients with cancer
- *Psychological distress and depression*
  - Botanical medicine—*St. John's wort* (mild to moderate depression): 300 mg extract standardized to 0.3% hypericin and 6% hyperforin three times daily; *Kava* (anxiety): 100 to 250 mg of a lipophilic extract standardized to 30% kavapyrones once to three times daily for daytime anxiety or 250 to 500 mg at bedtime; and *Valerian* (insomnia): 400 to 900 mg of a root extract standardized to 0.8% valerenic acid at bedtime.
  - Mind-body techniques: hypnosis, guided imagery, relaxation breathing, yoga, tai chi
  - Social support: from family friends and all health care workers involved in the patient's care

Resources for Persons with Cancer

Organization	Address/Telephone	Web Site	Notes
The Moss Report	718 636-4433	www.ralphmoss.com	Will search health information regarding cancer and alternative therapies for a fee (around $300).
Canhelp	3111 Paradise Bay Rd., Port Ludlow, WA 98365 360 437-2291	www.canhelp.com	Information on alternative therapies including interpretation of medical data.
Centerwatch	800 765-9647	www.centerwatch.com	Lists the ongoing clinical research trials for various cancer therapies.
Commonweal	P.O. Box 316, Bolinas, CA 94924 415 868-0970	www.commonweal.org	Provides retreats for people with cancer. Web site provides access to book by Michael Lerner: *Choices in Healing: Integrating the Best of Conventional and Complementary Approaches in Cancer.*[36]
National Center for Complementary and Alternative Medicine (NCCAM)	P.O. Box 8218, Silver Spring, MD 20907-8218 888 644-6226	http://nccam.nih.gov	A division of the National Institutes of Health. Provides fact sheets on complementary therapies used for cancer and reviews current research in complementary/alternative medicine and cancer therapy.
National Alliance of Breast Cancer Organizations (NABCO)	9 East 37th St., New York, NY 10016 212 889-0606	www.nabco.org	Offers contact information on breast cancer support groups throughout the United States as well as general breast cancer information.

References

1. Haskell CM: Introduction. In Haskell CM (ed): Cancer Treatment, 5th ed, Philadelphia, WB Saunders, 2001, pp 2–8.
2. Rettig M, Sawicki MP: Biology of cancer. In: Haskell CM (ed): Cancer Treatment, 5th ed. Philadelphia, WB Saunders, 2001, pp 9–29.
3. Cole WC, Prasad KN: Contrasting effects of vitamins as modulators of apoptosis in cancer cells and normal cells: A review. Nutr Cancer 29:97–103; 1997.
4. Hainsworth JD: Nausea and vomiting. In Abeloff MD, Armitage JO, Lichter AS, Niederhuber JE (eds): Clinical Oncology, 2nd ed, New York, Churchill Livingstone, 2000, pp 950–964.
5. King CR: Nonpharmacologic management of chemotherapy-induced nausea and vomiting. Oncol Nurs Forum 24:41–48, 1997.
6. Ernst E, Pittler MH: Efficacy of ginger for nausea and vomiting: A systematic review of randomized clinical trials. Br J Anaesth 84:367–371, 2000.
7. Moyad MA, Hathaway S, Ni HS: Traditional Chinese medicine, acupuncture, and other alternative medicines for prostate cancer: An introduction and the need for more research. Semin Urol Oncol 17:103–110, 1999.
8. Koh HL, Woo SO: Chinese proprietary medicine in Singapore: Regulatory control of toxic heavy metals and undeclared drugs. Drug Safety 23:351–362, 2000.
9. Steggles S, Maxwell, J, Lightfoot NE, et al: Hypnosis and cancer: An annotated bibliography 1985–1995. Am J Clin Hypn 39:187–200, 1997.
10. Troesch LM, Rodehaver CB, Delaney EA, Yanes B: The influence of guided imagery on chemotherapy-related nausea and vomiting. Oncol Nurs Forum 20:1179–1185, 1993.

11. Doblin RE, Kleiman MAR: Marijuana as antiemetic medicine: A survey of oncologists' experiences and attitudes. J Clin Oncol 9:1314–1319, 1991.
12. Renn E, Mandel S, Mandel E: The medicinal uses of marijuana. P&T; 25:536–540, 2000.
13. Taylor HG: Analysis of the medical use of marijuana and its societal implications. J Am Pharm Assoc 38: 220–227, 1998.
14. Meguid MM, Laviano A: Weight loss and cachexia. In Abeloff MD, Armitage JO, Lichter AS, Niederhuber JE (eds): Clinical Oncology, 2nd ed. New York, Churchill Livingstone, 2000, pp 579–596.
15. Grossman SA, Sheidler VR: Cancer pain. In Abeloff MD, Armitage JO, Lichter AS, Niederhuber JE (eds): Clinical Oncology, 2nd ed, New York, Churchill Livingstone, 2000, pp 539–554.
16. Joint Commission for Accreditation of Healthcare Organizations web site: *http://jcaho.org.*
17. Wisconsin Cancer Pain Initiative web site: *http://www.wisc.edu/wcpi.*
18. Kaiko RF, Foley KM, Grabinski PY, et al: Central nervous system excitatory effects of meperidine in cancer patients. Ann Neurol 13:180–185, 1983.
19. Speyer JL, Freedberg RS: Cardiac complications. In Abeloff MD, Armitage JO, Lichter AS, Niederhuber JE (eds): Clinical Oncology, 2nd ed. New York, Churchill Livingstone, 2000, pp 1047–1060.
20. Iarussi D, Auricchio U, Agretto A, et al: Protective effect of coenzyme Q10 on anthracyclines cardiotoxicity: Control study in children with acute lymphoblastic leukemia and non-Hodgkin lymphoma. Mol Aspects Med 15:S207–S212, 1994.
21. Pepping J: Coenzyme Q10. Am J Health Syst Pharm 56:519–521, 1999.
22. Weis M, Mortensen SA, Rassing MR, et al: Bioavailability of four oral coenzyme Q10 formulations in healthy volunteers. Mol Aspects Med 15:S273–S280, 1994.
23. Lenzhofer R, Ganzinger U, Rameis H, et al: Acute cardiac toxicity in patients after doxorubicin treatment and the effect of combined tocopherol and nifedipine pretreatment. J Cancer Res Clin Oncol 106:143–147, 1993.
24. Kobrinsky NL, Ramsay NK, Krivit W: Anthracycline cardiomyopathy. Pediatr Cardiol 3:265–272, 1982.
25. Legha SS, Wang YM, Mackay B, et al: Clinical and pharmacologic investigation of the effects of alpha-tocopherol on Adriamycin cardiotoxicity. Ann N Y Acad Sci 393:411–418, 1982.
26. McDonald CJ, Muglia JJ, Vittorio CC: Alopecia and cutaneous complications. In Abeloff MD, Armitage JO, Lichter AS, Niederhuber JE (eds): Clinical Oncology, 2nd ed, New York, Churchill Livingstone, 2000, pp 980–999.
27. McDaniel JS, Musselman DL, Nemeroff CB: Psychological distress and depression. In Abeloff MD, Armitage JO, Lichter AS, Niederhuber JE (eds): Clinical Oncology, 2nd ed, New York, Churchill Livingstone, 2000, pp 556–578.
28. Spiegel D, Bloom JR, Kraemer HC, Gottheil E: Effect of psychosocial treatment on survival of patients with metastatic breast cancer. Lancet 2:888–891, 1989.
29. Ruschitzka F, Meier PJ, Turina M, et al: Acute heart transplant rejection due to Saint John's wort. Lancet 355:548–549, 2000.
30. Piscitelli SC, Burstein AH, Chaitt D, et al: Indinavir concentrations and St. John's wort. Lancet 355:547–548, 2000.
31. Fugh-Berman A: Herb-drug interactions. Lancet 355:134–138, 2000.
32. Speca M, Carlson LE, Goodey E, Angen M: A randomized, wait-list controlled clinical trial: The effect of a mindfulness meditation-based stress reduction program on mood and symptoms of stress in cancer outpatients. Psychosom Med 62:613–622, 2000.
33. Walker LG, Walker MB, Ogston K, et al: Psychological, clinical and pathological effects of relaxation training and guided imagery during primary chemotherapy. Br J Cancer 80:262–268, 1999.
34. Chen KM, Snyder M: A research-based use of Tai Chi/movement therapy as a nursing intervention. J Holist Nurs 17:267–279, 1999.
35. Janakiramaiah N, Gangadhar BN, Naga Venkatesha Murthy PJ, et al: Antidepressant efficacy of Sudarshan Kriya Yoga (SKY) in melancholia: A randomized comparison with electroconvulsive therapy (ECT) and imipramine. J Affect Disord 57:255–259, 2000.
36. Lerner M: Choices in Healing: Integrating the Best of Conventional and Complementary Approaches to Cancer. Cambridge, Mass, MIT Press, 1998.
37. Hermann CP: Spiritual needs of dying patients: A qualitative study. Oncol Nurs Forum 28:67–72, 2001.
38. Green DM, D'Angio GJ: Second malignant neoplasms. In Abeloff MD, Armitage JO, Lichter AS, Niederhuber JE (eds): Clinical Oncology, 2nd ed, New York, Churchill Livingstone, 2000, pp 1082–1100.
39. Thomson CA: Antioxidants and cancer. Support Line 22:3–10, 2000.
40. Manson MM, Gescher A, Hudson EA, et al: Blocking and suppressing mechanisms of chemoprevention by dietary supplements. Toxicol Lett 112–113:499–505, 2000.
41. Kelloff GJ, Crowell JA, Steele VE, et al: Progress in cancer chemoprevention: Development of diet-derived chemopreventive agents. J Nutr 130:457S–471S, 2000.
42. Low Dog T, Riley D, Carter T: Traditional and alternative therapies for breast cancer. Altern Ther Health Med 7:36–42, 45–47, 2001.
43. McMichael-Phillips DF, Harding C, Morton M, et al: Effects of soy-protein supplementation on epithelial proliferation in the histologically normal breast. Am J Clin Nutr 68 (Suppl):1431S–1435S, 1998.
44. Prasad KN, Kumar A, Kochupillai V, Cole WC: High doses of multiple antioxidant vitamins: Essential ingredients in improving the efficacy of standard cancer therapy. J Am Coll Nutr 18:13–25, 1999.
45. Chan AC: Partners in defense, vitamin E and vitamin C. Can J Physiol Pharmacol 71:725–731, 1993.
46. Yang G, Zhou R: Further observations on the human maximum safe dietary selenium intake in a seleniferous area of China. J Trace Elem Electrolytes Health Dis 8:159–165, 1994.
47. Fleshner NE, Klotz LH: Diet, androgens, oxidative stress and prostate cancer susceptibility. Cancer Metastasis Rev 17:325–330, 1998–1999.
48. Kraus J, Franz G: Immunomodulating effects of polysaccharides from medicinal plants. Adv Exp Med Biol 319:299–308, 1992.
49. Harwood K, Pickett C: A Cancer Patient's Guide to Complementary and Alternative Medicine, 2nd ed, November 2000. Available at http://www.cancer.duke.edu/PatEd.

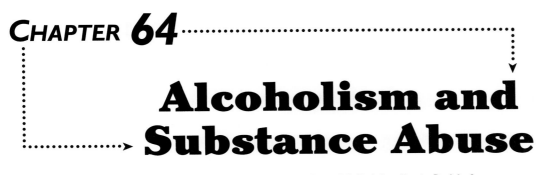

CHAPTER 64

Alcoholism and Substance Abuse

Don Warne, M.D., M.P.H., D.A.B.M.A.

The prevalence of alcoholism and substance abuse (SA) in the United States is significant. According to the 1999 National Household Survey on Drug Abuse conducted by the Substance Abuse and Mental Health Services Administration (SAMHSA), 8.2 million Americans are dependent on alcohol (3.7% of persons 12 years of age or older). In addition, there are an estimated 14.8 million users of illicit drugs in the United States. Of these, 3.6 million are considered dependent. Among youths aged 12 to 17 years, 10.9% are users of illicit drugs.[1] The management of addiction is complex owing to its behavioral, social, legal, public health, and biomedical components.

Alcoholism and SA have a negative impact on other chronic diseases managed in the primary care setting, as a result of the direct effects of the substances abused and issues related to compliance and self-care. Acute injury and illness resulting from alcohol abuse and SA are analogous with exacerbations of chronic conditions and therefore constitute issues of extreme importance in the arena of primary care. Unfortunately, many physicians do not routinely address these issues, and few conventional allopathic interventions are easily accessible and efficacious. This chapter examines the treatment options available to the primary care physician and also provides a source of information for appropriate referrals. A multitude of both illicit and prescribed substances are abused; the focus of this chapter is primarily on alcohol, tobacco, opiates, cocaine, and marijuana.

Drug or alcohol addiction should be treated as a chronic illness, not unlike diabetes mellitus or hypertension.[2] Like these disorders, addiction has behavioral components as well as underlying biochemical mechanisms. Also, within chronic addiction and recovery, there are exacerbations of abuse and relapses as well as chronic multiorgan system complications. Successful treatment of all chronic diseases requires good rapport between patient and provider, using a nonjudgmental approach.

PATHOPHYSIOLOGY

Alcoholism and SA have many dimensions, each with unique implications and standards of treatment. The processes of alcoholism and SA may be divided into broad categories including craving, active abuse, intoxication, withdrawal, detoxification, recovery, and relapse prevention.

A proposed mechanism of addiction for all substances of abuse involves the sudden release of dopamine in the "reward pathway" connecting the midbrain to the prefrontal cortex. This rush of dopamine is believed to cause a sense of euphoria and pleasure that is at the root of drug abuse. With extended drug use there is a profound alteration in brain chemistry. This change in central neurophysiology eventually causes a "switch" in the affected person from a state of drug abuse to addiction with uncontrollable cravings and dependence. The exact mechanisms of this process are as yet unknown.[3]

The process of addiction is, of course, not limited to brain chemistry. The impact of environmental, social, cultural, genetic, and behavioral factors is significant in the development of alcoholism and SA. These factors pose various degrees of importance in the development of addiction for each person. Addiction is therefore most accurately viewed as a complex illness with variable environmental and biochemical features.[4]

INTEGRATIVE APPROACH TO MANAGEMENT

Pharmaceuticals

Unfortunately, few effective pharmacologic options are available to the primary care physician to treat alcoholism and SA. Some of the most effective pharmaceutical agents are available only through licensed intensive outpatient and inpatient programs specializing in the treatment of addictions. Table 64–1 provides an overview of pharmaceutical treatments for alcoholism and SA. As noted, these treatments may be divided into broad categories of detoxification/withdrawal and craving/relapse prevention.

Management of Alcohol Withdrawal

The most common treatment for alcohol withdrawal is administration of diazepam or another benzo-

All material in this chapter is in the public domain, with the exception of any borrowed figures or tables.

Table 64–1. Pharmaceutical Agents Used for Treatment of Alcoholism and Substance Abuse

Substance	Detoxification/Withdrawal	Craving/Relapse Prevention	Other Uses
Alcohol	Benzodiazepines Phenobarbital	Naltrexone Acamprosate*	Disulfiram
Tobacco	Nicotine Bupropion	Nicotine Bupropion	
Opiates	Methadone Clonidine	Methadone LAAM Buprenorphine*	Naloxone
Cocaine	NA	TCAs SSRIs MAOIs Amantadine	
Marijuana	NA	NA	

* Not yet approved for use in the United States.

LAAM, levo-alpha-acetylmethadol; MAOI, monoamine oxidase inhibitor; NA, no accepted treatment available; SSRI, selective serotonin reuptake inhibitor; TCA, tricyclic antidepressant.

diazepine (BZ). The benefit of BZ treatment is relief of anxiety and sleep disturbances experienced during the withdrawal phase. A disadvantage of BZ therapy is the potential for producing dependence if the drug is not prescribed appropriately. BZ for detoxification should be prescribed only for a short period of time in a supervised setting. Phenobarbital or carbamazepine is occasionally used in managing withdrawal seizures. There is evidence that opioid receptors play a role in the physiologic response to alcohol. Naltrexone (ReVia), an opioid antagonist, has been shown to be effective in preventing alcoholic relapse. Acamprosate (calcium acetylhomotaurinate) is an amino acid derivative that modulates gamma-aminobutyric acid (GABA) in neurotransmission in the brain and shows potential for reducing alcohol cravings. However, it is not yet approved for use in the United States. Disulfiram (Antabuse) inhibits aldehyde dehydrogenase and produces unpleasant effects when alcohol is consumed, such as nausea, vomiting, and dizziness. Pharmacologic treatments for alcohol withdrawal generally work well and potentially can be used for outpatient withdrawal management if close follow-up is possible. Treatments for relapse prevention generally are not efficacious in the absence of comprehensive follow-up care.[5]

Dosage:
- Naltrexone (ReVia): 50 mg orally each day.
- Disulfiram (Antabuse): 250 to 500 mg daily.
- Benzodiazepine taper for withdrawal: The dosage is titrated to achieve a calming effect. High doses may be needed initially. An example is clonazepam (Klonopin), 1 mg 3 times daily with a gradual taper over 10 to 14 days.

Management of Nicotine Withdrawal: Smoking Cessation

Effective outpatient treatment regimens are avail-able for smoking cessation. Tapered nicotine replacement therapy is effective in the management of nicotine withdrawal and cravings. Bupropion (Zyban) also has been shown to be effective in managing symptoms of anxiety associated with nicotine withdrawal and craving. These medications can be used successfully in the outpatient primary care setting.[6]

Dosage. Buproprion (Zyban) 150 mg twice daily for 6 weeks, with a target quit date of 2 weeks after the start of therapy.

Management of Opiate Withdrawal

Acute opiate withdrawal is treated commonly with methadone, an opioid receptor agonist that can block withdrawal symptoms without producing the euphoria caused by heroin and other opiates. Owing to this effect, methadone is also commonly used in long-term maintenance programs for reducing cravings and risk of relapse. Clonidine has been shown to be effective in lessening opiate withdrawal symptoms and does not foster physiologic dependence. Levo-alpha-acetylmethadol (LAAM) is derived from methadone and acts in a fashion similar to that noted for methadone. The advantage of LAAM in maintenance therapy is that its effect lasts 72 hours, allowing for dosing every other day or 3 times per week. Buprenorphine is an opiate receptor partial agonist and is a promising agent for maintenance treatment, but approval for use in the United States is pending. Treatments for opiate dependence are used in the inpatient setting or in maintenance programs and are not available in the primary care setting, although administration of buprenorphine has the potential to become a primary care intervention for opiate addiction maintenance treatment. Naloxone is an opiate antagonist and is used for treating acute opiate overdose.[7]

Management of Cocaine Dependence

Cocaine withdrawal is associated with minimal symptoms. Several classes of pharmaceutical agents have been studied for their efficacy in treating cocaine dependence and relapse prevention, although none of these are approved by the Food and Drug Administration (FDA) for this purpose. Extensive abuse of cocaine can cause depression by depleting baseline levels of dopamine. Several antidepressants have been studied for their role in treating cocaine addiction including tricyclic antidepressants, selective serotonin reuptake inhibitors (SSRIs), and monoamine oxidase inhibitors; however, results are mixed and inconclusive. Amantadine, a dopamine agonist, has been studied for its role in cocaine dependence. In theory, dopamine agonist therapy should cause dopamine restoration and reduce the need for cocaine, but studies have not been convincing.[8]

In conclusion, with the exception of tobacco abuse, there are few effective pharmaceutical options available to the primary care provider for the treatment of alcoholism and SA. In the case of marijuana dependence, no accepted treatments are available.

Botanicals

Various herbs and combinations of herbs are reported to be effective in reducing cravings, but in general, no studies have been conducted to prove their effectiveness.

Kudzu

Kudzu, a traditional Chinese herb, has been used as an "anti-inebriation" treatment for hundreds of years. Its mechanism of action is not yet known.[9, 10]

Herbal Antidepressants/Anxiolytics

Because people who struggle with alcoholism and SA commonly have coexisting depression and anxiety, it is possible that herbal remedies used for these conditions may have a role in recovery and abstinence. Herbs such as *valerian* and *kava kava* that are effective in treating anxiety and insomnia might be helpful in managing anxiety associated with detoxification and cravings. Both of these herbs have been shown to enhance the levels and action of GABA, and therefore may also have a role in alcohol craving control and relapse prevention. These potential uses warrant further investigation. *St. John's wort* has a mechanism of action similar to that of SSRIs and has been shown to be effective in treating depression.[11] Its role in managing depression associated with alcoholism and SA has yet to be determined.

Other Herbal Remedies

Lobelia is described as a "respiratory stimulant" and has been used in homeopathic preparations as an aid to stop smoking. *Milk thistle (Silybum marianum)* has been studied for its hepatoprotective effects and appears to be a promising treatment for alcoholic cirrhosis.[12]

Acupuncture

Acupuncture is perhaps the most extensively studied and most promising integrative treatment for addictions. The practice of acupuncture was documented in Chinese literature as early as the Han dynasty in the second century BC, in the *Huang Di Nei Jing* ("Yellow Emperor's Classic of Medicine"). In acupuncture terms, the body is seen as having several energy channels, or meridians, that allow for the free flow of *qi* (pronounced "chee"), or energy. In a healthy or balanced state, qi flows smoothly throughout the body and provides for homeostasis. With disease, injury, or a state of imbalance, the normal movement of qi is obstructed or impaired. Acupuncture treatments are designed to unblock obstructions of meridians and to promote the healthy flow of energy.[13]

In 1973, Wen reported that opiate-addicted patients who were using electroacupuncture to treat postsurgical pain described relief from symptoms of withdrawal.[14] Omura brought the treatment protocol to Lincoln Hospital in New York in 1974, and Smith developed a five-point auricular acupuncture treatment protocol for addictions that is currently being taught and advocated by the National Acupuncture Detoxification Association (NADA).[15]

In acupuncture terms, SA can be seen as an attempt by the patient to self-treat an imbalance in the flow of qi. The "drug of choice" provides a temporary relief from energy imbalance, but unfortunately it also commonly causes further underlying imbalance. As a result, the baseline imbalance slowly worsens, and the need for more drugs slowly increases. The acupuncture treatment therefore provides energy balancing without the need for alcohol or drugs, and it provides relaxation and relief from cravings.[16]

NOTE

Acupuncture treatments influence the flow of qi to achieve energy balancing, relaxation, and reduction in cravings for alcohol, tobacco, and illicit drugs.

Another proposed mechanism of action is that the acupuncture needles stimulate peripheral nerves to cause release of endorphins in the brain, thereby causing relaxation and a sense of well-being; acupuncture thus can provide direct biochemical treatment of opiate and ethanol craving and withdrawal.[17] The NADA treatment protocol and certification course emphasizes the multifaceted nature of this modality and describes treatment benefits in the biochemical, psychological, and social realms as well as in the traditional Chinese paradigm.

The specific points used in the NADA protocol are *Shen Men* (spirit gate), *Sympathetic, Kidney, Liver,* and *Lung* (Fig. 64–1). These points have roles in balancing energy and calming as well as in regulating sympathetic nervous system function and specific organ function from the modern and traditional Chinese perspectives of physiology. The kidney, liver, and lung each have specific roles in the generation, regulation, and flow of qi. These organ-specific functions are described in acupuncture textbooks[18] and are beyond the scope of this chapter.

Auricular acupuncture has been studied in the treatment of addiction to various drugs including alcohol, cocaine, opiates, and marijuana. In 1989, Bullock reported that auricular acupuncture was effective in the treatment of recidivist alcoholics. In this study, eighty recidivist alcoholics who were enrolled in a treatment facility were randomized to receive either the appropriate treatment protocol (treatment group) or sham acupuncture at sites close to the appropriate points (control group). The outcomes measured included completion of the treatment program and self-reported abstinence at 1, 3, and 6 months following the treatment program. Of the 40 patients in the treatment group, 21 finished the program, whereas only 1 of 40 in the control group completed treatment. Information regarding self-reported drinking episodes was collected from all available subjects, including those who did not complete treatment. Fewer treatment group patients than control group patients reported drinking episodes at 1-, 3-, and 6-month follow-up evaluations.[19]

In 1998, Shwartz compared residential detoxification programs that used acupuncture with programs that did not.[20] In this retrospective study, 6907 patients completed non-acupuncture programs, and 1104 patients completed programs that used acupuncture as an adjunctive therapy. The study subjects were dependent on alcohol, cocaine, crack, heroin, or marijuana, or on a combination of these drugs. The primary outcome measured was readmission to a detoxification program in the 6 months following discharge. After the study was controlled for baseline differences in patients, those who completed programs offering acupuncture were readmitted to detoxification less frequently than were those from conventional programs.[20] A recent randomized controlled trial of auricular acupuncture for cocaine dependence studied 82 patients who were randomized to receive either appropriate acupuncture treatment, sham acupuncture, or relaxation therapy. Thrice-weekly urine screening for cocaine was conducted over an eight-week period. The patients who received the appropriate acupuncture protocol were less likely to test positive for cocaine on urine screening than were patients in the sham acupuncture control group or the relaxation control group.[21]

Auricular acupuncture has been shown by these studies to be a useful adjunct in treating alcoholism and SA. Further investigation in this area is warranted.

Mind-Body Therapies

As more is learned about the connection between thoughts and physiology, the field of mind-body medicine continues to grow and gain acceptance. Several commonly used therapies are classified as mind-body interventions, including meditation, biofeedback, hypnosis, guided imagery, yoga, and prayer. Research in this field appears promising for the effectiveness of mind-body medicine as an adjunctive intervention for alcoholism and SA.

NOTE

Mind-body therapies, including meditation, biofeedback, hypnosis, guided imagery, yoga, and prayer, use the power of the mind to influence the body. Relaxation and reduced physiologic responses to stress are helpful in the recovery process.

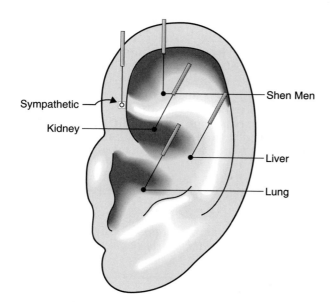

Figure 64–1. Acupuncture points for the National Acupuncture Detoxification Association (NADA) treatment protocol. (Courtesy of Joseph Helms, M.D., and Medical Acupuncture Publishers, Berkeley, Calif.)

Sympathetic
Kidney
Shen Men
Liver
Lung

Meditation

Meditation can be divided into three broad categories: concentrative, mindfulness, and transcendental. *Concentrative meditation* focuses attention on breathing, imagery, or sounds, and *mindfulness meditation* involves focused awareness on the passage of thoughts and images as they spontaneously appear. *Transcendental Meditation* (TM) is a technique brought to the United States by Maharishi Mahesh Yogi in the 1960s. TM was developed from the ancient East Indian Vedic belief system and helps practitioners of this technique to balance the physical, mental, emotional, and spiritual components of health.[22] Within this belief system, prolonged or excessive stress leads to holistic imbalance, which causes illness, including alcoholism and SA. The sense of balancing offered by TM allows for optimal function and decreases the need for drugs and alcohol.[23] Several studies and review articles have shown TM to be effective in the treatment of alcoholism and SA; however, most of these studies had flaws in design and methods without randomization, blinding, and appropriate control groups.[24] A randomized controlled trial indicated improvement in days of alcohol abstinence with the use of TM or biofeedback as compared with electronic neurotherapy and the Alcoholics Anonymous program or counseling.[25] TM has been shown to significantly increase serotonin levels and to decrease cortisol levels in as little as four months of practice.[26] This is a possible mechanism for improving the sense of balance and well-being and for reducing the effects of stress (see Chapter 94, Learning to Meditate). It should be noted, however, that there has been criticism of Maharishi Mahesh Yogi and the use of TM.[27]

Biofeedback

Biofeedback is a technique that uses electronic monitors, including those based on electroencephalography, electromyography, and electrocardiography, and also cutaneous thermometers and pulse oximeters to teach the patient how to consciously control measures of physiologic function such as respiratory rate, heart rate, skin temperature, and blood pressure. Conscious regulation of these functions is achieved through concentration, meditation, and the use of relaxation techniques. Biofeedback has been shown to be useful in managing stress-related disorders including hypertension, irritable bowel syndrome, pain, and substance abuse. Electromyographic biofeedback, which focuses on relieving muscle tension, has been shown to be an effective tool in treating alcoholism.[25] Unfortunately, there are limited studies on use of this intervention for treating addictions. The mechanism of action and the efficacy of biofeedback in managing alcoholism and substance abuse have not yet been determined.

Hypnosis

The German physician Franz Anton Mesmer introduced modern hypnotherapy in the eighteenth century as "mesmerism." The American Medical Association recognized hypnosis as a legitimate medical therapy in 1958, and it has been applied by various healthcare practitioners in the treatment of numerous disorders including alcoholism and SA. Hypnotherapy involves concentration, mental focusing exercises, relaxation techniques, guided imagery, and suggestion. Studies have shown that hypnosis improves memory and cognitive function[28] and can affect physiologic function by decreasing sympathetic nervous system activity, heart rate, blood pressure, and oxygen consumption.[29] Many techniques are utilized in hypnotherapy, making standardization difficult for research purposes; however, there are case reports of positive results in SA treatment and relapse prevention.[30] Controlled trials have not shown long-term benefits in the management of addictions. Some techniques used in hypnosis may be useful as adjunctive modalities in comprehensive recovery programs.

Guided Imagery

Guided imagery uses the power of the mind to directly affect physiologic function. Practitioners of this technique report improved insight into emotional and physical health. Imagery can modulate heart rate, blood pressure, oxygen consumption, and various other physiologic measures. Deeper insight into emotions, behaviors, and thoughts can assist patients to deal with the anxiety and depression associated with the recovery process.[31] (See Chapter 92, Guided Imagery and Interactive Guided Imagery.)

Yoga

Yoga is a traditional East Indian healing system that combines specific postures, breathing control, and meditation in order to reduce stress and to promote balance and a sense of well-being. Yoga, meaning "union," attempts to help its practitioners address and equilibrate the physical, mental, and spiritual forces that coalesce in the process of disease or disharmony. Yoga has been shown to have a beneficial effect on stress-related conditions including chronic pain and hypertension and in recovery from addiction.[32] There are, however, no randomized controlled trials specifically assessing the efficacy of yoga for management of addictions. The use of this technique may be beneficial as part of a comprehensive treatment program.

Spirituality

The role of spirituality in medicine and recovery has been steadily gaining acceptance by mainstream healthcare practitioners. Numerous studies on the role of spirituality in the recovery process from addiction have been conducted. Defining spirituality and religion and identifying interventions that exist within these realms are difficult. *Spirituality* is a subjective concept and can be considered to represent a person's connection with and relationship to a transcendent or higher power.[33] *Religion* can be defined in terms of a structured value and belief system with its own hierarchy, rituals, and practices.[34]

Commonly described practices in spirituality include prayer and meditation. The field of mind-body medicine often includes prayer with meditation as a synergistic tool to promote wellness and healing. Spirituality is addressed separately here because it transcends mind-body interventions and is not easily defined by objective markers. The role of spirituality—and, to some extent, religion—in the recovery process cannot be ignored. The regular practice of prayer and meditation is strongly correlated with recovery and abstinence from drugs of abuse.[35] Active participation in spiritual practices such as prayer appears to be more important in the recovery process than being prayed for by others.[36]

"Negative spirituality" may be at the root of addictions, and a "spiritual awakening" may be required before an affected person can genuinely recover from addiction.[37] Regular church attendance has been associated with negative perceptions of addiction and lower rates of alcoholism toward SA,[38] and tobacco use.[39] The extent of family religious practice also has an impact on youth attitudes toward SA.[40] Obviously, spirituality cannot be prescribed in the primary care setting, but it is important for the clinician to be aware of the patient's spiritual beliefs and value systems when identifying appropriate recovery programs for referral.

Twelve-Step Programs

Alcoholics Anonymous (AA) has helped millions of people in their approach to recovery from alcohol-ism worldwide since it began in 1935. The AA program of recovery is spiritually based, with frequent meetings, mentoring, and social support. The basic spiritual framework is described in the Twelve Steps of AA, presented in Table 64–2.

It should be emphasized that AA is rooted in spirituality and not in religion. The AA preamble, commonly recited at the start of meetings, states: "AA is not allied with any sect, denomination, politics, organization or institution." The belief in a "higher power" is seen as a point of connection for all AA members, no matter what each person calls his or her higher power. This generalized belief allows for a group/mutual connection to a transcendent power than can help in the healing and recovery process without the need for all members to share a common belief system or religion.

Meetings generally begin with reading the AA preamble and end with reading the "serenity prayer." Meetings may be open, in which anyone may attend, or closed, where only alcoholics may attend. There are AA meetings that serve specific populations including racial or ethnic groups, gays/lesbians, or specific professions, including doctors, nurses, or other healthcare providers. There are approximately 100,000 AA groups in nearly 150 countries that serve millions of members.

Several concepts used in AA add to the success of the program, including sponsorship, anniversaries, and social support. A new member of AA is mentored by another member, a sponsor, who is usually of the same gender and has been active in AA for a minimum of 1 year. New members are encouraged to contact their sponsors when they are considering drinking or are having difficulties with sobriety. This system of social support and mentoring has been shown to be beneficial both to the new member and to the sponsor. Cross showed that 91% of sponsors maintained their abstinence from alcohol after 10 years.[41]

Anniversaries of sobriety are emphasized in the AA model. Special events or parties are scheduled to

Table 64–2. The Twelve Steps of Alcoholics Anonymous

We:
1. Admitted we were powerless over alcohol; that our lives had become unmanageable;
2. Came to believe that a Power greater than ourselves could restore us to sanity;
3. Made a decision to turn our will and our lives over to the care of God as we understood Him;
4. Made a searching and fearless moral inventory of ourselves;
5. Admitted to God, to ourselves and to another human being the exact nature of our wrongs;
6. Were entirely ready to have God remove all these defects of character;
7. Humbly asked Him to remove our shortcomings;
8. Made a list of all persons we had harmed, and became willing to make amends to them all;
9. Made direct amends to such people wherever possible, except when to do so would injure them or others;
10. Continued to take personal inventory and, when we were wrong, promptly admitted it;
11. Sought through prayer and meditation to improve our conscious contact with God as we understood Him, praying only for knowledge of His will for us and the power to carry that out; and
12. Having had a spiritual awakening [experience] as the result of these steps, we tried to carry this message to alcoholics, and to practice these principles in all our affairs.

Reprinted with permission of Alcoholics Anonymous World Service, Inc. (AAWS). Permission to reprint this material does not mean that AAWS has reviewed or approved the content of this publication, or that AAWS agrees with the views expressed herein. AA is a program of recovery from alcoholism *only*—use of this material in connection with programs and activities which are patterned after AA, but which address other problems, or in any other non-AA context, does not imply otherwise.

coincide with the AA member's anniversary of sobriety. The arrangement encourages members to meet goals of prolonged abstinence as well as providing another avenue of social support. The social nature of these events also allows members to have fun and to make strong connections with others in the group without consuming alcohol. Primary care physicians should be aware of the AA groups in their geographic area, and they should know their patients' sobriety anniversaries in order to be supportive and acknowledge their accomplishments in the recovery process.

Several other twelve-step programs use models similar to that of AA, including Narcotics Anonymous (NA), Cocaine Anonymous, and Al-Anon. Family support groups like Al-Anon are available to family members and friends of alcoholics and substance abusers, with the understanding that people who are close to the addicted person are also deeply affected by substance abuse–related behaviors.

Traditional Native American Interventions

Native American Indians have the highest alcohol-related death rates and the highest prevalence of illicit drug use reported for any racial or ethnic group in the United States. According to Indian Health Service (IHS) data, the total age-adjusted alcohol-related death rate among Native Americans is 627% greater than that of the U.S. all-races population.[42] SAMHSA reports that 10.6% of Native Americans are illicit drug users. Although alcoholism and SA are common in many Native American communities, it must be remembered that there are significant differences between tribes from different regions, and that not all tribes are significantly affected by addiction.

Native American people have experienced an immense history of injustice over the last several hundred years. The theft of land, language, culture, and spirituality has created a sense of despair that continues today in many Native American communities. A detailed account of historical events is beyond the scope of this chapter, but it is important to recognize the relatively recent dramatic cultural changes that have occurred. I was fortunate to grow up in a family with many traditional healers and spiritual leaders of the Lakota tribe, and I incorporate this traditional philosophy into my medical practice.

The impact of the loss of land and culture on people of Native American heritage is recognized by many current traditional leaders. This sense of loss and mourning is at the root of why Native Americans experience high rates of depression, alcoholism, SA, and other chronic diseases. Ed McGaa, Eagle Man, states: "Native American Indians learned how to live with the earth on a deeply spiritual plane."[43] The loss of land resulted in a loss of spiritual tradition. The book by Arbogast and coauthors delineates the loss faced by many Nature Americans: "We need to understand that the primary reason our people are so afflicted with addiction, poverty, abuse and strife, is that our way of life was taken from us. Everything was taken. And nothing was replaced."[44] From a traditional perspective, not unlike that previously described for acupuncture and mind-body medicine, the use of alcohol and illicit drugs fills the void created by the loss of spirituality.

The *medicine wheel* is a symbol that has been used by numerous tribes to represent wholeness and balance. In order to be healthy, each person needs to achieve a balance between spiritual, mental, physical, and emotional forces (Fig. 64–2). This image provides a visual format for depicting the connection between spirituality and mental, physical, and emotional health. Another interpretation of the medicine wheel shows values, decisions, actions, and reactions as representing the spiritual, mental, physical, and emotional realms, respectively. From a spiritual perspective, in this interpretation, personal values (spiritual) are interpreted into decisions (mental). These decisions are then implemented into actions (physical), and the actions produce reactions (emotional). The emotions then provide feedback to the value system (spiritual). In this way, all decisions, actions, reactions, and emotions are rooted in the spiritual realm (Fig. 64–3).[45]

When the spiritual realm is weakened or broken, negative emotions such as depression, anger, and low self-esteem have no spiritual basis or value system in which to be processed. As a result, these negative emotions affect decision making and actions. For many American Indian people, the sense of a "broken spirit" and emotional despair is the reason why they experience high rates of alcoholism and SA (Fig. 64–4).

Within this model, healthcare practitioners can see the importance of addressing the concept of spiritual healing and promoting balance in treating addictions. Clearly, simple allopathic pharmacologic interventions are not enough to address addiction in

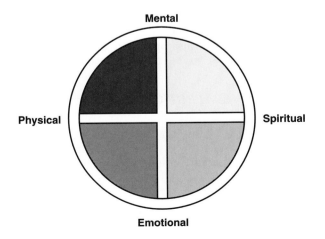

Figure 64–2. Traditional Lakota Indian medicine wheel.

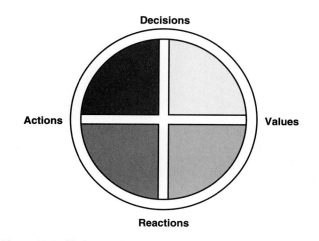

Figure 64–3. Medicine wheel showing spiritual values in decision making.

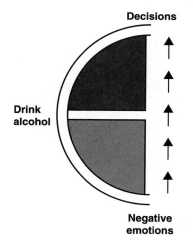

Figure 64–4. The "broken spirit" factor in alcoholism and substance abuse.

prayers in a culturally relevant and sacred manner. Anecdotally, most of my patients who participate in these healing rituals in the treatment of any chronic condition, including alcoholism and SA, find the traditional interventions to promote a sense of balance and wellness more effectively than anything offered by modern allopathic medicine.

Other Therapies to Consider

Nutrition

There may be a connection between nutritional deficiencies and addiction. Alcoholism is known to cause nutritional deficiencies, but it is not clear whether nutritional disorders lead to addiction. Preliminary studies of nutritional supplements appear promising in maintaining sobriety, reducing depression, and minimizing cravings.[46] Amino acid supplementation may be an effective adjunct in treating alcohol and cocaine addiction.

Homeopathy

Homeopathic remedies have been reported to be helpful in managing addictions, anxiety, and depression. The nature of homeopathy is such that the treatment regimen is formulated to address the individual patient's specific characteristics and complaints. Therefore, there is no specific "anti-addiction" homeopathic remedy. A skilled homeopathic physician may be able to prescribe remedies for specific patients that can aid in the recovery process.

this setting. Comprehensive programs that incorporate traditional cultural perspectives and philosophy with AA and other treatment methods are the most successful in treating SA in Native Americans.

Healing ceremonies such as the *sweat lodge* and *talking circle* are commonly used in Native American treatment programs. The *sweat lodge* is a traditional gathering for prayer, meditation, and purification. The *talking circle* is analogous to a support group, in which people share thoughts, emotions, and

---

NOTE

The most successful programs for treating addiction and promoting recovery utilize an integrative approach. Comprehensive programs address alcoholism and substance abuse in the spiritual, mental, physical, and emotional realms. Primary care practitioners need to be aware of the programs available in their geographic areas.

THERAPEUTIC REVIEW

The following is a summary of therapeutic options for alcoholism and SA. If a patient presents with a history and symptoms consistent with alcohol or SA withdrawal, immediate referral to a detoxification center is warranted.

Pharmaceutical Agents
- Alcohol: Benzodiazepines are commonly used for detoxification and withdrawal symptoms, and naltrexone has been effective in preventing relapse. Disulfiram promotes avoidance by producing unpleasant symptoms with alcohol consumption.

THERAPEUTIC REVIEW continued

- Tobacco: Tapered nicotine replacement and bupropion are effective in managing symptoms of withdrawal and cravings.
- Opiates: Methadone is the most commonly used pharmaceutical agent in relapse prevention and management of cravings.
- Cocaine: Antidepressant agents and amantadine have been used to decrease cravings and to prevent relapse with varying success.

Botanicals

- Valerian and kava kava are used for anxiety and insomnia and may be helpful in managing these symptoms in the recovery process. St. John's wort is used for depression, but its role in alcohol and SA recovery is yet to be determined.
- Kudzu is a traditional Chinese herb that has been used in alcohol recovery, but its efficacy and mechanism of action are not yet known.

Acupuncture

- Acupuncture is effective in producing relaxation and minimizing cravings for most substances of abuse.
- Treatment protocols typically involve five needles placed in each ear several times a week and are most effective as part of a comprehensive treatment program.
- Not all treatment facilities offer acupuncture, and referring physicians should be aware of treatment options available in their geographic area.

Mind-Body Therapies

- These therapies include meditation, biofeedback, hypnosis, guided imagery, yoga, and prayer. All of these interventions have been shown to be effective adjunctive therapies in treatment programs, but most of the studies conducted on these therapies have not been well controlled.

Spirituality

- Numerous studies have shown a benefit in the recovery process in persons who have a strong spiritual connection or actively participate in various religious practices. There is no correlation between any specific religion or belief system and recovery; the important factor appears to be any spiritual connection or practice.

Twelve-Step Programs

- Alcoholics Anonymous has proved to be successful in the alcoholism recovery process. The Twelve Steps are rooted in spirituality and social support.
- Other programs such as Narcotics Anonymous, Cocaine Anonymous, and Al-Anon use similar principles and focus on other substances of abuse and their effects on the abuser's family.
- Primary care physicians should be aware of the programs available in their geographic area.

Culturally Specific Interventions

- Various cultural and ethnic groups have been affected by alcoholism and SA to different degrees. In many cultures, including Native American cultures, cultural-specific interventions and practices can aid in the recovery process.
- Physicians should be aware of the patient's cultural background and belief system when making referrals to treatment facilities.

Further Resources

For more information regarding integrative approaches to treating alcoholism and substance abuse, the following agencies can be contacted:

National Acupuncture Detoxification Association (NADA)
P.O. Box 1927
Vancouver, WA 98668–1927

Alcoholics Anonymous World Services
475 Riverside Dr.
New York, NY 10115

National Institute on Alcohol Abuse and Alcoholism (NIAAA)
Office of Scientific Affairs
Willco Building
6000 Executive Blvd., Suite 409
Bethesda, MD 20892–7003

National Institute on Drug Abuse (NIDA)
6001 Executive Blvd., Room 5213
Bethesda, MD 20892

American Society of Addiction Medicine (ASAM)
4601 North Park Ave.
Suite 101, Upper Arcade
Chevy Chase, MD 20815

National Council on Alcoholism and Drug Dependence (NCCADD)
12 West 21st St.
New York, NY 10010

References

1. Substance Abuse and Mental Health Services Administration. Available at http://www.samhsa.gov
2. McLellan AT, Lewis DC, O'Brien CP, Kleber HD: Drug dependence, a chronic medical illness: Implications for treatment, insurance, and outcomes evaluation. JAMA 284:1689–1695, 2000.
3. Leshner AI: Drug abuse and addiction are biomedical problems. Hosp Pract Spec Rep April:2–4, 1997.
4. Barbutt JC, West SL, Carey TS, et al: Pharmacological treatment of alcohol dependence: A review of the evidence. JAMA 281:1318–1325, 1999.
5. Leshner AI, Adler MW, Barthwell AG, et al: Principles of Drug Addiction Treatment: A Research Based Guide. NIH Publication No. 99–4180. Bethesda, Md, 1999.
6. Wongwiwatthananukit S, Jack HM, Popovich NG: Smoking cessation: Part 2–pharmacologic approaches. J Am Pharmaceut Assn 38:339–353, 1998.
7. Stine SM, Meandzija B, Kosten TR: Pharmacologic therapies for opioid addiction. In Graham AW, Schultz TK (eds): Principles of Addiction Medicine, 2nd ed. Chevy Chase, Md, American Society of Addiction Medicine, 1998, pp 545–555.
8. Gorelick DA: Pharmacologic therapies for cocaine and other stimulant addiction. In Graham AW, Schultz TK (eds): Principles of Addiction Medicine, 2nd ed. Chevy Chase, Md, American Society of Addiction Medicine, 1998, pp 531–544.
9. Xie CI, Lin RC, Antony V, et al: Daidzin, an antioxidant isoflavonoid, decreases blood alcohol levels and shortens sleep time induced by ethanol intoxication. Alcohol Clin Exp Res 18:1443–1447, 1994.
10. Keung WM, Vallee BL: Daidzin and daidzein suppress freechoice ethanol intake by Syrian golden hamsters. Proc Natl Acad Sci 90:10008–10012, 1993.
11. Gruenwald J, Brendler T, Jaenicke C, et al: Physicians' Desk Reference for Herbal Medicines. Montvale, NJ, Medical Economics, 2000.
12. Aesoph L: Addictions. In Strohecker J, Trivieri L, Lewis D, et al (eds): Alternative Medicine: The Definitive Guide. Fife, Wash, Future Medicine Publishing, 1995, pp 485–493.
13. Helms JM: An overview of medical acupuncture. Altern Ther 4:35–45, 1998.
14. Wen JL, Cheung SYC: Treatment of drug addiction by acupuncture and electrical stimulation. Asian J Med 9:138–141, 1973.
15. Smith MO, Khan I: An acupuncture programme for the treatment of drug-addicted persons. Bull Narcot 40:35–41, 1988.
16. Auricular acupuncture for addiction treatment. In NADA Acupuncture Detoxification Specialist Trainee Manual. Vancouver, Wash, National Acupuncture Detoxification Association, 2000.
17. McLellan AT, Grossman DS, Blaine JD, Haverkos HW: Acupuncture treatment for drug abuse: A technical review. J Subst Abuse Treat 10:569–576, 1993.
18. Helms JM: Acupuncture Energetics: A Clinical Approach for Physicians. Berkeley, Calif, Medical Acupuncture Publishers, 1995.
19. Bullock ML, Culliton PD, Olander RT: Controlled trial of acupuncture for severe recidivist alcoholism. Lancet 1:1435–1439, 1989.
20. Shwartz M, Saitz R, Mulvey K, Brannigan P: The value of acupuncture detoxification programs in a substance abuse treatment system. J Subs Abuse Treat 17:305–312, 1998.
21. Avants SK, Margolin A, Holford TR, Kosten TR: A randomized controlled trial of auricular acupuncture for cocaine dependence. Arch Intern Med 160:2305–2312, 2000.
22. Shapiro D: Meditation. In Strohecker J, Trivieri L, Lewis D, et al (eds): Alternative Medicine: The Definitive Guide, Fife, Wash, Future Medicine Publishing, 1995, pp 339–345.
23. Walton KG, Levitsky D: A neuroendocrine mechanism for the reduction of drug use and addiction by Transcendental Meditation. In O'Connell DF and Alexander CN (eds): Self Recovery: Treating Addictions Using Transcendental Meditation and Maharishi Ayur-Veda. New York, Harrington Park Press, 1995.
24. Gelderloos P, Walton KG, Orme-Johnson DW, Alexander CN: Effectiveness of the Transcendental Meditation program in preventing and treating substance misuse: A review. Int J Addict 26:293–325, 1991.
25. Taub E, Steiner SS, Weingarten E, Walton KG: Effectiveness of broad spectrum approaches to relapse prevention in severe alcoholism: A long-term, randomized, controlled trial of Transcendental Meditation, EMG biofeedback and electronic neurotherapy. Alcohol Treat Q 11:187–220, 1994.
26. O'Connell DF, Alexander CN: Introduction: Recovery from addictions using Transcendental Meditation and Maharishi Ayur-Veda. In O'Connell DF, Alexander CN (eds): Self Recovery: Treating Addictions Using Transcendental Meditation and Maharishi Ayur-Veda. New York, Harrington Park Press, 1995.
27. Alexander CN, Chopra D, Singer MT, et al: Closing the chapter on Maharishi Ayur-Veda [letter]. JAMA 267:1337–1340, 1992.
28. Katz N: Hypnosis and the addictions: A critical review. Addict Behav 5:41–47, 1980.
29. Spiegel D, Bloom JR, Kraemer HC, Gottheil E: Effect of psychosocial treatment on survival of patients with metastatic breast cancer. Lancet 2:888–891, 1989.
30. Page R, Handley G: The use of hypnosis in cocaine addiction. Am J Clin Hypn 36:120–123, 1993.
31. Rossman ML: Guided imagery. In Strohecker J, Trivieri L, Lewis D, et al (eds): Alternative Medicine: The Definitive Guide. Fife, Wash, Future Medicine Publishing, 1995, pp 244–252.
32. Ballentine R, Munro R, Schatz MP: Yoga. In Strohecker J, Trivieri L, Lewis D, et al (eds): Alternative Medicine: The Definitive Guide. Fife, Wash, Future Medicine Publishing, 1995, pp 469–481.
33. Peterson EA, Nelson K: How to meet your client's spiritual needs. J Psychol Nurs 25:34–39, 1987.
34. Kurtz E, Ketcham K: The Spirituality of Imperfection: Modern Wisdom from Classic Stories. New York, Bantam Books, 1992.
35. Johnsen E: The role of spirituality in recovery from chemical dependency. J Addict Offend Couns 13:58–61, 1993.
36. Walker SR, Tonigan JS, Miller WR, et al: Intercessory prayer in the treatment of alcohol abuse and dependence: A pilot investigation. Altern Ther 3:79–86, 1997.
37. Warfield, RD, Goldstein MB. Spirituality: The key to recovery from alcoholism. Couns Values 40:196–205, 1996.
38. Miller WR: Researching the spiritual dimensions of alcohol and other drug problems. Addiction 93:979–990, 1998.
39. Spangler JG, Bell RA, Knick S, et al: Church-related correlates of tobacco use among Lumbee Indians in North Carolina. Ethn Dis 8:73–80, 1998.
40. Hardesty PH, Kirby KM. Relation between family religiousness and drug use within adolescent peer groups. J of Social Behavior and Personality 10:421–430, 1995.
41. Cross GM, Morgan CW, Mooney AJ, et al: Alcoholism treatment: A ten-year follow-up study. Alcohol Clin Exp Res 14:169–173, 1990.
42. Regional Differences in Indian Health 1998–99. Available at Indian Health Service web site: www.ihs.gov
43. McGaa EEM: Mother Earth Spirituality: Native American Paths to Healing Ourselves and Our World. San Francisco, Harper & Row, 1989.
44. Arbogast D, Two Dogs R, et al: Wounded Warriors: A Time for Healing. Omaha, Little Turtle Publications, 1995.
45. Warne DK: Traditional Healing and the Medicine Wheel. Educational Videotape. Western Washington University Productions, 2000.
46. Biery JR, Williford JH, McMullen EA: Alcohol craving in rehabilitation: Assessment of nutrition therapy. J Am Dietet Assn 91:463–466, 1991.

PART III

Disease Prevention

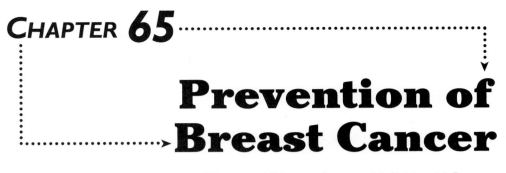

CHAPTER 65

Prevention of Breast Cancer

Bhaswati Bhattacharya, M.P.H., M.D.

EPIDEMIOLOGY

Because breast cancer is one of the leading causes of preventable mortality in the United States, it has been studied extensively. There are 180,000 new cases of breast cancer in the United States each year, and the annual mortality rate is about 30 per 100,000 women. Breast cancer accounts for approximately one third of all newly diagnosed cancers, making it the most common cancer diagnosed in women and still the leading cause of cancer death in women in most developed countries. Neoplasms of the breast can arise in the tissue composing the lobules of the breast, in the glandular or ductal tissue, or in the cells lining the ducts and channels that deliver milk. Accordingly, these neoplasms are referred to as lobular carcinoma, ductal carcinoma, or ductal carcinoma in situ and lobular carcinoma in situ, respectively. Breast cancer is considered more and more preventable as knowledge about risk factors and screening methods accumulates.

ETIOLOGY

The causes of breast cancer have been actively studied but remain unknown and are understood to be associated with certain risk factors. The commonly acknowledged risk factors are a history of previous breast cancer, a family history of breast cancer in a first-degree relative, long-term exposure to estrogen through either early menarche or late menopause or lack of childbirth to interrupt the estrogen cycle, age, high socioeconomic status within developed countries, and living in modernized societies.[1]

More recently, genetic studies have indicated that women carrying the *BRCA1* (chromosome 17), *BRCA2* (chromosome 13), and other genes such as the p53 tumor suppressor genes have an increased chance of developing early breast cancer. This association is based on the conclusion that 10% to 15% of all women with breast cancer have a genetic predisposition.

African American women have a lower incidence rate of breast cancer than that noted in European American women but have a twofold excess mortal-ity rate. The higher mortality has been postulated to be the result of differential exposure to toxic agents, socioeconomic factors, differences in access to mammography and to healthcare in general, and adiposity.

Prolonged exposure to organochlorine pesticides, polychlorinated biphenyls, chlorinated solvents, and ionizing radiation such as x-rays can increase the risk of breast cancer.[2] In addition, dietary factors evidently play a role in breast cancer, as high regular consumption of saturated fat, postmenopausal obesity, and daily alcohol consumption seem to be associated with an increased risk of breast cancer.

There is also strong evidence that estrogenic hormones can stimulate tissues predisposed to the development of cancer because of the presence of *BRCA* genes. In addition, women who bear children in later life or choose not to have children and do not use oral contraceptives experience longer periods of uninterrupted estrogen exposure. Women whose first menstrual period occurs before age 12 or whose last menstrual period occurs after age 55 are also at increased exposure risk.

NOTE

Despite the multitude of known risk factors, most breast cancer patients are women in whom no such factors have been identified.

SCREENING

Because 80% of breast cancers are diagnosed after a suspicious lump is found by a woman or her partner, routine breast self-examination is an important step in prevention. Worrisome, irregular, relatively well-defined, painless lumps that do not resolve after one menstrual cycle should be evaluated with a mammogram or ultrasound examination, or both. If needed, a biopsy should be done to evaluate the mass.

Agencies that have evaluated the issue of screening for breast cancer include the U.S. Preventive Services Task Force (USPSTF),[3] the American

Cancer Society (ACS) and the National Cancer Institute (NCI). The ACS recommends annual mammograms for patients older than 40 years of age, and the NCI recommends them biannually unless risk factors other than age are present.

Breast self-examination is still considered to be one of the most effective measures for preventing breast cancer, because although it has low sensitivity, this screening tool is inexpensive, involves the patient in her healthcare, and provides a consistent examiner.

INTEGRATIVE APPROACH TO PREVENTION

Lifestyle Interventions

Exercise

Exercise is a cornerstone of health maintenance. Aerobic exercise and regular toning of the musculoskeletal body are important for lymphatic flow, vascular maintenance, and hormone regulation. It is postulated that exercise with subsequent weight loss decreases serum concentrations of estrogens, insulin, and insulin-like growth factor-1 (IGF-1), thereby reducing breast cancer risk. Modifying a sedentary lifestyle has been shown to reduce the risk of breast cancer.[4–6] The patient should be supported in choosing an *enjoyable* form of aerobic exercise (walking, jogging, swimming), and a regimen of 30 minutes of activity 5 times a week should be implemented.

Stress Management

There is concrete evidence that chronic stress alters immune system function. This effect can lead to enhanced tumor growth and metastasis when the preventive functions of tumor suppression are altered. Direct associations between stress and the prevention of breast cancer are yet to be proved in biomedicine, but the beneficial effects of this therapy on general health, together with its low cost, support its use. Techniques for stress management include meditation, yoga, guided imagery, better financial management, good sleep hygiene, effective social support, and regular relaxation activities (see Chapter 91, Relaxation Techniques).

Limiting Exposure to Hormone-Disrupting Environmental Toxins

Decreasing exposure to xenobiotics and excess ionizing radiation prevents cellular mutagenesis and disruption of hormonal cycles. Sources of ionizing radiation include x-rays and ultraviolet radiation found in sunlight. Chemicals found in pesticides and plastics also make their way into the body from processed and packaged foods, leaching out of plastic wraps and cookware. For example, the pesticide dichlorodiphenyltrichloroethane (DDT) is metabolized to dichlorodiphenyldichloroethylene (DDE), which accumulates in breast and adipose tissue.[7] Although DDT was banned as a pesticide in the United States in 1973, it can still be found in significant quantities in soil and run-off water.

The patient can decrease exposure to unneeded chemicals by eating organic, whole, unprocessed foods. Drinking water should be filtered, and canned foods, herbicides, and pesticides should be avoided.

Cessation of Tobacco Use

Mutagens from cigarettes have been found in breast fluids of nonlactating women who smoke, and links have been established between cigarette smoking and cervical, pancreas, and bladder cancer. Breast cancer data are still equivocal but are being examined with regard to multiple confounding factors usually found with tobacco use.

Breast-Feeding

Breast-feeding suppresses estrogen. A study from the United Kingdom showed that the longer a woman breast-feeds and the more babies she nurses, the more she reduces her risk of breast cancer. The investigators also reported that postmenopausal women aged 50 to 79 years who had lactated for at least 2 weeks before 50 years of age were found to have a slightly lower risk of breast cancer than that noted in women in a control group.[8]

Limiting Alcohol Consumption

Kuper and associates have proposed that excess alcohol consumption increases the risk of breast cancer.[9]

Nutrition

Decreasing Saturated Fat Intake

Cross-cultural studies have shown that women from low-risk countries in Asia and Africa acquire the same high risk of breast cancer as their American counterparts when they move to the United States and adopt a Western diet. Probably the high fat content in concert with intake of processed foods poor in antioxidants is responsible for the increased morbidity by increasing circulating sex hormones. The absolute role of dietary fat in the development of breast cancer is a subject of ongoing debate.

Increasing Consumption of High-Fiber Foods

High-fiber diets suppress the activity of bacteria in the gut, reducing constipation, lowering the risk of colon cancer, and decreasing the amount of estrogen that is reabsorbed into the body, with excretion of excess amounts into the stool. A Canadian study of 57,000 women found that those who consumed high amounts of fiber had a 30% lower risk of breast cancer compared with those who consumed low amounts of fiber.

Patients should be encouraged to consume more fruits, vegetables, and whole grains.

Limiting Consumption of Well-Done Meat

Two recent studies proposed that consumption of well-done meat and the heterocyclic amines present in such meat was a factor in increasing breast cancer risk in some patients.[10, 11] Patients should be counseled to limit consumption of well-done meat.

Increasing Intake of Soy Products

Soy contains several phytoestrogens, including isoflavones and genistein. Isoflavone phytoestrogens appear to exert antiestrogenic effects in premenopausal women, who already have high levels of endogenous estrogen, and may lower the risk of breast cancer. In vitro and animal studies have shown that soybean phytoestrogens inhibit proliferation of breast cancer cells.

The current theory is that plant estrogens are protective because they bind weakly to estrogen receptors having about 1/200 the binding affinity of endogenous estrogens. Estrogen production is then down-regulated through a negative feedback loop involving the hypothalamic-pituitary axis. As yet, the decrease in estradiol and estrone levels due to phytoestrogens has not been shown to result in significant changes in breast cancer incidence or in serum levels of sex hormones.

Another theory postulates that isoflavones direct endogenous estrogen metabolism away from hydroxyestrone metabolites that are potentially carcinogenic. These genotoxic estrogens have been found in lower ratios in women who consume 65 to 132 mg of isoflavones daily.

The phytoestrogen genistein has gained attention for its role in cancer prevention. Human breast cancer cells incubated with genistein showed inhibited cell growth and increased differentiation, and genistein-treated cells behaved less aggressively when xenografted into nude mice. Genistein reduces tyrosine kinase and inhibits angiogenesis in tumors.

Women with *no* history of estrogen-driven breast cancer should consume more soy products—soy milk, nuts, beans, tofu, and tempeh, and nondairy soy desserts.

Dosage. The recommended dose is 1 or 2 ounces (24 to 50 mg) a day.

Precautions. For women with a history of estrogen-driven breast cancer, dietary moderation in natural phytoestrogen consumption is recommended; isolated isoflavone supplementation is discouraged.

Detoxification of the Body

Most American diets are filled with processed foods and preservatives, which burden the liver with additional toxins. Detoxification of the liver and gut is an important and often symptom-reducing step for patients with an unhealthy diet history. Programs for detoxification include reduction of processed sugars and a 6-week elimination of processed grains. In addition, milk thistle, available as an herbal supplement, can be used to fortify the liver and has been shown to regenerate hepatocytes in patients with hepatitis and other severe liver-debilitating conditions (see Chapter 98, Detoxification).

Botanicals

Seaweed

In 1981, Teas postulated that consumption of seaweed was the protective factor in Japanese women, who have the lowest incidence of breast cancer in the developed world. In addition, high urinary iodine levels were detected and attributed to a high dietary intake of seaweeds such as nori (*Porphyra* species), wakame (*Undaria* species), and kombu (*Laminaria* species). Subsequent studies have shown that low urinary iodine levels are associated with higher serum levels of follicle-stimulating and luteinizing hormones (FSH, LH) and thus high-estrogen states.[12]

In addition, seaweeds have been evaluated for their antitumor effects in animal studies and seem to immunopotentiate the host's overall defense mechanism. In addition, seaweeds have anticarcinogenic activity related to the high fiber content of these plants, which acts to reduce the absorption of carcinogens from the intestines. Nori seaweed in particular has been found to have antimutagenic activity, iodine content, and is an excellent source of vitamin B_{12}.

The patient should be counseled to introduce miso soup and traditional Japanese dishes with seaweed into the diet.

Rosemary

The traditional use of rosemary (*Rosmarinus officinalis*) for the treatment of cancer in Chile was documented in the 1980s and studied for antitumor effect in animals during the 1990s. Varied results have caused scientists to rule out any specific benefit, but more scrutinizing researchers have found that rosemary has varied effects depending on the types and amounts of lipids in the diet. Modern medical studies seem to misunderstand this herb and two of its constituents, ursolic acid and carnosol, and at present, traditional uses of rosemary are being reexplored alongside the biochemical data thus far accumulated.[12] Herbalists use rosemary as a topical and internal support in baths and wine decoctions to elicit its anti-tumor effects. Because it is a dietary herb and is not widely restricted as a medicinal herb, it is unregulated, and supportive evidence for a beneficial effect remains equivocal.

Dosage. 1 to 2 g of rosemary leaves in 150 mL of boiling water to make a tea; 1 cup is consumed two or three times daily; or liquid extract (1:1 in 45% alcohol), 2 to 4 mL three times a day.

Precautions. Undiluted rosemary oil should not be ingested owing to the risk of gastrointestinal intolerance, kidney damage, and seizures.

Green Tea

Green tea is the unfermented, dried version of black tea, *Camellia sinensis*, and has been consumed in large quantities in the Far East for centuries. The processing of green tea by steaming instead of fermenting alters enzymes in the leaves and concentrates polyphenolic antioxidants, which act in the liver to detoxify metabolites of carcinogens and are now known to be protective against cancer in humans.

The patient should be encouraged to substitute green tea for coffee.

Dosage. The consumption of 2 or 3 cups of green tea daily is recommended

Precautions. Green tea can cause gastrointestinal upset and constipation, although these effects are rare. Green tea contains caffeine, but decaffeinated forms are available.

Essiac

In the 1920s and 1930s, a Canadian nurse named Rene Caisse created a formula based on Native American traditional medicine of the Ojibwa tribe and gave it to nearly 400 women for treatment of breast cancer, many of whom experienced recovery. Although no toxicity was noted, the formula was "blacklisted" by allopathic physicians after their analysis and conclusion that the women who were cured were not definitively cured by essiac.

The original formula contained burdock root, slippery elm bark, Turkish rhubarb, and sheep sorrel and was subsequently altered for clinical studies at NCI to contain red clover, kelp, blessed thistle, and watercress. Because several of the patients who used

essiac achieved clinical stability or experienced recovery in the absence of conventional treatment, sale of essiac has continued despite the allopathic summaries.

Essiac sales exceed $8 million annually. A 1999 survey by the University of Texas found that among more than 5000 cancer patients, of whom the majority were women and 22% had breast cancer, 75% were using the formulation currently sold by Essiac International, known as Flor-Essence. Ongoing trials at the British Columbia Cancer Agency are evaluating essiac.[13]

Astragalus

A potent immunostimulant, astragalus (*Astragalus membranaceus*) is used regularly in the Asian diet and in traditional Chinese medicine for fatigue. Animal studies have shown that astragalus root stimulates the immune system; data from clinical trials are not yet available to validate whether it is useful for protecting against breast cancer. However, in view of the safety of regular usage of astragalus in cooked broth, many people choose to add astragalus to the diet as a supplement, especially around cold and flu season.

Dosage. The recommended daily dose is 1 to 1.5 g of the root, taken as 3 mL of a 1:5 tincture two or three times a day.

Precautions. Astragalus is generally safe, with no toxicity reported with daily doses of less than 25 g.

Milk Thistle

A potent hepatoprotectant, milk thistle (*Silybum marianum*) is also sold in the United States as silymarin, the constituent in the seed thought to be responsible for the herb's actions. Reports have shown that silymarin is beneficial in drug-induced hepatitis, and it is now commonly used alongside hepatotoxic medications such as chemotherapeutic agents, anti-HIV medication, and some antibiotics. Given the safety of this herb and its potential protective effect, many patients use it in anticipation of supportive evidence for its beneficial effect from ongoing trials.

Dosage. 240 to 420 mg per day of the herb taken as a standardized preparation containing 70% to 90% silymarin.

Precautions. Side effects are rare, and there are no known drug interactions. However, silymarin can have a laxative effect, and there is allergic potential.

American Ginseng

Unlike *Panax ginseng*, the Asian root (commonly called "panax"), American ginseng (*Panax quinquefolius*) is given to increase physical and mental strength, with long-term use. It has also been used traditionally to alleviate menopause symptoms. Found to suppress cell growth significantly and to have estrogenic properties at the estrogen receptor, American ginseng has been explored for its synergistic effect when given with chemotherapy agents such as tamoxifen, cyclophosphamide, paclitaxel, megestrol, and methotrexate.[12] Panax ginseng has been shown to lower overall cancer rates in Korea, and human studies with Panax and American ginseng are under way in international studies to explore the biochemical mechanism of an antiestrogenic effect.

Dosage. 0.25 to 0.5 mg of the root once or twice daily between meals.

Precautions. American ginseng is not as stimulating as other forms of ginseng such as Asian and Siberian (*Eleutherococcus*) ginseng and is thus less likely to cause hypertension and tachycardia.

NOTE

Because of overharvesting of wild American ginseng, Panax quinquefolius *has been declared an endangered species in the United States.*

Supplements

Vitamins

High-dose vitamin therapy, known as orthomolecular medicine, was founded by Linus Pauling on the theory that certain vitamins at high doses serve as antioxidants, which protect cells from free radicals. Studies have shown that carotenoids are associated with lower risk of breast cancer. To assess intake of vitamins A, C, and E, the Nurses' Health Study, comprising more than 83,000 women, showed that consumption of 5 or more servings of fruits and vegetables with these vitamins was associated with a modest decrease in the risk of premenopausal breast cancer and a larger decrease in this risk in women with a family history of breast cancer.

Wu and coworkers recently reported that low levels of vitamin B_{12} were found in postmenopausal women with breast cancer and have suggested an association.[14] A protective role for vitamin A was proposed after fenretinide, a vitamin A derivative, was found to significantly reduce the risk of contralateral breast cancer in premenopausal women with early breast cancer.

Patients should be reminded that the best source of vitamins is a healthy meal made with fresh vegetables, fruits, and grains. Multivitamins and supplements are meant to supplement, not substitute for, healthy meals.

Coenzyme Q10

As one of the most powerful antioxidants isolated from the mitochondria, coenzyme Q10 (CoQ10), or ubiquinone as it was originally called, is considered to be an important booster of the immune system, protecting normal tissues from free-radical damage. Endogenous CoQ10 acts as a proton-electron shuttle in mitochondrial production of adenosine triphosphate (ATP). Supplementation with CoQ10 has been proposed as an adjunctive cancer therapy. The studies done to date with CoQ10 supplementation for breast cancer prevention have been flawed methodologically, and the conclusions remain equivocal.

Dosage. The daily dosage used in most studies is 90 to 300 mg.

Precautions. CoQ10 can cause gastritis, nausea, loss of appetite, and diarrhea. Doses greater than 300 mg a day can cause elevation of serum aminotransferases.

Melatonin

Another antioxidant, melatonin, was first described as the hormone that works to provide an internal clock through the pineal gland in both animals and some plants. Although melatonin has been widely popularized as an agent to regulate sleep patterns, it has been shown in vitro to inhibit estrogen-responsive human breast cancer cells, via its antioxidation capacity and lipophilic nature, and to augment the action of antiestrogenic tamoxifen. Furthermore, decreased levels of melatonin were found in women with estrogen receptor–positive breast cancer.

Iodine

When seaweed in Japanese diets was analyzed for its protective effect against breast cancer, the Japanese women were found to have urinary iodine concentrations 10 times higher than those in American women. Further investigation of iodine's effects on the breast has shown that iodine supplementation apparently significantly reduces mastalgia and the prevalence of breast cysts, fibrous tissue plaques, and breast pain. In addition, low urinary iodine levels are associated with higher serum levels of FSH and LH and thus high-estrogen states. Because most of these studies have been done outside of the United States, in Europe, Russia, and Japan, the results have not been well publicized in the American medical literature. However, some experts argue that breast cancer mortality has not been altered with the introduction of iodized salt and suggest that in fact iodine is not the important factor in seaweed that gives its protective effect. Currently, the recommendation is to include more nori seaweed in the diet and to continue to use iodized salt.

Calcium D-Glucarate

Sold widely as supplements that may prevent estrogen-driven cancers, calcium D-glucarate is a precursor to a beta-glucuronidase inhibitor used clinically for phase 2 detoxification in the liver. Phase 2 detoxification accomplished via this inhibitor prevents conversion of tumor promoters into harmful active compounds. It also works by decreasing the absorption of estrogen hormones from the gut. Animal studies show reduction of beta-glucuronidase activity and a reduction in mammary cancer with an increase of calcium D-glucarate in the diet. Human clinical studies are being proposed to derive supportive evidence for the usage, but as this supplement is considered safe for human beings, many people continue to use calcium in this formulation.

Dosage. Calcium D-glucarate is found naturally in grapefruit, apples, oranges, broccoli, and Brussels sprouts. If a supplement is used, 200 to 400 mg is given for prevention, and 400 to 1200 mg is recommended for patients who have breast cancer.

Precautions. Although calcium D-glucarate is a very safe supplement with no major adverse effects, further research is needed to support its use.

Pharmaceuticals

Treatments offered by most biomedically trained physicians for the prevention of breast cancer include prophylactic mastectomy, hormone therapies, and some diet and nutrition counseling. For secondary prevention of estrogen receptor–positive cancers after surgery for primary breast cancer, tamoxifen (Nolvadex), aromatase inhibitors, and anastrozole (Arimidex) are being used.

Oral Contraceptive Pills/Estrogen

Hormone therapies such as prophylactic use of oral contraceptive pills (OCPs) are given to periodically interrupt estrogen exposure to breast, uterine, and ovarian tissues. Although OCPs have widely been considered protective in this role, the Collaborative Group on Hormonal Factors in Breast Cancer recently concluded that use of OCPs is in fact associated with a small increase in breast cancer, though at less advanced stages, among current users and in patients who stopped use in the past 10 years.[15]

Hormone replacement therapy (HRT) has also been shown to increase the risk of breast cancer by 35% in patients who have used HRT for 5 years or longer. The risk was shown to revert to normal 5 years after HRT cessation; this finding must be taken into account in weighing the risks and benefits of HRT for postmenopausal symptoms.

Tamoxifen

The use of antiestrogenic compounds such as tamoxifen is an option for the prevention of breast cancer in developed countries. Conflicting data make simplistic conclusions difficult, but most studies agree that tamoxifen significantly reduces the risk of invasive breast cancer in women receiving HRT and in those at greater risk of estrogen-positive tumors (e.g., those who are *BRCA1/BRCA2*-negative).[16, 17]

Likewise, selective estrogen receptor modulators (SERMs) such as raloxifene (Evista) have been shown to reduce the incidence of breast cancer in women taking it for osteoporosis. Its antiestrogenic effect on the breast and uterus is being investigated as a secondary end point in the MORE trial.[18]

Surgery

Prophylactic Mastectomy

Prophylactic mastectomy was recently shown to reduce breast cancer risk by 90% in a retrospective study at the Mayo Clinic and is most often considered by women who have the *BRCA* gene and a first-degree relative who experienced breast cancer at an early age. This choice warrants careful consideration and in-depth discussion before it is undertaken, as it is an irreversible option for the prevention of breast cancer.[19]

Mind-Body Medicine

Support Groups

Participation in breast cancer support groups has been shown to improve immune function as well as to enhance qualitative measures of hope, wellness, and quality of life. Social support and the expression of emotions and concerns in such settings also are proactive elements in the journey to self-care and health for women.

Biofeedback

Biofeedback and guided imagery were shown in a crossover study by Gruber in 1993 to improve immune function and to increase natural killer cell activity as well as blood lymphocyte counts.

Other Approaches

Additional approaches that are actively utilized in stress management and in teaching coping skills are yoga, music therapy, breathing exercises (pranayama), meditation, hypnosis, and prayer.

PREVENTION PRESCRIPTION

Preventive Measures

- *Patients at high risk for breast cancer (those with a history of previous breast cancer, family history of breast cancer in a first-degree relative, BRCA genes, or older age) should have mammograms annually and do breast self-examinations monthly, tracking any lumps or cystic changes with a physician.*
- *Patients without risk factors for breast cancer should have mammograms every 2 years after the age of 40 and should do breast self-examinations monthly.*
- *Healthy eating habits should be encouraged, to include consumption of whole foods, unprocessed high-fiber grains, and 5 to 6 servings of fruits and vegetables each day.*
- *A practical exercise routine should be incorporated into the patient's lifestyle.*
- *Stress management should be actively undertaken.*
- *Intake of soy products should be increased if the patient is not at risk for the development of estrogen receptor–positive cancer.*
- *Exposure to environmental toxins such as pesticides and petroleum wastes should be minimized.*
- *Tobacco products and excessive alcohol use are to be avoided.*
- *A diet low in saturated fats and in well-done meats should be encouraged.*
- *Herbs such as seaweed, green tea, and milk thistle and vitamins A, C, and E can be used as antioxidants.*
- *Use of astragalus and ginseng can be considered for their immunostimulant actions during illnesses that challenge the immune system.*
- *Patients who are at high risk for the development of breast cancer should avoid estrogen supplementation.*
- *Mind-body approaches such as guided imagery, meditation, and breathing exercises can be incorporated into the patient's array of coping strategies in order to maintain and reestablish balance in life.*

Further Resources[13, 20]

www.cancerbacup.org.uk/info/breast.htm
This British cancer support organization presents data to explain possible causes of breast cancer.

www.womens-wellness.com
Specific alternative treatments for breast cancer are presented under the cancer section in this web site.

www.cancerdecisions.com
This is the web site of Dr. Ralph Moss. Detoxification, nutrition, diet, and stress interventions are presented.

SHARE: Self-Help for Women with Breast Cancer (212) 382–2111

Breast Cancer Action (415) 922–8279

References

1. Goldman MB, Hatch MC: Women and Health. New York, Academic Press, 2000.
2. Boik J: Cancer and Natural Medicine: A Textbook of Basic Science and Clinical Research. Princeton, Minn, Oregon Medical Press, 1996.
3. Report of the U.S. Preventive Services Task Force. Guide to Clinical Preventive Services, 2nd ed. Baltimore, Williams & Wilkins, 1996, pp 73–87.
4. Kiningham RB: Physical activity and the primary prevention of cancer. Prim Care 25:515–536, 1998.
5. McTiernan A: Associations between energy balance and body mass index and risk of breast carcinoma in women from diverse racial and ethnic backgrounds in the US. Cancer 88:1248–1255, 2000.
6. Stoll BA: Western nutrition and the insulin resistance syndrome: A link to breast cancer. Eur J Clin Nutr 53:83–87, 1999.
7. Ellenhorn MJ: Ellenhorn's Medical Toxicology, 2nd ed. Baltimore, Williams & Wilkins, 1997.
8. Newcomb PA, et al: Lactation in relation to postmenopausal breast cancer. Am J Epidemiol 150:174–182, 1998.
9. Kuper H, Ye W, Weiderpass E, et al: Alcohol and breast cancer risk: The alcoholism paradox. Br J Cancer 83:949–951, 2000.
10. Deitz AC, Zheng W, Leff MA, et al: N-acetyltransferase-2 genetic polymorphism, well-done meat intake, and breast cancer risk among postmenopausal women. Cancer Epidemiol Biomarkers Prev 9:905–910, 2000.
11. Gertig DM, Hankinson SE, Hough H, et al: N-acetyl transferase 2 genotypes, meat intake and breast cancer risk. Int J Cancer 80:13–17, 1999.
12. Abascal K, Yarnell E: Herbs and breast cancer: Research review of seaweed, rosemary, and ginseng. Altern Complem Ther 7:32–36, 2001.
13. Low Dog T, Riley D, Carter T: CME: Traditional and alternative therapies for breast cancer. Altern Ther Health Med 7:36–47, 2001.
14. Wu K, Helzlsouer KJ, Comstock GW, et al: A prospective study on folate, B$_{12}$, and pyridoxal 5'-phosphate (B$_6$) and breast cancer. Cancer Epidemiol Biomarkers Prev 8:209–217, 1999.
15. Collaborative Group on Hormonal Factors in Breast Cancer: Breast cancer and hormone replacement therapy: Collaborative reanalysis of data from 51 epidemiological studies of 52,705 women with breast cancer and 108,411 women without breast cancer. Lancet 350:1047–1059, 1997.
16. Fisher B, Constantino JP, Wickerham DL, et al: Tamoxifen for the prevention of breast cancer: Report of the National Surgical Adjuvant Breast and Bowel Project P-1 Study, J Natl Cancer Inst 90:1371–1388, 1998.
17. Leris C, Mokbel K: The prevention of breast cancer: An overview. Curr Med Res Opin 16:252–257, 2001.
18. Cummings SR, Eckert S, Krueger K, et al: The effect of raloxifene on the risk of breast cancer in postmenopausal women: Results from the MORE randomized trial. JAMA 281:2189–2197, 1999.

19. Hartmann LC, Schaid DJ, Woods JE, et al. Efficacy of bilateral prophylactic mastectomy in women with a family history of breast cancer. N Engl J Med 340:77–84, 1999.

20. Mason R: WebWatch: Alternative and complementary resources on breast cancer. Altern Complem Ther 7:55–56, 2001.

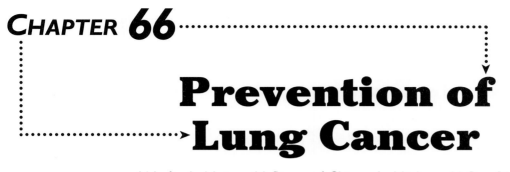

CHAPTER 66

Prevention of Lung Cancer

Wadie I. Najm, M.D., and Shiraz I. Mishra, M.D., Ph.D.

Lung cancer is the second most common cancer diagnosed in the United States and the leading cause of cancer death in both men (accounting for 31% of deaths due to cancer) and women (accounting for 25%). Lung cancer is classified into small cell lung cancer (SCLC) which constitutes 20% to 25% of all lung cancers, and non–small cell lung cancer (NSCLC), of which adenocarcinoma is the most common form. The incidence of new cases in men has decreased since the 1980s, with a decrease of 1.7% per year reported between 1990 and 1997. In women, the incidence of new cases has been stable since 1991 (13%). The 5-year survival rate is poor (15.8%) owing to the often late diagnosis.

ETIOLOGY

Tobacco Use

It is well documented that cigarette smokers have a higher risk of morbidity from cardiovascular disease, pulmonary disease, and various cancers. Approximately 85% to 90% of lung cancers are due to tobacco smoking. The risk for persons who smoke more than 20 cigarettes per day is 20 to 30 times higher than that for nonsmokers. The risk declines gradually after quitting, reaching nonsmokers' risk after 20 to 25 years. Epidemiologic studies indicate that the ultimate decrease in cancer risk in persons who smoke "ultralight" or reduced tar cigarettes is not proportional to the decrease in tar concentration.

Passive Smoking

Passive smoking has been the subject of intense discussion as an additional cause of lung cancer. Despite the low relative risk of passive smoking (1.5), the large number of people exposed raises its possible impact.

Other Environmental Carcinogens

Other environmental carcinogens that have been implicated in lung cancer include asbestos, arsenic, chromium, nickel, tar, mineral oils, mustard gas, ionizing radiation, and bis(chloromethyl)ether.

SCREENING

Chest Radiography

The sensitivity of chest radiography for lung cancer detection is dependent on the location and size of the lesion and the skill of the interpreting physician. Use of chest x-ray studies has a limited potential in screening for lung cancer, particularly in comparison with newer technologies with higher resolution. The 20-year Mayo Clinic lung project found that chest x-ray screenings at frequent intervals do not decrease the death rate from lung cancer.

Spiral (Helical) Computed Tomography

Spiral computed tomography (CT) is a low-radiation-dose radiologic modality in which multiple thin-slice (5-mm) images are obtained and then assembled into a three-dimensional model of the anatomic structures examined. Studies to evaluate its benefit for cancer screening are under way (i.e., the lung cancer screening study of the National Cancer Institute [NCI]). In an ongoing nonrandomized clinical trial (the Early Lung Cancer Action Project [ELCAP]), CT of the lungs significantly outperformed chest radiography in the detection of small pulmonary nodules[1].

Sputum Cytology

Sputum cytology was examined in a large multicenter lung cancer screening trial, but this modality did not positively predict lung cancer development. Results of the NCI cooperative trials showed no added benefit over chest radiography. Efforts to refine sputum cytology screening are continuing.

Laser Bronchoscopy

In laser technology, light of a special wavelength can be used to stimulate different intracellular components (fluoroflors, which include flavins, riboflavins, nucleic acids, and proteins) to emit a spectral pattern specific to that particular tissue. Utilizing this principle, laser bronchoscopy can be used to differentiate dysplastic from neoplastic tissue, which contains altered levels of fluoroflors. The usefulness of this technique for lung cancer screening is under evaluation.

Genetic and Other Biomarkers

Mutations of the *p53* gene have been found in approximately 50% of persons with NSCLC and in bronchial dysplasia. However, use of *p53* mutation as a biomarker is limited by technical difficulty and variability.

Another biomarker being investigated as a screening tool is the K *ras* gene. However, owing to its low prevalence in NSCLC (30% of the cases), K *ras* gene assay is not an effective screening method.

In up to 80% of smokers, evidence of loss of heterozygosity (loss of one chromosomal allele) or genomic instability (loss or gain of genetic material within a chromosomal region) in bronchial tissue can be demonstrated. Use of these markers as intermediate end point in lung cancer prevention studies is under investigation.

Another potentially useful biomarker is the retinoic acid receptor-beta (RAR-β), as levels are reduced in bronchial metaplasia, dysplasia, and NSCLC.

An increase in the level of the epidermal growth factor receptor (EGFR) has been noted in bronchial metaplasia, and proliferating cell nuclear antigen (PCNA) levels are increased in dividing cells and in NSCLC. Both EGFR and PCNA assays may therefore prove useful in lung cancer screening.

INTEGRATIVE APPROACH TO PREVENTION

Life Style Interventions

There is abundant evidence that smoking cessation is the single most important factor in decreasing the incidence of lung cancer. Patients should be counseled to abstain from smoking. Various products and programs, including acupuncture, to assist in smoking cessation are available, and the costs of these interventions are covered by many insurance providers.

Nutrition

A major limitation of assessment of nutritional approaches to the prevention of lung cancer is the low accuracy of dietary questionnaires and the poor specificity of instruments used to collect the information. Some evidence, however, points to a beneficial effect of some nutrients.

Consumption of *green leafy vegetables and carrots* has been strongly correlated with a reduction in the risk of lung cancer. The protective effect persisted after tobacco use was removed as a possible confounder.

Consumption of *cruciferous vegetables* (broccoli, Brussels sprouts, cauliflower, mustard greens, turnips, and rutabagas) has been suggested as having a protective effect against cancer of the aerodigestive tract, owing to the high content of glucosinolates in these vegetables. Prospective cohort studies and case control studies have yielded mixed results. However, consumption of *Brassica vegetables*, particularly cabbage, appeared to have an inverse association with cancer risk.

Other types of food—meat, fish, eggs, and legumes—have not been shown to have a protective effect. A cohort study conducted in the Netherlands found no relation between the consumption of onions, leeks, or garlic and a reduction in risk of lung cancer.[2] An observational study on the consumption of *black tea* did not show a protective effect against lung cancer.[3]

Botanicals

Green Tea

Animal studies point to a possible protective effect of polyphenolic fraction and water extract of green tea. However, results of epidemiologic studies on the role of green tea in lung cancer prevention remain inconclusive. Green tea has been shown to inhibit the formation of DNA strand and lipid peroxidation in cultured human lung cells,[4] and consumption with meals may inhibit the formation of nitrosamines. In animal studies, green tea reduced lung oncogene expression[5] and was very effective in inhibiting lung carcinogenesis induced by asbestos and benzo-[*a*]pyrene.[6] Controlled randomized studies are needed to evaluate the effect of green tea for cancer prevention. Although green tea is considered safe, precaution should be taken to limit intake in pregnant and lactating women owing to its significant caffeine content.

Ginseng

Animal studies suggest variable outcomes based on the type and age of ginseng used. The majority of studies have indicated a tendency for *Panax ginseng* to decrease the incidence of lung cancer. An acidic polysaccharide, ginsan, was found to be safe and effective in decreasing the incidence of lung cancer.[7] Human studies showed a dose-response inhibitory effect. Smokers who used ginseng had a decreased odds ratio (OR) of developing lung cancer compared with nonusers (OR: 2.0, 95% confidence interval [CI]: 1.3–3.2); these results were substantiated by a cohort study (relative risk: 0.3, 95% CI: 0.1–0.7). The available evidence points to a significant preventive effect against cancer for *Panax ginseng*.[8]

Chinese Herbs

Studies have focused mainly on the use of Chinese herbs in the treatment of persons with cancer. No lung cancer prevention studies were identified. The possible role of Chinese herbs in the prevention of lung cancer remains to be investigated.

Maitake Mushroom

Maitake mushroom has been used in tonics, soups, teas, and herbal formulas by Asian therapists to promote health. Laboratory studies indicate that it has an immune-enhancing effect and inhibits the spread of tumors.[26] These findings have not been verified by human studies.

Kombucha Tea

Kombucha tea is promoted to enhance and boost the immune system and to fight cancer in the early stages. There is no scientific evidence to support its use. The U.S. Food and Drug Administration has issued a warning to consumers to exercise caution when using this botanical, following two reports of Kombucha-related acidosis.

Supplements

Selenium

Selenium is not an antioxidant; however, it is essential for the production of two enzymes that affect the antioxidant network. It is not produced in the body and must be obtained through food. The amount of selenium in foods will vary depending on the soil where the food is grown. Foods rich in selenium are garlic, onions, broccoli, egg yolks, and wheat germ.

NOTE

Brazil nuts (the ones grown in Brazil) may contain up to 120 μg of selenium per nut. They are one of the few nuts obtained in the wild, and eating them not only provides abundant selenium but helps to preserve the rain forest where they are grown.

The exact mechanism by which selenium may prevent cancer is unclear. Proposed mechanisms are through inhibition of cell proliferation, an effect on immune response, and removal of toxic byproducts of lipid peroxidation by glutathione peroxidase.

Several cohort studies have evaluated the impact of selenium level on the development of lung cancer.[9, 10] Results are controversial, with a few studies showing an inverse relationship and others showing a direct relationship with lung cancer. Three randomized studies looked at the effect of selenium supplementation on lung cancer prevention.[11–13] Despite these encouraging reports, questions remain about the exact dose to be used, the population it protects (smokers versus nonsmokers, or persons with low levels versus normal levels of selenium), and the length of time needed to achieve the protective effect.

Vitamin A, Beta Carotene, and Retinoids

The term *vitamin A* is popularly used to indicate two different families of dietary factors: (1) retinyl esters, retinol and retinal (preformed vitamin A), and (2) beta-carotene and other carotenoids (pro–vitamin A) that serve as precursors to vitamin A.[14] The seven predominant carotenoids in human beings are beta-carotene, lycopene, lutein, alpha-carotene, alpha-cryptoxanthin, beta-cryptoxanthin, and zeaxanthin. Different carotenoids are concentrated in different organs. The circulating level of beta-carotene is influenced by retinol intake, or retinol suppresses its conversion to vitamin A.

Various theories have been proposed to explain the role of vitamin A in fighting cancer. Specific possible mechanisms of vitamin A activity include the following[15]:

- Vitamin A may have antioxidant properties in conditions of low oxygen tension.
- It may inhibit proliferation and induce differentiation of epithelial cells.
- It may modulate cytochrome P450.
- It may inhibit arachidonic acid metabolism.
- It may modulate immune function.
- It may induce gap junction communication.
- It may inhibit chromosome instability and damage.
- It may influence apoptosis.

Several studies evaluated the effect of beta-carotene on lung cancer. Diet, serum level, and supplement use were examined. Interest in vitamin A and beta-carotene for the prevention of lung cancer is based on initial animal and epidemiologic data, which suggested a protective effect in lung cancer.[16] Even with early-stage cancer, questions are raised about whether smoking status, type of food, and food ingredient (other than carotenoids) may influence the outcome.

Some of the early epidemiologic studies tried to determine whether the effect of vitamin A or carotenoids differs between genders. Two studies found similar results in both men and women, whereas other studies found a protective effect in men and an adverse effect in women.[17, 18]

Lung cancer risk was reduced with consumption of large quantities of vegetable and fruits. This association was found to be stronger in case-control studies than in cohort studies.[10] However, this effect was found to be stronger for vegetable and fruit intake than for beta-carotene intake. Prospective studies looking at the effect of dietary beta-carotene intake on decreasing the risk of lung cancer found a non-significant association.[19–21] Thus, the inverse relationship found with vegetable and fruit intake was not maintained in beta-carotene studies.

Plasma or serum beta-carotene levels were found to be lower in several studies exploring the prediagnostic level of beta-carotene in persons who developed lung cancer.[22, 23] However, interpretation of these studies was based on one measurement taken several years before the onset of cancer.

Other studies looking at the association of other carotenoids found an inverse association of lung cancer with dietary intake of lutein and alpha-carotene. Prospective studies, however, failed to establish such an association for lutein, alpha-carotene, and lycopene.[24]

Several multicenter double-blind controlled trials explored a possible role for beta-carotene supplements in the primary prevention of lung cancer. Two studies—the Alpha-Tocopherol and Beta-Carotene Cancer Prevention study (ATBC) and the Beta-Carotene and Retinol Efficacy Trial (CARET)—indicated a higher incidence of lung cancer among the group receiving beta-carotene supplementation. In contrast, the Physician's Health Study (PHS) reported no effect of beta-carotene supplementation on the incidence of lung cancer. The low number of smokers (11%) in the PHS study group may explain the discrepancy. In the ATBC and CARET studies, a higher incidence of lung cancer was noted among smokers. Persons smoking 20 or more cigarettes a day were at

higher risk. Above-average alcohol consumption was also noted to be a predisposing factor.

Vitamin E

The association between dietary intake of alpha-tocopherol and lung cancer was explored in a few studies, with variable results. In the ATBC study, in a cohort of persons receiving alpha-tocopherol (in a dose of 50 mg per day), protective effect for lung cancer was not demonstrated. Most cohort studies looking at serum concentrations of alpha-tocopherol showed no association, except for one study, which showed an inverse relation.

Vitamin C

Several prospective studies examined the effect of dietary vitamin C on the risk of lung cancer. Results showed no effect; more recent studies, however, indicate an inverse association. No controlled trials of vitamin C supplementation and lung cancer were identified for this review.

Melatonin

Melatonin is very popular as an antidote to jet lag and as a sleep aid. It also has antioxidant properties and acts to stimulate the main antioxidant of the brain, glutathione peroxidase. Recent in vitro studies reported a possible anticancer role. The proposed mechanism is an antiestrogenic activity and augmentation of the anticancer effect of interleukin-2. Melatonin (in a dose of 10 mg per day) has been studied in patients with metastatic NSCLC; results included an increased 1-year survival rate and disease stabilization.[25] The role of melatonin for the prevention of lung cancer is still to be determined.

Pharmaceuticals

Etretinate, a synthetic retenoid, was found in a nonrandomized study to decrease bronchial metaplasia in smokers. However, a randomized study failed to substantiate this benefit.

NOTE

Research does not support a role for beta-carotene alone in the prevention of lung cancer. In fact, beta-carotene supplementation seems to have an adverse effect, particularly among smokers and heavy alcohol users.

—*PREVENTION PRESCRIPTION*

- *Patients should be counseled to stop smoking, and to avoid smoke-filled areas.*
- *Appropriate precautions should be taken to prevent possible environmental exposure to known carcinogens and dusts.*
- *Use of green tea and ginseng (Panax ginseng) in moderate doses may have a preventive effect.*
- *Consumption of Brassica vegetables, particularly cabbage, is recommended.*

THERAPEUTIC REVIEW   continued

- *Intake of vitamin A and/or beta-carotene should be increased through dietary means by eating yellow, orange, and red fruits and vegetables.*
- *Smokers (particularly those who smoke more than 20 cigarettes per day) should avoid vitamin A and beta-carotene supplements.*

Resources

Cancer Trials
Web site: http://cancertrials.nci.nih.gov
Telephone: 1-800-4-CANCER
A great resource for up-to-date information on ongoing trials and preliminary results of ongoing studies.

National Center for Complementary and Alternative Medicine
Web site: http://nccam.nih.gov
An excellent resource for different complementary and alternative medicine information, research centers, and database, and as a connection to other relevant agencies in the National Institutes of Health.

American Cancer Society
Web site: http://www.cancer.org/alt_therapy
Telephone: 1-800-ACS-2345
A rich source of information on prevention and treatment options for professionals and consumers. A great site for national and local resources and for general information on some dietary supplements.

References

1. Henschke CI, McCauley DI, Yankelevitz DF, et al: Early Lung Cancer Action Project: Overall design and findings from baseline screening. Lancet 354:99–105, 1999.
2. Dorant E, Van den Brandt PA, Goldbohm RA: A prospective cohort study on *Allium* vegetable consumption, garlic supplement use, and the risk of lung carcinoma in the Netherlands. Cancer Res 54:6148–6153, 1994.
3. Goldbohm RA, Hertog MG, Brants HA, et al: Consumption of black tea and cancer risk: A prospective cohort study. J Natl Cancer Inst 88:93–100, 1996.
4. Leanderson P, Faresjo A, Tagesson C: Green tea polyphenols inhibit oxidant-induced DNA strand breakage in cultured lung cells. Free Radic Biol Med 23:235–242, 1997.
5. Hu G, Han C, Chen J: Inhibition of oncogene expression by green tea and (-)-epigallocatechin gallate in mice. Nutr Cancer 24:203–209, 1995.
6. Luo SQ, Liu XZ, Wang CJ: Inhibitory effect of green tea extract on the carcinogenesis induced by asbestos plus benzo(a)pyrene in rat. Biomed Environ Sci 5:54–58, 1995.
7. Lee YS, Chung IS, Lee IR, et al: Activation of multiple effector pathway of immune system by the antineoplastic immunostimulator acidic polysaccharide ginsan isolated from *Panax ginseng*. Anticancer Res 17:323–332, 1997.
8. Shin HR, Kim JY, Yun TK, et al: The cancer-preventive potential of *Panax ginseng*: A review of human and experimental evidence. Cancer Causes Control 11:565–576, 2000.
9. Knekt P, Jarvinen R, Seppanen R, Rissanen A, et al: Dietary antioxidants and risk of lung cancer. Am J Epidemiol 134:471–479, 1991.
10. Koo LC: Diet and lung cancer 20+ years later: More questions than answers? Int J Cancer 10(Suppl):22–29, 1997.
11. Yu S Y, Mao B L, Xiao P, et al: Intervention trial with selenium for the prevention of lung cancer among tin miners in Yunnan, China. A pilot study. Biol Trace Elem Res 24:105–108, 1990.
12. Blot W, Li J, Taylor P, et al: Nutrition intervention trials in Linxian, China: Supplementation with specific vitamin/mineral combinations, cancer incidence, and disease specific mortality in the general population. J Natl Cancer Ins 85:1483–1492, 1993.
13. Clark L, Combs G, Turnbull BW, et al: Effects of selenium supplementation for cancer prevention in patients with carcinoma of the skin. JAMA 276:1957–1963, 1996.
14. Omenn GS: Chemoprevention of lung cancer: The rise and demise of beta carotene. Annu Rev Public Health 19:73–99, 1998.
15. Pryor WA, Stahl W, Rock CL: Beta carotene: From biochemistry to clinical trials. Nutr Rev 58:39–53, 2000.
16. Ziegler RG, Mason TJ, Stemhagen A, et al: Carotenoid intake, vegetables, and the risk of lung cancer among white men in New Jersey. Am J Epidemiol 123:1080–1093, 1986.
17. Gregor A, Lee PN, Roe JC, et al: Comparison of dietary histories in lung cancer cases and controls with special reference to vitamin A. Nutr Cancer 2:93, 1980.
18. Hinds MW, Kolonel LN, Hankin JH, Lee J: Dietary vitamin A, carotene, vitamin C and risk of lung cancer in Hawaii. Am J Epidemiol 119:227–237, 1984.
19. Bandera EV, Freudenheim JL, Marshal JR, et al: Diet and alcohol consumption and lung cancer risk in the New York State cohort. Cancer Causes Control 8:828–840, 1997.
20. Yong LC, Brown CC, Schatzkin et al: Intakes of vitamins E, C, and A and risk of lung cancer. The NHANES I epidemiologic follow-up study. Am J Epidemiol 146:231–243, 1997.
21. Ocke MC, Bueno-de-Mesquita HB, Feskens EJM, et al: Repeated measurements of vegetables, fruits, β-carotene, and vitamins C and E in relation to lung cancer. Am J Epidemiol 145:358–365, 1997.
22. Comstock GW, Alberg AJ, Huang HY, et al: The risk of developing lung cancer associated with antioxidants in the blood; ascorbic acid, carotenoids, α-tocopherol, selenium, and total peroxyl radical absorbing capacity. Cancer Epidemiol Biomarkers Prevent 6:907–916, 1997.
23. Stahelin HB, Gey KF, Eichholzer M, et al: Plasma antioxidant vitamins and subsequent cancer mortality in the 12 year follow up of the prospective Basel study. Am J Epidemiol 133:766–775, 1991.
24. Steinmetz KA, Potter JD, Folsom AR: Vegetables, fruit, and lung cancer in the Iowa Women's Health Study. Cancer Res 53:536–543, 1993.
25. Lissoni P, Tisi E, Barni S, et al: Biological and clinical results of a neuroimmunotherapy with interleukin-2 and the pineal hormone melatonin as a first line treatment in advanced non-small cell lung cancer. Br J Cancer 66:155–158, 1992.
26. Nanbu H, Kubo K: Effect of maitake D-fraction on cancer prevention. Ann N Y Acad Sci 833:204–207, 1997.

CHAPTER 67

Preventing Prostate Cancer

Mark W. McClure, M.D., and David Rakel, M.D.

ETIOLOGY

Although the exact causes remain unknown, harmful eating habits, destructive lifestyle choices, and environmental toxins increase the risk of prostate cancer (Table 67–1). Perhaps the greatest risk factor for prostate cancer, however, is a family history. For instance, if one first-degree relative (brother or father) has prostate cancer, the risk is two to three times greater; with two first-degree relatives, the risk is five to six times greater; and with three, it is eight to eleven times greater. If a second-degree relative (uncle or grandfather, on either side of the family) has prostate cancer, there is still a one and a half to two times greater risk.[1] If two second-degree relatives have prostate cancer, the risk is nine times greater.[2] The risk is even greater for men with *hereditary* prostate cancer, which is suspected when there is a history of prostate cancer affecting family members within three generations (three first-degree relatives) or in two relatives before the age of 55. Men who inherit a dominant gene for prostate cancer have a 16 to 18 times greater chance of developing prostate cancer. This equates to an 80% to 90% chance of developing prostate cancer by age 85.[3] Other risk factors for prostate cancer are listed in Table 67–1.

Fortunately, selective lifestyle and dietary modifications can alter the initiation, promotion, and progression stages of prostate cancer. Because research has shown that a small percentage of teenagers have latent prostate cancer and that the incidence increases with age, preventive measures should be instituted as early as possible.[4]

Table 67–1. Risk Factors for Prostate Cancer

Age
Family history
African American race
Obesity
Smoking
High-fat diet
Occupational exposure (e.g., farming, lawn care, exterminator)

SCREENING

Although prostate-specific antigen (PSA) screening can detect prostate cancer at an early stage, professional medical organizations are divided on the value of prostate cancer screening. With the exception of the American Cancer Society and the American Urological Association, no other professional medical organization advocates routine PSA screening. Opponents claim that PSA screening often detects insignificant cancers, fails to impact overall survival, and may adversely impact quality of life. Just the same, they advise informed decision making for the individual patient. In contrast, proponents point out that 93% of PSA-detected prostate cancers are life threatening (if left untreated, the cancer progresses), and screening increases the chance for cure by detecting a greater percentage of organ-confined disease (86%, vs. 35% of cases in the pre-PSA era).[5, 6] At any rate, regardless of the controversy surrounding PSA screening for the general population, men in the high-risk group should begin screening at age 40. There are also certain other caveats to consider: Men with a PSA less than 2.5 can have a PSA drawn once every 2 years; normal PSA values may vary with age and race, and percentage-free PSA can help identify men with the greatest risk of harboring prostate cancer (see later).

Because PSA values vary according to age, some researchers recommend using the following age-specific PSA values[7]:

- Men aged 40 to 49—2.5 ng/mL or less
- Men aged 50 to 59—3.5 ng/mL or less
- Men aged 60 to 69—4.5 ng/mL or less
- Men aged 70 to 79—6.5 ng/mL or less.

Additionally, other researchers recommend separate age-specific PSA values for African American men as follows[8]:

- Men aged 40 to 49—2 ng/mL or less
- Men aged 50 to 59—4 ng/mL or less
- Men aged 60 to 69—4.5 ng/mL or less
- Men aged 70 to 79—5.5 ng/mL or less

Percentage-free PSA measures the ratio between total PSA (bound and unbound) and unbound or "free" PSA. This test is most useful for PSA values between 4 and 10 ng/mL. The lower the percentage, the higher the risk of prostate cancer.[9] For example, in men aged 50 to 64, if the percentage-free fraction is greater than 25%, there is a only a 5% risk of prostate cancer; however, if it is less than 10%, the risk of prostate cancer jumps to 56%.

NOTE

Percentage-free PSA is affected by manipulation of the prostate gland (unlike total PSA). Therefore, you should not order a percentage-free PSA test on the same day as a rectal examination or within 24 hours of intercourse.

LIFESTYLE

Exercise

According to one study, men younger than age 60 who are most fit are four times less likely to develop prostate cancer than those less fit.[10]

Exercise (e.g., walking, jogging, swimming) 30 minutes or longer at least three times weekly.

Xenobiotic Exposure

A xenobiotic is any chemical or toxin that is foreign to the body. Herbicides and pesticides are two common xenobiotics that increase prostate cancer risk by causing DNA damage and altering hormone metabolism.[11] According to the Environmental Protection Agency (EPA), *atrazine*—the most commonly used herbicide in the United States—is a "probable" cause of cancer.[12] (Atrazine is routinely used on corn, sorghum, and citrus crops.)

Endocrine disrupters—substances that mimic natural hormones—are xenobiotics that also increase prostate cancer risk by disrupting hormone metabolism. Common examples of endocrine disrupters include polychlorinated biphenyls, or PCBs (used to make plastic, ink, and electrical and electronic equipment), and plasticizers (substances used to make plastic food-wrap more pliable).

Finally, in addition to being high in fat, dairy and beef products are often contaminated with toxic pesticide and hormone residues.[13]

Reduce prostate cancer risk by washing all produce, peeling nonorganic produce (when applicable), and buying organic fruits and vegetables whenever possible; preserving and cooking food in glass containers instead of plastic ones; and limiting or eliminating meat and dairy consumption.

Hormone-Altering Medications and Supplements

Injudicious use of DHEA (dehydroepiandrosterone), androstenedione, human growth hormone, and testosterone may promote prostate cancer. Avoid them unless medically indicated, especially for men at increased risk for prostate cancer.

Alcohol

Men who drink more than 96 g of alcohol weekly (about 10 drinks) triple their risk of developing prostate cancer.[14] Avoid indiscriminate use of alcohol.

Smoking

Among other carcinogens, tobacco contains cadmium, a heavy metal that increases prostate cancer risk. Smoking also induces a more aggressive form of prostate cancer.[15]

NUTRITION

Animal Fat

Compelling data have associated saturated fat, particularly animal fat, with prostate cancer risk.[16] A typical American diet is high in saturated animal fat but low in fruits, vegetables, fish, and soy protein, whereas a typical Japanese diet is the reverse. According to epidemiologic researchers, these dietary differences may account for the 20-fold increased incidence of clinical (as opposed to latent) prostate cancer in American versus Japanese men.[17] As further evidence of the dietary connection, once Japanese males adopt a typical American diet, their incidence of prostate cancer jumps 10-fold.[18]

Saturated fat increases prostate cancer risk by increasing the production of an omega-6 essential fatty acid called *arachidonic acid (AA)*. Arachidonic acid is converted to inflammatory prostaglandin E_2 (PGE_2) molecules and series four leukotrienes. These messenger molecules enable prostate cancer cells to evade the immune system, inactivate natural killer cells and cytotoxic T cells, promote angiogenesis, and prevent apoptosis.[18] Research has shown that prostate cancer cells produce 10 times as much PGE_2 as surrounding benign cells.[19] Meat-based diets and most cooking oils (with the exception of canola and olive oils) increase AA formation.

Dairy products, which are loaded with saturated fat, also increase the risk of prostate cancer.[20] Furthermore, recombinant bovine growth hormone, a genetically engineered hormone that is used to increase milk production, increases the risk of prostate cancer by as much as eightfold because it increases the production of insulin growth factor-I (IGF-I).[21] IGF-I increases angiogenesis, prevents apoptosis, and stimulates prostate cancer cells to produce a tumor growth factor called *urokinase-type plasminogen activator.*[22, 23]

Decrease prostate cancer risk by limiting or eliminating food items that increase AA production (e.g., animal fat, hydrogenated oils, and dairy products).

Soy Protein

Derived from soybeans and rich in cancer-fighting substances called *isoflavones* (most notably genistein), soy protein dramatically inhibits prostate cancer cell growth.[24] Soy's anticancer properties can be traced to its abilities to inhibit estrogen-mediated cell growth, block the activity of 5-alpha reductase and tyrosine-specific protein kinase, and reduce angiogenesis.

Providing up to 3 mg of isoflavones per gram, soy protein is available in a variety of food items, including tofu, tempeh, soy milk, soy cheese, textured soy foods, and soy flour. In addition, soy protein provides five times as much protein as wheat, and 25 times as much as beef.

For prostate cancer prevention, consume enough soy protein to yield at least 80 mg of genistein daily (approximately 4 oz).[25] Drinking soy milk can provide additional protection. According to one report, men who drank several glasses of soy milk daily lowered their risk of prostate cancer by 70%.[26]

Lycopene

Lycopene is a cancer-fighting antioxidant vitamin that gives tomatoes, strawberries, and watermelon their rosy color. Other natural sources of lycopene include apricots, pink grapefruit, and guava juice. According to one report, men who consumed tomato products four times weekly reduced their prostate cancer risk by 20%, and those who ate 10 or more helpings weekly reduced their risk by 45%.[27] Cooking tomatoes and adding a little olive oil improves lycopene absorption.

Fruits and Vegetables

Packed with cancer-fighting vitamins, minerals, and fiber, fruits and vegetables decrease prostate cancer risk.[28] In fact, more than 100 research studies have shown that eating cruciferous vegetables decreases overall cancer risk.[29] This explains why the National Cancer Institute recommends eating five to nine servings of fruits and vegetables daily. Unfortunately, only 9% of Americans heed their advice.

SUPPLEMENTS

Vitamin E (Mixed Tocopherols)

According to scientific research, vitamin E decreases prostate cancer incidence and mortality.[30] Researchers theorize that vitamin E prevents prostate cancer by inhibiting the accumulation of toxic hydrogen peroxide byproducts within the prostate.[31] Natural vitamin E (*d*-alpha tocopherol) is more bioavailable than the synthetic form (*dl*-alpha tocopherol). Furthermore, "mixed" tocopherols (alpha, beta, and gamma tocopherol) may confer additional protection. Men younger than 50 should take 400 IU daily with meals; those 50 and older should take 400 IU twice daily.

Selenium

According to researchers at MD Anderson Cancer Center, men who supplement their diet with 200 μg of selenium daily can reduce their prostate cancer risk by two thirds. Selenium also slows the promotion and progression stages of prostate cancer.[32]

A potent antioxidant, selenium teams up with *glutathione peroxidase* to convert hydrogen peroxide to water, instead of toxic hydroxyl radicals. Hydroxyl radicals hamper the immune system and stimulate prostate cancer cell growth.[33, 34] Prostate cancer cells are deficient in both selenium and glutathione peroxidase.

Selenium is derived from the soil; therefore, foods that are grown in selenium-deficient regions of the country (Pennsylvania, Ohio, the eastern two thirds of Washington State and Oregon, northern California, the Atlantic Coastal Plain, and the Upper Mississippi river valley) are lacking in this cancer-protective micronutrient. On the other hand, foods that are grown in the Northern Great Plains usually contain sufficient amounts of selenium.[35]

Men who live in selenium-deficient areas of the country should supplement their diets daily with 200 μg of yeast-derived selenium (selenomethionine or selenocysteine [contained in selenoglutathione or selenodiglutathione preparations] may be substituted if they are allergic to yeast).[36] When in doubt, check a serum selenium level; if it is 200 μg or higher, additional selenium is not needed.

BOTANICALS

Green Tea (*Camellia sinensis*)

Researchers theorize that antioxidants found in green tea called *catechins* prevent prostate cancer by preventing DNA strand breaks, inhibiting cell proliferation, decreasing the contact of carcinogens with cells, blocking cancer initiation, and slowing cancer progression.[37] Green tea's cancer protective benefit is dose related. Drink 3 to 5 cups of decaffeinated green tea daily for prevention, or if cancer is present, take a standardized green tea extract, 500 mg twice daily (equivalent to 9 cups of tea).

PC- SPES

PC-SPES (*PC* stands for "prostate cancer," and *SPES* is Latin for "hope") is a proprietary over-the-counter alternative cancer medication that contains eight different herbs: *Isatis indigotica* (da qing ye), *Glycyrrhiza glabra* and *Glycyrrhiza uralensis* (gan cao), *Panax pseudoginseng* (san qi), *Ganoderma lucidum* (ling zhi, reishi), *Scutellaria baicalensis* (huang qin), *Denodrantherma (Chrysanthemum) morifolium*, *Rhabdosia rubescens*, and *Serenoa repens* (saw palmetto).[38] Although the exact mechanism of PC-SPES is unclear, researchers theorize that, by working synergistically, the herbs within PC-SPES inhibit angiogenesis, stimulate the immune system, induce an estrogenic effect, and inhibit 5-alpha reductase.[39] PC-SPES has been shown to prevent the promotion and progression of both androgen-sensitive and androgen-insensitive prostate cancer.[40]

Dosage must be individualized. The normal dose is six to nine 320-mg capsules daily. Because insurance doesn't cover the cost of PC-SPES, depending on the dosage, the out-of-pocket cost ranges between $300 and $400 monthly. Although not specified by the manufacturer, PC-SPES can cause a variety of adverse effects, some of which can be life threatening. These include skin rash, nausea, impotence, breast tenderness, fluid retention, and blood clots, including pulmonary embolus.[41]

PHARMACEUTICALS

Although results are still pending, a 10-year multicenter prospective trial is under way to determine whether finasteride (Proscar) can prevent prostate cancer.

Although not curative, androgen deprivation therapy (luteinizing hormone–releasing hormone agonists and/or antiandrogens) is used to treat men with metastatic prostate cancer. These medications can cause a variety of untoward effects such as anemia, hot flashes, fatigue, mood swings, liver damage, and osteoporosis. Integrative therapies can ameliorate some of these distressing adverse effects.

For instance, the risk of developing osteoporosis can be lessened by exercising regularly, making dietary modifications (eliminating junk food, refined sugar, red meat, dairy, caffeine, alcohol, and excess salt), eating soy protein, eliminating tobacco products, and taking a high-potency multivitamin.

Medication-induced liver damage can be reduced by avoiding acetaminophen and alcohol plus taking α-lipoic acid (300 mg), *N*-acetyl-L-cysteine (500 mg), and milk thistle *(Silybum marianum),* 150 mg daily.

Hot flashes can be reduced by eliminating bad habits (e.g., smoking, drinking alcohol, and consuming caffeinated beverages and foods), exercising regularly, eating soy protein, taking selective herbs (40 drops of a standardized extract of Chasteberry *[Vitex Angus-castus],* dong quai *[Angelica sinensis],* and damiana *[Turnera diffusa]* twice daily), taking vitamin E 400 IU daily and vitamin B complex 50 mg twice daily, and undergoing acupuncture.

MIND–BODY MEDICINE

Psychosocial interventions can improve the quality of life for cancer patients and significantly prolong survival. According to one study, men who were taught new coping skills (mental relaxation and imagery techniques, stress management, ways to develop self-esteem and spirituality, receptive imagery/intuition and problem solving, and how to create a personal health plan/goal) lived twice as long as men in the control group.[42]

PREVENTION PRESCRIPTION

- *For men at high risk, perform a digital rectal examination and PSA yearly after age 40.*
- *For men at normal risk, discuss the pros and cons of PSA screening and provide information on prostate cancer prevention.*
- *Encourage exercise for 30 minutes or longer at least three times weekly.*
- *Avoid hormone-altering medications such as DHEA, androstenedione, human growth hormone, and testosterone, unless medically indicated.*
- *Instruct patients to buy organic produce whenever possible. Wash all produce and peel when applicable. Drink filtered water, and cook and store food in glass containers.*
- *Advise patients to reduce or eliminate dairy and meat consumption.*
- *Instruct patients to use olive or canola oil instead of other vegetable oils.*
- *Emphasize that patients should avoid tobacco products and excessive alcohol consumption.*

PREVENTION PRESCRIPTION   *continued*

- *Teach patients to drink soy milk and eat at least 4 oz of soy protein daily.*
- *Encourage intake of 5 to 9 servings of fruits and vegetables daily.*
- *Instruct patients to drink 3 to 5 cups of decaffeinated green tea daily for prevention, or to take a standardized green tea extract, 500 mg, twice daily if prostate cancer is present.*
- *Advise patients to take vitamin E (mixed tocopherols), 400 IU, daily with meals for men younger than 50, and 800 IU daily for men 50 and older.*
- *Suggest that patients take 200 µg daily of yeast-derived selenium.*

Resources

Organizations

American Foundation for Urologic Disease (AFUD), 300 W. Pratt St., Suite 401, Baltimore, MD 21201; (800) 242-2383.

CaP Cure, 1250 Fourth St., Suite 360, Santa Monica, CA 90401; (310) 458-2873.

Prostate Cancer Research Institute, 5777 W. Century Boulevard, Suite 885, Los Angeles, CA 90045; (310) 743-2116.

US-TOO Prostate Cancer Survivor Support Groups, 930 N. York Rd., Suite 50, Hinsdale, IL 60521-2993; (630) 323-1002.

Internet Web Sites

CancerNet @ http://cancernet.nci.nih.gov/

American Foundation for Urologic Disease (AFUD) @ http://www.afud.org/

CaP Cure @ http://www.capcure.org

National Cancer Institute (NCI) @ http://www.nci.nih.gov

Prostate Cancer Infolink @ http://www.comed.com/prostate

Prostate Forum @ http://www.prostateforum.com/

Prostate Cancer Research Institute @ http://www.prostate-cancer.org

Newsletters

Prostate Forum Newsletter, P.O. Box 6696, Charlottesville, VA 22906; (800) 305-2432.

PCRInsights, Prostate Cancer Research Institute, 5777 W. Century Boulevard, Suite 885, Los Angeles CA 90045; (310) 743-2116.

Books and Booklets

Nutrition & Prostate Cancer: A Monograph from the CaP CURE Nutrition Project. CaP Cure, 1250 Fourth St., Suite 360, Santa Monica, CA 90401; (310) 458-2873.

Prostate Cancer Resource Guide. American Foundation for Urologic Disease (AFUD), 300 W. Pratt St., Suite 401, Baltimore, MD 21201; (800) 242-2383.

Myers CE, Steck SS, Myers RS: *Eating Your Way to Better Health: The Prostate Forum Nutrition Guide.* Charlottesville, VA, Rivanna Health Publications, Inc, 2000.

Oesterling JE, Moyad MA: *The ABCs of Prostate Cancer.* NY, Madison Books, 1997.

Kirby RS, Christmas TJ, Brawer M: *Prostate Cancer.* London, UK, Times Mirror International Publishers, Ltd, 1996.

Phillips RH: *Coping With Prostate Cancer.* Garden City Park, NY, Avery Publishing Group, 1994.

McClure MW: *Smart Medicine for a Healthy Prostate.* NY, Avery Publishing Group, 2001.

References

1. Myers CE Jr (ed): *Prostate Forum Newsletter,* November 1996:1–2.
2. Margolis S, Samet JM: The Johns Hopkins White Papers, Early Detection and Prevention of Cancer. New York, Medletter Assoc, Inc, 1998, p 34.
3. Carter HS, et al: Mendelian inheritance of familial prostate cancer. Proc Natl Acad Sci, 1992, pp 3367–3371.
4. Myers CE Jr (ed): *Prostate Forum Newsletter,* June 1996:1.
5. Richie JP: Screening for prostate cancer: Why the controversy? Contemp Urol 10:31, 1998.
6. Richie JP: Contemp Urol 10:31, 1998.
7. Morgan TO, et al: Age-specific ranges for serum prostatic-specific antigen in black men. N Engl J Med 335:304, 1996.
8. Oesterling JE, et al: Serum prostate-specific antigen in a community-based population of healthy men: Establishment of age-specific reference ranges. JAMA 270:860, 1993.
9. Catalona WJ, et al: Use of percentage of free prostate-specific antigen to enhance differentiation of prostate cancer from benign prostatic disease. JAMA 279:1542–1547, 1998.
10. Whittemore AS, et al: Prostate cancer in relation to diet, physical activity, and body size in blacks, whites and Asians in the United States and Canada. J Natl Cancer Inst 87:652–661, 1995.
11. Simone CB: Cancer and Nutrition, A Ten-Point Plan to Reduce Your Risk of Getting Cancer. Garden City Park, NJ, Avery Publishing Group, Inc, 1994, p 148.
12. Kerr RR (ed): In Brief. *Urology Times*, August 2000:3.
13. Robbins J: Diet for a New America, How Your Food Choices Affect Your Health, Happiness and the Future of Life on Earth. Walpole, NH, StillPoint Publ, 1987, pp 315, 331, 343.
14. Putnam SD, et al: Lifestyle and anthropometric risk factors for prostate cancer in a cohort of Iowa men. Ann Epidemiol 10:361–369, 2000.
15. Margolis S, Carter HB: The Johns Hopkins White Papers, Prostate Disorders. New York, Medletter Assoc, Inc, 1998, p 28.
16. Giovannucci E, et al: A prospective study of dietary fat and risk of prostate cancer. J Natl Cancer Inst 85:1571–1579, 1993.
17. Gillenwater JY, et al (eds): Adult and Pediatric Urology, 3rd ed. St. Louis, Mosby-Year Book, Inc, 1996, p 1577.
18. Myers CE, Steck SS, Myers RS: Eating Your Way to Better Health: The Prostate Forum Nutrition Guide. Charlottesville, VA, Rivanna Health Publications, Inc, 2000, pp 15–16.
19. Myers CE, Steck SS, Myers RS: Eating Your Way to Better Health: The Prostate Forum Nutrition Guide. Charlottesville, VA, Rivanna Health Publications, Inc, 2000, p 16.
20. Giovannucci E, et al: A prospective study of dietary fat and risk of prostate cancer. J Natl Cancer Inst 85:1571–1579, 1993.
21. Chan JM, et al: Plasma insulin-like growth factor-1 and prostate cancer risk: A prospective study. Science 279:563–566, 1998.
22. Miyake H, et al: Elevation of serum levels of urokinase-type plasminogen activator and its receptor associated with disease progression and prognosis in patients with prostate cancer. Prostate 39:123–129, 1999.
23. Nakao-Hayashi J, et al: Stimulatory effects of insulin and insulin-like growth factor 1 on migration and tube formation by vascular endothelial cells. Atherosclerosis 92:141–149, 1999.
24. Fair WR, Fleshner NE, Heston W: Cancer of the prostate: A nutritional disease? Urology 50:843, 1997.
25. Myers CE, Steck SS, Myers RS: Eating Your Way To Better Health: The Prostate Forum Nutrition Guide. Charlottesville, VA, Rivanna Health Publications, Inc, 2000, p 46.
26. Jacobsen BK, Knutsen SF, Fraser GE: Does high soy milk intake reduce prostate cancer incidence? The Adventist Health Study (United States). Cancer Causes Control 9:553–557, 1998.
27. Giovannucci E, et al: Intake of carotenoids and retinol in relation to risk of prostate cancer. J Natl Cancer Inst 87:1767–1776, 1995.
28. Hirayama R: Epidemiology of prostate cancer with special reference to the role of diet. NCI Monograph 53:149–155, 1979.
29. Fahey JW, Talalay P: The role of crucifers in cancer chemoprotection. In Gustine DL, Flores HE (eds): Phytochemicals and Health. American Society of Plant Physiologists, 1995, p 88.
30. Heinonen OP, et al: Prostate cancer and supplementation with

alpha-tocopherol and beta-carotene: Incidence and mortality in a controlled trial. J Natl Cancer Inst 90:440–446, 1998.
31. Myers CE Jr (ed): *Prostate Forum Newsletter*, June 1998:3–4.
32. Clark LC, et al: Effects of selenium supplementation for cancer prevention in patients with carcinoma of the skin. JAMA 276:1957–1963, 1996.
33. Myers CE Jr (ed): *Prostate Forum Newsletter*, November 1997:5.
34. Baker AM, et al: Expression of antioxidant enzymes in human prostatic adenocarcinoma. Prostate 32:229–233, 1997.
36. Myers CE, Steck SS, Myers RS: Eating Your Way To Better Health: The Prostate Forum Nutrition Guide. Charlottesville, VA, Rivanna Health Publications, Inc, 2000, p 28.
36. Myers CE Jr (ed): *Prostate Forum Newsletter*, January 2000:7.
37. Smith TJ, et al: How can carcinogenesis be inhibited? Ann NY Acad Sci 768:82–90, 1995.
38. Lewis J: The Herbal Remedy for Prostate Cancer. Westbury, NY, Health Education Literary Publisher, 1999, pp 34–37.
39. Halicka HD, et al: Apoptosis and cell cycle effects induced by extracts of the Chinese herbal preparation PC SPES. Int J Oncol 11:437–448, 1997.
40. Small EJ, et al: Prospective trial of the herbal supplement PC-SPES in patients with progressive prostate cancer. J Clin Oncol 18:3595–3603, 2000.
41. Small: Prospective Trial of the Herbal Supplement PC-SPES in Patients With Progressive Prostate Cancer, 3599–3600.
42. Shrock D, Palmer RF, Taylor B: Effects of a psychosocial intervention on survival among patients with stage 1 breast and prostate cancer: A matched case-control study. Altern Ther Health Med 5:49–55, 1999.

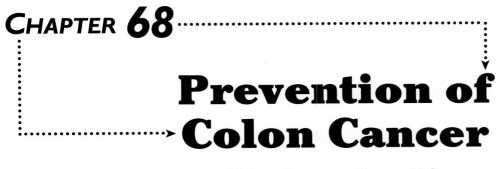

CHAPTER 68

Prevention of Colon Cancer

Melissa Constance Young, M.D.

ETIOLOGY

The majority of colorectal cancers arise from adenomatous polyps. Progression from normal colonic mucosa to adenomatous polyp to invasive cancer often takes a decade or more. Although hereditary factors clearly play a role, it is estimated that 75% of cases of colorectal cancer are a result of dietary and life style factors that can be modified. Researchers continue to explore the role of chemopreventive agents in combating the development of colorectal cancer and adenomas.

RISK FACTORS

The following risk factors for the development of colon cancer have been identified:

- Family history of colorectal cancer or polyps in a first-degree relative (a brother, sister, mother, or father) younger than 60 years of age, or in two first-degree relatives of any age
- Family history of colorectal cancer syndromes (familial adenomatous polyposis and hereditary nonpolyposis colon cancer)
- Personal history of ovarian, endometrial, or breast cancer
- Personal history of chronic ulcerative colitis or Crohn's colitis
- Obesity (abdominal)
- Smoking
- Sedentary lifestyle

> ### NOTE
>
> *It is estimated that 75% of cases of colorectal cancer are a result of dietary and life style factors that can be modified.*

SCREENING

Up to 90% of colorectal cancers are curable if detected and treated early. Regular screening is a key aspect of colon cancer prevention. There is a wide range of effective screening recommendations that include fecal occult blood testing (FOBT), sigmoidoscopy, barium enema, and colonoscopy. Physicians should determine the best screening procedures for each patient on the basis of individual risk factors and accepted screening recommendations. Colonoscopy is generally recommended for people of any age who are at higher-than-average risk for the development of colorectal cancer.

Guidelines for screening differ somewhat between professional organizations. The American Cancer Society and the National Cancer Institute recommend annual digital rectal examinations for all adults beginning at age 40 years and two tests for average risk persons beginning at age 50: annual FOBT with rehydration and flexible sigmoidoscopy every 3 to 5 years. In addition, colonoscopy is recommended for high-risk persons. The American

Table 68–1. Screening Recommendations for Colon Cancer

Patient Group	Age (yr)	Test
Asymptomatics	40	DRE, FOBT annually
Normal risk	50	DRE, FOBT annually
		Flexible sigmoidoscopy every 3–5 years, *or*
		Flexible sigmoidoscopy and double-contact barium enema every 3–5 years, *or*
		Colonoscopy every 10 years
High risk	35–40, or 10 years younger than age at diagnosis of youngest affected family member	DRE, FOBT annually *and/or*
		Flexible sigmoidoscopy or colonoscopy every 3–5 years.
Family history of familial adenomatous polyposis	10–12	Flexible sigmoidoscopy every 3–5 years

DRE, digital rectal examination; FOBT, fecal occult blood testing.

Gastroenterological Association and the American Society for Gastrointestinal Endoscopy concur. The American College of Obstetricians and Gynecologists suggests FOBT for all women 40 years and older as part of their annual examination.

The World Health Organization recommends starting at age 50 with annual FOBT and DRE, plus flexible sigmoidoscopy every 3 to 5 years, with colonoscopy following positive results on FOBT. For high-risk patients, annual FOBT and/or DRE and flexible sigmoidoscopy or colonoscopy every 3 to 5 years beginning at age 35 to 40 is recommended. Flexible sigmoidoscopy beginning at age 10 to 12 years is recommended for patients with familial adenomatous polyposis.

INTEGRATIVE APPROACH TO PREVENTION

Lifestyle Interventions

Body Mass Index

In the Health Professionals Follow-up Study of 47,723 men, body mass index (BMI) was shown to have a direct association with colon cancer risk independent of physical activity level. In particular, waist circumference and waist-to-hip ratio (an indicator of abdominal fat) were shown to be strongly associated with risk for colon cancer.[1]

In another study of 6000 older persons, researchers at the University of Pittsburgh found that abdominal fat doubled the risk of colon cancer in both men and women. As with physical inactivity, abdominal fat has been linked to increased insulin production and may promote tumor growth in the colon.[2]

Patients should be counseled to maintain a healthy body weight, within the standard weight guidelines for adults, with a BMI between 19 and 25, through combined diet and exercise. Weight gain during adulthood should be avoided.

Smoking Cessation

A recent 14-year study of more than 1 million adults shows strong evidence linking cigarette smoking and colorectal adenomatous polyps. Mortality rates from colorectal cancer were highest among current smokers and people who smoked for more than 20 years. The study also showed that among people who stopped smoking, mortality rates at 20 years were about the same as in people who had never smoked.[3]

Patients should be counseled to stop smoking. Regular screening for current and former smokers should be encouraged.

Alcohol

Case-control studies suggest a positive correlation between alcohol consumption and increased risk of colorectal cancer. Alcohol can lower levels of folic acid, a B vitamin that may help protect against damage to DNA and prevent polyp formation, and methionine, an amino acid that may block carcinogenesis.[4]

Patients should be counseled to limit alcohol consumption to two drinks a day in men and one in women. Folic acid supplementation in doses of 400 to 800 μg in persons who continue to drink is recommended. High-risk patients should consider abstaining from alcohol.

Exercise

A sedentary life style has been shown to be associated with increased risk of colorectal cancer. Studies have shown up to a 50% reduction in incidence of colon cancer in men and women who are physically active, independent of other risk factors such as diet and body weight.[5] Exercise may also favorably modify certain risk factors for colon cancer such as increased BMI, insulin resistance, and prostaglandin levels. An epidemiologic study in more than 4000 adults reported that people who were getting the most exercise had less than half the incidence of colon cancer of those getting little or no exercise.[6]

A study in Chinese men and women in western North America and China showed an elevation of colorectal cancer risk among men employed in sedentary occupations in both continents.[7]

Patients should be advised to engage in moderate to vigorous exercise of at least 30 minutes' duration for a minimum of 5 days a week (see Chapter 86, Writing an Exercise Prescription).

Nutrition

Several dietary modifications constitute an important aspect of colon cancer prevention.
- **Decrease consumption of red meat and animal fat.**
  Many studies show an association between consumption of red meat and an increased risk of colon cancer. In a prospective risk assessment study of 47,949 male health professionals in the United States, researchers found an elevated risk of colon cancer with meat consumption 5 or more times a week, in comparison with meat consumption less than once a month.[8]

  The Nurses' Health Study found that an increased incidence of colon cancer was associated with consumption of red meat and fat from animal sources.[9] The etiology of this association is unclear. Many studies show an increased risk of colon cancer with high intake of processed meats and with degree of "doneness" of the meat.[10] Processed meats and overcooked meat contain levels of carcinogenic compounds. Some persons may also be more susceptible genetically to these chemicals.[11] Another possible etiologic factor is the kind of fats found in meat.[12]

Meat eaters should limit intake to one serving of meat a day while increasing protein from other sources including fish, soy, and beans. Limiting meat intake to only several times a month is recommended.

- **Increase intake of fruits and vegetables.**

Numerous studies have shown diets high in fruit and vegetable intake to be associated with lowered risk of common cancers.[13] Fiber, vitamins, and antioxidants such as vitamin E, vitamin C, and beta-carotene have been proposed to have protective effects. It is unclear whether one substance in particular is the effective agent. It is also unclear whether an isolated single agent is protective, rather than consumption of a varied diet rich in whole foods.[14] Studies assessing the role of supplemental antioxidants in prevention of primary and secondary colorectal cancer have not shown clear benefit.

A varied intake of at least 5 to 7 servings of fruits and vegetables a day is recommended.

- **Decrease intake of simple sugars.**

Simple sugars are broken down quickly and easily in the body, leading to increased levels of glucose and insulin. Preliminary studies have shown an associated risk between increased sugar intake and risk for colon cancer. It is unclear whether this is a direct effect or may be an indicator of the need for life style and dietary changes.

Intake of simple carbohydrates, which include sugar (sucrose) and products made with "white" flour such as breads and pasta, should be decreased. Whole grains should be substituted as much as possible.

- **Increase dietary fiber.**

Results of studies on the role of fiber in the prevention of colorectal cancer are conflicting. Many mechanisms for the role of fiber in decreasing the risk of colorectal cancer have been proposed. Fiber may bind to bile acids that can irritate and damage the cells lining the colon or to carcinogens in the bowel lumen, thereby facilitating their elimination. The results of the Polyp Prevention Trial did not show that a diet high in fiber, fruit, and vegetables and low in fat prevented recurrence of colorectal adenomas.[15] Another recent study failed to show that a randomized trial of fiber supplementation protected against recurrence of colorectal adenomas.[16]

In contrast, initial (unpublished) results from the European Prospective Investigation of Cancer Study (EPIC) of over half a million people in 10 European countries show a strong protective effect of dietary fiber on colorectal cancer prevention. It was found that persons at lowest risk for colon cancer ate an average of 50% more fiber than persons at highest risk.

Although current recommendations do not include increased dietary or supplemental fiber for colorectal cancer prevention, the debate is ongoing. A high-fiber diet clearly has other important health benefits and may be protective in colorectal cancer. Thus, a diet high in fiber, fruits, vegetables, and whole grains is recommended.

Supplements

Folic Acid

Studies show an inverse relationship between the incidence of colon cancer and dietary intake of folate. In the Nurses' Health Study in nearly 90,000 nurses, women who took a daily multivitamin with 400 μg of folate over a 15-year period showed a 75% decrease in risk of colon cancer.[17] It is thought that the folate exerts its protective effect by reducing damage to DNA.

Dosage. 400 μg of folic acid daily. This dose is found in most multivitamins. Folate is also abundant in green leafy vegetables such as spinach, kale, and chard. Other sources include legumes, especially lentils, and broccoli, cabbage, and whole grains.

Precautions. Elevated serum folate levels may be associated with altered sleep patterns, irritability, vivid dreaming, lower seizure threshold, nausea, flatulence, and zinc depletion.

Calcium

Most human studies show an inverse relationship between calcium supplementation or high-calcium diets and the risk of colorectal cancer or colorectal adenomas. One large study showed a decreased risk of adenomatous polyps in people who took 1200 mg of supplemental calcium.[18] It is thought that calcium may bind to bile acids and fatty acids in the bowel lumen, thus decreasing proliferation of colonic epithelial cells and tumor formation.

Dosage. 1200 mg of supplemental calcium a day. Calcium citrate has been found to be best absorbed from the gastrointestinal tract, but most studies have used calcium carbonate, which is generally cheaper. The citrate form is best for patients older than 65 years of age.

Precautions. Oral calcium can cause constipation and gastrointestinal irritation.

Probiotics

Lactobacillus and *Bifidus* species are the "good" or beneficial bacteria that live in the colon. By producing lactic acid and hydrogen peroxide they inhibit the growth of "bad" bacteria. Several studies suggest that administration of bifidobacteria or lactobacilli alone can alter colonic microflora populations to decrease early preneoplastic lesions and tumors.[19] These probiotics are also being studied for their potential in inhibiting an enzyme activated by fatty foods that is thought to trigger malignant changes potentially leading to colon cancer.

Probiotics may be beneficial in high-fat diets but further research is needed.

Dosage. A supplement should contain at least 1 billion organisms and should be taken on an empty stomach.

A product called Culturelle provides viable *Lactobacillus* GG. It may be obtained on the producer's Web site: www.culturelle.com. The usual dose is 1 capsule daily (see Chapter 97, Prescribing Probiotics).

Precautions. Long-term use of these supplements needs further study. Probiotics may best be used after proper evaluation of the intestinal flora of the patient. Probiotics should be avoided in immune-compromised patients.

Pharmaceuticals

Aspirin and Other Nonsteroidal Anti-Inflammatory Drugs

It is thought that acetylsalicylic acid (ASA) and other nonsteroidal anti-inflammatory drugs (NSAIDs) may prevent tumor formation and growth by inhibiting prostaglandins. Experiments have shown that large amounts of prostaglandins, particularly prostaglandin E$_2$, are produced by colonic tumor cells.[20] Aspirin and other NSAIDs inhibit cyclo-oxygenase-1 (COX-1) and cyclo-oxygenase-2 (COX-2), enzymes involved in prostaglandin synthesis. Of particular interest, COX-2 expression has been shown to be elevated in up to 90% of sporadic colon carcinomas and in 40% of colonic adenomas but is not elevated in normal colonic epithelium.[21] Epidemiologic studies have reported decreased incidence of colon cancer with regular aspirin use. In an American Cancer Society study in over 600,000 people, the mortality rate was 40% lower for colorectal cancer in regular aspirin users.[22] Another prospective study also found a lower mortality rate with regular aspirin use.[23]

Patients with a family history of colorectal cancer or other risk factors should discuss aspirin/NSAID therapy with their doctor.

Dosage. The therapeutic dose to obtain benefit but minimize potential toxicity is unclear. In high-risk patients, one 325-mg tablet daily or every other day is recommended.

Precautions. Aspirin and the other NSAIDs should be avoided in patients with a history of gastric reflux or ulcer disease.

In addition, substances known to increase prostaglandins, such as evening primrose oil, borage oil, and black currant oil, should be avoided (see Chapter 84, The Anti-Inflammatory Diet).

Hormone Replacement Therapy

There is increasing evidence that hormone replacement therapy (HRT) reduces the risk of colorectal cancer in women. A Harvard study found a 20% lower incidence of colon cancer in postmenopausal women who had used HRT compared with women who had never used it. This association was strongest among women currently taking HRT.[24] Researchers postulate that estrogen decreases both bile acid production and levels of insulin-like growth factor, a hormone that has been associated with colon cancer.

Postmenopausal women considering HRT should be informed of the possible protective effects in colorectal cancer. However, HRT should be recommended only to a patient considering HRT for other reasons such as relief of postmenopausal symptoms and prevention of osteoporosis. The risks and benefits of therapy should be assessed on an individual basis.

―PREVENTION PRESCRIPTION―

- *Regular screening for colorectal cancer in average-risk patients after age 40 according to guidelines, with earlier screening in high-risk patients according to individual risk*
- *Maintainenance of a healthy weight and avoidance of excess weight gain in adulthood*
- *Incorporation of moderate to vigorous exercise into daily routine*
- *Limited alcohol consumption and use of tobacco products*
- *A diet low in animal fat, with intake of red meat limited to no more than 3 ounces a day*
- *Consumption of no more than 25% of calories from fat*
- *At least 5 to 7 servings of fruits and vegetables every day, selected from a wide variety of colors and types and including leafy green vegetables and legumes (beans and lentils) for folate content*
- *Decreased intake of simple carbohydrates including sugar, white bread, pasta, and processed products made with white flour*

PREVENTION PRESCRIPTION *continued*

- *Increased intake of fiber to at least 25 g a day in the form of whole grains, legumes, fruits, and vegetables for overall health*
- *A calcium-rich and calcium-fortified diet, supplemented with calcium for a total of 1200 mg a day*
- *Folate supplementation in a dose of 400 µg daily*
- *Aspirin 325 mg a day may be beneficial in high-risk patients.*

Resources

Further Information

http://cancer.med.upenn.edu A cancer-oriented Web server containing links to other oncology centers in the world.

http://ontumor.com/colorectal.htm A cancer-oriented Web server containing links to other oncology centers in the country.

http://cancer.org The American Cancer Institute Web site.

http://clinicaltrials.gov/ct/gui A comprehensive summary of clinical trials including colon cancer.

References

1. Giovannucci E, Ascherio A, Rimm EB, et al: Physical activity, obesity, and risk of colon cancer and adenoma in men. Ann Intern Med 122:327–334, 1995.
2. Schoen RE, Tangen CM, Kuller LH, et al: Increased blood glucose and insulin, body size, and incident colorectal cancer. J Natl Cancer Inst 91:1147–1154, 1999.
3. Chao A, Thun MJ, Jacobs EJ, et al: Cigarette smoking and colorectal cancer mortality in the Cancer Prevention Study II. J Natl Cancer Inst 92:1888–1896, 2000.
4. Giovannucci E, Stampfer MJ, Colditz GA, et al: Folate, methionine, and alcohol intake and the risk of colorectal adenoma. J Natl Cancer Inst 85:875–884, 1993.
5. Colditz GA, Cannusciocc CC, Frazier AL: Physical activity and reduced risk of colon cancer: implications for prevention. Cancer Causes Control 8:649–667, 1997.
6. Slattery ML, Edwards SL, Boucher KM, et al: Lifestyle and colon cancer: An assessment of factors associated with risk. Am J Epidemiol 150:869–877, 1999.
7. Whittmore AS, Wu-Williams AH, Lee M, et al: Diet, physical activity, and colorectal cancer among Chinese in North America and China. J Natl Cancer Inst 882:915–926, 1990.
8. Giovannucci E, Rimm EB, Stampfer MJ, et al: Intake of fat, meat, and fiber in relation to risk of colon cancer in men. Cancer Res 54:2390–2397, 1994.
9. Willet WC, Stampfer MJ, Colditz GA, et al: Relationship of meat, fat, and fiber intake to the risk of colon cancer in a prospective study among women. N Engl J Med 323:1664–1672, 1900.
10. Sinha R, Chow WH, Kulldorf M, et al. Well done grilled red meat increases the risk of colorectal adenoma. Cancer Res 59:4320–4324, 1999.
11. Vieneis P, McMichael A: Interplay between heterocyclic amines in cooked meat and metabolic phenotype in the etiology of colon cancer. Cancer Causes Control 7:479–486, 1996.
12. Willet WC: Diet and cancer. Oncologist 5:393–404, 2000.
13. Block G, Patterson B, Subar A: Fruit, vegetables, and cancer prevention: A review of the epidemiological evidence. Nutr Cancer 18:1–29, 1992.
14. Greenberg RE, Baron JA, Tosteson TD, et al: A clinical trial of antioxidant vitamins to prevent colorectal adenoma. N Engl J Med 331:141–147, 1994.
15. Schatzkin A, Lanza E, Corle D, et al: Lack of effect of low-fat, high-fiber on the recurrence of colorectal adenomas. N Engl J Med 342:1149–1155, 2000.
16. Alberts DS, Martinez ME, Roe DJ, et al: Lack of effect of high-fiber cereal supplement on the recurrence of colorectal adenomas. N Engl J Med 342:1156–1162, 2000.
17. Giovannucci E, Stampfer MJ, Colditz GA, et al: Multivitamin use, folate, and colon cancer in women in the Nurses' Health Study. Ann Intern Med 129:517–524, 1998.
18. Baron JA, Beach M, Mandel JS, et al: Calcium supplements for the prevention of colorectal adenomas. N Engl J Med 340:101–107, 1999.
19. Wollowski I, Rechkemmer G, Ool-Zobel BL: Protective role of probiotics and prebiotics in colon cancer. Am J Clin Nutr 73:451S-455S, 2001.
20. Garay CA, Engstrom F: Chemoprevention of colorectal cancer: Dietary and pharmacological approaches. Oncology 13:89–105, 1999.
21. Janne A, Mayer RJ: Chemoprevention of colorectal cancer. N Engl J Med 342:1960–1968, 2000.
22. Thun MJ, Namboordiri M, Heath CW: Aspirin use and reduced risk of fatal colon cancer. N Engl J Med 325:1593–1596, 1991.
23. Giovannucci E, Egan KM, Hunter DJ, et al: Aspirin and the risk of colorectal cancer in women. N Engl J Med 333:609–614, 1995.
24. Grodstein F, Newcomb A, Stamfer MJ: Postmenopausal hormone therapy and the risk of colorectal cancer: A review and meta-analysis. Am J Med 106:574–582, 1999.

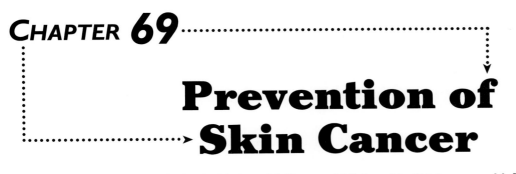

CHAPTER 69

Prevention of Skin Cancer

Wadie I. Najm, M.D., and Vivian M. Dickerson, M.D.

Skin cancer can be divided into two major groups: melanoma and nonmelanoma skin cancer (NMSC). Melanoma is a tumor derived from melanocytes in the basal layer of the epidermis. The incidence of melanoma varies in different populations. Whites have a higher (10-fold) incidence than nonwhites. NMSC encompasses different types of cancer, the two most common types being basal and squamous cell carcinomas. Basal cell carcinoma (BCC), the most common type of skin cancer, arises from basal cells found in the outer layer of the skin. Squamous cell carcinoma (SCC), the second most common type of skin cancer, originates from scaly cells on the surface of the skin. It is estimated that the incidence of nonmelanoma skin cancer is approximately equal to the combined incidence of all cancers.

ETIOLOGY

Skin cancer can occur in any individual. Exposure to ultraviolet light (UV) and sunburn increase the

Table 69–1. Risk Factors Associated with Malignant Melanoma

A multivariate analysis identified the following as independent risk factors that increase the incidence of malignant melanoma:

- Family history of malignant melanoma (first-degree relative)
- Having red or blond hair
- Marked freckles on upper back
- Three or more blistering sunburns before 20 years of age
- Three or more years of summer jobs during teenage years
- Actinic keratosis

Environment Factors
- Living near the equator
- Outdoor recreational habit
- Working outdoors

Phenotypic Factors
- Blue or green eyes
- Light complexion
- Inability to tan
- Blond or red hair
- Freckles
- Sun sensitivity

From Evans RD, Kopf AW, Lew RA, et al: Risk factors for the development of malignant melanoma: Review of case-control studies. J Dermatol Surg Oncol 14:393-408, 1988.

incidence of all skin cancers (Table 69–1). Approximately 90% of NMSC can be attributed to UV exposure.

SCREENING

The American Cancer Society screening guidelines recommend a regular skin self-examination for all adults. Pamphlets for self-examination of the skin are available from the American Cancer Society, the American Academy of Dermatology, and the Skin Cancer Foundation.

Clinical examination of the skin should be done annually, particularly for individuals at high risk.

People considered at high risk are those with a family history of skin cancer or melanoma; those with a personal history of skin cancer or precancer; and those with a high number of melanocytic nevi, xeroderma pigmentosum, and basal cell nevus syndrome.

Recognize early melanoma using the **ABCD** screening guideline:

Asymmetry
Border irregularity
Color variegation
Diameter greater than 6 mm

LIFESTYLE

The depletion of the ozone layer has increased peoples' exposure to ultraviolet light. To protect themselves, people should wear protective clothing; avoid acute exposure to sunlight, particularly at midday; and apply a broad-spectrum, high sun protection factor (SPF) sunscreen. These precautions are not limited to sunny days; the sun's rays can penetrate light clouds and mist, and they are reflected by snow (85%) and water (5%). Multiday exposure to sunlight significantly increases sensitivity of the skin to sun damage on the second day, particularly in susceptible individuals. When such exposure occurs, application of higher SPF sunscreen (30) is recommended. A major portion of UV exposure is received during childhood and adolescence; therefore, application of sunscreen during this time reduces considerably the incidence of NMSC. It should be cautioned that application of sunscreen may cause subjects to feel protected; hence, they may spend a longer period of time exposed to the sun and develop a higher risk of skin cancer.[3] Sunscreen should be reapplied every 2 hours if subjects decide to prolong their sun exposure.

NUTRITION

Dietary Fat

Preliminary studies in the early 1980s reported a possible association of fat intake with incidence of melanoma. Although this initial work was based mainly on a dietary questionnaire, a follow-up study indicated a higher content of polyunsaturated fat in the adipose tissue of subjects who developed melanoma compared with controls.[3] Studies on the effect of fat intake on nonmelanoma skin cancer reported a similar association between fat intake and the incidence of new cancer. Reduction of fat intake (but not total calories) decreased the incidence of new actinic keratosis (premalignant lesions) compared with a control group.[4]

Garlic and Onion

Garlic and onion oils were found to decrease the number of skin tumors in an animal study. Diallyl sulfide (DAS), a component of garlic, applied topically 1 hour before or after exposure to carcinogens, delays the onset of tumors and confers significant protection from skin carcinogenesis.[5] Translation of these results into human prevention studies is lacking.

Fish and Fish Oil

One study reported the protective effect of a diet rich in fish, suggesting a possible role for fish oil in the prevention of melanoma.[6]

Botanicals

Green Tea

Several animal studies investigating the oral and topical application of green tea to prevent skin cancer have suggested that green tea may reduce the risk of skin cancer induction in humans by UV radiation.[7] A randomized study is currently under way to evaluate the efficacy of green tea extract *Epigallocatechin gallate* (polyphenon E topical oil) in treating patients with actinic keratosis.

Panax Ginseng

Animal studies indicate a dose-dependent inhibitory effect on skin cancer, prolonging the latency and reducing the tumor number.

Thuja Standishii

Labdane diterpnoids, derived from the stem bark of *Thuja standishii* (Japanese name: Kurobe) and from marine sources have been found to demonstrate a variety of types of bioactivity, such as anti-inflammatory, antibacterial, antifungal, antileishmanial, cardiotonic, and cytotoxic activities.[9] A two-stage mouse skin carcinogenesis study reported an inhibitory effect on TPA-induced tumor promotion.[10] A potential role in the prevention or treatment of human skin cancer is yet to be established.

Supplements

Selenium

Despite early indications of a possible role of selenium in the prevention of skin cancers, randomized studies on the use of selenium for melanoma and nonmelanoma skin cancers do not show a protective effect.[8]

Beta-Carotene

Animal studies point to an inhibitory role of beta-carotene in UV-induced skin cancer. In addition, an inverse relationship between the level of serum beta-carotene and the incidence of skin cancer was noted.[11]

Nonmelanoma skin cancer: In large clinical trial, the protective effect of beta-carotene was not supported.[12]

Melanoma: High levels of retinol and carotenoids were not found to have a protective effect.[13]

Vitamin E

Animal studies indicate a possible protective effect of vitamin E. The effect was noted to be greater in vivo than in vitro. Vitamin E had a strong inhibitory effect on tumor promotion in a two-stage protocol following;[12] dimethylbenz anthracene (DMBA), application. To date, human studies do not show a protective effect from melanoma and NMSC with vitamin E supplementation; however, a consistent increased risk was noted in subjects with low vitamin E intake.

Vitamin C

Animal studies and laboratory studies report that vitamin C lowers the incidence of skin cancer in UV light–treated mice; it also has a photoprotective effect in human epithelial cells.[14]

PHARMACEUTICALS

Sunscreen

No randomized controlled trials (RCTs) have assessed the effect of sunscreens on the incidence of, or mortality from, malignant melanoma. Retrospective and observational studies indicate conflicting results, most probably due to variable exposure time. One RCT found that sunscreens reduced the incidence of solar keratosis. Despite the lack of prospective studies, use of sunscreens for the prevention of melanoma and other nonmelanoma skin cancer seems sensible and is highly recommended.

Vaccine Therapy

Trials are under way to evaluate the efficacy of vaccines (CD 34$^+$ derived) for treating patients with high-risk stage III or completely resected metastatic melanoma. Another trial is evaluating the efficacy of two different regimens of melanoma vaccine (mutated gp 100 melanoma vaccine in HLA-A 2.1) in treating subjects with nonmetastatic melanoma.

PREVENTION PRESCRIPTION

- *Avoid midday sunlight and prolonged sun exposure starting in childhood.*
- *Wear protective clothing and a wide-brimmed hat when exposed to sunlight.*
- *Apply a broad-spectrum high sun protection factor (SPF) sunscreen of 15 or greater. Reapply every 2 hours and as needed. Use of sunscreen does not mean that one can prolong exposure time.*
- *Perform yearly skin examinations and educate patients to do self-examination using the **ABCD** warning signs.*
- *A low-fat diet may have a beneficiary effect in the prevention of melanoma and nonmelanoma skin cancers.*
- *Consider an increase in fish or omega-3 fatty acids for subjects at high risk of melanoma.*

Resources

American Cancer Society 1-800-ACS-2345
http://www.cancer.org
Melanoma Patient's Information Page
http://www.mpip.org
Provides information, database, chat room, and a patient network with case profiles for people concerned about, or dealing with, melanoma. Also provides a list of, and information about, ongoing trials.
Melanoma Education Foundation
http://www.skincheck.com
Good resource for patients and healthcare workers, with pictures and useful link sites.
Guide to Internet Resources for Cancer
http://www.cancerindex.org/clinks2s.htm
Provides a wealth of information, resources, links, and database about skin cancer for both professionals and patients.

References

1. Evans RD, Kopf AW, Lew RA, et al: Risk factors for the development of malignant melanoma: Review of case-control studies. J Dermatol Surg Oncol 14:393–408, 1988.
2. Autier P, Dore J-F, Negrier S, et al: Sunscreen use and duration of sun exposure: A double-blind, randomized trial. J Natl Cancer Inst 91:1304–1309, 1999.
3. Mackie BS, Mackie LE, Curtin LD, Bourne DJ: Melanoma and dietary lipids. Nutr Cancer 9:219–226, 1987.
4. Black HS, Thornby JI, Wolf JE, et al: Evidence that a low-fat diet reduces the occurrence of non-melanoma skin cancer. Int J Cancer 62:964–969, 1995.
5. Singh A, Shukla Y: Antitumour activity of diallyl sulfide on polycyclic aromatic hydrocarbon-induced mouse skin carcinogenesis. Cancer Lett 131:209–214, 1998.
6. Bain C, Green A, Siskind V, et al: Diet and melanoma. Ann Epidemiol 3:235–238, 1993.
7. Mukhtar, H, Katiyar SK, Agarwal R: Green tea and skin—anticarcinogenic effects. J Invest Dermatol 102:3–7, 1994.
8. Clark LC, Combs GF, Turnbull BW, et al: Effects of selenium supplementation for cancer prevention in patients with carcinoma of the skin. A randomized controlled trial. Nutritional Prevention of Cancer Study Group. JAMA 276:1957–1963, 1996.
9. Singh M, Pal M, Sharma RP: Biological activity of the labdane diterpenes. Planta Med 65:2–8, 1999.
10. Tanaka R, Ohtsu H, Iwamoto M, et al: Cancer chemopreventive agents, labdane diterpenoids from the stem bark of *Thuja standishii* (Gord.) Carr. Cancer Lett 161:165–170, 2000.
11. Kune GA, Bannerman S, Field B, et al: Diet, alcohol, smoking, serum beta-carotene, and vitamin A in male nonmelanocytic skin cancer patients and controls. Nutr Cancer 18:237–244, 1992.
12. Greenberg ER, Baron JA, Stukel TA, et al: A clinical trial of beta carotene to prevent basal-cell and squamous-cell cancers of the skin. The Skin Cancer Prevention Study Group. N Engl J Med 323:789–795, 1990.
13. Stryker WS, Stampfer MJ, Stein EA, et al: Diet, plasma levels of beta-carotene and alpha-tocopherol, and risk of malignant melanoma. Am J Epidemiol 131:597–611, 1990.
14. Miyai E, Yanagida M, Akiyama J, Yamamoto I: Ascorbic acid 2-O-alpha-glucoside, as table form of ascorbic acid, rescues human keratinocyte cell line, SCC, from cytotoxicity of ultraviolet light B. Biol Pharm Bull 19:984–987, 1996.

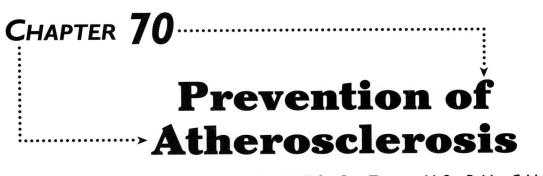

CHAPTER 70

Prevention of Atherosclerosis

Gregory A. Plotnikoff, M.D., M.T.S., Sue Towey, M.S., R.N., C.N.S., L.P.
and David Infanger, B.A.

PATHOPHYSIOLOGY

Heart disease due to atherosclerosis is the leading cause of mortality for both men and women in the United States. The mortality rate from atherosclerosis in the United States is nearly the highest for all Western countries and more than twice that in Japan. This remains true despite the decline over the past three decades in age-adjusted rates of death from coronary artery disease (CAD). For 2001, the American Heart Association (AHA) estimated the cost of atherosclerosis to be more than $298 billion, including $182 billion in direct medical expenses.[1]

Atherogenesis refers to the progressive accumulation of lipids and fibrous elements in arterial vessels. Atherosclerosis begins with the formation of "fatty streaks," which are found in the aorta by the age of 10 years, in the coronary arteries by age 20, and in the cerebral vasculature by age 40. The fatty streak is the start of the growth of atherosclerotic plaque, consisting of lipid-rich necrotic debris enclosed by a fibrous "cap" of smooth muscle cells and their secreted extracellular matrix.[2]

Classically, life-threatening heart disease was believed to follow from progressive atherosclerosis resulting in coronary artery occlusion. However, more than half of all myocardial infarctions originate in stenotic vessels with less than 50% occlusion.[3] Up to 25% of all sudden deaths from myocardial infarctions occur in persons with no previous manifestation of CAD.[4]

Well-known preventive interventions for normal persons include smoking cessation, blood pressure control, cholesterol management with special attention to levels of low-density lipoprotein cholesterol (LDL-C), increased physical activity, and weight management. Such interventions have been demonstrated to favorably alter the natural progression of atherosclerotic disease. Conventional preventive medicine focuses on these risk factors plus management of comorbid medical conditions such as diabetes.

However, these risk factors do not explain adequately why, even in the most successful clinical trials, less than 50% of cardiovascular events are prevented in the treatment groups.[5] In addition, although cholesterol management is aggressively promoted, most myocardial infarctions occur in patients who have normal cholesterol levels. Furthermore, more than 35% of patients with CAD have a total serum cholesterol level of less than 200 mg per dL.[6]

Emerging biologic data demonstrate that most myocardial infarctions follow from plaque rupture and secondary thrombosis. Autopsy studies show that plaques most likely to rupture are those with a soft lipid core covered by a thin and inflamed fibrous cap.[7] For these reasons, prevention of cardiac events requires more than cholesterol reduction; antioxidant, anti-inflammatory, and anti-thrombotic interventions all are essential.

Integrative medicine offers optional approaches to LDL-C reduction as well as additional interventions directed at preventing (1) LDL-C deposition, (2) LDL-C oxidation, (3) inflammation mediated plaque rupture, and (4) coronary thrombosis. Furthermore, integrative medicine approaches modify adverse cardiovascular stress responses through behavioral and psychosocial risk factor management.

The scientific rationale for these approaches is based on the pathophysiology of atherosclerosis, which can be divided into eight steps:

Step 1: Atherosclerosis is initiated by arterial uptake and deposition of LDL-C. By both passive diffusion and the action of specific receptors, LDL-C is trapped and accumulates in the subendothelial matrix. This is enhanced by elevated serum concentrations of LDL-C and the proinflammatory cytokine interleukin-1(IL-1).

Step 2: Trapped LDL-C is then exposed to reactive oxygen species and undergoes initial oxidation to what is termed *minimally oxidized LDL* (MM-LDL). This oxidative stress can result from normal vascular cell metabolism or elevated serum homocysteine, hypertension, smoking, or diabetes.

Step 3: The presence of MM-LDL initiates and promotes proinflammatory responses within the vascular wall. MM-LDL induces chemoattractant agents such as IL-8 and tumor necrosis factor alpha (TNF-α) to recruit monocytes and T lymphocytes to the arterial wall. These cells are then bound to the wall by induced adhesion molecules. MM-LDL–induced macrophage colony stimulating factor (M-CSF) stimulates the proliferation and differentiation of macrophages.

Step 4: MM-LDL is further oxidized to highly oxidized LDL (ox-LDL-C), whose uptake by either macrophages or vascular smooth muscle cells results in so-called foam cells. Oxidation occurs by endothelial cell, macrophage, and enzyme-generated highly reactive oxygen species. Specific "scavenger receptors" are up-regulated by proinflammatory cytokines. Special enzymes found in atherosclerotic lesions promote monocyte chemotaxis, LDL-C oxidation, and LDL-C binding to macrophage scavenger receptors.

Step 5: The death of foam cells results in the accumulation of subendothelial, extracellular cholesterol and other lipids as well as the production of a fibrous cap. This accumulated material is the soft lipid core and accompanying fibrous cap seen on microscopy. The fibrous cap follows from smooth muscle cell growth stimulation and extracellular matrix secretion. Factors that directly stimulate cell proliferation include macrophage cytokines and growth factors, T cell–produced interferon-gamma (IFN-γ), increased homocysteine, and increased angiotensin II found in hypertension. Both ox-LDL-C and homocysteine block release from endothelial cells of the smooth muscle cell proliferation inhibitor nitric oxide (NO).

Step 6: Accumulation of dead foam cells results in a lipid-rich atheromatous core covered with a thinned fibrous cap that is unstable and prone to rupture. Continued oxidant stress and inflammatory cytokine production from the dead foam cells result in inhibition of vascular smooth muscle cell extracellular matrix production, enhanced vascular smooth muscle cell apoptosis, and increased local release of matrix-degrading metalloproteinases (MMPs).

Step 7: Inflammation and/or hemodynamic forces precipitate an acute plaque ulceration or erosion with secondary thrombosis. This inflammation is important; lipid profiles are not the only predictors of cardiac risk. Inflammatory marker are both independent and additive (with unfavorable lipid profile) predictors of cardiovascular risk.[8] An important inflammatory marker is liver-generated C-reactive protein (CRP), which binds to ox-LDL-C and activates multiple complement components found within the arterial wall. CRP production in the liver results from stimulation by systemic cytokines such as TNF-α, IL-1β, and IL-6, which are themselves associated with known risk factors[9] including excessive adipose tissue and omega-3 fatty acid deficiency. Hemodynamic and mechanical forces include surges in, or excessive persistence of, sympathetic nervous system activity.

Step 8: Post-rupture thrombosis results from the exposure of procoagulant elements such as tissue factor (TF) to circulating elements of the coagulation cascade. Not all ruptured plaques result in thrombosis. TF concentration in coronary atherosclerotic plaques varies significantly. Both ox-LDL-C and CRP enhance production of TF.

Coronary artery thrombosis is also a function of platelet adhesion and aggregation. These actions are enhanced by risk factors such as stress, hostility, depression, anxiety, and smoking. Mediators include dietary or medication induced intracellular magnesium deficiency and endothelial injury–released factors such as the prothrombotic agent thromboxane A_2.

INTEGRATIVE APPROACH TO PREVENTION

LDL-C–Reducing Agents

Nutrition

Population and population migration studies document that diet plays a key role in serum LDL-C levels and cardiovascular disease risk. Important risk factors appear to be dietary cholesterol and saturated fat as well as obesity. The practical translation to recommended diets is very controversial. Ornish and colleagues have advocated a 10% fat whole foods vegetarian diet in the setting of life-style changes; their study documented regression of atherosclerosis and reduction of coronary events in the intervention group compared with the control group.[10] The recent Dietary Alternatives Study in 531 male Boeing employees with hypercholesterolemia demonstrated that fat reduction below 25% of total calories consumed with carbohydrate intake above 60% did not further lower LDL-C but lowered high density lipoprotein cholesterol (HDL-C) and raised triglyceride levels.[11] Further study is needed on genetic and other variables.

Given that the average American diet contains excessive amounts of saturated fats and processed foods, most patients need to modify the diet to include whole grains, dark green and yellow/red/orange vegetables and fruits, legumes, nuts, and seeds. In addition, a diet emphasizing high fiber and low glycemic index foods (see Chapter 83, The Glycemic Index) and excluding foods containing hydrogenated vegetable oils and high-fructose corn syrup may be very helpful.

Supplements

Niacin

Large doses of niacin (nicotinic acid) lower LDL-C, triglycerides, and lipoprotein(a) levels and also markedly raise HDL-C levels[12]. Niacin has been shown to significantly decrease cardiovascular and all-cause mortality.[13] A prominent side effect is flushing, which can be minimized by gradual increase in the dose and concomitant use of aspirin.

Soy Protein

Soybeans are a low-fat, no-cholesterol food that contains high-quality protein, isoflavones (phytoestrogens), and essential fatty acids. A diet fortified with soy protein has been shown to significantly lower total serum and LDL-C levels in hypercholesterolemic patients. A 1995 meta-analysis of 38 clinical trials (743 patients) concluded that 31 to 47 g of soy protein per day resulted in reductions of LDL-C by 13%, or –21.7 mg per dL (95% confidence interval [CI]: –31.7 to –11.2).[14] The U.S. Food and Drug Administration has granted approval for soy protein products to be marketed as foods (as are oat bran and psyllium) that help lower the risk of heart disease.

As a phytoestrogen, soy binds to estrogen receptors and is believed to have effects similar to those of other estrogens, which exhibit cholesterol-mitigating efficacy. However, this specific mechanism for soy remains unproved. Just as estrogen replacement increases prostacyclin and NO production and may inhibit LDL-C oxidation, soy may also play these additional roles in decreasing risk of CAD. Allergies to soy are atypical, and side effects are rare as well.

Chinese Red Yeast Rice (Cholestin)

Rice-fermented fungus *Monascus purpureus Went* is a traditional Chinese remedy for improving blood circulation and also a potent inhibitor of 3-hydroxy-3 methylglutaryl coenzyme A (HMG CoA) reductase activity. In one randomized controlled clinical study in 83 hyperlidemic subjects on the AHA step I diet, intake of 2.4 g of red yeast rice per day resulted in an 18% decrease in total cholesterol after 8 weeks compared with the placebo treatment group ($P < .001$).[15] Red yeast rice is available as a commercial product called Cholestin.

Oat Bran

Oat bran and oatmeal both have demonstrated LDL-lowering capability in hypercholesterolemic patients. Beta-glucan is the soluble fiber credited with the lipid attenuating efficacy of many oat products and is roughly twice as abundant in oat bran as in oatmeal. A 12-week, dose-controlled study in 140 hypercholesterolemic patients discovered that 56 g (2 ounces) of oat bran consumed daily reduced levels of LDL by 16%.[16] A meta-analysis evaluating 20 oat product studies concluded that substantial LDL reductions were obtained when 3 g of beta-glucan was consumed.[17]

Psyllium

Psyllium (*Plantago psyllium*) is an excellent source of soluble fiber, with up to 12% mucilage. One intervention trial in hypercholesterolemic patients demonstrated that after 4 months LDL-C levels decreased by 11 to 13 mg per dL.[18] Soluble fiber, by increasing volume, bulk, and viscosity of intestinal contents, is believed to alter metabolic pathways of hepatic cholesterol and lipoprotein metabolism, thereby lowering LDL-C levels. Common sources of psyllium include commercially available fiber-rich laxatives such as Metamucil.

Pharmaceuticals

3-Hydroxy-3-Methylglutaryl Coenzyme A Reductase Inhibitors

Lowering LDL-C levels reduces cardiovascular morbidity and mortality in patients with symptomatic CAD,[19, 20] as well as in asymptomatic patients at increased risk.[21] Meta-analysis of five randomized controlled trials with 30,817 participants has demonstrated that HMG CoA reductase inhibitors (statins) reduce the risk of CAD as well as all-cause mortality in men, women, and elderly and middle-aged persons. Specifically, treatment demonstrated a 28% reduction in LDL-C levels and a 5% increase in HDL-C levels. This result translates to a 31% risk in major coronary events (95% confidence interval [CI]: 26%–36%).[22]

Estrogen

Estrogen has multiple potentially antiatherogenic, vasodilatory, and anti-inflammatory effects on vessel walls. Estrogen therapy in postmenopausal women reduces LDL-C, increases HDL-C, and decreases serum lipoprotein(a) levels. Estrogen may block LDL-C oxidation. Estrogen supplementation partially reverses endothelial dysfunction by its stimulation of prostacyclin and NO production. Estrogen inhibits TNF-α–induced endothelial cell apoptosis, which may prevent plaque erosion and secondary thrombosis.

Postmenopausal hormone replacement therapy among 85,941 participants in the Women's Health Study was associated with decline in the incidence of CAD.[23] The meaning of this association was somewhat confounded by concurrent smoking cessation and dietary changes. Although large reductions of lipoprotein(a) have been shown to decrease the risk of recurrent cardiac events,[24] other estrogen intervention trials have not demonstrated positive benefits. The Heart and Estrogen/Progestin Replacement Study (HERS) demonstrated that 4 years of hormone replacement had no positive effect on the rate of cardiac events or death among postmenopausal women with known CAD. Paradoxically, a significantly increased risk of cardiac events was noted in the first year but declined afterward.[25] Definitive clinical trials evaluating the efficacy of hormone replacement for primary or secondary prevention of coronary events are ongoing.

Low-Density Lipoprotein Cholesterol Antioxidant Agents

Nutrition

Whole grains, nuts and seeds, and vegetables and fruits are excellent sources of many natural antioxidants such as the tocopherols, ascorbic acid, the carotenoids (including beta-carotene and lycopene), and the flavonoids. Several epidemiologic studies and one large clinical trial[26] have correlated consumption of these antioxidants with significant cardiovascular health benefits.

Supplements

Folic Acid and Vitamins B_6 and B_{12}

Owing to accumulating in vitro and epidemiologic evidence regarding hyperhomocysteinemia as a significant cardiac risk factor, in 1999 the AHA recommended to all patients with a family history of CAD to exceed recommended dietary allowance (RDA) values for folate and vitamins B_6 and B_{12}.[27] Supplementation with 400 μg of folic acid daily has reduced serum homocysteine levels by 5 μmol/per liter (equivalent to a 30% to 35% reduction).[28] Greatest attenuation is seen in patients with hyperhomocysteinemia.[29] Folic acid supplementation has also improved endothelial cell dysfunction in patients with established atherosclerosis.[30]

Elevated serum homocysteine levels are also associated with relative pyridoxine (vitamin B_6) and cyanocobalamin (vitamin B_{12}) deficiencies. Supplementation with B_{12} for a month (in a dose of 1 mg/per week) has been shown to reduce serum homocysteine by 35%.[31] Pyridoxine also exhibits similar efficacy at 2 mg per day, but results are most substantial when pyridoxine is taken concomitantly with folic acid.[32, 33] No prospective clinical trials on cardiovascular event reduction have been published, but nine such studies are under way, with greater than 53,000 patients scheduled to be enrolled.

Dosage:
- Folic acid (Folate) 4 mg orally daily.
- Vitamin B_6 (pyridoxine) 2 to 50 mg orally daily.
- Vitamin B_{12} at least 2.4 μg daily. Baseline serum levels should be checked.

Precautions. Folate consumption can mask signs of B_{12} deficiency. Dosages of B_6 above 500 mg per day have precipitated ataxia and sensory neuropathy.[34, 35] No side effects have been shown with B_{12} consumption.

Coenzyme Q10

Coenzyme Q10 (CoQ10) is a potent lipid-soluble inhibitor of LDL and lipid peroxidation. It is the first molecule to oxidize when LDL is subjected to a free radical environment. CoQ10 protects against postischemic reperfusion lipid peroxidation in cardiac and other tissues. Furthermore, CoQ10 may also aid in the redox rejuvenation of vitamin E.

Coenzyme Q is found naturally in beef and eggs. Lesser concentrations are also found in spinach, legumes, and grains. One open trial of CoQ10 supplementation with serum concentrations of 2.0 μg per mL in 424 cardiac patients demonstrated improvement by one New York Heart Association (NYHA) class in 58% of the patients and improvement by two NYHA classes in 28% of the patients.[36]

Dosage. 200 μg daily of CoQ10. The dose should be increased to 400 μg daily in patients taking an HMG CoA reductase inhibition because these drugs deplete CoQ10 levels.

Precautions. CoQ10 is virtually free of side effects and is considered safe.

Vitamin E

Alpha-tocopherol is a lipophilic antioxidant that has been shown in vitro to directly inhibit multiple atherogenic mechanisms including LDL oxidation, ox-LDL-C–induced apoptotic signaling pathways, monocyte–endothelial cell adhesion, IL-1 and TNF-α cytokine release, monocyte release of reactive oxygen species, platelet adhesion, and smooth muscle cell proliferation.

The Nurses' Health Study, conducted in 87,245 women over an 8-year period, demonstrated that women who consumed roughly 200 mg of vitamin E daily reduced their chances of major coronary artery disease by 40%.[37] Similar age-adjusted risk reduction was found in the nearly 40,000 men enrolled in the four-year Health Professionals' Follow-up Study.[38] Dosages of 100 to 400 international units (IU) per day in men have resulted in significant reductions in coronary artery lesion progression.[39]

These findings are supported by positive findings in the 2002-subject Cambridge Heart Antioxidant Study (CHAOS)[40] but not in the 9200-subject prospective Heart Outcomes and Prevention Evaluation (HOPE) study.[41] The HOPE study focused on patients with advanced atherosclerosis, who may benefit more from plaque stabilization and antithrombotic agents. The study was also confounded, however, by no measures of overall antioxidant intake, nor were there any objective measurements of supplementation.

Dosage. 400 IU of mixed tocopherols daily.

Precautions. Vitamin E should be administered with caution in patients receiving warfarin sodium or in those with low vitamin K concentrations.[42]

Beta-Carotene

In vitro studies have demonstrated beta-carotene oxidation preceding that of LDL-C when challenged with free radicals. In epidemiologic studies, lower indices of beta-carotene correlate with elevated CAD risk,[43] but clinical studies do not support this observation. The CARET study of beta-carotene and retinol was stopped prematurely because the treatment group had a 46% increased lung cancer mortality and a 26% increased cardiovascular mortality without serum lipid changes.[44] A 15-trial meta-analysis deduced that results are so varied that no clear recommendations can be made.[45]

Natural sources of beta-carotene and the hundreds of other carotenoids are found in yellow, red, and orange vegetables. Dietary inclusion of these foods may avoid harm from carotenoid dysequilibrium in beta-carotene supplementation.

Vitamin C

Vitamin C (ascorbic acid) is a water-soluble antioxidant, and supplementation correlates with a reduced risk of CAD mortality.[46, 47] Vitamin C depletion has been commonly seen in patients considered to be at elevated risk for cardiac events.[48–50] Additional antioxidant benefit has been observed in patients taking vitamin C and vitamin E concurrently, greater than with ingestion of either vitamin alone.[51, 52]

NOTE

After vitamin E and carotenoids, vitamin C may represent the next line of defense against lipid peroxidation and may regenerate the antioxidant activity of vitamin E.[53]

Dosage. 250 to 500 mg of vitamin C daily.

Precautions. Vitamin C supplementation is safe. However, patients with high iron concentrations who take large amounts of ascorbic acid may be at risk for iron toxicity.[54]

Selenium

Selenium is an essential trace element and a cofactor for glutathione peroxidase, a crucial enzyme for catalyzing the reduction of endothelial cell membrane oxidants such as lipid hydroperoxides to less reactive alcohols. Epidemiologic studies suggest an inverse relationship between serum selenium levels and both atherosclerotic disease[55] and cardiovascular mortality.[56] The U.S. Department of Agriculture has reported moderate to severe selenium deficiency in up to 42% of market cattle.[57] Subnormal whole blood selenium concentrations have been reported in the United States, Scandinavia, France, Germany, and China.[55] One study from the United Kingdom demonstrated that 25% of healthy volunteers and 50% of medical patients had serum selenium levels below those required for full expression of selenium-dependent antioxidant activity.[58] Several animal studies have shown positive effects on ather-

ogenesis with supplementation, but few clinical trials have been conducted. Dietary selenium supplementation at 0.2 mg per day for 6 renal transplant patients in a 6-month cross-over study led to an increase in red blood cell glutathione peroxidase and reductase activity by 64% and 57%, respectively. Selenium treatment also resulted in a 50% decrease in LDL levels and plasma lipid peroxidation. These values all returned to baseline after 3 months on placebo.[59]

Dosage. 200 mg of selenium daily.

Precautions. Symptoms of toxicity include nausea, vomiting, nail changes, fatigue, hair loss, white horizontal streaks on the fingernails, muscle tenderness, and tremor. Thrombocytopenia and hepatorenal dysfunction can also occur with toxic serum levels (greater than 2000 μg per liter).

Anti-Inflammatory Agents

Nutrition

Increasing use of vegetable oils in cooking and hydrogenated vegetable oils in prepared foods has significantly increased dietary intake of the omega-6 polyunsaturated fatty acids (n-6 PUFAs). Simultaneously, increased use of cereal-based livestock production has resulted in significant decreases in dietary n-3 fatty acids. The result has been an inordinate shift in the balance of the two essential fatty acids. This change has been documented by decreased concentrations of docosahexaenoic acid (DHA n-3) and increased concentrations of linoleic acid (n-6) in breast milk.[60] This shift is clinically important because n-3 and n-6 fatty acids are not interconvertible but are nonetheless crucial components of practically all cell membranes. Their balance directs eicosanoid metabolism, immune cell function, gene expression, and intercellular communication.

The ideal dietary ratio of n-6 to n-3 fatty acids is 1:1 to 2:1, but contemporary diets have shifted this balance to 10:1 to 25:1.[61] N-3 fatty acids in the form of alpha linolenic acid are found in soybean, canola, and particularly, flaxseed oils. Additional sources include ocean-harvested cold water fish (mackerel, herring, sardines, albacore tuna, and salmon), green leafy vegetables, and walnuts (see Chapter 84, The Anti-Inflammatory Diet).

Supplements

Omega-3 Fatty Acids

Dietary supplementation with omega-3 polyunsaturated fatty acids (n-3 PUFAs) suppresses production of the proinflammatory cytokines IL-1β, IL-1α, IL-6, IL-8, and TNF-α,[62–64] and of endothelial leukocyte adhesion molecules, as well as monocyte chemotaxis. In keeping with these anti inflammatory actions, *n*-3 PUFA supplementation would be expected to have antiatherogenic and plaque-stabilizing effects.

Two large clinical trials of *n*-3 PUFA supplementation confirm these theoretical benefits. First, the 2033 men enrolled in the prospective Diet and Reinfarction Trial (DART) were randomized to receive oily fish twice a week or usual cardiovascular care. Of the men randomized to fish, 25% refused and were instead given fish oil capsules 900 mg per day. Those who ate fish twice a week had a 29% reduction in overall mortality (*P* < .05).[65] Those who took the fish oil had a 62% reduction in cardiac deaths (*P* < .04) and a 57% reduction in total mortality (*P* < .03).[66]

Second, the 11,324-person, GISSI trial documented that in persons with a recent myocardial infarction or cerebrovascular accident, *n*-3 fatty acid supplementation at 850 mg per day resulted in a 45% reduction in risk of death in the supplementation group compared with the placebo group (95% CI: 24%–60%).[67] This reduction was considered especially significant because nearly all participants were already on a Mediterranean diet, and 90% were on aspirin, 44% on beta-blockers, and 50% on angiotensin-converting enzyme (ACE) inhibitors.

NOTE

Daily n-3 fatty acid supplementation has been calculated to save 20 lives per 1000 post–myocardial infarction patients, which is better than the benefit obtained with use of HMG CoA reductase inhibitors.[68]

Dosage. 1 to 4 g of fish or flax seed oil daily. The dose may be increased to up to 16 g per day in patients with elevated CRP levels. Vitamin E 400 IU a day should be added to reduce the pro-oxidant effect the metabolism of these fatty acids can produce.

Precautions. Dioxin and polychlorinated biphenyl (PCB) concentrations may be elevated in fish oil supplements. CRP levels should be monitored and dosage adjusted.

Pharmaceuticals

Thiazolidinediones

Thiazolidinediones are best known as insulin sensitizers. They exert their effect by activating PPAR-gamma, a member of the nuclear hormone receptor superfamily involved in insulin sensitivity, glucose homeostasis, and obesity. However, PPAR-gamma also regulates inflammatory responses. Endothelial cells treated with PPAR-gamma activators significantly inhibit expression of chemoattractants, synthesis of MMPs, and migration of vascular smooth muscle cells, as well as both macrophage activation and production of proinflammatory cytokines including TNF-α, IL-1β, IL-6, IL-8, and monocyte chemotactic protein-1 (MCP-1).[69–71] Prospective trials of thiazolidinediones in the presention of atherogenesis have not been published.

Antithrombosis Agents

Nutrition

Antithrombotic foods include garlic (*Allium sativum* L.) and onions (*Allium cepa* L.). Garlic has been promoted as a heart-healthy supplement because of studies suggesting lowered cholesterol and blood pressure, enhanced fibrinolytic activity, and inhibited platelet aggregation. However, these studies have been appropriately criticized for methodologic flaws. Most promising may be garlic's antithrombotic activity as a blocker of platelet thromboxane production. Onions also have antithrombotic actions secondary to their documented antiplatelet and fibrinolytic activities. Multiple animal and human studies suggest that garlic may also block atherosclerosis development.

Supplements

Magnesium

Magnesium treatment reduces intracellular calcium mobilization and inhibits platelet aggregation. Patients with low intracellular magnesium levels have significantly increased platelet-dependent thrombosis.[72] Magnesium supplementation inhibits platelet-dependent thrombosis by 35% in patients with CAD already receiving aspirin prophylaxis.[73]

Botanicals

Ginseng

Ginseng *(Panax ginseng)* has been asserted to have many beneficial effects on overall health and well being. Research has shown that a nonsaponin fraction in ginseng root inhibits thromboxane A$_2$ production, thereby inhibiting platelet aggregation.[74] Caution is indicated with the use of ginseng in patients with preexisting hypertension or diabetes.

Hawthorn

Proanthocyanidins found in the flower heads of hawthorn (*Crataegus oxycantha*) have been demonstrated to inhibit thromboxane A$_2$ biosynthesis.[75] Hawthorn's flavonoids may have hypocholesterolemic,[76] vasodilatory,[77] and increased coronary blood flow effects.[78] Hawthorn should be used cautiously with cardiac glycosides such as digoxin.

Ginkgo

Ginkgo (*Ginkgo biloba*) is a potent free radical scavenger as well as a vasodilator and an antagonist of platelet-activating factor. Ginkgo has been subjected to clinical trials for intermittent claudication and peripheral arterial disease but not for CAD.

Pharmaceuticals

Aspirin

Aspirin is an effective antiplatelet agent, and aspirin prophylaxis is considered the standard of care for prevention of myocardial infarction in men older than 50 years of age. Aspirin also protects endothelial cells from oxidative stress, possibly in a synergistic fashion with vitamin E.[79]

Selective Serotonin Reuptake Inhibitors

Serotonin is a key agent both in depression and in platelet function and vasoconstriction. For this reason, serotonin may be a link between increased cardiovascular morbidity and depression. Recently, the selective serotonin reuptake inhibitor (SSRI) paroxetine, in a controlled cross-over trial, was shown to decrease intraplatelet serotonin concentrations by 83%, to inhibit platelet plug formation by 31%, and to significantly lower expression of the platelet activation marker CD36. Clinically, these results translate to reduced aggregation in response to shear stress or thrombin-activating peptide.[80] Prospective clinical trials have not been conducted, and this class of agents remains indicated only for depression.

Angiotensin-Converting Enzyme Inhibitors

Clinical studies have documented clearly that antihypertensive ACE inhibitors reduce cardiovascular morbidity and mortality in patients with left ventricular dysfunction. The obverse antihypertensive agents, the angiotensin II (AT II) antagonists, are believed to also offer similar benefits. Recent studies have documented that both agents block or modulate expression of the procoagulant TF in monocytes and macrophages.[81, 82] Prospective clinical trials have not been conducted, and this class of agents remains indicated only for hypertension, congestive heart failure, and microalbuminuria.

Fibric Acid

Fibric acids are best known as agents for reducing the frequency of coronary events in men with CAD by raising HDL and lowering triglycerides. However, fibric acids also activate PPAR-alpha, thereby reducing TF expression and activity.[83] At much higher serum levels, PPAR-gamma activation occurs. Further study is required to understand the preventive role of fibrates in stabilizing plaque and preventing thrombosis.

LIFESTYLE INTERVENTIONS

Beyond the breakthroughs in cardiovascular molecular biology, biomedical research has also demonstrated the importance of behavioral and psychosocial factors in the prevention, development, and treatment of atherosclerosis.[84] Exercise and physical activity are already well-documented and well-known preventive interventions.[85] Two additional approaches involve therapes that modify excessive physiologic responses—termed "mind-body interventions"—and those that strengthen emotional resources—termed "psychosocial interventions." The remainder of this chapter is devoted to discussion of these important aspects of management and prevention of atherosclerosis.

Mind-Body Healing Interventions

Stress, anxiety, and depression are contributing factors in the development and progression of coronary artery disease.[86–88] These mental processes are linked to pathogenic cardiovascular, metabolic, hormonal, immune system, and autonomic nervous system functioning.[89–91] Hypotheses being tested today include autonomic nervous system dysfunction, hypothalamic-pituitary axis hyperactivity, and increased platelet reactivity. Even in the absence of clear mechanisms of action, numerous mind-body interventions appear to be both safe and effective.

Many psychiatric and somatic stress-related disorders represent variations of pathogenic arousal, also seen as limbicogenic neurologic hypersensitivity.[92] Mind-body interventions may facilitate reversing such "disorders of arousal." Activities or practices that modulate sympathetic nervous system arousal lower both blood pressure and serum levels of cortisol and catecholamines. The capability to induce such changes is important because a significant number of people are susceptible to prolonged physiologic responses to stress.[93] Training in autonomic nervous system modulation enables the self-regulation of the physiologic responses of the body, or limitation of such responses to more appropriate levels. For persons at risk for cardiovascular disease, such training may be crucial.[94]

Mind-body approaches to health and healing may include meditation, imagery, visualization, biofeedback, hypnosis, music, and prayer.[91] Although these methods are a few of the more commonly researched approaches, any activity found by an individual patient to enhance the ability of the body and mind to self-regulate the hyperarousal response may be of benefit to the cardiovascular system (see Chapter 91, Prescribing Relaxation Techniques).

Personal preferences and individualized intervention methods should be identified based on the patient's life style and ability to incorporate the practice into daily life. Meditation practices may include those that are either sendentary (sitting) or moving.

Meditation: Sedentary

Mindfulness Meditation

Mindfulness-Based Stress Reduction (MBSR), a revolutionary program developed by Kabat-Zinn[95] and Santorelli[96] and others at the University of Massachusetts Medical Center more than two decades earlier, has been used to help patients with the management of stress, anxiety, and chronic disease. Patients are taught methods to manage their negative physiologic responses incorporating mindfulness meditation (vipasana) and other forms of movement meditation. Existing clinical data are limited. However, in an 8-week, physician-referred outpatient group stress reduction intervention mindfulness program, all 20 participants demonstrated significant reductions in Hamilton and Beck Anxiety and Depression scores immediately following the intervention and at 3-month follow-up.[97]

Transcendental Meditation

Transcendental meditation (TM) is an ancient form of meditation that uses a mantra, repeated silently over and over, as the focus of attention to quiet the mind. Early medical research on the role of TM in cardiovascular disease found that regular use of this practice resulted in a reduction in high blood pressure and a decrease in serum cholesterol levels.[98]

Relaxation Response

Mental and physical relaxation can be elicited using any form of mental concentration that distracts the affected person from the usual cares or worries of the mind. Benson named this innate hypothalamic mechanism the *relaxation response*.[99]

In a study assessing sympathetic nervous system activity in experimental and control groups, participants were exposed to graded orthostatic and isometric stress during monthly hospital visits. After the first visit, participants in the experimental group practiced a technique that elicited the relaxation response. Their concentrations of plasma norepinephrine during subsequent graded stresses were significantly lower. No such changes were noted in the control group. These results were replicated in the control group in a cross-over experiment.[100]

Recommendations for meditation practice vary widely. Length of practice time may depend on the type of practice and the desired health outcomes.

Meditation practice once or twice daily for 20 to 60 minutes per session is often recommended (see Chapter 94, Learning to Meditate).

Meditation: Movement

Hatha Yoga

Hatha Yoga, a specific aspect of ancient yoga practice that originated in India and Pakistan, is a method of moving the physical body into specific positions, or asanas, to help create a physical energy balance in the body. In one study, the use of yoga training combined with dietary changes was found to reduce cholesterol levels by an average of 14 mg per dL after 3 weeks.[101]

Daily yoga practice for 30 to 60 minutes per session improves the function of the autonomic nervous system and improves regulation of heart rate control.[102]

Tai Chi and Qi Gong

Tai chi and qi gong are quite different in their practice. Tai chi is a rhythmic, nonaerobic form of exercise. Qi-gong exercises combine repetitions of coordinated physical motions with mental concentration and directive efforts to move lifeforce energy, termed "qi," in the body. Both of these Asian practices use focused breathing and movement as a form of meditation. Individual preference may vary, and either one of these practices may be helpful to self-regulate the body, decrease stress, and quiet the nervous system. As with the sitting meditations, the length of practice time may depend on the type of practice and the desired health outcomes. Also as with sitting meditation, practice once or twice daily for 20 to 60 minutes per session is often recommended.

Psychosocial Healing Interventions

Two stressors with important implications for cardiovascular health are social isolation and lack of control over one's environment.[103] Programs that meaningfully connect persons with others and that help an individual patient to cope with life crises, acute and chronic stress, hostility, anxiety, and depression provide significant cardiovascular benefits. A 1996 meta-analysis of 22 randomized controlled trials of psychosocial interventions in 3180 persons with cardiac disease demonstrated significant reductions in psychological distress (−0.34), systolic blood pressure (−0.24), heart rate (−0.38), and cholesterol level (−0.54). These results translated to a statistically significant odds ratio of 1.84 for morbidity (95% CI:1.12–2.99) and 1.70 for mortality (95% CI:1.09–2.64). In summary, psychosocial interventions have been documented to result in a 46% decline in morbidity and a 41% decline in mortality.[104] These findings have been confirmed in one recent prospective trial[105] and are being evaluated in a ongoing large psychosocial intervention trial.[106]

Individual and Group Psychotherapy and Social Support

Cognitive-Behavioral Therapy

Cognitive-behavioral therapy (CBT) is a form of psychotherapy that focuses on specific thoughts that affect emotions and behavior. Stress is defined by the perceiver, so that the response to any situation is determined by the perceptions of the person experiencing the event.[107] Perceptions resulting in hostility, depression, despair, anxiety, impatience, and stress have been linked to the development of CAD and may be modified through the use of this therapy.[108]

Supportive Therapy

Psychotherapy or supportive counseling enables the patient to manage the emotional aspects of a variety of life crises. Some examples of meaningful losses that represent CAD risk factors are divorce, bereavement, loss of a job, loss of economic status, or any change in major life areas, such as work or financial status.

Support groups may be helpful to decrease a sense of isolation and to promote a sense of belonging with others experiencing similar health-affecting issues. Grief support groups are particularly helpful for patients who are experiencing bereavement due to the death of a loved one and who desire emotional support to process the experience. Many cardiac treatment programs include the use of a support group as part of the program.

Identification and Promotion of Relationship, Community, and Spiritual Support

Persons with a high level of social support—that is, those who are connected to supportive, nurturing communities—have significantly lower morbidity and mortality rates.[109–112] Such lower rates were noted even among members of an isolated Pennsylvania community with hyperlipidemia and poor heart-health habits who also had strong extended family as well as community social ties.[113]

Individual needs and choices for community support will vary and may include family and friends, neighborhood, and church/synagogue/mosque, as well as the community created around a particular activity such as sports, hobbies, or care of children. Participation in religious organizations may offer additional benefits beyond those from increased social contact and support.[114, 115]

PREVENTION PRESCRIPTION

The goal of both primary and secondary prevention of CAD is accomplished by interventions aimed at reducing LDL-C, maximizing LDL-C anti-oxidation, minimizing inflammation, combating thrombogenesis, modifying pathogenic physiologic responses, and strengthening emotional resources. The relative importance of each intervention will vary depending on the patient's underlying disease.

Laboratory Testing

To establish baseline values, a fasting lipid panel and determination of serum homocysteine, vitamin B_{12}, CRP, and magnesium levels are indicated.

Nutrition

The ideal heart-healthy diet has not been defined. However, LDL-C reduction to 100 mg per dL or less appears to be indicated. This goal can be approached by including soy proteins, oat bran, and fiber in the diet and avoiding all saturated fats. LDL-C antioxidation can be accomplished through the inclusion of at least 6 servings of vegetables and fruits per day. Anti-inflammatory effects can be achieved by limiting omega-6 essential fatty acids (vegetable oils) in the diet and adding omega-3 essential fatty acids (fish, flaxseed, walnuts, canola oil). Antithrombotic foods include garlic and onions. "Slowfood" meals—that is, sit-down communal dining as opposed to eating fast food on the run—may have innumerable positive health effects.

Supplements

Significant LDL-C reduction can be accomplished through the following:

- *Niacin: 1500 mg orally twice daily with aspirin for flushing prophylaxis.*
- *Cholestin: 2.4 g per day with monitoring of liver functions.*

Significant LDL-C oxidation can be prevented by normalizing homocysteine serum levels, as well as by supplementing with antioxidant agents including the following:

- *Folate: 4 mg orally per day.*
- *Vitamin B$_6$: at least 2 mg orally per day and no more than 50 mg orally per day.*
- *Vitamin B$_{12}$: at least 2.4 μg orally per day. (Serum levels should be monitored to avoid hypovitaminosis B$_{12}$.)*
- *Coenzyme Q10: 200 μg orally per day. The dose should be doubled in patients receiving an HMG CoA reductase inhibitor.*
- *Vitamin E: 400 IU orally per day of mixed D-alpha-, delta-, and gamma-tocopherols. The dose should be doubled in patients receiving fatty acid supplementation in doses greater than 4 g of omega-3 fatty acids daily.*
- *Selenium: 200 μg orally per day.*

Suppression of counterproductive proinflammatory eicosanoids and cytokines can be achieved by supplementation with omega-3 essential fatty acids. The CRP serum level should be monitored, the goal being a serum level of less than 0.4 mg per dL.

- *Flaxseed oil: 4 to 16 g of refrigerated oil orally per day, depending on CRP levels. Flaxseed oil provides alpha linolenic acid (ALA).*
- *Fish oil: 4 to 16 g orally per day may be used instead of flaxseed oil, depending on CRP levels. Fish oil provides both the ALA elongated chains eicosapentaenoic acid (EPA) and DHA.*

Supplements for the inhibition of thrombosis include herbal therapies of unproven efficacy. These herbs have been studied with favorable results in patients with atherosclerosis.

- *Ginkgo biloba: up to 240 mg orally per day of a standardized preparation (EGB 761) in divided doses.*
- *Hawthorn leaf with flower: 160 mg orally per day of a standardized preparation (WS 1442).*

Pharmaceuticals

The use of pharmaceutical agents can be considered first-line therapy in patients with severe hyperlipidemia and other risk factors. Such therapies are passive in nature, however, and true prevention requires much more significant interventions.

Significant LDL-C reduction can be accomplished through the following:

- *HMG CoA reductase inhibitors such as pravastatin (Pravachol) or similar agents 10 mg orally per day, with increases dictated by serum cholesterol level responses. Supplementation with coenzyme Q10 at 200 μg orally per day may be considered for prevention of deficiency.*

Antithrombosis can be accomplished with the use of the following regimen:

- *Enteric-coated aspirin: 85 to 325 mg orally per day.*

Lifestyle Interventions

The patient should be encouraged to reach ideal body weight and to engage in some form of aerobic exercise daily.

Significant reduction of excessive sympathetic nervous system activity can be accomplished via training in numerous mind-body practices.

Enhancement of psychological and spiritual strength, with cardiovascular benefits, can be accomplished through support groups, cognitive-behavioral therapy, and/or inclusion in other relationship supports.

References

1. American Heart Association web site: *www.americanheart. org.* Accessed March 3, 2001.
2. Lusis AJ: Atherosclerosis. Nature 407:233–241, 2000.
3. Koenig W: Inflammation and coronary heart disease: An overview. Cardiol Rev 9:31–35, 2001.
4. Hennekens CH: Increasing burden of cardiovascular disease: Current knowledge and future directions for research on risk factors. Circulation 97:1095–1102, 1998.
5. Bittner V: Atherosclerosis and the immune system. Arch Intern Med 158:1395–1396, 1998.
6. Castelli WP: The new pathophysiology of coronary artery disease. Am J Cardiol 82:60T–65T, 1998.

7. Conti CR: Updated pathophysiologic concepts in unstable coronary artery disease. Am Heart J 141(2 Pt 2):12–14, 2001.

8. Ridker PM, Henneckens CH, Buring JE, Rifai N: C-reactive protein and other markers of inflammation in the prediction of cardiovascular disease in women. N Engl J Med 342:836–843, 2000.

9. Rader DJ: Inflammatory markers of coronary risk. N Engl J Med 343;1179–1182, 2000.

10. Ornish D, Scherwitz LW, Billings JH, et al: Intensive lifestyle changes for reversal of coronary artery disease. JAMA 280:2001–2007, 1998.

11. Knopp RH, Retzlaff B, Walden C, et al: One-year effects of increasingly fat-restricted, carbohydrate-enriched diets on lipoprotein levels in free-living subjects. Proc Soc Exp Biol Med 225:191–199, 2000.

12. Illingworth DR, Stein EA, Mitchel YB, et al: Comparative effects of lovastatin and niacin in primary hypercholesterolemia. Arch Intern Med 154:1586–1595, 1994.

13. Canner BL, Berge KG, Wenger NK, et al: Mortality in Coronary Drug Project patients during a nine year posttreatment period. Am Coll Cardiol 8:1245–1255, 1986.

14. Anderson JW, Johnstone BM, Cook-Newell ME: Meta-analysis of the effects of soy protein intake on serum lipids. N Eng J Med 333:276–282, 1995.

15. Heber D, Yip I, Ashley JM, et al. Cholesterol-lowering effects of a proprietary Chinese red yeast dietary supplement. Am J Clin Nutr 69:231–236, 1999.

16. Davidson MH, Dugan LD, Burns JH, et al: The hypocholesterolemic effects of beta glucan in oatmeal and oat bran: A dose-controlled study. JAMA 265:1833–1839, 1991.

17. Ripsin CM, Keenan JM, Jacobs DR, et al: Oat products and lipid lowering: A meta-analysis. JAMA 267:3317–3325, 1992.

18. Spreecher DL, Harris BV, Goldberg AC, et al: Efficacy of psyllium in reducing serum cholesterol levels in hypercholesterolemic patients on high- or low- fat diets. Ann Intern Med 119:599–605, 1993.

19. Scandinavian Simvastatin Survival Study Group: Randomized trial of cholesterol lowering in 4444 patients with coronary artery disease: The Scandinavian Simvastatin Survival Study (4S). Lancet 344:1383–1389, 1994.

20. Sacks FM, Pfeffer MA, Moye LA, et al, for the Cholesterol and Recurrent Events Trial Investigators: The effect of pravastatin on coronary events after myocardial infarction in patients with average cholesterol levels. N Engl J Med 335:1001–1009, 1996.

21. Shepard J, Cobbe SM, Ford I, et al, for the West of Scotland Coronary Prevention Study Group: Prevention of coronary heart disease with pravastatin in men with hypercholesterolemia. N Engl J Med 333:1301–1307, 1995.

22. LaRosa JC, He J, Vupputuri S: Effect of statins on risk of coronary disease: A meta-analysis of randomized controlled trials. JAMA 282:2340–2346, 1999.

23. Hu FB, Stampfer MJ, Manson JE, et al: Trends in the incidence of coronary heart disease and changes in diet and lifestyle in women. N Engl J Med 343:530–537, 2000.

24. Shlipak MG, Simon JA, Vittinghoff E, et al: Estrogen and progestin, lipoprotein(a), and the risk of recurrent coronary heart disease events after menopause. JAMA 283:1845–1852, 2000.

25. Hulley G, Grady D, Bush T, et al: Randomized trial of estrogen plus progestin for secondary prevention of coronary heart disease in postmenopausal women. JAMA 280:605–613, 1998.

26. De Lorgeril M, Salen P, Martin J-L, et al: Mediterranean diet, traditional risk factors, and the rate of cardiac complications after myocardial infarction: Final report of the Lyon Diet Heart Study. Circulation 99:779–785, 1999.

27. Malinow MR, Bostom AG, Krauss RM: Homocyst(e)ine, diet, and cardiovascular diseases: A statement for healthcare professionals from the Nutrition Committee, American Heart Association. Circulation 99:178–182, 1999.

28. Omenn GS, Beresford SAA, Motulsky AG: Preventing coronary heart disease: B vitamins and homocysteine. Circulation 97:421–424, 1998.

29. Selhub D, Jacques PF, Wilson PWF, et al: Vitamin status and intake as primary determinants of homocysteinemia in an elderly population. JAMA 270:2693–2698, 1993.

30. Title LM, Cummings PM, Giddens K, et al: Effects of folic acid and antioxidant vitamins on endothelial dysfunction with coronary artery disease. J Am Coll Cardiol 36:758–765, 2000.

31. Dierkes J, Domröse U, Ambrosch A, et al: Supplementation with vitamin B_{12} decreases homocysteine and methylmalonic acid but also serum folate in patients with end-stage renal disease. Metabolism 48:631–635, 1999.

32. Ellis JM, McCully KS: Prevention of myocardial infarction by vitamin B_6. Res Commun Mol Pathol Pharmacol 89:208–220, 1995.

33. Dierkes J, Krosen M, Pietrzik K: Folic acid and vitamin B_6 supplementation and plasma homocysteine concentrations in healthy young women. Int J Vit Nutr Res 68:98–103, 1998.

34. Schaumburg H, Kaplan J, Windebank A, et al: Sensory neuropathy from pyridoxine abuse: A new megavitamin syndrome. N Engl J Med 309:445–448, 1983.

35. Bernstein AL: Vitamin B_6 in clinical neurology. Ann N Y Acad Sci 585:250–260, 1990.

36. Langsjoen H, Langsjoen P, Langsjoen P, et al: Usefulness of coenzyme Q10 in clinical cardiology: A long-term study. Mol Aspects Med 15:S165–S175, 1994.

37. Stampfer MJ, Hennekens CH, Manson JE, et al: Vitamin E consumption and the risk of coronary disease in women. N Engl J Med 328:1444–1449, 1993.

38. Rimm EB, Stampfer MJ, Ascherio A, et al: Vitamin E consumption and the risk of heart disease in men. N Engl J Med 328:1444–1449, 1993.

39. Hodis HN, Mack WJ, LaBree L, et al: Serial coronary angiographic evidence that antioxidant vitamin intake reduces progression of coronary artery atherosclerosis. JAMA 273:1849–1854, 1995.

40. Stephens NG, Parsons A, Schofield PM, et al: Randomized controlled trial of vitamin E in patients with coronary disease: Cambridge Heart Antioxidant Study (CHAOS). Lancet 349:1715–1720, 1996.

41. The HOPE Investigators: Vitamin E supplementation and cardiovascular events in high risk patients: HOPE. N Engl J Med 342:154–161, 2000.

42. Bendich A, Machlin LJ: Safety of oral intake of vitamin E. Am J Clin Nutr 48:612–619, 1988.

43. Levy Y, Nseir W, Boulos M, et al: Relationship between plasma antioxidants and coronary artery disease. Harefuah 127:154–157, 1994.

44. Redlich CA, Chung JS, Cullen MR, et al: Effect of long-term beta-carotene and vitamin A on serum cholesterol and triglyceride levels among participants in the Carotene and Retinol Efficacy Trial (CARET). Atherosclerosis 145:425–432, 1999.

45. Kritchevsky SB: β-Carotene, carotenoids, and the prevention of coronary heart disease. J Nutr 129:5–8, 1999.

46. Enstrom JE, Kanim LE, Klein MA: Vitamin C intake and mortality among a sample of the United States population. Epidemiology 3:194–202, 1992.

47. Trout DL: Vitamin C and cardiovascular risk factors. Am J Clin Nutr 53:322S–325S, 1991.

48. Gey KF, Stähelin HB, Eichholzer M: Poor plasma status of carotene and vitamin C is associated with higher mortality from ischemic heart disease and stroke: Basel prospective study. Clin Inves 71:3–6, 1993.

49. Vollset SE, Bjelke E: Does consumption of fruit and vegetables protect against stroke? Lancet 2:742, 1983.

50. Singh RB, Niaz MA, Bishnoi L, et al: Diet, antioxidant vitamins, oxidative stress and risk of coronary artery disease: The Peerzada prospective study. Acta Cardiol 49:453–467, 1994.

51. Reaven PD, Khouw A, Beltz WF, et al: Effect of dietary antioxidant combinations in humans: Protection of LDL by vitamin E but not by β-carotene. Arterioscler Thromb 13:590–600, 1993.

52. Mosca L, Rubenfire M, Mandel C, et al: Antioxidant nutrient supplementation reduces the susceptibility of low density lipoprotein to oxidation in patients with coronary artery disease. J Am Coll Cardiol 30:392–399, 1997.

53. Simon HB: Patient directed, nonprescription approaches to

cardiovascular diseases. Arch Intern Med 154:2283–2296, 1994.

54. Gerster H: High-dose vitamin C: A risk for persons with high iron stores? Int J Vit Nutr Res 69:67–82, 1999.

55. Oster O, Prellwitz W: Selenium and cardiovascular disease. Biol Trace Elem Res 24:91–103, 1990.

56. Salonen JT, Alfthun G, Huttunen JK, et al: Association between cardiovascular death and myocardial infarction and serum selenium in a matched-pair longitudinal study. Lancet 2:175–179, 1982.

57. Dargatz DA, Ross PF: Blood selenium concentrations in cows and heifers on 253 cow-calf operations in 18 states. J Anim Sci 74:2891–2895, 1996.

58. Pearson DJ, Day JP, Suarez-Mendez VJ, et al: Human selenium status and glutathione peroxidase activity in north-west England. Eur J Clin Nutr 44:277–283, 1990.

59. Hussein O, Rosenblat M, Refael G, Aviram M: Dietary selenium increases glutathione peroxidase and reduces the enhanced susceptibility to lipid peroxidation of plasma and low density lipoprotein in kidney transplant recipients. Transplantation 63:679–685, 1997.

60. Sanders TA: Polyunsaturated fatty acids in the food chain in Europe. Am J Clin Nutr 71(1 Suppl):176S–178S, 2000.

61. Simopoulos AP: Human requirement for *n*-3 poluyunsaturated fatty acids. Poult Sci 79:961–970, 2000.

62. Endres S, Ghorbani R, Kelley VE, et al: The effect of dietary supplementation with *n*-3 polyunsaturated fatty acids on the synthesis of interleukin-1 and tumor necrosis factor by mononuclear cells. N Engl J Med 320:265–271, 1989.

63. DeCaterina R, Cybulsky MI, Clinton SK, et al: The omega-3 fatty acid docosahexaenoate reduces cytokine-induced expression of proatherogenic and proinflammatory proteins in human endothelial cells. Arterioscler Thromb 14:1829–1836, 1994.

64. DeCaterina R, Liao JK, Libby P: Fatty acid modulation of endothelial activation. Am J Clin Nutr 71:213S–223S, 2000.

65. Burr ML, Felihy AM, Gilbert JF, et al: Effects of changes in fat, fish and fiber intakes on death and myocardial reinfarction: Diet and Reinfarction Trial. Lancet 2:757–761, 1989.

66. Burr ML, Sweetham PM, Felihy AM: Diet and reinfarction. Eur Heart J 15:1152–1153, 1994.

67. Investigators G: Dietary supplementation with *n*-3 PUFA and vitamin E after myocardial infarction: Results of the GISSI-Prevenzione trial. Lancet 354:447–455, 1999.

68. Long-Term Intervention with Pravastatin in Ischemic Disease (LIPID) Study Group: Prevention of cardiovascular events and death in patients with coronary artery disease and a broad range of initial cholesterol levels. N Engl J Med 339:1349–1357, 1998.

69. Lee H, Shi W, Tontonoz P, et al: Role for peroxisome proliferator–activated receptor alpha in oxidized phosopholipid induced synthesis of monocyte chemotactic protein-1 and interleukin 8 by endothelial cells. Circ Res 87:516–521, 2000.

70. Ricote M, Li AC Willson TM, et al: The peroxisome proliferator–activated receptor-gamma is a negative regulator of macrophage activation. Nature 391:79–82, 1998.

71. Jiang C, Ting AT, Seed B: PPAR-gamma agonists inhibit production of monocyte inflammatory cytokines. Nature 391:82–86, 1998.

72. Schecter M, Merz CN, Rude RK, et al: Low intracellular magnesium levels promote platelet-dependent thrombosis in patients with coronary artery disease. Am Heart J 140:212–218, 2000.

73. Schecter M, Merz CN, Paul-Labrador M, et al: Oral magnesium supplementation inhibits platelet-dependent thrombosis in patients with coronary artery disease. Am J Cardiol 84:152–156, 1999.

74. Park HJ, Rhee MH, Park KM, et al: Effect of nonsaponin fraction from *Panax ginseng* on cGMP and thromboxane A$_2$ in human platelet aggregation. J Ethnopharmacol 49:157–162, 1995.

75. Vibes J, Lasserre B, Gleye J, Declume C: Inhibition of thromboxane A$_2$ biosynthesis in vitro by the main components of *Crataegus oxycantha* (hawthorn) flower heads. Prostaglandins Leukot Essent Fatty Acids 50:173–175, 1994.

76. Rajerdan S, Deepalakshmi PD, Paraskthy K, et al: Effect of

tincture of *Crataegus* on the LDL-receptor activity of hepatic plasma membrane of rats fed an atherogenic diet. Atherosclerosis 123:235–241, 1996.

77. Blesken R: [*Crataegus* in cardiology.] Fortschr Med 110:290–292, 1992.

78. Roddweig C, Hensel H: [Reaction of local myocardial blood flow in nonanesthesized dogs and anesthesized cats to the oral and parenteral administration of a *Crataegus* fraction (oligomere procyanidines).] Arzneimittelforschung 27:1407–1410, 1977.

79. Podhaisky HP, Abate A, Polte T, et al: Aspirin protects endothelial cells from oxidative stress—possible synergism with vitamin E. FEBS Lett 417:349–351, 1997.

80. Hergovich N, Aigner M, Eichler HG, et al: Paroxetine decreases platelet serotonin storiage and platelet function in human beings. Clin Pharmacol Ther 68:435–442, 2000.

81. Napoleone E, DiSanto A, Camera M, et al: Angiotensin-converting enzyme inhibitors downregulate tissue factor synthesis in monocytes. Circ Res 86:139–143, 2000.

82. Soejima H, Ogawa H, Yasue H, et al: Angiotensin-converting enzyme inhibition reduces monocyte chemoattractant protein-1 and tissue factor levels in patients with myocardial infarction. J Am Coll Cardiol 34:983–938, 1999.

83. Marx N, Mackman N, Schonbeck U, et al: PPAR alpha activators inhibit tissue factor expression and activity in human monocytes. Circulation 103:213–219, 2001.

84. US Department of Health and Human Services: National Heart, Lung and Blood Institute Report of the Task Force on Behavioral Research in Cardiovascular, Lung and Blood Health and Disease, 1998. Available at: *http://www.nhlbi.nih.gov/resources/docs/taskforce.htm*

85. Accessed March 5, 2001. Berlin JA, Colditz GA: A meta-analysis of physical activity in the prevention of coronary artery disease. Am J Epidem 132:612–628, 1990.

86. Bosma H, Marmot MG, Hemingway H, et al: Low job control and risk of coronary artery disease in Whitehall II (prospective cohort) study. BMJ 314:558–565, 1997.

87. Everson SA, Lynch JW, Chesney MA, et al: Interaction of workplace demands and cardiovascular reactivity in progression of carotid atherosclerosis: Population based study. BMJ 314:553–558, 1997.

88. Januzzi J, Stern T, Pasternak R, DeSanctis R: The influence of anxiety and depression on outcomes of patients with coronary artery disease. Arch Intern Med 160;1913–1921, 2000.

89. Chrousos GP, Gold PW: The concept of stress and stress system disorders: Overview of physical and behavioral homeostasis. JAMA 267:1244–1252, 1997.

90. McEwen BS: Protective and damaging effects of stress mediators. N Engl J Med 338:171–179, 1998.

91. Achterberg J, Dossey L, Gordon J: Mind-body interventions. In Berman B, Larson D (eds): Alternative Medicine: Expanding Medical Horizons. 1994; pp 3–43. (A report to the National Institutes of Health on Alternative Medical Systems and Practices in the United States.)

92. Everly GS, Benson HD: Disorders of arousal and the relaxation response: Speculations on the nature and treatment of stress-related diseases. Int J Psychosom 36:15–21, 1989.

93. Gerin A, Pickering TG: Association between delayed recovery of blood pressure after acute mental stress and parental history of hypertension. J Hypertens 13:603–610, 1995.

94. Kaplan JR, Pettersoson K, Manuck SB, Olsson G: Role of sympathoadrenal medullary activation in the initiation and progression of atherosclerosis. Circulation 84. (Suppl VI):VI23–VI32, 1991.

95. Kabat-Zinn J: Full Catastrophe Living: How to Use the Wisdom of Your Body and Mind to Face Stress, Pain and Illness. New York, Delta, 1991.

96. Santorelli S: Heal Thyself: Lessons on Mindfulness in Medicine. New York, Bell Tower, 2000.

97. Miller J, Feltcher K, Kabat-Zinn J: Three year follow-up and clinical implications of a mindfulness meditation–based stress reduction intervention in the treatment of anxiety disorders. Gen Hosp Psychiatry 17:192–200, 1995.

98. Cooper M, Aygen M: Effect of meditation on blood cholesterol and blood pressure. J Israel Med Assoc 95:1–2, 1978.

99. Benson H: The Relaxation Response. New York, Morrow, 1975.
100. Hoffman JW, Benson H, Arns PA et al: Reduced sympathetic nervous system responsivity associated with the relaxation response. Science 215:190–192, 1982.
101. Ornish D, Scherwitz RD, Doody, et al: Effects of stress management training and dietary changes in treating ischemic heart disease. JAMA 249:54–59, 1983.
102. Monaghan P, Viereck E. Meditation: The Complete Guide. Novato, Calif, New World Library, 1999.
103. Seeman TE, McEwen BS: The impact of social environment characteristics on neuroendocrine regulation. Psychosom Med 58:459–471, 1996.
104. Linden W, Stossel C, Maurice J: Psychological interventions for patients with coronary artery disease: A meta-analysis. Arch Intern Med 156:745–752, 1996.
105. Blumenthal JA, Wei J, Babyak M, et al: Stress management and exercise training in cardiac patients with myocardial ischemia: Effects on prognosis and on markers of myocardial ischemia. Arch Intern Med 157:2213–2223, 1997.
106. The ENRICHD Investigators: Enhancing Recovery in Coronary Heart Disease Patients (ENRICHD): Study design and methods. Am Heart J 139:1–9, 2000.
107. Lazarus RS, Folkman S: Stress, Appraisal and Coping. New York, Springer-Verlag, 1984.
108. Williams RB, Littman AB: Psychological factors: Role in cardiac risk and treatment strategies. Cardiol Clin 14:97–104, 1996.
109. Berkman LF, Syme SL: Social networks, host resistance and mortality: A nine-year follow-up study of Alameda County residents. Am J Epidemiol 109:186–204, 1979.
110. Blazer D: Social support and mortality in an elderly community population. Am J Epidemiol 115:684–694, 1982.
111. Broadhead WE, Kaplan BH, James SA, et al: The epidemiologic evidence for a relationship between social support and health. Am J Epidemiol 117:521–537, 1983.
112. House JS, Landis KR, Umberson D: Social relationships and health. Science 241:540–545, 1988.
113. Egolf B, Lasker J, Wolf S, Potvin L: The Roseto effect: A fifty-year comparison of mortality rates. Am J Epidemiol 125:186–204, 1992.
114. Strawbridge WJ, Cohen RD, Shema SJ, Kaplan GA: Frequent attendance at religious services and mortality over 28 years. Am J Public Health 87:957–961, 1997.
115. Gouldbourt U, Yaari S, Medalie JH: Factors predictive of long-term coronary heart disease mortality among 10,059 male Israeli civil servants and municipal employees. Cardiology 82:100–121, 1993.

CHAPTER 71

Prevention of Stroke

Lee D. Litvinas, M.D.

ETIOLOGY

Stroke is the third leading cause of death in the United States, after heart disease and neoplasm. There are about 500,000 new strokes yearly, resulting in approximately 160,000 deaths.[1] Stroke is the second most common cause of death worldwide.[2] Prevention focuses on minimizing the effects from the major modifiable risk factors of hypertension, smoking, diabetes mellitus, and elevated cholesterol. The contribution of these risk factors to the development of cerebral arteriosclerosis is well known. Additional risk factors include obesity, carotid stenosis, homocysteinemia, lack of fruits and vegetables in the diet, and a sedentary life style.[3, 4] Nonmodifiable risk factors include age over 55 years, male gender, black and Hispanic ethnicity, and a maternal or paternal family history of stroke.[17] Ischemic strokes account for 85% to 90% of all strokes in Western societies, with the remainder coming from intracranial hemorrhages.[5] Ischemic strokes are classified as thrombotic, embolic, vasoconstrictive, or veno-occlusive in etiology. Most hemorrhagic strokes are hypertensive in etiology.

SCREENING

Screening tests should focus first on identifying the presence and determining the severity of major risk factors. For hypertension screening programs, combined systolic and diastolic hypertension as well as isolated systolic hypertension should be easy to identify over the course of several blood pressure measurements. Diastolic blood pressure values consistently greater than 90 mm Hg and/or systolic blood pressure values consistently greater than 140 mm Hg indicate hypertension. Smoking and accompanying nicotine addiction are self-identifiable. Occult diabetes and insulin resistance can be found by looking for the usual elevations in glycohemoglobin, fasting glucose, and triglycerides, as well as low levels of high density lipoprotein (HDL) cholesterol. Elevation of low density lipoprotein (LDL) cholesterol levels, particularly in association with atherosclerotic heart disease, increases stroke risk and should be addressed.[6, 7]

After identification of major risk factors, screening for other potentially modifiable risk factors is warranted. Nonfasting levels of homocysteine normally range from 5 to 12 μmol per liter.[8] Homocysteine values above this range and high-normal values in patients with comorbid disease indicate the need for B complex supplementation.[9, 10] Screening for obesity is usually done using the usual parameters of body mass index greater than 27 and waist hip ratio greater than 1.0 for men and 0.8 for women. Dietary patterns need to be reviewed for consumption of fruits, vegetables, and types of fats; intake can be determined via a patient's food diary or by a questionnaire. Exercise patterns should also be easily self-identifiable. The association of hormone replacement therapy (HRT) and stroke risk continues to be researched, with most studies showing insignificant or equivocal risks, although the Framingham Heart Study found a 2.6-fold increase in the relative risk of stroke in HRT users versus nonusers.[3, 11] Of note, often in clinical practice women are counseled to discontinue HRT after a cerebrovascular event regardless of the current evidence. Benefits and risks of HRT need to be carefully reviewed and individualized with each patient, taking into account any underlying tendencies toward osteoporosis, breast cancer, or hypercoagulable state.

Primary prevention of stroke must also include discussion of screening for asymptomatic carotid artery stenosis. Although studies are clear that endarterectomy is beneficial for symptomatic patients with high-grade stenosis, it is still an area of controversy for those with asymptomatic stenoses, as reviewed in the literature.[3, 12–15] In asymptomatic carotid artery stenosis, the risk for stroke increases in direct proportion to severity of the stenosis. A decision to intervene surgically appears acceptable for asymptomatic high-grade stenosis with greater than 70% occlusion in patients with few comorbid conditions and if endarterectomy is performed by a surgeon having a less than 3% morbidity and mortality rate.

INTEGRATIVE APPROACH TO PREVENTION

Nutrition

It is now recognized that atherosclerosis is a disease of chronic inflammation; therefore, basic diet modification should focus on eliminating foods with proinflammatory effects.[16] Accordingly, foods containing trans fatty acids—in particular, partially hydrogenated fats—should be avoided. Likewise, adherence to a diet rich in omega-3 fatty acids will improve cardiovascular and cerebrovascular health. Omega-3 fatty acids as a class have anti-inflammatory properties, and food sources include salmon and flaxseed oil[17] (see Chapter 84, The Anti-Inflammatory Diet). A diet that supplies most fat calories from monounsaturated fats such as olive oil appears to be less atherogenic. Daily red meat consumption also increases stroke risk and should be avoided.

Basic recommendations to improve diet for control of diabetes should be followed. These include eating low glycemic index foods (see Chapter 83, The Glycemic Index) with high fiber content, such as legumes, whole grains, and vegetables. Whole grain consumption has recently been shown to be associated with lower risk for stroke in women.[18]

Ischemic stroke risk can be decreased significantly by consuming more fruits and vegetables.[4] Cruciferous vegetables (broccoli, cauliflower, cabbage, and watercress, among others), green leafy vegetables, and citrus fruits have the most effect. An increment of one serving per day of fruits or vegetables has been reported to be associated with a 6% lower risk of ischemic stroke.

Homocysteine blood levels can be decreased by eating foods rich in folic acid, vitamin B_6, and vitamin B_{12}. Folic acid sources include green leafy vegetables, mushrooms, dried beans, and whole wheat bread. Vitamin B_6 (pyridoxine) is found in greatest concentration in whole grain products, nuts, beans, spinach, and lean meat. Good sources of vitamin B_{12} are milk, eggs, fish, cheese, and some cooked sea vegetables.

Lifestyle Interventions

Exercise

Aerobic exercising 30 to 45 minutes a day lowers hypertension, improves lipid profiles, combats insulin resistance, and enhances elasticity of arteries supplying the brain. The practice of Qi gong has been impressively shown to decrease hypertension and related conditions such as stroke.[19]

Alcohol

Alcohol should be limited to no more than 2 drinks per day, as with consumption of higher amounts its protective effect for ischemic stroke is surpassed by an increased risk for hemorrhagic stroke. Protective effects from alcohol can be achieved with consumption of only 1 drink per week.[20]

Weight Loss

In obese patients, weight loss via a balanced approach that combines common sense caloric restriction with an exercise program will decrease stroke risk substantially.

Supplements and Botanicals

If dietary goals are not achievable, then use of supplements should be considered. The effect of additional intake of vitamins E, C, and carotenoids on stroke risk has been studied, but the results are often difficult to interpret.[21–25] In general the reported studies suggest that vitamin C tends to decrease risk for hemorrhagic stroke and may also decrease risk for ischemic stroke, vitamin E tends to increase the risk for hemorrhagic stroke while decreasing the risk for ischemic stroke, and beta-carotene likewise tends to increase risk for hemorrhagic stroke and decrease risk for ischemic stroke. Such evidence seems to dictate caution in the use of vitamin E and beta-carotene supplementation in patients with difficult-to-control hypertension. The carotenoid lutein (yellow pigment) has been shown to be associated with decreased risk for both hemorrhagic and ischemic stroke and is therefore worth considering as a supplement.[21] In addressing the relation between antioxidant consumption and stroke risk, there appears to be no substitute for a diet rich in fruits and vegetables.

Supplementing with a B100 complex vitamin daily gives added assurance against high homocysteine levels and is without significant side effect.

It is important to emphasize that supplement and botanical recommendations should be directed to the appropriate risk factor identified in the patient. Other chapters in this book focus specifically on diabetes, hypertension, atherosclerosis, and hyperlipidemia. In general, minced raw garlic tends to lower cholesterol, acts as a mild blood thinner, and may relax smooth muscle of arteries. Supplementing with calcium carbonate or calcium citrate in a dose of about 1500 mg daily improves blood pressure. Magnesium oxide in a dose of about 500 mg daily in divided doses helps to control both hypertension and diabetes. Diabetes management can be further enhanced by chromium supplements. Guggulipid can lower cholesterol, thereby decreasing stroke risk, especially in patients with atherosclerotic heart disease.

Protecting the brain against hypoxemic injury has been shown to be one of the actions of *Ginkgo biloba*, so this botanical is worth considering as a supplement.[26] Loss of intellectual function associated with cerebrovascular disease has been shown to be minimized with consumption of the Chinese herbal mix yi zhi capsules; use of this botanical under physician guidance is also worth considering.[27]

Table 71–1. Approved Medical Therapies for Stroke

Name	Mechanism of Action	Daily Dose	Administration	Major Adverse Effects	Indications
Aspirin	Antiplatelet, CO pathway inhibitor	81–325 mg	81–325 mg PO qd	GI upset, bleeding	AIS, stroke prophylaxis
Dipyridamole-ASA combination, slow-release (Aggrenox)	Antiplatelet, PDE and CO pathway inhibitor	ASA 50 mg + DP 400 mg	ASA 25 + DP 200 PO bid	Headache, diarrhea, GI irritation	Stroke prophylaxis, I/F other antiplatelets
Clopidogrel (Plavix)	Antiplatelet, ADP pathway inhibitor	75 mg	75 mg PO qd	Rash, diarrhea, GI irritation	Stroke prophylaxis, I/F other antiplatelets
Ticlopidine (Ticlid)	Antiplatelet, ADP pathway inhibitor	500 mg	250 mg PO bid	Diarrhea, rash, neutropenia (CBC q 2 wk × 6)	Stroke prophylaxis, I/F other antiplatelets
Warfarin (Coumadin)	Anticoagulant, limits gamma-carboxylation of factors II, VII, IX, and X and proteins C and S	Adjusted dose	PO adjusted dose to INR target	ICH, systemic bleed, drug interactions	Stroke prophylaxis, INR 2–3 for most cardioembolisms, INR 3–4.5 for prosthetic valves
Heparin, unfractionated, high-dose	Anticoagulant, catalyst for thrombin-antithrombin binding	Adjusted 1000 IU/h infusion, no bolus	Adjusted IV infusion, target PTT 1½–2 times control	ICH, systemic bleeding, immune thrombocytopenia	Large-vessel stenosis or cardioembolism
Recombinant t-PA (Activase)	Thrombolytic, plasminogen activator	0.9 mg/kg (max 90 mg)	10% dose IV bolus, 90% dose IV infusion × 1 h	ICH, systemic bleeding	AIS ≤3 h onset

Abbreviations: ADP=adenosine diphosphate; AIS=acute ischemic stroke; ASA=acetylsalicylic acid (aspirin); CBC=complete blood count; CO=cyclo-oxygenase; DP=dipyridamole; GI=gastrointestinal; ICH=intracerebral hemorrhage; I/F=intolerance/failure; INR=International Normalized Ratio; PDE=phosphodiesterase; PTT=partial thromboplastin time; t-PA, tissue plasminogen activator.

From Rakel RE, Bope ET (eds): Conn's Current Therapy. Philadelphia, WB Saunders, 2001, p 903.

Pharmaceuticals

Statins are a class of pharmaceuticals that inhibit the rate-limiting step in hepatic cholesterol biosynthesis. One of these drugs, pravastatin (Pravachol) has been shown to significantly decrease the risk of stroke in patients with underlying coronary artery disease.[6, 7, 28] This benefit is probably generalizable to other drugs in the same class.

Anticoagulants are often used after an initial stroke and range from aspirin alone, to aspirin with dipyridamole (Aggrenox), to thienopyridines such as clopidogrel (Plavix), to the strongest anticoagulant warfarin (Coumadin). Indications for therapy are based on the clinical status of the individual patient (see Table 71–1).

A "baby aspirin" 81 mg daily is recommended in patients with any risk factors for stroke and with no bleeding tendencies.

As always, pharmaceuticals for control of hypertension, diabetes, and hyperlipidemia are selected according to the individual needs of the patient.

Mind-Body Medicine

Stress reduction is essential and should be pursued with whatever works well for the patient. Options include meditation, simple breathing techniques, listening to relaxing music, going for walks, engaging in yoga or tai chi, spending more time in nature, trying a news-free holiday, and pursuing a mindful approach to daily activities. Developing a social network with persons who have a similar philosophy toward health and lifestyle should be encouraged.

 — *PREVENTION PRESCRIPTION*

- *The warning signs of stroke should be review with patients. In addition, patients should be counseled to seek immediate medical attention for unexplained paralysis, numbness, slurred speech, severe headache, confusion, or dizziness.*
- *Any risk factors for stroke should be identified and appropriate interventions instituted to control modifiable risk factors such as hypertension, diabetes, smoking, elevated cholesterol, atherosclerosis, elevated homocysteine, and obesity.*

PREVENTION PRESCRIPTION *continued*

- *A diet rich in fruits, vegetables, and fiber is recommended, as an increment of one serving daily decreases the risk for ischemic stroke by 6%.*
- *Patients with any risk factors, modifiable or nonmodifiable, should consider taking one "baby aspirin" (81 mg) daily. Contraindications include any bleeding tendencies and concurrent anticoagulant therapy.*
- *Patients should exercise aerobically daily for 30 to 45 minutes if possible.*
- *Dietary fat consumption should be altered to include more omega-3 fatty acids and monounsaturated fats.*
- *Saturated, hydrogenated, and trans fats should be avoided.*
- *Alcohol consumption should be limited to 1 or 2 drinks per day at most, preferably 1 a week.*
- *Older, at risk adults may be screened for asymptomatic high-grade carotid stenosis (i.e., greater than 70% occlusion).*
- *Stress reduction techniques such as meditation, breathing exercises, or nature walks should be practiced regularly.*
- *Development of a social network that promotes a healthy lifestyle should be encouraged.*
- *The following basic mix of vitamins and supplement is recommended: vitamin C 250 mg twice a day, a B 100 complex daily, vitamin E 400 IU daily, calcium citrate or carbonate 1500 mg daily, selenium 200 μg daily, and mixed carotenoids 10,000 to 25,000 IU daily.*

References

1. American Heart Association Stroke Statistics web site: http://americanheart.org/statistics/stroke.html
2. Barnett HJ, Eliasziw M, Meldrum HE: Evidence based cardiology: Prevention of ischaemic stroke. BMJ; 318:1539–1543, 1999.
3. Goldstein LB, Adams R, Becker K, et al: Primary prevention of ischemic stroke: A statement for healthcare professionals from the Stroke Council of the American Heart Association. Stroke 32:280–299, 2001.
4. Joshipura J, Ascherio A, Manson J, et al: Fruit and vegetable intake in relation to risk of ischemic stroke. JAMA; 282:1233–1239, 1999.
5. Easton JD, Hauser S, Martin J: Cerebrovascular diseases. In Harrison TR, Fauci AS (eds): Harrison's Principles of Internal Medicine, 14th ed. New York, McGraw Hill, 1998.
6. White HD, Simes RJ, Anderson NE, et al: Pravastatin therapy and the risk of stroke. N Engl J Med 343:317–326, 2000.
7. Herbert PR, et al: Cholesterol lowering with statin drugs, risk of stroke, and total mortality. JAMA 278:313–321, 1997.
8. Eikelboom JW, Lonn E, Genest J, et al: Homocyst(e)ine and cardiovascular disease: A critical review of the epidemiologic evidence. Ann Intern Med 131:363–375, 1999.
9. Bostom A, Rosenberg IH, Silbershatz H, et al: Nonfasting plasma total homocysteine levels and stroke incidence in elderly persons: The Framingham Study. Ann Intern Med 131:352–355, 1999.
10. Selhub J, Jacques PF, Rosenberg IH, et al: Serum total homocysteine concentrations in the Third National Health and Nutrition Examination Survey (1991–1994): Population reference ranges and contribution of vitamin status of high serum concentrations. Ann Intern Med 131:331–339, 1999.
11. Simon JA, Hsia J, Cauley JA, et al: Postmenopausal hormone therapy and risk of stroke: The Heart and Estrogen Progestin Replacement Study (HERS). Circulation 103:638–642, 2001.
12. Fieschi C, Fisher M (eds): Prevention of Ischemic Stroke. London, Martin Dunitz, 2000.
13. Gubitz G, Sandercock P: Regular review: Prevention of ischaemic stroke. BMJ 321:1455–1459, 2000.
14. Cina CS, Clase CM, Haynes RB: Carotid endarterectomy for symptomatic carotid stenosis (Cochrane Review). Available at http:/cochrane.org/cochrane/revabstr/ab001081.htm
15. Ingall TJ, Dodick DW, Zimmerman RS: Carotid endarterectomy. Which patients can benefit? Postgrad Med 107:97–100, 104–106, 109, 2000.
16. Gariballa SE: Nutritional factors in stroke. Br J Nutr 84:5–17, 2000.
17. Weil A: Eating Well for Optimum Health. New York, Alfred A Knopf, 2000.
18. Liu S, Manson JE, Stampfer MJ, et al: Whole grain consumption and risk of ischemic stroke in women: A prospective study. JAMA 284:1534–1540, 2000.
19. Cohen K: The Way of Qi Gong. New York, Ballantine Books, 1997.
20. Berger K, Ajani UA, Kase CS, et al: Light-to-moderate alcohol consumption and the risk of stroke among U.S. male physicians. N Engl J Med 341:1557–1564, 1999.
21. Ascherio A, Rimm EB, Hernan MA, et al: Relation of consumption of vitamin E, vitamin C, and carotenoids to risk for stroke among men in the United States. Ann Intern Med 130:963–970, 1999.
22. Leppala JM, Virtamo J, Fogelholm R, et al: Vitamin E and beta carotene supplementation in high risk for stroke. A subgroup analysis of the Alpha-tocopherol, Beta-carotene Cancer Prevention Study. Arch Neurol 57:1503–1509, 2000.
23. Hirvonen T, Virtamo J, Korhonen P, et al: Intake of flavonoids, carotenoids, vitamins C and E, and risk of stroke in male smokers. Stroke 31:2301–2306, 2000.
24. Yochum LA, Folsom AR, Kushi LH: Intake of antioxidant vitamins and risk of death from stroke in postmenopausal women. Am J Clin Nutr 72:476–483, 2000.
25. Pearce KA, Boosalis MG, Yeager B: Update on vitamin supplements for the prevention of coronary artery disease and stroke. Am Fam Physician 62:1359–1366, 2000.
26. Logani S, Chen MC, Tran T, et al: Actions of *Ginkgo biloba* related to potential utility for the treatment of conditions involving cerebral hypoxia. Life Sci 67:1389–1396, 2000.
27. Xu H, Shao N, Cui D, et al: A clinical study of yi zhi capsules in prevention of vascular dementia. J Tradit Chin Med 20:10–13, 2000.
28. Byington RP, Davis BR, Plehn JF, et al: Reduction of stroke events with pravastatin: The Prospective Pravastatin Pooling (PPP) project. Circulation 103:387–392, 2001.

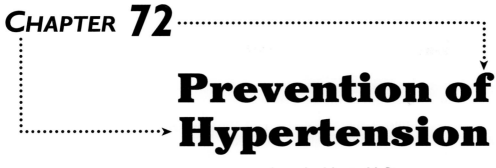

CHAPTER 72

Prevention of Hypertension

Jane L. Hart, M.D.

ETIOLOGY

Lifestyle behaviors, genetic predisposition, and environmental factors may contribute to the onset and evolution of primary or essential hypertension. The exact etiology of primary hypertension, however, remains unknown. Complex interactions among the sympathetic nervous system, the vasculoendothelial system, sodium transport mechanisms, and the renin-angiotensin-aldosterone system contribute to and maintain elevated arterial pressure. Secondary hypertension may result from a defect of renal, endocrine, or cardiovascular origin or from the adverse effects of drugs.

With an estimated 50 million hypertensive people in the United States, hypertension remains a major public health problem and contributes significantly to cardiovascular morbidity and mortality.[1] Modification of lifestyle behaviors has gained increasing attention as an important focus for both the prevention and treatment of hypertension. In the quest to prevent hypertension, patient education must focus on maintaining optimal body weight, getting enough exercise, reducing excessive alcohol consumption, and adopting dietary patterns that increase fruit and vegetable intake and decrease fat.

NOTE

At-risk populations—such as patients with a positive family history for hypertension, African Americans, diabetic patients, the elderly, the obese, and pregnant women—warrant special informative attention.

SCREENING

Early detection of hypertension is imperative. The benefits of treating hypertension have been proved and treatment reduces the morbidity and mortality of cardiovascular disease. The sixth report of the Joint National Committee on Prevention, Detection, Evaluation, and Treatment of High Blood Pressure

(JNC VI) recommends routine blood pressure monitoring at each healthcare encounter.[2] The report of the United States Preventive Services Task Force advises that clinical discretion is important in determining the optimal interval for blood pressure screening with patients.[3]

The JNC VI report defines optimal blood pressure (Table 72–1). In general, elevated blood pressure should be confirmed on three separate occasions at least 2 months apart, but higher degrees of elevation—greater than 160/90—may require more vigilant monitoring.[4] Follow-up of abnormal blood pressure readings is in part dictated by the degree of abnormality, previous blood pressure values, and concomitant risk factors that may exist. Various factors can contribute to incorrect measurement of blood pressure, and physicians should always perform the standard sphygmomanometry technique to verify values reported by other sources.

Although the U.S. Preventive Services Task Force acknowledges that the evidence is less strong for the screening of children and adolescents, periodic checks of blood pressure in this population are recommended primarily to identify secondary causes of hypertension.[5]

LIFESTYLE

Weight Loss

Maintaining a healthy body weight is a crucial factor in preventing hypertension. A direct relationship between body weight and blood pressure has

Table 72–1. Defined Blood Pressure Values

Optimal <120/80
Normal <130/85
High Normal 130–139/85–89
Hypertension ≥140/90

* Confirm elevation on 3 separate occasions at least 2 mo apart for borderline values.

From sixth report of the Joint National Committee on prevention, detection, evaluation, and treatment of high blood pressure. Arch Intern Med 157: 2413–2446, 1997.

been well documented, and the relative risk of developing hypertension increases as body mass index (BMI) increases.[6] Weight loss may reduce blood pressure in overweight individuals with high normal diastolic blood pressure.[7] A recent review of the Trials of Hypertension Prevention (TOHP) phase II revealed that a 10-lb weight loss can result in a significant reduction in blood pressure in persons with high normal blood pressure. Additionally, losing weight and then gaining it back may still reduce the mortality and morbidity from cardiovascular disease compared with those who never lose weight. However, maintenance of weight loss is important in maintaining ongoing beneficial effects. Weight loss may not prevent age-related increases in systolic blood pressure.[8]

Compliance with diet is difficult for many overweight patients, and realistic goals need to be set and monitored. Ongoing educational support and nutritional guidance to help patients lose weight and maintain weight loss are critical aspects of this population's patient care (see Chapter 30, Obesity).

Exercise

A sedentary lifestyle may increase the risk for hypertension. A large observational study found that among 14,000 Harvard alumni, those who did not participate in vigorous sports activity had a 35% greater risk of hypertension compared with men who did, and this was true for a wide range of ages.[9] Another study followed normotensive men and women over a 1- to 12-year period and determined that persons with lower levels of physical fitness had a relative risk of 1.52 for developing hypertension compared with persons engaging in higher levels of fitness.[10]

Thirty minutes of moderate activity (such as dancing, brisk walking, or mowing the lawn) most days of the week is recommended to help prevent hypertension and maintain general health.[11] Further increases in activity, such as aerobic exercise, may have additional benefit in preventing hypertension.[12]

Additional studies examining the benefits of exercise in specific populations are needed.

Alcohol

Alcohol may have both beneficial and adverse effects on health, but when consumed in excess, alcohol may increase the risk of hypertension. Experimental and observational studies have demonstrated a significant association between alcohol and blood pressure and show that a reduction in alcohol use can lead to a reduction in blood pressure.[13] One study demonstrated that reducing alcohol intake in moderate to heavy drinkers can lead to reduced blood pressure in both normotensive and hypertensive individuals.[14] In the Prevention and

Treatment of Hypertension study (PATHS), however, lowered alcohol consumption in moderate drinkers did not lead to statistically significant reductions in blood pressure.[15] The discrepancy between the two studies may be dose related, with a difference in the amount of alcohol reduction among participants. In the prospective Nurses' Health Study, women drinking more than 35 g of alcohol (about three drinks) per day had a relative risk of developing hypertension of 1.9 (95% CI 1.6 to 2.2) compared with nondrinkers. Women drinking 50 g or more of alcohol per day had a relative risk of 2.7 (95% CI 2.0 to 3.5).[16]

The consensus for drinking guidelines is that 1 to 2 drinks per day is probably safe and may help prevent cardiovascular disease.

Stress

Although the association between stress and hypertension appears to be strong, the specific psychosocial factors contributing to hypertension are less clear. The Framingham Study evaluated baseline anxiety and anger traits in 1126 normotensive men and women and followed them over 18 to 20 years for the onset of hypertension. Middle-aged men who developed hypertension had higher baseline anxiety compared with those who remained normotensive. In this study, anger was not a predictor of hypertension.[17]

Evidence is emerging to support the role of stress management and relaxation techniques in the treatment of hypertension; however, scientific evidence to support the use of stress management for the prevention of hypertension is lacking. The TOHP phase I study examined the use of stress management in persons with high normal diastolic blood pressure and did not find stress management efficacious in preventing hypertension.[18]

However, as stress contributes to anxiety and illness (particularly cardiovascular disease), it is appropriate to address stress reduction as a part of any general health and prevention plan. Relaxation techniques such as progressive muscle relaxation, meditation, deep abdominal breathing, and biofeedback have all proved to help reduce stress and may attenuate the blood pressure response (see Chapter 91, Prescribing Relaxation Techniques).

Caffeine

Ingestion of caffeine may lead to an acute increase in blood pressure. Several studies suggest that caffeine's pressor effects may be more pronounced in hypertensive individuals than in normotensive individuals.[19]

Still, the long-term effects of caffeine ingestion and the risk of hypertension are not known, and further studies are needed to evaluate this issue.

Smoking

Smoking is an independent risk factor for cardiovascular disease, and when smoking is combined with hypertension, that risk increases significantly. Patients should be advised to quit smoking and should be directed toward educational support to accomplish that end.

Medications

Multiple drugs can contribute to high blood pressure, including oral contraceptives, steroids, cocaine, sympathomimetics, nonsteroidal anti-inflammatory agents, and others. Licorice root, if taken on a regular basis, can cause hypertension as well. A thorough history with all patients is important for uncovering the use of both prescribed and over-the-counter medications so that their blood pressure may be appropriately monitored.

NUTRITION

Dietary Patterns

Results of the Dietary Approaches to Stop Hypertension (DASH) and DASH-Sodium trials suggest that specific dietary patterns may be effective for both prevention and treatment of hypertension (see Chapter 85, The DASH Diet).[20, 21]

Both normotensive and hypertensive DASH participants consuming a diet composed predominantly of fruits, vegetables, low-fat dairy, and reduced total and saturated fat experienced statistically significant blood pressure reductions compared with those consuming a typical American diet.[22] The DASH-Sodium trial revealed that this diet in combination with reduced sodium intake may have even greater effects on blood pressure reduction.[23] The JNC VI report and the American Heart Association (AHA) guidelines now recommend a diet similar to this as part of any plan to prevent and treat hypertension.[24, 25]

Various epidemiologic and human trials have suggested that a vegetarian diet may lower blood pressure in normotensive patients.[26, 27] Whether this relates to higher intakes of specific nutrients, lower body weights, or other factors among vegetarians is not clear; further studies are warranted. (Please see the following section regarding specific nutrients and their role in the prevention of hypertension.)

Sodium Intake

Reducing dietary salt intake in salt-sensitive hypertensive patients may lead to a reduction in blood pressure and may lessen the need for medications in certain populations. The long-term clinical benefits for normotensive individuals of significantly reducing their dietary salt intake is a point of ongoing controversy.[28] The recent DASH-Sodium trial supported data that suggest that salt reduction is an independent factor in blood pressure reduction and may have additive effects when combined with a diet such as the DASH diet as opposed to a typical diet. This effect, however, was more pronounced in hypertensive participants, black participants on the control diet, and women participants on the DASH diet. Overall, actual reductions in individual blood pressure were small, and even smaller in normotensive individuals.[29]

Generalizations that all Americans should reduce their salt intake are controversial because the long-term clinical benefits of doing this are unknown. However, studies have suggested that diastolic reductions as small as 2 mm Hg can reduce the risk of hypertension and other cardiovascular disease.[30] Additional large, controlled studies are needed to determine the long-term clinical benefits of dietary salt reduction in normotensive individuals.

Relatives of salt-sensitive hypertensives should pay particular attention to avoiding excessive salt intake. Otherwise, both the JNC VI report and the AHA guidelines recommend less than 6 g of dietary salt intake per day for general health.[31, 32]

Fat

Studies have failed to demonstrate that alterations in dietary fat significantly affect blood pressure. Patients should be encouraged to maintain a healthy body weight, and dietary fat should be limited to less than 30% of calories.

Fiber

Although increasing fiber in the diet may have many beneficial effects, changing the amount of fiber in the diet has not been proven to help prevent hypertension.

SUPPLEMENTS

Potassium Intake

Although dietary potassium and supplemental potassium may help reduce blood pressure in hypertensive patients, potassium supplementation for the prevention of hypertension is controversial.[33, 34] Epidemiologic data support the notion that high dietary intake of potassium may have protective effects against hypertension.[35] A meta-analysis of randomized, controlled trials examining the effects of supplemental potassium suggests that supplemental potassium may be of benefit in the prevention and treatment of hypertension.[36] Clinical studies, however, have been inconsistent.[37] Inadequate dietary potassium may leave certain populations particularly vulnerable to hypertension; therefore, adequate dietary potassium is important for all patients. Patients who are prone to hyperkalemia must be warned about excessive potassium intake, and they must be monitored.

Calcium

Data examining the effects of calcium on blood pressure have been inconsistent, and further clinical trials are needed to examine this issue. In the TOHP phase I study, 445 normotensive individuals were given 1 g of calcium or placebo for 6 months, and no significant effect on blood pressure was seen.[38]

The initial Nurses' Health Study suggested that increased calcium intake reduced the risk of hypertension, but a follow-up report refuted these effects.[39]

Adequate dietary calcium is important for maintaining general health.

Magnesium

Inconsistent data with conflicting results and limited clinical trials do not support the use of supplemental magnesium for the prevention of hypertension.[40] Adequate dietary magnesium is important for maintaining general health.

Omega-3 Fatty Acids

Data at this time do not support the use of fish oil for the prevention of hypertension. A meta-analysis revealed that high daily doses (approximately 3 g/d) of omega-3 polyunsaturated fatty acids did not result in statistically significant reductions in blood pressure in normotensive individuals.[41] The TOHP phase I study also demonstrated no blood pressure effects from fish oil in normotensives.[42]

Vitamin C

Ascorbic acid may lower blood pressure, as has been demonstrated in epidemiologic studies. Large controlled clinical trials are needed to further evaluate this effect.[43]

BOTANICALS

Garlic

Human and animal studies have revealed that garlic may lower blood pressure.[44] Supplemental garlic may lower blood pressure in normotensive individuals, but this indication has not been fully investigated. The significance of dietary garlic intake and its effect on the development of hypertension are also unknown.[45]

PREVENTION PRESCRIPTION

- *Strive for optimal body weight. As little as 10 lb of weight loss can have a significant impact on reducing blood pressure.*
- *Exercise at a moderate capacity for at least 30 minutes a day most days of the week. Further increases in intensity and duration of exercise may improve risk reduction for various diseases, including hypertension.*
- *Avoid excessive alcohol intake. Limit intake to 1 to 2 drinks (or fewer) per day.*
- *Be mindful of dietary patterns. Increase fruit and vegetable consumption and reduce fat intake. Consider the DASH diet (see Chapter 85).*
- *Make lifestyle choices that reduce stress. Perform relaxation exercises that fit your lifestyle. Stress can lead to illness, anxiety, and depression.*
- *Obtain adequate levels of vitamins and minerals from your diet. Consider referral to a nutritionist for further assessment and education.*

Additional Information

www.americanheart.org
www.nhlbi.nih.gov/health/public/heart/index.htm

References

1. Sixth report of the Joint National Committee on prevention, detection, evaluation, and treatment of high blood pressure. Arch Intern Med 157:2413–2446, 1997.
2. Sixth report of the Joint National Committee on prevention, detection, evaluation, and treatment of high blood pressure. Arch Intern Med 157:2413–2446, 1997.
3. U.S. Preventive Services Task Force. Guide to Preventive Services, 2nd ed. Baltimore, Williams and Wilkins, 1996, pp 39–51.
4. Sixth report of the Joint National Committee on prevention, detection, evaluation, and treatment of high blood pressure. Arch Intern Med 157:2413–2446, 1997
5. U.S. Preventive Services Task Force. Guide to Preventive Services, 2nd ed. Baltimore, Williams and Wilkins, 1996, pp 39–51.
6. McCarron DA, Reusser ME: Nonpharmacologic therapy in hypertension: From single components for overall dietary management. Prog Cardiovasc Dis 41:451–460, 1999
7. The Trials of Hypertension Prevention Collaborative Research Group: The effects of nonpharmacologic interventions on blood pressure of persons with high normal levels. Results

of the Trials of Hypertension Prevention, Phase I. JAMA 267:1213–1220, 1992.

8. Stevens VJ, Obarzanek E, Cook NR, et al: Long-term weight loss and changes in blood pressure: Results of the trials of hypertension prevention (TOHP), Phase II. Ann Intern Med 134:1–11, 2001.

9. Paffenbarger RS, Wing AL, Hyde RT, Jung DL: Physical activity and incidence of hypertension in college alumni. Am J Epidemiol 117:245–57, 1983.

10. Blair SN, Goodyear NN, Gibbons LW, Cooper KH: Physical fitness and incidence of hypertension in healthy normotensive men and women. JAMA 252:487–490, 1984.

11. U.S. Department of Health and Human Services: Physical activity and health: Areport of the surgeon general. Atlanta, U.S. Department of Health and Human Services, Centers for Disease Control and Prevention, National Center for Chronic Disease Prevention and Health Promotion, 1996.

12. Kelley GA: Aerobic exercise and resting blood pressure among women: A meta-analysis. Prev Med 28:264–275, 1999.

13. National High Blood Pressure Education Program: Working Group Report on Primary Prevention of Hypertension. Arch Intern Med 153:186–208, 1993.

14. Puddey IB, Parker M, Beilin LJ, et al: Effects of alcohol and caloric restrictions on blood pressure and serum lipids in overweight men. Hypertension 20:533–541, 1992.

15. Cushman WC, Cutler JA, Hanna E, et al: Prevention and treatment of hypertension study (PATHS): Effects of an alcohol treatment program on blood pressure. Arch Intern Med 158:1197–1207, 1998.

16. Witteman JCM, Willett WC, Stampfer MJ, et al: Relation of moderate alcohol consumption and risk of systemic hypertension in women. Am J Cardiol 65:633–637, 1990.

17. Markovitz JH, Matthews KA, Kannel WB, et al: Psychological predictors of hypertension in the Framingham study. JAMA 270:2439–2443, 1993.

18. The Trials of Hypertension Prevention Collaborative Research Group: The effects of nonpharmacologic interventions on blood pressure of persons with high normal levels. Results of the Trials of Hypertension Prevention, Phase I. JAMA 267:1213–1220, 1992.

19. Hartley TR, Sung BH, Pincomb GA, et al: Hypertension risk status and effect of caffeine on blood pressure. Hypertension 36:137–141, 2000.

20. Appel LJ, Moore TJ, Obarzanek E, et al: A clinical trial of the effects of dietary patterns on blood pressure. N Engl J Med 336:1117–1124, 1997.

21. Sacks FM, Svetkey LP, Vollmer WM, et al: Effects on blood pressure of reduced dietary sodium and the dietary approaches to stop hypertension (DASH) diet. N Engl J Med 344:3–10, 2001.

22. Appel LJ, Moore TJ, Obarzanek E, et al: A clinical trial of the effects of dietary patterns on blood pressure. N Engl J Med 336:1117–1124, 1997.

23. Sacks FM, Svetkey LP, Vollmer WM, et al: Effects on blood pressure of reduced dietary sodium and the dietary approaches to stop hypertension (DASH) diet. N Engl J Med 344(1):3–10, 2001.

24. Sixth report of the Joint National Committee on prevention, detection, evaluation, and treatment of high blood pressure. Arch Intern Med 157:2413–2446, 1997

25. Krauss RM, Eckel RH, Howard B, et al: AHA Dietary Guidelines Revision 2000: A statement for healthcare professionals from the Nutrition Committee of the American Heart Association. Circulation 102:2284–2299, 2000.

26. Austin S, Yarnell E, Gaby A, Brown D: Clinical applications of complementary and alternative medicine: Hypertension. Part One: Dietary and lifestyle changes. HNR 7(1):48–58, 2000.

27. Rouse IL, Armstrong BK, Beilin LJ, Vandongen R: Blood-pressure-lowering effect of a vegetarian diet: Controlled trial in normotensive subjects. Lancet 1:5–9, 1983.

28. Taubes G: A DASH of data in the salt debate. Science 288:1319. 2000.

29. Sacks FM, Svetkey LP, Vollmer WM, et al: Effects on blood pressure of reduced dietary sodium and the dietary approaches to stop hypertension (DASH) diet. N Engl J Med 344:3–10, 2001.

30. Greenland P: Beating high blood pressure with low-sodium dash. N Engl J Med 344:53–55, 2001.

31. Sixth report of the Joint National Committee on prevention, detection, evaluation, and treatment of high blood pressure. Arch Intern Med 157:2413–2446, 1997.

32. Krauss RM, Eckel RH, Howard B, et al: AHA Dietary Guidelines Revision 2000: A statement for healthcare professionals from the Nutrition Committee of the American Heart Association. Circulation 102:2284–2299, 2000.

33. Whelton PK, He J, Cutler JA, et al: Effects of oral potassium on blood pressure. JAMA 277:1624–1632, 1997.

34. Burgess E, Lewanczuk R, Bolli P, et al: Recommendations on potassium, magnesium and calcium. CMAJ 160(Suppl 9):S35–S45, 1999.

35. Langford HG: Dietary potassium and hypertension: Epidemiologic data. Ann Intern Med 98(part 2):770–772, 1983.

36. Whelton PK, He J, Cutler JA, et al: Effects of oral potassium on blood pressure. JAMA 277:1624–1632, 1997.

37. Burgess E, Lewanczuk R, Bolli P, et al: Recommendations on potassium, magnesium and calcium. CMAJ 160(Suppl 9):S35–S45, 1999.

38. The Trials of Hypertension Prevention Collaborative Research Group: The effects of nonpharmacologic interventions on blood pressure of persons with high normal levels. Results of the Trials of Hypertension Prevention, Phase I. JAMA 267:1213–1220, 1992.

39. Burgess E, Lewanczuk R, Bolli P, et al: Recommendations on potassium, magnesium and calcium. CMAJ 160(Suppl 9):S35–S45, 1999.

40. Burgess E, Lewanczuk R, Bolli P, et al: Recommendations on potassium, magnesium and calcium. CMAJ 1999;160(Suppl 9):S35–45.

41. Appel LJ, Miller ER, Seidler AJ, et al: Does supplementation of diet with fish oil reduce blood pressure? A meta-analysis of controlled clinical trials. Arch Intern Med 153:1429–1438, 1993.

42. The Trials of Hypertension Prevention Collaborative Research Group: The effects of nonpharmacologic interventions on blood pressure of persons with high normal levels. Results of the Trials of Hypertension Prevention, Phase I. JAMA 267:1213–1220, 1992.

43. Duffy SJ, Vita JA: Correspondence. Lancet 355:1272–1274, 2000.

44. Murray MT: Garlic. In The Healing Power of Herbs. Prima Publishing, 1995, pp 126–127.

45. Austin S, Yarnell E, Gaby A, Brown D: Clinical applications of complementary and alternative medicine: Hypertension. Part Two: Nutritional supplements and botanicals. HNR 7:48–58, 2000.

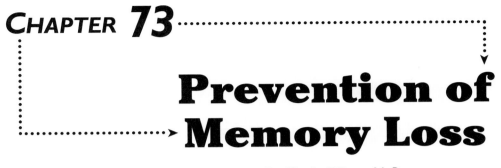

CHAPTER 73

Prevention of Memory Loss

Raffaele Filice, M.D.

Optimizing cognitive function has become a preoccupation for many in our society, from the concerned parent to the increasingly health-conscious "baby boomer." Many specific interventions have been identified to prevent or at least minimize age-related decline in mental functioning. The availability of such options reflects, at least in part, our refusal to accept cognitive decline as an inevitable part of aging. There is a growing number of centenarians who are quite vital both physically and cognitively. Furthermore, our understanding of the general functioning of the brain, the mind, and memory has been evolving in a dramatic fashion over the past two decades. Our knowledge about the causative factors for a decline in brain functioning has also been in a state of flux. A new paradigm about human memory is emerging.

Mind-body medicine research has provided growing evidence that neither the mind nor memories are contained expressly within the brain. Evidence strongly suggests that a person's conscious awareness is extracorporeal. Parts of the brain—the hippocampus, midbrain, prefrontal cortex, and related tracts—have been shown to be specifically involved in memory formation and retrieval, but the thinker of the thoughts has awareness beyond the immediate activity of the brain. In essence, the brain is the instrument through which thoughts are manifested, not their source. Furthermore, there is growing acceptance of the belief that memory is a function of the *whole* body. Memories are just as likely to be triggered by the manual manipulation of a limb as they are by an electrode introduced directly into the prefrontal cortex.

ETIOLOGY AND PREDISPOSING FACTORS

Decline in cognitive function is a multifactorial problem (Table 73–1). There is a spectrum of severity ranging from simple forgetfulness to frank dementia. The most prevalent form of dementia is Alzheimer's disease (AD). Considerable epidemiologic and clinical data have been published; although the evidence derives mostly from study of AD, it can be extrapolated to overall cognitive functioning.

Table 73–1. Risk Factors for Cognitive Decline

Chronic stress
Atherosclerotic disease
Diet high in saturated fat, low in omega-3 fatty acids
Lack of physical and cognitive exercise
History of head trauma
Poor education

Stress, as with many other ailments, has been shown in both animal and human models to have a significant impact on cognitive functioning. Extensive research has elucidated that stress results in increased levels of circulating cortisol, which in turn has both direct and indirect neurotoxic effects. High cortisol levels have been found in human studies to result in hippocampal atrophy measurable by magnetic resonance imaging (MRI), as well as in progressive memory deficits, in some cases eventuating in Alzheimer's-type dementia.[1] An association has been found between atherosclerotic disease and AD.[2] The type of dietary fat consumed has also been found to have some bearing on the development of AD. A diet high in saturated fat increases risk, whereas consumption of fish oils (containing omega-3 fatty acids) confers a protective effect.[3] Physical and cognitive exercise can reduce the chance of cognitive decline, whereas watching television may actually be a risk factor.[4] An association has also been found between previous significant head trauma with loss of consciousness and subsequent increased incidence of cognitive dysfunction and dementia.[5] The risk of dementia decreases with the number of years of formal education. In view of these influences on cognitive function, an integrative approach incorporating life style and nutritional modifications, including some basic dietary supplementation and stress management, would be expected to have a significant effect on reducing or even preventing memory loss and other cognitive disturbances.

Lifestyle Interventions

Adequate Rest/Sleep

Advice to get adequate rest and sleep seems almost trite. However, chronic fatigue and sleep disturbance are rampant in today's society. Shift work is a modern invention that while increasing productivity has had human costs. The ramifications of neglect of the diurnal rhythms cannot be over-estimated. I encourage all of my patients to be mindful of the importance of establishing a daily routine, which should include regular eating times, as well as early bed times and early rising times. Furthermore, I suggest to my patients to look critically at all of the responsibilities that they are shouldering. I have them prepare a type of cost-benefit analysis of all endeavors in which they are involved. Almost invariably, people unwittingly take on more than is reasonably possible to accomplish. The goal is to help people simplify their lives and to respect the body's call for rest.

Physical Exercise

Does anything more need to be said about the importance of regular physical activity for the maintenance of health? Virtually any physical activity can confer benefit as long as it is done on a regular basis.[6] Most often recommended is a daily early morning walk, in keeping with the adage that "a healthy body means a healthy mind." There is now growing evidence that weight training, at virtually any age, improves overall health.[7] Practices such as yoga, tai chi and Qi gong have historically been recommended for improving cognitive as well as physical functioning.

Cognitive Exercise

Like muscle, the brain needs conditioning. The regular performance of intellectually challenging tasks helps to enhance cognitive functioning. Adults with hobbies that exercise the brain such as reading, working jigsaw puzzles, or playing chess were found to be 2.5 times less likely to develop AD. Intellectual activity has been shown to increase dendritic sprouting as well as to enhance neuronal plasticity.[8, 9] These changes may translate into increased cognitive ability and efficiency.

Keeping engaged cognitively is the key. Higher education is protective against memory decline. Although watching television is passive, a discussion about the implications or importance of the program watched is a more active process. Also recommended is maintaining social interactions, preferably combined with active thinking, as in a book club or bridge club. In addition, specific memory techniques such as use of mnemonics, associations, and repetition can be learned and practiced (see Further Resources and Internet-Based Resources at the end of the chapter).

Mind-Body Medicine for Stress Management

As discussed earlier, stress can have both acute and chronic effects on cognitive functioning. A deliberate strategy for coping with stress is therefore strongly recommended. I usually recommend several tools to maximize success in this area.

Exercise

Regular physical exercise has been found to be an effective means of not only alleviating stress but also for enhancing the ability to tolerate stress. Mind-body practices such as yoga can be particularly effective.

Breathing Exercises

Learning one or two deep-breathing techniques and practicing them regularly can be the foundation for a successful stress management program. These exercises can be done at any place and at any time, as needed (see Chapter 88, Breathing Exercises).

Basic Meditation

Meditation has been found to have numerous benefits on the whole person: physical, mental, and spiritual. There are many different meditation traditions. From an evidence-based medicine perspective, Transcendental Meditation is probably the most validated technique. Efficacy has been shown in reducing stress, improving health care procedure outcomes, and reducing health care costs, as well as improving cognitive functioning. Electroencephalographic studies have demonstrated increased brain wave coherence, particularly with the advanced technique of the Transcendental Meditation Sidhi Program. Mindfulness Meditation has also shown clinical efficacy in many areas of health. As with exercise, the best practice is the one that the patient can do regularly. The patient should be encouraged to keep a broad perspective to facilitate overcoming potential barriers to learning a meditation technique, such as financial, philosophical, cultural, or religious. In general, patients usually find the method that best suits them. It should be noted that simple progressive relaxation techniques, while helpful, have not generally been found to have the same efficacy as that of more formal meditation practices[10] (see Chapter 94, Learning to Meditate).

Advanced Meditation

Once a regular meditation practice is established, learning more advanced techniques should be encouraged. There is growing evidence that the

Table 73–2. Nutritional Recommendations for Memory Protection

- Reduce total caloric consumption (2000–3000 calories per day)
- Reduce saturated fats; favor monounsaturated fats (olive oil)
- Avoid partially hydrogenated vegetable oils
- Increase omega-3 essential fatty acids (fish, nuts, flaxseed)
- Favor whole cereals and grains
- Increase fruit and vegetable consumption
- Reduce meat intake
- Avoid artificial sweeteners, additives, and preservatives

effects of meditation can be augmented by some advanced practice (as noted in Khalsa's *Meditation as Medicine*). Vocal intonations, more complex mantras, yogic postures (mudras), and exercises (kriyas) all can enhance cerebral functioning (see Chapter 6, Alzheimer's Disease).

Nutrition

There is little question that nutrition has a bearing on cognitive functioning, (Table 73–2). Improved performance has been seen in schools in which breakfast programs have been instituted. Optimizing diet obviously has a bearing on overall health. One of the most comprehensive studies of the dietary links to AD demonstrated that the incidence of AD is affected by diet, with risk factors including alcohol consumption, saturated fat intake, refined carbohydrates, dietary salt, and total calorie consumption. Preventive factors identified include antioxidants, essential trace minerals, estrogen for postmenopausal women, fish and fish oils, and anti-inflammatory therapeutic agents.[3] Subsequent studies have also found other omega-3 fatty acids, as occur in nuts and seeds (flaxseed), to be slightly protective.[11] Although AD is an extreme case of memory loss, extrapolating these findings to suggest a memory-protective diet seems reasonable. Some of the aforementioned factors have also, of course, been implicated in other diseases, such as coronary artery disease and cancer.

Supplements

Vitamins

Oxidative stress and inflammation have been implicated in many disease states and as a cause of aging.[12] Some vitamin deficiencies are known to affect cognitive functions directly, for example, vitamin B$_1$ deficiency causes Korsakoff's psychosis. A recent study of elderly persons with no cognitive dysfunction showed improved performance on tests of cognitive functioning including memory, abstraction, and visuospatial processing in those who had taken a vitamin supplement, compared with those who had not.[13] A review of antioxidant therapy for AD concluded that there was reasonable evidence of

efficacy for vitamin E.[14] Vitamin supplementation is therefore recommended as both an enhancing and a preventive measure. The exact vitamins to supplement are somewhat controversial, but I generally recommend the antioxidant vitamins A, E, and C, as well as the B-complex vitamins. Lecithin has also been found to enhance learning and memory.

Coenzyme Q10

Ubiquinone, or coenzyme Q10, also has antioxidant activity and is found in both neuronal cell membranes and mitochondria. There is laboratory evidence for its potential use as a neuroprotective agent.[15]

Phosphatidyl Serine

Phosphatidyl serine (PS) is a naturally occurring phospholipid found in cell membranes throughout the body, most abundantly in the brain. In neurons, PS seems to facilitate conduction of nerve impulses and the release of adequate amounts of neurotransmitters. Improvement in cognitive functioning has been found in persons with mild cognitive impairment as well as in those with early AD.[16–18]

Dosage. PS may be utilized at a lower dose of 100 mg per day to optimize cognitive function and at a higher dose of 300 mg per day for memory-impaired persons.

Acetyl L-Carnitine

Acetyl L-carnitine (ALC) is a metabolic cofactor for the conversion of fatty acids into energy within the mitochondria of neurons, thereby helping to keep them supplied with energy. It is also involved in the synthesis of the neurotransmitter acetylcholine. ALC has been studied primarily as a therapeutic agent in varied disorders of cognition: AD, stroke, dementia of chronic alcoholism, and age-associated memory impairment. In most cases, ALC has shown some efficacy.[19] ALC has also been shown to improve membrane phospholipid metabolism.[20] It is therefore theoretically possible that ALC and PS taken together may have a synergistic effect. ALC is a relatively expensive supplement.

Dosage. Most of the clinical trials used doses ranging from 1500 to 3000 mg per day. As a preventive agent ALC in a dose of 250 to 500 mg per day should suffice.

Botanicals

Ginkgo

Ginkgo is among the most researched of herbs. The extract used clinically is derived from the leaves of the *Ginkgo biloba* tree. It is widely used for improving circulation and cognitive functions. There appear to be multiple mechanisms of action, including modulation of blood vessel tone, decreasing blood viscosity, free radical scavenging, and neurotransmitter modulation. Again, most of the studies have focused on application to clinically significant problems such as dementia. One well-known study found significant improvement in cognitive and behavioral performance in patients with mild to severe dementia who were given 120 mg of a *Ginkgo biloba* extract (EGb) daily (specifically, EGb 761).[21] It should be noted that not all extracts of *Ginkgo biloba* are created equal. Although this is true of most herbal extracts, it is particularly pertinent for ginkgo. I recommend to my patients to use the same extracts as those used in the clinical trials.

Precautions. *Ginkgo biloba* should not be used in combination with anticoagulants. Careful monitoring is required with use of ginkgo in patients taking medicines that have antiplatelet activity.

Ginseng

Various animal studies have demonstrated improvement in cognitive functioning with use of gingseng. The mechanism whereby ginseng produces these results seems in part to relate to its acetylcholine agonist activity.[22] Ginseng is, of course, one of the most widely used herbs in the elderly by practitioners of traditional Chinese medicine. More clinical research, however, is needed to evaluate the cognition enhancing properties of ginseng in humans.

Huperzine A

Huperzine A is an alkaloid isolated from the Chinese club moss *Huperzia serrata*. Its traditional use is in the treatment of fever, inflammation, and irregular menses. More recently, the extract has been found to be a potent anticholinesterase inhibitor. In comparison tests with tacrine, it was found to be more potent, more selective, and longer lasting and to have fewer side effects.[23] There is considerable interest in this compound by the U.S. military in its use as a protective agent against organophosphate chemical weapons. Laboratory testing confirmed huperzine A to be more effective and longer lasting than physostigmine. One 3-month open-label trial in Alzheimer's disease patients showed a dose-related response to huperzine A treatment.[24] A Chinese study in adolescent students performed using a double-blind protocol found enhanced memory and learning performance after just 4 weeks of treatment. Huperzine A is available as a dietary supplement and is a component of a number of memory-enhancing formulas.

Dosage. 100 μg twice daily.

Pharmaceuticals

Acetylcholinesterase Inhibitors

Acetylcholinesterase inhibitors indicated for the treatment of dementia are the following:

- tacrine (Cognex)
- donepezil (Aricept)
- rivastigmine (Exelon)

Hormone Replacement Therapy

Hormone replacement therapy (HRT) is an area of both great interest and great controversy; a thorough discussion is beyond the scope of this chapter. Nevertheless, the following hormones used in HRT have been suggested to be useful in memory protection:

- estrogen
- testosterone
- growth hormone
- dehydroepiandrosterone (DHEA)/pregnenolone
- melatonin
- thyroid hormone

Estrogen has been found to specifically maintain verbal memory and may prevent or forestall the deterioration in short-term and long-term memory. Also, there is evidence that estrogen decreases the incidence of AD.[26] The Women's Health Initiative Memory Study is now well under way and should yield important information about the beneficial effects of HRT in women. There is a trend toward use of full HRT replacement therapy for both women and men as an anti-aging strategy. In keeping with the current interest in this area of research, more comprehensive hormone replacement protocols are expected to emerge. There is also evidence of cognitive benefit from the use of both pregnenolone and DHEA.

Frontier Approaches

Electroencephalographic Neurofeedback

EEG neurofeedback may ultimately contribute to increasing conscious control over brain wave patterns to facilitate optimal states of learning and functioning.

Beta-Amyloid Vaccinations

Several recent laboratory studies have reported memory loss prevention in mice using a vaccination against beta-amyloid, the protein moiety associated with the neural plaques found in AD.[27, 28] Human trials are being planned.

Secretase Enzyme Blockers

Secretase enzyme blockers are a new class of drugs that are in the early phases of clinical trials. These drugs inhibit the enzymes that cleave amyloid precursor protein into $A\beta$ peptide and then finally into the beta-amyloid found in the plaques of AD.

Antifibrillogenic Drugs

Antifibrillogenic drugs are being studied for their ability to interfere with the formation of neurofibrillary tangles in the brain that potentially contribute to the development of dementia.

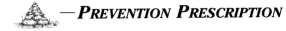 — ***PREVENTION PRESCRIPTION***

- *Daily routine*
  - AM: Patients are counseled to awaken at or around sunrise and to take a 20- to 30-minute walk and practice meditation.
  - Lunch: Patients should make lunch the main meal of the day.
  - PM: Patients should practice meditation, eat a light supper, and go to bed no later than 10:30.
- *Exercise: A brisk 20- to 30-minute early-morning walk is a good way to get started. This can be increased or supplemented, depending on the patient's fitness level. Weight training should also be considered if possible.*
- *Stress management: Regular use of 2 or 3 breathing exercises and practice of basic meditation 10 to 30 minutes twice daily are recommended.*
- *Nutrition: Some guidelines are presented in Table 73–2.*
- *Basic supplements, included as preventive measure*
  - Multivitamin dosage ranges
    Vitamin E as mixed tocopherols: 400 to 800 IU per day
    Vitamin C: 500 mg per day in divided doses
    Vitamin A: 10,000 IU per day
    Vitamin B_1: 50 mg per day
    Vitamin B_6: 50 mg per day
    Vitamin B_{12}: 100 to 1000 μg per day
    Folate: 400 μg per day
  - Coenzyme Q10: 30 to 100 mg per day
- *Advanced supplements, to be considered in patients who have some memory dysfunction*
  - Phosphatidyl serine: prevention: 100 mg per day; therapeutic: 100 mg 3 times a day
  - Acetyl L-carnitine: prevention: 250 to 500 mg per day; therapeutic: 1500 to 3000 mg per day
  - Possible synergistic effect of these supplements used in combination
- *Botanicals*
  - *Ginkgo biloba*: prevention: 60 to 120 mg per day; therapeutic: 120 to 240 mg per day
  - Ginseng: variable
  - Huperzine A: prevention: 50 to 100 μg per day; therapeutic: 100 to 300 μg per day

ACKNOWLEDGMENT

My writing of this chapter would not have been possible if not for the guidance and encouragement of Dr. Dharma Singh Khalsa. It was through his books, seminars, and personal instruction that I came to an awareness of the possibilities for preventive measures in the area of memory and cognitive function.

Further Resources

Penfield W: The Mystery of the Mind. Princeton, Princeton University Press, 1975.

Hutchison M: Megabrain. New York, Ballantine Books, 1991.
Khalsa DS: Meditation as Medicine. Pocket Books, 2001.
Khalsa DS: Brain Longevity. Warner Books, New York, 1997.
Sapolsky RM: Why Zebras Don't Get Ulcers. New York, WH Freeman & Co, 1998.

Internet-Based Resources

Memory techniques and excellent links: www.premiumhealth.com/memory
Cognitive brain exercises using ThinkFast, available at www.brain.com
Think Fast is a web-based neurocognitive tool created by Josh Reynolds, Cognitive Care Inc. (telephone 949-718-1111, ext. 106; josh@brain.com). This technology has the potential for clinical

application. The participants' test results are saved on the system so that test performance can be evaluated over time. The website is for the commercial branch of Cognitive Care Inc.

References

1. Lupien SJ, deLeon M, deSanti S, et al: Cortisol levels during human aging predict hippocampal atrophy and memory deficits. Nat Neurosci 1:69–73, 1998.
2. Hofman A, Ott A, Breteler MM et al: Atherosclerosis, apolipoprotein E and prevalence of dementia and Alzheimer's disease in the Rotterdam Study. Ann Neurol 42:776–782, 1997.
3. Grant WB: Dietary links to Alzheimer's disease. Alz Dis Rev 2:42–55, 1997.
4. Friedland RP: AD. Proc Natl Acad Sci U S A. 2001.
5. Graves ABB, White E: The association between head trauma and Alzheimer's disease: Am J Epidemiol 131:491, 1990.
6. Kramer AF, Hahn S, Cohen NJ et al: Ageing, fitness and neurocognitive function. Nature 400: 418–419, 1999.
7. Smith AL, Cole R, Smyth KA, et al: Protective effects of physical exercise on the development of AD. Neurology 50:A89–A90, 1998.
8. Diamond MC, Lindner B, Johnson R, Bennett EL: Differences in occipital cortical synapses from environmentally enriched, impoverished and standard colony rats. J Neurosci Res 1:109–119, 1975.
9. Cotman C: Synaptic plasticity, neurotropic factors and transplantation in the aged brain. In Schneider EL, Rowe JW (eds): Handbook of the Biology of the Aging. New York, Academic Press, 1990, pp 255–274.
10. Alexander CN, Chandler HM, Langer EJ, et al: Transcendental meditation, mindfulness and longevity. J Personality Soc Psych 57:950–964, 1989.
11. Grant WB. Dietary links to Alzheimer's disease: 1999 update. J Alz Dis 1:197–201, 1999.
12. Harman D: Aging: Minimizing free radical damage. J Anti-Aging Med 2:15–36, 1999.
13. LaRueA, Koehler KM, Wayne SJ, et al: Nutritional status and cognitive functioning in a normally aging sample: A 6 year reassessment. Am J Clin Nutr 65:20–29, 1997.
14. Pitchumoni SS, Doraiswamy PM: Current status of antioxidant therapy for Alzheimer's disease. J Am Geriatr Soc 46:1566–1572, 1998.
15. Beal MF: Coenzyme Q-10 administration and its potential for treatment of neurodegenerative diseases. Biofactors 9:261–266, 1999.
16. Caffarra P, Santamaria V: The effects of phosphatidyl serine in patients with mild cognitive decline. Clin Trials J 24:109–114, 1987.
17. Amaducci L, Crook TH, Lippi A, et al: Use of phosphatidylserine in Alzheimer's disease. Ann NY Acad Sci X:245–249, 1991.
18. Crook TH, Tinklenberg J, Yesavage J, et al: Effects of phosphatidylserine in age-associated memory impairment. Neurology 14:644–649, 1991.
19. Kidd PM: A review of nutrients and botanicals in the integrative management of cognitive dysfunction. Altern Med Rev 4:144–161, 1999.
20. Pettegrew JW, Klunk WE, Panchlingam K, et al: Clinical and neurochemical effects of acetyl L-carnitine in Alzheimer's disease. Neurobiol Aging 16:14, 1995.
21. LeBars PL, Katz MM, Berman N, et al: A placebo-controlled double-blind randomized trial of an extract of *Ginkgo biloba* for dementia. JAMA 278:1327–1332, 1997.
22. Benishin CG, Lee R, Wang LCH, Liu HJ: Effects of ginsenoside Rb1 on central cholinergic metabolism. Pharmacology 42:223–229, 1991.
23. Cheng DH, Tang XC: Comparative studies of huperzine A, E2020 and tacrine on behavior and cholinesterase activities. Pharm Biochem Behav 60:377–386, 1998.
24. Mazurek A: An open label trial of huperzine A in the treatment of Alzheimer's disease. Altern Ther 5:A97–A98, 1999.
25. Sun QQ, Xu SS, Pan JL, et al: Huperzine A capsules enhance memory and learning performance in 34 pairs of matched adolescent students [abstract]. Acta Pharm Sinic 20:601–603, 1999.
26. Sherwin BB: Can estrogen keep you smart? Evidence from clinical studies. J Psychiat. Neurosci 24:315–321, 1999.
27. Janus C, Pearson J, McLaurin J, et al: Aβ peptide immunization reduces behavioral impairment and plaques in a model of Alzheimer's disease. Nature 408:979–982, 2000.
28. Morgan D, Diamond DM, Gottschall PE, et al: Aβ peptide vaccination prevents memory loss in an animal model of Alzheimer's disease. Nature 408:982–985, 2000.

The Prevention of Diabetes Mellitus

Jeffrey A. Morrison, M.D.

DIABETES MELLITUS

CHAPTER 74

Epidemiology

In the United States, 16 million people are estimated to have diabetes mellitus (DM). The World Health Organization (WHO) estimates that 28% of 45- to 74-year-olds are affected by diabetes or impaired glucose tolerance. It is the leading cause of end-stage renal disease,[1] and the seventh leading cause of death in the United States.

Etiology

Diabetes mellitus is a metabolic disease caused by an absolute or relative deficiency of insulin. As a result, carbohydrate utilization is reduced, and lipid and protein utilization is enhanced. There are two major categories of DM: type 1 DM (insulin-dependent diabetes mellitus [IDDM]) and type 2 DM (non–insulin-dependent diabetes mellitus [NIDDM]).

Type 1 Diabetes Mellitus

Although the exact cause of type 1 DM is unknown, current theory suggests that it results from injury to the insulin-producing beta cells, coupled with some defect in tissue regeneration capacity. Antibodies for beta cells are present in 75% of all cases of type 1 DM, compared with 0.5% to 2% of nondiabetic patients. It is possible that antibodies to beta cells develop as a result of both genetic and environmental factors (e.g., viral, chemical, free radical exposure, food allergies).

Type 2 Diabetes Mellitus

About 90% of all patients with DM fall into the category of type 2. Their insulin and blood sugar levels are typically elevated during a 2-hour glucose-tolerance test (GTT), which indicates a loss of insulin sensitivity by the cells of the body. Obesity and a diet high in sugars are major contributing factors.[3] In many cases, achieving an ideal body weight is associated with restoration of normal blood sugar levels in these patients.

Other Types of Diabetes

Diabetes can also be the result of secondary causes such as pancreatitis and hemochromatosis, which destroy insulin-producing pancreatic beta cells. Acromegaly, Cushing syndrome, and hyperthyroidism are endocrine causes of diabetes. Certain drugs such as oral contraceptives, steroids, and thiazide diuretics can also predispose to this condition. Additionally, during pregnancy, women may develop gestational diabetes, which typically resolves after delivery; however, it is an indication that these women are at higher risk for developing diabetes later in life.

Screening

Approximately 800,000 new cases of diabetes are diagnosed each year in the United States. Criteria for screening have been established by the National Diabetes Data Group and the International Expert Committee on the Diagnosis and Classification of Diabetes Mellitus of the American Diabetes Association (ADA). Professional organizations that provide research and education for screening guidelines include the National Institutes of Health (NIH) Diabetes and Kidney Diseases Organization, the American Diabetes Association, and the Joslin Diabetes Centers. Current consensus for the diagnosis of diabetes includes:

- Fasting plasma glucose above 126 mg/dL
- 2-hour glucose tolerance test with glucose level greater than 200 mg/dL
- Random plasma glucose concentration of 200 mg/dL or greater
- Glycosylated hemoglobin (HbA_{1C}) greater than 6.0% can also be used to screen, but if it is elevated, one of the tests described previously should be done to confirm the diagnosis.

Risk factors for *type 1 DM* include:

- Free radical damage in the pancreas
- Viral infections in the pancreas
- Autoimmune reactions directed against the pancreas

Risk factors for *type 2 DM* include:

- Family history of diabetes
- Age older than 45 years
- Obesity
- Lack of regular exercise
- HDL-cholesterol less than 35 mg/dL
- Triglyceride level greater than 250 mg/dL
- Belonging to certain racial and ethnic groups (e.g., African Americans, Latinos, Asian and Pacific Islanders, and Native Americans)
- In women, the development of gestational diabetes (a form of diabetes occurring in 2% to 5% of all pregnancies) or giving birth to a baby weighing 9 pounds or more at birth
- Hypertension

High-risk individuals should be screened every 3 years or tested when any of the following symptoms of DM are noted: polyuria, polydipsia, polyphagia, frequent infections, blurred vision, cuts/bruises that are slow to heal, tingling/numbness in the hands or feet, or recurring skin, gum, or bladder infections.

PREVENTION OF DIABETES MELLITUS

The Diabetes Control and Complications Trial (DCCT) is a clinical study conducted from 1983 to 1993 by the National Institute of Diabetes and Digestive and Kidney Diseases (NIDDK).[44] The study showed that keeping blood sugar levels as close to normal as possible slows the onset and progression of eye, kidney, and nerve diseases caused by diabetes. In fact, it demonstrated that any sustained lowering of blood sugar helps, even if the person has a history of poor control. The following recommendations will help patients reduce their risk of developing DM and will assist those with DM to control their blood sugar through the use of lifestyle modifications and nutritional and dietary supplements.

Lifestyle

Exercise

Exercise is recommended for both type 1 DM and type 2 DM; it is vital in helping to prevent type 2 DM. Some of the benefits include enhanced insulin sensitivity with a resultant diminished need for exogenous insulin, improved glucose tolerance, reduced total serum cholesterol and triglycerides with increased HDL levels, and improved weight loss in obese diabetics.[4, 5]

- Exercise (e.g., walk, jog, swim) for 30 minutes or longer at least three times per week. (See Chapter 86, Writing an Exercise Prescription.)

Stress Management

Concrete evidence reveals that chronic stress alters immune function and cortisol function, which in turn affects insulin sensitivity. Regular meditation and stress management training can lower chronic cortisol output and reduce chronic output of insulin. (See Chapter 91, Prescribing Relaxation Techniques, and Chapter 94, Learning To Meditate.)

Environmental Factors

Many chemicals in foods and in the environment have been implicated in the damage done to beta cells of the pancreas, thereby causing type 1 DM.[12] These chemicals typically damage the pancreas by acting as free radicals, which destroy the cellular components and the functional ability of the beta cells. Foods that are smoked, cured, or preserved with nitrosoamine compounds may cause the most damage in susceptible individuals.

NOTE

Children at risk for developing DM should avoid or limit smoked foods in their diets.

Alcohol

Alcohol is known to decrease insulin sensitivity in normal subjects.[16] However, if a patient's diabetes is well controlled, the blood glucose level will rarely be affected by the use of alcohol in moderation.[17]

- Alcohol may be used in moderation in patients with well-controlled DM, but excessive amounts should be avoided in those at risk of developing diabetes.

Nutrition

Tight control of blood glucose has been correlated with a lower incidence of the common complications of diabetes in the DCCT (Diabetes Control and Complications Trial). To achieve this goal, patients with DM should make a number of essential choices.

Sugar and Refined Carbohydrates

Two studies in 1998 illustrated the effects of carbohydrate restriction on improving glycemic control among patients with type 2 DM and gestational DM. They found that a significant relationship exists between carbohydrate restriction and reduction of the need for glycemic agents such as insulin or sulfonylurea drugs.[6, 7]

- Eliminate all refined sugars (including fructose) and refined carbohydrates from the diet.

Fiber

Fiber is the indigestible part of the plants we eat. It is believed to be beneficial for decreasing cholesterol levels and decreasing the risk of bowel cancer. However, it is less well known that fiber improves all aspects of diabetes control. The usual sources of fiber are vegetables, whole grain cereals, nuts, seeds, fruits, and beans. It appears that legumes (i.e., beans such as peas, soy, and green beans) provide the greatest benefit.[8] The reason for this may be because beans supply about 8 g of fiber in a half cup cooked versus most vegetables, which supply 2 to 3 g of fiber in a half cup cooked.

- Improve glycemic control by eating 50 to 100 g of fiber daily.

Fat

A great deal of research has linked a diet that is high in fat with heart disease and stroke. For this reason, the American Heart Association has recommended a diet in which less than 30% of calories are derived from fat. The worst fats are those that are saturated (fats that are solid at room temperature) or *trans*-fatty acids (essentially most processed foods, like margarine and shortening). The *trans*-fatty acids interfere with the body's ability to use the good essential fatty acids.

The role of fat in the diabetic diet is controversial. At one time, a high-fat, low-carbohydrate diet was recommended for dietary management of DM. However, it has been found that a diet high in saturated fats is associated with type 2 DM.[13] In addition, an editorial in *JAMA* suggested that fat has a negative impact on glycemic control and may increase the risk of atherosclerosis.[11] However, substituting saturated fat with polyunsaturated and monounsaturated fat may be preferable to replacing it with complex carbohydrates because this substitution avoids inducing the deleterious effects on carbohydrate and lipoprotein metabolism caused by a low-fat, complex-carbohydrate diet.[14]

- Replace saturated fats and *trans*-fatty acids with monounsaturated fat or non-partially hydrogenated polyunsaturated fat.

Cow's Milk

A critical review and analysis of the medical literature indicates that early cow's milk exposure may increase a person's risk of developing type 1 DM by 1.5 times.[15] Patients with type 1 DM were more likely to have been breast-fed for less than 3 months and to have been exposed to cow's milk before the age of 4 months. In addition, cow's milk protein can be found in mother's breast milk.

NOTE

In children with a family history of DM, mothers should avoid cow's milk while breast-feeding and children should not be fed cow's milk before 4 months of age.

The Glycemic Index

In 1981, David Jenkins described the "glycemic index" as a method of estimating the rise of blood glucose after the consumption of particular foods.[30] He set the standard value at 100, based on the rise in serum glucose after the ingestion of glucose. The rise in insulin parallels the rise in glucose among patients who do not have DM.

The glycemic index is a powerful tool to help guide patients with DM to select carbohydrate sources that will have a less drastic effect on their serum glucose and insulin levels (Table 74–1). Essentially,

Table 74–1. Glycemic Index of Some Common Foods
....

Food	Glycemic Index
Sugars:	
• Glucose	100
• Honey	75
• Sucrose	60
• Fructose	20
Fruits:	
• Apples	39
• Bananas	62
• Oranges	40
• O.J.	46
• Raisins	64
Vegetables:	
• Beets	64
• Carrot, raw	31
• Carrot, cooked	36
• White potato	98
Grains:	
• Bread, white	69
• Cornflakes	80
• Oatmeal	49
• Pasta	45
• Rice, white	70
• Wheat cereal	67
Legumes:	
• Beans	31
• Lentils	29
• Peas	39
Other Foods:	
• Nuts	13
• Sausages	28

patients with DM are advised to select foods that have a low glycemic index, such as nuts, and to avoid foods with a high glycemic index, like white potatoes. (See Chapter 83, The Glycemic Index.)

- Patients with DM should be encouraged to select foods with a glycemic index lower than 50.

Supplements

The following information documents the usefulness of specific nutrients in the treatment of diabetes. However, it is important to remember that supplements must be used as part of a comprehensive approach in which diet is the primary focus. In addition, all supplements should be taken under the supervision of a health care provider who has experience in the use of nutritional supplements.

Chromium

Chromium is an essential mineral in the treatment of diabetes because of its effect on glucose uptake by insulin-sensitive cells. Chromium is a necessary component of glucose tolerance factor (GTF), a substance present in brewer's yeast that is known to improve glucose tolerance in laboratory animals by potentiating the effect of insulin on carbohydrate metabolism. In one study, patients with type 2 DM significantly improved their fasting glucose level, 2-hour postprandial glucose level, insulin level, glycosylated hemoglobin level, and cholesterol level with chromium picolinate 500 mcg two times per day.[18]

Niacin (Vitamin B$_3$)

Niacin-containing enzymes play an important role in energy production and in fat, cholesterol, and carbohydrate metabolism. Like chromium, niacin is an essential component of GTF, making it a key component in the treatment of DM. One of niacin's most exciting roles is its potential to prevent type 1 DM.[19] The mechanism of action appears to work through its antioxidant role by preventing damage to the beta cells by the immune system.[20]

Dosage. The daily dose of niacinamide may be based on body weight in children: 25 mg/kg/day or up to 100 to 200 mg/day. In adults, up to 300 mg three times per day may be used. Most patients prefer the safe, nonflush inositol hexaniacinate.

Precaution. Slow-release niacin is not recommended because of its potential to cause liver toxicity.[21]

Alpha-Lipoic Acid (ALA)

Alpha-lipoic acid is a relatively newly discovered nutrient that is unusual because it is both a fat-soluble and a water-soluble antioxidant. Its major role for patients with diabetes seems to be in the treatment of patients with peripheral neuropathy. In one study of 328 patients with diabetic peripheral neuropathy, a significant improvement in symptoms was accomplished using ALA 600 mg intravenously per day in 3 weeks.[22] Another study using 600 mg of ALA orally three times per day concluded that it improved symptoms and deficits resulting from polyneuropathy in patients with type 2 diabetes, without causing significant adverse reactions.[23]

Dosage. 600 mg PO tid for established peripheral neuropathy. Limited data are available for preventive use.

Biotin

Biotin is a nutrient that functions in the manufacturing and utilization of carbohydrates, fats, and amino acids. It is manufactured in the intestine by bacteria, and a vegetarian diet has been found to enhance the synthesis and absorption of biotin. Studies have demonstrated that abnormalities of biotin metabolism occur in diabetics and that administration of biotin 9 mg per day corrects hyperglycemia in patients with biotin deficiency without affecting serum insulin levels.[24, 25]

Dosage. 9 mg/day.

Zinc

Zinc is a mineral that is involved in virtually all aspects of insulin metabolism; it has a protective effect against beta-cell destruction. Patients with DM have significantly greater urinary zinc excretion than do control subjects; supplementation has been shown to improve insulin levels among both type 1 and type 2 diabetic patients.[26, 27]

Dosage. Zinc supplementation should be provided at a dose of 30 to 45 mg/day.

Coenzyme Q10 (CoQ10, ubiqinone)

CoQ10 can be found in every cell of the body. It functions as an antioxidant and helps the mitochondria produce energy for the cell. CoQ10 is important for patients with DM because it has been found to increase insulin synthesis and secretion and to promote peripheral glucose utilization, thereby facilitating control of blood sugar levels.[28, 29]

Dosage. Patients with DM may take CoQ10 100 to 200 mg/day.

Essential Fatty Acids (EFAs)

Essential fatty acids are an essential part of the diabetic diet. The two major EFAs are omega-3 fatty acids, which are usually found in cold-water fish or flaxseed oil, and omega-6 fatty acids, which occur in higher concentration in evening primrose oil and borage oil.

In one study, patients with type 2 DM who took 8 g of omega-3 fatty acids had been shown to decrease total cholesterol levels by 11% and triglycerides by 33% in 8 weeks.[31] In another study on omega-6 fatty acids, 4 g of evening primrose oil daily was found to significantly improve diabetic neuropathy after 6 months.[32] Essential fatty acid supplementation should be given to patients with diabetes to help prevent and possibly reverse diabetic neuropathy and atherosclerosis. However, when high doses of fish oil (4 to 10 g/day) are given to patients, vitamin E should be given simultaneously, to prevent increased membrane peroxidation and cellular damage.[33]

Dosage. For the prevention of DM, 1 to 2 g of an omega-3–rich oil (flax or fish oil) may prove beneficial. The patient should at least replace saturated fat (red meat, dairy) with omega-3–rich foods such as fish and nuts. (See Chapter 84, The Anti-Inflammatory Diet.)

Botanical Medicines

Before the pharmaceutical industry discovered how to synthesize insulin, DM was treated with plant medicines. Many of the herbs discussed later have blood sugar–lowering properties, but it is important to remember that the natural treatment and prevention of diabetes integrate diet, nutritional supplements, and lifestyle with botanical medicines.

Garlic (*Allium sativum*) and Onion (*Allium cepa*)

Garlic and onions have blood sugar–lowering capabilities. The principal mechanism of action is believed to be the sulphur-containing compounds—allyl propyl disulphide (APDS) in onions and diallyl disulphide oxide (allicin) in garlic. The APDS and allicin lower glucose levels by competing with insulin for insulin-inactivating sites in the liver, thereby increasing circulating free insulin levels.[34]

Dosage. Recommend that your patient add 1 to 7 oz of fresh onion, or 1 to 3 cloves of fresh garlic, to the daily diet.

Bitter Melon (*Momordica charantia*)

Bitter melon is a gourdlike tropical fruit that is widely cultivated in Asia, Africa, and South America. The blood sugar–lowering action of the fresh juice or extract of the unripe fruit has been studied with favorable results in clinical trials.[35, 36]

The antidiabetic properties of bitter melon are from *Charantin* and *Momordica*. *Charantin* works like a hypoglycemic agent and may be more potent than the oral hypoglycemic drug tolbutamide. *Momordica* contains an insulin-like polypeptide, which has been found to lower blood sugar levels when injected like insulin into type 1 diabetics.[36]

The oral administration of bitter melon in patients with type 2 diabetes was found to have good clinical results. In one study, 15 g of aqueous extract of bitter melon produced a 54% decrease in after-meal blood sugar levels and a 17% reduction in glycosylated hemoglobin in 6 patients.[35]

Dosage. Unfortunately, the taste of bitter melon lives up to its name; it is rather bitter. However, patients who would like to try this may use 1 to 2 oz of fresh juice three times per day.

Gymnema sylvestre

A plant native to the tropical rainforest of India, *Gymnema* has long been used as a treatment for diabetes. Scientific investigation has substantiated its effectiveness in the treatment of both type 1 and type 2 DM.[37, 38] The mode of action seems to be the regeneration of insulin-producing beta cells in the pancreas.

An extract of the *Gymnema* leaves given to a group of patients with type 1 DM, on insulin therapy, was shown to reduce insulin requirements and fasting blood sugar levels, and to improve blood sugar control.[37] In a group of type 2 DM patients taking oral hypoglycemic agents, *Gymnema* extract was found to improve blood sugar control, allowing a significant number of patients to decrease their drug dosage.[38] Interestingly, *Gymnema* given to healthy volunteers does not cause hypoglycemia.

Dosage. For both type 1 and type 2 DM patients, the dose of *Gymnema sylvestre* is 400 mg/day. There are no known side effects from this herb.

Fenugreek (*Trigonella foenum-graecum*)

Patients with type 1 or type 2 DM may benefit from fenugreek. In insulin-dependent diabetics, a 50-g twice-daily dose of defatted fenugreek seed powder was found to significantly reduce fasting blood sugar levels and to improve glucose tolerance test results.[39] In non–insulin-dependent diabetics, 15 g of fenugreek seed powder soaked in water significantly reduced postprandial glucose levels during a meal tolerance test.[40]

Salt Bush (*Atriplex halimu*)

Salt bush is a branchy, woody shrub especially common around the Jordan Valley. In Israel, human studies demonstrated improved blood glucose regulation and glucose tolerance in patients with type 2

DM.[41] Salt bush is noted to be high in chromium, which may partially account for its beneficial effects.

Dosage. The dosage used in human studies was 3 g/day.

Bilberry (*Vaccinium myrtillus*)

Bilberry is a shrubby plant that is native to Europe. It is similar in appearance to the American blueberry, differing only in the color of its blue-black fleshy pulp. The anthocyanosides of the bilberry fruit provide many benefits to the patient with DM. Anthocyanosides have been found to have an affinity for the blood vessels of the retina where they function as powerful antioxidants, decrease the breakage of small blood vessels, and improve circulation.[42] It has been found to be clinically effective for diabetic retinopathy and has been prescribed for this condition in France since 1945.

Dosage. The standard dose is 80 to 160 mg three times per day.

Ginkgo biloba

Ginkgo has primarily been used to treat cerebrovascular insufficiency; however, it is also an important treatment for peripheral vascular disease caused by diabetes. In a double-blind trial, *ginkgo* was found to be superior to placebo in improving pain-free walking distance and increasing blood flow through the affected extremity via Doppler measurements in patients with intermittent claudication.[43]

Dosage. The dose of *Ginkgo biloba* extract should be standardized to contain 24% *ginkgo* flavoglycosides at 40 to 80 mg three times per day.

Precaution. *Ginkgo* should not be used with any patient who is taking blood-thinning medications owing to the increased risk of hemorrhage.

Pharmaceuticals

It cannot be overemphasized that diet, exercise, and nutrition are the three most important factors necessary for treatment and prevention of DM. However, medications are necessary when a patient's blood sugar cannot be kept under good control with the previous options.

Insulin is used as a first-line agent for patients with type 1 DM, but it should be kept as a last resort for patients with type 2 DM. Patients with type 2 DM usually have a problem with insulin resistance and may be successfully treated with biguanides, like metformin (Glucophage). Thiazolidinediones, like pioglitazone (Actos) or rosiglitazone (Avandia), also improve insulin resistance, but are associated with liver toxicity; so liver function tests must be monitored before treatment is started, and then every 2 months for the first year. Some of the risk of hepatic toxicity may be mitigated with the use of natural supplements that improve liver function capabilities, such as milk thistle *(Silybum marianum)* and alpha-lipoic acid.

Sulfonylureas as a class are known to increase pancreatic insulin production in patients with type 2 DM. This approach should be kept as a last resort for the same reason as exogenous insulin. Patients with type 2 DM typically have a problem with decreased insulin sensitivity, so delivering more insulin into the system does not take care of their underlying insulin resistance problem.

Additional information on conventional treatments for DM is beyond the scope of this chapter, but this information may be found online at the American Diabetes Association web site at *www.diabetes.org.*

Therapies to Consider

Acupuncture

Acupuncture is a procedure that involves the insertion of needles into designated points on the skin by a trained practitioner. It has been shown to offer relief from chronic pain; for this reason, acupuncture may be useful for patients with diabetic neuropathy, the painful nerve damage of diabetes.

Biofeedback

Biofeedback is a technique that helps a person become more aware of, and learn to deal with, the body's responses to pain. This alternative therapy emphasizes relaxation and stress-reduction techniques. *Guided imagery* is a relaxation technique that some professionals who use biofeedback do. With guided imagery, a person thinks of peaceful mental images, such as ocean waves. A person may also include the images of controlling or curing a chronic disease, such as diabetes. People using this technique believe their condition can be eased with these positive images.

Magnet Therapy

People have used *magnets* for years as a safe nonpharmaceutical approach for treating refractory pain. In a study of 24 patients with painful diabetic peripheral neuropathy, a significant improvement in pain levels using multipolar magnetic foot insoles was achieved over a 4-month period. In addition, none of the diabetic patients in this study had worsening of their neurologic examination during the 4-month treatment period.[46]

PREVENTION PRESCRIPTION

- *All individuals age 45 and older should be tested for diabetes; if the test is normal, they should be retested every 3 years. Testing should be conducted at earlier ages and carried out more frequently in high-risk individuals.*
- *Children at risk for developing DM should avoid or limit smoked foods in their diets.*
- *Exercise for 30 minutes or longer at least three times weekly.*
- *Eliminate all refined sugars and refined carbohydrates from the diet.*
- *Eat 50 to 100 g of fiber daily.*
- *Replace saturated fats and trans-fatty acids with monounsaturated fat or non-partially hydrogenated polyunsaturated fat in the diet.*
- *Children with a family history of DM should not be fed cow's milk before 4 months of age.*
- *Patients with a family history of type 2 DM should be encouraged to select foods with a glycemic index less than 50.*

FURTHER INFORMATION

Internet Websites

- American Diabetes Association at *www.diabetes.org*
- Joslin Diabetes Center at *www.joslin.harvard.edu*
- National Institute of Diabetes and Digestive and Kidney Diseases at *www.niddk.nih.gov*
- National Center for Complementary and Alternative Medicine at *www.nccam.nih.gov*
- NIH Office of Dietary Supplements at *www.dietarysupplements.info.nih.gov*

Books and Booklets

- Guthrie DW, Guthrie RA: Alternative and Complementary Diabetes Care: How to Combine Natural and Traditional Therapies. New York, John Wiley and Sons, 2000.
- Nutrition Recommendations and Principles for People with Diabetes Mellitus, American Diabetes Association. Diabetes Care 23(suppl 1):S43–S46, January 2000. Available from American Diabetes Association. 1701 North Beauregard Street, Alexandria, VA 22311. Telephone: (800) 232–3472. Website: www.diabetes.org

References

1. Centers for Disease Control and Prevention: National Diabetes Fact Sheet, November 1998.
2. Murray M, Pizzorno J: Encyclopedia of Natural Medicine, 2nd ed. Rocklin, Calif., Prima Publishing, 1998, pp 401–430.
3. Gutierrez M, et al: Utility of a short-term 25% carbohydrate diet on improving glycemic control in type 2 diabetes mellitus. J Am Coll Nutr 17:595–600, 1998.
4. Koivisto V, et al: Exercise in the treatment of type II diabetes. Acta Endocrinol 262:107–111, 1984.
5. Selby J, et al: Environmental and behavioral determinants of fasting plasma glucose in women: A matched co-twin analysis. Am J Epidemiol 125:979–988, 1987.
6. Major D, et al: The effects of carbohydrate restriction in patients with diet-controlled gestational diabetes. Obstet Gynecol 91:600–604, 1998.
7. Gutierrez M, et al: Utility of a short-term 25% carbohydrate diet on improving glycemic control in Type 2 diabetes mellitus. J Am Coll Nutr 17:595–600, 1998.
8. Simpson H, et al: A high carbohydrate leguminous fibre diet improves all aspects of diabetic control. Lancet 1:1–5, 1981.
9. Nicholson A, et al: Toward improved management of NIDDM: A randomized, control, pilot intervention using a low fat, vegetarian diet. Prev Med 29:87–91, 1999.
10. Kolata G: Dietary dogma disproved: Nutritionists find that some complex carbohydrates act like simple sugars and vice versa. Science 487:220, 1983.
11. Steiner G: Editorial: From an excess of fat, diabetics die. JAMA 262(3):398–399, 1989.
12. Leslie R: Early environmental events as a cause of IDDM. Diabetes 43:843–850, 1994.
13. Marshall J, et al: High-fat, low-carbohydrate diet and the etiology of non-insulin-dependent diabetes mellitus: The San Luis Valley Diabetes Study. Am J Epidemiol 134:590–603, 1991.
14. Garg A, et al: Comparison of a high-carbohydrate diet with a high-monounsaturated-fat diet in patients with non-insulin-dependent diabetes mellitus. N Engl J Med 319(13):829–834, 1988.
15. Gerstein H: Cow's milk exposure and type I diabetes mellitus: A critical review of the clinical literature. Diabetes Care 17:13–19, 1994.
16. Avogaro A, et al: Alcohol impairs insulin sensitivity in normal subjects. Diabetes Res 5:23–27, 1987.
17. Franz M: Diabetes mellitus: Considerations in the development of guidelines for the occasional use of alcohol. J Am Diet Assoc 83:147–152, 1983.
18. Anderson R, et al: Beneficial effect of chromium for people with type II diabetes. Diabetes 45(suppl 2):124A/454, 1996.
19. Pocoit F, et al: Nicotinamide: Biological actions and therapeutic potential in diabetes prevention. Diabetologia 36:574–576, 1996.
20. Anderson H: Nicotinamide prevents interleukin-1 effects on accumulated insulin release and nitric oxide production in rat islets of Langerhans. Diabetes 43:770–777, 1994.
21. Henkin Y, et al: Rechallenge with crystalline niacin after drug-induced hepatitis from sustained-release niacin. JAMA 264:241–243, 1990.
22. Ziegler D, et al: Treatment of symptomatic diabetic peripheral neuropathy with the anti-oxidant alpha-lipoic acid. Diabetologia 38:1425–1433, 1995.
23. Ruhnau K, et al: Effects of 3-week oral treatment with the antioxidant thioctic acid (alpha-lipoic acid) in symptomatic diabetic polyneuropathy. Diabet Med 16:1040–1043, 1999.
24. Coggeshall J, et al: Biotin status and plasma glucose in diabetics. Ann NY Acad Sci 447:389, 1985.
25. Maebashi M, et al: Therapeutic evaluation of the effect of biotin on hyperglycemia in patients with non-insulin dependent diabetes mellitus. J Clin Biochem Nutr 14:211–218, 1993.

26. Pidduck H, et al: Hyperzincuria of diabetes mellitus and possible genetical implications of this observation. Diabetes 19:240–247, 1970.

27. Hegazi S, et al: Effect of zinc supplementation on serum glucose, insulin, glucagon, glucose-6-phosphatase, and mineral levels in diabetics. J Clin Biochem Nutr 12:209–215, 1992.

28. Shimura Y,et al: Jpn J Clin Exp Med 58:1349–1532, 1981. (Japanese)

29. Kihara A, et al: Diagnosis Treatm 66:2327–2332, 1978. (Japanese)

30. Jenkins D, et al: Glycemic index of foods: A physiological basis for carbohydrate exchange. Am J Clin Nutr 24:362–366, 1981.

31. Friday K, et al: Omega-3 fatty acid supplementation has discordant effects on plasma glucose and lipoproteins in type II diabetes [abstract]. Diabetes 36(suppl 1):12A, 1987.

32. Jamal G, et al: Treatment of diabetic neuropathy with gamma-linolenic acid (GLA) as evening primrose oil. J Am Coll Nutr 6:86, 1987.

33. Laganiere S, et al: High peroxidaizability of subcellular membrane induced by high fish oil diet is reversed by vitamin E. Clin Res 35:A565, 1987.

34. Sharma K, et al: Antihyperglycemic effect of onion: Effect on fasting blood sugar and induced hyperglycemia in man. Ind J Med Res 65:422–429, 1977.

35. Srivastava Y, et al: Antidiabetic and adaptogenic properties of *Momordica charantia* extract: An experimental and clinical evaluation. Phytotherapy Res 7:285–289, 1993.

36. Welihinda J, et al: The insulin-releasing activity of the tropical plant *Momordica charantia*. Acta Biol Med Germ 41:1229–1240, 1982.

37. Shanmugasundaram E, et al: Use of *Gymnema sylvestre* leaf extract in the control of blood glucose in insulin-dependent diabetes mellitus. J Ethnophamacol 30:281–294, 1990.

38. Baskaran K, et al: Antidiabetic effect of a leaf extract from *Gymnema sylvestre* in non-insulin dependent diabetes mellitus patients. J Ethnophamacol 30:295–305, 1990.

39. Sharma R, et al: Effect of fenugreek seeds on blood glucose and serum lipids in type I diabetes. Eur J Clin Nutr 44:301–306, 1990.

40. Mada Z, et al: Glucose-lowering effect of fenugreek in non-insulin dependent diabetics. Eur J Clin Nutr 42:51–54, 1988.

41. Earon G, et al: Successful use of *Atriplex halimus* in the treatment of type II diabetic patients: Controlled clinical research report on the subject of *Atriplex*. Unpublished study conducted at the Hebrew University of Jerusalem, Israel.

42. Caselli L: Clinical and electroretinographic study on activity of Anthocyanosides. Arch Med Intern 37:29–35, 1985.

43. Rudofsky V: The effect of ginkgo biloba extract in cases of arterial occlusive disease: A randomized placebo controlled double-blind cross-over study. Fortschr Med 105:397–400, 1987.

44. Results of the DCCT. Reported in N Engl J Med 329(14), September 30, 1993.

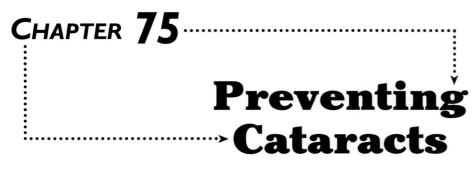

CHAPTER 75

Preventing Cataracts

Robert Abel, Jr., M.D.

ETIOLOGY

The lens is one of the body's most solid tissues, being approximately 36% solid. It is composed of mostly proteins (crystalline fibers and enzymes) and some carbohydrate and polyunsaturated fatty acids. The lens curvature and the alignment of the fibers are designed for the bending of light rays in the visual spectrum and absorbing radiation above and below that spectrum. A *cataract* is any opacification of the normally clear crystalline lens of the eye. Oxidation of lens fibers, catalyzed by short, phototoxic ultraviolet (UV) wavelengths of light, destroys the sulfhydryl protein bonds. Breaking of these bonds leads to a denaturation and clumping of the protein, with consequent loss of lens clarity.

The eye is a remote outpost that relies on good nutrition, liver function, circulation, and breathing. The lens, in particular, has no direct vascular or neurologic supply and therefore must rely for delivery of nutrition and removal of toxins on the circulation of the small amount of aqueous humor going from the ciliary body out through the trabecular meshwork.

The aqueous humor has very high levels of water-soluble compounds, such as ascorbic acid, glutathione, and its key amino acid, cysteine, which are the major diet-derived antioxidants that protect lens clarity.

However, the eye is not an isolated organ; it is connected to the brain and the cardiovascular and digestive systems. It requires protection from bright illumination, provided by the lids, lashes, watery tear film, and cornea. Cataract formation is often symptomatic of deeper abnormalities and systemic imbalances. In a common clinical scenario, the ophthalmologist tells the patient that he or she has a cataract, followed by reassurance of its nonacute nature: "Don't worry, I'll see you in six months." Six months later the patient is told: "It's time to operate!" Earlier interventions directed at the disturbances underlying cataract formation can halt or significantly retard this inevitable progression.

Central or nuclear cataracts are often related to aging, lifelong solar exposure, and smoking. Cortical cataract changes, as shown in the Chesapeake Waterman's study, are often due to UV light exposure as well.[1] Posterior subcapsular cataract forma-tion often occurs in younger people and can be rapidly progressive. The posterior subcapsular variety may result from corticosteroid administration, trauma, diabetes, and unusual retinal diseases. Biochemical alterations in sulfhydryl groups and lens epithelial cells' permeability account for changes in lens curvature, clarity, and refractive error.

Vision provides up to 80% of our sensory input and is to be preserved at any cost. This chapter reviews the recent evidence correlating antioxidant deficiency with the prevalence of cataract formation, as well as the administration of specific antioxidants reduce the incidence of lens opacification.

NOTE

Cataracts are the leading cause of vision impairment in both developed and developing countries and are the major cause of blindness worldwide.

SCREENING

Changes in Vision

Subtle cataract development leads to unrecognized loss of color interpretation and fine detail and to difficulty with contrast and distance vision. In younger patients, fluctuating vision is often related to refractive error, computer use, diminishing accommodation, and even medications. As reported by mature adults, the following visual symptoms may indicate early cataract formation and can serve as the basis for questioning the patient during a general medical history and physical examination:

- Blurred vision
- Difficulty with reading road signs and distance vision
- Trouble reading
- Loss of depth perception
- Difficulty following the golf ball
- Difficulty with night driving
- Glare, especially at night
- Double vision
- Reduced vision

NOTE

Patients may not volunteer information about decreasing vision because they do not notice the gradual decrement, or they may fear losing a driver's license or are anxious about having their eyes examined.

Primary Care Diagnosis

The new small-pupil Welsh-Allyn ophthalmoscope enables primary care physicians to look at the fundus to detect diabetic and other changes. The device is focused by a simple rotary movement of the thumb. It is possible to assess lens transparency as well as to observe the fundus.[2]

Ophthalmologic Referral

The definitive diagnosis of cataract is made by ophthalmologic referral and slit lamp examination. Distance visual acuity, near vision, and depth perception can be evaluated, as well as contrast sensitivity and peripheral vision. Glare testing may also approximate real-world conditions and may corroborate functional impairment.

Documentation of Progression

Because cataracts are slowly progressive, and phacoemulsification removal with intraocular lens implantation is an elective procedure, most ophthalmologists choose to wait for patients to volunteer information about level of inconvenience or significant loss of function. The mere appearance of early cataract changes alone rarely warrants surgical intervention.

Cataract Surgery

Cataract surgery is the number one item on the Medicare budget, with roughly 2 million procedures performed annually. The subsequent laser treatment of an opacified capsule ranks among the 10 most frequent surgical procedures. With appropriate history and physical examinations and regular eye examination, early cataract formation can be detected long before functional visual loss develops.

NOTE

Cataract is the number one expense item in the Medicare budget. Delaying cataracts for 10 years would result in tremendous cost savings.

Table 75–1. Major Stressors to the Eye and Lens

....

Ultraviolet light (sunlight)
Inadequate nutrition
Lifestyle habits
Stress
Chronic disease

RISK FACTORS

The incidence of cataract formation varies with a number of risk factors (Table 75–1). Cataract formation is not inevitable with age. It is not unusual to find men and women in their 80s and 90s with relatively clear lenses who have had healthy life style habits. The following risk factors for cataract formation have been identified:

- Age
- Sunlight exposure
- Stress
- Medications
- Smoking
- Alcohol excess
- Obesity
- Chronic disease
- Malnutrition
- Saturated fat diet
- Heredity
- Trauma
- Congenital disorders
- Inborn errors of metabolism
- Dehydration
- Diabetes
- Vitamin deficiencies
- Low estrogen

INTEGRATIVE APPROACH TO PREVENTION

Lifestyle Interventions

Ultraviolet Light–Blocking Sunglasses

Increased solar exposure and high altitudes have long been known to increase the frequency of cataracts in all decades of life. UV light, especially in the presence of oxygen, contributes strongly to the denaturation of lens protein, which results in cataract formation; this phenomenon was known to occur even before the deterioration of the ozone layer.

There currently are anecdotal veterinary reports of increased incidence of cataract in rabbits in Patagonia and in dogs in Australia. Beachgoers and sunlamp users must be counseled to always wear adequate eye protection. Parents should encourage their children, including infants, to wear sunglasses and other forms of eye protection.

Appropriate protective lenses should also be used in occupations such as welding and ironwork, in which workers are exposed to prolonged amounts of hazardous radiation, even above and below the visual spectrum of 400 to 700 nm. Use of hats and visors has been the recommendation of several long-term epidemiologic and longitudinal studies. UVA (also called near-UV) light and UVB (far-UV) light constitute toxic radiation, and the long-term effects are cumulative. Near-UV light penetrates the cornea and is generally absorbed by the lens, whereas far-UV light is more damaging but is usually absorbed by the cornea, but not entirely. For this reason, astronauts have been known to take large amounts of *N*-acetyl cysteine (3000 mg), a glutathione booster, while on space missions.

Stress Management

Stress depresses immune function, alters sleep patterns, impairs gastrointestinal absorption, and reduces available antioxidants. Stress also stimulates the sympathetic nervous system, causing vasoconstriction, increasing muscle tension, and, over long periods of time, decreasing microcirculation through the ophthalmic artery and its tributaries. A direct correlation between stress and cataract formation remains to be proved in humans, but there is ample evidence that stress, smoking, nutritional deficiency, radiation, and corticosteroids increased cataractogenesis in animal models.

Medications

More than 300 common medications are known to be photosensitizing agents. Many antibiotics, diuretics, anti-hypertensives, botanicals (St. John's wort), psoralens, and other agents increase the sensitivity of lens protein to UV damage. Therefore, it is important to advise all people taking medicine to wear sunglasses and to ask their pharmacist about whether their medications are photosensitizers. Many medications also require hepatic excretion and may interfere with normal nutritional biochemistry in the liver. For instance, many cholesterol-lowering agents decrease the production of coenzyme Q10 and glutathione in the liver. Glutathione, a sulfur-containing tripeptide, is a major free radical scavenger in the human lens.

Corticosteroids

Corticosteroids by any route of administration (topical, oral, intranasal, inhalable, or intravenous) are known to increase the incidence of both cataracts and glaucoma in susceptible persons. This adverse effect is most frequent with topical corticosteroids used in treating ocular inflammation and allergies. Therefore, it is advisable for patients who are prescribed ocular steroids for allergies not to have refills without appropriate ophthalmologic supervision. There are other ways to treat ocular allergy, such as with topical antihistamines, mast cell stabilizers, and the administration of oral vitamin C (1000 mg) and the eucalyptus bioflavonoid preparation quercetin (1000 mg).

Often, the patient who sees many physicians develops a polypharmacy, which is perpetuated. Chinese and Ayurvedic healers tend to use a mixture of herbal remedies for a limited time; they then re-evaluate the patient within 2 weeks and readjust the formula. This approach is a good one to incorporate into contemporary Western medicine.

Smoking

Smoking not only reduces available ascorbic acid and alpha tocopherol but also has a direct toxic effect on the lens of the eye. The longitudinal Physicians' Health Study and Nurses' Health Study have shown a significant increase in cataract formation in smokers, with twice the incidence in the male physicians' study and two-thirds more cataract operations in the women who smoked.[3, 4] Many pack-a-day smokers will develop a yellow-brown cast to the nucleus over 20 years.

Alcohol

Excess alcohol is known to increase the incidence of cataract formation, probably via loss of some of the B and fat-soluble vitamins and possible alteration of liver function.

Lack of Exercise

Exercise stimulates breathing and parasympathetic activity. This effect is especially desirable in persons with chronic glaucoma conditions and macular degeneration. A group of University of Oregon investigators found that 30 to 40 minutes of walking, 4 times weekly, lowered intraocular pressure and also decreased stress. Improved aqueous flow is important to the health of the crystalline lens of the eye as well.

Overweight

Obesity or an unfavorable waist-to-hip ratio has been associated with increased incidence of cataract formation.[5] This association is yet another reason why it is important to encourage maintenance of ideal body weight and moderation of caloric intake.

Management of General Medical Conditions

Patients with diabetes have 3 to 5 times the risk of cataract formation noted in the general poipulation.[6] Effective management of diabetes is important to avoid both the highs and lows of serum glucose. An elevation in blood sugar causes an influx of fluid into the lens of the eye, significantly changing the refractive error. This change in permeability ultimately enhances protein decomposition and cataract formation via the sorbitol pathway. Quercetin, a preparation of naturally occurring eucalyptus bioflavonoids, inhibits the aldose reductase pathway. Several recent studies indicate that hypothyroidism is also more frequent in persons with cataracts. Hypertension and Cushings' syndrome are also associated with cataract formation.

Female Gender

Some studies have indicated a higher incidence of cataracts in females that cannot be accounted for solely by the slight preponderance of women in the general population older than 65 years of age. Replacement estrogen therapy is correlated with a protective effect; therefore, the use of natural or synthetic estrogens may be appropriate in patients without contraindications.

Aging

Because the incidence of cataract rises every decade past the age of 45 years, it is important to screen this age group for general health and driving ability. Several studies in the orthopedic literature have indicated that visual disability is one of the risk factors for hip fracture. The loss of depth perception makes people particularly vulnerable to falls because they assume that they can see well with one eye yet may be likely to miscalculate steps and distances.

Lack of Sleep

Patients should be advised to get plenty of sleep. Darkness is a time when the eyes, especially the retina, get a chance to rest and replenish. The lens and intraocular structures are bombarded by light, with the formation of free radicals, all day; sleep provides an opportunity for the liver and circulation to replenish the necessary antioxidants and minerals to the lens and other ocular tissues.

Nutrition

Fruits and Vegetables

Ascorbic acid, carotenoids, tocopherol, and glutathione are present in the lens epithelium and lens fibers. Proteolytic enzymes that act to remove damaged protein are also present in the lens and are spared by glutathione and other free radical scavengers. In general, the colored bioflavonoids and carotenoids are nature's protectors and should be part of a balanced diet. Multiple studies have identified green leafy vegetables as being preventive of cataract as well as of age-related macular degeneration (AMD). The Australian Blue Mountains Study, which included 3654 persons, found that subjects with a diet high in protein, fiber, vitamin A, niacin, thiamine, and riboflavin had a decreased incidence of nuclear cataract. Persons whose diet had higher levels of polyunsaturated fatty acids had a significant reduction in cortical cataract formation.[7]

Vitamin C

Citrus fruits and many other fruits and vegetables contain high levels of ascorbic acid, which is a major antioxidant in the lens of the eye. The lens and aqueous humor concentrate ascorbic acid in amounts more than 10 times those found in human plasma. Ascorbate is richer in the cortical fibers than in the older, nuclear fibers. Higher blood levels seem to confer some protection against cataract. Persons with higher than average vitamin C intake appear to have a decreased risk of nuclear cataract, and those younger than 60 years have a decreased risk of cortical opacities, with intake range of 150 to 300 mg per day.[8]

Lutein-Containing Foods

Spinach, kale, collard greens, guava, and even corn and eggs contain lutein, which has been found to be protective against cataract formation. Among persons who consume high levels of green leafy vegetables and whose serum lutein levels are in the highest quintile, risk of cataract formation is reduced by approximately 20%.[9, 10] In both the Physicians' Health Study and Nurses' Health Study, cataract surgery was associated with lower intake of foods such as spinach, which are rich in lutein and zeaxanthin carotenoids rather than beta-carotene.

Avoidance of Saturated Animal Fat

By reducing saturated fats, the patient will find it easier to reach and maintain an ideal body weight.

Hydration

The patient should be encouraged to drink plenty of water. The lens of the eye is a dehydrated tissue much like a fingernail, another avascular ectodermal structure. Drinking 6 to 8 glasses of filtered water a

Table 75–2. Tips for Prevention of Dry Eyes
••

- Adequate hydration can be promoted by drinking 6 to 8 glasses of water daily.
- It is important to remember to blink, especially in work with computers and other tasks requiring visual concentration.
- The beneficial fats in the tear film can be reinforced with DHA supplementation and fat-soluble nutrients such as vitamin A and lutein. DHA produces amazing improvement in comfort within a week.
- Use of eye drops and ointments as moisturizers is recommended. Tears Again, a liposomal vitamin A and E spray, can be applied externally on the lid and appears to penetrate the eye quickly, providing relief.
- Mechanical problems with the lower lids should be ruled out, especially in patients who may be sleeping with their eyes open. When observing the patient, the clinician should check to see whether the lower lid moves during routine blinking.
- A humidifier should be kept in the bedroom.
- Periodic evaluation of the patient's medication profile is recommended.

DHA, docosahexaenoic acid.

day is an excellent way to increase aqueous humor circulation, which supports lens health. Tips for preventing dry eyes are presented in Table 75–2.

Sulfur-Containing Foods

Glutathione is a major antioxidant in the lens and is found in such foods as onions, garlic, avocados, cruciferous vegetables, asparagus, and watermelon. Glutathione and its boosters are thiol compounds, which scavenge free radicals. These include L-cysteine, lipoic acid, and methanyl sulfonylmethane (MSM). Glutathione also spares proteolytic enzymes in the cortical lens fibers. In studies from the late 1960s, extracted mature cataracts were demonstrated to contain very low levels of glutathione and ascorbic acid; this finding was considered to represent a secondary aspect of cataract formation. In retrospect, this deficiency appears to be a preliminary event and one that may be nutritionally managed.

Algae-Eating Fish

Single-cell algae are at the bottom of the food chain. When the early hominids began eating fish, their brains developed further, approaching human dimensions. The traditional Japanese diet appears to protect against cataract formation because of the inclusion of cold-water fish and algae, both of which are rich in docosahexaenoic acid (DHA). (Examples of such fish are tuna, mackerel, salmon, sardines, and cod.) Currently, fish such as salmon are being farm raised. Because farm raised fish are fed grain instead of algae, they contain less DHA and provide less benefit to the eyes and body.

Supplements

See Chapter 76, Preventing Age-Related Macular Degeneration, for a more complete listing of supplements that promote eye health.

Lutein and Zeaxanthin

The Physicians' Health Study and Nurses' Health Study have indicated an approximately 20% protection against cataract formation among persons with serum lutein values in the highest quintile.[9, 10] Lutein and its isomer, zeaxanthin, are present in high levels in ocular tissues including the lens. Their importance may lie in the fact that they absorb and reflect the phototoxic blue and UV wavelengths. The carotenoids present in the lens turn out to be lutein and zeaxanthin more than beta-carotene. A daily dose of 2.4 mg of lutein has been shown to double the serum level.

Dosage. Patients with early cataracts should take 6 mg a day for the first month and then 2 mg as part of their daily multivitamin.

Vitamin C

Numerous studies have shown that increased vitamin C consumption (60 to 600 mg) over many years protects against cataracts. In one study, the 5-year risk for the development of any cataract was 60% lower among 3634 participants, aged 43 to 86, who had been taking a multivitamin that included vitamin C for 10 years.[11] Another study showed a 45% protection rate against cataract surgery in women who had consumed vitamin C supplements for 10 years. The investigators found that women with a mean intake of 359 mg of vitamin C a day for 10 years had a 77% lower prevalence of earlier lens opacities.[12]

Dosage. The authors of the study on vitamin C supplementation recommend approximately 300 mg of vitamin C daily, although I recommend 1000 mg daily.

Vitamin A

Hankinson found a 39% reduction in the incidence of cataract formation in more than 50,000 nurses who had an adequate intake of vitamin A over an 8-year period.[13] This association has been reported in other studies as well. Vitamin A or beta carotene is included in most good multivitamins.

Multivitamins

Multivitamins have been observed to reduce the risk for cataracts by approximately 20% to 60%, depending on the content of ascorbic acid. *d*-Alpha tocopherol is also protective, as found by numerous studies. Robertson found that vitamin C (300 to 600 mg) and vitamin E (400 international units [IU]) had a 50% protective effect.[14]

The 10-year randomized, controlled Age-Related Eye Disease Study (AREDS) was concluded early. It supported the use of a multivitamin with A, C, E, and zinc in macular degeneration.

Dosage. Taking a multivitamin is a convenient way to get a daily amount of beta carotene or vitamin A, trace minerals, lutein, and other essential nutrients in 1 or 2 capsules or tablets.

Vitamin E

As noted, people who took 400 IU of vitamin E with 300 mg of vitamin C experienced a 50% reduction in the incidence of cataract formation.[14] The Eye Disease Case Control Study has also confirmed that alpha tocopherol is protective against lens opacity.[15] Another study from Linxian, China, also found vitamin E to be protective against cataract formation in persons older than 45 years of age.[16]

B Vitamins

The B vitamins, especially riboflavin, thiamine, and niacin, have been found to be protective in both the Blue Mountains Study in Australia and in another study from Linxian, China.[7, 16]

Glutathione Boosters

Glutathione is a major protector against oxidation in lens fibers and the lens epithelium. Glutathione boosters such as MSM (1000 mg), alpha lipoic acid (250 mg twice daily), *S* adenosyl methionine (SAMe) (200 mg twice daily), and most important, *N*-acetyl cysteine (NAC), have not been studied, but would intuitively seem to be useful.

Dosage. As an option, NAC 600 mg can be used once or twice daily by people with early cataracts. Use of a 5% MSM eye drop solution has a variable effect on arrest of cataract progression.

Docosahexaenoic Acid

DHA, the end product of omega-3 fatty acid metabolism, is known to protect cell membranes in thiol groups. DHA is an important constituent of retina and brain and has also been found in the lens of the eye. With its presence in all cell membranes and its six double bonds, replenishment of this compound is important. The DHA in breast milk has been documented to reduce learning disabilities in children and to improve head size and growth in the first

year of life. The Crete Diet has a 1:1 omega 3 to omega 6 fatty acid ratio, whereas in the average American diet the ratio is closer to 1:6 to 1:20.

Dosage. A supplemental regimen of 200 to 800 mg of DHA daily is helpful for almost all persons.

Minerals

Minerals are important as cofactors with cell enzymes and vitamins. These include selenium, zinc, copper, and magnesium.

Pyruvate

Animal studies have shown that pyruvate, a normal breakdown product of glucose metabolism, quenches free radicals and protects the lens against cataract formation. Pyruvate definitely blocks the formation of cataracts after exposure to selenite in laboratory animals. Studies in humans have not yet been performed.

Botanicals

Numerous herbs are known to improve blood flow to the eye and to strengthen liver function. Bioflavonoids in certain berries have been proved to enhance capillary formation; however, their effect on night vision is inconclusive. Astragalus, milk thistle, (silymarin), oleander, turmeric root, garlic bulb in oil, and wheat sprouts are botanicals that strengthen liver function.[17] Some supplements are used to improve and support liver function, such as SAMe and silymarin.

Turmeric

Curcuman, a constituent of turmeric (*Curcuma longa*), is a spice included in Indian curry dishes. This compound is an effective antioxidant known to induce the glutathione-linked detoxification pathways in rats. It significantly reduces the rate of cataract formation in laboratory rats.

Cineraria

Cineraria maritima or *senecio cinerario* (silver ragwort) has been used for centuries as an eye drop preparation for the treatment of conjunctivitis and early cataract. Homeopathic preparations have also been employed, but they have not been subjected to controlled studies.

Bioflavonoids

The eucalyptus bioflavonoid preparation querce-tin has been found in multiple laboratory studies to inhibit the formation of steroid, diabetes, and radiation induced cataracts.

PREVENTION PRESCRIPTION

- *Annual eye examination for people over 50 and persons at risk. Use of preventive measures is appropriate even in patients with early cataract*
- *Use of sunglasses, with side shields as necessary, as well as hats or visors and sunblock in persons whose occupation or interests dictate spending time outdoors*
- *A balanced diet including 5 or 6 servings of fruits and vegetables as well as grains, nuts, berries, and organic eggs for amino acids, with consumption of cold-water fish 2 or more times a week*
- *Lutein rich foods such as spinach three times weekly, as these foods are especially important for ocular protection*
- *Adequate hydration, with intake of 6 to 8 glasses of filtered water daily, and reduction in intake of soft drinks and artificial sweeteners*
- *A daily multivitamin including taurine, zinc, lutein, an additional 1000 to 2000 mg of vitamin C, 400 IU of vitamin E, and 5000 to 10,000 IU of vitamin A palmitate*
- *Maintenance of an appropriate body weight and avoidance of animal fat in the diet*
- *Healthful lifestyle habits including stretching, exercise, moderate alcohol intake, and a regular sleep pattern, with cessation of smoking*
- *Maintenance of a positive attitude and optimism*
- *Periodic review of prescription and other medications for ophthalmologic effects*
- *Regular physical examinations and vision testing*

NOTE

Do we want to wait for unassailable proof of nutrition protection for the ocular lens, or shall we develop preventive strategies for ocular health now?

References

1. West S, et al: Sunlight exposure and risk of lens opacity in a population-based study. JAMA 280:714–718, 1998.
2. Bresnick G, Mukamel D, Dickinson J, et al: A screening approach to the surveillance of patients with diabetes for the presence of vision threatening retinopathy. Ophthalmology 107:19–24, 2000.
3. Hankinson SE, Willett WC, Colditz GA, et al: A prospective study of cigarette smoking and risk of cataract surgery in women. JAMA 268:994–998, 1992.
4. Cristen WG, Manson JA, Seddon JM, et al: A prospective study of cigarette smoking and risk of cataract surgery in men. JAMA 268:989–993, 1992.
5. Shamburg DA, Glynn RJ, Christen WG, et al: Relations of body fat distribution and height with cataract in men. Am J Clin Nutr 72:1495–1502, 2000.
6. Bunce G: Animal studies on cataract. In Taylor A (ed): Nutritional and Environmental Influences on the Eye. Boca Raton, Fla, CRC Press, 1999, pp 105–115.
7. Cumming RG, Mitchell P, Smith W: Diet and cataract. The Blue Mountains Eye Study. Ophthalmology 107:450–456, 2000.
8. Taylor A: Nutrition and cataract risk. Ophthalmol Clin 40:27, 2000.
9. Chasan-Taber L, Willett WC, Seddon JM, et al: A prospective study of carotenoid and vitamin A intakes and risk of cataract extraction in U.S. women. Am J Clin Nutr 70:509–516, 1999.
10. Brown L, Rimm ER, Seddon JM, et al: A prospective study of carotenoid intake and risk of cataract extraction in U.S. men. Am J Clin Nutr 70:517–524, 1999.
11. Mares Perlman JA, Lyle BJ, Klein R, et al: Vitamin supplement use and incident cataracts in a population-based study. Arch Ophthalmol 118:1556–1563, 2000.
12. Jacques PF, Taylor A, Hankinson SE, et al: Long-term vitamin C supplement use and prevalence of early age related lens opacities. Am J Clin Nutr 66:911–916, 1997.
13. Hankinson SE, Stampfer MJ, Sedden JM, et al: Nutrient intake and cataract extraction in women: A prospective study. BMJ 305:335–339, 1992.
14. Robertson JM, Danner AP, Trevithick JR: A possible role for vitamin C and E in cataract prevention. Am J Clin Nutr 53:346S–351S, 1991.
15. Leske MC, Chylack LT, Wu SY: The Lens Opacities Case-Control Study: Risk factors for cataract. Arch Ophthalmol 109:244–251, 1991.
16. Sperduto RD, Milton RC, Zhao JL, et al: The Linxian cataract studies. Arch Ophthalmol 111:1246–1253, 1993.
17. Tillotson AK: The One Earth Herbal Sourcebook. New York, Kensington, 2001.

Suggested Reading

Taylor A (ed): Nutritional and Environmental Influences on the Eye. Boca Raton, Fla, CRC Press, 1999.
Friedlander MH (ed): Nutrition. Int Ophthalmol Clin 40:1-122, 2000.

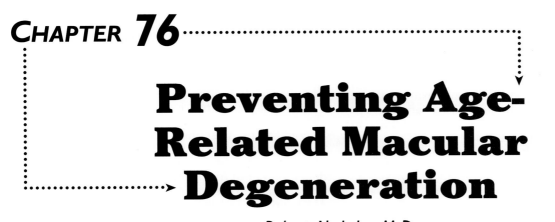

CHAPTER 76

Preventing Age-Related Macular Degeneration

Robert Abel, Jr., M.D.

Nowhere has there been so much scientific documentation about nutritional prevention as in the case of macular degeneration. The irony lies in the fact that this information is often virtually ignored by the very specialists who manage patients with the disease.

ETIOLOGY

Age-related macular degeneration (AMD) is the scourge of the golden years. People 65 years of age and older constitute the fastest-growing segment of the population in developed countries; the risk and impact of AMD will only become greater in the future. There is a tremendous need to develop preventive strategies to counter AMD and to arrest early cases before the loss of useful vision.

Retinal photoreceptors are subjected to oxidative stress from the combined exposure to light and oxygen on a daily basis. The body's ability to resupply the photoreceptors and its underlying pigment epithelium with essential nutrients is the basis for the maintenance of good vision throughout life. Diseases of the retina are the leading cause of blindness throughout the developed countries of the world. Among these diseases, macular degeneration is the most common, and it is increasing in incidence as the population ages. Population-based studies propose that approximately 30% of persons 75 years of age and older demonstrate early signs of the disease, and 7% have late signs of disease.[1]

Free radicals are thought to attack the rod and cone cell membranes, and the retinal pigment epithelium (RPE), a monolayer beneath the retina, fails to keep up with the removal of lipid debris, which accumulates as drusen (yellow spots of different sizes.) The melanin pigment protects the retina from radiation, but the amount of this pigment decreases with age, smoking, and low serum lutein levels. When the RPE cells drop out, pigmentary defects can be noted by ophthalmoscopy and by retinal photography. Drusen and progressive RPE atrophy characterize the dry form of macular degeneration, which accounts for 90% of the cases of AMD.

The other 10% of cases are attributable to the exudative or vascular type of AMD. A hyaline membrane (i.e., Bruch's membrane) separates the choroidal blood supply from the RPE and overlying retina. Degeneration of Bruch's membrane, retinal anoxia, and impairment of choroidal circulation are believed to be factors that induce the vascular ingrowth characteristic of this form of the disease; these fragile new vessels grow rapidly and may bleed spontaneously.

Most ophthalmologists agree that oxidative stress combined with failure to fortify the retinal photoreceptors is a major pathophysiologic mechanism in this disease, which currently affects 14 million to 20 million elderly Americans. Many of these physicians also consider vision loss from macular degeneration to be inevitable, believing that nothing can be done for the dry form, and that perhaps only laser therapy is useful for treatment of the wet form of macular degeneration, if it is detected in time. However, considerable evidence is available to indicate that nutritional approaches play a major part in prevention and management of this age-related disease. Cumulative photo-oxidative stress, other systemic diseases, and nutritional deficiencies contribute to the onset and progression of this degenerative disorder. With aging, the protective cellular-derived enzymes—catalase, superoxide dismutase (SOD), and glutathione peroxidase—decrease, as does the ability to absorb the diet-derived antioxidants.

SCREENING

Owing to the growing ranks of the elderly, the number of persons with macular degeneration is increasing. Routine dilated-eye examinations are fundamental to early detection and management of AMD. The onset is often so gradual as to go unnoticed.

Use of an Amsler grid, a 4 × 4-inch checkerboard square with a central dot for fixation, is an excellent way to diagnose AMD and allows home monitoring of the condition. This approach to management is especially useful in patients with the slowly progressive, dry form of the disease (see Fig. 76–1).

Primary care physicians should know the AMD risk profiles in order to alert patients about preventive steps and the need for periodic eye examinations. Patients with multiple systemic diseases are at greatest risk. Early detection offers greater flexibility in using complementary therapies.

Referral to an ophthalmologist is indicated for dilated funduscopic examination and retinal photography (fluorescein angiography), which can clearly document stages of AMD. Occasionally, retinal specialists will be needed to perform laser surgery.

Primary care physicians should help patients to coordinate the various medicines used in managing underlying and concurrent diseases. Periodic review of medications is important, as polypharmacy may contribute to the risk for AMD.

NOTE

Primary care physicians should know the risk profiles of AMD and can use an eye chart and Amsler grid as part of a routine medical examination.

INTEGRATIVE APPROACH TO PREVENTION

Risk Factors

The following risk factors for AMD have been identified:

- Age
- Sunlight exposure
- Previous cataract surgery
- Light colored irises/fair complexion
- Obesity
- Female gender/parity
- Postmenopausal status
- Smoking
- Physical inactivity
- Elevated cholesterol levels
- Hypertension
- Nocturnal hypotension
- Poor digestion/use of antacids
- Hypothyroidism/use of thyroid hormones
- Family history
- Low dietary intake of carotenoids/low serum carotenoids
- Low macular pigment density
- Low serum zinc levels
- Hyperopia

Age

The National Health and Nutrition Examination Survey demonstrated that in 65- to 70-year-old respondents, the chance of developing AMD was nearly 5 times that in the 45- to 54-year-old age group.[2]

Sunlight

Reduced exposure to sunlight by using hats and sunglasses has been stressed in numerous studies.[3] A University of Wisconsin study in 3684 persons between the ages of 43 and 84 years found a positive correlation between daily sun exposure and the development of AMD. Persons who spent more than 5 hours a day in the sun were twice as likely to develop AMD as those with less than 2 hours of sun exposure.[4]

Gender

The incidence of AMD in postmenopausal women is at least 3 times greater than that in men of similar age. Two studies have indicated that hormone replacement therapy (HRT) significantly reduces this risk, whereas another study failed to find any correlation. Apparently, women require more lutein than men, because it is preferentially deposited in fat tissue rather than the retina.[5] Obstetricians and gynecologists should inform their patients about early prevention and participate in decisions about HRT where appropriate.

Smoking and Other Factors

Numerous investigators have determined that current smokers, especially those who smoke 1 pack a day or more, have a significantly elevated risk of developing AMD over that in persons who have given up smoking 10 years previously, or that in nonsmokers. The Nurses' Health Study indicated that women who smoked 25 or more cigarettes a day were more than twice as likely as nonsmokers to develop AMD.[6] The Physicians' Health Study also showed a greater than twofold incidence in men who smoked 20 or more cigarettes daily.[7] One study indicated an association between smoking, low serum selenium levels, and the development of AMD. Smoking has been shown to contribute to decreased levels of circulating antioxidants, as well as to decreased levels of the lutein pigment in the macular area.

The Age-Related Eye Disease Study (AREDS) found that smoking was associated with three of its five stages of macular degeneration.[8] This multicenter, randomized controlled trial has also found that hypertension, obesity, hyperopic refractive error, white race, and increased use of thyroid hormones and antacids were indicators of the most severe stages of the disease.

Risk Summary

Retinal health is dependent on remote nutrition, liver health, good cardiovascular status, normal gastrointestinal function, and protection against photo-toxic ultraviolet (UV) and blue light. The patient can be evaluated for risk factors for AMD as part of a general medical history and physical examination.

NOTE

Smoking, increasing age, light-colored irises, and low serum carotenoid levels all have been associated with decreased macular pigment density. It has been suggested that increased macular pigment may retard age-related decline in visual function.[9]

Lifestyle Interventions

Sunglasses, Hats, and Visors

The need to wear sunglasses with light protection, hats, and visors should be emphasized as early as childhood. People with dilated pupils, sunstarers, and those who frequent tanning beds may be at a higher risk of developing macular degeneration. Microscope light during cataract surgery is another source of phototoxicity. Sun exposure is a known causative factor in the progression of the hereditary disorder retinitis pigmentosa.

Stress Management

Hormonal imbalance and lack of sleep contribute to debilitation of retinal health. Depression contributes to food habituation, overeating, and abnormal sleep patterns. Ocular health remains in a sensitive balance between oxidative stress and antioxidant support of cell membranes. Therefore, smoking and inadequate nutrition both tip the scale toward increased or imbalanced free radical activity.

Limiting Alcohol Intake

Alcohol excess has been associated with cardiovascular and liver disorders. The Beaver Dam Eye Study documented an association between beer consumption and risk of RPE degeneration. Two recent studies have indicated that 1 or 2 glasses of red wine daily can confer a 40% to 50% AMD risk reduction. However, the Physicians' Health Study and Nurses' Health Study, conducted between 1980 and 1994, could not confirm any significant benefit. Red wine has a protective effect on cardiovascular health and may improve retinal and choroidal blood flow. Apparently, white wine, which lacks the high levels of grape skin bioflavonoids, does not confer as much ocular protection.

Recognition of Medication Effects

Numerous medications, including phenothiazines, hydroxychloroquine, and ethambutol, may affect the RPE. Other agents may alter digestion or liver function. The liver not only filters out all of the nutrients and toxins from the gastrointestinal tract but also stores fat-soluble vitamins, activates the B vitamins, and manufactures glutathione. Chinese and Ayurvedic physicians have known for millennia that the liver is essential to good vision.

NOTE

Antacid usage has been positively correlated with the development of AMD. The lack of gastric acidity reduces the stimulus for secretion of pancreatic and biliary enzymes into the duodenum.

Hydration

Drinking 6 or more glasses of good water a day hydrates the body, flushes the liver and kidneys, and decreases appetite. Patients should be counseled against immoderate caffeine and soft drink consumption.

Exercise

Exercise plays a role in cardiovascular health and in stimulating the parasympathetic nervous system. Physical activity also plays a part in relaxation of the mind, decreasing intraocular pressure, and increasing ocular blood flow.

Breathing

Deep breathing relaxes the mind, strengthens the diaphragm, and improves blood flow to the eye. Conscious attention to breathing is the foundation of meditation and stress-reduction practices.

Whole Body Health

Management of concurrent medical conditions is essential. Regulating blood pressure and cholesterol, controlling diabetes, supporting necessary weight reduction, and managing cardiovascular health are important to the long-term maintenance of good vision. It is wise to remember that the eye is intimately connected to the rest of the body.

Estrogen

Females are more likely to develop AMD than males. Several studies have demonstrated that postmenopausal women who are taking HRT exhibit a lower incidence of macular degeneration, especially the wet form of the disease.[10] However, one study was unable to determine any significant effect of estrogen replacement therapy.

Familial History of Age-Related Macular Degeneration

People with a familial history of AMD or who have fair skin or are of northern European ancestry are the most susceptible to AMD.

Sleep

Sleep is crucial to restoration of photoreceptor and ocular health. The eye requires darkness to restore photoreceptor integrity and to replenish nutrients consumed during the daylight hours, when UV wavelengths and bright light are constantly bombarding the eye.

Attitude

Adopting a positive attitude is the first step in lifestyle modification. The placebo effect is another demonstration of the "power of positive thinking." Sixty-eight percent of persons who took a multivitamin for 6 months showed an improvement in macular appearance on the electroretinogram; however, 32% of the placebo group also showed improvement. Similarly, in an initial study of photodynamic therapy to control retinal bleeding, approximately 50% of people demonstrated some benefit, compared with 28% of the placebo group. This nearly 30% placebo effect, which contributed to the cessation of retinal bleeding, is a demonstration of the power of positive thinking.

Nutrition

Fruits and Vegetables

Fruits and vegetables contain vitamins A, C, and E and beta-carotene. The yellow-orange vegetables such as carrots and sweet potatoes are important for daytime vision.

Lutein-Containing Foods

Spinach, collard greens, kale, guava, and many other green and yellow fruits and vegetables contain lutein and its isomer, zeaxanthin. These two carotenoids are concentrated in the macular pigment; their accumulation is directly dependent on dietary intake and serum level.

Table 76–1. Top 10 Foods for Sight Preservation

- Cold-water fish (sardines, cod, mackerel, tuna)—an excellent source of DHA, which provides structural support to cell membranes and is recommended for dry eyes, treatment for macular degeneration, and sight preservation (see Chapter 84, The Anti-Inflammatory Diet)
- Spinach, kale, and green leafy vegetables—rich in carotenoids, especially lutein and zeaxathin; lutein, a yellow pigment, protects the macula from sun damage and from blue light
- Eggs—rich in cysteine, sulfur, lecithin, amino acids, and lutein; sulfur-containing compounds protect the lens of the eye from cataract formation
- Garlic, onions, shallots, and capers—rich in sulfur, which is necessary for the production of glutathione, an important antioxidant for the lens of the eye, and the whole body
- Soy—low in fat, rich in protein; has become a staple in vegetarian diets; contains essential fatty acids, phytoestrogens, vitamin E, and natural anti-inflammatory agents
- Fruits and vegetables—contain vitamins A, C, and E and beta-carotene; the yellow vegetables, such as carrots and squash, are important for daytime vision
- Blueberriers and grapes—contain anthocyanins, which improve night vision; a cupful of blueberries, huckleberry jam, or a 100-mg bilberry supplement may improve dark adaptation within 30 minutes
- Wine—Known to exert a cardioprotective effect; has many important nutrients that protect vision, heart, and blood flow (as with any alcohol, moderation is always important)
- Nuts and berries—nature's most concentrated food sources; grains such as flaxseed are high in the beneficial omega-3 fatty acids, which help to lower cholesterol and to stabilize cell-membranes
- Extra virgin olive oil—a monounsaturated oil; a healthy alternative to butter and margarine

DHA, docosahexaenoic acid.

The complete name of the visually sensitive center of the retina is *macula lutea*, because of its yellow color (Latin *luteus*, "yellow"). Lutein and zeaxanthin are known to be responsible for the yellow color. The normal retina is capable of concentrating these carotenoids to a level several orders of magnitude greater than the serum level.

In one study, persons consuming lutein-rich foods 5 times a week were 8 times less likely to develop AMD than those consuming such foods once per month.[11] In addition, persons with serum lutein values in the highest quintile had a 43% lower risk for AMD. Another study demonstrated that consumption of 4 to 8 ounces of spinach daily for 4 months was shown to result in increased macular pigment density. The vitamin K content in spinach may interfere with blood-thinning agents such as warfarin sodium. Preliminary data have demonstrated improvement in visual function in patients with the dry form of AMD whose diet was modified to provide an abundance of dark green vegetables.[12]

Avoidance of Saturated Fats

Patients should be advised to decrease their intake of saturated fats.[13]

Cold-Water Fish

Docosahexaenoic acid (DHA), found in cold-water, deep-dwelling fish, is an essential ingredient for good brain and retinal function. The flesh of algae-eating fish is high in DHA, which is important in building and protecting photoreceptor membranes. In one study, persons consuming cold-water fish more than once a week were half as likely to develop macular degeneration as those consuming fish less than once a month.[14] The same study found a 2.7-fold greater incidence of AMD in persons consuming high levels of cholesterol in the diet.

Wine in Moderation

Most researchers agree that consumption of moderate amounts of red wine decreases the risk of macular degeneration. In addition, many studies report that moderate wine consumption is associated with lengthened life span.

Glutathione

An important study found that glutathione and related precursor amino acids are protective against damage to human RPE cells, which underlie the macula. Foods that contain the tripeptide glutathione are onions, garlic, avocadoes, asparagus, watermelon, and cruciferous vegetables.

SUPPLEMENTS

Multivitamins

Many studies indicate the protective effect of antioxidants on retinal photoreceptors and the RPE. Some studies have demonstrated an association between vitamin or mineral deficiencies (e.g., zinc, tocopherol, carotenoids, taurine) and an increased risk of AMD. Ascorbate, as well as lipoic acid, helps to recycle tocopherol in retinal tissue. AMD patients in general were found in one study to have a decreased intake of tocopherol, magnesium, zinc, pyridoxine, and folic acid. In an important Veterans Affairs study, AMD patients taking an antioxidant capsule (containing 19 ingredients) twice daily maintained better vision than that determined in the placebo control group.[15]

The 10-year randomized, controlled Age-Related Eye Disorder Study (AREDS) was concluded early. It demonstrated that the combination of Vitamins C and E, beta-carotene, and zinc significantly reduced the progression of macular degeneration.[16] Ophthalmologists regard this as a landmark study acknowledging the effect of supplementation on macular degeneration. Proof of specific benefits of a balanced diet and broader nutrient supplementation has exciting implications.

Lutein

Carotenoids are powerful antioxidants. Lutein and zeaxanthin have been precisely identified in high levels in the retina, particularly in the macular area. They have also been identified in significant concentrations in the iris, choroid, and lens (all of which are needed to reflect UV light and blue light). Increased lutein consumption is directly associated with elevated serum levels and an increased macular pigment density. Investigators[17] studying 23 pairs of donor eyes found that the eyes with lower lutein and zeaxanthin levels were the ones with histopathologic signs of AMD. Another study evaluated lutein and zeaxanthin levels in 56 donor eyes affected by AMD and 56 donor eyes known to be without the disease. Donor eyes with the highest amounts of lutein and zeaxanthin were 82% less likely to exhibit the signs of macular degeneration.[18]

As little as 2.4 mg daily of lutein can double the serum level. A dose of 6 mg a day produced a 43% lower prevalence of AMD.[11]

Dosage. Healthy persons should select a multivitamin containing 2 mg of lutein, and patients already diagnosed with AMD should take 6 to 10 mg daily for several months to build up their plasma and macular levels.

Beta-Carotene, Vitamin A, and other Carotenoids

Investigators have confirmed in both laboratory and clinical studies that carotenoids such as vitamin A protect retinal cell membranes from light damage. Vitamin A is required to provide adequate levels of rhodopsin for optimal rod function. Severe vitamin A deficiency causes keratomalacia, xerophthalmia, and impaired vision. Vitamin A administration has been helpful in patients suffering from retinitis pigmentosa. An early study documented an association between low vitamin A levels and macular degeneration and encouraged the inclusion of yellow fruits and vegetables in the diet.[2] A more recent study discovered a positive association between beta-carotene intake and number of drusen.[19] Beta-carotene is the precursor to vitamin A and in healthy persons should confer the same protective effect. Only one study indicated a specific beneficial effect of the carotenoid lycopene on the macula.[13]

Tocopherols

Tocopherols protect against lipid peroxidation in cell membranes. Multiple studies have shown a powerful protective effect of *d*-alpha-tocopherol against macular degeneration. Some of these studies indicate a similar protective effect of plasma ascorbic acid and beta-carotene as well. High serum levels of *d*-alpha-tocopherol have been associated with decreased prevalence of early (appearance of drusen[19, 20]) and late macular degeneration. French researchers examined 2500 patients and found that those with the highest serum levels of vitamin E had an 82% decreased prevalence of AMD.[20] Gamma-tocopherol and tocotrienol may prove superior to d-alpha-tocopherol.

Vitamin C

Ascorbic acid reduces the loss of rhodopsin and photoreceptor cell nuclei occurring on exposure to light. Vitamin C also rejuvenates vitamin E– and cell membrane–related enzymes. In several of the major studies that showed a protective effect for multivitamins against AMD, the multivitamin included at least 60 mg of vitamin C. Ocular tissues, especially the lens, contain high levels of vitamin C and glutathione.

Alpha-Lipoic Acid

Alpha-lipoic acid is an important nerve stabilizer and reduces insulin resistance in diabetics. It may protect the remaining ganglion cells and nerve fibers in glaucoma patients. Additionally, alpha-lipoic acid helps to regenerate the reduced form of ascorbic acid.

B Vitamins

Pyridoxine deficiency has been identified in two observational studies in AMD populations. Folate deficiency has been identified in one of the studies. The B vitamins in general are important for nerve conduction, and the methylators (B_4, B_6, and B_{12}) reduce homocysteine levels.

Glutathione

Glutathione has been reported as being protective against damage to human RPE cells. Glutathione is manufactured in the liver after ingestion of the appropriate amino acids and sulfur-containing foods. This underappreciated water-soluble compound serves as an antioxidant and regenerator of vitamin E and carotenoids, as well as an intracellular enzyme. Because glutathione is hydrolyzed in the stomach, supplementation with glutathione boosters is recommended. These compounds are N-acetyl cysteine (NAC) 600 mg twice a day, methanyl sulfonylmethane (MSM) 1000 mg, S-adenosyl methionine (SAMe) 200 mg twice a day, and alpha-lipoic acid 250 mg twice daily.

Bioflavonoids

Studies show that quercetin, a preparation of eucalyptus bioflavonoids, facilitates vitamin E protection of bovine and rat retina from induced lipid peroxidation. It also exerts an antihistaminic effect that may be beneficial for patients with chronic allergies.

Taurine

Taurine, the only nonbound circulating amino acid, is a stabilizer of biologic membranes and protects rod outer segments, supports cardiovascular function, and modulates nerve transmission. Isolated taurine deficiency has been documented to cause retinal degeneration, and taurine administration has been shown in several studies to stabilize retinal changes.[21]

Zinc and Copper

Zinc is found in high concentrations in the retina, RPE, and choroid. This trace mineral serves as a cofactor with many important retinal enzymes, including superoxide dismutase (SOD), catalase, carbonic anhydrase, retinol dehydrogenase, and protein phosphorylase and also releases vitamin A from the liver. A 2-year study demonstrated that 100 mg of zinc sulfate daily significantly slowed the progression of AMD compared with the course of the disease in controls.[22] A study utilizing a dietary intake questionnaire found a significant inverse association between zinc consumption and number of drusen.[19] Copper is adversely affected by prolonged elevation of zinc levels (50 mg or more) and needs to be supplemented as well. A good multivitamin for long-term use will include 15 to 30 mg of zinc and 2 mg of copper. Both copper and zinc are needed to synthesize SOD and act with other retinal enzymes to scavenge free radicals.

Other Minerals

Magnesium

Magnesium is important in nerve conduction and it dilates blood vessels. Magnesium is important for maintaining blood flow to the eye and brain in elderly persons with macular degeneration or diabetes at a time of decreased blood pressure because they are lying down. The dose is 400 to 500 mg at bedtime.

Chromium

Chromium is helpful in regulating blood sugar. The supplement dose should be no more than 200 mg daily.

Selenium

Selenium (maximum dose 200 mg) is a cofactor for vitamin E and glutathione enzymes. Low serum selenium levels and smoking both have been associated with AMD.

Intravenous Supplementation

In anecdotal reports of uncontrolled studies, short-term improvement has been obtained in persons with AMD by giving intravenous vitamins C and E, magnesium, zinc, and selenium (e.g., Jonathan Wright, M.D., personal communication, 2001). Controlled studies and photodocumentation are necessary to support these findings.

Chelation Therapy

Disodium ethylenediaminetetraacetic acid (EDTA) chelation therapy has been reported to be effective in patients with early and moderate forms of AMD, but again, controlled studies are lacking. The concept of removing calcium from blood vessels as well as the retina is intuitively sound. Many advocates alternate intravenous nutritional supplementation on alternate visits with intravenous EDTA chelation therapy.

Digestive Enzymes

Hypochlorhydria increases with age and with chronic administration of certain medications such as nonsteroidal anti-inflammatory drugs (NSAIDs). Giving medications to reduce gastric acidity effectively eliminates the initial hydrolysis of food. An acid pH in the food bolus in the duodenum is necessary for the normal release of pancreatic and biliary enzymes. Antacids therefore interfere with the entire digestive process and the availability of nutrients. Digestive enzymes rapidly improve the digestion much more effectively than antacid preparations can. Betaine HCl is the most commonly used digestive enzyme; others are protease, amylase, and lipase. These enzymes should be taken on a full stomach.

Docosahexaenoic Acid (DHA)

The primary source of DHA is algae and the cold-water, deep-dwelling fish that eat them. DHA not only supports retinal health in general but also improves hand-to-eye coordination, sharpens night-driving ability, and stabilizes cell membranes throughout the body. With its six unsaturated double bonds, it composes 30% to 50% of the "good" fat in the outer segments of the retinal photoreceptors. Because people are undersupplied with DHA from infancy, it is important to incorporate DHA capsules in the diet. The suggested supplementation amount is 200 to 500 mg per day.

NOTE

Alpha-linolenic acid (present in flaxseed oil, among others) is the parent omega-3 fatty acid. It takes 20 to 30 of these 18-carbon molecules to make one 22-carbon DHA molecule, which is a building block for every cell membrane in the body.

Botanicals

Ginkgo

The ginkgo tree is the sole survivor of a family of trees that flourished before the Ice Age. *Ginkgo biloba*, which increases cerebral blood flow, has been demonstrated to improve retinal blood flow by 23% and is prescribed regularly by certain glaucoma specialists. For vasodilation, I recommend either 15 drops of a ginkgo solution (24% ginkgosides) in water twice daily or magnesium 500 mg at bedtime (when nocturnal hypotension occurs).

Sage

Sage (*Salvia officinalis*) also improves circulation, but unlike ginkgo, which has an excitatory effect, it has a calming effect. A controlled study from Hunan Medical College in China indicated that *Salvia miltorrhizae* as part of a four-herb formula improved visual field in a third of a glaucoma population receiving the formula for over 19 months. Herbalists recommend 2 g orally twice daily. More studies are necessary, however.

Bilberry

Bilberry (*Vaccinium myrtillus*) has been said to improve night vision; with the exception of one preliminary French study, however, it has not proved effective in stabilizing AMD.

Milk Thistle

Silymarin, from the herb milk thistle (*Silybum marianum*), is a major liver support and is the only known treatment for chronic active hepatitis and for alcoholic cirrhosis. The liver is the key organ for maintenance of eye health, because the fat-soluble vitamins and glutathione are stored and the B vitamins are activated in the liver. The usual dose of milk thistle is 150 mg 2 to 3 times daily. An alternative is SAMe in a dose of 200 mg twice daily.

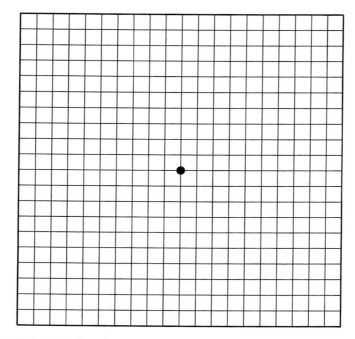

Figure 76–1. Using an Amsler grid. This checkerboard-patterned square has parallel vertical and horizontal lines. The patient looks at the central dot with one eye covered and notes the pattern of the lines. If any line in any direction is missing or wavy, the patient marks it in with a pencil or makes a note. The Amster grid can be used to determine whether there is a disorder of the optic nerve or macula; in particular, use of the grid is an excellent way to follow macular degeneration to determine whether it is stable or progressing.

NOTE

The eye is subjected to bright light throughout the day, and the important ingredients for molecular repair are stored in the liver. When the liver is overburdened, eyesight will be compromised.

Coleus forskohlii, Pilocarpus jaborandi, and Triphala

Coleus forskohlii, Pilocarpus jaborandi, and Triphala have been successful in lowering the intraocular pressure (via parasympathetic stimulation) in glaucoma patients. Triphala—composed of Emblica officinalis, Terminalia belerica, and Terminalis che-

bula—has long been used in Ayurvedic medicine for this purpose and has a generalized calming effect, which may be valuable in certain persons with AMD.

Chinese Herbs for Age-Related Macular Degeneration

Experienced herbalists report that tien chi root, dang gui root, triphala, lycium fruit, ginseng root, cooked and raw rehmannia, shilajatu, wild asparagus root, and elderberry have been used in ancient formulas to treat vascular disease inside the eye.[23] None of these remedies have been used in controlled studies, although there is ample anecdotal evidence in the Chinese literature of success as measured by nonprogression over 3 years.

— *PREVENTION PRESCRIPTION* —

- *Adoption of a positive attitude and awareness of risk factors and potential medication effects*
- *Sunglasses and other sun protection*
- *Increased consumption of green leafy vegetables*
- *Diet rich in polyunsaturated fatty acids and low in saturated fats*
- *Multivitamins with zinc, taurine, and lutein*
- *Use of supplements, with attention to overall good dietary nutrition*
- *Digestive enzymes instead of antacids*
- *Regular exercise*
- *Deep-breathing exercises on a regular basis*
- *Use of Amsler grid and periodic eye examination*
- *Use of low vision aids for persons with vision loss*

> ## NOTE
>
> *Early intervention after recognition of macular degeneration is crucial. The performance of an Amsler grid examination is recommended in all patients (Fig. 76–1). It is important to remember that the retina can be rebuilt.*

References

1. Klein R, Klein BE, Linton KI: Prevalence of age-related maculopathy. The Beaver Dam Eye Study. Ophthalmology 99:933–943, 1992.
2. Goldberg J, Flowerdew G, Smith E, et al: Factors associated with age-related macular degeneration. Am J Epidemiol 128:700–710, 1988.
3. Cruickshank KJ, Klein R, Klein BE: Sunlight and age related macular degeneration. The Beaver Dam Eye Study. Arch Ophthalmol 111:514–518, 1993.
4. Cruickshank KJ, Klein R, Klein BE, et al: Sunlight and the 5-year incidence of early age-related maculopathy. Arch Ophthalmol 119:246–250, 2001.
5. Johnson EJ, Hammond BR, Yeum KJ, et al: Relation among serum and tissue concentrations of lutein and zeaxanthin. Am J Clin Nutr 71:1555–1562, 2000.
6. Seddon JM, Willett WC, Speizer FE, et al: A prospective study of cigarette smoking and risk of age-related macular degeneration in women. JAMA 276:1141–1146, 1996.
7. Christen WG, Glynn RJ, Manson JE, et al: A prospective study of cigarette smoking and risk of age-related macular degeneration in men. JAMA 276:1147–1151, 1996.
8. Age-Related Eye Disease Study Research Group: Risk factors associated with age-related macular degeneration. Ophthalmology 107:2224–2232, 2000.
9. Hammond BR, Johnson EJ, Russell RM, et al: Dietary modification of human macular pigment density. Invest Ophthalmol Vis Sci 38:1795–1801, 1997.
10. Eye Disease Case-Control Study Group: Risk factors for neovascular age-related macular degeneration. Arch Ophthalmol 110:1701–1708, 1992.
11. Seddon JM, Ajani UA, Sperduto RD, et al: Dietary carotenoids, vitamins A, C, and E, and advanced age-related macular degeneration. JAMA 272:1413–1420, 1994.
12. Richer S: Part II: ARMD Pilot (case series) environmental intervention data. J Am Optom Assoc 70:24–36, 1999.
13. Mares-Perlman JA, Brady WE, Klein R, et al: Serum antioxidants and age-related macular degeneration in a population-based case-control study. Arch Ophthalmol 113:1518–1523, 1995.
14. Smith W, Mitchell P, Leeder S: Dietary fat and fish intake and age-related maculopathy. Arch Ophthalmol 118:401–404, 2000.
15. Richer S: Multicenter ophthalmic and nutritional age-related macular degeneration study—part 2: Antioxidant intervention and conclusions. J Am Optom Assoc 67:30–49, 1996.
16. AREDS Investigators: A randomized placebo-controlled clinical trial of high dose supplementation with Vitamins C and E, beta-carotene and zinc for age-related macular degeneration and vision loss. Arch Ophthalmol 119:1417–1436, 2001.
17. Bone RA, Landrum JT, Dixon Z, et al: Lutein and zeaxanthin in the eyes, serum and diet of human subjects. Exp Eye Res 71:239–245, 2000.
18. Bone RA, Landrum JT, Mayne ST, et al: Macular pigment in donor eyes with and without AMD. Invest Ophthalmol Vis Sci 42:235–240, 2001.
19. VandenLangenberg GM, Mares-Perlman JA, Klein R, et al: Associations between antioxidant and zinc intake and the 5-year incidence of early age-related maculopathy in the Beaver Dam Eye Study. Am J Epidemiol 148:204–214, 1998.
20. Delcourt C, Cristol JP, Tessier F, et al: Age-related macular degeneration and antioxidant status in the POLA Study. Arch Ophthalmol 117:1384–1390, 1999.
21. Lombardini JB: Taurine: Retinal function. Brain Res Rev 16:151–169, 1991.
22. Newsome DA, Swartz M, Leone NC, et al: Oral zinc in macular degeneration. Arch Ophthalmol 100:192–198, 1988.
23. Tillotson AK: One Earth Herbal Sourcebook. New York, Kensington, 2001.

Suggested Reading

Snodderly DM: Evidence for protection against age-related macular degeneration by carotenoids and antioxidant vitamins. Am J Clin Nutr 62:1448S–1461S, 1995.

CHAPTER 77

Prevention of Otitis Media

Marcey Shapiro, M.D.

ETIOLOGY

The term *otitis media* (OM) refers to middle ear effusion, or the presence of fluid in the middle ear space. *Acute otitis media* (AOM) denotes acute inflammatory symptoms, such as pain, fever, and malaise that accompany the fluid in the middle ear. Often, a viral or bacterial pathogen that has tracked from the nasopharynx during an acute upper respiratory infection is the culprit. *Serous otitis media,* or *otitis media with effusion* (OME), refers to the presence of fluid in the middle ear without inflammatory symptoms. Serous OM may be a sequela of acute otitis or may occur idiopathically.

In children, OM is especially common, as the immature eustachian tube is small and narrow.[1] It is easily closed in the presence of inflammation, preventing drainage of fluids. In fact, OM is the second most common reason for a child to visit a physician, after well-child checkups.

SCREENING

Screening of the tympanic membranes is performed in routine well-child checkups, as well as in well-adult physical examinations. An otoscopic examination with insufflation can assess the mobility of the tympanic membrane and evaluate whether there is fluid behind it.

INTEGRATIVE APPROACH TO PREVENTION

Primary versus Secondary Prevention

Primary prevention of OM is an admirable goal. However, in most cases, prevention of OM is not considered unless there has been at least one episode of AOM. Modalities that are effective in primary prevention include osteopathy, smoking cessation in the home and workplace, adequate hydration, and dietary and nutritional modifications including identification of food sensitivities.

Secondary prevention is more commonly the norm. Physicians and patients or their parents are concerned about how to prevent recurrences of AOM. This chapter, then, deals mostly with secondary prevention, but much of the information included here may apply to primary prevention as well.

Lifestyle Interventions

Breast-feeding

Breast-feeding for longer than 4 months has been shown to decrease risk of AOM.[2] This effect is due in part to the passive immunity conferred by immune-enhancing constituents of breast milk such as secretory immunoglobulin (IgA) and lactoferrin.[3] The benefits noted may also be due to delayed introduction of more allergenic cow's milk, as most infant formulas are cow's milk–based. Furthermore, breast-feeding appears to enhance protection against AOM and other childhood illnesses for years after breast-feeding has ceased.[4] Breast-feeding protects babies even in the day care setting, where infants who are formula-fed are twice as likely as breast-fed infants to develop AOM.[5]

Pacifiers

Use of pacifiers has been demonstrated to increase the risk of AOM, at least in children who attend day care programs.[6] Up to 25% of cases of recurrent OM in children younger than 3 years of age who attend day care programs can be attributed to pacifier use.

Day Care

Early attendance at day care centers is associated with increased risk of AOM, whereas care at home reduces risk.[5] Although it is not feasible for all parents, ideally children should not be introduced to the day care setting until at least the age of 6 months or older. If this is not possible, then small-group care, with fewer than 6 infants, minimizes risks.

Nutrition

A diet high in nutritious foods, with daily intake of several servings of fresh fruits and vegetables, is advised. Inclusion of whole grains, beans, lean meats, and fish that are freshly prepared is also advised. These foods are rich in vitamins and minerals and contain many natural immune-enhancing substances such as bioflavonoids, proanthocyanidins, and antioxidants. Daily consumption of a variety of fresh fruits and vegetables allows the body to maximally develop natural host resistance to a variety of illnesses. A diet high in bioflavonoids helps to decrease allergic and inflammatory responses as well.

On the other hand, processed foods and sweets should be minimized, as these provide empty calories. Consumption of foods containing preservatives and other chemicals may strain the body's detoxification mechanisms, decreasing its ability to eliminate pathogens early on. Trans fats, found in many fast foods, especially those that are fried, activate proinflammatory prostaglandin cascades and may have an especially deleterious effect on the body's detoxification mechanisms. (see Chapter 84, The Anti-Inflammatory Diet).

Good hydration is key for prevention of any upper respiratory ailment. Dry mucous membranes do not clear debris well, leading to impaired lymphatic drainage, and serve as a potential locus for infections to take hold.

Allergies

Food Allergies

Dietary triggers are important to investigate in cases of chronic recurrent or persistent OM. Food allergies can cause increased mucus in the respiratory tract, potentially leading to episodes of AOM. The most common culprits are wheat and dairy products; however, corn, citrus, and soy each may be the offending food in a large number of children. Processed foods, sugar, and sweets and fast foods are also frequently problematic. However, virtually any food may be a trigger in a sensitive person. (see Chapter 81, Food Allergy).

An allergy elimination diet (see Chapter 82) is therefore always a good idea in children or adults with recurrent upper respiratory tract ailments such as OM. Typically, the diet is instituted during a period of time convenient for the patient or if the patient is a child, for the parents. Holidays and birthdays are usually not the best times to begin.

The likely triggers, as listed earlier, are completely avoided for 6 weeks, while all other foods are rotated. This means that no food is given more frequently than every 4 days, although a food may be given twice or three times on its rotation day. A diary is kept, usually by the parents, of the foods eaten and the symptoms noted. The diet during this period should emphasize fresh fruits and vegetables, whole grains, and legumes, as well as unprocessed meats and fish—which ideally should be free of hormones and antibiotics. Processed foods should also be avoided. Usually, the patient again visits the practitioner at the end of 6 weeks for evaluation of the results of the initial phase, and any improvement or lack thereof is noted. Often, all persons involved in the trial of the elimination diet will note significant benefits, with reduction in symptoms and resolution of any persistent effusion. The results of the rotation diet are analyzed, and other individual trigger foods are eliminated.

If the patient has improved, the potential trigger foods are reintroduced, one at a time on the rotation schedule. Resumption of symptoms, such as increase in rhinitis or nasal stuffiness, should be noted, and foods that caused the symptoms should again be eliminated. If the patient has not improved, it is worthwhile to try expanding the restrictions, especially of grains. The patient should remain off the offending foods, once identified, for at least 6 months and preferably 1 year. At this time the foods can be gradually reintroduced, often without the previous symptoms. (See Chapter 82 for further discussion of the elimination diet.)

Environmental Allergies

Seasonal allergens such as tree, flower, or grass pollens can produce nasal congestion in sensitive persons, leading to blockage of the eustachian tube with the potential for OM. Early treatment of allergies with botanicals, homeopathic remedies, or pharmaceuticals can prevent later episodes of AOM.

Affected persons may also be sensitive to molds in the home or to dust mites in the bedding. Visible molds should be removed as soon as possible. A moldy smell in the home should lead to further investigation and eradication of the sources. For dust mite allergies, frequent vacuuming and cleaning are advised. Wood floors are best, with no covering, or only low-pile area rugs. Air circulation is helpful, achieved either by opening windows for fresh air or with use of an HEPA filter in the bedroom. Dust mite covers are available for all bedding, but such coverings must be cleaned frequently to be effective in preventing exposure to dust mites.

Smoking Cessation

Smoking by the parents is best stopped. Cigarette smoke is strongly associated with increased risk of upper respiratory infection, OM, and asthma.[7] If parents must smoke, it is best done outdoors. Blowing smoke out of an open window in the home is not adequate. Wood-burning fireplaces and stoves also deposit a significant amount of particulate matter in the home and are a major cause of indoor air pollution. Burning wood contains many carcinogens and toxins. Despite the beauty of fireplaces and wood-burning stoves, they are best not used by persons trying to prevent OM.

Osteopathy

Ideally, every infant should have a cranial osteopathic evaluation before 6 months of age. Such an evaluation is indicated particularly if there has been a difficult labor or forceps delivery, or if the infant had any problems with breast-feeding, formula allergies, or colic. Implementation of this preventive measure is supported by the developmental anatomy. In infants and children up to 7 years of age, the cranium is not fully developed and the bones of the skull are not yet fused. For example, at birth until approximately 6 months of age, the occiput consists of 4 separate bones. With appropriate early treatment, before these bones fuse in a pathologic or strained pattern, a lifetime of health sequelae of these strain patterns in the cranium can be avoided. If a restriction is treated early, an otherwise susceptible individual may not go on to develop OM or other health problems. Even in older children and adults with previous OM, osteopathic treatment can be of great benefit in releasing restrictions and eradicating the source of acute and recurrent illness.

Osteopathic physicians consider more than one episode of AOM in a child under 1 year of age to be diagnostic of a cranial osteopathic restriction. Clearing these pathologic patterns through manual medicine prevents the onset of repeated episodes and is thought to assist in optimizing overall health. It may prevent later problems with sinuses and allergies as well as hearing loss secondary to recurrent OM. Practitioners with appropriate training in these techniques can be found through the American Academy of Osteopathy.

Lymphatic Drainage

Lymph drainage therapy is an important adjunct in treatment of otitis. Although it may be helpful in the acute setting, its greatest value is in the resolution of chronic or serous otitis, and in the prevention of recurrent otitis. In persons, including children, for whom this gentle technique is most appropriate, palpation of anterior, posterior cervical, or posterior auricular lymph nodes will reveal congestion or "shotty" adenopathy. In proper lymph drainage treatment, the upper thorax is generally treated first, as all lymph will need to drain through the lymphatic vessels of the upper thorax, especially the thoracic duct. These vessels, of course, drain the lymph into the circulatory system, where cellular debris and waste matter can be cleared for excretion by the liver and kidneys.

After any central congestion in the lymphatic system is cleared, the neck including the involved lymph nodes, followed by other areas of the head, can be treated. The lymphatic system can often use this assistance, because there is no central pump that moves lymphatic circulation as the heart moves the blood. Instead, movement of lymph relies on fluid pressure gradients and muscular contraction. When lymph nodes and vessels become congested during and after illness, scavenger cells such as macrophages are inhibited in removing waste matter and products of inflammation from affected tissues, and stagnation in the lymphatic chains may result. The risk for such stagnation is especially high if there is excessive debris, or when the detoxification mechanisms of the body are slowed because of dietary or lifestyle choices. As a result of this stagnation, the body's immune response to new pathogens may be impaired, as the debris of old pathogens persists in the tissues. Assisting the body in removal of waste by this gentle technique, along with some support of detoxification mechanisms of the liver or kidney, may restore immune function.

Most osteopathic practitioners are familiar with lymph drainage techniques, as are persons trained in the Vodder method of manual lymph drainage or the Chikly method of lymph drainage therapy.

Botanicals

Astragalus

When there is frequent upper respiratory infection leading to otitis media, the herb of choice for prevention is astragalus (*Astragalus membranaceus*). Because of its ability to enhance the immune system, astragalus is one of the most well-known and widely studied of the herbs used in traditional Chinese medicine. It is used specifically to strengthen resistance to upper respiratory tract infections and OM in babies, children, and adults.

According to recent studies, several fractions of this plant, including the saponins and polysaccharides, are immunostimulating. In Chinese research, astragalus has been demonstrated to activate macrophages and to improve the size and weight of the mouse spleen,[8] to increase production of interleukin-2, and to augment the activity of natural killer cells in a manner similar to the activity of alpha-interferon.[8] Astragalus enhances splenic lymphocyte activity and modulates splenic, hepatic, and blood levels of cyclic guanosine monophosphate and cyclic adenine monophosphate.

In traditional Chinese medicine, astragalus is typically used in persons younger than 30 years of age, including children. It is the preferred herb for strengthening the spleen and immunity in this age group and has been used safely and effectively for thousands of years. It is used most often between episodes of AOM and can be given during serous OM to strengthen resistance to pathogens.

Dosage. Astragalus is usually given as a tincture or decoction. Tincture: In infants, 2 to 3 drops per 5 pounds of body weight three times daily; in children (older than 3 years of age), 0.5 to 2.0 mL three times daily. Decoction: In infants, 1 teaspoon per 5 pounds of body weight three times daily; in children, 2 to 4 tablespoons three times daily.

Precautions. No adverse effects or contraindications are known.

Hearing Testing

Hearing can be tested in all children older than 6 months of age. If any problem is suspected, hearing should be tested by a qualified audiologist.

Pharmaceuticals

Pharmaceuticals are not prescribed for primary prevention of OM but are often used for weeks at a time when clear serous fluid is present behind the tympanic membrane (i.e., in OME), to prevent AOM outbreaks. Amoxicillin is most frequently used. Although the practice of using prolonged courses of antibiotics in OME is common, it is no longer advised. The Pediatric URI Consensus team has advised limiting use of antibiotics to episodes of AOM alone.[9]

Surgery

Myringotomy

When multiple courses of antibiotics have failed to clear repeated episodes of OM, myringotomy, or surgical placement of drainage tubes through the tympanic membrane, is often performed. This procedure is often advised in children in whom persistent middle ear effusion is interfering with hearing and thus language development. Myringotomy will usually prevent recurrent episodes of AOM, but risks include reaction to anesthesia, failure to prevent recurrent OM, and scarring of the tympanic membrane.

Adenoidectomy

Adenoidectomy is often performed either alone or with myringotomy when OME fails to resolve. The adenoids are thought to serve as a possible reservoir for infection and may also physically obstruct the eustachian tube.[10]

 — PREVENTION PRESCRIPTION

- *Breast-feeding for infants should be encouraged to at least 4 months of age.*
- *Mucus-forming foods such as wheat, dairy, and orange juice should be avoided during episodes of upper respiratory tract infection.*
- *Food allergies should be identified. Eliminate consumption of offending foods from the diet.*
- *Environmental allergies should be identified and removed if possible.*
- *All smoking in the environment must be stopped.*
- *Wood-burning stoves and fireplaces should not be used.*
- *Use of a pacifier should be avoided.*
- *When possible, home care of the infant rather than day care is advised.*
- *A diet high in nutritious foods such as fresh fruits and vegetables, whole grains, lean meats, and fish is recommended. Intake of processed foods and of mucus-forming foods should be limited.*
- *Cranial osteopathic evaluation and treatment if indicated are ideal before the age of 6 months, but if that is not feasible, these should certainly be performed for any child who has had recurring episodes of AOM.*
- *Immune-strengthening botanicals such as astragalus tincture given as 2 drops per pound of body weight two times daily for 6 weeks can be used after an acute bout of OM, when other household members are ill, and in persons prone to recurrence.*

Resources

American Academy of Osteopathy. Telephone: (317) 879-1881.
American Botanical Council. www.herbalgram.org, Telephone: (512) 926-4900
American Academy of Medical Acupuncture. www.medicalacupuncture.org

References

1. Suzuki C, Balaban C, Sando I, Sudo M, et al: Postnatal development of eustachian tube: A computer-aided 3-D reconstruction and measurement study. Acta Otolaryngol (Stockh) 118:837–843, 1998.
2. Duncan B, Ey J, Holberg CJ, et al: Exclusive breast-feeding for at least four months protects against otitis media. J Pediatr 120:856, 1992.
3. Qui J, Hendrixson DR, Baker EN, et al: Human milk lactoferrin inactivates two putative colonization factors expressed by *Haemophilus influenzae*. Protocols Natl Acad Sci USA 95:12641–12646, 1998.

4. Hanson LA: Breastfeeding provides passive and likely long-lasting active immunity. Ann Allergy Asthma Immunol 81:522–533, 1998.
5. Duffy LC, Faden H, Wasielewski R, et al: Exclusive breast-feeding protects against bacterial colonization and day care exposure to otitis media. Pediatrics 100:E7, 1997.
6. Niemela M, Uhari M, Mottonen M: A pacifier increases the risk of recurrent acute otitis media in children in day care centers. Pediatrics 96:884, 1995.
7. Etzel RA, Patishall EN, Haley NJ, et al: Passive smoking and middle ear effusion among children in daycare. Pediatrics 90:228, 1992.
8. Tang W, Eisenbrand G: Chinese Drugs of Plant Origin. Springer-Verlag 1992, p. 197.
9. Dowell SF, Schwartz B, Phillips WR: Appropriate use of antibiotics for URIs in children: Part 1. Otitis media and acute sinusitis. Am Fam Physician 58:1113–1118, 1123, 1998.
10. Wright ED, Pearl AJ, Manoukian JJ: Laterally hypertrophic adenoids as a contributing factor in otitis media. Int J Pediatr Otorhinolaryngol 45:207–214, 1998.

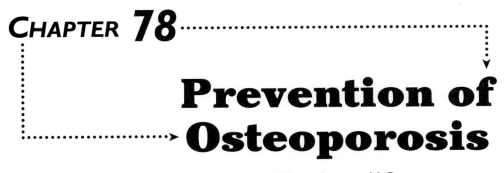

CHAPTER 78

Prevention of Osteoporosis

Alison Levitt, M.D.

Osteoporosis is a skeletal disease characterized by a reduction in bone mass per unit volume. Bones become thinner and more porous, leading to enhanced bone fragility and increased risk of fracture.

Osteoporosis is the most common metabolic bone disease, affecting approximately 25 million Americans. It is associated with 1.5 million fractures annually; of this total, about 300,000 are hip fractures, the most serious complication of osteoporosis. In the year following a hip fracture, 20% of the affected patients will die, 25% will be confined to long-term care facilities, and 50% will experience long-term loss of mobility. The medical and social cost of this disease is estimated to be 6.1 billion annually. Osteoporosis is no longer simply a disease—it has become an epidemic!

Osteoporosis can be a debilitating, devastating disease. Fortunately, it is also preventable. Therefore, it is vitally important for clinicians to be knowledgeable about this condition and to be able to educate patients on how to prevent osteoporosis and its consequences. With early screening and intervention, the pain, suffering, and death caused by osteoporosis can be greatly reduced.

ETIOLOGY

Bone is a dynamic tissue that is constantly undergoing remodeling. This turnover is necessary for bone maintenance, growth, and repair and occurs throughout the life span. *Resorption*, or the breakdown of bone, is accomplished by cells known as *osteoclasts*. The formation of bone is done by cells known as *osteoblasts*. It is the balance between these two different types of cells and their rate of activity that determines the bone turnover rate and the associated risk of development of osteoporosis. Any changes in remodeling rate that result in a rate of bone resorption faster than that of bone formation can lead to a decrease in bone mass.

Until about the age of 40 years, the process of breaking down and building up bone by osteoclasts and osteoblasts is a nearly perfectly coupled system, with one phase stimulating the other. In both genders, between the ages of 40 to 50 years there is a slow rate of bone loss. The reason for age-related bone loss is still unknown. In some cases, turnover rate of bone is very high, in others, the turnover rate is very gradual, but the breakdown of bone eventually overtakes the buildup. The loss of bone that accompanies aging proceeds faster in women, with a trend toward accelerated loss before menopause.

The activity of osteoclasts and osteoblasts is controlled by a variety of factors, including levels of hormones such as estrogen and parathyroid, as well as other nutritional and blood factors that affect cell growth. Changes in levels of any of these substances may play a role in uncoupling the balance between these two cell lines, thereby contributing to the development of osteoporosis.

SCREENING

With a precision of measurement of 1% and a radiation dose of less than 5 mrem, dual-energy x-ray absorptiometry (DEXA) is currently the best modality for measuring bone mineral density. It provides the most reliable measurement of bone density and has the advantage of using very low levels of x-rays, exposing the patient to very little radiation. It measures bone density throughout the body within 2 to 4 minutes. Osteoporosis should be distinguished from osteopenia (Table 78–1).

Simpler techniques such as single-energy x-ray absorptiometry measure density in the forearm and heel. Ultrasound techniques measure bone density in heel, finger, and leg bones. Dental x-ray films of bone may also be helpful. A new device called a

Table 78–1. Diagnosis of Osteoporosis and Osteopenia

Disease	Diagnosis Based on Bone Mineral Density
Osteopenia	1–2.5 SD below the mean
Osteoporosis	2.5 SD below the mean

Note: For each standard deviation (SD) decrease in bone density from the young adult mean, there is a twofold to threefold increased risk of fracture.

Sahara Clinical Bone Sonometer can be used to assess the risk for osteoporosis in about 1 minute. None of these methods are as precise as standard DEXA in establishing a diagnosis, but they are still effective, inexpensive, and portable.

LABORATORY TESTING

Osteoporosis is a preventable disease that usually goes undetected for decades until a fracture occurs. Therefore, it is important to be able to make an early diagnosis of bone loss. Diagnosing osteoporosis with a bone density scan is effective if the patient already has the disease. Attention, however, should be directed at prevention. This approach is the most effective way to put an end to the epidemic of this disease.

A urine test may indicate increased risk for hip fracture if it reveals high levels of the chemicals deoxypyridonoline and *C*-telopeptide. These substances are produced when bone is broken down. Another urine test, Osteomark-NTX, measures bone loss by detecting a substance called *N*-telopeptide. This compound is linked to bone breakdown, thereby indicating bone loss. This test can be used to monitor the rate of bone loss and the success of therapy. These tests can be performed on persons who are at increased risk for osteoporosis.

Early screening is important. The risk factors listed in Tables 78–2 and 78–3 should be reviewed for each patient, and appropriate tests and therapies selected and implemented before the disease develops and advances to the fracture stage.

INTEGRATIVE APPROACH TO PREVENTION

Lifestyle and Bone Health

Exercise

Numerous studies have demonstrated that regular weight-bearing exercise is a major determinant of bone density. Exercise stimulates osteoblast-mediated bone formation and can increase bone mass in postmenopausal women. Prolonged immobilization, on the other hand, increases the rate of calcium excretion, resulting in a negative calcium balance.

Exercise is very important for slowing the progression of osteoporosis. Women should begin exercising before adolescence, because bone mass

Table 78–2. Risk Factors for Osteoporosis

Factor	Comment/Example
Age	The risk of developing osteoporosis increases with age.
Gender	Women are at greater risk for developing osteoporosis.
History of fractures as an adult	Family history and personal history increase the risk of developing osteoporosis.
Race	Caucasian and Asian women are more likely to develop osteoporosis.
Bone structure and body weight	Small-boned, short, slender, blond, blue-eyed, fair-skinned, and thin women (weight less than 127 pounds) are at greater risk for development of osteoporosis.
Menopause/menstrual history	Normal or early menopause, history of amenorrhea, oligomenorrhea, late menstrual onset, nulliparity, and anovulation increase the risk of developing osteoporosis.
Eating disorders	Anorexia nervosa and bulimia increase the risk of developing osteoporosis.
Chronic diseases	Rheumatoid arthritis, diabetes mellitus, hyperthyroid, Cushing's syndrome, hyperparathyroidism, dental conditions, stress fractures, and prolonged immobilization increase the risk for osteoporosis.
Digestive problems	Risk of developing osteoporosis increases with maldigestion or malabsorption.

Table 78–3. Lifestyle Factors That Promote Osteoporosis

Factor	Comment
Smoking	Smoking causes bone depletion of calcium.
Alcohol	Consumption of moderate or greater amounts of alcohol causes bone depletion of calcium.
Caffeine	Studies have demonstrated an increased loss of calcium in the urine after ingestion of caffeine.
Cola ingestion	Soft drinks and other high-phosphorus beverages have been implicated in the development of osteoporosis. They increase the level of phosphates, thereby promoting calcium loss from bone; further research is needed.
Depression	Studies have found an association among major depression, stress, and low bone mineral density. In one study, women who suffered from major depression had low bone density, comparable to that of postmenopausal women, which may contribute to increased risk for developing osteoporosis.

increases during puberty and reaches its peak between ages 20 and 30 years. Weight-bearing exercise can increase bone density by as much as 2% to 8% a year. High-impact weight-bearing exercise in premenopausal women is very protective. However, in elderly patients, it increases the risk for osteoporotic fractures. Regular brisk, long walks can also improve bone density. Exercises specifically targeted to strengthen the back help to prevent fractures later on in life and can be beneficial in improving posture and reducing kyphosis. Low-impact exercises that improve balance and strength, particularly yoga and tai chi, have been found to decrease the risk of falling. In one study, practice of tai chi reduced the risk by almost half.

Nutrition

Soy and Isoflavones

Soybeans are essentially the unique dietary source of isoflavones. These substances have chemical structures similar to those of estrogen, and they are also a rich source of potassium. Animal studies have shown that isoflavones, mainly diadzein and genestein found in soy, act directly to stop bone demineralization. In studies on soy protein isolates, soy protein was found to conserve body calcium by diminishing calcium excretion in the urine.

In one study, bone density increased in postmenopausal women who ate foods rich in soy protein and low in fat. Tofu fortified with calcium may be particularly beneficial; 3 ounces of tofu supplies 60% of daily calcium requirements.

Ipriflavone, a synthetic derivative of isoflavones, has been shown to prevent bone loss. Studies also report a positive effect on bone density, with only very mild side effects (mostly gastrointestinal).

Dosage
- Isoflavones: 25 to 45 mg daily.
- Ipriflavone: 200 mg 3 times a day.

Omega-3 Fatty Acids

Essential fatty acids increase calcium absorption from the gut, reduce urinary excretion of calcium, and increase calcium deposition in bone. Animal studies have demonstrated that rats deficient in essential fatty acids are more prone to osteoporosis. Supplementation with essential fatty acids in elderly persons produced an increase in bone density. This effect may be potentiated by concurrent supplementation with gamma-linoleic acid (GLA). Evening primrose oil and borage seed oil are two sources of GLA. Omega-3 fatty acids are found in most cold-water fish like salmon, tuna, sardines and mackerel.

Alkaline Ash Diet

A diet high in animal protein and low in fruits and vegetables—typically, the average American diet—produces a lot of acid, mainly in the form of sulfates and phosphates. The kidneys then respond with a net excretion of acid. The skeleton supplies buffer through active resorption of bone, which increases calcium excretion.

The addition of exogenous alkali buffers to a diet rich in animal protein results in a less acidic urine and, ultimately, decreased excretion of calcium. Acid ash-forming foods to avoid include fish, poultry, shellfish, eggs, wheat, corn, barley, rye, rice, lentils, buckwheat, cranberries, plums, cane sugar, and cheese. Alkaline ash-forming foods to include in the diet are milk, almonds, chestnuts, coconut, all vegetables except corn and lentils, and most fruits except plums and cranberries.

Limiting Sodium Intake

High sodium intake interferes with calcium retention. The higher the level of sodium, the more calcium the body needs to meet its daily requirements.

Limiting Dietary Protein

Studies have demonstrated that excessive dietary protein may promote bone loss. Animal protein in particular causes an increase in urinary excretion of calcium.

Green Vegetables

Vegetables such as asparagus, broccoli, Brussels sprouts, cabbage, collards greens, romaine lettuce, and other green leafy vegetables all contain vitamin K. Vitamin K mediates the carboxylation of glutamyl residues on several bone proteins, notably osteocalcin. Vitamin K is essential for the formation, remodeling, and repair of bone.

Increased consumption of vitamin K was shown to be associated with a lower risk for hip fractures but not with an increase in bone density. One study indicated that 1 mg of additional vitamin K (10 times the U.S. recommended dietary allowance [RDA]) reduced urinary calcium loss by 33% in postmenopausal women.

Limiting Refined Sugar Intake

Refined sugar may also reduce calcium content in bone. Following sugar intake, there is enhanced calcium excretion in urine.

Avoiding Undesirable Fats

Saturated fat and *n*-6 polyunsaturated vegetable fats, found in most vegetable oils and "fast foods," may slow bone growth and adversely affect calcium and magnesium metabolism. In contrast, the ingestion of olive oil appears to be positively associated with bone mineral density. More studies, however, are needed.

Supplements

Calcium

In postmenopausal women, calcium supplementation has been shown to decrease bone loss by as much as 50% at nonvertebral sites. The effects were greatest in women who were calcium deficient. Effective supplementation dosages were 1000 to 1500 mg daily. Because skeletal calcium depletion is noted in only 25% of osteoporotic women, it is clear that calcium supplementation alone is not enough.

Calcium supplements exist in different compounds, such as calcium carbonate, calcium citrate, calcium gluconate, and calcium lactate. All of these provide calcium with different concentrations and absorption capabilities. Supplements should be taken after meals. If these compounds are taken with large amounts of antacids, absorption of calcium can be impaired.

Calcium-rich foods include milk fortified with vitamin D, dark green vegetables (broccoli, kale, turnip greens), shrimp, salmon or sardines, blackstrap molasses, calcium-fortified tofu, and almonds.

Dosage. 1000 to 1500 mg daily.

Vitamin D

Vitamin D improves bone strength mainly by increasing intestinal calcium absorption and reabsorption of calcium by the kidney. Several intervention studies demonstrated in humans that vitamin D can improve bone status as measured by bone density.

Vitamin D deficiencies are more commonly seen in elderly persons secondary to decreased sun exposure, decreased dietary intake, and malabsorption. Vitamin D is found in foods such as liver, fish, eggs, and fortified dairy products.

Dosage. The recommended dose is 400 international units (IU) of vitamin D daily.

Vitamin K

Recent research also points to a role of vitamin K in bone metabolism. As noted previously, vitamin K mediates the carboxylation of glutamyl residues on several bone proteins, notably osteocalcin, and it is essential for the formation, remodeling, and repair of bone. Epidemiologic studies and results from first intervention trials consistently suggest that vitamin K may improve bone health. Vitamin K is found in many green leafy vegetables and may also be supplemented if necessary.

Magnesium

Magnesium is essential to numerous biochemical reactions that take place in bone. Deficiencies are associated with abnormal calcification of bone and may contribute to the development of osteoporosis. Magnesium is found in wheat bran, spinach, kelp, wheat germ, cashews, almonds, walnuts, filberts, pecans, beet greens, tofu, rye, millet, sole and halibut, buckwheat, and brewer's yeast. It can also be taken as a supplement.

Dosage. The recommended dose is between 400 and 800 mg of magnesium daily.

Precautions. Excessive magnesium may be harmful in people with diabetes or kidney disease.

Vitamin B$_6$, Folic Acid, and Vitamin B$_{12}$

Vitamin B$_6$ (pyridoxine), folic acid, and vitamin B$_{12}$ are important in the conversion of methionine to cysteine. A deficiency in these vitamins can lead to an excess of homocysteine, a methionine metabolite that is believed to promote osteoporosis. Low levels of vitamin B$_6$, folic acid, and vitamin B$_{12}$ are unfortunately quite common, especially in the elderly population.

In addition, menopause has been associated with decreased serum folate levels. Tobacco smoking, alcohol use, and oral contraceptives also tend to promote folic acid deficiency.

Dosage. The recommended dose of vitamin B$_6$ is 50 mg per day and of folic acid, 400 mcg per day.

Vitamin C

Vitamin C is considered an essential cofactor in collagen formation. Epidemiologic studies report a positive association between vitamin C intake and bone density. Intervention studies on the effect of vitamin C on bone status are, however, lacking.

Dosage. The recommended dose is 500 mg of vitamin C twice a day.

Trace Minerals

Zinc

Zinc is needed for normal bone formation. It enhances the biochemical actions of vitamin D. It is required for the formation of osteoblasts and osteoclasts and is necessary for the synthesis of various proteins in bone tissue. Low zinc levels have been found in elderly people with osteoporosis. Because the typical American diet is low in zinc, deficiency of this mineral is common and should be addressed in osteoporosis prevention programs.

Dosage. The recommended dose is 30 to 45 mg per day.

Boron

Boron plays a role in calcium and magnesium metabolism as well as in hormonal stabilization. In postmenopausal women, boron supplementation was shown to reduce urinary excretion of calcium and magnesium and to increase serum concentrations of 17 beta-estradiol and testosterone. Boron appears to exert an estrogenic effect without exposing the body to dangerous amounts of estrogens.

Dosage. The recommended dose is 3 to 5 mg of boron per day.

Manganese

Manganese is required for bone mineralization. Deficiencies can cause a reduction in the amount of calcium laid down in bone.

Dosage. The recommended dose is 3 mg of manganese per day.

Copper

Copper deficiency is a known cause of abnormal bone development in children. In rats fed a copper-deficient diet, bone mineral content and bone strength both are reduced. Copper supplementation also has been noted to inhibit bone resorption in vitro. Copper deficiency may contribute to development of osteoporosis. The mechanism of action is still unknown.

The typical American diet contains only about 50% of the RDA for copper (i.e., 2 mg per day), so deficiencies of this mineral may be quite common.

Silicon

Silicon is found concentrated in the body's calcification sites. It appears to strengthen the connective tissue matrix. In animals fed a silicon-deficient diet, abnormal skull development and bone growth retardation resulted.

Other Related Factors

Hydrochloric Acid Deficiency

Hydrochloric acid deficiency may inhibit calcium absorption.

Table 78–4. Medications or Supplements That Increase Calcium Loss

Drug	Comment
Corticosteroids	Long-term use leads to calcium loss.
Furosemide (Lasix)	
Antiseizure medications	
Antacids with aluminum	
Immunosuppressive drugs	
Antibiotics	Excessive use affects vitamin K–producing bacteria in the gut.
Thyroid hormone	Calcium loss occurs with excessive doses only. Adjusting the dose can offset this effect.
Warfarin sodium	
Cholestyramine	

Aluminum Toxicity

Aluminum inhibits bone mineralization. The greater the aluminum exposure, the higher the risk for fracture. Calcium supplementation may be effective in reversing the effects of aluminum-induced metabolic bone disease.

Medications or Supplements That Increase Calcium Loss

Table 78–4 lists agents that may increase loss of calcium from the body.

Pharmaceuticals and Hormones

Hormone Replacement Therapy

Estrogen replacement therapy (ERT) or hormone replacement therapy (HRT) is known to be beneficial in the prevention of osteoporosis (Table 78–5). HRT that includes estrogen, with or without progesterone, has been shown to reduce osteoclast activity, decrease bone loss, reduce spine and hip fractures, and prevent loss of height. In one study, the risk for hip fracture decreased by 4% for every year of HRT without progesterone and by 11% for each year of HRT with progesterone. Both oral and transdermal formulations decrease bone loss, reduce the incidence of fractures, and prevent height loss.

Published studies have raised concerns among many women about an association between HRT and an increased risk of breast cancer. The American Medical Association and the National Cancer Institute have concluded that the use of estrogen increases the average woman's risk of breast cancer and that use of a combination of estrogen-progestin increases that risk even more. Estrogen also increases the risk of uterine cancer, although the addition of progesterone to the regimen significantly reduces this danger. Hormone therapy with or

Table 78–5. Estrogen Regimens for Postmenopausal Woman and Dose Equivalents for Moderate to Severe Osteopenia or Documented Osteoporosis

Estrogen*	Standardized Regimens For Postmenopausal Women	Dose-Equivalent Estrogens for Moderate-to-Severe Osteopenia or Documented Osteoporosis
Estradiol		
Estrace	0.5 mg/day	1 or 2 mg/day
Estraderm	0.05-mg patches used biweekly	0.1 mg biweekly
Esterified estrogens Estratab	0.3 mg/day	0.625 to 1.25 mg/day
Ethinyl estradiol	5 μg/day	10 μg/day
Estrone		
Ogen	0.625 mg/day	1.25 mg/day
Conjugated estrogens Premarin	0.625 mg/day	0.625 or 0.9 mg/day

*Studies suggest that lower-dose estrogen treatment is better than no estrogen treatment to preserve bone mass.

without progesterone increases the risk for blood clots, and studies indicate some risk for breast cancer with long-term estrogen use.

In addition, it appears that estrogen must be taken life long for maximum protection against osteoporosis. Women who take ERT and then stop begin to lose bone density until, after 5 years, all protection is lost. The benefits of the use of estrogen must be weighed against the risk in each patient. Thus, treatment protocols should be established on an individual basis.

Dosage. Esterified estrogens (ESE) are available as an oral preparation to be used in a dose of 0.3 mg for the prevention of osteoporosis. Climara (estradiol transdermal system), available as an 0.025-mg patch, has been approved by the U.S. Food and Drug Administration for the prevention of osteoporosis.

Natural Hormones

Much attention has been given to the use of natural hormones for the treatment of menopausal symptoms as well as for the prevention of osteoporosis. Natural estrogens are mainly derived from wild Mexican yam and soy.

Studies have shown that when progestins are administered alone, bone density is preserved, and there is a decrease in the level of biochemical markers of bone remodeling. In a study from the University of Columbia, female marathon runners who were anovulatory were found to develop osteoporosis despite having high estrogen levels. Other evidence indicated that progesterone receptors exist in osteoblasts, which are likely to enhance new bone formation.

Transdermal natural progesterone has been claimed to actively increase bone mass and bone density. The lack of progesterone has been postulated to be the primary pathophysiologic factor in the development of osteoporosis.

Dosage. The recommended minimum daily dose of *conjugated estrogens* for the prevention of osteoporo-

sis is 0.625 mg per day. With use of natural estrogens, therefore, the equivalent doses of estrone and estradiol should add up to this amount because interconversion of these hormones occurs. The dose of oral micronized *progesterone* documented in the PEPI trials is 100 mg twice a day. There are, however, a variety of forms of natural progesterone and estrogen currently available, including oral, transdermal, micronized, and topical creams. A compounding pharmacist can be consulted for assistance in the formulations. (See Chapter 44, Menopause.)

Androgens

The use of exogenous androgens for the treatment of osteoporosis still needs further investigation. In vitro androgens have been noted to stimulate osteoblast activity. Although only a few studies, which were of limited duration, on the use of androgens have been conducted, the data suggest that the use of androgens is associated with some protection against fractures.

Bisphosphonates

Bisphosphonates are nonhormonal drugs for osteoporosis prevention and treatment that reduce bone resorption by inhibiting osteoclast activity. Available evidence suggests that these drugs are at least as effective as HRT in preventing bone loss and reducing the risk of fractures. Concerns include gastrointestinal intolerance and risk of esophageal ulcer, especially if these drugs are taken incorrectly. Alendronate (Fosamax) and risedronate (Actonel) are approved for use in glucocorticoid-induced osteoporosis in both men and women.

The Fracture Intervention Trial (FIT) and other large clinical trials show that alendronate effectively increases bone density and reduces the risk of hip and vertebral fractures by approximately half within the first 12 to 18 months (Table 78–6). Alendronate is also effective for preventing bone loss in early post-

Table 78–6. Alendronate* Doses for Treatment and Prevention of Osteoporosis

Alendronate Dose		
Treatment of Osteoporosis	*Prevention of Osteoporosis*	**Comment**
10 mg/day, or 70 mg/wk, for 3 years	5 mg/day or 35 mg/wk	To be taken with 6 to 8 ounces of water, on arising, at least 1 half-hour before breakfast.

*Calcium supplements and antacids interfere with absorption of alendronate. Safety of treatment for longer than 4 years has not been studied.

menopausal women. In one study, risedronate increased bone density by 5% in the spine and hips of postmenopausal women, and there was no increase in gastrointestinal side effects. More studies are needed, however.

Other bisphosphonates currently being evaluated for clinical use in postmenopausal osteoporosis, include the following:

- Clodronate
- Pamidronate (oral form)
- Risedronate (in phase III clinical trials)
- Tiludronate (in phase III clinical trials)
- Ibandronate (in phase III clinical trials)

The use of these drugs should be considered in patients who are at high risk for developing osteoporosis or have severe osteoporosis, who are nonresponsive to other interventions, or in whom hormonal therapy was not tolerated or is contraindicated.

Selective Estrogen Receptor Modulators

Commonly called "designer estrogens," selective estrogen receptor modulators (SERMs) imitate the beneficial effects of estrogen on bone density and serum cholesterol but do not have the negative effect of increasing the risk of breast cancer and uterine cancer. In many cases, the positive effects of SERMs are weaker than those of estrogen. Although the beneficial effect on bone density of SERMs is weaker than that of HRT, studies indicate that SERMs work just as well as HRT in reducing spine fractures. The data on hip fractures are still pending. SERMs, however, also carry the same risk of blood clots as for HRT and produce hot flashes in some women.

Tamoxifen is the best-known SERM. A recent study reported that low-dose tamoxifen reduces the risk for fractures. The drug is also being studied for protection against breast cancer, although results to date are conflicting. Unlike estrogen, tamoxifen appears to offer little protection against heart disease.

In a preliminary report to the National Osteoporosis Foundation, one group of investigators observed that treatment with raloxifene (Evista), 30 to 150 mg daily, plus calcium supplementation at 500 mg daily, resulted in a 2% to 4% bone mass increase over that obtained with placebo. Raloxifene also produced a 10% decrease in low-density lipoprotein (LDL) cholesterol levels and a 6% decrease in total cholesterol levels. Treatment was associated with little risk of uterine bleeding. Both raloxifene and tamoxifen increase the risk for blood clots.

Droloxifene and tibolone (Livial) are other SERMs under investigation that appear to protect against bone loss without increasing cancer risks.

Calcitonin

Calcitonin is a peptide hormone that inhibits bone resorption. It has been demonstrated to be effective in the prevention of bone fractures and is currently used for treatment of osteoporosis. Calcitonin derived from salmon (Calcimar, Miacalcin) slows bone loss progression and reduces spinal fractures. Its effect on the hip is not yet known. It also helps to relieve bone pain associated with established osteoporosis. Calcitonin may be an alternative for patients who cannot take alendronate or estrogen. It is available as a nasal spray and in injection form.

Dosage. Calcitonin regimens vary. A suggested dose is one spray (200 IU) per day, in alternating nostrils.

Precautions. Potential adverse effects include headache, dizziness, anorexia, diarrhea, skin rashes, and edema. The most common adverse effect experienced with calcitonin injection is nausea, with or without vomiting; this occurs less often with the nasal spray. The nasal spray may cause nose bleeds, sinusitis, and inflammation of the membranes in the nose. Also, because calcitonin is a protein, a large number of people taking the drug develop resistance or allergic reactions after long-term use.

PREVENTION PRESCRIPTION

- *The patient's individual risk for osteoporosis should be assessed.*
- *For women at high risk, bone mineral density should be assessed, and nutritional, lifestyle, and appropriate supplement, hormone, or drug interventions should be instituted.*
- *Bone mineral density testing also may be warranted in premenopausal women who have significant risk factors such as prolonged amenorrhea, eating disorders, corticosteroid treatment, or renal disease.*
- *Patients with low risk should receive nutritional and lifestyle counseling on the prevention of osteoporosis.*
- *An exercise routine should be incorporated into the lifestyle of all patients. Weight-bearing exercise such as jogging, walking, tai chi, yoga, and aerobics is particularly important for the prevention of osteoporosis.*
- *A high-potency multivitamin and mineral complex should be taken daily.*
- *Judicious supplementation of minerals is recommended.*
  - *Calcium: 800 to 1200 mg per day.*
  - *Vitamin D: 400 IU per day.*
  - *Magnesium: 400 mg per day.*
  - *Boron: 3 mg per day.*
  - *The need for a daily B complex vitamin should also be assessed.*
- *A diet low in animal fat is advised.*
- *Intake of soy-based foods should be increased, to 1 or 2 ounces a day.*
- *Abundant fruits and vegetables should be included in the diet, with 5 to 6 servings daily, focusing specifically on green leafy vegetables and alkaline fruit, as described.*
- *Intake of omega-3 fatty acids and olive oil should be increased, while ingestion of saturated hydrogenated, and* trans *fatty acids should be decreased.*
- *Salt, sugar, caffeine, and soft drinks should be avoided in the diet.*
- *Use of tobacco products and excessive consumption of alcohol are contraindicated.*

Internet Resources

nof.com
Medscape.com
Osteoporosis.ca
vicus.com
webmd.com

References

1. Abelow BJ, et al: Cross cultural association between dietary animal protein and hip fractures: A hypothesis. Calcif Tissue Int 50:14–18, 1992.
2. Adams JS, Lee G: Gains in bone mineral density with resolution of vitamin D intoxication. Ann Intern Med 127:203–206, 1997.
3. Amdur MO, et al: The need for magnesium in bone development in rats. Proc Soc Exp Biol Med 59:254–255, 1945.
4. Andon M, et al: Effects of dietary copper and manganese restrictions on serum mineral concentrations and femoral shaft bone density in rats. J Am Coll Nutr 11:600, 1992.
5. Atik OS: Zinc and senile osteoporosis. J Am Geriatric Soc 31:790–791, 1983.
6. Bjamason NH, Bjamason K, Haarbo J, et al: Tibolone: Prevention of bone loss in late postmenopausal women. J Clin Endocrinol Metab 81:2419–2422, 1996.
7. Gaby A: Nutrients and Bone Health. Review 1988.
8. Gamble CL: Osteoporosis: Making the diagnosis in patients at risk for fracture. Geriatrics 50:24–33, 1995.
9. Gutin B, Kasper MJ: Can vigorous exercise play a role in osteoporosis prevention? Osteoporosis Int 2:55–68, 1992.
10. Breslau NA: Calcium, estrogen, and progestin in the treatment of osteoporosis. Rheum Dis Clin North Am 20:691–716, 1994.
11. Cummings SR, Kelsey JL, Nevitt MC, et al: Epidemiology of osteoporosis and osteoporotic fractures. Epdemiol Rev 7:178–208, 1985.
12. Calhoun, et al: The effects of zinc on ectopic bone formation. Oral Surg 39:698–706, 1975.
13. Hollingbery PW, et al: Effects of caffeine and aspirin on urinary calcium and hydroxyproline excretion in pre- and postmenopausal women. Fed Proc 44:1149, 1985.
14. Hudson T: Osteoporosis: An overview for clinical practice. J Naturopath Med 7:27–34, 1999.
15. Infant-Rivard C, et al: Folate deficiency amongst institutionalized elderly. J Am Geriatric Soc 34:211–214, 1986.
16. Kanis JA, Melton LJ, Christiansen C, et al: The diagnosis of osteoporosis. J Bone Miner Res 9:1137–1141, 1994.
17. Liberman UA, Weiss SR, Broll J, et al: Effect of oral alendronate on bone mineral density and the incidence of fractures in postmenopausal osteoporosis: The Alendronate Phase II Osteoporosis Treatment Study Group. N Engl J Med 333:1437–1443, 1995.
18. Licata AA: Prevention and osteoporosis management. Cleve Clin J Med 61:451–460, 1994
19. Lindsay R, Tohme JF: Estrogen treatment of patients with established postmenopausal osteoporosis. Obstet Gynecol 76:290–295, 1990.
20. Mahoney AW, et al: Role of gastric acid in the utilization of dietary calcium by the rat. Nutr Metab 16:375–382, 1974.
21. Melton LJ, Atkinson EJ, O'Fallon WM, et al: Long-term fracture prediction by bone mineral assessed at different skeletal sites. J Bone Miner Res 8:1227–1234, 1993.
22. Melvyn R, Warbuach: Osteoporosis. In Textbook of Nutritional Medicine. 1999, pp 581–595.
23. Merendez-Avila, et al: Caffeine, moderate alcohol intake and risk of fractures of the hip and forearm in middle-aged women. Am J Clin Nutr 54:157–163, 1991.
24. Overgaard K, Hansen MA, Jensen SB, et al: Effect of salcatonin given intranasally on bone mass and fracture rates in estab-

lished osteoporosis: A dose response study. BMJ 305:556–561, 1992.

25. New tests for osteoporosis. Vicus.com Online 2000.

26. Notelovitz M: Osteoporosis: Screening, prevention, and management. Fertil Steril 59:707–725, 1993.

27. Osteoporosis prevention, diagnosis, and therapy. NIH Consensus Statement Online 27–29; 17:1–36, March 2000.

28. Recker RR: Calcium absorption and achlorhydria. N Engl J Med 313:70–73, 1985.

29. Rosen CJ, Chestnut CH, Mallinak NJS: The predictive value of biochemical markers of bone turnover for bone mineral density in early postmenopausal women treated with hormone replacement or calcium supplementation. J Clin Endocrinol Metab 82:1904–1910, 1997.

30. Spencer M, et al: Alcohol osteoporosis. Am J Clin Nutr. 41:847, 1985.

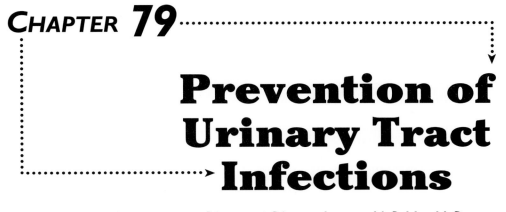

CHAPTER 79

Prevention of Urinary Tract Infections

Bhaswati Bhattacharya, M.P.H., M.D.

EPIDEMIOLOGY

Over 90% of urinary tract infections (UTIs) occur in women. This gender predilection exists because most infections are thought to arise from organisms ascending from the flora-rich perineum into the sterile bladder, and because the urethra is shorter in women than in men.

Statistics show that 10% to 20% of all women experience a UTI at least once a year; 37.5% of women with no history of UTI will have an infection within 10 years. In random samples, 2% to 4% of healthy women have elevated urinary levels of bacteria. Recurrent bladder infections can be a significant problem for some women, with eventual involvement of the upper urinary tract and kidneys. Recurrent kidney infection is associated with progressive damage of tissue, resulting in scarring and, rarely, in kidney failure.

UTI in males usually presents in infancy, with a male-to-female ratio of 1.5:1.[1] The occurrence of UTI in males generally indicates an anatomic abnormality or a prostate infection, or follows rectal intercourse. By the time children reach reproductive age, the male-to-female ratio of UTIs has reversed, to 1:50.[1]

With the change in the mid-1990s to over-the-counter self-treatment of yeast infections using vaginal creams such as clotrimazole and miconazole, the epidemiology of yeast infection–induced UTI is less certain, as many patients no longer report each infection to healthcare practitioners.

Other factors associated with the development of UTIs include pregnancy, when UTIs are twice as frequent, sexual intercourse, homosexual activity, mechanical trauma or irritation, and structural abnormalities of the urinary tract that block the free flow of urine, such as an enlarged prostate, kidney stones, or presence of a catheter. Complicated UTIs are more likely among men, immunosuppressed patients, people with diabetes, and pregnant women.

ETIOLOGY

UTIs occur when the transitional epithelium of the urinary tract becomes inflamed as a result of bacterial invasion. UTIs may be classified as follows: cystitis, occurring in the urinary bladder; ureteritis, occurring in the ureter; or pyelitis, occurring in the renal pelvis.

Because urine remains sterile on its journey from the kidneys, where it is secreted, to the urethral opening, infection requires introduction of bacteria by ascension from the urethra or, less commonly, the blood stream. Usually, fecal contamination or an increase in vaginal secretions is a factor in creating ascending infections. In addition, anatomic or functional obstructions to flow, such as with the presence of indwelling catheters, and immune system dysfunction are thought to play a role. Thus, free urinary flow, complete emptying of the bladder, and good hygiene are important in the prevention of UTI, as is maintenance of optimal immune defense. Pooling of urine in the bladder in men with enlarged prostates also contributes to the development of UTI.

Although most UTIs are benign, care must be taken to recognize recurrent UTIs because of the risk of overgrowth of organisms resistant to the antibiotics used in therapy of these infections and because of the risk of sepsis in patients with urinary tract morphologic abnormalities.

SCREENING

The standard procedure for screening is the triad of assessing clinical symptoms, doing a physical examination, and performing a urinalysis on a clean-catch or catheterized specimen.

Clinical symptoms of UTIs in adults include urinary frequency, dysuria (burning pain on urination), nocturia, lower abdominal pain, and turbid, foul-smelling, or dark urine. Physical examination may also reveal mucosal edema, redness, and occasionally, ulcerations around the urethra. Urinalysis should be done and often shows significant pyuria and bacteriuria. By convention, the presence of greater than 10,000 microorganisms per mL of clean-catch urine taken for urinalysis is considered to be definitive of a UTI.

Chronic interstitial cystitis, due not to infection but rather to a persistent inflammation of the interstitium along the lining of the bladder wall, can predispose patients to UTIs and is frequently responsible for subclinical symptoms. Food allergies have been implicated as a cause of chronic cystitis.

The diagnosis of UTIs has been somewhat empirical, because clinical symptoms and the presence of significant number of bacteria in the urine often have not been found to correlate well. In one study, only 60% of women with classic symptoms actually had a significant degree of bacteriuria.[1] Every screening test should end with counseling on preventive measures for UTIs, especially in patients with a predisposition to UTI, frequent recurrences, or chronic cystitis.

NOTE

Only two groups of patients are known to benefit from screening for and treatment of asymptomatic bacteriuria: pregnant women, for prevention of pyelonephritis and the risks of premature delivery, and patients scheduled for urologic surgery, to prevent postoperative complications.[4]

INTEGRATIVE APPROACH TO PREVENTION

Whereas most conventional methods of treating UTIs involve the use of antibiotics to combat the bacterial infection, or of surgical intervention to correct an anatomic abnormality, the holistic approach to UTI involves prevention through enhancing normal host protective measures and giving pathologic epithelium a chance to heal. Emphasis is placed on enhancing the flow of urine through proper hydration and urine production; promoting a urinary pH that will inhibit the growth of microorganisms; preventing bacterial adherence to the endothelial lining of the bladder; and enhancing the immune system. Antimicrobial botanical medicines are utilized only when needed. When the risk-benefit ratio for withholding antibiotics becomes unfavorable, only then are antibiotics used.

Lifestyle Interventions

Exercise

Exercise is generally known to keep muscles toned and to improve lymphatic flow. Pelvic muscles and an intact pelvic floor help to maintain the anatomy of the urinary tract. In men, maintenance of strong abdominal wall musculature prevents development of pressure-related hernias through the abdominal wall. In women, Kegel exercises, which are designed to tone the vaginopelvic voluntary muscles, improve tone and prevent bladder prolapse and urethral obstruction.

Hydration

Increasing urine flow is an important, safe, and inexpensive measure for prevention of UTIs. Drinking more fluids, especially cranberry juice, herbal teas, and clean filtered water, promotes good flow through the kidneys. Avoidance of liquids such as soft drinks, concentrated fruit drinks, coffee, and alcohol is advised. Care must obviously be taken in patients who have compromised renal function, as well as in patients with prerenal abnormalities such as congestive heart failure, edematous tendencies due to hypo-osmotic states, or hypertension. Patients should be counseled specifically to drink 6 to 8 glasses of water daily.

Stress Management

There is concrete evidence that chronic stress alters immune function, with a deleterious effect on host defenses. Accordingly, stress management techniques are recommended to fortify the body. (See Chapter 91, Prescribing Relaxation Techniques.)

Hygiene

One of the most difficult topics to address with adult patients is the issue of personal hygiene. Because most people are taught toileting habits at a young age, these second-nature behaviors are conditioned and difficult to alter. They are also difficult to assess in an office setting. Care and tact must be taken in covering the basics of cleaning after bowel movements, how to wash the perineum, the importance of preventing fecal-orofacial contact, handwashing, and the importance of changing underclothing daily. Review of proper bath products is also essential. A helpful tool is a diagram of the perineal area, with review of how to wipe front to back, the detailed anatomy of the labia in females and scrotum in males, and the basics of where flora tends to reside in the perineal area. A compassionate but not pedantic approach is of utmost importance.

Sexual Hygiene

Sexual hygiene is another difficult topic to address with adult patients. Discussion of this topic may be even more uncomfortable for patients of certain cultures, and it is a subject almost never taught during youth. A portion of the world's population has culture-based values concerning touch and exploration of sexual organs that are difficult for American physicians to appreciate. "Honeymoon cystitis"—UTI associated with increased frequency of intercourse—is a common complaint and can often be prevented with specific practices.

Basic issues include the importance of urinating after intercourse, handwashing, avoiding genital intercourse immediately after anal intercourse, techniques for safe anal-genital contact, washing the perineum carefully after mechanical trauma, techniques for clean but fulfilling oral-genital contact, and discussion of the basic flora that tends to reside in the vagina and around the scrotum. A diagram of the male and female genitalia is an important tool, as is reassurance that exploration of one's own body is important for understanding proper mind and body function.

Patients should be advised that the use of spermicides with or without a diaphragm promotes vaginal colonization with uropathogens and increases the frequency of UTIs. Especially in postmenopausal women who use lubricants during intercourse, it is important to emphasize that lubricants can alter the vaginal flora. Perhaps the details of some of these topics are not immediately relevant for each sexually active patient with a predisposition to UTIs, but the physician should be prepared to explore such issues with the patient.

NOTE

Estrogen deficiency leads to (1) a decrease in the frequency of vaginal colonization with Lactobacillus organisms, (2) a higher vaginal pH, and (3) increased frequency of colonization with E. coli. Topical application of estriol is a common remedy for estrogen-deficient women.

Diet and Nutrition

Food allergies may produce cystitis in some patients; therefore, many naturopathic practitioners use food elimination to cure or prevent UTIs. In addition, excessive sugar consumption and nutritional deficiencies can contribute to the development of UTIs. It is recommended that patients predisposed to UTIs avoid all simple sugars and refined carbohydrates in the diet and dilute any fruit juices consumed, as bacteria tend to thrive in high-sugar environments. Eating plenty of watermelon is also recommended, as it acts as a natural diuretic. Eating liberal amounts of garlic and onion, which have antimicrobial properties, is also highly recommended.

Cranberry Juice

Much attention has been given to cranberries and cranberry juice since clinical trials showed its effectiveness both in resolving active UTI and in preventing recurrence of bladder infection. The action of cranberry juice was previously thought to occur by its acidification of the urine and through the antibacterial effects of the hippuric acid present in the berry. However, naturopaths have noted that greater than 1 liter of pure juice would have to be consumed at one time in order to acidify the urine effectively, whereas beneficial effects are seen with consumption of a half-liter per day. Subsequently, studies focused on components in cranberry juice that reduce the ability of bacteria to adhere to the lining of the bladder and urethra, and this effect is now considered the most likely mechanism of action. A study in nursing home residents showed that drinking 4 to 6 ounces of cranberry juice almost daily for 7 weeks prevented UTIs in two-thirds of the patients.[3] Unfortunately, some studies have shown an increased recurrence rate once regular prophylaxis is discontinued.

Dosage. The recommended amount of unsweetened cranberry juice for prevention of UTIs is 0.5 liter (approximately 16 ounces) per day.

Precautions. Care must be taken to avoid juice products, most of which have added sugar and are diluted to contain as little as 10% cranberry juice. Only sweetening with apple or grape juice is permissible. Simultaneous consumption of citrus and other acidic juices is not recommended.

Acid versus Alkaline pH

There has been debate regarding urinary acidity and frequency of infections. Alkaline urinary pH is noted in chronic UTIs caused by microorganisms that produce urease, such as *Proteus* and *Klebsiella* organisms. Because it is difficult to acidify the urine, owing to the presence of abundant buffers in the nephron to prevent acidification, many researchers have noted the impracticality of maintaining acidified urine as a protective measure.

Alkalinization of the urine is a common approach for prevention of UTIs and can be achieved with citrate salts such as potassium citrate or sodium citrate, which work without affecting gastric pH or producing laxative effects. These salts are excreted partly as carbonate, thus raising the pH of the urine, and have long been used in the treatment of lower UTIs.[7] In addition, many of the herbs used to treat UTIs, such as goldenseal and *Arctostaphylos uva ursi*, work best in an alkaline environment.

Enhancing the Immune System

The healthy body has several defenses to prevent bacterial growth in the urinary tract. In addition to urine flow, which washes away bacteria, the surface of the bladder has antimicrobial properties in the smooth epithelial cell structure, and the pH of the urine inhibits the growth of many organisms. In addition, prostatic fluid has antimicrobial substances. Finally, the body quickly secretes white cells in the pelvis at the first sign of bacterial invasion.

Healing the Epithelium

In addition to the use of herbs such as gotu kola, which promote health of connective tissue, practical issues such as discontinuing the use of indwelling catheters may be relevant for some patients.

Botanicals

Goldenseal

Goldenseal (*Hydrastis canadensis*), although an endangered plant and thus discouraged for use for casual immunostimulation, has long been regarded as a powerful antimicrobial, working especially against *Escherichia coli* and *Klebsiella*, *Proteus*, and *Staphylococcus* species, as well as *Enterobacter aerogenes* and *Pseudomonas* species. Berberine, its active component, is known to work better in alkaline urine. Women who tend to develop bladder infections associated with sexual intercourse should wash the labia and urethra with a strong tea of goldenseal (2 teaspoons of the herb per cup of water) before and after intercourse, if possible.

Dosage. The recommended dosage is 4 to 6 mL of a 1:5 tincture or 250 to 500 mg of powdered solid extract standardized to 8% alkaloids.

Precautions. Prolonged oral use of goldenseal can cause gastrointestinal upset, constipation, and excitatory states. Toxic doses can cause hypotension and inhibit cardiac activity.

Gotu kola

Especially in chronic interstitial cystitis, disruption of the integrity of the bladder interstitium is a major pathologic feature in UTI. Extracts of *Centella asiatica*, or gotu kola, have been shown to have strong wound-healing activity through the herb's triterpene compounds (asiatic acid, madecassic acid, asiaticoside, and madecassoside), stimulating collagen synthesis and normal connective tissue matrix when taken orally.[5] Historically, gotu kola is well documented in the surgical text of Ayurveda, the *Sushruta Samhita*, and has been used internally and externally by surgeons and by people of Java and other islands of Polynesia for the female genitourinary tract to aid in epithelial healing. Clinically, Centella has also been used for treatment of burns, cellulite, cirrhosis of the liver, keloids, scleroderma, and perineal lesions. For preventing UTIs, Centella

can improve the integrity of the interstitium as well as healing ulcerations of the bladder.[6]

Dosage. The daily dose is 60 to 120 mg of a standardized extract containing 40% asiaticoside, 29% to 30% asiatic acid, 29% to 30% madecassic acid, and 1% to 2% madecassoside. Tinctures (1:5) can be used in amounts of 10 to 20 mL per day.

Precautions. When used orally, gotu kola can cause pruritus, photosensitivity, and elevated blood pressure. Pregnant women should not use this botanical. It may also increase the risk of miscarriage.

Arctostaphylos uva ursi

Research on *Arctostaphylos uva ursi*, also known as bearberry or upland cranberry, has shown that a powerful antiseptic component, aubutin, composes 7% to 9% of the leaves. Arbutin is hydrolyzed to hydroquinone, which alkalinizes the urine. Because crude plant extracts have been shown to be more effective than isolated arbutin, recent clinical trials focusing on the use of standardized uva ursi extract found that it was effective for recurrent cystitis.

Dosage. 4 to 6 mL of a 1:5 tincture, or 250 to 500 mg of solid plant extract standardized to 10% arbutin.

Precautions. Care must be taken to avoid toxicity, as small amounts of dried leaves have shown that pure uva ursi has a narrow therapeutic window. Toxic signs include tinnitus, nausea, vomiting, shortness of breath, and later, convulsions.

Garlic

Garlic (*Allium sativum*) has long been acknowledged as a powerful antimicrobial against the organisms commonly causing UTIs, such as *E. coli*, Proteus species, Klebsiella, and staphylococcal and streptococcal species. Fresh garlic chopped and combined with oil for use in cooking is optimal and preferred to garlic supplement formulations, although the hallmark odor often deters patients from use in plentiful amounts.

Dosage. 2 to 3 cloves of freshly chopped garlic daily.

Precautions. Garlic in large amounts can enhance the effects of warfarin.

Probiotics

Acidophilus

Probiotics are preparations aimed at supplementation of bacteria known to live in the human body that exert a protective effect on tissues where they reside, such as the gut, vagina, and bladder. *Lactobacillus* species are known as "friendly bacteria." Replacing friendly flora killed by antibiotic usage helps to boost immunity, to prevent colonization by pathogenic bacteria, and to maintain the health of bladder epithelium.

Dosage. The recommended dose of live-acidophilus *Lactobacillus* preparation is 1 capsule in the morning and right before bedtime. Use of vaginal *Lactobacillus* suppositories is especially helpful in addition to oral therapy immediately after an antibiotic course is completed. (See Chapter 97, Prescribing Probiotics.)

Precautions. Use of probiotics is contraindicated in immunocompromised patients.

Conventional Treatments

Antibiotics

Patients with persistently positive results on urine cultures or who experience recurrent UTIs without treatment should consider a course of 4 to 6 weeks of antibiotics for cure. Men may have an upper tract or prostatic source of infection and benefit greatly from 4 to 6 weeks of systemic antibiotic treatment. Trimethoprim-sulfamethoxazole and ciprofloxacin are the usual agents used, as they provide coverage against *E. coli*, *Staphylococcus saprophyticus*, and *Klebsiella*, as well as *Enterococcus*. Treatment of UTI secondary to systemic infection often requires stronger agents.

Pessaries

If pessaries are fitted to normalize the urinary tract and to approximate morphology allowing normal urinary flow, these devices can be useful and reassuring to help women with vaginal prolapse to maintain a more anatomic position of the vagina, as the prolapsed position predisposes patients to UTIs.

Other Therapies to Consider

Homeopathy

Homeopathic remedies, though they do not fit within the theories of the biomedical scientific model of analysis, have been shown to be some of the most effective agents for treatment of diseases involving inflammation or infection. Although homeopathic remedies are specifically tailored to symptoms of illness, Staphysagria 6C can be used especially for honeymoon cystitis and for recurrent infections, and Cantharis 6C can be used on the first days of burning pain during urination. From 3 to 5 pellets can be placed under the tongue 3 or 4 times a day when the symptoms first appear.

 ── *PREVENTION PRESCRIPTION* ──────────────────

- *Good hygiene consists of regular and complete emptying of the bladder and not holding urine for prolonged periods of time.*
- *Catheter use should be discontinued if possible.*
- *The perineal area should be cleansed properly and regularly.*
- *A healthy immune system should be maintained through effective stress management, so that host defenses can quickly combat developing infections.*
- *An exercise regimen should be incorporated into the daily routine, to help keep pelvic muscles and bladder support strong.*
- *During acute infections, avoid activities such as prolonged motorcycle rides, horseback riding, and bicycling.*
- *The use of perfumed bath products, toilet papers, sanitary napkins, douches, and strong washing detergents should be avoided, as they may add chemical irritation to the perineal area.*
- *Underclothing should be changed daily; thongs or tight underpants and leotards made of nylon or synthetic fabrics are best avoided. Cotton and silk are the best fabrics for people who are predisposed to UTIs.*
- *Urination before and after sexual intercourse is recommended. Sexual practices that do not spread or exacerbate infection should be identified for the patient.*
- *Drinking water, green tea or herbal tea, and diluted unsweetened fruit juices in plentiful amounts is highly recommended.*
- *Consumption of 16 ounces of unsweetened pure cranberry juice daily for prophylaxis is also recommended.*
- *Removal and regular cleaning of pessaries if used are recommended.*
- *Goldenseal tea can be used to wash the genitals, and uva ursi or garlic in a compounded mixture can be given as a natural antibiotic if needed.*
- *Prophylactic gotu kola may help to augment healing of bladder epithelium, especially in chronic cystitis patients.*
- *Acidophilus should be taken twice a day to promote healthy bacteria in the bladder, especially after a course of antibiotics.*

PREVENTION PRESCRIPTION continued

- *Nutritional supplements can be used to generally enhance function of the immune system and to increase antioxidant protection: vitamin C 500 mg every 2 hours for the first day of infection, bioflavonoids 1 g per day, vitamin A 25,000 IU per day, zinc 30 mg per day, and choline 1 g per day.*
- *Homeopathic remedies can be taken to curtail onset of UTI. When symptoms first appear, 3 to 5 pellets are placed under the tongue three or four times a day. Staphysagria 6C is given for honeymoon cystitis, and Cantharis 6C on the first days of burning pain during urination. (See Chapter 103, Therapeutic Homeopathy.)*

Internet Resources

www.garynull.com
  Chronicles the online reports of Gary Null, Ph.D., and contains excerpts from the *Clinician's Handbook of Natural Healing.*
www.urologychannel.com/uti/alternativetreatment.shtml
  Gives a nontechnical overview of natural treatments for UTIs; however, the focus is mostly on cure, not prevention.

References

1. Pizzorno JE, Murray MT: Cystitis. In Pizzorno JE, Murray MT (eds): Textbook of Natural Medicine, New York, Churchill Livingstone, 1999, pp 1183–1188.
2. Rubin RH: Infections of the urinary tract. In Dale DC: Scientific American Medicine, New York, Scientific American, 1997.
3. Gibson L, et al. Effectiveness of cranberry juice in preventing urinary tract infections in long-term care facility patients. J Naturop Med 2:45–47, 1991.
4. Reves RR: Urinary tract infections. In Mladenovic J (ed): Primary Care Secrets, Philadelphia, Hanley & Belfus, 1995, pp 223–226.
5. Bonte F, Dumas M, et al: Influence of asiatic acid, madecassic acid, and asiaticoside on human collagen I synthesis. Planta Med 60:683–688, 1994.
6. Etrebi A, Ibrahim A, Zaki K: Treatment of bladder ulcer with asiaticoside. J Egypt Med Assoc 58:324, 1975.
7. Spooner JB: Alkalinization in the management of cystitis. J Int Med Res 12:30–34, 1984.
8. Avorn J, Monan M, et al: Reduction of bacteriuria and pyuria after ingestion of cranberry juice. JAMA 271:751–754, 1994.

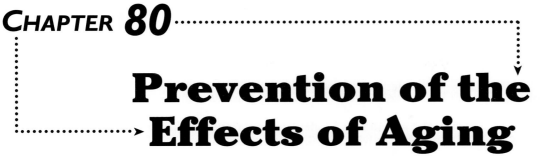

CHAPTER 80

Prevention of the Effects of Aging

Evan W. Kligman, M.D.

PATHOPHYSIOLOGY

With marked increases anticipated in both life expectancy and life span in the 21st century, clinicians need to be increasingly aware of the effects of aging on the provision of treatment modalities, especially to persons surviving into extreme old age. By the middle of this century in the United States alone, over 1 million people are expected to live to age 100 or beyond.[1]

As humans age, all functions and characteristics are modified. However, there is no clear consensus about what aging actually is—what "naturally" occurs with the passage of time—versus the effects of disuse and disease. Optimal health management requires not only an understanding of aging processes that are assumed to be natural and inevitable but also knowledge of the most accepted theories of how and why we age prematurely, usually owing to the presence of certain reversible risk factors. Although at present there is a significant emphasis on development of new technologies, especially in the area of human genomics and stem cell research, to provide greater clarity on genetic and cellular aging mechanisms,[2] adaptation of both traditional allopathic and complementary and alternative integrative modalities to reflect current understanding of the effects of aging, and of how to postpone or prevent premature aging,[3] is now possible.

Several earlier longitudinal studies attempted to identify the effects of natural or normal aging free of disease as distinct from the development of age-related diseases such as cancer, cardiovascular disease, diabetes, osteoporosis, and neurodegenerative diseases such as Alzheimer's disease. Results from such studies[4] suggest that the effects of aging are extremely "plastic" and variable from person to person. McEwen's concept of the "allostatic load" suggests that each person's signature of aging is a result of interactions among genetic make-up, lifestyle, diet, and environmental challenges.[5] Thus, a combination of holistic parameters can be used to assess cumulative physiologic and psychological challenges over the life span and to predict how today's health care practitioners will respond not only to new challenges such as management of age-related conditions and application of treatment mo-

dalities in old age but also to longevity itself. Accordingly, a broader pattern of aging processes or biomarkers should be considered in determining how "well" a particular person is aging and how to customize interventions to reduce the effect of a chronic condition, thereby preventing certain processes from leading to the development of one or more ailments that are more likely to appear in old age.

NOTE

Appropriate interventions individualized to the patient can help to "compress morbidity" by shortening the period of functional decline common in old age. Thus, the "health span" will come closer to matching the life span.

However, the science of identification of biomarkers of human aging remains in its infancy.[6] Table 80–1 lists various physiologic biomarkers found more often with suboptimal aging.[7] Another finding, from longitudinal studies, is that normal aging appears to be a phenomenon of gradual rather than precipitous change. Rapid decline is more likely to occur with the onset of a specific age-related pathologic process.

Table 80–1. Biomarkers of Aging

Loss of strength
Reduced flexibility
Decreased cardiovascular endurance
Increased body fat (and resultant loss of lean muscle mass, or sarcopenia)
Reduced resting energy expenditure
Lower kidney clearance
Reduced cell-mediated immunity
Increased hearing threshold
Reduced vibratory sensation
Compromised near vision and dark accommodation
Reduced taste and smell acuity
Altered hormone levels
Increased autoantibodies

Adapted from Evans W, Rosenberg IH: Biomarkers: The 10 Keys to Prolonged Vitality. New York, Fireside, 1991.

Biologic and Holistic Factors in Aging

Biologic and holistic determinants of life span, or of general health, follow basic biologic concepts—theories and principles—common to most mammals. These concepts include cell doubling (with a maximum of 90 doublings for most human cells over a period of 120 years); telomere shortening; loss of VO_2 max or oxygen-carrying capacity (the rate of loss being variable and related to level of aerobic activity, at least beyond the age of 30 years, with universal decline beyond the minimum of 0.5% a year becoming more pronounced only in the ninth decade of life); caloric restriction (proven in nonprimate mammals to extend life span by 30%, or potentially to age 120 years in humans, with a 30% reduction in caloric intake); longevity genes, found in extremely long-lived persons; morphic resonance; and "allostatic load." These determinants predict to a large extent how any person is aging and thus may be considered at least surrogate clinical biomarkers of aging. These determinants and biomarkers, listed in Table 80–1, allow an appreciation of the heterogeneity of the effects of aging processes. These biomarkers are associated with a loss of organ reserve (see Table 80–2) and a higher likelihood that the affected

Table 80–2. Common Changes Associated with Normal Aging

System/Structure Affected	Age-Related Change	Change in Function
Overall	Decrease in height and weight Decreased total body water Decreased lean muscle mass	
Skin	Increased wrinkling Atrophy of sweat glands	
Cardiovascular	Elongation of arteries and aorta Arterial wall thickening Arterial fibrosis Valvular sclerosis Decrease in blood flow to kidneys, liver, and brain	Decreased cardiac output Decreased heart rate response to stress Decreased maximum heart rate (no change in resting heart rate)
Kidney	Increase in abnormal glomeruli Decreased ability of kidneys to clear toxins and to metabolize most drugs	Decreased creatinine clearance
Lung	Decreased elasticity Decreased cilia activity	Decreased vital capacity Decreased maximal oxygen uptake Decreased cough reflex
Gastrointestinal	Decreased hydrochloric acid Decreased saliva flow Fewer taste buds Decreased ability of liver to clear toxins and to metabolize drugs	
Musculoskeletal	Loss of bone, cartilage, and collagen	
Eye/vision	Decreased pupil size Increase in lens opacities	Decreased accommodation Hyperopia Decreased visual acuity Decreased color sensitivity Decreased depth perception
Ear/hearing	Degenerative ossicles Increased eustachian tube dysfunction Atrophy of external auditory meatus Atrophy of cochlear hair cells Loss of auditory neurons	Decreased high-frequency perception Decreased pitch discrimination
Immune system	Decrease in natural killer cell activity to fight infection and carcinogenesis	Decreased T cell activity
Nervous system	Decreased brain weight Decreased cortical cell count	Increased motor response time Slower psychomotor performance Decreased intellectual performance Decreased complex learning ability Decreased hours of sleep, especially rapid eye movement sleep
Endocrine	Decreased triiodothyronine (T_3) Decreased sex hormones Increased insulin Decreased glucose tolerance Increase in fasting glucose levels	

Adapted from The aging body. In Merck Manual 2001. Section 1: Fundamentals. Available at www.merck.com; and Kane R, et al: Essentials of Clinical Geriatrics, 3rd ed. New York, McGraw-Hill, 1994.

Table 80–3. Leading Causes of Mortality in Persons Older Than 65 Years of Age

....

1. Diseases of the heart
2. Malignant neoplasms
3. Cerebrovascular disease
4. Chronic obstructive pulmonary disease
5. Pneumonia and influenza
6. Diabetes mellitus
7. Accidents
8. Atherosclerosis
9. Nephritis and nephrosis
10. Septicemia

From National Center for Health Statistics.

person will suffer from common chronic conditions that appear to be age-related (see Tables 80–3 and 80–4). Integrative therapies may be able to control or prevent their occurrence.

Although the biomarkers and the physiologic and anatomic changes presented in Table 80–2 are common and found universally among human populations, the rate of change or decrease in capacity is probably dependent on the *allostatic load*—the interaction of genetic with environmental and lifestyle factors. Indeed, these changes occur within the web-like network of the individual person's "mind-body-spirit" integrity—or lack thereof.

In general, decline in physiologic function begins after age 30 years, when human performance peaks. The rate of decline varies, ranging from 0.5% a year in person with an optimal life style to as high as 3% a year in sedentary and overweight persons. By age 85, even master athletes begin to experience a straight-line decline of greater trajectory in cognitive and physical performance. Nevertheless, most physiologic function remains adequate for the healthy

person surviving even into extreme old age (to age 100 or older). This preservation of function is due to redundancy in systems and functional reserve capacity. Disease and disuse, rather than normal aging, account for the greater portion of functional decline in old age (age older than 85 years). As a result of this inevitable decline (especially in persons older than 85 years of age, who constitute the fastest-growing age group in the United States), the likelihood of drug-drug or drug-nutrient interactions, as well as of adverse effects from environmental exposures and infections, is far greater, suggesting that health promotion and disease prevention become even more important with old age.

NOTE

Disease and disuse are far more likely explanations for functional decline and the onset of common chronic conditions in older persons than is "true" natural or normal aging.

Recent research in various fields, including the emerging discipline of *functional medicine*,[10] has led to an understanding of modifiable factors that contribute to premature aging and, through their control or prevention, to optimal aging. Interventions to reduce the impact of these factors should be the underlying rationale for integrative approaches to health promotion and disease management in the aging population.

The most fundamental understanding of aging appears to be impairment of cell membrane perme-

Table 80-4. Common Chronic Conditions in Persons Older Than 65 Years of Age Modifiable by Lifestyle

....

Condition	Lifestyle Intervention
Osteoarthritis	Exercise, diet, weight reduction
Hypertension	Exercise, stress reduction, diet, weight reduction, no alcohol
Hearing impairment	Decrease exposure to loud noises and medications toxic to the auditory nerve
Heart disease	Control of hypertension, no tobacco, exercise, supplements, reduction in lipids
Cataracts	Antioxidants, sunglasses to reduce ultraviolet light exposure, no steroids
Orthopedic impairment	Muscle (especially resistance) training
Chronic sinusitis	Elimination of allergens, nasal lavage
Diabetes	Exercise, reduction weight, low-glycemic-index diet, stress control
Visual impairment	Antioxidants to reduce risk of macular degeneration, corrective lenses, cataract surgery
Varicose veins	Horse chestnut, support hose
Cancer	No tobacco, increased antioxidants, exercise, reduction in dietary fat, minimization of radiation exposure
Osteoporosis	Adequate calcium, manganese, magnesium, boron intake; no tobacco, weight-bearing exercise, hormone replacement therapy
Congestive heart failure	DASH diet, coenzyme Q10 up to 300 mg daily
Depression	B vitamins, psychotherapy, conventional pharmaceuticals, SAMe
Cognitive decline	Phosphatidylserine up to 500 mg daily, ginkgo, vitamin E, NSAID
Gait disorders	Physical therapy, mind-body modalities
Urinary incontinence	Kegel exercises
Constipation	Psyllium, natural vegetable laxatives, adequate water, physical activity
Adverse drug reactions	Consider alternative botanicals, herbs, or other modalities
Vascular insufficiency	*Gingko biloba*

Data from Hazzard W, et al: Principles of Geriatric Medicine and Gerontology, 2nd ed. New York, McGraw-Hill, 1990; and Kligman EW: Preventive geriatrics. Geriatrics 47:39–50, 1992.
DASH, Dietary Approaches to Stop Hypertension; NSAID, nonsteroidal anti-inflammatory drug.

Table 80–5. Common Reversible Functional Causes of Premature Aging
....

Oxidative stress and impaired mitochondrial function
Glycation (dysglycemia) and insulin resistance
Chronic inflammation
Altered methylation reactions
Lipid atherogenesis
Compromised detoxification capacity
Poor immune function
Chronic stress response
Hormone imbalance
Physical and mental inactivity

---

ability, leading to dysfunction in cellular communication and consequent functional decline. Underlying processes that result in membrane permeability problems are cumulative and include oxidative stress, dysglycemia, chronic inflammation, imbalanced methylation reactions, chronic stress response, lipid atherogenesis, impaired detoxification capacity, poor immune function, hormone imbalance, and, physical and mental inactivity. The presence or progression of all these processes in any one aging person is not inevitable; indeed, much of what is observed as aging effects is a result of disuse and other suboptimal life styles, rather than inexorable decline to be experienced by all persons.

Oxidative Stress

Oxidative stress is a fact of life for all organisms requiring oxygen for energy and growth. Damaging free oxygen radicals are continuously created during cell respiration. Although each person has a unique pattern of endogenous antioxidants and consumes varying levels of dietary antioxidants, unrepaired damage—from the mitochondrial level to the organ level—accumulates with aging. Human research has identified a number of degenerative disorders adversely influenced by oxidative stress (atherosclerosis, hypertension, diabetes, osteoarthritis, dementia, Parkinson's disease). Furthermore, at least in animal studies, antioxidant supplementation and higher levels of antioxidant enzymes, and reduced causes of oxidative stress, have been shown to be associated with an extended life span.

Dysglycemia

Dysglycemia is another unavoidable intrinsic aging process. A complex series of glucose reactions leads ultimately to protein cross-linking, causing blood vessel wall and connective tissue hardening, especially among persons with a high intake of refined carbohydrates, and consequent sustained high fasting insulin levels, with the resultant development of insulin resistance in many cases. This more serious sequela is certainly not inevitable with age, yet insulin resistance may occur even in young adults,

although it is preventable with lifestyle modifications including optimization of diet, increased physical activity, and stress reduction practices. Signs and symptoms of insulin resistance (i.e., metabolic syndrome or syndrome X), which occur with increased frequency with advancing age, include a ratio of triglycerides to high-density lipoproteins (HDLs) of greater than 5, elevated uric acid level, "hard" central adiposity, hypertension or some elevation of blood pressure, hypoglycemic episodes, glucose intolerance (fasting blood sugar level of 110 to 124 mg/dL), and elevated fasting insulin levels. Dysglycemia contributes to a number of chronic conditions (e.g., atherosclerosis, type 2 diabetes mallitus, connective tissue disorders and other autoimmune diseases, vascular dementia). Elevated insulin levels may be a major promoter of atheroma development and the progression of atherogenesis[11] (see Chapter 26, Insulin Resistance Syndrome).

Chronic Inflammation

Chronic inflammation occurs with age primarily because of an imbalance between the amounts of omega-6 and omega-3 essential fatty acids. In prehistoric diets, the ratio of these fatty acids was close to 1:1; now, it is about 45:1. This imbalance is believed to contribute to increased inflammatory disease in the brain, gut, coronary arteries, skin, muscles, and other tissues. Furthermore, inflammation leads to rigid cell membranes and impaired cellular communication, and a higher risk for cancer and autoimmune and cardiovascular disease. In summary, chronic inflammation contributes to the development and progression of rheumatoid arthritis and osteoarthritis, asthma, atherosclerosis, dementia, eczema, inflammatory bowel disease, and irritable bowel syndrome (see Chapter 84, The Anti-inflammatory Diet).

Altered Methylation

Altered methylation reactions occur with age primarily as a result of deficiencies in vitamins B_6 and B_{12} and folic acid. Methylation defects involve the transfer of methyl and sulfur molecules between compounds. A deficiency of beneficial compounds, such as S-adenosyl methionine (SAMe), and an excess of harmful compounds, such as homocysteine, results. Deficiencies in the B vitamin cofactors (due to diet or inadequate absorption) necessary for adequate methylation and the resultant production of excess homocysteine can contribute to a variety of common conditions seen in premature aging, including coronary artery disease, cerebrovascular disease, deep vein thromboses, type 2 diabetes mellitus, rheumatoid arthritis, osteoporosis, dementia, and depression and other psychiatric conditions. Impaired methylation reactions with alterations in

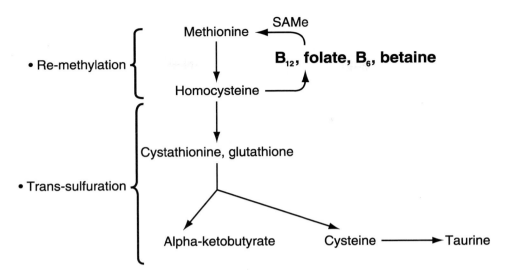

Figure 80–1. Homocysteine metabolism. Betaine is a source of trimethylglycine, a cofactor for converting homocysteine into methionine. SAMe, *S*-adenosyl methionine.

the folate cycle (Fig. 80–1) can also impair the effectiveness of certain genes, such as the estrogen receptor gene, thus reducing the beneficial effects of hormone replacement, and may also increase the risk of cancer.[10] Inadequate folate intake and serum levels have been associated with increased frequency of nucleic acid misincorporation and chromosome breaks in genetically susceptible persons.

Lipid Atherogenesis

Lipid atherogenesis is now considered to be the end result of a cascade of physiologic aberrations including plaque development from elevated cholesterol, atheroma development secondary to insulin resistance, inflammation caused by certain infective agents and inadequate intake of omega-3 essential fatty acids, and excessive coagulation due to high ferritin levels. Furthermore, depression, anxiety, and hostility have been associated with a greater risk for atherosclerosis. The relative risk in selected studies of these behavioral factors in causing ischemic heart disease ranges from 1.5 to 4.5.

Compromised Detoxification Capacity

Compromised detoxification capacity secondary to exposure to toxins, multiple medications using cytochrome P450 enzymes in redox reactions during phase I detoxification, food and drug allergens, pollutants, and even stress from "toxic" interpersonal relationships can also accelerate the aging process. The liver and gastrointestinal tract are the primary sites of detoxification in the body. However, an overload of toxic exposures can lead to gastrointestinal imbalances and a "leaky gut," with diminished absorption of important nutrients, and functional bowel disorders such as irritable bowel disease.

Poor Immune Function

Poor immune function can result from genetic predisposition, immune senescence due to changes in the helper T cell/suppressor T cell ratio caused by environmental influences, inadequate nutrition, or physical inactivity, which results in further decrease in the body's natural killer cell activity. Also, a leaky gut from impaired detoxification capacity can lead to lower serum levels of secretory immunoglobulin A (sIgA), hypochlorhydria, and maldigestion. Food allergies contribute to weakening of the immune system. The rise in food allergies in recent decades may be associated with earlier weaning; limited and less diverse diets; intolerance to repeatedly used foods such as cow's milk, whey, caramel, and artificial colors and flavorings; and medications that irritate the gut mucosa, an organ of the immune system.

Chronic Stress Response

Chronic stress response may evolve in persons who have difficulty dealing with excessive daily stress from various sources, such as emotional (fear, anxiety, worry), environmental (extreme heat or cold, noise, toxic exposures, disrupted light cycles), or physiologic (pain, hunger, inflammation, hunger, infection, poor sleep, excessive exercise or food intake, hypoglycemia) stress. Prolonged stress leads to sustained and chronic elevations of cortisol; prolonged exposure of the brain to high cortisol levels impairs neuron-neuron connections, furthering cognitive decline and increasing the incidence of depression.

Hormone Imbalance

Hormone imbalance is universal with aging; declines in all age-related hormones, except cortisol and possibly insulin, are seen. Hormones affected include adrenal (DHEA), pituitary (insulin-like growth factor-1 [IGF-1]), pineal gland (melatonin), and sex (estradiol, progesterone, testosterone) hormones. Thyroid hormone levels often decline after 55 years, in women especially. Men may actually experience an increase in progesterone with age. Natural menopause usually has its onset in women in their mid-40s to early 50s, and for male andropause the average age at onset is about 50. Changes in hormonal balance result from neuroendocrine dysfunction and insensitivity of the hypothalamus to feedback mechanisms in the endocrine system.

Nevertheless, the neuroendocrine dysfunction associated with natural aging may protect older persons from cancer and atherosclerosis. New studies suggest that growth hormone replacement in animals, for instance, may increase the risk of cancer and insulin resistance. However, decreased estradiol levels in men as well as in women are associated with greater risk of osteoporosis and fractures. Male andropause may include symptoms such as fatigue (in 80% of men studied), depression (in 70%), irritability and anger (in 60%), reduced libido and erectile dysfunction (in up to 80%), diminished lean muscle mass, and other subtle signs and symptoms of premature aging. Low testosterone levels in men and women have been associated with increased risk of atherosclerosis, low muscle mass, and weight gain from an increased percentage of body fat. Common signs and symptoms of female menopause include decreased libido, depression, fatigue, hot flashes, poor memory, subjective loss of motivation, and appearance of fine wrinkles in the skin.

Physical and Mental Inactivity

Physical and mental inactivity is common with aging. Sedentary older persons will benefit greatly from a regular exercise program and from daily activities that stimulate brain function. Increased activity is probably the single most important lifestyle intervention for reducing the risk of cognitive decline, the primary health fear most people have as they age, and heart disease, the leading cause of premature death. Maintaining an active lifestyle is the best way to ensure maintenance of the cells' oxygen-carrying capacity (Vo_2 max).

INTEGRATIVE APPROACH TO DISEASE PREVENTION AND FUNCTIONAL MAINTENANCE

Many geriatricians have come to realize that "modern medicine does not work well for old people."[15] Clinicians often fail to recognize that the goal of therapy, especially for people of old age, should be to relieve suffering and to improve function. All too often, the health care system "medicalizes" aging, placing a higher priority on accurate diagnoses, and delivering irrational care based on conventional therapies carrying significant risk.

In order to broaden healing opportunities through use of integrative therapies, the clinician's objective in working with older persons should be to normalize or enhance cellular communication by improving cell membrane permeability. Recommended interventions may alter many common reversible causes of decline, morbidity, and mortality with age.

As suggested by the allostatic load hypothesis, these therapies must be inherently holistic, because premature aging is itself a result of the impact of lifestyle, environment, and disease on genetic expression and potential. The interaction of the mind, body, and spirit dimensions of health with cellular function increases in significance with aging. Thus, it is appropriate to consider the following categories of interventions for the control as well as prevention of the effects of both normal, or natural, and premature aging:

- Biochemical: pharmaceutical, botanical, supplements for nutrient enhancement
- Biomechanical: surgery, osteopathy, massage
- Bioenergetics: traditional Chinese medicine, reiki, healing touch
- Mind-body therapies: hypnosis, guided imagery, counseling
- Lifestyle: body—physical activity and exercise; nutrition—diet and nutritional tailoring; mind—behavior modification for stress reduction; emotion and spirit—spiritual direction and counseling on purposeful living

Foundation Lifestyle

As recommended by Ballentine,[16] a sound foundation in lifestyle modification—nutrition, detoxification, and movement and exercise—can serve as a framework for the individual patient to build on using additional control measures as described subsequently. "Lifestyle medicine" is expected to have a significant impact, by reducing the magnitude of age-related changes and slowing the rate of aging processes that lead to both premature aging and the onset of a variety of common chronic conditions seen in old age.

Interventions to Control Effects of Aging and Reverse Common Conditions Leading to Premature Aging

For prevention of many of the reversible effects of premature aging, the older patient may be counseled to implement the following interventions.

Reduction of Oxidative Stress and Increased Antioxidant Intake

(see Chapter 96, Prescribing Antioxidants)

- Avoidance of overeating or weight reduction as appropriate
- Buildup of the immune system to decrease infection risk
- Appropriate resistance exercise training to increase efficiency of antioxidative processes in mitochondria by up-regulating enzymes and oxidative capacity of muscle
- Avoidance of excessive exercise, or increase in antioxidant intake to compensate
- Inclusion in the diet of 8 to 10 servings of fruits and vegetables daily (best dietary and liquid antioxidants: carrots, cooked tomatoes, broccoli, apples, spinach, oranges, bananas, blueberries, red peppers, sweet potatoes, strawberries, Brussels sprouts, green tea, red wine, red grape juice, dark beer and ale)
- Supplements such as vitamin C, mixed and natural tocopherols, selenium, coenzyme Q10, lutein, and lycopene
- Dark chocolate (1½ ounces daily) for fun and antioxidant phytophenols
- Low-glycemic-index diet (see Chapter 83, The Glycemic Index)
- Reduced intake of trans fatty acids and other saturated fats, which contribute to high oxidative stress

Laboratory Tests to Consider:

Oxidative stress protection factors (exogenous): ascorbate (vitamin C), coenzyme Q10, selenium

Carotenoids (alpha- and beta-carotene, lutein, lycopene, retinol); tocopherols (alpha-, delta- gamma-tocopherols)

Oxidative stress damage factors, with direct damage measured using serum and urine peroxide levels and indirect damage measured using serum copper, ferritin, glucose, fructosamine, and iron levels

Elimination of Dysglycemia and Insulin Resistance

- Low-glycemic-index carbohydrate diet
- Avoidance of aggressive caloric restriction in obese persons, which has minimal impact and leads primarily to loss of lean tissue
- Implementation of routine physical activity as the priority, especially weight-lifting and resistance exercise training, to increase lean muscle mass, boost metabolic rate, decrease abdominal girth and fat, maintain ideal body weight and prevent further weight gain, and decrease insulin levels
- Regular food intake, as skipped meals lead to increased epinephrine, cortisol, and insulin levels
- Balanced snacks and meals including protein, complex unrefined carbohydrates, and essential fatty acids or monounsaturated fats

- Elimination of caffeine, which reduces insulin sensitivity
- Stress management to control cortisol levels, as high levels reduce insulin sensitivity
- Stress reduction practices for 20 minutes every morning (and evening if possible)
- Adequate hormone replacement (see later on)
- Adequate antioxidant intake as noted previously
- Glucose tolerance factor (GTF) chromium 200 to 1000 μg daily to improve glucose metabolism (GTF chromium does not contain picolinate, which may build up, resulting in toxic effects)
- Fiber 30 to 40 g daily in divided doses
- Omega-3 essential fatty acids provided as cold water fish, flaxseed, walnuts, and liquid or gel cap supplements 1000 to 6000 mg daily
- Alpha-lipoic acid and alpha-linolenic acid
- Vanadium 30 to 60 mg three times a day
- Vitamin E up to 800 international units (IU) daily of mixed and natural tocopherols
- Avoidance of very-low-calorie diets, which lead to loss of lean muscle tissue and increased cortisol
- Avoidance of use of tobacco and oral contraceptives (or imbalanced hormone replacement therapy) with high androgenic activity, which contribute to insulin resistance
- Metformin (Glucophage) and thiazolidinediones (Avandia, Actos) to reduce insulin resistance

Laboratory Tests to Consider:

Markers of glycation and dysglycemia: fasting blood glucose, glycosylated hemoglobin

Fasting insulin level determination

Serum triglyceride levels (greater than 149 mg/dL is abnormal)

HDL cholesterol level (less than 40 mg/dL is abnormal)

Elevated uric acid levels

Reversal of Chronic Inflammation

- Omega-3 essential fatty acids 1000 to 6000 mg daily
- Consumption of 3 to 5 servings of cold water fish weekly
- Other natural anti-inflammatory agents—curcumin (in turmeric curry), ginger, *Boswellia*
- Caloric restriction (to reduce inflammatory response in brain)
- Green tea
- Pycnogenol (pine bark extract) for inflammatory skin disorders
- Statins and angiotensin-converting enzyme (ACE) inhibitors for their anti-inflammatory properties, especially in the vascular system

Laboratory Tests to Consider:

Omega-3–omega-6 ratio

C-reactive protein level

Serum fibrinogen level

Enhancement of Methylation Reactions

- Folic acid 2 mg daily
- Vitamin B_6 100 mg daily
- Vitamin B_{12} 100 units daily
- Trimethylglycine 750 mg daily
- Estradiol/progesterone replacement for women
- Diet rich in leafy greens, whole grains, fortified cereals, and beans

Laboratory Tests to Consider:

Homocysteine; vitamins B_6 and B_{12} and folic acid if there is difficulty in reducing homocysteine with a B-100 complex

Prevention/Reversal of Lipid Atherogenesis

- Optimization of lipid profile (see Chapter 31, Hyperlipidemia)
- Routine physical activity, especially aerobic exercise and resistance training, to raise HDL level, increase lean muscle mass, and so on (see Chapter 86, Writing an Exercise Prescription)
- Addition of red wine or red grape juice
- Niacin in sustained-release formulations 1500 to 3000 mg daily if tolerated
- Red yeast rice 400 mg twice a day
- Anti-inflammatory diet (see Chapter 84)
- Reduction of coagulation markers by donation of 1 pint of blood every 2 months, especially if ferritin or fibrinogen levels are elevated
- Aspirin daily if tolerated and/or garlic to reduce platelet aggregation
- Decrease in homocysteine levels to less than 8 with folic acid supplementation
- Stress reduction to reduce cortisol and insulin and to combat depression, anxiety, and negative emotional response (hostility) through mind-body interventions such as deep-breathing exercises, biofeedback, meditation, yoga or tai chi or gi gong, guided imagery, progressive muscle relaxation, hypnotherapy
- With elevated C-reactive protein levels, evaluation for infectious etiology with antibiotics as appropriate
- Reduction in insulin levels and insulin resistance (see earlier)
- Reversal or prevention of central adiposity
- Attainment/maintenance of ideal body weight and composition
- Statin medication to optimize lipid profile and decrease C-reactive protein (CRP) levels

Laboratory Tests to Consider:

Cardiovascular protection factors: apolipoprotein A_1, HDL cholesterol, heart rate variability
Cardiovascular risk factors: apolipoprotein B, total cholesterol, low-density lipoprotein (LDL) cholesterol, lipoprotein(a), triglycerides, high-sensitivity CRP, and homocystine.

Improvement of Detoxification Capacity

- Intake of eight 8-oz glasses of water daily
- Elimination or rotation diet to reduce food allergies
- Removal of known pathogens and toxic exposures
- Use of high-energy particulate air (HEPA) filter to reduce environmental allergens
- Inclusion in the diet of 8 to 10 servings of fruits and vegetables daily, especially cruciferous vegetables with phytonutrients (e.g., sulforaphrane in broccoli) and carotenes to support phase II detoxification
- Antioxidants from vegetables and herbs—flavones, flavonones, flavonols, anthocyanidins, and proanthocyanidins—and *Ginkgo biloba*
- Reduction of animal protein in the diet
- Use of prescription medications (especially antibiotics) only when necessary to maintain a healthy cytochrome P450 system
- Replacement of digestive enzymes
- Re-innoculate with beneficial gut flora and probiotics such as lactobacilli and bifidibacteria (see Chapter 97, Prescribing Probiotics)
- Limiting encounters with "toxic" persons and ending "toxic" relationships
- Reinforcement of childlike qualities in experience of life, such as humor, inquisitiveness, exploration, spontaneity, optimism, playfulness (anthropologists use the term *neotony* to describe elders in various cultures who age successfully and express these qualities)
- Daily tooth flossing and use of coenzyme Q10 in chewing gum or supplement to promote gingival health
- Cessation of smoking and use of all tobacco products
- Consumption of no more than 1 (women) or 2 (men) servings of alcoholic beverages daily in persons with normal results of liver function tests
- Regular exercise to improve detoxification ability of liver
- Limiting harmful estrogenic exposures from pesticides, toxins, certain medications (including conjugated estrogens [Premarin] in women)

Laboratory Tests to Consider:

Liver function tests
Blood urea nitrogen/serum creatinine
Comprehensive digestive stool analysis (CDSA)

Enhancement of Immune Function

- Elimination of food and environmental allergies whenever possible
- Use of prescription medications only when necessary
- As indicated, use of certain supplements such as extra vitamin C, astragalus, echinacea, spirulina,

garlic, and St. John's wort, which act as immune modulators
- Routine physical activity to increase natural killer cell activity
- Diverse dietary intake of fruits and vegetables with minimal animal protein
- Elimination from the diet of all foods containing artificial colors and flavorings
- Complete avoidance of tobacco products

Laboratory Tests to Consider:

- SIgA
- Helper T cell/suppressor T cell ratio
- Natural killer cell activity
- IgG
- Interleukin-2

Control of Stress and Prevention of Chronic Stress Response

- Stress reduction practices for 20 minutes twice a day (see Chapter 91, Prescribing Relaxation Techniques)
- Other relaxation interventions such as yoga, meditation, deep breathing, and progressive muscle relaxation
- At least 8 hours of sleep every 24 hours
- Enjoyment of living with meaning and purpose
- Maintenance of optimistic attitude and positive outlook
- Celebration of successes, with acceptance of lessons learned from failures
- Connection with inner spiritual direction and purpose

Laboratory Tests to Consider:

Serum or salivary cortisol and dehydroxyepiandrosterone (DHEA) levels
Insulin and glucose levels

Rebalance of Age-Related Hormones and Minimization of Fluctuations

- Physical activity, especially weight-bearing and resistance exercises to maintain lean muscle mass and bone density
- Acupressure, acupuncture, and various massage therapies to help maintain sex hormone levels
- Low-glycemic-index diet to reduce insulin elevations (see Chapter 83, The Glycemic Index)
- Reduction of stress to decrease high cortisol levels
- Treatment of hypothyroidism with levothyroxine or natural thyroid hormone

- Cautious approach to supplementation with human growth hormone until further studies on safety and efficacy are available
- Evaluation of role of individualized natural hormone replacement (estradiol, progesterone, testosterone, DHEA) from compounded highly concentrated phytoestrogen sources such as soy (see Chapter 44, Menopause)

Laboratory Tests to Consider:

- Sex hormones: estradiol, progesterone, testosterone
- Thyroid hormones: triiodothyronine (T_3), thyroxine (T_4)
- Pituitary hormones: (IGF-1), thyroid-stimulating hormone (TSH)
- Pancreatic hormone: insulin
- Adrenal hormones: DHEA sulfate, cortisol
- Pineal gland hormone: melatonin

Maintenance of Regular Physical and Mental Activity

- "Blended" physical activity for 30 minutes every day: with weight-bearing activity plus resistance exercise training (using a weight that produces muscle fatigue after 10 to 13 repetitions) every other day (see NIA web site for exercise recommendations)
- "Cross-training" of cognitive performance skills through dual hemispheric activity (e.g., learning artistic and musical skills in persons with mostly left-brain daily activity)
- Key interventions to maintain mental or cognitive vitality: lifelong learning, exercise, routine daily activities, stress reduction, averaging 8 hours of sleep nightly, maintenance of emotional stability, and adequate nutritional intake of B vitamins to reduce homocysteine
- Statins to decrease the risk of developing both vascular dementia and Alzheimer's disease
- Adequate protein intake for building muscle mass
- Adequate testosterone levels and reversal of causes of premature male andropause and poorly controlled female menopause, for maintenance of lean muscle mass and prevention of sarcopenia (in most patients)

Laboratory Tests to Consider:

- Body composition assay (percent body fat and lean muscle tissue)
- DexaScan to measure bone density

PREVENTION PRESCRIPTION

- *Daily stress reduction practices*
- *Daily physical activity*
- *8 to 10 servings of fruits and vegetables daily*
- *64 ounces of water daily*
- *3 servings of cold water fish weekly*
- *10 servings of cooked tomatoes weekly*
- *Reinforcement of childlike experience of life*
- *At least 8 hours of sleep every day*
- *Appropriate dental hygiene program, with daily tooth flossing*
- *Use of baby aspirin if tolerated*
- *No tobacco products*
- *Consumption of no more than 1 serving (in women) or 2 servings (in men) of alcoholic beverages daily*
- *Continued social connection with family and friends of different generations*
- *Meaningful communication with family and friends, especially sharing wisdom with young people*
- *Celebration of successes in life*
- *Maintenance of optimism and positive outlook*
- *Routine cancer and cardiovascular disease screening*
- *Supplementation with B vitamins and antioxidants*
- *Conscious enjoyment of living with meaning and purpose*
- *Maintenance of physical, mental, emotional, and spiritual balance with a relatively stable and disciplined daily regimen*

NOTE

Functional decline is inevitable but can be slowed down. Lifelong physical activity and moderately high-quality caloric monitoring are two lifestyle measures most likely to extend the "health span."

Resources

www.aging.arizona.edu

www.intellihealth.com

www.nih.gov/nia/health/pubs/nasa-exercise/intro

Kligman EW, Hewitt MJ, Crowell DL: Recommending exercise to healthy older adults: The preparticipation evaluation and exercise prescription. Physician Sports Med 27:42–62, 1999.

Bland JS: Genetic Nutritioneering. Lincolnwood, Ill, Keats Publishing, 1980.

Bland JS: The 20-Day Rejuvenation Diet Program. Lincolnwood, Ill, Keats Publishing, 1990.

Sapolsky R: Why Zebras Don't Get Ulcers. New York, WH Freeman, 1998.

Functional Medicine Update web site: www.fxmed.com

Rowe JW, Kahn RL: Successful Aging. New York, Pantheon Books, 1998.

www.realage.com

www.med.harvard.edu/programs/necs/ (New England Centenarian Study)

References

1. Cassel CK: Successful aging: How increased life expectancy and medical advances are changing geriatric care. Geriatrics, 56:35–39, 2001.
2. Kirkwood TB, Austad SN: Why do we age? Nature 408:233–238, 2000.
3. The aging factor in health and disease: The promise of basic research on aging. Workshop report International Longevity Center–USA, Ltd, February 1999.
4. Brody JA, Schneider EL: Diseases and disorders of aging: An hypothesis. J Chron Dis 39:871–876, 1986.
5. McEwen B: www.macses.ucsf.edu/Research/wgal.htm
6. Biomarkers of aging: From primitive organisms to man. Workshop report. International Longevity Center–USA, Ltd. October 2000. Available online at www.ikusa.org.
7. Evans W, Rosenberg IH: Biomarkers: The 10 Keys to Prolonged Vitality. New York, Fireside, 1991.
8. The aging body. Merck Manual 2001. Section 1: Fundamentals. Available at www.merck.com.
9. Kane R, et al: Essentials of Clinical Geriatrics, 3rd ed. New York, McGraw-Hill, 1994.
10. Bland JS: The use of complementary medicine for healthy aging. Altern Ther Health Med 4:42–48, 1998.
11. Schwarzbein D: The Schwarzbein Principle.
12. National Center for Health Statistics.
13. Hazzard W, et al: Principles of Geriatric Medicine and Gerontology, 2nd ed. New York, McGraw-Hill, 1990.
14. Kligman EW: Preventive geriatrics. Geriatrics 47:39–50, 1992.
15. Goodwin JS: Geriatrics and the limits of modern medicine. N Engl J Med 340:1283–1285, 1999.
16. Ballentine R: Radical Healing. New York, Harmony Books, 1999.

PART IV

Tools for Your Practice

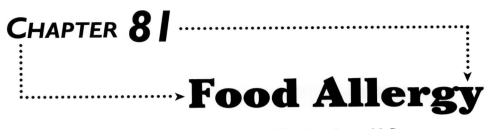

CHAPTER 81

Food Allergy

Bill Manahan, M.D.

Writing a chapter on food allergy is a labor of love for me. During the course of my active family practice, I became increasingly intrigued by the fact that many of my patients' problems and diseases have responded to simple dietary solutions. Often, I have found that merely eliminating a single food from the diet has alleviated a symptom or cured a disease that had been troubling the patient for months or even years.

For example, I was immensely gratified when I convinced a man who had experienced years of intermittent headaches to try eliminating coffee for 2 weeks. After he followed this advice his headaches disappeared. Another patient was both angry and happy when he discovered that the three glasses of milk he was drinking each day to help his heartburn and indigestion were actually making it worse. His heartburn and abdominal pains went away completely following a 2-week dairy elimination diet. He was angry because he had never been told that milk increases acid output in the stomach and may actually be harmful to some people with gastritis.

Over the past three to four decades, more and more information has been provided in the medical literature regarding food allergy. In fact, a recent look at the National Library of Medicine's *PubMed* Web site revealed 6671 articles on food allergy. Despite this enormous volume of literature about food allergy, present-day medical students and residents receive no more training about it than I did in the 1960s. Physicians have generally remained somewhat uninterested and uninformed about food allergy for reasons that I do not understand. I do know that the majority of patients are interested in the subject. Many realize that accurate nutritional knowledge can help them eliminate serious, painful, and debilitating health problems. I have found that people outside the medical establishment are "hungry" for nutritional information and an understanding of its relationship to disease. My hope is that after reading this chapter, clinicians will develop an appreciation for the role that hidden food allergies can play in the health and disease of many of their patients.

WHAT IS FOOD ALLERGY?

Allergy can be defined as an adverse response to a substance that does not cause an adverse response in most people. It is the exaggerated reactivity of a living organism to a foreign substance which sometimes occurs after exposure to the substance. *Food allergy is an altered or different reaction to substances ingested.* Part of the disagreement about food allergy comes from the belief of many in the medical system that the term *allergy* should be limited and applied only to those conditions in which an immunologic mechanism can be demonstrated. A patient who develops hives and laryngeal edema after eating peanuts is almost certainly manifesting an immunoglobulin E (IgE) response.

Immunologic mechanisms are extremely important in the explanation of allergic diseases, but they do not tell the entire story. Some people have an inability to assimilate and use specific foods in a normal manner which is often not IgE mediated. Lactose (milk), alcohol, and caffeine are three foods that can cause some individuals to have adverse reactions not mediated by IgE.

Even though the terms *intolerance* and *allergy* are not technically identical, in this chapter the term *food allergy* is used as the overall term meaning "all types of adverse reactions or responses to food," whether reactions are immune mediated or not.

NOTE

Many adverse food reactions should, be more appropriately labeled food intolerance or sensitivity, rather than food allergy.

THE IMPORTANCE OF FOOD ALLERGY TO CLINICIANS

The type of food allergy with which most clinicians are familiar is the immediate, food-induced anaphylaxis also known as acute or overt food allergy. This type of allergy is mediated by IgE antibodies and usually causes a reaction soon after the incriminating food is ingested. Actual fatalities from food-induced anaphylaxis tend to occur in atopic people with multiple prior anaphylactic episodes. *JAMA* has published an interesting article on seven deaths from food anaphylaxis; four deaths were caused by peanuts, one by pecans, one by crab, and one by cod.[1]

The other type of food allergy discussed in this chapter has been the subject of medical controversy for many decades. This type of allergy is referred to as delayed, hidden, masked, cyclic, or covert food allergy, and it tends to occur over hours to days rather than minutes to hours. It frequently is not immune mediated, so laboratory testing ranges from difficult to impossible. The symptoms are often chronic and low grade in nature, making diagnosis by history difficult.

It has taken medical science many years to discover that caffeine can be a trigger for headaches, that alcohol can cause fetal alcohol syndrome, that milk can cause multiple gastrointestinal symptoms, and that tobacco can cause lung cancer. Although these problems are not IgE mediated, they are adverse responses to an ingested substance (a food). Likewise, proponents of the food allergy and disease connection contend that multiple food allergies are often overlooked, and that multiple chronic symptoms and disorders may have a significant food allergy component.

NOTE

Many medical practitioners have observed that these delayed food allergies are a common cause of a wide range of physical, mental, and behavioral diseases and problems.

CLINICAL TOOLS FOR FINDING HIDDEN FOOD ALLERGIES

Detailed history taking is the most important ingredient in finding hidden food allergies. Pertinent historical information includes whether the patient has a history of atopic problems; hay fever; childhood allergy; colic as an infant; recurrent ear, throat, sinus, or lung problems; an excessive number of colds or respiratory problems; unusual reactions to prescribed medications; numerous gastrointestinal complaints; easy fluctuation of body weight; or a family history of allergies.

Four key questions should be asked of patients when one is searching for possible food allergies (Table 81–1). Caffeine can be used as a good example of why these four questions are important in detecting food allergy. Clinicians are aware that caffeine

Table 81–1. Key Questions to Ask Patients Who May Have Food Allergies
....

1. What foods do you frequently eat?
2. What foods do you crave?
3. What foods make you feel better?
4. What foods would be difficult for you give up or go without?

can at times cause or trigger a wide variety of symptoms such as anxiety, diarrhea, fatigue, headaches, heartburn, heart palpitations, hyperlipidemia, insomnia, restlessness, tachycardia, tinnitus, and tremors. In other words, caffeine is an example of a food that can cause adverse reactions in some of the people who consume it. Yet caffeine rarely causes IgE-mediated illness, so it is a good example of what I am describing as hidden food allergy.

Regarding caffeine consumption, what happens if we ask the four questions listed in Table 81–1? It is easy to see that some individuals take caffeine frequently and often crave it; caffeine helps these people to feel better, and it is difficult for many of them to completely stop consuming it. This illustrates how the relationship between ingestion of certain foods and the development of symptoms is often complicated by the tendency of people to become addicted to the foods to which they are allergic. This is called the *allergy-addiction syndrome* and appears to be consistent with Selye's[2] description of the general adaptation response to stress. Patients often experience short-term relief after ingesting foods that are later demonstrated to be the cause of their chronic symptoms. For example, after the patient drinks a cup of coffee, the headache or fatigue may disappear for a while.

There are multiple foods similar to caffeine that may cause many people to react in the manner just described. Many foods that cause delayed allergy problems are the ones most commonly consumed (Table 81–2). There are, of course, other foods besides these that cause problems in some people.

FACTORS PROMOTING FOOD ALLERGY

A number of factors appear to trigger or increase the incidence of delayed food allergy. It is not uncommon in my practice for a patient to tell me that he or she consumes more than a quart of milk each day, cheese at least six times a week, ice cream three times a week, and occasionally yogurt. It is not surprising that after many years of a large amount of dairy intake, that person may develop some medical and health problems related to dairy products.

Table 81–2. Foods That Are the Most Common Causes of Delayed Allergy Problems
....

Milk and milk products
Wheat and corn (corn syrup is found is many sugar products)
Chocolate and caffeine
Eggs, citrus, soy, and beef
Refined sugar
Food colorings and food chemicals such as citric acid (found in most sweets, soft drinks, fruit juices, tomatoes, and potatoes) and aspartic acid (found in the artificial sweetener aspartame)

NOTE

The most significant trigger of food allergy is excessive and prolonged consumption of a particular food.

Another common trigger of food allergy is physical or emotional stress. Following a bad viral infection, a significant injury, a divorce, or the loss of a job, it is not uncommon for people to develop food intolerances that did not previously exist. The opposite also is true. While on vacation, people can occasionally enjoy foods that previously caused them some sort of distress.

Other food allergy triggers include malnutrition (such as occurs in anorexia or alcoholism), altitude variations, seasonal changes, and menstrual periods.

DIAGNOSTIC TESTS FOR FOOD ALLERGY

The usual way to identify food allergies is by recording the history (as was mentioned earlier) and initiating an elimination diet followed by individual food challenges. Double-blind, placebo-controlled challenges are preferable, but these usually are not feasible in the typical outpatient setting. Therefore, open challenges are usually used. The elimination diet involves not eating for 10 to 14 days the foods that by history (1) are eaten frequently, (2) craved, (3) make the patient feel better, and (4) are difficult for the patient to stop eating. On day 11 or 15, the patient begins to reintroduce into the diet every 2 or 3 days one of the foods that had been eliminated. The patient pays careful attention to how she or he feels during the 24 hours after beginning an elimination food. More detailed information is presented in an extensive discussion of elimination diets and food challenges (see Chapter 82).

I encourage readers to take their own food history; if a few foods produce "yes" answers to three or four questions listed in Table 81–1, try an elimination diet. Remember that some of the common foods to which many people have adverse reactions include milk and milk products, wheat, corn, refined sugar, chocolate, caffeine, eggs, citrus, soy, beef, food colorings, and food chemicals.

Several blood tests are available that measure antibodies to individual food extracts. Measuring IgE antibody levels may be helpful for identifying classical food allergy reactions, but these measurements do not appear to be reliable indicators of hidden or delayed food allergy problems. An IgG enzyme-linked immunosorbent assay (ELISA) test is available that measures food-specific IgG4 antibodies. Symptom-provoking antibodies are included within the IgG4 fraction, which also appears to con-

tain blocking antibodies that may prevent allergic reactions. Consequently, the theoretical basis for measuring IgG4 antibodies is open to question.[3]

Another blood test known as ALCAT (www.alcat.com) has been shown to be fairly reliable for identifying reactions to food additives, but it has not been accurate in testing for other food allergies. Provocative food testing involves intradermal or sublingual administration of various dilutions of food extracts. The efficacy of food extract injection therapy has been demonstrated in a double-blind study,[4] but other studies have failed to show a beneficial effect.[5] Provocative food testing remains a controversial technique.

In conclusion, regarding diagnostic tests for hidden or delayed food allergy, laboratory testing remains somewhat unproven and controversial.

NOTE

The gold standard of food sensitivity testing at this time remains the food elimination diet and rechallenge.

SCIENTIFIC BASIS OF DISEASE CAUSED BY FOOD ALLERGY

As was mentioned earlier, almost 7000 articles and research papers on food allergy can be explored in the National Library of Medicine's *PubMed* Web site. Some of these studies are excellent, some are average quality, and some are not worth reading. In the following sections, I review a few of the studies (involving four different diseases) as examples of available literature regarding the relationship between food allergy and disease.

Recurrent Serous Otitis Media

Recurrent serous otitis media (SOM) in children is one of the frustrating problems with which family physicians and pediatricians commonly contend. Once physicians begin to use food elimination diets in children with recurrent otitis, they frequently find that the number of children needing long-term antibiotics or ear tubes decreases dramatically.

A number of studies have explored this problem; I mention only one of them here. The purpose of this study was to examine the prevalence of food allergy among children with recurrent SOM. A total of 104 children ages 1 to 9 with recurrent SOM were evaluated for food allergy by means of skin-prick testing, IgE testing, and food challenge. Those found to be allergic to food(s) underwent an elimination diet of the specific offending food(s) for a period of 16 weeks. The middle ear effusion was monitored and assessed by tympanometry. Of the 104 children, 81 had a significant statistical association between food allergy and SOM. The elimination diet led to a significant amelioration of SOM in 70 of 81 (86%) patients as assessed by clinical evaluation and tympanometry. The children were then placed back on the offending food(s) which provoked a recurrence of SOM in 66 of 70 patients (94%). The conclusion was that food allergy should be considered as a possible cause in all children with recurrent serous otitis media. For those interested in recurrent SOM, this article provides 31 other references for the reader to investigate.[6]

Migraine Headache

As early as 1930, food allergy was reported in the medical literature as a cause of migraine headache.[7] In a study of 55 migraine patients, avoidance of allergenic foods resulted in complete or nearly complete freedom from symptoms in 29 patients (53%) and partial improvement in 21 (38%), for a total of 91% of patients helped by this intervention. In another study published in 1935, 66% of 127 migraine patients experienced partial or complete relief of symptoms after following an elimination diet.[8]

Evidence suggests that perhaps 40% of migraine headaches are food induced.[9] Even this estimate may be too conservative, according to a study in *Lancet* which found that 93% of a group of 88 children with severe migraines responded to a food elimination diet. Note the intriguing title of the article—"Is Migraine Food Allergy?"[10]

Clinicians have been aware for many years that certain chemicals and food substances can trigger migraines in susceptible individuals (Table 81–3). What often is not appreciated is the number of commonly ingested foods that can trigger migraine headaches. For instance, in a blinded aspartame study, Koehler and Glaros found that the overall number of migraines increased from 1.55 in patients on placebo to a mean of 3.55 during the aspartame phase—a change of more than 100%. One of America's most commonly ingested liquids—diet soft drinks—may be causing some people significant headaches.[11]

Table 81–3. Food Chemicals and Foods That May Trigger Migraine Headaches

Tyramine	Found in aged cheeses and certain red wines
Phenylethylamine	Found in chocolate and some cheeses
Histamine	Found in fish, cheese, wine, and beer
Nitrates	Found in preserved meats such as hot dogs, bacon, and pepperoni
Monosodium glutamate	Naturally present in mushrooms, kelp, and scallops; found frequently in preserved meats, and often used for cooking Chinese food
Foods	Wheat, oranges, eggs, chocolate, caffeine, milk, and beef

Other foods that may trigger headaches include wheat, orange, eggs, chocolate, coffee, milk, and beef. In a study of 60 patients with migraines over 20 years, a food elimination diet resulted in improvement in all 60 patients, whereas 85% of them became headache free. The aggregate number of headaches in the group fell from 402 per months to 6 per month. Some of the common offenders were wheat (78%), oranges (65%), eggs (45%), coffee and chocolate (40%), milk (37%), and beef (35%).[12] The most difficult aspect of identifying the food(s) causing the headaches is that there are frequently numerous offenders. This study found that the mean number of offending foods was 10 per patient, with a range from 1 to 30 foods. It is evident that patient compliance regarding diet is most important.

Irritable Bowel Syndrome

Irritable bowel syndrome (IBS) is an example of a medical problem that conventional doctors struggle to treat, whereas alternative practitioners often enjoy a fair amount of success. Although the psychosocial influences on IBS are fairly well documented and not really controversial,[13] there remains debate as to the degree that food allergy plays a part in this disease. In my practice, I use a combination of mind-body interventions (such as meditation, counseling, biofeedback, hypnotherapy, or affirmations) plus food elimination diets to treat irritable bowel syndrome.

In a 1989 study, 189 patients with IBS were placed for three weeks on an elimination diet consisting of 10 foods, and 91 improved (48%).[14] The number of food intolerances ranged from 1 to 19 per person, with half of the patients reacting to 2 to 5 foods. The foods that most commonly caused problems were dairy products (41%), onions (35%), wheat (30%), chocolate and coffee (25%), and eggs (23%). Of the 91 patients who improved, 73 of them continued to avoid the foods that caused them problems, and 72 of them (98.6%) remained well for longer than one year. Of the 98 patients who did not improve with food elimination, only 3 of them were well at 15-month follow-up. My clinical experience matches that of the study in that about one half of the IBS patients seem to have a food allergy component as a cause of their symptoms.

Another study actually undertook double-blind food challenges in some patients with IBS.[15] Specific foods were found to provoke IBS symptoms in 14 of 21 patients (67%). Elimination of the offending foods caused the IBS symptoms to disappear. In the six patients who were challenged by double-blind testing, intolerance to certain foods was confirmed. Offending foods in descending order of frequency included wheat, corn, dairy products, coffee, tea, and citrus.

The conclusion of the authors of another study was that dramatic clinical improvement can result from the introduction of an adequate exclusion diet.[16] Using an elimination diet with blind provocation, they found that in 14 of 24 IBS patients, one or several foods were shown to induce the typical symptoms of IBS. Interestingly, in nine of the cases (all atopic individuals), an IgE-mediated mechanism could be incriminated.

It makes sense that for some patients with bowel problems, what is deposited in the gastrointestinal tract through the foods they eat makes a difference in how they feel. I encourage clinicians to try an elimination diet for patients with irritable bowel syndrome.

Rheumatoid Arthritis

The evidence is substantial that food intolerance affects some types of arthritis. I have found about 50 studies investigating the association between food allergy and rheumatoid arthritis (RA). The majority of these studies reveal a positive relationship of arthritis to diet, with improvement in arthritic symptoms when food elimination was attempted. Yet until recently, most medical authorities continued to deny that there was any connection between arthritis and food. In one study, 27 rheumatoid arthritis patients underwent a partial fast followed by individual food challenges.[17] A control group of RA patients ate an ordinary diet. After four weeks, the diet group showed a significant improvement in eight measured parameters such as grip strength sedimentation rate, and pain score. Only pain scores improved in the control group. The author's conclusion was that a diet omitting symptom-provoking foods is of value in the treatment of RA.

Darlington reported two controlled studies in which dietary manipulation was shown to be of real value in the control of RA over a prolonged period. The conclusion of one blinded, placebo-controlled study on dietary manipulation therapy in patients with RA was that there was "significant objective improvement during periods of dietary therapy compared with the periods of placebo treatment."[18] In a second study, Darlington treated 70 RA patients by identifying and eliminating symptom-provoking foods.[19] Of these 70 patients, 19% remained well and required no medication during follow-up periods ranging from 1 to 5 years.

Of the 24 studies I reviewed in which a relationship between food and arthritis was explored, only two resulted in no improvement. Even one of the statistically negative studies concluded that 2 of the 26 patients completing the study "improved notably on the experimental diet, continued to improve, and noted exacerbations of disease upon consuming certain foods."[20] The authors of that study concluded that their data "were not inconsistent with the possibility that individualized dietary manipulations might be beneficial for selected patients with rheumatic disease."

It is clear that certain foods affect some people who suffer with inflammatory arthritis. Clinicians must work with patients to discover who might benefit from dietary manipulation.

SUMMARY

There is a large body of medical literature indicating that hidden food allergy is a frequent and important cause of (or triggering factor for) multiple physical and mental diseases. Some other diseases not mentioned that have been responsive to food elimination diets are asthma, aphthous ulcers, atopic dermatitis, attention deficit/hyperactivity disorder, chronic respiratory system problems, enuresis, fatigue, inflammatory bowel disease, psoriasis, rhinitis, and urticaria.

The range of patient problems helped by the elimination of certain foods is impressive. The routine use of a good dietary history and an elimination diet in clinical practice can markedly improve the response rate of many patient problems that appear difficult to treat. Hidden food allergy is a hidden bit of information that, when brought to light, can improve the lives of many of our patients.

References

1. Yunginger JW, Sweeney KG, Sturmer WQ, et al: Fatal food-induced anaphylaxis. JAMA 260:1450–1452, 1988.
2. Selye H: Stress Without Distress. New York, JB Lippincott, 1974.
3. Gaby AR: The role of hidden food allergy/intolerance in chronic disease. Altern Med Rev 3:90–100, 1998.
4. Miller JB: A double-blind study of food extract injection therapy: A preliminary report. Ann Allergy 38:185–191, 1977.
5. Lehman CW: A double-blind study of sublingual provocative food testing: A study of its efficacy. Ann Allergy 45:144–149, 1980.
6. Nsouli TM, Nsouli SM, Linde RE, et al: Role of food allergy in serous otitis media. Ann Allergy 73:215–219, 1994.
7. Balyeat RM, Brittain FL: Allergic migraine. Am J Med Sci 80:212–221, 1930.
8. Sheldon JM, Randolph TG: Allergy in migraine-like headaches. Am J Med Sci 190:232–236, 1935.
9. Mansfield LE: Food allergy and migraine: Whom to evaluate and how to treat. Postgrad Med 83:46–55, 1988.
10. Egger J, Wilson J, Carter CM, et al: Is migraine food allergy? A double-blind controlled trial of oligoantigenic diet treatment. Lancet 2:865–869, 1983.
11. Koehler SM, Glaros A: The effect of aspartame on migraine headache. Headache 28:10–14, 1988.
12. Grant ECG: Food allergies and migraine. Lancet 1:966–968, 1979.
13. Whorwell P: Use of hypnotherapy in gastrointestinal disease. Br J Hosp Med 45:27–29, 1991.
14. Nanda R, James R, Smith H, et al: Food intolerance and the irritable bowel syndrome. Gut 30:1099–1104, 1989.
15. Jones VA, McLaughlan P, Shorthouse M, et al: Food intolerance: A major factor in the pathogenesis of irritable bowel syndrome. Lancet 2:1115–1117, 1982.
16. Petitpierre M, Gumowski P, Girard JP: Irritable bowel syndrome and hypersensitivity to food. Ann Allergy 54:538–540, 1985.
17. Kjeldsen-Kragh J, Haugen M, Borchgrevink CF, et al: Controlled trial of fasting and one-year vegetarian diet in rheumatoid arthritis. Lancet 338:899–902, 1991

18. Darlington LG, Ramsey NW, Mansfield JR: Placebo-controlled, blind study of dietary manipulation therapy in rheumatoid arthritis. Lancet 1:236–238, 1986.

19. Darlington LG, Dietary therapy for arthritis. Rheum Dis Clin North Am 17:273–285, 1991.

20. Panush RS, Carter RL, Katz P, et al: Diet therapy for rheumatoid arthritis. Arthritis Rheum 4:462–470, 1983.

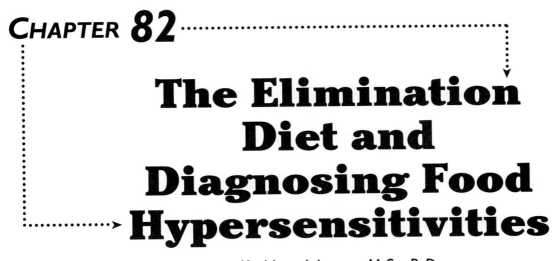

The Elimination Diet and Diagnosing Food Hypersensitivities

Kathleen Johnson, M.S., R.D.

Food hypersensitivities or allergies and food intolerances are being considered in managing a variety of symptoms from headaches to atopic dermatitis to autoimmune disorders.[1–3] An elimination diet has been traditionally considered a treatment strategy for food hypersensitivities, but it can also be successfully used as a diagnostic strategy.[4–6] Whereas there are laboratory tests that are of some usefulness in diagnosing food hypersensitivities or allergies, the "gold standard" is still considered to be the elimination/challenge diet. Different approaches to elimination diets as diagnostic strategy have been described. This chapter briefly describes those approaches and discusses some of the considerations important to the diet's success.

WHAT IS FOOD ALLERGY?

A food allergy involves an immune-mediated response to some component of food.[7]

The term *food allergy* has become controversial and is no doubt overused by the general public. Allergists confine the use of the term to people who have a true immunoglobulin E (IgE)–mediated reaction to food, including anaphylaxis. Examples include reactions to peanuts, walnuts, or shellfish. Allergists prefer to use the term *food hypersensitivity* to describe the various immune-mediated reactions including the classic IgE response. Reactions that do not involve the immune system have also been described. These are called *food intolerances*.

VARIOUS TYPES OF FOOD HYPERSENSITIVITIES AND INTOLERANCES

Several types of food hypersensitivities are recognized. They include those mediated by IgE antibodies, those mediated by IgA, IgG, or IgM antibodies, and those that do not involve antibodies at all.[4] Regardless of the mechanism involved in the reaction, an elimination diet strategy is helpful in diagnosing the specific foods involved.

IgE antibodies are produced by B cell lymphocytes. An IgE reaction involves mast cell degranulation leading to atopic symptoms such as wheezing, urticaria, angioedema, pruritus, rhinitis, bronchospasm, tachycardia, gastrointestinal symptoms, and anaphylaxis. The hypersensitivity is initiated by an asymptomatic initial exposure to the antigen, followed by subsequent symptomatic exposures. Reactions are usually immediate, occurring within a few minutes to hours. These are considered the classic allergic reactions.

Non–IgE-mediated reactions to foods may involve IgA, IgG, or IgM antibodies. These reactions typically involve T cell lymphocytes. Although the antibodies can be measured in serum, there is still controversy about whether or not they are associated with clinically significant symptoms. This type of reaction triggers an inflammatory response through the complement cascade and the formation of antigen-antibody complexes. Immediate or delayed reactions (up to 3 days after exposure) may be seen. Antibody levels are thought to be related to extent of exposure. The symptoms believed to be associated with this type of reaction are varied and range from typical atopic symptoms to more systemic ones.

Food intolerances are adverse reactions to foods or components of foods that are not immune mediated. The symptoms are diverse and the mechanisms responsible are not well understood. Intolerances include reactions to substances, such as salicylates or nitrates, and problems like lactose intolerance.

Table 82–1. Problems Associated with Food Hypersensitivity

General
  Anaphylactic shock
  Vasculitis
Skin
  Atopic dermatitis
  Urticaria
  Angioedema
  Pruritus
  Dermatitis herpeteformis
  Contact dermatitis
Respiratory Tract
  Asthma
  Allergic or perennial rhinitis
  Rhinorrhea
  Conjunctivitis
  Serous otitis media
  Laryngeal edema
  Heiner's syndrome
Digestive Tract
  Nausea
  Vomiting
  Diarrhoea
  Constipation
  Abdominal bloating
  Abdominal pain and cramping
  Reflux
  Indigestion
  Colitis
  Infantile colic
  Belching

Nervous System
  Migraine
  Other headache
  Hyperactivity
  Listlessness
  Lack of concentration
  Tension fatigue syndrome
  Irritability
  Chilliness
  Dizziness
Other
  Urinary frequency
  Bed wetting
  Hoarseness
  Muscle aches
  Low-grade fever
  Excessive sweating
  Pallor
  Dark circles around the eyes ("allergic shiners")

> ### NOTE
>
> *The main goal in food hypersensitivity is identifying offending foods and managing symptoms by reducing or eliminating exposure to the foods. The specific type of reaction is not as important as identifying the foods involved. Elimination diets are useful in diagnosing all the various types of food hypersensitivities and intolerances.*

Problems That May be Associated with Food Hypersensitivity or Intolerance

Table 82–1 shows the many problems that have either been documented to be associated with food hypersensitivity or intolerance or been suspected to be.

Table 82–2. Foods that Account for Hypersensitivity Reactions

Eggs	Milk and dairy products
Wheat	Other gluten-containing grains (oats, rye, barley)
Citrus	Soy
Peanuts	Tree nuts (walnuts, pecans, almonds)
Shellfish	Fish

Most Common Food Allergens

The foods implicated in hypersensitivity reactions vary tremendously from individual to individual. Nonetheless, a few foods are implicated more than others. Table 82–2 shows the foods that account for at least 80% of food hypersensitivity reactions.[2]

Substances Involved in Food Intolerance

The substances noted in Table 82–3, which either occur naturally in food or are used as additives, have been implicated in symptoms of food intolerance.[4]

Table 82–3. Substances Implicated in Food Intolerance

Lactose
Biogenic amines (histamine, tyramine)
Other disaccharides
Preservatives (benzoates, BHA, BHT, sulfites)
Artificial colors, especially tartrazine
Salicylates
Monosodium glutamate and other artificial flavors
Nitrates

BHA, butylated hydroxyanisole; BHT, butylated hydroxytoluene.

Table 82–4. Factors Associated with Hypersensitivity
....

Family history of allergic reactions
Frequency of exposure
Other allergic reactions (e.g., inhalant allergies)
Increased intestinal permeability to allergens ("leaky gut")
Vigorous exercise
Concurrent consumption of alcohol
Hormone levels
Stress

Factors Associated with Food Hypersensitivities

Certain factors seem to increase the likelihood of food hypersensitivities in individuals who are genetically predisposed (Table 82–4).[4]

THE ELIMINATION DIET

An elimination diet is largely a diagnostic tool to identify specific foods involved in hypersensitivity or intolerance reactions. The entire process involves an initial dietary history, the elimination phase, the challenge phase, and the development of a final diet. Several different approaches to an elimination diet have been utilized, with variations found in each step.

Steps in the Elimination Diet Protocol

Assessment

The process is most effective when it begins with a comprehensive medical and dietary history. This should focus on both symptoms and diet. First, collect information about frequency of symptoms thought to be associated with food hypersensitivity or intolerance. Then ask key questions regarding food frequency and cravings (Table 82–5). Finally, have the patient keep a diary that includes a systematic recording of foods consumed and symptoms experienced on those days. Critical in this first step is listening to the patient. Often, she or he has suspicions about the foods that trigger the symptoms. The information is used to make decisions about the likelihood of a relationship between symptoms and specific foods and to plan the second step, the elimination diet. This first step will allow the clinician to individualize the whole process.

Table 82–5. Key Questions to Ask Patients Who May Have Food Allergies
....

What foods do you frequently eat?
What foods do you crave?
What foods make you feel better?
What foods would be difficult to give up or go without?

Elimination

The second step in the process is the elimination diet itself, followed carefully for 2 to 4 weeks. The extent of foods eliminated is based on the information gathered in the first step and any food allergy tests that have been done. Allergy tests cannot be considered conclusive, but they can inform the decision about which foods to eliminate. The options for the range of foods to elimination include:

- One food only. If only one food is suspected or if eliminating many foods is too difficult for a patient, this approach can be used.
- Few foods. The most common approach is to eliminate all or some of the most common allergens (see Table 82–2). The most commonly eliminated foods in that list include milk and other dairy products and wheat and other gluten-containing grains. Another constellation of foods may be chosen, however, if the history indicates. This is the approach used most often by clinicians today.
- Many foods. An approach used in the past was to eliminate all foods commonly eaten by the patient, substituting foods never eaten. Another approach in a Scandinavian study on rheumatoid arthritis used essentially a fast with the patients consuming only vegetable tea. Some practitioners use an oligoantigenic food supplement to provide calories, protein, and other nutrients during this step. Eliminating many foods has the best chance of eliminating the allergens but may be the most difficult to follow. The help of a registered dietitian or nutritionist may be useful in this phase to help plan a diet that provides adequate nutrition, variety, and other needs of the patient.

Challenge

The next step in the process is the challenge phase. Some allergists believe that the only valid protocol is a double-blind, placebo-controlled food challenge using food or placebo in gelatin capsules with a clinician closely monitoring reactions. The main drawback to this approach is that the small amount of food in several capsules may not be enough to elicit symptoms and that a variety of other factors (including other foods) not controlled may augment the reactions in real life.

In a more open approach to this step, foods are added back one at a time and symptoms are tracked systematically in a diary or log. The challenge food is eaten for only 1 day. It should be as pure a form of the food as possible. One approach to this step is a sequential incremental dose challenge in which a small amount is consumed early in the day, followed by two increasingly larger amounts later in the day. This may allow a dose-response analysis, but will be meaningful only if symptoms emerge within a couple of hours. Another approach is to consume the food a couple of times during the day in moderate amounts.

Delayed response may be seen when non–IgE-immune-mediated reactions (specifically IgG-related) are involved. For this reason, symptoms should be tracked over a 3-day period and other foods should not be added back until after that period. After a food is challenged, it should be eliminated again until all foods are challenged. The elimination diet should be followed throughout the challenge period.

NOTE

A symptomatic response may occur over a 3-day period, following an individual food challenge. Thus, new food challenges should occur every 3 days.

Final Diet

After the challenge phase has been analyzed, a final diet can be planned. There are variations on this step as well. Foods that elicited symptoms in the challenge phase can be eliminated completely from the diet, or they may be eliminated for 3 to 6 months and then incorporated into a rotation diet. A rotation diet may be implemented from the beginning. Rotation diets include the suspect food on an infrequent but consistent basis from every 4 days to once a month. The rationale for a rotation diet is that levels of non-IgE antibodies will fall with reduced exposure to the antigen and will not rise again if exposure is infrequent.

Once again, the help of a registered dietitian or nutritionist may be useful in planning a nutritionally sound diet that meets all the needs of the patient.

Blood Tests

Blood tests that identify either IgE or IgG_4 antibodies using RAST (radioallergosorbent methodology) or ELISA (enzyme-linked immunosorbent assay) are used extensively by complementary and alternative medicine (CAM) practitioners.

These tests may provide a starting point for identifying reactive foods. Very often, however, individuals show elevated antibody levels with no accompanying symptoms. There continue to be concerns about the reliability of the tests as well.

A carefully monitored elimination diet continues to be the gold standard for identifying problematic foods.

NOTE

Many food allergy tests are available but their usefulness is limited. Skin tests are designed to identify immunoglobulin E (IgE) reactions to allergens, but there appears to be a great deal of cross-reactivity and nonspecific reactions when testing foods.

General Guidelines

Considering the energy and time put into the process of an elimination diet, following these general steps is important to maximize the potential for patient improvement.

The elimination diet itself should be followed for no more than 4 weeks. One concern is that following the diet for longer may reduce the chances of eliciting a symptom response. Antibody levels (other than IgE) and antigen-antibody complexes may decrease with decreased exposure to the antigen to the point that symptoms cannot be elicited in the challenge phase. Another concern is that nutritional inadequacies may develop, especially with a diet that has eliminated many foods. In fact, the elimination diet phase should be planned to ensure adequate nutrition if at all possible. A final concern is that sensitivity to antigens may actually increase during an elimination diet. Individuals who were asymptomatic, but had elevated IgE levels to certain foods, became symptomatic during an elimination diet.[8]

Care must be taken to avoid any exposure to the foods eliminated. Failure to do so may result in being unable to clearly define adverse reactions during the challenge step.[9] For the most common allergens, this means close scrutiny of ingredient labels to identify hidden sources.

If the elimination phase of the protocol does not result in a decrease in symptoms, it may be because food hypersensitivity or intolerance is not the cause of the symptoms. It may also be because the symptoms are related to some food still being consumed or that some other factor in addition to the food contributes to symptoms.

Table 82–6 contains a short list of ingredients on food labels that may indicate the presence of a hyperallergenic food. More extensive lists are found in the recommended resources.

It is important for the patient to understand that you are using the elimination diet as a diagnostic tool rather than a treatment, and that the challenge phase is extremely important. This may reduce the likelihood of the elimination phase of the diet being followed for long periods of time, a risk if the patient feels better on the diet. There should be no need to eliminate a food permanently if it cannot be implicated in symptoms.

Table 82–6. Food Label Ingredients That May Signal Hyperallergenic Foods

Dairy	Wheat	Soy
Casein, caseinate	Semolina	Hydrolyzed vegetable protein
Lactalbumin	Durum	
Milk solids	Modified food starch	Textured vegetable protein
Whey		
	Malt, malt syrup	Miso
		Lecithin

Resources

Several excellent resources are available to practitioners who are interested in utilizing elimination diet protocols in their practices. These will provide forms and logs for patients to use in charting their diets and reactions to foods. Perhaps the most comprehensive and well referenced is the *Food Allergy Handbook* by Janice Vickerstaff Joneja. Another strategy that utilizes a vegan, hypoallergenic diet is found in *Foods that Fight Pain* by Neal Barnard, M.D., Harmony Books, 1998.

References

1. Gaby AR: The role of hidden food allergy/intolerance in chronic disease. Altern Med Rev 3:90–100, 1998.
2. Kemp AS, Schembri G: An elimination diet for chronic urticaria of childhood. Med J Aust 143:234–235, 1985.
3. Lunardi C, Bambara LM, Biasi D, et al: Elimination diet in the treatment of selected patients with hypersensitivity vasculitis. Clin Exp Rheumatol 10:131–135, 1992.
4. Hedges HH: The elimination diet as a diagnostic tool. Am Fam Physician 46(Suppl):77S–84S, 1992.
5. Rancé F, Kanny G, Dutau G, Moneret-Vautrin DA: Food hypersensitivity in children: Clinical aspects and distribution of allergens. Pediatr Allergy Immunol 10:33–38, 1999.
6. Vatn MH, Grimstad IA, Thorsen L, et al: Adverse reaction to food: Assessment by double-blind placebo-controlled food challenge and clinical, psychosomatic and immunologic analysis. Digestion 56:421–428, 1995.
7. Joneja JV: The Food Allergy Handbook. 1995.
8. Larramendi CH, Martín Esteban M, Pascual Marcos C, et al: Possible consequences of elimination diets in asymptomatic immediate hypersensitivity to fish. Allergy 47:490–494, 1992.
9. Faulkner-Hogg KB, Selby WS, Loblay RH: Dietary analysis in symptomatic patients with coeliac disease on a gluten-free diet: The role of trace amounts of gluten and non-gluten food intolerances. Scand J Gastroenterol 34:784–789, 1999.
10. Fuglsang G, Madsen G, Halken S, et al: Adverse reactions to food additives in children with atopic symptoms. Allergy 49:131–137, 1994.

PATIENT HANDOUT
THE ELIMINATION DIET

Special diets called *elimination diets* are sometimes used to discover whether food allergies or sensitivities are related to symptoms you might be having. The goal of an *elimination diet* is to identify problem foods. The diet is temporary and must be followed very carefully so that a permanent diet to help you feel better can be planned.

The **steps** in an *elimination diet*:

1. **Decide which foods might be causing problems**. This step involves describing your diet for your doctor and sharing your ideas about what foods might be causing problems. Sometimes, food allergy tests are used to help with the decision.
2. **Avoid the foods completely for 2 to 4 weeks**. This is the actual elimination step. This step involves the greatest restrictions in your diet.
   *The foods need to be avoided completely for symptoms to be noticeable when the foods are added back.
   *Foods should be avoided both in their whole form and as ingredients in food.
   *Keeping track of how you feel during this step is important. It is useful to keep a written record. You may feel worse before you feel better but that should last only 1 or 2 days. If you feel worse for longer, please call your doctor.

3. **Add the foods back one at a time**. This is called the *challenge* step. It allows you to learn which foods, if any, are causing symptoms.
   *Decide with your doctor which food to add back first.
   *Keep track of how you feel throughout this step with a written record.
   *On the day a food is added, eat that food twice. For the next 2 days, do not eat that food again, but continue to follow the elimination diet. You can have a reaction up to 3 days after a food is eaten.
   *Add a new food every 3 days, because you can have a reaction up to 3 days after the challenge food is eaten.
   *If the food does not cause a reaction, that food "passes" and can be added back to your diet when the entire process is over. Do not eat the foods you have added back, even if they "passed," until you have tested all the foods.

After following the elimination diet carefully, you and your doctor will have a better picture of which foods, if any, are causing your problems. Remember that problems with foods can be intermittent, and it is sometimes difficult to tell exactly whether foods are a problem.

CHAPTER 83

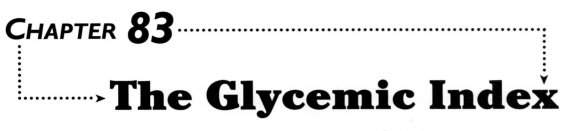

The Glycemic Index

Kathleen Johnson, M.S., R.D.

In the past, planning and evaluation of foods and diets were based primarily on macronutrient composition, a largely quantitative approach. Nutrient density, a qualitative concept, was introduced to focus on the quantity of micronutrients per calorie. Glycemic index is another tool that can be used to broaden understanding of the functional aspects of food and diet. Although it is a concept that can easily be misinterpreted, it is relevant to a number of health conditions, including diabetes, hypoglycemia, insulin resistance, hypertriglyceridemia and hypercholesterolemia, and obesity.

WHAT IS GLYCEMIC INDEX?

Glycemic index (GI) is a ranking of foods based on their postprandial blood glucose response compared with a reference food. It provides a means of understanding the body's functional response to a food as opposed to just knowing its nutrient composition. A high glycemic index food raises blood sugar levels to a greater degree over a 2- to 3-hour period than a low glycemic index food.

NOTE

Glycemic index is an indicator of how rapidly and to what degree blood sugar levels rise after a food is eaten.

Glycemic index reflects a comparison of the postprandial glucose curve for a food compared with a reference food, either glucose or white bread. It is basically a reflection of how rapidly a carbohydrate containing food is absorbed into the bloodstream.

HOW IS GLYCEMIC INDEX DETERMINED?

The definition of glycemic index is based on a well-defined method for determining the glycemic response to a given food. A consistent use of the method is essential so that foods tested in different laboratories can be compared.

Generally, a small group (most studies use between 5 and 20 subjects) is used for a glycemic index study. The subjects, who have fasted overnight, are fed a portion of a reference food (either glucose or white bread) that provides 50 g of carbohydrate. Serum glucose is plotted over a 2- to 3-hour postprandial period. On subsequent days, various other foods are administered in the same manner. The areas under the curves are calculated and expressed as a percentage of the area under the curve for the reference food. That percentage is the glycemic index of the food. The reference food always has a glycemic index of 100.[1]

When using a glycemic index, is important to know whether values in the table are based on a glucose or white bread standard. Using a different standard reference food does not change the relative ranking of a food, but changes the number by a factor of about 30. It is possible to compare the glycemic index values of foods tested using glucose as the reference food with those tested using white bread. Generally, adding 30 to the glycemic index of foods tested with glucose allows comparison with foods tested with white bread. The table included in this chapter is based on a glucose reference (see Table 83–1).

A noteworthy aspect of the postprandial response to a high glycemic index food is that within 2 to $2^{1}/_{2}$ hours, because of the insulin response to the glycemic rise, the blood sugar level drops to below fasting level. This may result in symptoms of fatigue. The flatter glycemic response to lower glycemic index foods does not cause the precipitous drop in blood sugar (Fig. 83–1).

The glycemic index values of most foods tested in different laboratories are consistent. A difference of 10 to 15 points is within the error expected with the test. When larger differences are found, they are usually the result of cooking method, cooking time, processing, ripeness, or the varieties of plants tested.[2, 3]

Glycemic index can be measured only in foods that contain carbohydrate.

WHAT FACTORS INFLUENCE THE GLYCEMIC INDEX OF A FOOD?

The glycemic index of a food simply reflects the rates of gastric emptying, digestion, and absorption of the food. Factors that influence this include the following:

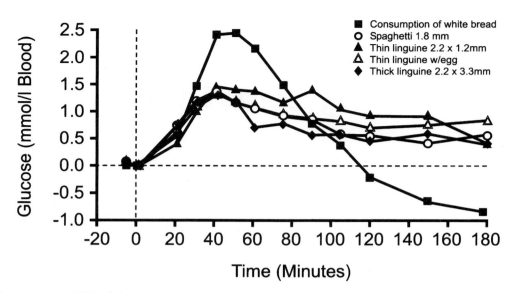

Figure 83–1. Mean incremental blood glucose responses in healthy subjects, 65 to 70 years of age. (Adapted from Bjorck I, Granfeldt Y, Liljeberg H, et al: Food properties affecting the digestion and absorption of carbohydrates. Am J Clin Nutr 59[suppl]:699S–705S, 1994.

Soluble Fiber

Although the amount of total dietary fiber is not a good predictor of glycemic index, the amount of soluble fiber is a fair one. Soluble fiber reduces the glycemic index.

Types of Sugars Present

Glucose is absorbed very quickly and raises blood glucose levels similarly; fructose raises blood glucose levels quite slowly by comparison. A fruit or vegetable with a higher percentage of fructose to glucose has a lower glycemic index.

Antinutrients

Antinutrients are substances in food that reduce the bioavailability of nutrients in foods. They include substances such as lectins, phytates, and enzyme inhibitors, which affect digestion. The actual effect of these substances on glycemic index is somewhat questionable, especially in cooked foods, although they need to be acknowledged.

Characteristics of Starch

Amylose versus amylopectin: The starch amylose is a long, unbranched polysaccharide chain of glucose molecules that is digested more slowly than amylopectin. Amylopectin, by contrast, is branched and digested more quickly. White, sticky rice is higher in amylopectin and has a higher glycemic index than basmati rice, which is higher in amylose.

Cooking causes starch gelatinization (i.e., swelling of starch granules in the presence of heat and water). This increases susceptibility to enzymatic digestion. One example is the boiled potato. Starch may also take on a more crystalline structure after being cooked and then cooled, which decreases the rate of digestion. An example is parboiled, or "converted," rice as opposed to regular long grain rice.

Particle Size and Method of Processing

Flour, with its powdery particle size, has a higher glycemic index than less finely ground grains such as cracked wheat. The whole version of a grain has the lowest glycemic index of all the possible foods made from that grain. Puffed grains have a higher glycemic indeed than whole, unprocessed grains. Parboiled rice has a lowe glycemic index than does regular white rice.

Density of the Food and Method of Preparation

Pasta made from semolina flour has a lower glycemic index than bread made from the same flour. Pasta cooked *al dente* (translates from Italian as "to the tooth," referring to pasta cooked only until it offers slight resistance when bitten into, and is not soft or overdone) has a lower glycemic index than does well-cooked pasta.

Specific Varieties of Plants

Different varieties of a fruit, vegetable, legume, or grain may have different glycemic index values. These differences probably reflect genetic variation in the amount and types of fiber, sugars, and starches.

Degree of Ripeness and Postharvest Changes

Changes in the amount and type of carbohydrate occur during ripening and after harvest. These can affect glycemic index. As an example, underripe bananas have a lower glycemic index than do over-ripe bananas.

Presence of Protein or Fat in the Food

The presence of both protein and fat in a food or meal can affect glycemic index. Protein triggers the release of insulin. Fat ingestion results in an increase in gastric inhibitory polypeptide, which enhances postprandial glucose-induced insulin secretion. Interestingly, this polypeptide may also decrease the insulin response to carbohydrate during the next meal, consumed hours later. Increased circulating insulin from protein or fat immediately begins moving absorbed glucose into cells, resulting in a lower postprandial curve.[3]

Fat is known to slow gastric emptying but it isn't clear whether this actually reduces glycemic response.

Presence of Acid in the Food

The presence of acid in a food slows gastric emptying. For this reason, sourdough bread has a lower glycemic index than a similar regular bread. The addition of lemon juice or vinegar to a meal results in a lower meal glycemic index.[4]

WHAT GENERALIZATIONS CAN BE MADE ABOUT THE GLYCEMIC INDEX OF FOODS?

1. Legumes have a lower glycemic index than grains. Barley, however, has a very low glycemic index.
2. Whole grains eaten as such (e.g., wheat berries) have a lower glycemic index than whole grain products (e.g., whole wheat bread or cereal) made from flour. Particle size is probably the biggest factor.
3. Tropical fruits have higher glycemic index values than fruits grown in temperate climates.

WHAT GENERALIZATIONS CANNOT BE MADE ABOUT THE GLYCEMIC INDEX OF FOODS?

It is not true that complex carbohydrates (starches) are absorbed more slowly and have lower glycemic index values than simple carbohydrates (sugars). Table sugar or sucrose, an equal mix of glucose and fructose, has a moderate glycemic index, lower than that of many starchy foods.

It is not true that all refined products have high glycemic index values, or that all whole grains or whole grain products have low glycemic index values. Pasta made from white flour has a relatively low glycemic index when cooked *al dente*. The glycemic index of bread made from whole wheat flour is not significantly different from that of bread made from white flour; brown rice glycemic index is not significantly different from that of white rice.

GLYCEMIC INDEX OF MIXED FOODS OR MEALS

The glycemic index of mixed foods or meals has been an area of controversy in the clinical application of glycemic index. It appears that the glycemic index of a mixed food or meal can be calculated by weighting the proportion of carbohydrate from each food within the meal with that food's glycemic index.[5]

WHAT IS THE CLINICAL RELEVANCE OF GLYCEMIC INDEX?

Blood Glucose Levels

A lower glycemic index diet compared with a higher glycemic index diet followed for two weeks resulted in a 37% lower 12-hr blood glucose level, a 16% lower day-long glucose level, a 9% lower glycosylated hemoglobin level, and a 7% lower fructosamine level.[6]

A low glycemic index meal has been shown to result in a lower glycemic response to the next meal. This "second meal effect" has been noted between breakfast and lunch, as well as between dinner and breakfast.[3]

Insulin Levels

The higher the glycemic index of a single food, the greater the insulin response to that food. The insulin response to mixed foods or meals, however, is not so straightforward. In mixed foods or meals, the insulin response is increased by the presence of fat and protein. This generally reduces the glycemic index of the mixed food or meal but may result in a higher postprandial insulin level.

Nonetheless, a mixed food or meal with a high glycemic index food results in a greater insulin response than one with a low glycemic index food. Lower glycemic index foods, eaten alone or as part of a mixed meal, result in a lower insulin response than higher glycemic index foods. This is relevant for the dietary management of patients with insulin resistance.[3, 7]

Satiety

A low glycemic index meal was associated with consumption of less food at the next meal in overweight adolescent boys. Low glycemic index foods were associated with increased serum cholecystokinin, which is known as a "satiety peptid.[8, 9]"

Glycemic index may be an important factor in designing weight loss diets.[10]

Energy Levels

A low compared with a high glycemic index pre-performance meal resulted in an additional 20 minutes of exercise to exhaustion on a cycling ergometer in endurance-trained athletes. Glycemic index may be an important factor in designing diets for sports performance or maintaining optimal levels of functioning during the day.[11, 12]

Serum Lipid Levels

Low glycemic index compared with high glycemic index diets have resulted in reductions in total cholesterol, low-density lipoprotein cholesterol, and triglycerides. It has been commonly believed that high triglyceride levels reflect a high fat intake. However, high triglyceride levels are now understood to be related to high carbohydrate levels, especially in individuals who are insulin resistant. The mechanism may be related to the release of free fatty acids that is part of the counterregulatory response of a rapid drop in blood sugar levels, which occurs with a high glycemic index food.[13, 14]

NOTE

Moderating glycemic response to meals is a useful approach to designing diets for individuals with non-insulin dependent diabetes mellitus, insulin resistance, hypertriglyceridemia, hypoglycemia, and obesity.

Modifying the diet to include low glycemic index foods, reducing high glycemic index foods, and eating smaller, more frequent meals is helpful.

WAYS GLYCEMIC INDEX MAY BE MISUSED

Many currently popular diet books, especially those advocating high-protein diets, discuss glycemic index. Some of those discussions give the impression that a high glycemic index food is a bad food. Labeling a food as "good" or "bad" is an oversimplification and should be avoided in most circumstances, but particularly when considering a food's glycemic index. The labeling of carrots and beets as "undesirable" foods is a good example of this.

These books rarely mention the concept of glycemic load. Small amounts of high glycemic index foods in the context of a mixed meal are not as significant as large amounts.

NOTE

Glycemic load combines the amount of carbohydrate food eaten with its glycemic index. It is probably more important than glycemic index alone. Two cohort studies have shown an association between glycemic load and a patient's risk of developing diabetes. Others have shown no such association.

Glycemic index does not reflect the nutrient content of a food. A food may have a high glycemic index but still provide significant amounts of vitamins and minerals. Fructose, although it has a low glycemic index, is not necessarily a desirable sweetener. It has been shown to increase insulin resistance, even though its effect on postprandial glycemic response is low.

The shape of the postprandial glucose curve may be an important factor that has not been a topic of research to date. Orange juice, a surprise with its relatively low glycemic index, may well show an early peak because of its rapid absorption of glucose, even though the area under the entire curve is significantly less than that of other foods.

References

1. Wolever TM, David JA, Jenkins et al: The glycemic index: Methodology and clinical applications. Am J Clin Nutr 54:846–54, 1991.
2. Bjorck I, Granfeldt Y, Liljeberg H, et al: Food properties affecting the digestion and absorption of carbohydrates. Am J Clin Nut 59(suppl):699S–705S, 1994.
3. Wolever TM: The glycemic index. Aspects of some vitamins, minerals and enzymes in health and disease. World Rev Nutr Diet, 62:120–185, 1990.
4. Brand-Miller J, Wolever T, Colagiuri S, Foster-Powell K: The Glucose Revolution.
5. Chew I, Brand J, Thorburn AW, Truswell AS: Application of glycemic index to mixed meals. Am J Clin Nutr 47:53–65, 1988.
6. Miller JC: Importance of glycemic index in diabetes. Am J Clin Nutr 59(suppl):747S–752S, 1994.
7. Frost G, Leeds A, Trew G, et al: Insulin sensitivity in women at risk of coronary heart disease and the effect of a low glycemic diet. Metabolism 47:1245–1251, 1998.
8. Holt S, Brand-Miller J, Saveny C, Hansky J: Glycemic index, satiety, and the cholecystokinin response. Am J Clin Nutr, 59(suppl):787S, 1994.
9. Ludwig DS, Majzoub JA, Al-Zahrani A, et al: High glycemic index foods, overeating, and obesity. Pediatrics 103:E26, 1999.
10. Spieth LE, Harnish JD, Lenders CM, A low-glycemic index diet in the treatment of pediatric obesity. Arch Pediatr Adolesc Med 154:947–951, 2000.
11. Kirwan JP, O'Gorman D, Evans WJ: A moderate glycemic index meal before endurance exercise can enhance performance. J Appl Physiol 84:53–95, 1998.
12. DeMarco HM, Sucher KP, Cisar CJ, Butterfield GE: Pre-exercise carbohydrate meals: Application of glycemic index. Med Sci Sports Exerc.
13. Luscombe ND, Noakes M, Clifton PM: Diets high and low in glycemic index versus high monounsaturated fat diets: Effects on glucose and lipid metabolism in NIDDM. Eur J Clin Nutr 53:473–478, 1999.
14. Järvi AE, Karlström BE, Granfeldt YE, et al: Improved glycemic control and lipid profile and normalized fibrinolytic activity on a low-glycemic index diet in type 2 diabetic patients. Diabetes Care, 22:10–18, 1999.

PATIENT HANDOUT
HOW TO USE THE GLYCEMIC INDEX

By making careful food choices, you can influence your hunger and energy as well as blood sugar, cholesterol, and triglyceride levels (see Table 83–1). If you have problems controlling how much food you eat, or if you have hypoglycemia, diabetes, or high triglyceride and cholesterol levels, considering glycemic index in your food choices may be helpful.

Blood sugar levels are raised after foods contain-ing carbohydrates (sugars and starches) are eaten. Different carbohydrate-containing foods affect blood sugar levels differently.

The glycemic index of a food refers to its effect on blood sugar levels. The number is a comparison with a reference food, in this case the sugar, glucose. Glucose is a very basic sugar that is not the same as table sugar. A high glycemic index may be con-

Table 83–1. Glycemic Index of Common Foods

Remember that glycemic index can only be measured on foods that contain carbohydrate. Glycemic index values have not been determined on all foods; however, more extensive lists can be found in the resources listed below. The reference food for this table is glucose.

Food	Glycemic Index
Breads	
Bagel	72
Kaiser roll	73
White bread	70
Whole wheat bread	69
Sourdough bread	52
Whole grain pumpernickel	51
Cereals	
Corn Flakes	83
Rice Krispies	82
Grapenuts Flakes	80
Total	76
Cheerios	74
Puffed Wheat	74
Shredded Wheat	69
Grapenuts	67
Cream of Wheat	66
Oatmeal	61
Special K	54
All Bran	42
Grains	
Instant rice	87
Millet	71
White rice	56
Brown rice	55
Bulgur	48
Converted rice	47
Barley	25
Snacks	
Rice cakes	82
Jelly beans	80
Soda crackers	74
Corn chips	72
Chocolate bar	68
Rye crispbread	63
Power Bar	57
Popcorn	55
Potato chips	54
Peanuts	14

Food	Glycemic Index
Pasta	
Spaghetti	41
Whole wheat spaghetti	37
Beans	
Baked beans	48
Chickpeas	33
Cooked beans	29
Lentils	29
Soy beans	18
Vegetables	
Baked potato	85
Beets	64
New potato	62
Sweet corn	55
Sweet potato	54
Carrots	49
Green peas	48
Fruit	
Watermelon	72
Pineapple	66
Raisins	64
Mango	55
Orange juice	52
Canned peach	47
Orange	43
Unsweetened apple juice	41
Apple	36
Pear	36
Peach	28
Grapefruit	25
Milk and Yogurt	
Chocolate milk	34
Low-fat fruit yogurt	33
Skim milk	32
Whole milk	27
Sugars	
Glucose	100
Honey	58
Sucrose (table sugar)	65
Fructose	43

More information on glycemic index can be found in *The Glucose Revolution* by Jennie Brand-Miller, Thomas M.S. Wolever, Stephen Colagiuri, and Kaye Foster-Powell, and on the website www.mendosa.com/gilists.htm

sidered to be a number between 70 and 100; medium range is between 50 and 70; and low values are those under 50.

If you think that considering glycemic index in your diet would be helpful, follow these guidelines.

1. Eat low and medium glycemic index food, such as beans, oatmeal, and pasta, regularly but in moderate quantity. Eat high glycemic index foods, such as bread, bagels, English muffins, baked potato, and snack foods, rarely and only in very small quantities.
   - Use beans as a side dish instead of rice or potatoes. Use beans like hummus eaten with raw vegetables as a snack food instead of chips, crackers, or rice cakes.
   - Cook pasta to the *al dente* state. *Al dente* translates from Italian as "to the tooth," and it refers to pasta cooked only until it offers slight resistance when bitten into, and is not soft or overdone. Serve one cup of cooked pasta with at least one cup of vegetables and a sauce of your choice.
   - Focus on lower glycemic index fruits such as apples, pears, berries, and citrus rather than on higher glycemic index fruits such as melon, pineapple, and raisins.
   - Choose a cereal with a low glycemic index, such as All Bran or oatmeal.
   - Have sugary foods such as candy, soda, and other sweetened beverages in small quantities and with a meal.
2. Eat smaller, more frequent meals.
   - Try including a snack, both at midmorning and at midafternoon.
   - Have a moderate-sized lunch and a smaller dinner, such as a salad, a bowl of soup, or a small portion of fish, chicken, or meat and vegetables.

CHAPTER 84

The Anti-Inflammatory Diet

David Rakel, M.D.

WHY IS INFLAMMATION A CONCERN?

Inflammation is at the root of many chronic medical conditions including coronary artery disease, autoimmune disorders, arthritis, Alzheimer's disease, and cancer. Improving the diet to reduce this process can have a major impact on health and the prevention of disease.

WHAT ARE ESSENTIAL FATTY ACIDS?

Essential fatty acids are fats that the human body is unable to make on its own. Humans must ingest them by eating plants or by eating the animals that eat the plants. Plants make fatty acids from triglycerides.

WHY ARE FATTY ACIDS ESSENTIAL?

Fatty acids are needed to maintain cell membrane integrity and chemical transport that is involved in proper development of the central nervous system, energy production, cell communication, oxygen transport, and regulation of inflammation.

HOW ARE FATS CLASSIFIED?

The three types of fats are:

1. Saturated: beef fat, dairy
2. Monounsaturated (omega-9 family): olive oil, canola oil
3. Polyunsaturated (essential fatty acids): many different sources. *Omega-6 family:* linoleic acid (LA); gamma-linolenic acid (GLA); arachidonic acid (AA). *Omega-3 family:* alpha-linolenic acid (ALA); eicosapentaenoic acid (EPA); docosahexaenoic acid (DHA).

Sources of fat contain a combination of the three types but some foods have a higher amount of one type than another.

WHAT DOES "SATURATION" HAVE TO DO WITH HOW FATS ARE CLASSIFIED?

A fat is a chain of carbon atoms with a methyl group (CH_3) on one end and a carboxyl group (COOH) on the other (Fig. 84–1). Saturation describes how many hydrogen (H) atoms are connected to the carbon atom. If the fat is completely saturated with hydrogen, there will be no double bonds and the fat will be called a *saturated fat*. If there is only one double bond (one carbon unsaturated with hydrogen), the fat is called a *monounsaturated fat*. The essential fatty acids are polyunsaturated and have multiple double bonds (many carbon atoms unsaturated with hydrogen).

NOTE

The more saturated the fat, the more stable it will be at room temperature.

If we take a liquid sample of each fat (bacon grease, olive oil, and flaxseed oil) and put them in the refrigerator, we can see how their saturation can affect their physical state. The saturated fat quickly

Omega 3 Fatty Acid

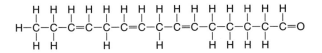

Omega 6 Fatty Acid

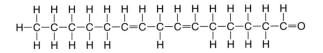

Figure 84–1. Atomic makeup of a fat: a chain of carbon atoms with a methyl group on one end and a carboxyl group on the other.

turns to a more stable solid; the olive oil also turns solid but may need a colder temperature than the bacon fat. In contrast, the flaxseed oil stays liquid despite the cold temperature. The fact that polyunsaturated fats stay liquid at more extreme temperatures helps explain why cold-water fish are a good source of omega-3 fatty acids. Their high percentage of polyunsaturated omega-3 fatty acids helps keep their cell membranes functioning in cold waters. They incorporate this into their system by eating omega-3–rich foods such as algae. Unfortunately, the instability of these polyunsaturated fats also means that they will spoil quickly if left at room temperature for extended periods of time.

WHAT DOES OMEGA MEAN IN THE NAMING OF FATTY ACIDS?

Omega describes where the first double bond is located. If we look at Figure 84–1 we can see that in omega-3 fatty acids, the first double bond is after the third carbon; in omega-6 fatty acids, it is after the sixth.

WHAT ARE PARTIALLY HYDROGENATED OILS AND HOW ARE THEY RELATED TO TRANS-FATTY ACIDS?

Back in the 1950s when we started to realize that saturated fats were harmful, scientists started to think of ways we could use less dangerous fats in our cooking (e.g., polyunsaturated). The problem was that polyunsaturated fats were unstable at room temperature, and if they were used to make crackers or chips, they would spoil quickly. The challenge was to manipulate these fats so they would be more stable at room temperature. Scientists did this through the process of hydrogenation. A large amount of polyunsaturated fat, such as vegetable oil, is placed in a large metal vat that is connected to a source of hydrogen and heated. Heating the oil does two things. It changes the fat from its natural cis form (Fig. 84–2) to a more stable trans form in which the methyl and carboxyl groups are on opposite sides of the carbon chain. It also breaks double bonds in the carbon chain, allowing the hydrogen gas to partially hydrogenate the oil. Partially hydrogenating (saturating) the oil and creating a transfatty acid allowed these oils to maintain "freshness" when used in foods such as Twinkies that now could be preserved on shelves for prolonged periods of time. Partially hydrogenated rich foods such as vegetable oil and margarine dramatically increased the intake of omega-6 fatty acids in industrialized countries.

HOW DOES THIS PROMOTE INFLAMMATION?

Partially hydrogenated oils are a major source of omega-6 fatty acids that are subunits of the body's main inflammatory precursor, arachidonic acid (AA). AA leads to the production of the main proponents of the inflammatory cascade, prostaglandins of the two family (PGE_2) and leukotrienes (Fig. 84–3). In contrast, omega-3 fatty acids have a more beneficial influence on inflammation. Omega-3 fatty acids lead to the production of less inflammatory prostaglandins of the one and three families (PGE_1 and PGE_3) and less inflammatory leukotrienes. The more omega-6 fatty acids in the body, the less we are able to utilize the beneficial influences of the omega-3 fatty acids. In the early 1900s, the ratio of omega-6 to omega-3 fatty acids in the Western diet was 4:1. This dramatically increased to greater than 25:1 by the end of the 20th century. One of the main goals in changing the diet is to try to reduce this ratio back to near 4:1. The change from a free-range diet in the early 20th century to one of more saturated fats and processed foods may play a role in the high incidence of chronic inflammatory conditions we see in the 21st century.

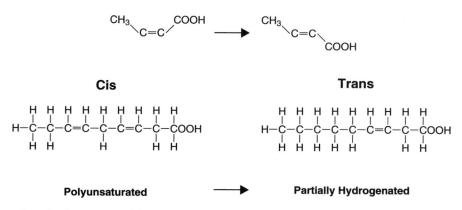

Figure 84–2. Hydrogenation of polyunsaturated fat.

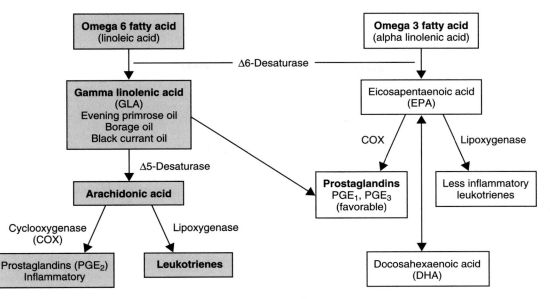

Figure 84–3. Influence of omega-6 fatty acids and omega-3 fatty acids on inflammation.

> ### NOTE
>
> *Omega-6 fatty acids increase inflammation and platelet aggregation, and omega-3 fatty acids reduce inflammation and platelet aggregation.*

Owing to their stable configuration, trans-fatty acids require more energy for the body to metabolize as a source of energy. This results in greater free radical production that increases the mobilization of AA from the cell membrane. High levels of trans-fatty acids not only raise harmful low-density lipoprotein (LDL) cholesterol and lower beneficial high-density lipoprotein (HDL) cholesterol but also may play a role in worsening inflammation.

WHAT ARE OTHER SOURCES OF ARACHIDONIC ACID AND WHAT MEDICINES ARE USED TO INHIBIT ITS INFLUENCE?

Besides partially hydrogenated oils, saturated fats including meat and dairy are major sources of AA. Research has shown that those people with chronic inflammatory diseases, such as rheumatoid arthritis, are less symptomatic on a vegetarian diet. The pharmaceutical industry has spent great amounts of money developing beneficial drugs that inhibit the influence of AA for diseases such as arthritis, asthma, and inflammatory bowel disease (Fig. 84–4). However, they should not be taken without the conscious effort to change the diet to reduce the load of AA in the first place instead of simply blocking its effects. Changing to a less inflammatory diet

may help us decrease our dependence on these medications.

WHAT IS GAMMA-LINOLENIC ACID?

GLA is an omega-6 fatty acid that includes evening primrose oil, black current oil, and borage oil. These are often used for treatment of dermatologic and gynecologic inflammatory conditions. Their benefit is thought to be due in part to GLA's ability to stimulate the production of less inflammatory PGE_1 (see Fig. 84–3). Unfortunately, GLA has a greater influence on the stimulation of the more inflammatory AA. Our goal is to try to improve the ratio of omega-6 to omega-3 fatty acids; therefore, it would be best to use these oils only therapeutically for the short term until more is known about their mechanism of action. Increasing omega-3 sources of fatty acids will have more beneficial long-term effects.

WHAT IS DELTA 6-DESATURASE ENZYME AND WHAT IS ITS SIGNIFICANCE?

Delta 6-desaturase is the main enzyme that both omega-6 and omega-3 fatty acids use in the cascade of events that leads to the production of prostaglandins and leukotrienes (see Fig. 84–3). Certain situations influence this enzyme to shift toward the omega-6 pathway, resulting in more inflammatory mediators. These include excessive alcohol, diabetes, stress, and a high omega-6 to omega-3 ratio. This may help explain why these conditions are associated with a high risk for inflammatory complications.

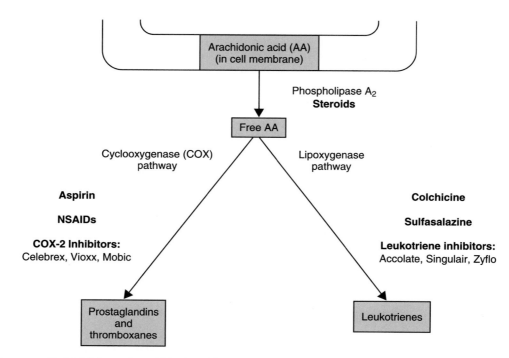

Figure 84–4. Pharmaceutical inhibitors of arachidonic acid.

WHAT ARE GOOD SOURCES OF OMEGA-3 FATTY ACIDS?

As mentioned previously, cold-water fish including salmon, mackerel, sardines, herring, and albacore tuna are excellent sources. Fish oils are sources of both EPA and DHA. These have beneficial effects on inflammation without the need for delta 6-desaturase enzyme. Unlike other omega-3 sources that require this enzyme to have beneficial effects on inflammation, fish oil has a more direct effect. This may partly explain its positive effect in heart disease.

One of the richest sources of omega-3 fatty acids is flaxseed. Flax can be used in different ways. It can be ground in a coffee grinder and sprinkled on cereals and salads. The oil can be used alone or on foods. The best way to store flax is in the seed form. Once it is ground or oil is made, the product can spoil; therefore, it should be refrigerated and used promptly.

Other sources of omega-3 fatty acids include nuts (particularly walnuts), dark green leafy vegetables, soybeans, algae, and hemp seeds.

IS THERE ANYTHING I SHOULD WATCH FOR WHEN BUYING FISH OR FISH OIL?

Not all fish products are the same. If able, buy wild fish from Northern waters and avoid farmed fish. The problem with most farm-raised fish is that they are fed foods such as cornmeal that have low amounts of omega-3 fatty acids. Wild fish eat a lot of algae, which is a rich source of omega-3 fatty acids.

HOW LONG WILL IT TAKE BEFORE A POSITIVE CHANGE OCCURS?

It can take up to 6 months for this type of diet to change the omega-6 to omega-3 ratio and have a noticeable clinical effect. This should be viewed as a positive change that is not simply used for a short period of time but incorporated into the daily lifestyle.

ARE THERE OTHER FOODS (BESIDES THOSE RICH IN OMEGA-3 FATTY ACIDS) THAT BENEFIT INFLAMMATION?

Just as pharmaceuticals can focus on influencing enzymes in the inflammatory cascade, so can some foods (see Fig. 84–4). For example, the phytonutrient quercitin (found in onions and apples) has been found to inhibit phospholipase A_2, cyclooxygenase, and lipoxygenase, reducing AA, prostaglandin, thromboxanes, and leukotrienes. Other nutrients that inhibit cyclooxygenase include curcumin (turmeric), capsaicin (red pepper), and ginger. Nutrients that inhibit lipoxygenase include carnosol (rosemary) and boswellic acid *(Boswellia)*. Using these foods and spices for cooking may enhance the effects of omega-3 fatty acids in reducing the inflammatory response. See Healthcomm International (www.healthcomm.com/research/tech-bul/index.html) for a technical bulletin on the subject.

IF I WANT TO SUPPLEMENT WITH OMEGA-3 FATTY ACIDS, HOW MUCH SHOULD I TAKE?

If treating an active inflammatory process, 2 to 4 g/day of ALA oil is recommended. For prevention of heart disease and other inflammatory conditions, 1 g/day is sufficient. Sources would include fish oils (EPA/DHA) or flaxseed oil. It is important to remember that more is not better and taking an excess amount of omega-3 fatty acids can worsen inflammation. When our body metabolizes fat to make energy, free radicals are produced that are usually handled by our body without trouble. But if excessive amounts of fatty acids are used, a large amount of free radicals will overwhelm the body's antioxidants and increase the mobilization of AA, worsening inflammation. For this reason, antioxidants should be taken by those using high doses of omega-3 fatty acids for prolonged periods of time. A recommended regimen would include vitamin E 400 IU, vitamin C 200 mg, and selenium 200 μg each day.

WHAT EFFECT DO LOW-CARBOHYDRATE DIETS HAVE ON INFLAMMATION?

Low-carbohydrate diets (Atkins) are helpful for lowering weight when used for short periods of time. Unfortunately, these diets are very high in foods rich in AA, such as animal products. Staying on this type of diet for extended periods of time would not be wise, particularly for those who have an active inflammatory condition.

WHAT DOES SOME OF THE RESEARCH TELL US ABOUT ESSENTIAL FATTY ACIDS AND HEALTH?

There is not enough space to cover all the research on this subject, but a few key studies are worth mentioning. Research in this area was initially triggered by an epidemiologic study of the Greenland Inuit Eskimos, who were found to have a significant reduction in the number of heart attacks versus Western controls. This was attributed to the high amount of fish products they consumed. O'Keefe and Harris[1] reviewed over 4500 studies.

Regarding heart disease, an Italian study (GISSI)[2] was done of over 11,000 people. The investigators found that those patients who took 850 mg/day of an omega-3–rich oil had 15% fewer cardiac events, 20% lower mortality, and a 45% decrease in incidence of sudden cardiac death compared with controls.

A group of patients with rheumatoid arthritis who consumed 1.8 g/day of EPA was found to have a decrease in the amount of morning stiffness and tender joints compared with controls.[3]

In a small Duke University study of men with active prostate cancer,[4] those who supplemented with flaxseed and maintained a low-fat diet had a decrease in the biomarkers of prostate cancer growth.

And finally, in a study of risk factors for asthma in preschool children,[5] it was found that a diet high in polyunsaturated fats (margarine and foods fried in polyunsaturated vegetable oil) doubled the risk of developing asthma.

References

1. O'Keefe JH Jr, Harris WS: From Inuit to implementation: Omega-3 fatty acids come of age. Mayo Clin Proc 75:607–114, 2000.
2. Dietary supplementation with n-3 polyunsaturated fatty acids and vitamin E after myocardial infarction: Results of the GISSI-Prevenzione trial. Gruppo Italiano per lo Studio della Sopravvivenza nell' Infarto miocardico. Lancet 354:447–455, 1999.
3. Kremer JM, Bigauouette J, Michalek AV, et al: Effects of manipulation of dietary fatty acids on clinical manifestations of rheumatoid arthritis. Lancet 1:184–187, 1985.
4. Denmark-Wahnefried W, Price DT, Polascik TJ, et al: Pilot study of dietary fat restriction and flaxseed supplementation in men with prostate cancer before surgery: Exploring the effects of hormone levels, prostate-specific antigen, and histopathologic features. Urology 58:47–52, 2001.
5. Haby MM, Peat JK, Marks GB, et al: Asthma in preschool children: Prevalence and risk factors. Thorax 56:589–595, 2001.

PATIENT HANDOUT: HOW THE "WESTERN" DIET PROMOTES INFLAMMATION

Saturated Fats (Source of Arachidonic Acid)

Over the past 100 years, the American diet has changed (Fig. 84–5). We now eat a higher percentage of animal products that include meat and dairy. One of the major building blocks of inflammatory agents in the body comes from AA, which we consume in the form of animal foods. Studies of inflammatory conditions such as rheumatoid arthritis have shown improvement of symptoms in those who ate small amounts of meat and dairy (vegetarian diet).

Polyunsaturated Fats (A Shift from Natural to Synthetic)

Essential fatty acids (omega-6 and omega-3) cannot be made in the human body and are required in our diets for proper function. Both are involved in the inflammatory process. Omega-6 fatty acids, in general, lead to the production of more inflammatory chemicals and omega-3 fatty acids result in less inflammatory chemicals. The ratio of omega-6 to omega-3 fatty acids in our diet has greatly increased owing to the introduction of vegetable oils and food preservation. In order to reduce the amount of saturated fats in our diet, the food industry created more stable polyunsaturated fats in the form of transfatty acids and partially hydrogenated oils. The introduction of these oils has led to longer shelf life for many baked products (crackers, chips) and has increased the amount of omega-6 fatty acids in our diet. The breakdown of transfatty acids also leads to free radical formation, which can lead to damage of blood vessels and to the production of more inflammatory agents. A diet high in omega-6 fatty acids prevents the body from using the less inflammatory omega-3 fatty acids. To help improve inflammation, the ratio needs to be reduced back to 4:1.

CHANGING TO A LESS INFLAMMATORY DIET

Reduce Amount of Saturated Fats (Arachidonic Acid)

- Animal products (except cold-water fish)
- Dairy products

Reduce Amount of Omega-6 Fatty Acids

- Margarine
- Corn oil, cottonseed oil, grapeseed oil, peanut oil, safflower oil, sesame oil, soybean oil, sunflower oil, partially hydrogenated oils. (Use monounsaturated oils, such as olive or canola oil, for cooking.)
- Any products that have a long shelf life (crackers, pastries, chips)

Increase Amount of Omega-3 Fatty Acids

- Cold-water fish (salmon, mackerel, sardines, herring)
- Flaxseeds or oil (go bad quickly, so keep refrigerated and use promptly)
- Nuts (particularly walnuts)
- Green leafy vegetables

Avoid Prolonged Use of Low-Carbohydrate Diets (High in Fat)

- Atkins

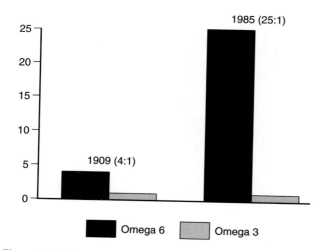
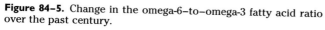

Figure 84–5. Change in the omega-6–to–omega-3 fatty acid ratio over the past century.

CHAPTER 85

The DASH Diet

David Rakel, M.D.

WHAT IS THE DASH DIET?

DASH stands for Dietary Approaches to Stop Hypertension. It consists of a type of diet that has been found to help lower blood pressure[1] as well as homocysteine levels.[2] It is a way of eating that is low in animal and dairy fat and rich in fruits and vegetables. It is a well-balanced diet that can be followed by everyone to help lead a healthy lifestyle (Table 85–1).

HOW MUCH CAN I EXPECT MY BLOOD PRESSURE TO COME DOWN?

A medical study[1] divided subjects into three groups. The first group ate a normal American diet, the second group a diet similar to the American diet but with more fruits and vegetables, and the third group ate the DASH diet. In those who did not have high blood pressure to begin with, the average systolic (top number) dropped 5.5 points and the diastolic (bottom number) dropped 3 points for those eating the DASH diet. African Americans had a slightly better response than whites. For those who already had high blood pressure, the systolic dropped by 11.6 points and the diastolic by 5.3. The blood pressure also dropped for group 2 (increase in fruits and vegetables) but not as much. These changes occurred after just 2 weeks on the diet.

This is a significant amount considering that a drop of just 5 points in systolic blood pressure can decrease complications related to heart disease.

WHAT IS HOMOCYSTEINE AND WHAT EFFECT DOES THE DASH DIET HAVE ON IT?

Homocysteine is a building block of protein (an amino acid) that, when elevated, can lead to hardening and clogging of the arteries by promoting the growth of atherosclerosis in the blood vessels. This can worsen high blood pressure and lead to the development of strokes and heart attacks. Homocysteine is reduced by eating foods rich in the B vitamins (particularly B_6 and B_{12}) and folic acid, which include grains, cereals, beans, and green leafy vegetables. Remember that folic acid comes from the word *foliage,* which consists of green leafy plants. The DASH diet is high in these food groups.

When homocysteine levels were measured in the three groups tested, it was found that the group eating the DASH diet had reduced homocysteine levels and the levels in the other two groups rose (the American diet levels rose more than levels with the American diet plus fruits and vegetables).[2]

WHAT IS DIFFERENT ABOUT THIS DIET?

The DASH diet can be most closely compared with a Mediterranean-type diet.

To summarize, it consists of foods that are
- High in fruits and vegetables
- Low in dairy, animal meat, and saturated fat
- High in nuts, seeds, and beans
- Low in snacks and sweets

HOW DO THESE FOODS REDUCE BLOOD PRESSURE AND THE RISK OF HEART DISEASE?

- The diet is high in potassium, calcium, and magnesium. Each of these nutrients have been found to reduce blood pressure and are found in a diet rich in vegetables and fruits.
- The diet is low in cholesterol and saturated fat. These fats are found to increase the risk of atherosclerosis and should be replaced with more healthy types of fats that are found in nuts and cold-water fish.
- The diet is low in snacks and sweets. Snack foods, such as chips and crackers, are high in partially hydrogenated fats, which preserve them on shelves for long periods of time. These types of fats are sources of trans-fatty acids, which play a major role in increasing the risk of heart disease. Sweets are mainly composed of simple carbohydrates. When consumed, they cause a rapid rise in the body's sugar levels. This triggers higher levels of insulin to try to store the energy that is not used. Over time, progressive elevation of insulin levels results in the body becoming less responsive to its

Table 85–1. The DASH Diet

Food Group	Daily Servings	Serving Sizes	Examples and Notes	Significance of Each Food Group to the DASH Eating Plan
Grains and grain products	7–8	1 slice bread 1 oz dry cereal* ½ c cooked rice, pasta, or cereal	Whole wheat bread, English muffin, pita bread, bagel, cereals, grits, oatmeal, crackers, unsalted pretzels, and popcorn	Major sources of energy and fiber
Vegetables	4–5	1 c raw leafy vegetable ½ c cooked vegetable 6 oz vegetable juice	Tomatoes, potatoes, carrots, green peas, squash, broccoli, turnip greens, collards, kale, spinach, artichokes, green beans, lima beans, sweet potatoes	Rich sources of potassium, magnesium, and fiber
Fruits	4–5	6 oz fruit juice 1 medium fruit ¼ c dried fruit ½ c fresh, frozen, or canned fruit	Apricots, bananas, dates, grapes, oranges, orange juice, grapefruit, grapefruit juice, mangoes, melons, peaches, pineapples, prunes, raisins, strawberries, tangerines	Important sources of potassium, magnesium, and fiber
Low-fat or fat-free dairy foods	2–3	8 oz milk 1 c yogurt 1.5 oz cheese	Fat-free (skim) or low-fat (1%) milk, fat-free or low-fat buttermilk, fat-free or low-fat regular or frozen yogurt, low-fat and fat-free cheese	Major sources of calcium and protein
Meats, poultry, fish	2 or less	3 oz cooked meats, poultry, or fish	Select only lean; trim away visible fats; broil, roast, or boil instead of frying; remove skin from poultry	Rich sources of protein and magnesium
Nuts, seeds, dry beans	4–5 per week	1.5 oz or ⅓ c nuts ½ oz or 2 tbsp seeds ½ c cooked dry beans and peas	Almonds, filberts, mixed nuts, peanuts, walnuts, sunflower seeds, kidney beans, lentils	Rich sources of energy, magnesium, potassium, protein, and fiber
Fats, oils†	2–3	1 tsp soft margarine 1 tbsp low-fat mayonnaise 2 tbsp light salad dressing 1 tsp vegetable oil	Soft margarine, low-fat mayonnaise, light salad dressing, vegetable oil (such as olive, corn canola, or safflower)	DASH has 27% of calories as fat, including that in or added to foods
Sweets	5 per week	1 tbsp sugar 1 tbsp jelly or jam ½ oz jelly beans 8 oz lemonade	Maple syrup, sugar, jelly, jam, fruit-flavored gelatin, jelly beans, hard candy, fruit punch, sorbet, ices	Sweets should be low in fat

* Equals ½–1¼ c, depending on cereal type. Check the product's nutrition label.

† Fat content changes serving counts for fats and oils: for example, 1 tbsp of regular salad dressing equals 1 serving; 1 tbsp of a low-fat dressing equals ½ serving; 1 tbsp of a fat-free dressing equals 0 servings.

From Dietary Approaches to Stop Hypertension. Joint National Committee on Prevention, Detection, Evaluation, and Treatment of High Blood Pressure and the National High Blood Pressure Education Program Coordination Committee: The Sixth Report of the Joint National Committee on Prevention, Detection, Evaluation, and Treatment of High Blood Pressure. Arch Intern Med 157: 2413–2446, 1997.

effect. High amounts of insulin result in more inflammation and a more rapid progression of heart disease.

- The diet is rich in B vitamins and folic acid. Vitamins B_6 and B_{12} and folic acid help reduce homocysteine levels that reduce the risk of heart disease.
- The diet is based on 2000 calories a day. One of the biggest problems of our Western diet is the size of our portions. Combining 2000 calories a day with a regular exercise routine will result in weight loss with benefits beyond the reduction of blood pressure.

COULD THE DASH DIET BE IMPROVED ON?

Cooking Oils

The type of fat may prove to be more important than the amount of fat we eat. The DASH diet does not differentiate between the types of cooking oils. Many vegetable oils consist of partially hydrogenated oils that are a major source of trans-fatty acids. When possible, use monounsaturated oils, such as olive or canola, for cooking.

Butter or Margarine?

For this same reason, using a small amount of butter may be even safer than using the same amount of margarine. Margarine is very high in polyunsaturated fats and butter is high in saturated fats. But if a small amount of each is used, butter may actually be healthier because it has less transfatty acids. More research is needed for a definitive answer.

More Fish Than Red Meat and Poultry

When eating meat, you may have greater benefit if you try to eat fish more than meat or poultry. Fish (particularly cold-water fish like salmon, herring, mackerel, and tuna) is rich in omega-3 fatty acids. These fats have been found to reduce the incidence of heart disease, probably by reducing inflammation that can lead to atherosclerosis.

HOW CAN SOMEONE GET MORE INFORMATION ABOUT THE DASH DIET?

- The National Heart, Lung, and Blood Institute (NHLBI) is a part of the National Institutes of Health (NIH). You can get free information mailed to you or view it over the Internet by visiting: www.nhlbi.nih.gov/health/public/heart/hbp/dash
- This site sponsored by Harvard Medical School is also an excellent source of information: http://dash.bwh.harvard.edu
- Consulting with a nutritionist can provide valuable information on how to incorporate this diet into your lifestyle.

References

1. Appel LJ, Moore TJ, Obarzanek E, et al: A clinical trial of the effects of dietary patterns on blood pressure. N Engl J Med 336:1117–1124, 1997.
2. Appel LJ, Miller ER 3rd, Jee SH, et al: Effect of dietary patterns on serum homocysteine: Results of a randomized, controlled feeding study. Circulation 102:852–857, 2000.

CHAPTER 86

Writing an Exercise Prescription

Michael J. Hewitt, Ph.D.

Regular physical activity, whether recreation, sport, labor, or participation in a structured exercise program, has been demonstrated to enhance function, reduce or prevent age-related physiologic decline, and reduce the risks of a sedentary lifestyle.[1] Most physicians recognize the benefit of exercise and most medical groups recommend regular physical activity.[2] However, because few medical training programs include even an overview of exercise physiology, and few clinical rotations address exercise prescription, it is a rare physician who has experience in the decision-making process associated with recommending physical activity. Practically, prescribing exercise is no different from prescribing medications or therapy; it is a thoughtful compromise between the potential benefits of a treatment and its potential adverse effects.[3]

BASIC PRINCIPLES

Two principles form the framework for making exercise recommendations: the overload principle and the concept of specificity of exercise. The overload principle, based on Hans Selye's general adaptation syndrome model, suggests that the body or physiologic system repeatedly exposed to a stressor of appropriate intensity ultimately adapts to that stressor. To scientists who specialize in exercise, this principle underlies the adaptations that occur after cardiorespiratory conditioning or strength training. Generally, there is an inverted J-curve relationship between the intensity of the stimulus and the physiologic adaptation. For example, resistance or strength work with light weights brings about modest increases in muscular strength, but work with heavier loads results in greater strength gains. Too much load, however, is often associated with injury.

NOTE

The challenge for physicians and their patients is to determine the appropriate exercise intensity for safe achievement of optimal functional enhancement.

Specificity of exercise refers to the relationship between the type of physiologic adaptation and the type of activity performed. It is widely accepted that strength training is beneficial, some say essential, to enhanced performance in most sports. Few collegiate athletic teams do not have a strength coach. However, if one wishes to become a competitive swimmer or an Alpine skier, strength training alone is woefully inadequate. One must spend time in the pool or on the mountain. For similar reasons, sprinters train differently than middle- or long-distance runners. The implication for physicians is that cardiorespiratory health concerns and osteoporosis require different modes of exercise therapy.

THE FIVE COMPONENTS OF FITNESS

- Cardiorespiratory fitness
- Muscular strength and endurance
- Flexibility
- Body composition
- Balance and agility

A useful model for exercise programming is one that addresses five components of fitness: cardiorespiratory or aerobic fitness, muscular strength and endurance, flexibility, body composition, and balance/agility. One could make an argument to include muscular power (i.e., the explosive application of strength), but lack of power is rarely a clinical limitation. Cardiorespiratory condition refers to the ability of the heart, lungs, and vascular network to deliver oxygen to the working muscles. Muscular strength is defined as the maximal ability of the musculoskeletal system to move a heavy load, and muscular endurance is the ability to move that load repeatedly. Flexibility is an index of joint range of motion. Body composition typically refers to the level of body fat, but a measure of fat-free body mass (FFB) is of equal clinical significance. Measurement of bone mineral content is another important component of body composition assessment. Balance and agility are the most frequently overlooked parts of physical function, but they have significant implications for fall prevention and mobility and therefore are very important to aging patients.

There is typically an age-related decline in each of these components (with the exception of percent body fat, which increases with age) that can be attenuated or reversed by appropriate physical activity. In fact, much of the functional decline associated with aging can be more specifically called *disuse atrophy*.

Body Composition

Body composition is the one component of fitness that does not require a specific exercise recommendation. Body composition changes as a consequence of cardiorespiratory exercise and strength training, as well as nutrient intake. However, assessment of body composition is a highly useful tool for determining the way in which patients should devote their limited exercise time. For instance, a man with greater than 25% body fat and a woman with greater than 38% body fat are in a group with a statistically greater risk of heart disease, type 2 diabetes, hyperlipidemia, and hypertension.[4] Exercise programming should attempt to specifically address those risks as well as help reduce the level of body fat.

Quantifying FFB further refines the exercise prescription. Many adults are at an appropriate weight based on height/weight scales or body mass index (BMI: height in m^2/weight in kg), but are *underlean*, as indicated by a lower than optimal FFB. Generally, cardiorespiratory exercise results in a reduction of percent body fat, but has limited impact on FFB. In contrast, strength training increases FFB (as well as muscular strength) and metabolic rate, ultimately resulting in a reduction in percent body fat. Most morbidly obese patients have developed adequate FFB simply to transport themselves and gain limited benefit from strength training, but they respond favorably to cardiorespiratory activity. Smaller individuals who fall within height/weight guidelines but who also have excess body fat benefit most by combining cardiorespiratory and strength programs.

The determination of bone mineral content (BMC, g) or bone mineral density (BMD, g/cm^2) allows for a superior level of exercise programming, in terms of both efficacy and safety. Dual-energy x-ray absorptiometry (DEXA) is considered the new gold standard for simultaneously determining percent body fat, FFB, and BMC. Its drawbacks are that the technique requires expensive equipment, and patients experience a small radiation exposure. However, DEXA is fast, accurate, and reliable, and it is not dependent on patient skill (as is underwater weighing). Several other field techniques can be effectively administered in a physician's office; these provide useful body composition data, but each method has its own limitations. A discussion of body composition assessment methodology is beyond the scope of this text, but readers are referred to three excellent summaries.[4–6]

> **NOTE**
>
> *Dual-energy x-ray absorptiometry (DEXA) determines percentage of body fat, fat-free body mass (FFB), and bone mineral content (BMC).*

THE FITT PRINCIPLE FOR EXERCISE PROGRAMMING

For cardiorespiratory conditioning, strength training, flexibility, and balance/agility training, a simple exercise prescription tool is the FITT principle. FITT is an acronym for:

- Frequency
- Intensity
- Type
- Time (duration)

These are the four variables of physical activity that must be considered in exercise programming. Physicians who recommend exercise should consider these factors, and should write a prescription specifically addressing each (Table 86–1). For example, individuals with elevated risk for heart disease should be encouraged to improve their cardiorespiratory condition. The *type* of exercise can include walking, jogging, or running, either outdoors or on a treadmill, bicycling, swimming, hiking, aerobics, use of any of a variety of aerobic machines (stairclimbers, rowing machines, cycle ergometers, etc.), dance, tennis, and so forth. The possibilities go on and on. The decision is affected by geographic concerns (cycling in the Midwest during January is difficult) and economic limitations (the patient who cannot afford a treadmill or the cost of participation in a fitness center), but the primary factor is patient preference. Equipment manufacturers often promote their devices based on the efficiency and effectiveness of the workout they provide. In reality, much of the inherent advantage of one type of exercise device over another is irrelevant when patients miss exercise sessions because they simply do not like the activity! The very best cardiorespiratory exercise is one that the patient will do. Of course, a patient with knee limitations may not tolerate distance running, and a woman with severe osteoporosis should not be advised to take up ice skating.

In 1998, the American College of Sports Medicine (ACSM) published a position stand on the recommended quantity and quality of exercise[7] that is an excellent reference and should be in the library of any health professional who recommends physical activity. In this position stand, *quantity* refers to the frequency and duration, and *quality* to the intensity, of physical activity.

CARDIORESPIRATORY TRAINING

The frequency of cardiorespiratory training is more often limited by patient compliance than by physiol-

Table 86–1. Exercise Prescription

Fitness Component	Type(s)	Frequency	Duration	Intensity
Cardiorespiratory Fitness	_____	_____ d/wk	_____ min	___ to ___ beats/min
	_____			___ to ___ RPE
Strength	___ Free weights		_____ min	
	___ Machines	_____ d/wk		_____ reps
	___ Floor work		_____ sets	
	___ Elastic resistance bands			
Flexibility	Static stretch	_____ d/wk	_____ sec	Hold below pain threshold
			_____ reps	
Balance and agility	_____	_____ d/wk	_____ min	_____
	_____			

Comments/progression: _____

_____

_____ Signature: _____

Key: RPE, rating of perceived exertion

ogy. It is not inappropriate for one to exercise daily, but few people do. The ACSM recommends a frequency of 3 to 5 days per week for cardiorespiratory fitness and body composition enhancement, and a duration of 20 to 60 minutes of continuous or intermittent exercise. Intermittent exercise is described as a minimum of 10-minute bouts accumulated throughout the day. In healthy adults, the recommended intensity is from 65% to 90% of maximum heart rate (HR_{max}); this recommended range is 55% to 64% in very unfit individuals. The challenge, of course, is to know maximal heart rate. Graded exercise tests rarely continue to exhaustion; therefore, they do not provide a true HR_{max}, and prediction equations for HR_{max} (e.g., 220 − age) lack sufficient precision to be clinically useful. A maximal or submaximal exercise tolerance test performed by an exercise physiologist can provide a useful estimate of HR_{max} and a target heart range (HR). It should be noted that graded exercise stress tests can identify hypertensive responses to activity and clinically significant electrocardiogram (ECG) abnormalities with exercise, and are thereby highly useful for providing a safe and effective cardiorespiratory exercise intensity range for at-risk patients. In healthy adults, heart rate is not essential for monitoring exercise intensity. The Borg scale[8] (Table 86–2) has been demonstrated to be an effective tool for monitoring cardiorespiratory exercise intensity. Healthy adults should maintain a subjective rating of perceived exertion (RPE) of "moderate" to "heavy," or about 13 to 15 on the scale. Beginners can improve compliance by limiting intensity to "Light" to "Moderate" (RPE: 11–13). It is not uncommon for athletes to reach "very, very heavy" (RPE: 19–20) for short bursts, particularly during interval training such as wind sprints and line drills, but there is little reason to recommend these levels for patients.

Another approach to recommending appropriate cardiorespiratory exercise intensity is based on the measured energy cost of the activity, reported in metabolic equivalents (METs). One MET is defined as the energy expenditure of sitting quietly, about 1 kcal · kg body weight^{-1} · hr^{-1}, and requires about 3.5 mL of oxygen · kg body weight^{-1} · min^{-1}.[10] Level walk-

Table 86–2. Borg Scale of Perceived Exertion

Number	Exertion Level
6	
7	Very, very light
8	
9	Very light
10	
11	Light
12	
13	Moderate
14	
15	Heavy
16	
17	Very heavy
18	
19	Very, very heavy
20	

From Borg GA: Psychophysical bases of perceived exertion. Med Sci Sports Exerc 14(5):377–381, 1982.

ing on a firm surface at 3.5 mph is rated at 3.5 METs, and running at 7 mph (8.5 miles · min⁻¹) is 11.5 METs. A listing of the MET level of more than 400 recreational and occupational activities has been compiled.[10] This compendium provides a simple comparison of the energy costs of activity and allows physicians to suggest several equivalent options. Its utility is further enhanced if a graded exercise test has been performed to quantify the patient's effective and maximal MET capacity.

RESISTANCE TRAINING

The same FITT principle can be applied to resistance (weight) training. The ACSM suggests that one set of 8 to 10 weight exercises that work all major muscle groups should be performed 2 to 3 days per week. A weight load that causes muscular fatigue in 8 to 12 repetitions is recommended. Older or frail individuals may find lighter weights that allow 10 to 15 repetitions to be more appropriate.[7] A second or third set may be advantageous if time and patient interest permit, but the majority of the benefit is derived in the first set.[9] Although many physicians refer patients for an initial session with an exercise physiologist, physical therapist, or personal fitness trainer to get the specifics of a strength training program, a program can be designed based on general advice.[11] Flexibility and balance/agility recommendations also follow the FITT principle.

LEVELS OF EXERCISE PRESCRIPTION

When prescribing exercise, it is useful for the health care provider to determine the patient's desired outcome. Strategies exist to help patients overcome their physical and psychological barriers to exercise compliance.[12] Individuals hoping to reduce disease risk may have a different level of

Table 86–3. Basics of Exercise Prescription for a Range of Health and Fitness Goals

Fitness Component	Disease Prevention	Basic Health	Enhanced Fitness	Performance
Cardiorespiratory fitness	Accumulate 30+ min of physical activity most days	Large-muscle repetitive exercise@ 20+ min, 3+ times/wk	Aerobic exercise or equivalent sports activity 40–60+ min, 4–6 times/wk	Add competition and/or interval training
Strength	Include weight-bearing activity	"Core Four" or equivalent program. One set, 2 times/wk, 8–12 or 12–15 reps to challenge weight*	Balanced whole-body free weight or machine program 1–3 sets, 8–12 reps to functional failure†	Add ascending or descending pyramids,‡ muscle endurance, or power training, Pilates work
Flexibility	Bend and stretch in daily activities	Perform 2–4 stretches after activity, 1 rep, hold ∼ 30 sec	Perform 6–10+ whole-body stretches before and after activity, 1–2+ repetitions	Add yoga, Pilates, and/or facilitated stretches with a partner
Body composition Men:		≥ 5%–≤ 25% fat Maintain fat-free body mass at ≥ 125–150+lb	12%–20% fat	8%–15% fat
Women:		≥ 14%–≤ 38% fat Maintain fat-free body mass at ≥ 90–110+lb	20%–30% fat	17%–25% fat
Balance and agility		"Act like a child," balance line, "Don't step on a crack"; brush teeth while standing on one foot	Recreational sports (e.g., tennis, biking); tai chi; social dance; therapy ball training	Agility or skill sports (e.g., skiing, skating, surfing); martial arts; performance dance; agility drills

* Challenge weight: The weight is difficult; just one or two additional repetitions could be accomplished.
† Functional failure: Unable to complete another repetition without sacrificing lifting form.
‡ Ascending pyramids: More weight is added after each set to cause fatigue in fewer repetitions. Descending pyramids: Weight is removed after each set to allow more repetitions until fatigue.

From Kligman EW, Hewitt MJ, Crowell DL: Recommending exercise to healthy older adults: The preparticipation evaluation and exercise prescription. Physician Sportsmed 27(11):42–62, 1999.

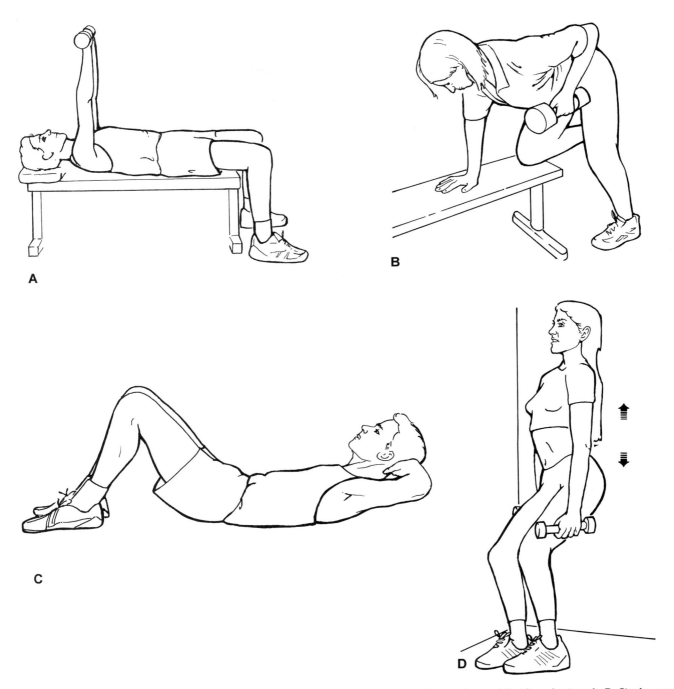

Figure 86–1. Core Four exercises. A, Supine bench press (pectoralis major and minor, anterior deltoid, and triceps). B, Single arm dumbbell row (trapezius, latissimus dorsi, and biceps). C, Abdominal crunch (rectus abdominis). D, Dumbbell squat (quadriceps, hamstrings, and gluteals).

commitment than others who seek physical fitness or athletic performance. Table 86–3 summarizes exercise recommendations for several levels in the cardiorespiratory, strength, flexibility, body composition, and balance/agility areas.[3] General recommendations for body fat and FFB at each level are also reported; however, body composition standards are subject to significant individual variation. A useful approach is to encourage patients to perform at least the recommended activity for the pre-

vention of disease, and to strive to consistently exercise at the "Basic Health" level. When these patterns become habitual, one should encourage physical activity at the level to achieve "Enhanced Fitness" (see Table 86–3).

Effective exercise programming provides guidelines for variety and allows for a progression of activity. The programs of long-term participants bear little resemblance to those of new exercisers. Compliance is enhanced if the initial program is broad enough and sufficiently challenging to effect measurable improvement, but compact enough to fit within a patient's busy schedule. An experienced physician or exercise physiologist will develop a small starting program and suggest a progression over a specific time frame. One may start with a 10-minute walking or bicycle ergometer program three times weekly, and progress to 20 minutes four times each week within 2 or 3 months, ultimately striving for 40 minutes or longer on most days.

THE "CORE FOUR" STRENGTH PROGRAM (Fig. 86–1)

In strength work, a simple starting program such as the "Core Four"[3] allows a basic whole-body strength workout to be completed in less than 10 minutes. Few patients have an effective argument for why they cannot find 10 minutes for strength work twice a week. The Core Four can be performed using weight machines, inexpensive handheld dumbbells, or even elastic resistance bands, making equipment and space limitations moot. The four exercises are the double-leg press machine or dumbbell squat (quadriceps, hamstrings, gluteals), which can be performed against the wall for additional support; the chest press machine or supine dumbbell bench press (pectoralis major and minor, anterior deltoid, triceps brachii); either the lateral pulldown or seated row machine or the single-arm dumbbell row (trapezius, latissimus dorsii, and biceps brachii); and the abdominal crunch (rectus abdominis). These four exercises work approximately 85% of the muscular system. Although body-builders might scoff at a basic program such as the Core Four, even smaller series of lifts have been demonstrated to rapidly improve strength, muscle mass, and mobility in older adults,[13, 14] and these core exercises form the framework for more sophisticated lifting regimens.

BALANCE AND AGILITY

Balance and agility are the most often overlooked components of fitness, yet poor balance and its associated fall risk are potentially the greatest health concerns for many older adults. Balance and agility require a rapid central nervous system response to signals from the inner ears (vestibular signals), eyes (visual signals), and postural muscles in the legs and back (proprioceptive signals). Although some deterioration in the quality of these signals occurs with age, it is primarily a slower rate of integration and response by the central nervous system (CNS) that appears to cause the loss of function (disuse atrophy). Function loss is insidious. Low function results in reduced confidence, which leads to avoidance of balance challenges; further reduction in function follows in a destructive cycle. Even highly skilled athletes lose function rapidly if they fail to practice. Balance and agility can be restored by safely challenging the system with appropriate exercises. Tai chi, dance, and simple balance exercises such as standing on one foot while brushing teeth or hair provide effective signals to stimulate CNS adaptation. In severe cases, ai chi, a form of tai chi performed in a swimming pool, provides a no-falling-risk stimulus to the balance control system. Sports such as tennis or bicycling are greater challenges, and are associated with both greater risk and greater potential for improvement. High-level activities, including skiing, skating, and martial arts, are appropriate for a select group of patients.

— *THERAPEUTIC REVIEW* —

The ACSM provides guidelines[15] that illustrate the standard of care and prove invaluable for clinicians and physiologists who make exercise recommendations. Additionally, the College provides a resource manual to support the guidelines, which includes background summaries in applied anatomy, exercise physiology, exercise testing and programming, emergency procedures, terminology, and more.[16]

A comprehensive exercise program has a synergistic effect. Improved strength in the postural muscles is reflected in improved balance because those muscles can better respond to signals from the balance centers. Better cardiorespiratory conditioning allows for a more challenging strength-training program, and improved body composition allows greater range of motion for more effective stretching. Equally important, enhanced function allows for greater participation, usually resulting in better compliance. Exercise prescription need not be complicated; virtually any activity has positive effects. The key is to gently challenge each of the physiologic systems in such a way as to allow patients to experience enhanced function and then encourage patients to modestly increase the stimulus.

References

1. U.S. Department of Health and Human Services: Physical Activity and Health: A Report of the Surgeon General. Atlanta, Centers for Disease Control and Prevention, 1996.
2. U.S. Preventative Services Task Force: Guide to Clinical Preventive Services, 2nd ed. Baltimore, Williams and Wilkins, 1996.
3. Kligman EW, Hewitt MJ, Crowell DL: Recommending exercise to healthy older adults: The preparticipation evaluation and exercise prescription. Physician Sportsmed 27:42–62, 1999.
4. Lohman TG: Advances in Body Composition Assessment. Champaign, Ill, Human Kinetics, 1992.
5. Lohman TG, Roche AF, Martorell R: Anthropometric Standardization Reference Manual. Champaign, Ill, Human Kinetics, 1988.
6. Lohman TG, Houtkooper L, Going SB: Body fat measurement goes high-tech; not all are created equal. ACSM Health Fitness J 1:30–35, 1997.
7. ACSM: Position stand on the recommended quantity and quality of exercise for developing and maintaining cardiorespiratory and muscular fitness and flexibility in healthy adults. Med Sci Sports Exerc 30:975–991, 1998.
8. Borg GA: Psychophysical bases of perceived exertion. Med Sci Sports Exerc 14:377–381, 1982.
9. Pollock ML, Abe T, De Hoyos DV, et al: Muscular hypertrophy responses to 6 months of high- or low-volume resistance training. Med Sci Sports Exerc 30:S116, 1998.
10. Ainsworth BE, Haskell WL, Leon AS, et al: Compendium of physical activities: Classification of energy costs of human physical activities. Med Sci Sports Exerc 2:71–80, 1992.
11. Fleck SJ, Kraemer WJ: Designing Resistance Training Programs. Champaign, Ill, Human Kinetics, 1987.
12. Dunlap J, Barry HC: Overcoming exercise barriers in older adults. Physician Sportsmed 27:69–75, 1999.
13. Fiatarone MA, Evans WJ: Exercise in the oldest old. Top Geriatr Rehabil 5:63–77, 1990.
14. Fiatarone MA, Marks EC, Ryan ND, et al: High-intensity strength training in nonagenarians: Effects on skeletal muscle. JAMA 263:3029–3034, 1990.
15. ACSM Guidelines for Exercise Testing and Prescription, 6th edition. Indianapolis, Lippincott, Williams & Wilkins, 2000.
16. Roitman JL (ed): Resource Manual for Guidelines for Exercise Testing and Prescription, 4th ed. Indianapolis, Lippincott, Williams & Wilkins, 1998.

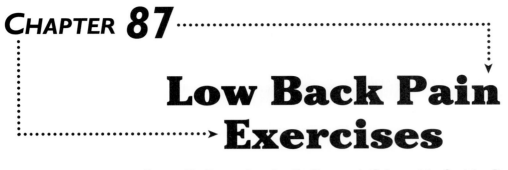

CHAPTER 87

Low Back Pain Exercises

Brian F. Degenhardt, D.O., and Coleen M. Smith, D.O.

EXERCISE IN LOW BACK PAIN

Patients who seek treatment for low back pain can be difficult to manage for any practitioner. The etiology can be from the skin, soft tissue, or skeletal components. Low back pain can be referred from other sources, even visceral structures, or can be secondary to postural decompensation.

The history and physical examination should guide the practitioner to further evaluation and treatment. Multidisciplinary treatment approaches are often necessary to facilitate healing for the patient with low back pain. Understanding the patients' belief systems about their low back pain may be an important component of their recovery.[1] A treatment plan may include an exercise prescription. The benefit of exercise in recovery from acute lumbar back pain is questionable, whereas the use of strengthening and flexibility exercises in patients with chronic lumbar back pain has demonstrated benefit.[2]

NOTE

Back pain may herald other diseases. Listen to the patient and perform a complete examination to make the most accurate diagnosis for the underlying cause of the pain syndrome.

The traditional exercise prescription includes a written description of the exercise, including the number of repetitions per set, number of sets per session, and frequency of sessions. This format is specific for strength exercises and has been applied to flexibility exercises. Many traditional exercise routines are assigned and performed too literally, without recognition of the subtle changes the patient experiences from day to day in a healing exercise program. The goal of any complementary exercise recommendation is to encourage a dynamic interchange between the patient's mind and body. With appropriate education, the patient can become more sensitive to information being generated from the body and can perform the exercise program in a much more precise, safe, and effective manner. Attention to the body's feedback mechanisms should be encouraged to allow the patient to modify any portion of the exercise prescription. This allows the patient to achieve optimal outcomes from the rehabilitation program. The outcomes of an exercise plan are to enhance flexibility, minimize or eliminate pain by reducing muscle tension, and improve strength, thereby encouraging joint stability. A complementary exercise plan for a person with lumbar back pain should include the following approaches:

1. Breathing and Relaxation Training
2. Flexibility Training
3. Strength Training
4. Coordination Training

Breathing and Relaxation Training

Flexibility and relaxation techniques are often great starting points in a patient's exercise prescription. They calm the patient and foster awareness of information from the body that helps guide and individualize the exercise prescription. These exercises enhance diaphragmatic function and improve oxygenation, lymphatic flow, and autonomic nervous system regulation. To begin this component of the exercise prescription, the patient should get into a comfortable position and minimize distraction, perhaps by listening to soothing background music. While taking a slow, deep breath, the patient needs to use the abdominal diaphragm, and, as inspiration continues, both the diaphragm and the rib cage (see chapter 88, Breathing Exercises). The number of repetitions is likely to vary from day to day because stress and tightness also vary daily. The patient needs to learn how to recognize when the body is relaxed and ready to move on to other components of the exercise prescription. Once relaxation and focus have been obtained, participants should use deep breathing throughout all cycles of the exercise plan.

> ### NOTE
> *Encouraging patients to pay attention to messages within their body during their exercise session will empower them to perform the most precise, effective, and safe exercise program.*

Flexibility Training

The flexibility portion of an exercise plan uses stretching to promote increased range of motion in all planes. Properly performed, stretching allows for better neuromusculoskeletal function, promoting less pain and more motion. To stretch properly, the patient needs to go to the point of tension and perform deep breaths to gently stretch the tight tissue. It is important to go slowly and gently in and out of stretches. There are other models describing how to stretch, but this approach minimizes the chance of exacerbating the patient's back pain by overstretching. Although an outline of a stretch gives the patient a guide for promoting flexibility for specific areas of the body, the patient listens each day to the information the body is generating to determine where the tightness is present. This allows the patient to modify a stretch and maximize its effectiveness each day. The stretch is considered complete only after the patient appreciates a change in the tension while holding the stretch. This can occur after only one or two repetitions, or it may need more repetitions as determined by the patient via attention to the body's feedback system. It must be emphasized that patients stay within pain limitations to prevent reflex muscle tightening and injury.

In most chronic low back pain patients, specific instruction is necessary for hip flexors and extensors. Achieving increased flexibility as well as a balance of flexibility between the same muscles on both sides of the body and between reciprocal muscles, particularly with the hamstring, iliopsoas, and piriformis muscles, is also important for recovering muscle tightness and decreasing pain.

Strength Training

Strengthening exercises encourage active use of muscle groups and lead to increased muscle tone and strength. It is important not to sacrifice flexibility for strength; the two are equally important for proper lumbar mechanics in patients with low back pain. Evaluation of strength can be performed clinically by having the patient perform isometric contractions against a physician's resistance to determine whether there is gross asymmetry of strength. Asymmetry of strength may lead to hypertonicity in one muscle group and weakness in opposing muscle groups. Once strength asymmetry or weakness has been diagnosed, specific instructions

must be given to first stretch the hypertonic muscles and then motivate the patients to exercise the weakened muscles. Patients are often unaware of this local muscle weakness. In many exercise programs, patients focus on rote repetition of exercises that strengthen hypertonic muscles rather than conditioning weakened muscle groups. In the case of hypertonic lumbar extensors, it can be beneficial to have patients perform abdominal curlups to strengthen weakened antagonistic abdominal muscles after stretching the lumbar erector spinae. Both exercises will lead to a decreased hypertonicity in the lumbar extensor muscle group.

In many cases of lumbar back pain, strengthening activities must start as isometric exercises instead of typical isotonic exercises, because isometric exercises are safer. Isometric stretching allows the origin and insertion of the involved muscle to remain in constant position while the patient presses against a resisting force that is equal to the patient's force. An example of an isometric exercise is pushing against a solid wall without moving. Isometric exercises are often useful for patients who have arthritis in which joint movement causes pain and limitation.

Coordination Training

Differences in proprioception exist in individuals with and without back pain. Coordination training in low back pain patients is based on the observation that the response of a patient's spine to stress causes the postural muscles to tighten and the antagonist muscles to react by inhibition, weakness, and atrophy.[3] Coordination training is imperative for improving overall postural balance in the patient with lumbar back pain. Proprioceptive education of patients with low back pain begins with improving ankle, knee, and pelvic coordination. Having the patient use a wobble board or fitness ball can achieve this. Remind the patient of safety precautions when coordination training is initiated. Usually, basic coordination exercises can be taught in the office and performed by the patient independently. Advanced proprioceptive training usually requires supervision to ensure correct technique and safety.

> ### NOTE
> *Encourage the patient to use all treatment modalities for recovery from low back pain.*

Further Resources

Stretching by Bob Anderson is an excellent resource for complete stretching advice. www.enteract.com is a Web source for patients, which describes specific stretches for all body regions.
Pain Free: A Revolutionary Method for Stopping Chronic Pain by Pete Egoscue has many stretches described for the lay person.
Foundations for Osteopathic Medicine, edited by Robert Ward, D.O.,

is a text on exercise and neuromusculoskeletal system retraining.

Exercise in Health and Disease by Michael Pollock, Ph.D., and Jack Wilmore, Ph.D., is a comprehensive text about exercise.

Exercise and Osteopathic Manipulative Medicine: The Janda Approach by P. Jones, D.O., and M. Tomski, M.D. (Physical Medicine and Rehabilitation: State of the Art Reviews vol/14, (1) Philadelphia, Hanley and Belfus, 2000.) is a concise article on rehabilitation exercises for each back muscle group.

References

1. Pfingsten M, Hildebrandt J, Leibing E, et al: Effectiveness of a multimodal treatment program for chronic low-back pain. Pain 222–223, 1998.
2. Van Tulder, Maurits, Malmivaara, et al. Exercise therapy of low back pain: A systemic review within the framework of the Cochrane collaboration back review group. Spine 25:2784–2796, 2000.
3. Pollock ML, Wilmore JH: Exercise in Health and Disease, 2nd ed. Philadelphia, W.B. Saunders, 1990.

Exercise Program for Low Back

1. Listen to your body signals; the dose of exercise may vary from day to day. Always stay within pain limitations when performing exercises.
2. It is important to breathe properly and into your abdomen during all aspects of your exercise program.
3. Move slowly and gently during stretching exercises. Do not bounce!
4. Repeat the stretch until you perceive relaxation in the intended muscle group.
5. If you experience pain during or after a specific exercise, the dose and frequency should be reduced.

BREATHING AND RELAXATION EXERCISES

Breathing and Body Stretch (Fig. 87–1)

1. Lie on your back. Place your hands on your abdomen.
2. Breathe deeply into your abdomen so that your hands rise and fall with each breath.
3. Repeat slowly and gently for 2 minutes.
4. Place your arms above your head and reach upward as you point your toes downward.
5. Hold the stretch for 5 slow, deep breaths.
6. Slowly return to the starting position and repeat the stretch twice.

STRETCHING EXERCISES

Pelvic Tilt Exercise (Fig. 87–2)

1. Lie on your back. Bend your knees and place your feet flat on the floor, allow your knees to touch.
2. Rock your pelvis backward by flattening your lower back against the floor.
3. Hold this position for 20 to 40 seconds, or until fatigued, while breathing slowly and deeply.
4. Release slowly. Repeat twice.

Low Back Flexion Exercise (Fig. 87–3)

1. Sit. Roll your head, neck, chest, and low back

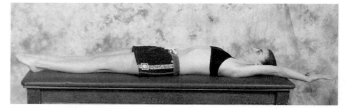

Figure 87–1

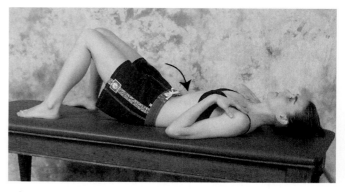

Figure 87–2

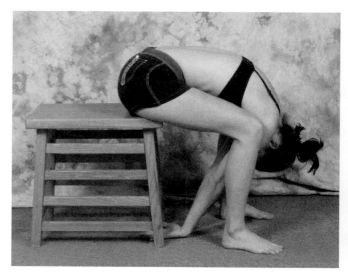

Figure 87–3

forward between your knees. Roll as far forward as is comfortable and painless.
2. Hold position through 3 deep breaths or until fatigue is noted.
3. Gently return to a sitting pose.
4. Repeat 2 times.

Low Back Extension Exercise (Fig. 87–4)

1. Lie on your stomach, with feet separated the width of the shoulders and toes pointing downward.
2. Bring the elbows under your shoulders to support your weight.
3. Gently raise your head and slowly arch your back. Go only as far as is painless until your muscles are more flexible.
4. Hold the position and breathe into the abdomen for at least three deep breaths or until the tightness in your back releases.
5. Repeat 2 times.

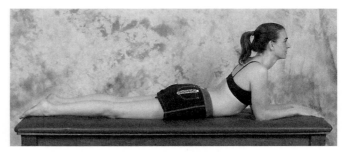

Figure 87–4

Cat/Dog Stretch Exercise (Fig. 87–5)

1. Kneel on the floor with your knees apart the width of the hips. Place your hands apart on the floor the width of the shoulders, with palms down.
2. Slowly arch your back from the tailbone to your upper back as a cat stretches. Allow your head to lower comfortably. Hold this position for three slow breaths.
3. Slowly release the stretch in the reverse order.
4. Once in the starting position, lift your buttocks upward, let your stomach sag to the floor, and slowly look toward the ceiling.
5. Hold this position for three breaths and gradually return to the starting position.
6. Repeat gently two times.

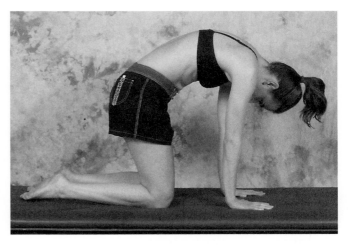

Figure 87–5

Hip Flexor Stretch Exercise (Fig. 87–6)

1. Kneel on one knee. Bend your other knee to 90 degrees and place your hands on it for balance.
2. Lean your trunk forward while keeping your low back straight.
3. Hold this position for three slow breaths and slowly return to the starting position.
4. Repeat two times.

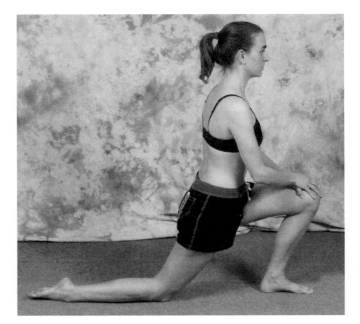

Figure 87–6

Piriformis Exercise (Fig. 87–7)

1. Lie on your back with your legs straight. To stretch the left side, bend your left knee and place your left ankle over your right knee with the left foot on floor.
2. Place your left hand on the left side of the pelvis and your right hand on your left knee.
3. Slowly pull your left knee across the right leg, feeling the stretch in your left buttock. Keep your pelvis from rotating with your left hand.
4. Hold this position for at least three slow, deep breaths.
5. Slowly and gently return to the resting position.
6. Repeat steps one through six two times.
7. Repeat on the opposite side.

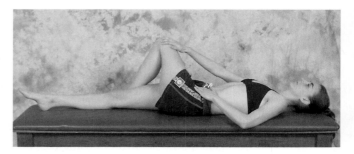

Figure 87–7

Hamstring Exercise (Fig. 87–8)

1. Lie on your back with your legs straight.
2. Gently bend your knee and grasp behind the thigh. Do not lift your pelvis or other knee off the floor during this exercise.
3. Straighten your knee. Go only as far as your flexibility comfortably allows and hold this position for three slow breaths.
4. Slowly lower your leg to the floor and repeat for the opposite leg.
5. Repeat each side three times.

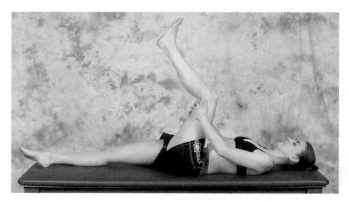

Figure 87–8

STRENGTH EXERCISES

Abdominal Curl-Up Exercise (Fig. 87–9)

1. Lie on your back with your knees comfortably bent and your arms placed across your chest.
2. Keeping your neck and shoulders relaxed, lift your rib cage from the table. Move only as far as your body allows without pain. Hold this position for three deep breaths.
3. Slowly and gently return to resting position.
4. Repeat two times and increase repetitions as tolerated.

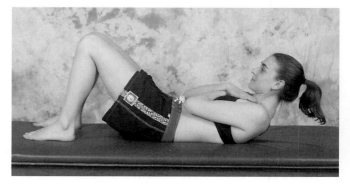

Figure 87–9

Gluteus Maximus Exercise (Fig. 87–10)

1. Lie on your stomach with your toes pointing downward.
2. Slowly raise your straight leg as far as is comfortable. Keep your pelvis flat on the floor and keep your buttocks tight.
3. Hold this position for three deep breaths or until your muscles feel fatigued.
4. Gently return to the resting position.
5. Repeat two times and increase repetitions as tolerated.

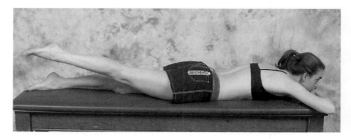

Figure 87–10

Gluteus Medius Exercise (Fig. 87–11)

1. Lie on your side. Press your upper arm to the floor for stability, if necessary.
2. Raise your upper leg as far as is comfortable and painless.
3. Hold this position for three slow breaths and slowly return your leg to the resting position.
4. Repeat two times and increase repetitions as tolerated.

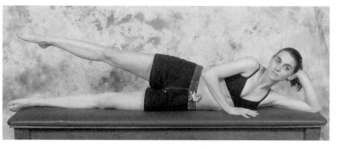

Figure 87–11

COORDINATION EXERCISES

Standing on One Leg Exercise

1. Stand on one leg and maintain your balance. Keep your back straight and your arms across your upper chest.
2. Hold this position 1 minute while continuing to take slow, deep breaths.
3. Gently return to resting position and repeat two times.
4. After mastering this exercise, perform step 2 with your eyes closed.

Rocker Board Exercise (Fig. 87–12)

1. Place your feet parallel on the rocker board and maintain your balance.
2. Close your eyes and maintain your balance
3. Hold this position for 1 minute while continuing to take slow breaths.
4. Gently step off the board.

Advanced Rocker Board Exercise

1. Place your feet parallel on the rocker board.
2. Hold this position for 1 minute while continuing to take slow breaths.
3. Arrange your feet so that one is in front of the other by a half step.
4. Hold this position for 1 minute while continuing to take slow breaths.
5. Gently step off the board.
6. After mastering this exercise perform steps 2 and 5 with your eyes closed.

Ball Coordination Exercise

1. Sit on a large ball with your feet on the floor and maintain your balance.
2. Hold this position comfortably for 1 minute while adjusting to changes that you feel.
3. Lift your foot for 20 to 40 seconds while remaining relaxed and maintaining your balance.
4. Repeat for the other foot.
5. Gently rise from the ball.

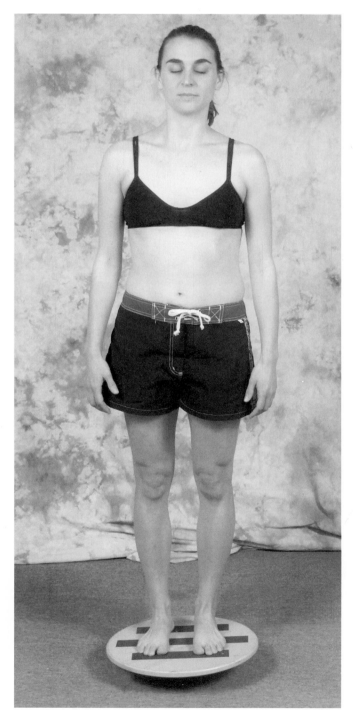

Figure 87–12

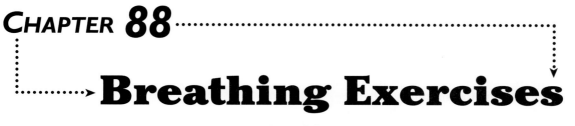

CHAPTER 88

Breathing Exercises

David Rakel, M.D.

BREATHING AS A BRIDGE

It is thought by many cultures that the process of breathing is the essence of being. A rhythmic process of expansion and contraction, breathing is one example of the consistent polarity we see in nature—night and day, wake and sleep, seasonal growth and decay, and ultimately, life and death. In yoga, the breath is known as *prana* or a universal energy that can be used to find a balance between the body-mind, the conscious-unconscious, and the sympathetic-parasympathetic nervous system. Unlike other bodily functions, the breath is easily used to communicate between these systems, which gives us an excellent tool to help facilitate positive change. It is the only bodily function we do both voluntarily and involuntarily. We can consciously use breathing to influence the involuntary (sympathetic nervous) system that regulates blood pressure, heart rate, circulation, digestion, and many other bodily functions. *Pranayama* is a yoga practice that literally means the control of life or energy. It uses breathing techniques to change subtle energies within the body for health and well-being. Breathing exercises can act as a bridge into those functions of the body over which we generally do not have conscious control.

AN EXAMPLE OF HOW LIFE AFFECTS PHYSIOLOGY

During times of emotional stress, our sympathetic nervous system is stimulated and affects a number of physical responses. Our heart rate rises, we perspire, our muscles tense, and our breathing becomes rapid and shallow. If this process happens over a long period of time, the sympathetic nervous system becomes overstimulated, leading to an imbalance that can affect our physical health resulting in inflammation, high blood pressure, and muscle pain, to name a few. Consciously slowing our heart rate, decreasing perspiration, and relaxing muscles is more difficult than simply slowing and deepening breathing. The breath can be used to directly influence these stressful changes, causing a direct stimu-lation of the parasympathetic nervous system, resulting in relaxation and a reversal of the changes seen with the stimulation of the sympathetic nervous system. We can see how our bodies know to do this naturally when we take a deep breath or sigh when a stress is relieved.

THE BREATHING PROCESS CAN BE TRAINED

Breathing can be trained for both positive and negative influences on health. Chronic stress can lead to a restriction of the connective and muscular tissue in the chest, resulting in a decreased range of motion of the chest wall. Owing to rapid, more shallow breathing, the chest does not expand as much as it would with slower, deeper breaths, and much of the air exchange occurs at the top of the lung tissue, toward the head. This results in "chest" breathing. You can see if you are a chest breather by placing your right hand on your chest and your left hand on your abdomen. As you breathe, see which hand rises more. If your right hand rises more, you are a chest breather. If your left hand rises more, you are an abdomen breather.

Chest breathing is inefficient because the greatest amount of blood flow occurs in the lower lobes of the lungs, areas that have limited air expansion in chest breathers. Rapid, shallow, chest breathing results in less oxygen transfer to the blood and subsequent poor delivery of nutrients to the tissues. The good news is that, similar to learning to play an instrument or ride a bike, you can train the body to improve its breathing technique. With regular practice, you will breathe from the abdomen most of the time, even while asleep.

NOTE

Using and learning proper breathing techniques is one of the most beneficial things that can be done for both short-term and long-term physical and emotional health.

THE BENEFITS OF ABDOMINAL BREATHING

Abdominal breathing is also known as diaphragmatic breathing. The diaphragm is a large muscle located between the chest and the abdomen. When it contracts, it is forced downward, causing the abdomen to expand. This produces a negative pressure within the chest, forcing air into the lungs. The negative pressure also pulls blood into the chest, improving the venous return to the heart. This leads to improved stamina in both disease and athletic activity. Like blood, the flow of lymph, which is rich in immune cells, is also improved. By expanding the lung's air pockets and improving the flow of blood and lymph, abdominal breathing also helps prevent infection of the lung and other tissues. But most of all, it is an excellent tool to stimulate the relaxation response that results in less tension and an overall sense of well-being.

Abdominal Breathing Technique

Breathing exercises such as this one should be done twice a day or whenever you find your mind dwelling on upsetting thoughts or when you are experiencing pain.

- Place one hand on your chest and the other on your abdomen. When you take a deep breath in, the hand on the abdomen should rise higher than the one on the chest. This ensures that the diaphragm is pulling air into the bases of the lungs.
- After exhaling through the mouth, take a slow deep breath in through your nose, imagining that you are sucking in all the air in the room, and hold it for a count of 7 (or as long as you are able, not exceeding 7).
- Slowly exhale through your mouth for a count of 8. As all the air is released with relaxation, gently contract your abdominal muscles to completely evacuate the remaining air from the lungs. It is important to remember that we deepen respirations not by inhaling more air but through completely exhaling it.
- Repeat the cycle four more times for a total of five deep breaths.

Once you feel comfortable with this technique, you may want to incorporate words that can enhance the exercise. Examples would be to say to yourself the word "relaxation" (with inhalation) and "stress" or "anger" (with exhalation). The idea being to bring in the feeling/emotion you want with inhalation and release those you do not want with exhalation.

In general, exhalation should be twice as long as inhalation. The use of the hands on the chest and abdomen is needed only to help you train your breathing. Once you feel comfortable with your ability to breathe into the abdomen, they are no longer needed.

Abdominal breathing is just one of many breathing exercises. But it is the most important one to learn before exploring other techniques. The more it is practiced, the more natural it will become, improving the body's internal rhythm.

Using Breathing Exercises to Increase Energy

If practiced over time, the abdominal breathing exercise can result in improved energy throughout the day, but sometimes we are in need of a quick "pickup." The bellows breathing exercise (also called the stimulating breath) can be used during times of fatigue that may result from driving over distances or when you need to be revitalized at work. It should not be used in place of abdominal breathing but in addition as a tool to increase energy when needed. This breathing exercise is opposite that of abdominal breathing. Short, fast, rhythmic breaths are used to increase energy, which are similar to the chest breathing we do when under stress. The bellows breath re-creates the adrenal stimulation that occurs with stress and results in the release of energizing chemicals such as epinephrine. As with most bodily functions, this serves an active purpose, but overuse results in adverse effects, as discussed previously.

The Bellows Breathing Technique (The Stimulating Breath)

This yogic technique can be used to help stimulate energy when needed. It is a good thing to use before reaching for a cup of coffee.

- Sit in a comfortable upright position with your spine straight.
- With your mouth gently closed, breath in and out of your nose as fast as possible. To give an idea of how this is done, think of someone using a bicycle pump (a bellows) to quickly pump up a tire. The upstroke is inspiration and the downstroke is exhalation, and both are equal in length.
- The rate of breathing is rapid, with as many as two to three cycles of inspiration/expiration per second.
- While doing the exercise, you should feel effort at the base of the neck, chest, and abdomen. The muscles in these areas will increase in strength the more this technique is practiced. This is truly an exercise.
- Do this for no longer than 15 seconds when first starting. With practice, slowly increase the length of the exercise by 5 seconds each time. Do it as long as you are comfortably able, not exceeding 1 full minute.
- There is a risk for hyperventilation that can result in loss of consciousness if this exercise is done too

much in the beginning. For this reason, it should be practiced in a safe place such as a bed or chair.

This exercise can be used each morning on awakening or when needed for an energy boost.

Further Resources

An excellent book to help explore more advanced breathing techniques is *Conscious Breathing* by Gay Hendricks (New York, Bantam, 1995).

An excellent audiotape, *Breathing: The Master Key to Self Healing*, by Andrew Weil, discusses the health benefits of breathing and directs the listener through eight breathing exercises (Sounds True, 1999).

The reader is encouraged to enroll in a yoga class through a local community or fitness center. Most well-trained instructors will educate students on how the breath is used to enhance well-being with yoga practice.

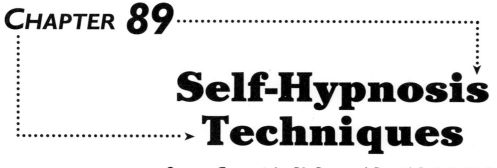

CHAPTER 89

Self-Hypnosis Techniques

Steven Gurgevich, Ph.D., and David Rakel, M.D.

OVERVIEW

Hypnosis is a system or collection of methods that allows us to enhance the communication and sharing of information between and within the mind and the body. We can do this entirely by ourselves, with the help of others, and by using learning materials such as books, videotapes, and audiotapes. But whether someone helps us (e.g., a trained therapist) or we do it alone, all hypnosis is self-hypnosis.

One method of hypnosis is trance. A hypnotic trance is a state of consciousness in which an individual's focus of awareness allows great absorption in the experience and sensation of ideas.

A daydream is a good example of a trance. In a daydream, there is awareness of locale and of what one is doing, but, at the same time, one is very absorbed in the experience and sensations of the thoughts, ideas, and images of the daydream. In other words, hypnotic trance and daydreaming are the same process. Most daydreams arise out of boredom or when we have too little to think about actively. And *trance* becomes the daydream state of consciousness when we deliberately set it into being. Hypnosis includes many different ways of calling up the "daydream", or trance, state of mind. These include what we call induction techniques, imagery methods, focusing concentration, and forms of passive relaxation and meditation. If you think of a daydream as a trance, then you have experienced trance states every day in many ways.

Learning to use this exquisite tool to enhance mind–body communication for healing, greater performance, comfort, and relaxation is easy and very beneficial. The word *learning* is a key to understanding hypnosis and trance. For once you discover how to achieve the results you want, you have also taught that achievement to your body and mind, and you own those abilities for as long as you practice them. What kinds of abilities can be learned in this way? Overcoming anxiety on an airplane, relaxing smooth muscle of the intestines for more comfortable digestion, relieving pain or producing one's own anesthesia, improving sleep patterns, changing habits, improving concentration skills, and alleviating nausea associated with chemotherapy are just a few abilities that can be developed by use of hypno-sis. In essence, hypnosis is a system of methods for accessing and using the unconscious influence of the mind on the body.

Although there are many different techniques for accessing subconscious influence on the body, for practical purposes this chapter focuses on one tool that primary care providers can use and modify to meet the needs of their patients. This tool requires five main principles (Table 89–1): 1. Education, 2. tailoring to the patient's beliefs or interests, 3. trance induction, 4. utilization of trance directed toward a specific goal, and 5. realerting (coming out of trance).

EDUCATION

To remove fear and misunderstanding, time must be taken to educate the patient about hypnosis. The first task is to dispel the myths and misconceptions about hypnosis. The most predominant misconceptions are:

1. *Subjects lose consciousness and conscious control.* This statement is incorrect because at all times, subjects are consciously aware of where they are and what they are doing.
2. *Subjects can be made to do things or reveal things that they ordinarily would not do in a waking state.* Subjects are very much aware of everything and always in control of what they are choosing to experience.
3. *Subject must be gullible or weak-minded to be hypnotized.* On the contrary, research has shown that some of the best subjects are those with great intellectual capacity, open-mindedness, and creativity.

Table 89-1. Summary of the Hypnotic Process

Education to remove preconceived fears
Tailoring to match the suggestions to the patient's beliefs
Induction
    Thumb-and-finger release technique to trigger trance
    Staircase technique to help with progressive muscle relaxation and deepening of trance
Utilization of trance for a specific purpose (e.g., headache, warts)
Realerting to bring the patient out of trance

The next task is to define trance. This is a heightened state of consciousness in which the individual is prone to suggestion. Emphasize to the patient that everyone has experienced trance many times. An example is daydreaming. Another is a driving trance after which the individual arrives home unable to remember the drive because the mind was focused on other thoughts. Being absorbed in a good movie offers another excellent example. While the viewer is focusing on the film, there is less awareness of things happening near by and more responsiveness to suggestions that are offered on the screen. The viewer may jump if startled, or cry if saddened. The movie's ability to provoke these physical responses usually correlates with how well it does at the box office. The viewer is always in control and can decide to go and get popcorn.

A good movie or a good hypnosis session involves three factors: absorption, dissociation, and suggestibility. Through an induction technique, the subject becomes fully absorbed in the matter at hand, resulting in dissociation from various distractions. This creates a heightened state of awareness that allows the person to be more receptive to suggestions that can influence physical and behavioral change. Educating the patient regarding the purpose of hypnosis helps to remove fear and confusion and results in a better clinical response.

TAILORING

The talented therapist tailors the hypnotic technique to each individual's unique needs. Because most practitioners who use this reference do not have this experience, the chapter focuses on a few questions that can easily be remembered, helping to tailor the hypnosis to the patient's beliefs and interests. The more the technique relates to these beliefs, the more acceptable and useful it is for the individual. In contrast, if the technique used encourages an image associated with anger or fear, or one that is simply foreign to the subject, the process will be counterproductive. Think of tailoring as the therapist's effort to make the hypnotic experience *personally familiar* to the subject.

Statements and questions that help to tailor or personalize hypnosis are as follows:

• Name a favorite place that brings comfort and a sense of peace to your mind.
• What is your favorite color?
• What are some of your favorite activities and pastimes?
• What kinds of events and activities give you the greatest pleasure?

TRANCE INDUCTION

The practitioner performs trance induction for the first hypnosis session to familiarize the patient with the procedure. It is helpful if the therapist walks the patient through the process so that the patient will subsequently feel comfortable doing it alone. Children learn the procedure very easily, but adults often need a little practice.

There are many different techniques for trance induction. It is helpful to use a trigger to tell the body it is time to relax and focus. Each time the individual uses or rehearses the hypnosis with that particular method of induction, the trigger cues, or signals the associated responses and the body becomes conditioned. This creates a more automatic response to the trigger and trance becomes easier to initiate the more it is used. The thumb-and-finger technique is one that is easy to perform.

Thumb-and-Finger Technique To Induce Trance

Instruct the patient to gently press the tips of the thumb and index finger together making the "OK" sign. When the patient is ready, have them take a deep breath and hold it while you count to five. With each increasing number, tell the patient to deliberately increase some acceptable anxiety and to make it a physical experience by pressing the thumb and index finger more tightly together. Let the patient know that they are in control of this form of tension and anxiety, and when the count of five is reached, the breath should be exhaled and released and the thumb and finger relaxed. Tell the patient to keep the eyes closed, to permit the hand to relax, and to allow the breathing to become very calm and regular. You may tell the patient that this action is a cue for relaxing and going into trance. This cue can be used at any time by the patient for self-hypnosis. With repetition, a conditioned response is created, which facilitates a more rapid and easier induction.

NOTE

Do not be afraid to use your voice to convey the message you intend. That is, use inflections, pauses, tone, and volume, and accent your tone to emphasize your message.

Imagining a Staircase to Induce Relaxation and Deepen Trance

Imagining a beautiful staircase with 10 steps allows each step to be used to help focus on relaxing a different part of the body as the patient descends to a favorite place. In the {} brackets, insert patient preferences that were asked about during tailoring, such as favorite place or color. The process may be something like the following scenario:

Imagine a beautiful {favorite color} staircase that has 10 steps. These 10 steps lead to a peaceful and relaxing {favorite place}. In a moment, I am going to start counting backwards from 10 to 1. With each step, you can notice your body relaxing more comfortably, allowing you to gently relax deeper and deeper with each step. It will be so nice to discover which parts of your body relax more quickly and easily as tension is automatically released.

As you start at the top of the staircase, allow each exhalation to release any tension or strain in your body. Let each breath now be a relaxing breath.

10—Relax your face and jaw, letting tongue gently rest on the floor of your mouth.

9—Relax your temples, eyes, and eyelids as you step down to. . .

8—Relax the back of your neck and shoulders, simply letting go.

7—Relax your arms, knowing that there is nothing for them to do.

Sometimes you will notice that your body is already getting ahead of my voice and the numbers, and sometimes it feels so comfortable when your body catches up to your relaxation.

6—Relax your chest with each rise and fall of the breath.

5—Relax your abdomen, setting the muscles free.

4—Relax your pelvis, allowing it to sink into the chair.

Sometimes your body may be so heavy that you feels as if you are sinking, and other times you feel so light that you may seem to be floating. Whatever you experience is correct for you; let it happen.

3—Relax your legs, giving them the day off, with nothing to support.

2—Relax your toes as we arrive at {favorite place}.

1—Continue past zero as you feel comfortable and at ease with this very relaxed form of concentration.

Exploring the Favorite or Peaceful Place

Taking a few moments to allow exploration of the peaceful place allows deepening of the trance and more vivid imagery and sensory recruitment. It also allows the individual time to become more familiar with any alterations in perception. If time is limited, you can jump right to utilization.

With the mind's eye, have the patient explore the surroundings.

- What do you see, such as colors or objects?
- Do you notice any scents or smells?
- What do you hear?
- Ask the patient if it would be all right for them to feel comfortable here, suggesting that they now find "a comfortable place" to settle down or sit.

It is now time to use the trance for a specific goal.

UTILIZATION

This is the process of using focused attention for an active purpose such as symptom relief. Following are scenarios that may be used for some common problems seen in the primary care setting.

Abdominal Pain (Assuming a Pathologic Condition Has Been Ruled Out)

Balloon Technique

Tailor the experience by asking the following questions:

- What color would best describe your pain?
- What is your favorite color?

Focus your attention on your pain. Now, imagine your discomfort to be a large {insert pain color} balloon. Your discomfort is a large {pain color} balloon. Now, imagine that you can watch this bright {pain color} balloon get smaller and smaller as it slowly loses air. Imagine the color of the balloon beginning to lighten, slowly changing to a soft {insert favorite color} color as it gets smaller. As you watch the balloon become smaller and smaller, you feel less and less discomfort. The balloon gets smaller and you feel less discomfort. You begin to feel better and better. You feel better as you watch the balloon lose air and become smaller. Now, watch the pale {favorite color} balloon become tinier and tinier, smaller and smaller. The balloon is shrinking to a small {favorite color} dot, a small {favorite color} dot. Now, watch it simply disappear, and when it disappears, you feel much, much better. You feel better, more comfortable. You feel better, more comfortable. You feel completely comfortable.

Headache

Cool Breeze Technique

Cooling the head helps to facilitate vasoconstriction. This is accompanied by imagery of warming the hands, which directs greater circulation to the extremities and helps to reduce pressure and pain in the head (particularly the pain of migraine headache).

The induction technique mentioned often reduces pain by facilitating relaxation. Further time spent on relaxation of the head is warranted, because tension is often involved in the pathogenesis of headaches.

Feel the muscles in your temples relax. Focus your attention on your eyes and forehead and let them relax with each breath exhaled. With each breath, let the muscles relax more and more. Now, follow the muscles through the scalp to the base of the skull and relax this area. Exhale and feel the whole head relax.

Imagine walking along a snowy path in the mountains, with a cool breeze blowing across your face and cooling your head, your face, your eyes. Imagine a cool and soothing sensation across your forehead and above each eye. Your hands are tucked in your pockets. They are warming, and now they are warm. Your hands are warm and comfortable while a cool breeze and cold air make your head feel cooler, soothing and relaxing every muscle, releasing any tightness, any stress.

Just feel a calm sensation flowing through your eyes and forehead. You are calm and comfortable and relaxed. Just notice the cool breeze of each breath coming in your nose and softly blowing up and onto your forehead, and the air warmed by your hands and body is now being exhaled. Cool air in, soothing your head—warm air out, relaxing your body. (Repeat if needed.)

Localized Pain from Injury or Preparation for a Painful Procedure

Glove Anesthesia Technique

This technique involves creating numbness in one of the patient's hands, which can then be transferred from the hand to any part of the body for pain relief.

Tailor by asking the patient's favorite color.

Focus your attention on one of your hands, directing all of your attention to that hand. Begin to imagine the hand becoming numb. Recall a time when your hand fell asleep and how wooden your hand felt. As you numb your hand, imagine it gradually turning {insert favorite color}. Your hand is turning {favorite color}, and as it does, there is a tingling in your fingertips and warmth flows through your hand. Soon, all the feeling will drain out of your hand as it turns a deeper {favorite color}. Soon all the feeling will drain out of your hand, and it will turn a beautiful {favorite color}. Let go, let the feeling drain from your hand. The hand is feeling so numb, so very numb. The hand feels heavy, and it feels as if it were made of wood. Let all the feeling drain from the hand, which now begins to glow a beautiful {favorite color} color. Let the hand feel numb, let it feel numb as it glows brighter, glows like a beautiful {favorite color} light bulb. Your hand is now completely numb and filled with {favorite color} light. Now, place your numb {favorite color} hand on your {insert part of body with pain—knee, jaw}, place your hand on {body part}, and now let the numbness and the {favorite color} light drain into your {body part}. Feel your {body part} become numb and watch as the numbing {favorite color} light slowly leaves your hand and covers your {body part}, becoming numb, woodlike, heavy, numb, numb, thick, as if it were made of wood. When all the {favorite color} light has left your hand, numbing

your {body part}, place your hand back down into a comfortable position {pause}. You can keep your {body part} numb for as long as you need to, as long as you need to. When you have completed, just let go and feel the numbness and the {favorite color} light drain away, drain away. Your {body part} returns to normal. When you no longer need it to be numb, it returns to normal.

Warts

Hand Tracing Technique (Best Used for Children with Warts)

- Have the patient trace both hands on a piece of paper (the patient may also draw other parts of the body that contain warts).
- Have the patient draw the location of the warts on the tracing (see Fig. 89–1).

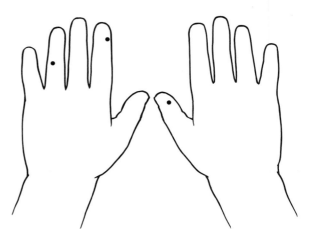

- Tailor by asking about the patient's favorite place and color.
- Have the patient go to a favorite place. Children are able to do this quickly and easily, but adults may have to use the induction technique discussed earlier.

Imagine that you are miniaturized, small enough to get into a beautiful {favorite color} space ship and travel through your body to where your warts are. Look at the roots of the wart and see what they are like. What would you like to do to prevent the roots from getting any nourishment from your body? Would you like to spray them or paint them with a powerful chemical that only warts can feel? Or would you like to cap them off with a plastic bubble, or cut them off and take them out of your body?

- As the patient invents a method to "treat" the roots of the warts, you may give some brief suggestions that reinforce the patient's power to do this from inside.

Go ahead and do that now, and make sure that you treat all your warts.

Do you need more time to work on the warts?

- When the patient says that the process is finished, ask for "one more thing" to ensure that these warts do not stand a chance.

Your body will continue to work on these warts even while you are sleeping. How long do you think it will take your body to remove these warts? I wonder how quickly your body will get the job done for you.

- Ask the patient to return to a normal size and come out of the body. Offer encouragement on a job well done. Mention how powerful the images seem and how well the body heard everything it needed to do the job.
- After the patient comes out of trance, ask for the warts to be erased on the tracing that was created. Have the patient erase the warts or paint them with whiteout.
- Have the patient do this imagery once more at home. Success with wart resolution has been found after two or three imagery sessions.

REALERTING

The process of realerting involves not only speech but also tone of voice. As you get closer to having the patient open the eyes, the tone of your voice should rise accordingly. Realerting can simply be a reversal of the induction technique—climbing up the staircase with energy coming back into the relaxed muscles. Effort should be taken to empower the patient to feel comfortable with using the technique when it may be needed in the future.

In a moment, we will climb the staircase, counting each step. Afterward, you will be happy that you have found this medium and pleased because you realize that you can visit this place whenever you wish, knowing you have the power to influence your condition whenever you need it.

As you proceed up the first step, allow the energy to reenter your body, starting at your toes. . .

2. And now allow it to flow up your legs. . .

3. and into your pelvis as you feel it press down into the chair,

4. travelling to your abdomen. Feel your body come alive.

5. Take in this energy with each rise of the chest. Your voice is becoming stronger as you return to a more normal pattern of speech,

6. as you feel the energy travel into your arms,

7. going up to a the shoulders and the neck,

8. into the temples, eyes and eyelids. Your voice should now be the normal one you use in your waking state.

9. Feel your tongue, your jaw, and the muscles of your face energize, and allow your eyes to open when you are ready to feel wonderfully refreshed and energized.

HOMEWORK FOR THE PATIENT

The scenario discussed above should first be done with the practitioner in the clinic to help show the patient how this process can be done alone. Think of the hypnotic work as a rehearsal for what you want the patient to practice alone at home. However, for warts, experience shows that only one or two sessions are needed, and further sessions may hinder the process. For conditions such as pain, there is no limit to the frequency of use, and the tool can be used to abort such pain as headache. You educate patients to use this tool on their own by practicing what they have experienced with you in the clinic or office. Review the steps from beginning to end, reminding the patients that their body hears everything they say, that it hears, thinks, and imagines, and that it uses their thoughts and ideas as instructions for the inner work to be achieved. You may also ask patients to tell you where they plan to practice at home, and what are they going to say or think to themselves to make it happen. Provide instructions as necessary to set them in motion for a positive experience at home.

NOTE

Inducing and suggesting hypnosis is an art that takes time and practice. Simple techniques such as those discussed should be used to enhance the experience in the primary case setting, but for more complicated cases, referral should be made to a licensed practitioner.

WHAT TO LOOK FOR IN A CONSULTANT

When selecting a therapist to offer hypnosis to your patient, review qualifications for treating the condition. A good rule of thumb for therapists is to use hypnosis only for conditions that they have qualifications to treat. There are many so-called certified hypnotherapists advertising their services. Frequently, their certification is given by a lay school of hypnosis, which teaches only the techniques of hypnosis and does not provide instruction practicing medicine, psychology, dentistry, or social work at the clinical level. Choose a practitioner who is licensed in a clinical specialty that is also certified by the American Society of Clinical Hypnosis. This professional organization provides extensive and comprehensive training and requires supervised practice before granting certification. Both the American Society of Clinical Hypnosis and the American Psychotherapy and Medical Hypnosis Association provide referrals to qualified practitioners. They are listed below.

FURTHER TRAINING

- The American Society of Clinical Hypnosis (ASCH) offers excellent workshops that lead to certification. The telephone number is 312–645–9810 and the web site address is *WWW.asch.net/*
- Another resource is the American Psychotherapy and Medical Hypnosis Association. A referral service is available through their website at *http:// APMHA.com*

Bibliography

Crasilneck H, Hall J: Clinical Hypnosis: Principles and Applications, 2nd ed. Orlando, Fla, Grune & Stratton, 1985.

Hadley J, Staudacher C: Hypnosis for Change, 3rd ed. New York, MJF Books, 1996.

Hammond DC: Handbook of Hypnotic Suggestions and Metaphors. New York, WW Norton, 1990.

Hammond DC: Hypnotic Induction and Suggestion. Chicago, American Society of Clinical Hypnosis, 1998.

Meyer RC: Practical Clinical Hypnosis: Techniques and Applications. New York, Lexington Books, Macmillan, 1992.

Olness K, Kohen DP: Hypnosis and Hypnotherapy with Children, 3rd ed. New York, Guilford Press, 1996.

Temes R: Medical Hypnosis: An Introduction and Clinical Guide. Medical Guides to Complementary and Alternative Medicine. Philadelphia, Churchill Livingstone, 1999.

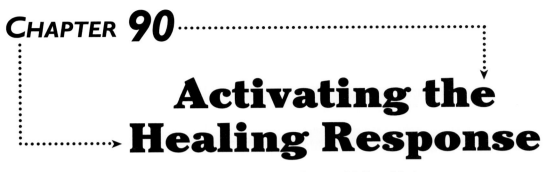

Activating the Healing Response

Opher Caspi, M.D., M.A.

You are in the middle of an appointment with a recently married, 24-year-old woman who has been referred to you for evaluation. She has suffered from fatigue, malar rash, and polyarthralgia for quite some time, and recently she miscarried. Her blood work supports the diagnosis of systemic lupus erythematosus (SLE). In a very compassionate way, you tell her that you think you know the common source of her multiple complaints. You explain to her what SLE is. Shocked, she starts crying. You are quiet. After a few moments of silence, she asks you for her prognosis. You struggle with how much to tell her now. Your heart is pounding. Once again, you must break bad news. Bursting into tears anew, she asks: "Will I ever be a mom? Am I going to need dialysis? Why me?" You, of course, do not know the answers—medicine is notoriously practiced in uncertainty. You are quiet again.

The case of another patient comes to mind—a young man who, a few years back, participated in a double-blind, randomized, controlled study evaluating a new treatment for Crohn's disease. He has been completely healed since undergoing the treatment. You remember clearly how astonished you were when the study code was broken and you learned that he had received a placebo. Your intuition had misled you; on the basis of his response, you had been sure that he was getting the real medication. You remember how relieved you felt when he refused to learn what he was receiving, because you were concerned that disclosing the truth would be harmful.

Now, however, you keep searching for what to say to this woman. Her next question brings you back into the encounter at once: "Can I be cured?" she asks, this time determined to get an answer.

After years in practice, you know that your answer to that seemingly simple question will almost certainly govern her attitude and mindset for years to come. As a responsible physician, you feel that your duty is to first educate her about the disease, yet you sense her misery, and your primary instinct is to comfort her. "Of course," you say—and she smiles for the first time.

The foregoing scenario is only one of many in which the art of medicine interfaces closely with its science. This chapter presents practical and proven approaches to activation of the healing response, mainly through the placebo effect. To put these two constructs—healing response and placebo effect—

in context, it must be remembered that the two share a fundamental characteristic—they both originate from within. Accordingly, I suggest that all health care providers should realize that their role must evolve *primarily* from activating those internal processes that lead to healing and homeostasis.

NOTE

Contrary to the current belief that the placebo effect "just happens," the premise of this chapter is that the placebo effect can and should be triggered proactively.

The placebo effect appears to be a contextual, situational phenomenon more than the result of an enduring personality trait (Fig. 90–1).[1] An entire line of research aimed at characterizing patients as either "placebo responders" or "nonresponders" failed to identify a difference, and it is now commonly agreed that each person has the inherent capacity to experience the placebo effect.[2] The question, therefore, is not which patients can enjoy the placebo effect but rather how it can be triggered in everyone.

THE PLACEBO EFFECT AND HEALING

The power of placebo draws on the innate ability of the body to heal itself spontaneously.[3] That innate capacity is best represented in the fundamental biologic principle of homeostasis that is believed to exist in all living beings. Evidence exists that self-repair occurs at all levels of physiology and anatomy.[4] Nonetheless, like many other scientific concepts, healing remains a theoretical construct that cannot be directly observed but can only be inferred. In other words, certain manifestations are observed that are hypothesized to be related to the mechanism of healing—such as wound healing and DNA repair—but may also originate in processes distinct from that mechanism. This difference is extremely important to appreciate because the placebo effect

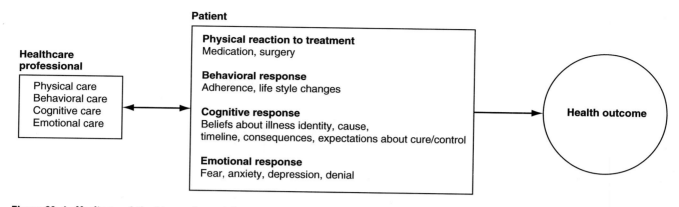

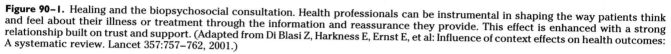

Figure 90–1. Healing and the biopsychosocial consultation. Health professionals can be instrumental in shaping the way patients think and feel about their illness or treatment through the information and reassurance they provide. This effect is enhanced with a strong relationship built on trust and support. (Adapted from Di Blasi Z, Harkness E, Ernst E, et al: Influence of context effects on health outcomes: A systematic review. Lancet 357:757–762, 2001.)

is also an inferential construct—that is, a label. The sugar pill's positive effect may be called placebo, but the process of how healing was triggered involves much more than just the pill. Misattribution of cause and effect, especially when placebos are involved, poses an important methodologic challenge that requires great attention and critical thinking. Thus, it is entirely possible that the same biologic events are being labeled by different observers as spontaneous remission, spontaneous healing, or placebo effect depending on the observer's viewpoint, belief system, and context.

The common theme of this chapter is that the placebo effect is believed to promote health and healing. *Healing* refers to the process of restoring the patient's perception of connectedness, indestructibility, and control.[5] It is a journey rather than a destination.[6] Proponents of this viewpoint regard the activation of the placebo effect as a powerful method that should be exploited rather than discarded.[3, 7, 8] *Health* is that state of spiritual, emotional, cognitive, physical, social, and environmental functioning that facilitates the person's development—that is, the balanced, coherent, and integrated adjustment of, and accommodation to, internal and external events.[9]

THE MEDICAL ENCOUNTER AND THE THERAPEUTIC RELATIONSHIP: SPECIFIC AND NONSPECIFIC EFFECTS OF THERAPY

Placebo effect and *nonspecific* treatment are often used interchangeably, reflecting some confusion regarding cause and effect of therapy.[10] The popular definition of placebo as a "nonspecific" element of therapy is not entirely accurate, as placebo effects are typically highly specific. They include effects such as pain reduction,[11] healing of a peptic ulcer,[12] bronchodilation in asthmatics,[13] and so on. Nonspe-

cific effects, on the other hand, refer to the features common to *all* therapeutic interventions regardless of theoretical orientation, such as the therapeutic relationship and the patient's expectations.[14] Thus, the distinction is not just a matter of semantics but is made to support the assertion that unlike clinical research that seeks to tease apart cause and effect, the medical encounter offers multiple opportunities to improve patients' outcomes through subtle, yet powerful interventions that elicit the placebo effect and trigger healing.

Specific, defining, or characteristic elements of therapy[15] are those therapeutic maneuvers derived from a particular theoretical orientation as being necessary for the amelioration of a symptom or disorder. By definition they are well defined, theoretically derived, intentional actions or intervention strategies of the physician that are unique to a specific therapy. The application of these techniques is believed to be causally responsible for the outcome.

Nonspecific or incidental elements of therapy,[15] on the other hand, are those unspecified variables that accompany the characteristic elements but that are not necessary components of the specified therapy. They happen in conjunction with and after the therapy, and would not have happened if the therapy had not been given. Examples of these nonspecific elements are the patient–physician interaction, individual patient and physician characteristics during therapy, and elements of the treatment structure, change processes, and strategies.[16]

Closely related to these nonspecific elements are the preliminary elements of therapy.[17] These, in turn, may affect patients' outcomes *even before* treatment is eventually offered. The diagnostic process, for instance, may include elements that are perceived as meaningful to the patient and thus may trigger healing well before any medical advice is given.[18, 19]

The placebo effect is considered to arise mainly from the incidental and preliminary elements of therapy. The effect depends on the interaction among the clinician, the treatment process, and the patient.[20] The patient's perception of that interaction often ignites the healing/placebo process. Thus, the clinician is a therapeutic agent, and the medical encounter is the playing field.[21, 22]

NOTE

"The physician is a vastly more important institution than the drug store" (T. Findly).[23]

THE THERAPEUTIC RELATIONSHIP AND THE PLACEBO EFFECT

The experience of the therapeutic relationship has been shown to facilitate change. Evidently there is a set of desired qualities that imbue the practitioner or the patient with some sort of special power. But it is the relationship, not the individual person, that provides the framework for change.[9]

Optimal care of patients requires that the placebo effect be maximized.[7] Research suggests that the placebo effect is more likely to occur in the clinic when the patient regards the clinician as experienced, competent, and optimistic[17, 24] and when the clinician expects the treatment to help.[25, 26] An attempt to formalize these qualities into a systematic clinical approach led recently to the development of the "sustained relationship" model between physicians and patients[27] as a way to enhance the effect of therapy, probably through maximizing the placebo effect.[28]

Benson and Epstein[29] suggested that the placebo effect occurs only when both patients and physicians are of like mind. According to that supposition, both need to share positive beliefs and expectations and to perceive that they have a good relationship. Thomas[21] conducted a study on the impact of the physician's positive attitude on the patient's outcome and found that the physician's advice was a more effective placebo intervention than the administration of a placebo prescription medication. In a systematic analysis of all placebo-controlled studies in ulcerative colitis,[30] only one variable, the number of clinic visits, was shown to predict increased placebo effect. A plausible explanation is that the more frequent the contacts with the healthcare provider in a supportive setting, the higher the chances that the patient will respond. One of the major elements in this perception of support relates to the physician's ability to attend to the needs of the patient.[17] Indeed, the derivation of the word *therapy* is from the Greek word meaning "to attend."[9] Furthermore, motivational enhancement is among the most effective therapeutic techniques available.[31, 32] It depends on the clinician's skills of empathy and providing feedback in a nonjudgmental manner. This in turn suggests that the clinician's

skills may well interact with treatments to enhance their effectiveness. Relationship skills appear to enhance the effectiveness of interventions rather than substitute for them.

Patients are not "innocent bystanders"—passive recipients of treatment—but rather should be treated as full partners. Consistent with the ethical principles of patient-centered care,[33] the integrative approach to healthcare is based on a partnership of patient and practitioner within which conventional and alternative modalities are used to stimulate the body's innate healing potential. The principles of integrative medicine maintain that the experience of a therapeutic relationship facilitates the healing process. The physician emphasizes the patient's participation and responsibility and recognizes the patient's preferences and self-knowledge when designing a treatment plan.[34]

The foregoing approach characterizes, in essence, "holistic" medical practice. A recent observational study showed that patients prefer a patient centered approach over a biomedical one.[35] Some investigators have demonstrated that patients' perceptions of the patient-centeredness of the medical interaction were a strong predictor not only of health outcomes but also of the efficacy of healthcare.[36]

PATIENT-RELATED ATTRIBUTES IN ACTIVATION OF THE HEALING RESPONSE

Specifically what can be done in the therapeutic relationship to activate the healing response? Evidence exists to support the claim that healing can be purposely and effectively activated.

Hope

In the clinical scenario presented at the beginning of the chapter, was it justifiable to suggest to the patient that SLE is curable? To what extent should the clinician use hope as an anchor for change? Are clinicians allowed to activate healing at all expense? For example, is the instillation of false hope ethical? Although the answers to many of these questions seem to be very complex, it has been proposed that hope is the primary mechanism of change in folk traditions of healing, as well as in psychotherapy. Frank[37–39] proposed that all healing endeavors share the following features: (1) a patient in distress, (2) a clinician who is perceived as an expert in dealing with the patient's distress, (3) an acceptable explanation or "myth" provided by the clinician, and (4) some sort of healing ritual conducted by the clinician that serves to instill hope and positive expectations in the patient. Thus, according to one viewpoint, the specific ingredients of the clinician's technical interventions are important only because they provide a shared belief system between the patient and the clinician, give form to prescribed rituals, and create positive expectations.

Expectancy

A recent review by Crow and associates[40] found that patients' expectancy was positively correlated with healthcare outcomes. Some important areas of healthcare in which expectancy has been studied are preparation for medical procedures, management of chronic illness, and medical treatment.

- In studies evaluating preparation for medical procedures, skill training to reduce stress in complying with medical procedures (e.g., relaxation training) that increased self-efficacy, either alone or in combination with information about the medical procedures, was more effective than information alone. The main health outcomes were less anxiety and reduced use of pain medication.
- In studies evaluating the management of chronic illness, training with regard to the management of the disorder that increased self-efficacy resulted in reduction in the patient's symptoms (e.g., improved mood, less anxiety, reduced pain, control of asthma) and improvement in the patient's disease status (e.g., lowered blood pressure, immunologic changes, better metabolic control).
- In studies of medical treatment, when positive outcome expectancies were stated by the clinician, rather than cautious or skeptical expectancies, most studies provided evidence that positive outcome expectancies enhanced medical outcomes. The improvements, however, were primarily patient self-reported reductions in anxiety, pain, and distress, rather than objective physiologic outcomes.

Expectations may be altered by even small variations in instructions and experimental designs in clinical research. For example, Kirsch and Weixel[41] found that differences between double-blind and deceptive administration of placebos can produce different outcomes. In a study of response expectancies about coffee, subjects were administered decaffeinated coffee under two different instructional sets. In one design, subjects were given the usual double-blind administration as used in clinical trials, in which they were told that they would receive either caffeinated or decaffeinated coffee. Neither the subject nor the experimenter knew which beverage was being administered. In the other design, subjects were told that they would receive caffeinated coffee, when in fact they received decaffeinated coffee—a procedure more akin to what might happen in a clinical setting. The authors proposed that deceptive administration would have stronger effects on outcome than double-blind administration because in double-blind administration, the subjects would be less certain about whether they actually were receiving caffeinated coffee. The results were complex but did confirm that the different protocols produced different effects.

Attribution

Expectancy, however, is only one of many cognitive constructs that have been investigated to explain healing and placebo effects. An important line of research in social cognition has focused on how people attach meaning and make causal inferences about their experiences. Attribution theorists have proposed that self-attributed behavior change has a greater probability of being maintained over time than that noted for behavior change attributed to an external source such as a drug[42] (see Chapter 95, Motivational Interviewing Techniques). In a creative test of this hypothesis, Davison and colleagues[43] administered a treatment package for insomnia that consisted of chloral hydrate (a hypnotic), a brief relaxation training procedure, and instructions to schedule and regularize bedtime behaviors. Subjects who demonstrated improvement in sleep onset latencies from this treatment regimen were told after they improved that they had received either an optimal dose of the drug or a dose that previous research indicated was ineffective. Subjects who were led to attribute their improvement to their own efforts, rather than to the drug, maintained their improvement after the drug was withdrawn. Subjects led to attribute their improvement to the drug returned to their baseline levels of sleep disturbance. Patients with many disorders may attribute their improvement to salient medical interventions. These attributions may make patients more vulnerable to relapses when the interventions are withdrawn.

Meaning and Mastery

Attribution theory is one way of understanding how people give meaning to their experiences. *Meaning*, as an explanatory concept, has received increased recent attention in the placebo literature. Brody[44] has proposed that "an encounter with a healer is most likely to produce a positive placebo response when it changes the meaning of the illness experience for that individual in a positive direction." According to Brody, three conditions are associated with this change in meaning: (1) the patient is listened to and receives an explanation for the illness that makes sense, (2) the patient feels care and concern being expressed by the healer and others in the environment, and (3) the patient feels an enhanced sense of mastery or control over the illness or its symptoms. *Mastery*, in turn, not only is an important element in the placebo effect but also leads to patient empowerment, which results in better health outcomes.[45] In a recent hypothesized causal account of the placebo response, Brody[28] suggested that meaning precedes other causal mechanisms such as conditioning and expectancy. It should be emphasized, however, that the assignment of meaning to health problems and therapeutic rituals by the patient provides a summary context of the operation of a number of causal variables. I believe that these variables (such as conditioning, expectancy, information from the clinician, and feedback through changes in the internal and external environment) affect each other reciprocally and recursively.

Meaning is also used as a central explanatory construct in another but related literature. In an impressive set of studies, Pennebaker and other linguistics investigators have found that writing about one's deepest thoughts and feelings on a specific number of 20- to 30-minute occasions has health consequences even months later (for a summary of this literature, see the article by Pennebaker[46]). In examining changes in how people expressed their thoughts and feelings across the assigned occasions, Pennebaker[46] found that increases in causal and insight words are associated with improved health. He proposed that the construction of stories or narratives may be an important way in which human beings integrate emotional experiences into their lives. An alternative explanation of the beneficial effects of writing about emotional experiences is that the writing assignment may produce extinction of negative emotional associations through repetition and exposure.[47] If extinction of emotional reactivity associated with thoughts of events is an important part of the process, then the linguistic changes that Pennebaker observed may be consequences, rather than causes, of changes in emotional reactivity.

A CONCEPTUAL MODEL FOR THE PLACEBO EFFECT WITHIN THE THERAPEUTIC PROCESS

A biomedical model that seeks to understand the mechanisms by which the placebo effect occurs has largely dominated research on this intriguing phenomenon in the last few decades. Although findings in that line of research can help in understanding the "mind-body connection,"[48] another aspect still needs to be explored: how does the placebo effect fit into the therapeutic process?

Based on the foregoing discussion, I proposed a conceptual model for the placebo effect within the therapeutic process (Fig. 90–2). Two theoretical assumptions underlie this model. First, the placebo effect is not static. It constantly evolves and changes in response to other biologic and psychologic signals that play a role in the therapeutic process. In other words, the placebo effect is a dependent variable that is affected by various other independent variables, both internal and external to the individual.

The second assumption is that the placebo effect always interacts—in a synergistic rather than in an additive way—to an unpredictable degree with other elements of the therapeutic intervention, such as biologic and psychologic treatments.

The core concept of the proposed model is the recognition that clinician-patient interaction not only results in the generation of a treatment plan by the clinician but also influences the patient's formulation of health status meaning, as explained earlier. The clinician's treatment plan can be in the form of a one-line prescription or a comprehensive multistep multidimensional program. For example, a patient with SLE may be advised to take several medications from now on, or the medication regimen may be prescribed as part of a more general program that requires extensive lifestyle modifications.

It is proposed that the assignment of meaning by the patient is at times equally important in determining the outcome as the recommended biologic treatment itself. For example, the patient with SLE may be devastated by her recent diagnosis if this was preceded by good health, or she may be grateful for being diagnosed at an early stage of the disease, knowing that lupus is often associated with significant morbidity if left untreated. Reality perception is a complex phenomenon in itself that is highly influenced by sociocultural and ecologic factors, patient belief systems, and the like. Yet information and suggestions provided by a physician who is perceived as competent and confident may also play a role in the creation of meaning. Thus, the patient-physician interaction provides an excellent opportunity in which to positively reframe the meaning of any medical condition.

The patient's outlook has limited implications when it is considered merely in positive versus negative (favorable versus unfavorable) terms, but the implications may be expanded with cognitive reframing. Such reframing may lead to (1) the placebo effect through the creation of positive or negative expectations and (2) the development of coping strategies that will determine the patient's future health-related behavior. That behavior not only is manifested in adherence and compliance but also leads to other patient-initiated activities that join the physician-initiated recommended treatment to form the total package of care. Thus, for instance, the physician may recommend steroids for the patient with SLE, but the patient may add to that any number of other self-initiated interventions, such as stress reduction, a healthier diet, physical activity, and the like that may influence the clinical outcome.

According to the proposed conceptual model, the placebo effect can potentially affect the medical outcome in three different ways:

1. *Directly*—through the activation of innate homeostatic healing processes, often referred to as spontaneous healing regardless of what the biologic treatment may be. For instance, in the case

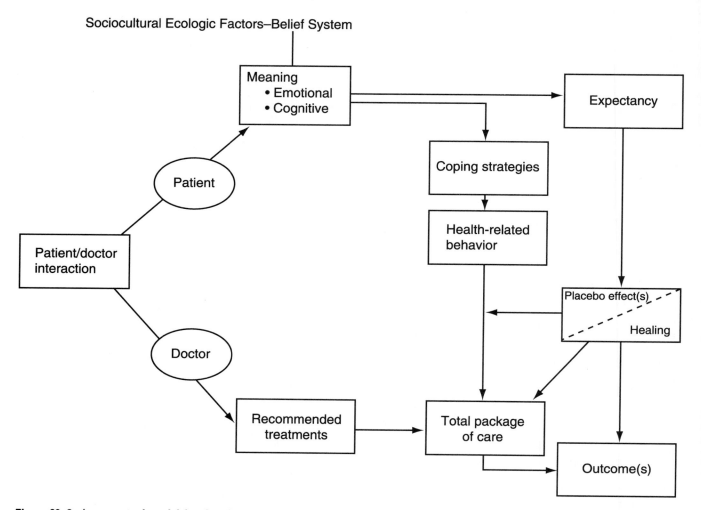

Figure 90–2. A conceptual model for the placebo effect within the therapeutic process. The model outlines the potential role of the placebo effect and healing in causing health outcomes and suggests that the therapeutic process is complex rather than linear. Furthermore, the model emphasizes the importance of meaning and expectations in activating the healing response.

of viral pharyngitis, antibiotics may be ineffective, yet certain elements associated with the characteristic aspects of drug therapy may trigger the placebo effect. Thomas[24] refers to the inability to acknowledge the ineffectiveness of antibiotics as a "therapeutic illusion" produced by the effectiveness of the placebo effect.

2. *Indirectly*—through patient behavior as a mediating variable. For instance, Horwitz and Horwitz[49] found that patients who adhered more closely to the placebo treatment, in clinical trials across various conditions, had better outcomes than those in patients who did not. One plausible explanation is that patients who adhered to the treatment protocol may also have engaged in other health promoting activities, and that the incidental element of adhering to the treatment protocol may have affected the outcomes.

3. Through interaction of active and indirect effects

with the total package of care, as noted earlier. That is, treatments may be more or less effective depending on the interaction of meaning with active change ingredients.

In summary, this conceptual model has two advantages over a framework that focuses merely on individual components. First, it is hypothesized that the model better represents how individual components interact to produce change. Cause and effect are seldom linear and unifactorial. The model emphasizes the multidimensional and interactive aspects of change. Second, the model provides a framework on which to integrate the complex knowledge about placebo effects and healing. As stressed throughout the chapter and emphasized by the integrative conceptual model, the interplay between the patient, the disorder, and the clinician is important.

— THERAPEUTIC REVIEW —

Key Points

- *The power of placebo draws on the innate ability of the body to heal itself spontaneously.*
- *Optimal care of patients requires that the placebo effect be maximized.*
- *Patients are not passive recipients of treatment but rather should be treated as full partners.*
- *The placebo effect appears to be a contextual, situational phenomenon more than the result of an enduring personality trait.*
- *The capacity to elicit the placebo effect is probably inherent in all persons.*
- *The placebo effect is considered to arise mainly from the incidental and preliminary elements of therapy. The effect depends on the interaction among the clinician, the treatment process, and the patient. The patient's perception of that interaction often ignites the healing/placebo process.*
- *The experience of the therapeutic relationship has been shown to facilitate change. It is the relationship, not the individual person, that provides the framework for change.*
- *Patients' expectancy, meaning, and mastery not only are important elements of the placebo effect but also lead to patient empowerment, which results in better health outcomes.*

Acknowledgment

I wish to thank Richard R. Bootzin, Ph.D., for his help in conceptualizing many of the ideas included in this chapter.

References

1. Di Blasi Z, Harkness E, Ernst E, et al: Influence of context effects on health outcomes: A systematic review. Lancet 357:757–762, 2001.
2. Spiro H: Clinical reflections on the placebo phenomenon. In Harrington A (ed): The Placebo Effect: An Interdisciplinary Exploration. Cambridge, Mass, Harvard University Press, 1997.
3. Bennet P: Placebo and healing. In Pizzorno JE, Murray MT (eds): Textbook of Natural Medicine. New York, Churchill Livingstone, 1999.
4. Weil A. Spontaneous Healing. New York, Fawcett Columbine, 1995.
5. Cassell EJ: The Healer's Art. Philadelphia, JB Lippincott, 1978.
6. Maizes V, Caspi O: The principles and challenges of integrative medicine. West J Med 171:148–149, 1999.
7. Ernst E, Herxheimer A: The power of placebo: Let's use it to help as much as possible. BMJ 313:1569–1570, 1996.
8. Benson H, Friedman R: Harnessing the power of the placebo effect and renaming it "remembered wellness." Annu Rev Med 47:193–199, 1996.
9. Mitchell A, Cormack M: The Therapeutic Relationship in Complementary Health Care. Edinburgh, Churchill Livingstone, 1998.
10. Kaptchuk TJ: Powerful placebo: The dark side of the randomized controlled trial. Lancet 351:1722–1725, 1998.
11. Amanzio M, Pollo A, Maggi G, Benedetti F: Response variability to analgesics: A role for nonspecific activation of endogenous opioids. Pain 90:201–215, 2001.
12. Moerman DE: General medical effectiveness and human biology: Placebo effects in the treatment of ulcer disease. Med Anthropol Q 14:3–16, 1983.
13. Luparello TJ, Leist N, Lourie CH, Sweet P: The interaction of psychologic stimuli and pharmacologic agents on airway reactivity in asthmatic subjects. Psychosom Med 32:509–513, 1970.
14. Arkowitz H: Integrative theories of therapy. In Wachtel PL, Messer SB (eds): Theories of Psychotherapy: Origins and Evolution. Washington, DC, American Psychogical Association, 1997.
15. Grünbaum A: Explication and implications of the placebo concept. In White L, Schwartz GE, Tursky B (eds): Placebo: Theory, Research and Mechanisms. New York, Guilford Press, 1985.
16. Grencavage LM, Norcross JC: Where are the commonalities among the therapeutic common factors? Profess Psychol Res Pract 21:372–378, 1990.
17. Barfod TS: Placebo therapy in dermatology. Clin Dermatol 17:69–76, 1999.
18. Brody H: "My story is broken; can you help me fix it?" Medical ethics and joint construction of narrative. Lit Med 13:79–92, 1994.
19. Brody H, Waters DB: Diagnosis is treatment. J Fam Pract 10:445–449, 1980.
20. Oh VM: The placebo effect: Can we use it better? BMJ 309:69–70, 1994.
21. Thomas KB: General practice consultations: Is there any point in being positive? BMJ 294:1200–1202, 1987.
22. Houston WR: The doctor himself as a therapeutic agent. Ann Intern Med 11:1416–1425, 1938.
23. Findley T: The placebo and the physician. Med Clin North Am 37:1821–1826, 1953.
24. Thomas KB: The placebo in general practice. Lancet 344:1066–1067, 1994.
25. Evans FJ: The placebo response in pain reduction. In Bonica JJ (ed): Pain. Adv Neurol 4, 1974.
26. Gracely RH, Dunbar R, Deeter WR, Wolskee PJ: Clinician's expectations influence placebo analgesia [letter]. Lancet 1:43, 1985.
27. Leopold N, Cooper J, Clancy C: Sustain partnership in primary care. J Fam Pract 42:129–137, 1996.
28. Brody H: The placebo response: Recent research and implications for family medicine. J Fam Pract 49:649–654, 2000.
29. Benson H, Epstein MD: The placebo effect: A neglected asset in the care of patients. JAMA 232:1225–1227,1975.
30. Bernstein CN: Placebos in medicine. Semin Gastrointest Dis 10:3–7, 1999.
31. Miller WR, Brown JM, Simpson TL, et al: What works? A methodological analysis of the alcohol treatment outcome literature. In Hester RK, Miller WR (eds): Handbook of Alcoholism Treatment Approaches: Effective Alternatives, 2nd ed. Boston, Allyn & Bacon, 1995.
32. Miller WR, Andrews NR, Wilbourne P, Bennett ME: A wealth of alternatives: Effective treatments for alcohol problems. In

Miller WR, Heather N (eds): Treating Additive Behaviors, 2nd ed. New York, Plenum Press, 1998.

33. Brown J, Stewart M, Tessier S: Assessing Communication between Patients and Doctors: A Manual for Scoring Patient-Centered Communication. (Working Paper Series 95-2). London, Thames Valley Family Practice Research Unit, 1995.

34. Gaudet TW: Integrative medicine: The evolution of a new approach to medicine and to medical education. Integ Med 1:67–73, 1998.

35. Little P, Everitt H, Williamson I, et al: Preferences of patients for patient-centered approach to consultation in primary care: observational study. BMJ 322:468–472, 2001.

36. Stewart M, Brown JB, Weston WW, et al: Patient-centered Medicine Transforming the Clinical Method. Thousand Oaks, Calif, Sage Publications, 1995.

37. Frank JD: Persuasion and Healing. Baltimore, Johns Hopkins University Press, 1961.

38. Frank JD: Therapeutic factors in psychotherapy. Am J Psychother 25:350–361, 1971.

39. Frank JD: Therapeutic components shared by all psychotherapies. In Hawey JH, Parks MM (eds): Psychotherapy Research and Behavior Change. Washington, DC, American Psychological Association, 1981.

40. Crow R, Gage H, Hampson S, Hart J, et al: The role of expec-tancies in the placebo effect and their use in the delivery of health care: A systematic review. Health Technol Assess 3:3, 1999.

41. Kirsch I, Weixel LJ: Double-blind versus deceptive administra-tion of a placebo. Biomed Ther XVI:242–246, 1988.

42. Valins S, Nisbett RE: Attribution Processes in the Development and Treatment of Emotional Disorders. Morristown, NJ, Gen-eral Learning Press, 1971.

43. Davison GC, Tsuimoto RN, Glaros AG: Attribution and the maintenance of behavior change in falling asleep. J Abnorm Psychol 82:124–133, 1973.

44. Brody H: The Placebo Response. New York, Harper Collins, 2000.

45. Greenfield S, Kaplan S, Ware JE: Expanding patient involve-ment in care: Effects on patient outcomes. Ann Intern Med 102:520–528, 1985.

46. Pennebaker JW: Writing about emotional experiences as a therapeutic process. Psychol Sci 8:162–166, 1997.

47. Bootzin RR: Examining the theory and clinical utility of writing about emotional experiences. Psychol Sci 8:167–169, 1997.

48. Dienstfrey H (ed): Placebo and health. Adv Mind-Body Med 16:6–46, 2000.

49. Horwitz RI, Horwitz SM: Adherence to treatment and health outcome. Arch Intern Med 153:1863–1868, 1993.

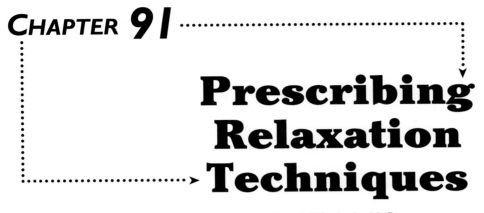
Prescribing Relaxation Techniques

David Rakel, M.D.

HISTORICAL PERSPECTIVE

In the early 20th century, the physiologist Walter Cannon discovered that when subjects were exposed to a number of physical and mentally stressful events, they secreted a large amount of epinephrine, which prepared them for action. He later coined the term "fight-or-flight response" to describe this physical reaction to stress. On the other side of the coin was the Nobel Prize–winning Swiss physiologist, Walter Hess. In the 1930s, Hess found that by stimulating certain areas of the brain of laboratory animals, he was able to induce a physical reaction that was opposite to that seen with the fight-or-flight response. One area triggered signs of relaxation that included reduced muscle tone, breathing, and heart rate. Herbert Benson, working from the same laboratory as Cannon did years earlier, helped pioneer this field when he described the "relaxation response" and how meditation could be used to decrease the response of the sympathetic nervous system. Meditation was found to reduce heart rate, respiratory rate, plasma cortisol, and pulse rate, and to increase electroencephalogram alpha waves associated with relaxation.[1] Evidence was accumulating to support the fact that lifestyle practices can have a direct influence on disease and its prevention.

STRESS AND RELAXATION AND THEIR EFFECTS

It has been well established that stress has damaging effects on health and the immune system caused by dysregulation of the autonomic nervous system and the hypothalamic-pituitary-adrenal axis.[2] As can be seen in Figure 91–1, stress triggers emotions that release chemicals through these sites to stimulate somatic changes that can lead to poor health. Chronic stress results in a continuous activation of cycle A, which helps explain the association between chronic stress and increased susceptibility to infection.[3]

In this age of multitasking, it is not uncommon to see someone driving a car while talking on a phone and jotting down a message. It takes time for our minds to change focus from one topic to another. The more we divert our attention, the less we are able to concentrate on any one task well. If we are constantly being distracted by multiple thoughts, our fight-or-flight response is triggered owing to fear of not being able to address them all. (I am sure many readers can relate.) Giving attention to lifestyle changes that reduce triggers and practicing techniques that activate the relaxation response (cycle B) can have significant health benefits. It is important to remember that the relaxation response can be learned, but it takes practice for the body to benefit. Regular use results in long-term physiologic changes that last throughout the day, not only during the time that the relaxation technique is being practiced.[4]

NOTE

Relaxation techniques are tools that help one to balance the effects of stress, but they are not substitutes for exploring problems that may be causing it.

THE EVIDENCE FOR RELAXATION

There are more than 3000 studies that show the beneficial effects of relaxation on health. It would be foolish to think that we could discuss all of them here. Table 91–1 lists common conditions in which relaxation has been found useful. Many studies document the value of relaxation exercises such as meditation, regulated breathing, and progressive muscle relaxation. Beneficial effects have been shown in tension headaches,[5] anxiety,[6] insomnia,[7] psoriasis,[8] blood pressure,[9, 10] cardiac ischemia and exercise

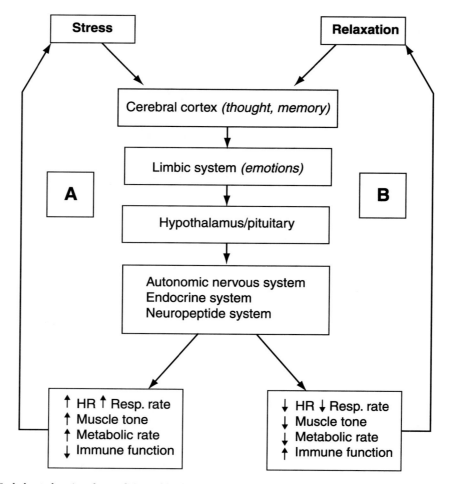

Figure 91–1. A simplified chart showing the cyclic mind-body and body-mind influences of stress (A) and relaxation (B) on health. As our body experiences the physical responses to stress and relaxation, our central nervous system remembers them, causing a continuation of the cycle and resulting in long-term positive or negative physical consequences. HR, heart rate; Resp., respiration.

tolerance,[11] cardiac arrhythmia,[12] premenstrual syndrome,[13] infertility,[14] longevity and cognitive function in the elderly,[15] use of medical care,[16] medical costs in treating chronic pain,[17] smoking cessation,[18] and serum cholesterol.[19] Recommending relaxation

Table 91–1. Conditions that Benefit from Relaxation Exercises
••••••••••••••••••••••••••••••••

Anxiety, anger, and hostility
Depression
Infertility
Pain, headaches
Irritable bowel syndrome
Essential hypertension
Asthma
Dermatologic disorders
Raynaud's disease
Rheumatoid arthritis
Temporal mandibular joint disease
Diabetes
Chronic dyspepsia
Premenstrual syndrome
Cardiac arrhythmias
Smoking cessation
Cognitive function

therapy is very important in the primary care setting because more than 60% of all physician visits are stress related.

WHAT RELAXATION EXERCISES HAVE IN COMMON

It is the mind's thoughts that trigger the physiologic changes that can result in poor health. Working to get "my mind off it" involves focusing on something other than thoughts that cause stress. Mental focus is what all relaxation techniques have in common. Meditation may focus on a mantra; yoga may focus on a body posture (asana) or the breath; guided imagery focuses on an image; and progressive muscle relaxation focuses on the muscles. Relaxation does not need to include these traditional mind–body therapies and may simply involve focusing on a hobby such as painting, playing an instrument, or gardening. Whatever task is used, the mind has a tendency to wander. If this happens, we can simply accept it and bring attention back to the activity at hand. Using a more structured technique helps emphasize the importance of this. Focus frees the mind from its usual stressful thoughts such as worrying, planning, thinking, and reasoning and dampens the production of adrenergic catecholamines that stimulate the limbic system, which, in turn, inhibits immune activity.

RELAXATION AND AEROBIC EXERCISE

We usually do not associate relaxation with exercise, but Herbert Benson and colleagues found that the relaxation response could also be elicited during aerobic exercise. Compared with a control group, volunteers who focused their thoughts on a word or phrase while riding a stationary bike reduced both their oxygen consumption and their metabolic rate, resulting in improved efficiency.[20]

Few may have the time to meditate for 20 minutes twice a day, exercise for 30 minutes, spend quality time with their family, and make a living while still getting 8 hours of sleep each night. Combining relaxation and exercise into one activity uses time more efficiently.

MATCHING THE TECHNIQUE TO THE INDIVIDUAL

Relaxation techniques are similar to ice cream flavors. Once an individual finds a pleasing flavor, there is a tendency to think everyone should try it. The important thing is not to get everyone to meditate but to match a technique that best suits each person's lifestyle. In fact, it has been shown that various relaxation techniques, such as medita-

tion, biofeedback, hypnosis, guided imagery, or progressive muscle relaxation, induce the same physiologic response.[21] There are many different ways to arrive at the desired outcome. Matching the technique to the individual leads to greater success in inducing relaxation; also, with this approach, the technique is used more often. For example, a body-vigilant woman with breast cancer may not respond well to progressive muscle relaxation, because this requires focus on specific parts of the body. An anxious, type A individual may do better with this technique because it gives an active mind a focal point.[22] A relaxation exercise should be as individualized as a medication prescribed for hypertension.

> ### NOTE
> *The most important task for the medical provider is to match the relaxation technique to the patient's personality, beliefs, and lifestyle.*

Relaxation exercises are a low-cost, well-tolerated therapy that can be recommended for many problems seen in the primary care setting. It may be most useful in treating patients suffering from anxiety, heart disease, recurring pain syndromes, and chronic illness, but it will also be beneficial in helping patients find a balance, which results in the best medicine of all—prevention. Table 91–2 provides a brief summary of various relaxation exercises.

Table 91–2. Relaxation Techniques

Relaxation Technique	Summary	Further Resources
Breathing exercise (see Chapter 88, Breathing Exercises.)	The foundation of most relaxation techniques. Have the patients place one hand on the chest and the other on the abdomen. Instruct the patient to take a slow deep breath, as if sucking in all the air in the room. While doing this, the hand on the abdomen should rise higher than that on the chest. This promotes diaphragmatic breathing that increases alveolar expansion in the bases of the lungs. The patient should hold the breath for a count of 7 and then exhale. Exhalation should take twice as long as inhalation. This process should be repeated for a total of 5 breaths. Encourage patients to do this three times a day.	*Conscious Breathing* by Gay Hendricks is one of many good resources on the use of breathing for relaxation and health.
Meditation (see Chapter 94, Learning to Meditate)		
Transcendental meditation (TM)/The relaxation response	To prevent distracting thoughts, the subject repeats a mantra (a word or sound) over and over again while sitting in a comfortable position. If a distracting thought comes to mind, it is accepted and let go with the mind focusing again on the mantra.	www.mindbody.harvard.edu or *The Relaxation Response* by Herbert Benson. www.tm.org for information on transcendental meditation.

Table 91–2. Relaxation Techniques (Continued)

Relaxation Technique	Summary	Further Resources
Mindful meditation	Represents the philosophy of living in the present or the moment. The **body scan** is one technique whereby the subject uses breathing to obtain a relaxed state while lying or sitting. The mind progressively focuses on different parts of the body where it feels any and all sensations intentionally but nonjudgmentally before moving onto another part of the body. A patient with back pain may focus on the quality and characteristics of the pain as if to better understand it and bring it under control.	*Full Catastrophe Living* by Jon Kabat-Zinn describes this technique in full and the program for stress reduction at the University of Massachusetts Medical Center.
Centering prayer	A form similar to TM that has a more religious foundation. The subject repeats a "sacred word" similar to a mantra. As thoughts come to mind, they are accepted and let go, clearing the mind to become more centered on the spirit within. It is as if the mind's preoccupied thoughts are the layers of an onion that are peeled away, allowing better understanding of the spirit at the core.	www.centeringprayer.com Look under "method of centering prayer" for a nondenominational discussion.
Progressive muscle relaxation (PMR)	A form of relaxation whereby the subject is attuned to the difference in feelings when the muscles are tensed and then relaxed. The subject chooses a comfortable position and starts by tensing the whole body from head to toe. While doing this, feelings of tightness are noted. A deep breath should be taken in, and as it is let out, the tension is released and the muscles relax. This is followed by progressive tension and relaxation throughout the body. One may start by clenching the fists and then tensing the arms, shoulders, chest, abdomen, hips, legs, and so on, with each step followed by relaxation.	www.uaex.edu/other_Areas/ publications/HTML/FSHEI-28.asp is a good review of PMR as well as other relaxation exercises. It is sponsored by the University of Arkansas. *You Must Relax* is a book by the founder of this technique, Edmund Jacobson.
Visualization/self-hypnosis (see Chapter 92, Guided Imagery and Interactive Guided Imagery, and Chapter 89, Self-Hypnosis Techniques)	The subject uses visualization to call up images that create a relaxed state. For example, if a person is anxious, visualizing images of a place and time that were peaceful and comforting would help induce relaxation. This is best used in conjunction with a breathing exercise.	There are many audiotapes available to guide people through a visualization "script", with resultant relaxation. Emmett Miller is one well-known author.
Autogenic training	A physiologic response is induced by use of simple phrases. For example, "My legs are heavy and warm" is meant to increase the blood flow to this area, resulting in relaxation. This is done progressively from head to toe with the use of deep breathing and repetition of the phrase. After completing this process, attention should be focused on any body part that may still be tense. The breath and phrase are focused on that area until the whole body is relaxed.	The British Autogenic Society, www.autogenictherapy.org.uk is a good resource for more information.
Exercise/movement		
Aerobic exercise	While performing an aerobic exercise, the subject focuses attention on a phrase, sound, word, or prayer and passively disregards other thoughts that may enter the mind. Some may focus on their breathing, by saying to themselves "in," with inhalation and "out," with exhalation, or by repeating "one two, one two" with each step while jogging. Doing this helps the mind focus and prevents other thoughts that may cause tension.	*Beyond the Relaxation Response* by Herbert Benson includes discussion on his research on inducing the relaxation response while exercising.
Yoga	Has been practiced for thousands of years in India. In America, it has been divided into three aspects: breathing (pranayama yoga), bodily postures or asanas (hatha yoga), and meditation to maintain balance and health. Regular practice induces relaxation.	For this and the following therapies, it is best to encourage patients to take a class at a local community center or gym and to pick up an introductory book at a library or bookstore.
Tai chi	An ancient Chinese martial art that uses slow, graceful movements combined with inner mindfulness and breathing techniques to help bring balance between the mind and body.	As above.
Qi gong	A traditional Chinese practice that uses movement, meditation, and controlled breathing to balance the body's vital energy force, chi.	As above.

References

1. Shapiro D: Meditation. In Strohecker J, Trivieri L, Lewis D, Florence M (eds): Alternative Medicine: The Definitive Guide, Fife, Wash, Future Medicine Publishing, 1995, pp 339–345.
2. Stanford SC, Salmon P: Stress: From Synapse to Syndrome. London, Academic Press, 1999.
3. Everly GS, Benson H: Disorders of arousal and the relaxation response: Speculations on the nature of treatment of stress-related diseases. Int J Psychosom 36:15–21, 1989.

4. Hoffman JW, Benson H, Arns PA, et al: Reduced sympathetic nervous system responsivity associated with the relaxation response. Science 215:190–192, 1982.
5. Blanchard EB, Nicholson NL, Taylor AE, et al: The role of regular home practice in the relaxation treatment of tension headache. J Consult Clin Psychol 59:467–470, 1991.
6. Eppley KR, Abrams AL, Shear J: Differential effects of relaxation techniques on trait anxiety: A meta-analysis. J Clin Psychol 45:957–974, 1989.
7. Jacobs GD, Benson H, Friedman R: Perceived benefits in a behavioral-medicine insomnia program: A clinical report. Am J Med 100:212–216, 1996.
8. Kabat-Zinn J, Wheeler E, Light T, et al: Influence of a mindfulness meditation-based stress reduction intervention on rates of skin clearing in patients with moderate to severe psoriasis undergoing phototherapy and photochemotherapy. Psychosom Med 60:625–632, 1998.
9. Alexander CN, Schneider RH, Staggers F, et al: Trial of stress reduction for hypertension in older African Americans. II. Sex and risk subgroup anaylysis. Hypertension 28:228–237, 1996.
10. Stuart E, Caudill M, Leserman J, et al: Nonpharmacologic treatment of hypertension: A multiple-risk-factor approach. J Cardiovasc Nurs 1:1–14, 1987.
11. Zamarra J, Schneider RH, Bessighini I, et al: Usefulness of the transcendental meditation program in the treatment of patients with coronary artery disease. Am J Cardiol 77:867–870, 1996.
12. Benson H, Alexander S, Feldman CL: Decreased premature ventricular contractions through use of the relaxation response in patients with stable ischemic heart disease. Lancet 2:380–382, 1975.
13. Goodale IL, Domar AD, Benson H: Alleviation of premenstrual syndrome symptoms with the relaxation response. Obstet Gynecol 75:649–655, 1990.
14. Domar AD, Seibel M, Benson H: The mind/body program for infertility: A new behavioral treatment approach for women with infertility. Fertil Steril 53:246–249, 1990.
15. Alexander C, Chandler HM, Langer EJ, et al: Transcendental meditation, mindfulness, and longevity: An experimental study with the elderly. J Personal Soc Psychol 57:950–964, 1989.
16. Orme-Johnson D: Medical care utilization and the transcendental meditation program. Psychosom Med 49:493–507, 1987.
17. Caudill M, Schnable R, Zuttermeister P, et al: Decreased clinic use by chronic pain patients: Response to behavioral medicine interventions. Clin J Pain 7:305–310, 1991.
18. Royer-Bounour P: The transcendental meditation technique: A new direction for smoking cessation programs. Dissertation Abstr Int 50:3428B, 1989.
19. Cooper M, Aygen M: Effect of meditation on blood cholesterol and blood pressure. Isr Med Assoc 95:1–2, 1978.
20. Benson H, Dryer T, Hartley LH: Decreased VO$_2$ consumption during exercise with elicitation of the relaxation response. J Hum Stress 4:38–42, 1978.
21. Delmonte MM: Physiological concomitants of meditation practice. Int J Psychosom 31:23–36, 1984.
22. Rakel DP, Shapiro DE: Mind-body medicine. In Rakel RE (ed): Textbook of Family Practice, 6th ed. Philadelphia, WB Saunders, 2002, pp. 52–64.

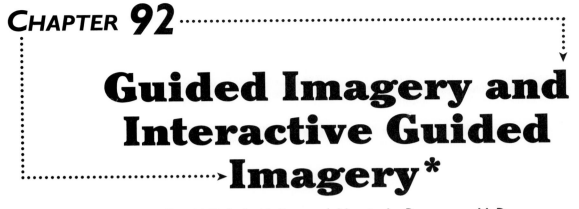

CHAPTER 92

Guided Imagery and Interactive Guided Imagery*

David Rakel, M.D., and Martin L. Rossman, M.D.

Imagination is more important than knowledge.
                                        Albert Einstein

Imagery is simply a form of sensory-based thinking that is an extremely effective tool for accessing and influencing the subconscious mind. Imagery not only can cause direct changes in the physical body but also can act as an avenue for the expression of subconscious feelings. This expression can lead to resolution of fear, guilt, anger, or grief that may have been directly affecting physical health. Guided imagery can help patients to prepare for surgery and can relieve pain, reduce anxiety, and stimulate healing responses in the body.

Interactive Guided Imagery is a specific technique that helps patients to develop insight regarding illness and to use their inner resources more effectively to facilitate healing. In this modality, a trained practitioner guides the patient to discover and work with personal imagery regarding a symptom or illness, to clarify any issues that may be involved, and to use the mind to support the healing process.

Guided imagery uses the mental equivalents of the five senses to allow communication with physiologic and emotional processes usually out of the realm of awareness. Imagery is sometimes referred to as a "right brain" type of thinking because it tends to be synthetic, creative, and emotional. This type of thinking contrasts with the more familiar "left brain" type of linear, logical thinking. To illustrate the difference between these two types of thinking, imagine watching a train go by. From the left brain perspective, the train is seen from the ground in a linear array in which each car goes by, one by one. From the right brain perspective, the train is viewed from above, as a single entity. The visualization incorporates where it is going and where it has been.

Imagery-based thinking can often reveal perspectives that demonstrate how life events, emotions, and physical symptoms are connected. For example, in one patient with lumpy breasts, guided imagery revealed the lumps to be like pearls—formed in response to irritation. She further imagined: "They are trying to protect me. They want me to reduce the stress I've been living with, and the caffeine I've been using to try to keep up."

Guided imagery, especially Interactive Guided Imagery, is a tool that can empower patients to help themselves. Having a better understanding of what the subconscious mind may be signaling through symptoms can often result not only in symptom resolution but in a more balanced overall approach to health maintenance. These benefits are possible whether the patient has a diagnosed illness or a group of symptoms that cannot be further classified (Table 92–1).

PRECAUTIONS AND CONTRAINDICATIONS

Although directed guided imagery sessions—in which a patient is the passive recipient of suggested images from a recording or practitioner—are generally quite safe in the hands of a skilled practitioner, it is important to realize that Interactive Guided Imagery—in which the patient is in active discussion with the practitioner guide to explore images and their meaning—can be a powerful tool that can connect people with emotional material very quickly. Primary care providers who have well-established

Table 92–1. Indications for Guided Imagery

Intervention for acute stress or anxiety (pediatric and adult patients)
To prepare for surgery or a procedure
To help reduce or manage side effects of medications or procedures
To help patients and practitioners better understand symptoms
To help fight illness through working with the body's own healing processes
To help manage anxiety, fear, and pain
To help people prepare for changes including life style, habits, adaptation to illness, and even death

---

*Interactive Guided Imagery is a particular approach taught by the Academy for Guided Imagery.

Table 92-2. Contraindications to Guided Imagery
....

Strong religious beliefs proscribing the use of imagery
Disorientation, dementia, or impaired cognition due to
   pharmacologic or other agents
Inability to hold a train of thought for at least 5 to 10 min
Potential litigation—guided imagery may be considered a form
   of hypnosis, which affects the legal status of information
   obtained with its use

Table 92-3. Cautions in Using Guided Imagery*
....

History of physical or sexual abuse
Active psychosis or prepsychotic state
Diffuse dissociative disorders
Post-traumatic stress disorder/anxiety disorders
Personal history of suicide attempt(s), or family history of
   suicide/suicide attempts
Unstable medical problems such as severe asthma, heart
   disease, or pain

*Practitioners treating people in these categories should be
very well versed in both the treatment of the underlying
disorder and the use of guided imagery.

Table 92-4. Common Interactive Guided Imagery Phrases
....

"Allow an image to form."
"What do you notice about it?"
"What are you aware of?"
"What are you experiencing?"
"What would you like to do now?"
"What feelings do you notice yourself having?"
"What would you like to say to it?"
"What sensations are you aware of?"
"Let me know when you are ready to move on."

relationships with patients will generally know which persons have the resiliency to tolerate the affect and insight that can come from an Interactive Guided Imagery session (Table 92–2). The practitioner should proceed with caution, however, with patients who have a history of serious childhood abuse or psychiatric disease (Table 92–3).

The practitioner should be sufficiently versed in guided imagery skills to be able to recognize potentially problematic situations and to remedy them if encountered unexpectedly.

THE BASICS OF A GUIDED IMAGERY SESSION

Before a session of guided imagery, it is important to educate the patient about what guided imagery is and then to obtain the patient's verbal consent to participation. The practitioner should give the patient an idea of what will happen in the session. For example, in explaining the technique to a patient with chronic pain, the practitioner may state:

"We will first lead you into a state of relaxation. Here you will be able to focus inward, allowing your subconscious to easily access images. After you are relaxed, you will be asked to focus on a safe and comfortable place. This may be a place you've been before or a place that just exists in your imagination. Once you feel comfortable in this place, you will progress to allowing an image to form that represents your pain. You will then get to know this image and learn how it relates to your pain and what information it can bring you."

Once it has been established that the use of guided imagery is safe and appropriate, and after the patient's consent has been obtained, the practitioner may select a scripted guided imagery process or tape or may choose to use Interactive Guided Imagery if

he or she is qualified to do so. It is important to realize that the role of an Interactive Imagery guide is that of a facilitator. The practitioner does not provide specific content for the patient, but rather creates opportunities that allow the patient to explore his or her own images.

For the practice of Interactive Guided Imagery, use of a specific language will allow the patient to explore and learn from the experience most effectively. The questions should be open-ended and content-free. The practitioner guide helps the patient to notice the character of the imagery using all five senses. The practitioner must also feel comfortable using pauses of silence to allow the patient's mind to investigate its image. Some samples of common guiding phrases are listed in Table 92–4. The practitioner must also be careful not to use words conducive to negative thoughts or suggestive of failure. Phrases such as "try to" and "can you" are to be avoided, whereas the use of open, engaging words such as "allow" and "you may" is desirable. The goal is to use language that is noninvasive and allows the patient to have complete freedom in exploring the experience.

OUTLINE OF A GUIDED IMAGERY SESSION

Table 92–5 outlines a basic guided imagery session. Discussion of the specific components follows.

Assessment

The assessment is similar to taking a history. The practitioner asks about previous experience with imagery, hypnosis, or relaxation. The problem that will be addressed with imagery is identified, and the patient is asked what he or she would like to get out of the session. For example, the patient's main complaint may be back pain, and the desired result is symptom relief. This information can then be used to help the patient interact with the image in order to gain a better understanding of how he or she can decrease the pain. For example, the patient may give the pain an image of a nail in the back. The practitioner will then facilitate dialogue, or conversation, with the nail that may lead to an understanding of why it is there and what it may "need." This under-

Table 92–5. Components of a Guided Imagery Session
....

1. Assessment
   • Ask what symptom, illness, or thoughts the patient would like to explore.
   • Ask what the patient wants to get out of the session.
   • Ask the patient to narrow the problem down to one or two words.
   • How does the patient best relax?
   • Help the patient to formulate a one-sentence summary of goals.
   • Obtain the patient's consent.

2. Relaxation
   • Deep breathing with body contacts, body scan, or golden light.
   • Patients can use a relaxation technique of their own.

3. Helping the patient to conceptualize a "special place"
   • "Allow yourself to imagine a comfortable and peaceful place. It might be a place that you have been before or something that's just coming into your imagination now. If you imagine several places coming to mind, allow yourself to pick just one to explore now."
   • "Describe the place with regard to sensations. What do you see, hear, smell, feel, and taste? Why does it make you feel comfortable?"
   • "Find a comfortable place to settle down."

4. Imagery dialogue
   • **Form an image** that represents the illness or symptom.
   • **Describe** the image in detail. (Have the patient describe at least three characteristics, such as appearance, character, and emotions of the image.)
   • **Identify qualities** that the image portrays.
   • **Explore feelings** toward the image.
   • **Express these feelings** to the image and allow it to respond.

   Other questions

   "How do you feel about that?"
   "What is the meaning of that?"
   "Why is it there?"
   "How might it help you?"
   "Do you have any questions you would like to ask it?"
   "What does the image want or need?"
   "What does it want you to know?"
   "What does it need from you?"
   "What does it have in common with you?"
   "What does it have to offer?"

   • Ask the image what it can tell you about the **problem**.
   • Ask the image what it can tell you about the **solution**.
   • Go back to the safe place; then return from the inner place.

   Summary

   Facilitate communication between the patient and the image. If the patient appears frightened, ask if she or he feels safe; if not, the patient mentally returns to the safe place, or the patient is asked to identify what he or she needs to feel safe. Repeat key phrases the patient uses to encourage further exploration of the image.

5. Evaluation
   • Explore the **meaning**. (What did the session tell the patient about the symptom or illness?)
   • Identify the **next steps** to be taken. (The practitioner assists the patient to explore options based on what she or he has learned.)

standing can lead to decreased symptoms or a behavioral change that will help control the pain.

The practitioner then summarizes what the goals of the guided imagery will be in one or two sentences and obtains consent from the patient to participate in the process.

Relaxation

In order to be able to focus on the imagery, it is important for the patient to achieve a relaxed state. Some patients may be able to do this quickly and easily; for others it will take much longer. The practitioner asks whether the patient has a specific way to relax; if so, the patient describes the method used. Then the patient is simply invited to use that method and to state when he or she is comfortable and relaxed.

If the patient does not know a way to relax, the practitioner can teach a relaxation method such as one of the following methods.

Body Scan. This is done by having the patient focus on each body part in turn, starting at one end of the body, and allowing each to relax as it is named in sequence. The sequence can progress in either the caudal or cephalic direction. This technique takes more time but is useful for persons who may have trouble relaxing.

Golden Light. The patient is directed to imagine a ball of golden energy at the base of the spine. With each inhalation, it is pictured as moving up the spine to the head; with exhalation, it spills over, causing the body to go deeper into a relaxed state.

Points of Contact. After focusing on breathing, the patient concentrates on the parts of the body that are in contact with the chair or bed or other support surface. The patient can also focus on parts of the body that are in contact with each other, such as in interlacing of the fingers. This method is the fastest and is best used in persons who are able to relax well.

After one of these relaxation scenarios is completed, the patient is asked to raise a finger or nod the head when he or she feels completely relaxed and is ready to go on.

Conceptualizing a Special Place

The "special place" is an image that brings comfort and peace. It serves as a place of safety to which the patient can return at any time if he or she feels threatened or in danger. It also sets the stage for further exploration into the subconscious.

In assisting the patient to develop an image of a special place, the practitioner may state:

"Allow yourself to imagine a comfortable, peaceful place. It may be a place you've been before or something that's just coming into your imagination now. If you notice several places coming to mind, allow yourself to pick just one to explore now. When you are there, describe it to me."

In describing this place, the patient characterizes the qualities in relation to the senses. What does the patient see, hear, smell, feel, or taste? The patient also describes the feelings he or she is experiencing and why the place feels so comfortable. Once the patient has explored the surroundings, he or she settles down in one place and relaxes.

Interactive Imagery Dialogue

The dialogue between the patient and the symptom or illness as imaged is the heart of the session. It allows communication to take place between the patient and the image conjured up to represent the problem. The practitioner may state:

"Allow an image to form that represents your back pain, and when you are ready, describe it to me."

The patient is encouraged to describe the qualities of the image in depth. The practitioner uses phrases such as "Go on" or "Tell me more" to assist the patient to stay connected to this image. The patient should describe the image at three different levels, such as appearance, character, and emotions. Next, the patient describes his or her feelings about the image. Then it is time to facilitate communication between the patient and the image. The patient is directed to express his or her feelings to the image itself, allowing the image to respond. As the patient learns more about the image through this dialogue, the practitioner helps the patient to address the questions he or she was concerned about in the assessment. For example, with back pain, the practitioner may have the patient ask the image why it is causing him or her so much pain.

After the communication has occurred, it is time to end the session. The patient should be encouraged to take any information learned with him or her. The practitioner assists the patient to go back to the safe place and to relax there for a few breaths, and then to return to the outer world by having the patient slowly become aware of the physical self. The patient is directed to move the toes, feet, legs, and arms and to stretch and open the eyes.

Evaluation

For the evaluation, the practitioner asks the patient what he or she learned from the imagery. It is not the practitioner's job to interpret the patient's experience. Rather, the patient is assisted to explore the meaning of the session and then to identify the "next steps" based on what has been learned. Some patients may learn what they need to know after just one session, but most will need further sessions to better understand their condition. The practitioner takes notes during these sessions for reference during any subsequent visits.

TRAINING

This chapter is merely an introduction to a very useful tool for exploring the mind-body influence on health. Guided imagery requires practice and training, just as with any other modality. Further training can be obtained from the following institutions.

- Academy for Guided Imagery
  Offers training that leads to certification in Interactive Guided Imagery.
  P.O. Box 2070
  Mill Valley, CA 94942
  (415) 389-9325 or (800) 726-2070
  www.interactiveimagery.com

- Imaginative Medicine
  Offers training for health professional groups.
  (509) 533-9481 (based in Washington)

Resources for Guided Imagery Recordings

Although prerecordings do not allow for individualization and interaction with images, they can be helpful tools in helping to facilitate healing. Some respected resources for imagery tapes and compact discs are listed. All of these web site listings include disease-specific recordings as well as more recordings on general topics such as surgery preparation and recovery, immune support, and cancer therapy.

- Emmett Miller, M.D.
  Dr. Miller has spent many years studying and practicing psycho-physiologic medicine.
  www.docmiller.com
  (800) 528-2737

- Steven Gurgevich, Ph.D.
  On the faculty of the Integrative Medicine program at the University of Arizona, Dr. Gurgevich uses the art of hypnotherapy to provide tapes for many medical conditions.
  www.tranceformation.com
  (520) 886-1700

- Belleruth Naparstek, LISW
  Many of this practitioner's recordings have been used in medical research.
  www.healthjourneys.com
  (800) 800-8661

- The Imagery Store
  A service of the Academy for Guided Imagery.
  www.interactiveimagery.com
  (800) 726-2070

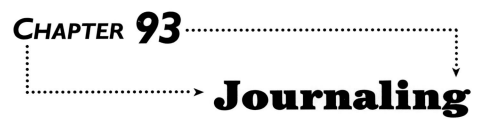

CHAPTER 93 Journaling

David Rakel, M.D.

I find, by experience, that the mind and the body are more than married, for they are most intimately united; and when one suffers, the other sympathizes.

Lord Chesterfield

DISCLOSURE

The pathologist William Boyd was quoted as saying at the turn of the 19th century, "The sorrow that hath no vent in tears, may make other organs weep." The expression of emotionally upsetting experiences by writing or talking has been found to improve physical health, enhance immune function, and result in fewer medical visits.[1] For example, simply writing about past stressful life experiences has been found to result in symptom reduction in patients with asthma and rheumatoid arthritis. One hundred and seven patients with these diseases were assigned to write either about the most stressful event of their lives (study group) or about daily events (control group) for just 20 minutes over 3 consecutive days. Four months after journaling, the asthma patients in the treatment group showed a 20% improvement in lung function versus no improvement in the control group. The patients with rheumatoid arthritis who wrote about stressful events showed a 28% reduction in disease severity, whereas the control group showed no change.[2] These are excellent results requiring only paper, pencil, and 60 minutes of the patient's time. Another study showed that there were increased incidences of infectious diseases and cancer in gay men who concealed their homosexual identity when compared with those who were open.[3]

To understand the pathophysiology behind the positive clinical effects of disclosure, we review a study by James Pennebaker, a pioneer in the field. He interviewed polygraphers (operators of lie detectors) who worked for the FBI and CIA. In doing these tests, the polygraphers would look for changes in parameters of the autonomic nervous system, such as heart rate, blood pressure, respiratory rate, and skin conductance, for clues of validity. He described what was called "the polygraph confession effect," in which readings in these areas significantly dropped after a person confessed. These changes were consistent with those seen with relaxation. It is thought that to actively inhibit one's thoughts, feelings, and behaviors requires physical work, work that can result in a chronic low-grade stress to the autonomic nervous system that may result in disease.[4] This inhibition can also lead to dysregulation of the hypothalamic-pituitary-adrenal axis (HPA) that results in hypercortisolemia and immune suppression.[5]

Disclosing stressful events transfers repressed thoughts from the unconscious to the conscious level where they can be organized and controlled. This removes the need for chronic low-grade stress to stimulate the autonomic nervous system and the HPA that can lead to disease and somatic symptoms. Disclosing allows our mind to interpret this new information from the subconscious, unlocking emotions that can stimulate positive physical results. In trying to understand how a stressor is stored in the mind, think of a money machine that you may have seen at a fair. A lucky person wins a chance to enter the booth and grab as much paper money as possible while a fan blows it all around. When our mind stores a stressful event, it is not organized and stored as a concrete thought, but rather as a chaotic accumulation of a multitude of images, sensations, and emotions similar to the money in the booth. It is not until we grab the money, hold it in our hand, and count it that we are aware of what we have. Disclosing is the process of organizing chaotic thoughts, allowing us to interpret and evaluate the stressor. In doing so, the chronic somatic stress improves.

It is important to keep in mind that the process of disclosure may improve physical but not always mental health.[6] Our minds suppress these traumatic events for a reason, and uncovering them can be difficult for the conscious mind to handle, especially in children. Disclosure has been found to be beneficial for those who have endured traumatic events (e.g., holocaust survivors) but has not been found beneficial for those with documented post-traumatic stress disorder (PTSD) without simultaneous coping skills training.[7] In many cases, it is important to work closely with a licensed therapist so the patient can continue to heal from this expression.

The primary care provider is in an ideal position to help patients heal through disclosure because people are more likely to discuss these stressful events with someone who is accepting and whom they trust.[8] This relationship takes time to develop to a point at which the patient feels comfortable revealing secrets. It takes an average of 1 month for children to disclose an abusive event to a psychotherapist.[9] The patient does not need to disclose verbally to another human being. The healing process can occur by writing down the thoughts, a process commonly known as *journaling*. The idea is that the patient is able to organize the thoughts of the stressful event through verbal or written words that can then be reflected on and be kept confidential if the patient wishes. Directions for your patients on how to journal to improve health are given in the Patient Handout.

References

1. Berry DS, Pennebaker JW: Nonverbal and verbal emotional expression and health. Psychother Psychosom 59:11–19, 1993.
2. Smyth JM, Stone AA, Hurewitz A, Kaell A: Effects of writing about stressful experiences on symptom reduction in patients with asthma or rheumatoid arthritis. JAMA 281:1304–1309, 1999.
3. Cole SW, Kemeny ME, Taylor SE, Vischer BR: Elevated physical health risk among gay men who conceal their homosexual identity. Health Psychol 15(49):243–251, 1996.
4. Pennebaker JW: Opening Up: The Healing Power of Expressing Emotions. New York, Guilford, 1997.
5. Kiecolt-Glaser JK, Glaser R, Cacioppo JT, Malarkey WB: Marital stress: Immunologic, neuroendocrine, and autonomic correlates. Ann N Y Acad Sci 840:656–663, 1998.
6. Pennebaker JW, Mayne TJ, Francis ME: Linguistic predictors of adaptive bereavement. J Pers Soc Psychol 72:863–871, 1997.
7. Gidron Y, Peri T, Connolly JF, Shalev AY: Written disclosure in posttraumatic stress disorder: Is it beneficial for the patient? J Nerv Ment Dis 184:505–507, 1996.
8. Fox SG, Strum CA, Walters HA: Perceptions of therapist disclosure of previous experience as a client. J Clin Psychol 40:496–498, 1984.
9. Gonzales LS, Waterman J, Kelly RJ, et al: Children's patterns of disclosures and recantations of sexual and ritualistic abuse allegations in psychotherapy. Child Abuse Negl 17:281–289, 1993.

PATIENT HANDOUT
USING JOURNALING TO AID HEALTH

What Is Journaling?

Journaling is the process of writing about times in our lives that were stressful or traumatic. It provides an avenue for the expression of thoughts and memories that may have been internalized, worsening physical symptoms. A quote by William Boyd, a pathologist at the turn of the 20th century, describes this process well. He said, "The sorrow that hath no vent in tears, may make other organs weep." Journaling is one type of therapy that can be used to aid this process.

How Does It Work?

Studies have found that if we express feelings about a time in our lives that was very traumatic or stressful, our immune function strengthens, we become more relaxed, and our health may improve. Writing about these processes helps us organize our thoughts and create closure to an event that our minds have a tendency to want to suppress or hide. This can be done in the privacy of the home and requires only pen and paper.

Does Anybody Need to Read It?

No. You can share your writings with others if you desire but no one needs to read what is written. The most benefit comes from writing the document; the words can be thrown away if desired. In fact, burning or destroying the document can ceremonially bring closure to a difficult time in your life. Others prefer to keep their writings private to look back on and see how they have grown from the events.

Are There Any Side Effects or Things I Should Be Aware Of?

Recalling stressful memories can make you feel uncomfortable for a few days. If this were not the case, the body would not use so much energy trying to repress them. The benefits from journaling become most apparent weeks to months after writing.

This process can bring back to mind some frightening events that may need the help of a licensed counselor. Please notify your medical provider if you develop feelings that would benefit from further discussion. This is often the first step toward creating an environment that will promote healing from within.

How Is It Done?

There are many different ways to express emotions. Journaling is simple and inexpensive and can be done independently. It would be beneficial to keep a regular journal to write about events that bring anger, grief, or joy. But if that is unlikely and you just want to deal with a specific event or see whether this will help your condition, follow these steps.

- Find a quiet place where you will not be disturbed.
- Using pen, pencil, or computer, write about an upsetting or troubling experience in your life: something that has affected you deeply and that you have not discussed at length with others.
- First describe the event in detail. Write about the situation, surroundings, and sensations that you remember.
- Then describe your deepest feeling regarding the event. Let go and allow the emotions to run freely in your writing. Describe how you felt about the event then and now.
- Write continuously. Do not worry about grammar, spelling, or sentence structure. If you come to a block, simply repeat what you have already written.
- Before finishing, write about what you may have learned or how you may have grown from the event.
- Write for 20 minutes daily for at least 4 days. You can write about different events or reflect on the same one each day.
- Consider keeping a regular journal if the process proves helpful.

How Can I Learn More?

An excellent resource for more information on this subject can be found in the book, *Opening Up: The Healing Power of Expressing Emotions* by James Pennebaker, Ph.D. (Guilford Press, 1997).

www.journaltherapy.com is a comprehensive web site on the subject.

CHAPTER 94

Learning To Meditate

David Rakel, M.D.

WHAT IS IT?

"Meditation is simplicity itself. . . . It's about stopping and being present, that is all." This quote by Jon Kabat-Zinn sums up the process nicely. In our culture, many of us are on autopilot in which thoughts are focused on memories of the past or desires of the future. We may drive home from work a thousand times and not notice the objects that we pass because our minds are somewhere else. Meditation helps us quiet the mind of these distracting thoughts so that we can live more in the present moment. It is here that we can explore our inner selves and bring peace. For the peace is already there once you stop disturbing it.

Meditation involves focusing the mind and paying attention. This attention may be directed toward a word, sound, picture, prayer, or the breath. This focus allows the mind to settle into the present moment, decreasing the many stressful thoughts that bring us into the past or future. An analogy can be made with a radio dial. The static represents numerous thoughts of the day that preoccupy the mind. Meditation is a tool that allows fine-tuning of the dial so that the music and thoughts of the inner self can be heard more clearly.

There are many methods of meditating; the important thing is to find the one that best fits you.

WHAT CAN IT DO?

It has been well established that long-term stress has damaging effects on health and the immune system through creating an imbalance of the chemicals in the brain that control function.[1] Benson and coworkers pioneered this field when they described the "relaxation response" and how meditation could be used to decrease the response of the sympathetic nervous system, or what was termed the fight-or-flight response.[2] Meditation was found to reduce heart rate, oxygen consumption, respiratory rate, plasma cortisol, and pulse rate and to increase alpha brain waves that are associated with relaxation.[3] Relaxation exercises such as meditation have shown beneficial effects on the severity of tension headaches,[4] anxiety,[5] psoriasis,[6] blood pressure in African Americans,[7] cardiac ischemia and exercise tolerance,[8] longevity and cognitive function in the elderly,[9] use of medical care,[10] medical costs in treating chronic pain,[11] smoking cessation,[12] and serum cholesterol.[13]

Meditation not only results in improvement and prevention of chronic disease but also can lead to deeper spiritual understanding. Harvard's Benson found that patients who were taught meditation for stress reduction often reported feeling more spiritual, more connected to all people and things. It is an excellent tool that may open the door to infinite possibilities of exploring the spirit. Whether we know it or not, we are all on a spiritual journey. We are looking for a better, more meaningful way of life. Quieting the mind can be the first step to help us find that inner voice that rings true in this world of cluttered thought and expectations.

Many of the major religions would agree. Years ago, when practitioners of Christianity, Islam, Buddhism, Judaism, and Hinduism developed meditation techniques, their primary goal was not relaxation, but direct insight into the nature of God and the universe. Meditation was a means of letting go of the self or ego and of cultivating an understanding of love and compassion. Christian teachings claim, "The path leading to heaven is that of complete stillness." The Jewish Psalm urges, "Be still and know that I am God." The Buddha teaches, "May you develop mental concentration . . . for whosoever is mentally concentrated, sees things according to reality."

HOW IS IT DONE?

Quieting the mind can be done successfully in many ways. For ease of demonstration we focus on a mantra meditation that is similar to Transcendental Meditation (TM).

- First pick a word or phrase (mantra) that has meaning to you. This can be anything that brings you comfort. A neutral word may be "peace," "joy," "one," or "love." A religious example might include "God," "Shalom," or "the Lord is my shepherd."
- Find a quiet place to sit where there are few distractions.
- Commit to a set amount of time. Time yourself by periodically glancing at a clock, if needed, but do not set an alarm.

- Sit in a comfortable position that you can maintain with your back straight but not stiff.
- Close your eyes and relax.
- Allow yourself to notice your breath as you inhale and exhale. Breathe slowly and naturally. As you exhale, repeat your word or phrase. If you have a long phrase, feel free to divide it into half with inhalation and half with exhalation.
- When you notice your mind wandering, simply and gently return to your focus word. You will have thoughts of daydreams, tasks, worries, passions, and the like, but simply say to yourself, "oh well" or "that's interesting," and return to the repetition.
- Assume a passive attitude and do not worry whether you are doing it right or wrong. Some find it helpful to use the analogy of swimming in the ocean. The idea is to drop 4 or 5 feet below the surface and observe the waves of thoughts as they go by. As you focus on your word or phrase, the sea will calm.
- At the end of your meditation, sit comfortably for a minute or two and stand slowly when ready.

TIPS

- Meditate on an empty stomach. Food has been found to inhibit the beneficial physiologic effects on the body.
- If able, meditate with a friend, spouse, or relative.

EXPECTATIONS

The process of quieting the mind is unique for each individual, and having a goal to reach contradicts the mission of the activity. With continued practice, though, you may find it helpful to learn of the various experiences and benefits meditation may bring.

- The experienced practitioner will find it easier to quiet the mind. Whereas the beginner may have hundreds of thoughts during meditation, with time these will become fewer and fewer.
- Some may enter what is called "the gap," which is void of thought and mantra—a time for simply being present in the moment.
- Some may experience an increased sense of control in the world instead of being a passive "victim."
- Some may develop less focus on self or ego, which enhances a sense of love and compassion.
- There may be a deepening of spiritual life and/or religious experience.
- There may be a feeling of being more connected to all people and things.

A simple Russian peasant who lived around the middle of the 19th century sums up the journey of a meditative practice nicely: "At first, spiritual practitioners feel that the mind is like a waterfall, bouncing from rock to rock, roaring and turbulent, impossible to tame or control. In midcourse, it is like a great river, calm and gentle, wide and deep. At the end its boundaries expand beyond sight and its depth becomes unfathomable as it dissolves into the ocean, which is both its goal and Source."[14]

PRECAUTIONS

Meditation does not create unpleasant feelings. But quieting the mind may make you more aware of ones that are already there. This can be a very important step in healing but often requires the help of a professional counselor to make sure that these thoughts and feelings are dealt with in a constructive and educational way. If you experience any strong or disturbing emotions, please discuss them with your medical care provider.

> ### NOTE
>
> *Quieting the mind can make one aware of preexisting stressors or memories that may require the aid of a counselor to deal with these emotions in a constructive way.*

THE DOSE

Meditate for 15 to 20 minutes once or twice a day. Meditating for shorter periods of time each day is better than 1 hour once a week.

Further Resources

Meditation: An Eight-Point Program by Eknath Easwaran is a straightforward introduction to the subject.
How to Meditate: A Guide to Self Discovery by Lawrence LeShan reviews different types of meditation and gives direction for practice.
The Miracle of Mindfulness: A Manual on Meditation by Thich Nhat Hanh is an excellent, short, and practical guide.
Wherever You Go, There You Are and *Full Catastrophe Living* by Jon Kabat-Zinn are excellent reviews on being mindful and mindfulness meditation.
Essential Spirituality by Roger Walsh, M.D., Ph.D., is an excellent review of how the great religions teach similar exercises for spiritual growth.
Centering prayer is a form of meditation similar to TM but has a more religious foundation: www.centeringprayer.com
The best way to learn is to find a class that is offered in your community. Check with a local hospital, community college, or the YMCA for classes.

References

1. Stanford SC, Salmon P: Stress: From Synapse to Syndrome. London, Academic, 1998.
2. Benson H, Kotch JB, Crassweller KD: The relaxation response:

A bridge between psychiatry and medicine. Med Clin North Am 61:929–938, 1977.

3. Shapiro D: Meditation. In Strohecker J, Trivieri L, Lewis D, Florence M (eds): Alternative Medicine: The Definitive Guide. Fife, Wash: Future Medicine Publishing, 1995, pp 339–345.

4. Blanchard EB, Nicholson NL, Taylor AE, et al: The role of regular home practice in the relaxation treatment of tension headache. J Consult Clin Psychol 59:467–470, 1991.

5. Eppley KR, Abrams AL, Shear J: Differential effects of relaxation techniques on trait anxiety: A meta-analysis. J Clin Psychol 45:957–974, 1989.

6. Kabat-Zinn J, Wheeler E, Light T, et al: Influence of a mindfulness meditation–based stress reduction intervention on rates of skin clearing in patients with moderate to severe psoriasis undergoing phototherapy and photochemotherapy. Psychosom Med 60:625–632, 1998.

7. Alexander CN, Schneider RH, Staggers F, et al: Trial of stress reduction for hypertension in older African Americans. II. Sex and risk subgroup analysis. Hypertension 28:228–237, 1996.

8. Zamarra J, Schneider RH, Bessighini I, et al: Usefulness of the transcendental meditation program in the treatment of patients with coronary artery disease. Am J Cardiol 77:867–870, 1996.

9. Alexander C, Chandler HM, Langer EJ, et al: Transcendental meditation, mindfulness, and longevity: An experimental study with the elderly. J Pers Soc Psychol 57:950–964, 1989.

10. Orme-Johnson D: Medical care utilization and the transcendental meditation program. Psychosom Med 49:493–507, 1987.

11. Caudill M, Schnable R, Zuttermeister P, et al: Decreased clinic use by chronic pain patients: Response to behavioral medicine intervention. Clin J Pain 7:305–310, 1991.

12. Royer-Bounour P: The transcendental meditation technique: A new direction for smoking cessation programs. Dissertation Abstr Int 50(8):3428-B, 1989.

13. Cooper M, Aygen M: Effect of meditation on blood cholesterol and blood pressure. Isr Med Assoc 95:1–2, 1978.

14. Walsh R: Essential Spirituality. New York, John Wiley & Sons, 1999, pp 170–171.

CHAPTER 95

Motivational Interviewing Techniques

David Rakel, M.D.

Much of the time and effort spent on research and clinical experience is wasted if the patient is unable to change a particular behavior that relates to a medical recommendation. The days of the patient listening to advice and doing whatever is recommended by the authoritative physician are gone. It is important to learn how to facilitate change that will result in improved health. This is closely tied to the art of medicine and relies on a sound rapport with the patient that fosters trust and compassion. Most of all, it demands the most sincere form of flattery—listening.

PRIMARY GOALS OF MOTIVATIONAL INTERVIEWING

1. For patients to look inward and reflect on why they act in a specific way (to get them thinking about their behavior)
2. To encourage patients to do most of the talking while the physician does most of the listening
3. To help patients go through the process (the practitioner does not argue for one side or the other)

HOW TO CONDUCT MOTIVATIONAL INTERVIEWING

- Build rapport and trust.

Take time to get to know the patient. Save motivational interviewing for the second or third visit. Approaching this topic too soon may result in resistance (Table 95–1). Assess readiness to change.

After interviewing the patient, the practitioner should develop an idea of how great is the motivation for change. This can be simply plotted on a linear continuum (Fig. 95–1). If you talk to patients as if they were farther along this scale than they really are, they may become defiant and move in the opposite direction.

- Use paraphrases and open-ended questions to assess patients' relationship to their behavior.

Table 95–1. Points That May Push the Patient in the Wrong Direction

Discussing change when the patient is not ready
Discussing change before rapport and trust are established
Arguing with or preaching to the patient

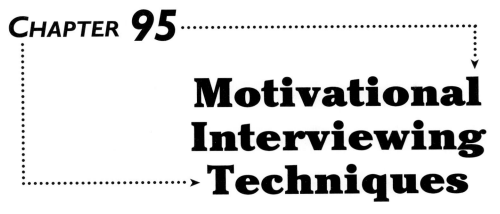

Precontemplation	Contemplation	Action
Not even considering a change	Thought of change has entered the mind	Ready to work on changing

Figure 95–1. Readiness for change levels.

An example of a paraphrase would be to repeat a sentence that the patient uses in the form of a question. For example, "You say that drinking helps ease the pain?" This encourages them to explore the meaning of their statement.

Open-ended questions provide room for self-exploration. An example would be, "What role does eating play in the way you handle stress?"

TYPES OF MOTIVATIONAL TECHNIQUES

Techniques for Precontemplators

Lifestyle, Stresses, and Behavior

Ask an open-ended question regarding the patient's main stressors and how they may affect the patient's lifestyle. Then raise a question regarding the concerned behavior, such as, "Where does your use of _____ fit in?" The response will allow you to understand the context in which the behavior is used.

A Typical Day

Have the patient discuss a typical day from morning to evening. Ask (nonjudgmentally) where the specific behavior fits into the day.

> **NOTE**
>
> *Techniques used for precontemplation allow the practitioner to learn about the patient's lifestyle, which places the behavior in context.*

Techniques for Precontemplators and Contemplators

Before using this technique for precontemplators, acquire an understanding of the specific behavior by using one of the techniques presented earlier.

Good Things, Not So Good Things

This is the most useful tool in motivational interviewing. It allows individuals to look inward in relation to the behavior and why they may want to change it, based on their own comments.

Find a piece of paper and draw a line vertically down the middle. On the left side, have the patient list "Good Things" about the specific behavior, and on the right, "Not So Good Things." If you need to step out of the room, you can have the patient fill the

Table 95–2. Sample Chart Used in "Good Things, Not So Good Things" Technique

Good things about smoking	Not so good things about smoking
I enjoy it	Smoking annoys my wife
It helps me relax	I was told it could worsen my child's asthma
I like the taste	Cigarettes are expensive
I like smoking with friends at work	Smoking increases my insurance premiums
	It is a hassle to find a place to smoke
	It is not good for my health

chart out while you are away. This allows time for contemplation. Verbally summarize what was written in the "Good Things" column; follow with a summary of the "Not So Good Things." Then leave time for the patient to react or respond (Table 95–2).

An example of the summary would be to say, "I see that you enjoy smoking because of _____ (good things). On the other hand, smoking annoys your wife and _____ (not so good things)." This is followed by a pause for the patient to respond.

The main points to remember for the "good things, not so good things" technique are the following:

- Ask what are some of the "good things" regarding the behavior.
- Ask what are some of the "not so good things" regarding the behavior.
- Summarize the good and not so good things and leave time for the patient to react.

> **NOTE**
>
> *The key to motivational interviewing is allowing the patients to explore their own ambivalence for change. Patients' attitudes are shaped by their own words, not by those of the practitioner. This process allows for internal examination that can be a powerful trigger for change.*

Like/Dislike

If you don't have enough time to have them write down the responses, you can simply ask, "What do you like/dislike about your use of _____?" Follow the same steps for summarizing after discussing the two sides.

Technique for Contemplators

The Future and the Present

This allows the patient to focus on the discrepancy between present circumstances and the way the patient would like things to be in the future.

This process involves three questions:

1. "How would you like things to be different in the future?" After clarifying future aspirations, you can then focus on the present.
2. "What's keeping you from doing these things you want to do?" This opens discussion of sources of current dissatisfaction, which allows focus on exploration of behavioral change.
3. "How does your current behavior fit into these future goals?"

In summary, ask patients what goals they want to reach in the future and how their current behavior will help or hinder their ability to reach them.

Technique for Those Ready for Action

Giving Advice and Support.

Giving advice is what we are comfortable doing. An example of this is discussing a relaxation exercise or pharmaceuticals that may help with anxiety during nicotine withdrawal for smoking cessation. Giving advice too early can be futile and may hinder the process of positive change.

References

Rollnick S, Heather N, Bell A: Negotiating behavior change in medical settings: The development of brief motivational interviewing. J Ment Health 1:25–37, 1992.

Rollnick S, Mason P, Butler C: Health Behavior Change. A Guide for Practitioners. Edinburgh, Churchill Livingstone, 1999.

Russell M, Wilson C, Baker C, Taylor C: Effect of general practitioners' advice against smoking. Br Med J 2:231–235, 1979.

Stott N, Pill R: "Advise yes, dictate no." Patients' views on health promotion in the consultation. Fam Pract 7:125–131, 1990.

Stott N, Rollnick S, Rees M, Pill R: Innovation in clinical method: Diabetes care negotiating skills. Fam Pract 12:413–418, 1995.

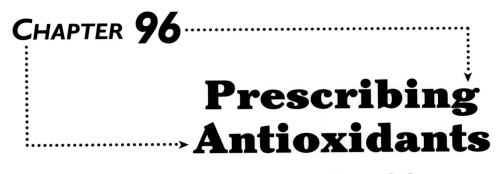

CHAPTER 96

Prescribing Antioxidants

Karen L. Mutter, D.O.

For the past 50 years it has been known that many diseases, from malignancy to cardiovascular disease and dementia, are caused by oxidative stress.[1] Free radicals—electrically unstable molecules generated by oxidative stress—cause cellular damage and have been implicated in more than a hundred disease conditions in humans. Antioxidants, both intrinsic and from food and supplement sources, act as potent scavengers of free radicals to keep cellular damage to a minimum and to inhibit neoplastic processes. Antioxidants can be utilized to act not only as preventive but also as therapeutic agents in the treatment of disease. This chapter provides basic information on the concepts of free radicals, oxidation, and antioxidant agents and their practical application along with a regimen for clinical use (Tables 96–1 and 96–2).

FREE RADICALS AND OXIDATION

Oxidative stress, or *oxidation*, in the body is caused by oxygen free radicals. A free radical is an atom or a group of atoms that contains at least one unpaired electron. Unpaired electrons are unstable and can easily steal electrons from other atoms or molecules, making them, in turn, less stable. In this

Table 96–1. Antioxidant Regimen for Patients at High Risk for Osteoporosis

Low-fat diet including a variety of green, red, and yellow fruits and vegetables with a minimum of 5 servings per day
Vitamin C 500 mg daily, ideally with bioflavonoids added to the formula
Vitamin E (*d*-alpha-tocopherol) 800 IU once daily with food
Mixed carotenes (e.g., lutein, beta carotenes, lycopenes) 25,000 IU daily
Selenium 200 mg daily, best taken with vitamin E to enhance absorption
Lipoic acid 100 mg twice daily
Oligomeric proanthocyanidins (in the form of Pycnogenol or grape seed extract, or combination formulas available in health food stores) 50–200 mg daily
Coenzyme Q10 75–100 mg twice daily
Elimination of sources of oxidant stress or toxicity (e.g., tobacco use, alcohol excess, environmental exposures)

manner, a chain reaction is initiated eventuating in damage to cellular proteins and DNA. Although a free radical may exist for only a fraction of a second, the cellular damage it leaves behind can be dramatic and irreversible.[2] It is important to remember that free radicals in small numbers are normally present in the body and can have a beneficial effect. For example, oxygen free radicals are manufactured in the body both as part of normal metabolic processes such as activation of the body's immune system and also following exposure to radiation, pollution, viruses or other infectious agents, and drugs and medications including alcohol and cigarettes.[3]

NOTE

Free radicals in small numbers are normally present in the body and serve beneficial functions.

Diet also contributes to the formation of oxygen free radicals when energy is created from the breakdown of food products. A diet that is high in fat can increase free radical formation because oxidation occurs more readily in fat molecules than in carbohydrates or protein molecules. Cooking fats heated to high temperatures, particularly as occurs with frying foods in oil, can produce large numbers of free radicals. Thus, environmental exposures and dietary choices play a significant role in the development of disease and the aging process.

To prevent widespread damage from excessive free radicals, there is a potent and diverse antioxidation system in all cells. When this system is overwhelmed or depleted, disease can occur.

THE ROLE OF ANTIOXIDANTS

Substances known as *antioxidants* neutralize free radicals by donating one of their own electrons, ending the electron "stealing" reaction. Through this process antioxidants act as free radical scavengers helping to prevent cell and tissue damage that

Table 96–2. Antioxidants

Antioxidant	Benefits	DV and Higher-Strength Doses	Food Source	Toxicity	Comments
Vitamin C (ascorbic acid) Water-soluble	Collagen synthesis (in wound healing); helps iron absorption, immunity (shortens common cold duration); cataract prevention; regenerates vitamin E and beta-carotene; protects LDL	75 mg in women, 90 mg in men 500–6000 mg in div. doses	Fresh fruits and vegetables: spinach, broccoli, red bell peppers, snow peas, tomato juice, kiwi, mango, citrus fruits, strawberries, kale, collard and turnip greens	Mouth ulcers, diarrhea, gas and bloating with doses of >1000–2000 mg qd Toxicity reversible with discontinuation of drug or decrease in dose	Best taken in combination with flavonoids and vitamin E Maximum 1000 mg/dose; more needed by smokers. Take with or without food
Vitamin E (tocopherols, tocotrienols) Fat-soluble	Cardiovascular protection; protects LDL and cell membranes; reduces risk of cancer, cataract, macular degeneration; for skin problems, impotence, Alzheimer's disease, MS, menopausal discomfort, chronic inflammatory disease	30 IU 400–800 IU daily	Soybean, corn, and canola oils, wheat germ, tofu, sunflower seeds, almonds, avocado, sweet potatoes, shrimp, cod, spinach, turnip and mustard greens	Possible increased risk of hemorrhagic stroke or bleeding, usually with higher doses Caution with warfarin (Coumadin)	Take with fat-containing foods Best taken with vitamin C, selenium; natural form, *d*-alpha-tocopherol, more desirable than synthetic *dl*-tocopheryl acetate
Carotenoids Vitamin A activity as beta-carotene Both fat-soluble water-soluble forms	Cancer protection, heart disease, immune support, eye diseases, reduce risk of DM, Alzheimer's disease, sunburn, exercise-induced asthma	Vitamin A: 5000 IU; beta-carotene DV: none Mixed carotenes containing up to 25,000 IU of vitamin A activity	Orange and yellow vegetables, dark leafy greens, carrots, squash, broccoli; 5 servings of fruits and vegetables daily	Beta-carotene: orange discoloration of skin. Some evidence for increased risk of lung cancer in smokers	Best taken as mixed carotenoid complex. Synthetic, water-soluble form more potent than food sources
Bioflavonoids Water-soluble **OPCs**	Enhance Vitamin C absorption; anti-inflammatory, antihistamine, antiviral; protection of blood vessels, LDL, and circulation; Alzheimer's, disease; potentially cancer-protective; others (see text)	DV: none 50–200 mg d	Wide range of food sources Grape seeds and skins, wine, green and black tea, beans, red and purple berries	None known	Take with or without foods Usually costly Helpful for menopausal symptoms
Soy Isoflavones (genistein)		30–45 mg d	Soy foods	Possible soy allergy or sensitivity	
Quercetin		200–400 mg bid–tid	Onions, beans, apples, black tea, leafy greens	Possible headache or extremity tingling	Best in combination with bromelain
Ginkgo biloba		60–120 mg, bid standardized to 6% terpenes, 24% flavones	*Ginkgo biloba* extract (from tree leaves)	Mild upset stomach, headache, dizziness, palpitations, or skin allergy	Use caution with anticoagulant, antiplatelet drugs

could lead to changes associated with the aging process and disease. Numerous synthetic and natural antioxidants have been demonstrated to exert beneficial effects on human health and disease prevention. This chapter covers only a small number of the many known antioxidants. For purposes of discussion, antioxidants can be divided into two categories: (1) intrinsic enzyme antioxidants and (2) phytonutrients from foods, which include vitamins, minerals, and herbs.

Table 96–2. Antioxidants (Continued)

Antioxidant	Benefits	DV and Higher-Strength Doses	Food Source	Toxicity	Comments
Alpha-lipoic acid Fat- and water-soluble (universal antioxidant)	Used in cellular metabolism and energy production Enhances antioxidant function of vitamins C and E, glutathione; may prevent diabetic complications, glaucoma, hepatic cirrhosis	DV: none 150–800 mg qd in div. doses	Limited data: beef, spinach, potatoes Made in the body	Rare; skin rash and potential for hypoglycemia in diabetics	May be important supplement for vegetarians Endorsed by ADA with vitamin E for diabetics Take on an empty stomach
Coenzyme Q10 (ubiquinone, CoQ10)	Cardiac support in patients with angina, arrhythmias, CHF, lipid disorders, hypertension; immune stimulant; strengthens gums, protects nerves, generation of ATP in mitochondria	DV: none 20–120 mg bid, depending on condition	Oily fish, organ meats, whole grains Made in the body	Rare; possible slight decrease in effectiveness of warfarin (Coumadin)	Depleted by statin drugs and some oral hypoglycemic agents Best taken as gelcaps in oil base Take with food
Selenium Water-soluble	Cancer prevention, heart disease, degenerative eye disorders, thyroid hormone synthesis, cold sores and shingles	55–70 μg 100–400 μg/day	Brazil nuts, grains, meats, seafood, poultry Content dependent on soil levels (ingestion of too much unlikely from dietary sources)	Depression, anxiety, garlicky odor to breath and perspiration In megadoses, hair loss, nausea, vomiting, nail changes	Most effective when taken with vitamin E Avoid doses > 600 μg for any extended periods

ADA, American Dietetic Association; ATP, adenosine triphosphate; CHF, congestive heart failure; div., divided; DM, diabetes mellitus; DV, daily value; IU, international units; LDL, low-density lipoprotein; MS, multiple sclerosis; OPCs, oligomeric proanthocyanidins.

Enzyme Antioxidants

Enzyme antioxidants are manufactured in the body and include superoxide dismutase, catalase, and peroxidase. These three enzymes play similar roles in removing hydrogen peroxide, a common byproduct in antioxidation. They rely on copper, zinc, and manganese for their function.[4] Glutathione, a key component of the enzyme glutathione peroxidase, and its amino acid precursor cysteine are powerful detoxifiers of alcohol, tobacco smoke, and environmental pollutants. To regenerate glutathione peroxidase, glutathione can be taken in supplement form but is not well absorbed. Instead, cysteine in the form of *N*-acetyl cysteine (NAC) is utilized. NAC has been used for years as a mucolytic and in the treatment of acetaminophen overdose. Studies showing its powerful disease-modifying role as an antioxidant have focused on treatment of respiratory diseases, human immunodeficiency virus infection and viral replication, influenza, lipid protection, and Parkinson's disease.

Dosage. The average dose of NAC is 500 mg three times daily, but this varies depending on the condition treated.

Precautions. Higher-than-recommended doses may cause vomiting or rash with fever. Regular supplementation may increase excretion of copper. Thus in patients taking NAC for extended periods, copper 2 mg and zinc 30 mg daily are recommended.

Phytonutrient Antioxidants

Phytonutrients with prominent antioxidant effects are numerous and diverse. The major phytonutrient antioxidants are vitamin C, vitamin E, selenium, carotenoids (the orange-red pigment in fruits and vegetables), bioflavonoids (including soy isoflavones, proanthocyanidins, Quercetin, and *Ginkgo biloba*), alpha-lipoic acid, and coenzyme Q10.

Vitamin C

Vitamin C (ascorbic acid), a water-soluble compound made famous by its role in the treatment and prevention of scurvy, provides the first line of defense against free radicals generated in metabolic processes. It acts in the plasma to scavenge free radicals before they can react with biologic membranes and lipoproteins. Vitamin C is required for collagen formation and tissue repair as well as a wide variety of metabolic processes and immune function. Ascorbic acid enhances iron absorption and has the ability to regenerate the activity of lipid-soluble antioxidants, such as vitamin E and beta-carotene (discussed later).

There appears to be an inverse relationship between vitamin C intake and mortality from cardiovascular disease. In addition, vitamin C affects other potential risk factors associated with cardiovascular disease by lowering total cholesterol levels as well as decreasing blood pressure—possibly by influencing prostaglandin synthesis.[5] Other areas of use include reduction of cancer risk, prevention of preeclampsia in high-risk pregnancies, control of exercise-induced asthma, and reversal of photoaging changes in facial skin.[6]

Vitamin C is abundant in fresh fruits and vegetables, especially citrus fruits.

Dosage. The recommended dietary allowance (RDA) or daily value (DV) for vitamin C is a dose of 90 mg in adult men and 75 mg in adult women. Tobacco users should take an additional 35 mg per day. To enhance iron absorption, 200 mg of vitamin C per 30 mg of iron should be given. The upper limit is set at 2000 mg, based on the adverse effect of osmotic diarrhea. Despite a DV of 90 mg, which is easily supplied by a diet that includes fruits and vegetables, it is estimated that one in every four Americans gets less than this daily requirement.

Precautions. Adverse reactions to vitamin C are dose-related and usually resolve quickly with reduction in dose. They include nausea, vomiting, esophagitis, heartburn, abdominal cramps, gastrointestinal obstruction, fatigue, flushing, headache, insomnia, sleepiness, diarrhea, hyperoxaluria, and the precipitation of urate, oxalate, or cysteine stones in the urinary tract.[6]

Certain drugs are known to increase elimination of vitamin C from the body: barbiturates, estrogen and oral contraceptives, nicotine, and tetracyclines.

Vitamin E

Vitamin E is a fat-soluble antioxidant that consists of tocopherols and tocotrienols. Although alpha-, beta-, delta-, and gamma-tocopherols have been recognized, alpha-tocopherol is the most abundant and the most potent form in this group. Tocotrienols are possibly more potent antioxidants but are present in much smaller quantities. Vitamin E has been touted to be the most effective antioxidant for reducing lipid peroxidation, specifically of low-density lipoprotein LDL.[5] Despite the large variability in the data on benefits of vitamin E in heart disease, evidence exists to support supplementation with vitamin E to inhibit the progression of atherosclerosis in persons already suffering from heart disease. Specifically, the Cambridge Heart Antioxidant Study (CHAOS) published in 1996 showed that patients with existing coronary atherosclerosis who took vitamin E had a 77% lower risk of subsequent non-

fatal myocardial infarction than that in patients who took a placebo.[7] It appears that vitamin E supplementation can lower the risk of heart disease in healthy people as well; however, studies are still ongoing. Because vitamin E also has the ability to prevent clot formation and to minimize the inflammatory process involved in the development of atherosclerosis, it may also be beneficial in the prevention of stroke. Other research indicates that the protective effect of vitamin E on cell membranes plays an important role in preventing certain cancers such as prostate cancer in male smokers. Cataracts and macular degeneration may also be prevented or delayed with higher blood levels of vitamin E. Alzheimer's disease and memory problems in elderly persons may be the result of free radical damage to nerve fibers. High dosages (2000 international units [IU] per day) have been shown to slow the progression of Alzheimer's disease.[8] Immune function support, repair of cell membrane damage as seen in the aging process, formation of red blood cells, healing of burns and eczema or other skin problems, and reduction in symptoms of premenstrual syndrome all have been found to be enhanced by supplementation with vitamin E.

Vitamin E is available in natural and synthetic forms, although the natural forms seem to be superior to the synthetic forms. Natural forms are designated with a "d," as in d-alpha. Synthetic forms are designated with a "dl," as in dl-alpha. Because only the alpha-tocopherol form of vitamin E is maintained in plasma and thought to be therapeutically beneficial,[6] supplementation with the d-alpha form is preferred. Food sources include polyunsaturated plant oils (soybean, corn, and canola oils), wheat germ, sunflower seeds, tofu, avocado, sweet potatoes, shrimp, and cod. Vitamin E supplements should be taken with foods that contain fat to promote absorption.

Precautions. Adverse reactions are rare, but high doses may increase the risk of bleeding in patients taking anticoagulant or antiplatelet drugs.

Selenium

Selenium is a trace mineral and antioxidant that is both synergistic with vitamin E and an essential component of the antioxidant enzyme glutathione peroxidase. It is an immune system booster and is involved in thyroid hormone synthesis. Cancer research has demonstrated a reduction in total cancer mortality and total cancer incidence in patients taking 200 μg of selenium daily. Patients with cancer and low selenium levels had a higher likelihood of recurrence and shorter survival times. Selenium may also have a cardioprotective role as an anticoagulant and by increasing the proportion of high-density lipoprotein HDL to LDL. Other benefits include protection against cataracts and macular degeneration, healing of cold sores and shingles, and anti-inflammatory action in patients with lupus, psoriasis, eczema, and rheumatoid arthritis. Selenium is found in many foods, although amounts will vary with soil content. Grains, meats, seafood, and poultry are good sources.

Dosage. Selenium is safe when taken in doses up to 400 μg daily. Selenium is better absorbed when taken with vitamin E.

Precautions. Acute toxicity can develop with use of higher-than-recommended doses, manifested as nausea, vomiting, fatigue, and irritability.

Beta-Carotene and the Carotenoids

Carotenoids are the pigments that color fruits and vegetables red, orange, and yellow. Although more than 600 carotenoids have been identified in foods, only a handful have been researched and recognized as powerful antioxidants in the body. These compounds include alpha-carotene, lycopene, lutein, zeaxanthin, cryptoxanthin, and beta-carotene. Several of these are converted into vitamin A as the body needs it[9]; thus, beta-carotene is often called provitamin A. Like vitamin E, the carotenoids, including beta-carotene and lycopene, are fat-soluble and carried within lipoprotein particles. Carotenoids have been shown to reduce the risk of certain types of cancer—namely, premenopausal breast cancer and cervical, prostate, digestive tract, and lung cancers. In smokers, however, some evidence suggests an increase in lung cancer in persons taking supplemental beta-carotene.[10] Lycopene and beta-carotene taken in conjunction with vitamins C and E may help to protect the body against toxic effects of chemotherapy or radiation therapy. Other benefits include protection against heart disease, cataracts, and macular degeneration, improvement in glucose tolerance, protection of nerve cells and their deterioration as seen in Alzheimer's disease, and protection of sperm in the treatment of male infertility.

Ideally, carotenoid supplements should contain a mixture of naturally occurring carotenoids. Supplements containing carotenoids or carotenes should be very orange to red in color and should be taken with food if they contain the fat-soluble form. Although the positive relationship between high dietary intake of carotene-containing foods and lower incidence of certain cancers has been well documented, most Americans ingest well below the recommended levels. Supplementation with mixed carotenoids, and certainly consumption of 5 servings per day of fruits and vegetables, is desirable to provide the widest scope of protection. Best sources of the five major carotenoids are canned pumpkin, carrots, sweet potatoes, apricots, leafy greens such as spinach, melons, parsley, citrus fruits, red pepper, and tomatoes. There is no toxicity associated with the use of beta-carotene, unlike that reported with the use of vitamin A.

Bioflavonoids

Bioflavonoids (flavonoids, flavones) are another group of plant-based substances that contain antioxidant compounds. These compounds are responsible for the color and numerous health benefits of fruits, vegetables, and herbs. More than 4000 flavonoids have been identified; many are available as nutritional supplements. The bioflavonoids discussed here include the oligomeric proanthocyanidins (OPCs), specifically, pine bark extract and grape seed extract; soy isoflavones (genistein); Quercetin; and *Ginkgo biloba*. Bioflavonoids enhance vitamin C absorption and thus are frequently formulated in combination preparation.

Oligomeric Proanthocyanidins

Oligomeric proanthocyanidins (OPCs) are found in many different plants, the two most common being pine bark extract (Pycnogenol) and grape seed extract. These compounds have powerful antioxidant capabilities and excellent bioavailability. Clinical studies suggest that the antioxidant potency or OPCs may be as much as 50 times that of vitamin E and 20 times that of vitamin C. Grape seed extract has demonstrated cytotoxicity toward human breast, lung, and gastric adenocarcinoma cells, while enhancing the growth and viability of normal human gastric mucosal cells.[11] OPCs have been shown to be of benefit in chronic venous insufficiency. Pycnogenol or pine bark extract may also reduce atherogenesis and thrombus formation. Research also suggests an improvement in T cell and B cell function. OPCs have no known toxictiy.

Dosage. Maintenance doses for grape seed extract are 40 to 80 mg per day, with a range of 75 to 300 mg per day. The maintenance dose for pine bark extract is typically 50 mg daily but may range from 25 to 150 mg per day.

Soy Isoflavones

Soy isoflavones, which include genistein and daidzein, are phytochemical constituents of soybeans. They are antioxidants and protect DNA from oxidative damage. They possess estrogen-type properties and are sometimes referred to as phytoestrogens. The mild estrogenic activity may ease menopause symptoms and may help to regulate hormone levels in premenopausal women. Soy isoflavones have been shown both to prevent atherosclerosis by suppressing LDL oxidation and also to exert an anticarcinogenic effect by protecting DNA from oxidative damage as seen in tumor formation.[12] A review study of soy research found that 65% of 26 animal-based cancer studies showed a protective effect of soy or soy isoflavones.[13] Soy's effect in women with breast cancer is still not clear; some preclinical studies show breast cancer protection, whereas others suggest increased breast cell proliferation.

Studies have also determined that soy isoflavones can help to prevent bone loss when calcium is deficient, and they can improve blood lipid profiles, thus reducing the risk of heart disease.

Dosage. Although the optimal dosage for soy is not known, the recommended amount is 40 to 60 mg of isoflavones, or one serving of soy foods per day. Food sources include roasted soy nuts, tofu, tempeh, soy milk, miso, and soy protein powders. These provide about 30 to 40 mg per serving. Soy sauce and soy oil do not contain isoflavones.[14]

Precautions. Soy products are generally safe, even in large amounts, unless the patient has a soy allergy. Soy allergy may present as constipation, bloating, nausea, skin rash, pruritus, or asthma.

Quercetin

Quercetin is a water-soluble preparation of naturally occurring bioflavonoids that act as an antihistamine and has potent anti-inflammatory properties. It inhibits oxidation of LDL, much like vitamin E does, and has been linked to protection against cardiovascular disease. Preliminary studies suggest inhibitory effects on various cancer types, and it may also have antiviral properties. Its most well-known use is in the treatment of seasonal allergies because of its histamine-blocking effects. Quercetin has also been shown to be effective in improving quality of life in the treatment of chronic nonbacterial prostatitis.[15] Food sources include onions, apples, red wine, black tea, leafy green vegetables, and beans. It is often taken with bromelain (a protein-digesting enzyme from pineapples) to increase its absorption.

Dosage. Dosage is usually 600 to 1500 mg of Quercetin daily in divided doses.

Precautions. Adverse effects may include headache and extremity tingling. No clear toxicity has been identified with oral dosing.

Ginkgo

Ginkgo biloba is a powerful plant antioxidant best known for its ability to enhance circulation and preserve nerve function. Medicinal use of gingko can be traced back almost 5000 years in Chinese herbal medicine. The active ingredients of *Ginkgo biloba* extract (GBE), the flavone glycosides and the terpene lactones, are responsible for their antioxidant activity, their ability to inhibit platelet aggregation, which helps to prevent circulatory diseases such as atherosclerosis, and their support of the brain and central nervous system. GBE increases circulation to both the brain and the extremities. It also regulates the tone and elasticity of blood vessels. It has been used to reverse selective serotonin receptor inhibitor (SSRI)-induced sexual dysfunction, to treat vertigo or tinnitus, and for the prevention of altitude sickness. Its antioxidant activity may help to prevent age-related decline in brain function, especially that seen in Alzheimer's disease.[16] This protection extends to nerve cells in the CNS that are damaged during periods of ischemia such as a stroke.

Dosage. The usual dose is 120 to 160 mg of GBE standardized to contain 6% terpenes and 24% flavone glycosides in divided doses given 2 or 3 times per day. Amounts of 120 to 240 mg per day are used in patients with cerebrovascular insufficiency, confusion, memory loss, and resistant depression.

Precautions. Adverse effects with therapeutic dosages may include mild stomach upset, headache, dizziness, palpitations, and allergic skin reactions.

Alpha-Lipoic Acid

The antioxidant alpha-lipoic acid is classified as a coenzyme and is synthesized by the body. It is soluble in both fat and water and helps to neutralize the effects of free radicals by enhancing the antioxidant functions of vitamin C, vitamin E, and glutathione. Alpha-lipoic acid has been most often researched for its benefits in persons with diabetes owing to its role in carbohydrate metabolism. It enhances glucose uptake in non–insulin-dependent diabetes, inhibits glycosylation, and has been used to combat diabetic nerve damage and neuropathic pain.[17] In Germany it is used in high dosages for the treatment of diabetic neuropathy. Preliminary data suggest a protective effect in brain or neuronal injury, cardiac reperfusion injury, liver disease, and HIV infection.[6] Although alpha-lipoic acid is only about 30% absorbed from food, good sources are yeast and liver, as well as spinach, broccoli, potatoes, and kidney.

Dosage. The average antioxidant dose is 20 to 50 mg per day, but doses of 600 mg 3 times daily have been used without toxicity and with positive clinical benefit in patients with diabetes and peripheral neuropathy.[18]

Precautions. Adverse effects are rare but may include skin rash and the potential for hypoglycemia in diabetic patients. Alpha-lipoic acid should be taken on an empty stomach.

Coenzyme Q10

The antioxidant coenzyme Q10 (CoQ10) was first identified in 1957 and is widely used in Japan for the treatment of cardiovascular disease. It is synthesized by the body and found in all cells. CoQ10 is most highly concentrated in heart muscle because of high energy needs there. It is utilized to support the body's bioenergetic functions—particularly in the mitochondria, to assist in the generation of adenosine triphosphate (ATP). After the age of 30 years, natural levels of CoQ10 begin to diminish. Further loss is exacerbated by stress, illness, and some medications such as the HMG-CoA reductase inhibitors (cholesterol-lowering, "statin" agents), certain oral hypoglycemic agents, and beta blockers. Research suggests that CoQ10 may be of benefit in almost any disease related to the heart, including angina, arrhythmias, congestive heart failure, lipid disorders, hypertension, and cardiotoxicity associated with doxorubicin (Adriamycin) chemotherapy. It has been shown to enhance immune function in AIDS and to improve blood sugar control in diabetes.[19] It has been used topically in the treatment of periodontal disease.[20]

Dosage. Doses range from 50 to 200 mg of CoQ10 daily, depending on the condition being treated. Typical doses for heart failure or angina are 50 mg 2 or 3 times daily. CoQ10 is best taken in gel capsule with oil for better absorption.

Precautions. CoQ10 can cause gastritis, anorexia, nausea, and diarrhea and, if taken in doses greater than 300 mg per day, can elevate serum levels of aminotransferases.

▲ — *THERAPEUTIC REVIEW* —

- *Health, in the context of basic biochemical functions, is always about balance, a major aspect of which is the balance between oxidative stress and the ability of the body to provide adequate antioxidation.*
- *Each cell has antioxidant capability to manage ongoing free radical production. When this system is overwhelmed, cellular damage and disease can result.*
- *The best source of antioxidant nutrients for health maintenance is still the whole food source, with use of concentrated supplements for repletion and treatment of the diseased state.*
- *When supplementation is indicated, use of combined antioxidants, even in lower dosages, appears to be more beneficial, with synergistic effects, than single antioxidant usage.*
- *Supplementation with antioxidants is generally safe at recommended doses.*
- *Healthy choices regarding diet and life style habits have the power to decrease the body's oxidant stress load and hence potential disease manifestations.*

References

1. Parke DV: Nutritional antioxidants and disease prevention: Mechanisms of action. In Basu TK, Temple NJ, Garg M (eds): Antioxidants in Human Health and Disease. CABI Publishing, 1999, p 1.
2. Balch J, Balch A: Prescription for Nutritional Healing: Antioxidants. Avery Publishing Group, 1997, pp 43–46.
3. Bland J: The 20 Day Rejuvenation Diet Program. Keats Publishing, 1997, pp 81–97.
4. Thomas JA: Oxidative stress and oxidant defense. In Shils ME (ed): Modern Nutrition in Health and Disease, 9th ed. Baltimore, Williams & Wilkins, 1999, pp 751–758.
5. Basu TK: Potential role of antioxidant vitamins. In Basu TK, Temple NJ, Garg M (eds): Antioxidants in Human Health and Disease CABI Publishing 1999, pp 19–22.
6. Jellin JM, Grogory P, Batz F, et al: Pharmacist's Letter/Prescriber's Letter Natural Medicines Comprehensive Database, 3rd ed. Stockton, Calif., Therapeutic Research Faculty; 2000, pp 40–42, 1067–1069, 1077–1079.
7. Stephens NG, Parsons A, Schofield PM, et al: Randomised controlled trial of vitamin E in patients with coronary disease: Cambridge Heart Antioxidant Study. Lancet 347:781–786, 1996.
8. Sano M, Ernesto C, Thomas RG, et al: A controlled trial of selegiline, alpha-tocopherol, or both as treatment for Alzheimer's disease. The Alzheimer's Disease Cooperative Study. N Engl J Med 336:1216–1222, 1997.
9. Gissen AS: Carotene confusion: Choosing a carotenoid supplement. VRP Newsletter, December 1993.
10. Omenn GS: Chemoprevention of lung cancer: The rise and demise of beta-carotene. Annu Rev Public Health 19:73–99, 1998.
11. Bagchi D, et al: Free radicals and grape seed proanthocyanidin extract: Importance in human health and disease prevention. Toxicology 148:187–97, 2000.
12. Zheng G, Zhu S: Antioxidant effects of soybean isoflavones. In Basu TK, Temple NJ, Garg M (eds): Antioxidants in Human Health and Disease. CABI Publishing, 1999, pp 123–128.
13. Messina MJ, et al: Soy intake and cancer risk: A review of the in vitro and in vivo data. Nutrl Cancer 21:113–131, 1994.
14. United Soybean Board: Soyfoods and isoflavones. Available at www.talksoy.com
15. Shoskes DA, Zeitlin SI, Shahed A, et al: Quercetin in men with category III chronic prostatitis: A preliminary prospective, double-blind, placebo-controlled trial. Urology 54:960–963, 1999.
16. Oken BS, et al: The efficacy of Ginkgo biloba on cognitive function in Alzheimer disease. Arch Neurol 55:1409–1415,1998.
17. Packer L, Witt EH, Tritschler HJ: Alpha-lipoic acid as a biological antioxidant [review 1]. Free Rad Biol Med 19:227–250, 1995.
18. Zeigler D, Hanefeld M, Ruhnau K, et al: Treatment of symptomatic diabetic polyneuropathy with the antioxidant alpha-lipoic acid: A 7-month multicenter randomized controlled trail (ALADIN III Study). Diabetes Care 22:1296–1301, 1999.
19. Coenzyme Q10. Mol Aspects Med 15(Suppl):S257–S263,1994.
20. Hanioka T, Tanaka M, Ojima M, et al: Effect of topical application of coenzyme Q10 on adult periodontitis. Mol Aspects Med 15(Suppl):S241–S248, 1994.

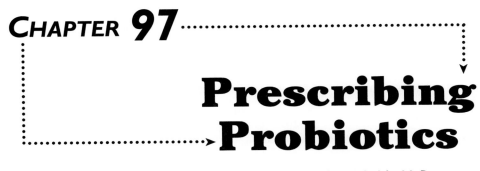

CHAPTER 97

Prescribing Probiotics

Russell H. Greenfield, M.D.

WHAT IS A PROBIOTIC?

A precise definition remains elusive, but most experts would agree in principle that a probiotic is a preparation or product containing a defined single or mixed culture of live microbes that exert beneficial effects on health by altering the gastrointestinal microbiota (a term preferable to "intestinal flora").[1-3]

In order for a food or supplement to be considered a probiotic, certain specifications must be met:

1. It must contain live organisms capable of colonizing the gastrointestinal tract.
2. The organisms contained therein must be able to withstand exposure to gastric acid and bile salts.
3. It should improve the health and well-being of the host.
4. The organisms contained therein should not be pathogenic (GRAS—generally recognized as safe).
5. Host-specific strains of organisms should be used (human vs animal).

HOW DO PROBIOTICS WORK?

Theories abound but no consensus exists as yet regarding the mechanism of action of probiotics. It is likely that a number of processes are at work, including:

- Stimulation of host immune response
- Competition with indigenous microbial pathogens for a limited number of receptor sites
- Increased production of mucin, resulting in blockage of mucosal adhesion of pathogenic organisms
- Interference with bacterial toxins
- Competitive consumption of nutrients

WHAT ARE PREBIOTICS AND SYNBIOTICS?

Also known as "probiotic enhancers" or "colon food," prebiotics are nondigestible nutrients that selectively stimulate the growth and activity of one or more colonic microorganisms that act to promote the health and well-being of the host.[4] The prebiotics developed thus far are nondigestible oligosaccharides (prototypes of which include inulin [a chicory fructan]), and fructo-oligosaccharides (which occur naturally in onions, asparagus, chicory, banana, and artichoke).[5] Inulin and oligofructose stimulate the growth of bifidobacteria at the expense of bacteroids, clostridia, or coliforms, which are then maintained at low levels.[4] Chicory fructans have been shown to enhance the absorption and balance of dietary calcium.[6, 7] Other oligosaccharides show promise as prebiotics as well, including xylose, maltose, and mannose.

In vitro studies suggest that prebiotics and synbiotics could play a role in colon cancer chemoprevention by reducing the incidence of aberrant crypt foci, as has been shown in rat studies in which intestinal changes were induced by known carcinogens.[8-10] Synbiotics contain both probiotics and prebiotics in a single product, theoretically improving the odds that live microbes will be implanted in the gastrointestinal tract. The combination may improve survival during transit through the upper gastrointestinal tract and may selectively stimulate microbial metabolism and growth of beneficial microbes, both within the supplement and in the gastrointestinal tract. This should result in enhanced gastrointestinal colonization by the beneficial organisms.

NOTE

Synbiotics are products that contain both prebiotics and probiotics.

WHAT IS THE SCIENTIFIC RATIONALE BEHIND THE USE OF PROBIOTICS?

Most lay people consider the gastrointestinal tract a closed tube through which foodstuffs and then waste products pass. Healthcare providers understand that microorganisms and a wide variety of molecules regularly pass into and out of the gastrointestinal tract, so that the mucosal system that begins in the mouth and ends at the anus is in fact a permeable one. If the previous statement is accepted as true, one is left with the realization that what people eat can significantly impact health, the development of disease, and symptom severity as a consequence of exposure to microbes (microbial translocation) and other dietary antigens that leach from the gastrointestinal tract into the systemic circulation and tissues.

The enteric microbiota account for 95% of the total number of cells in the human body. Four to five hundred different species of microorganisms inhabit the gut (mostly anaerobes such as *Bacteroides*), but there is a predominance of perhaps 30 to 50 species. Consider that 80% of the human immune system is found in the gastrointestinal tract,[11] and it is easy to see the fundamental underpinnings of probiotic therapy: The microbiota of the gastrointestinal tract play an integral role in human health by helping to resist colonization by pathogens and by enhancing the activity of the immune system. Thus, gut health is one of the more important determinants of overall health and wellness. One article[12] posited that the gut microbiota may actually help shape human physiology through their influence on expression of genes critical to intestinal development and function, including the following:

- Nutrient absorption and metabolism
- Integrity of the mucosal barrier
- Metabolism of toxic compounds
- Gut maturation and angiogenesis

Gastrointestinal physiology and the makeup of the microbiota are affected by individual host factors but can also be adversely impacted by a number of commonly experienced factors, including:

- Poor eating habits
- Chronic physical and emotional stress
- Lack of exercise
- Insufficient rest
- Overuse of antibiotics
- Geographic factors

The judicious use of probiotics may counteract these factors and help promote gut health, thereby promoting overall health and wellness. The idea is not to change the entire makeup of the microbiota, which is not possible at present, but to add "good" bacteria in the hope of limiting colonization by pathogens and maximizing beneficial metabolic and immune processes. This is not a new idea; Metchnikoff, during the early years of the 20th century, first proposed the idea of ingesting carefully selected live microbes to optimize the balance between gastrointestinal pathogens and nonpathogens.[13]

HOW DO HUMAN MICROBIOTA BECOME ESTABLISHED?

Every individual's microbiota are initially determined at birth, specifically by the mode of delivery. A child who is delivered vaginally seeds its gastro-intestinal tract with organisms from the mother's vagina, and the gut of a child delivered via cesarean section is populated by organisms from the surrounding environment of the delivery suite.[14–16] Other factors in the neonatal period play a role in the type of gut microbiota a child ultimately develops:

> Breast versus bottle feeding (a higher concentration of potentially beneficial *Lactobacilli* and *Bifidobacteria* are found in the gut when babies are breast-fed)
> Term versus preterm birth
> Administration of antibiotics
> Degree of sanitation
> Socioeconomic status
> Geographic factors

The microbiota resist new colonization and protect against overgrowth of potentially pathogenic organisms. Once established, the intestinal microbiota are relatively constant and difficult to alter over the long term.

HOW MIGHT A PROBIOTIC BENEFIT HUMAN HEALTH?

Research data and clinical observations have contributed to this list of potentially health-promoting actions of probiotics:

- Maintenance of balance between pathogenic organisms and nonpathogens (especially after antibiotic therapy)
- Lessened systemic antigenic exposure/decreased allergic sensitization (nonallergic children have higher concentrations of lactobacilli and bifidobacteria than children with allergies)
- Enhanced local (increased gut-associated lymphoid tissue [GALT] activity, levels of immunoglobulin A [IgA], and interferon) and perhaps systemic immune function
- Decreased intestinal inflammation and enhanced mucosal integrity (normalization of gut permeability)
- Possible cancer chemopreventive effects

The World Health Organization has gone so far as to recommend the use of probiotic therapy (also termed microbial interference treatment [MIT], or, simply, bacterial interference) as an alternative to antibiotic therapy whenever possible.

WHAT ARE POTENTIAL CLINICAL INDICATIONS FOR PREBIOTIC AND PROBIOTIC USE?

Research supports the use of probiotics in preventing and treating rotaviral infectious diarrhea, diarrhea due to *Clostridium difficile* infection, antibiotic-associated diarrhea, traveler's diarrhea, and allergic colitis. Benefit is suggested for patients with

Table 97–1. Potential Indications for Probiotic Use
....

Prevention and treatment of diarrheal illnesses (rotaviral, antibiotic-associated, traveler's, and infantile)[18–25]

> Especially notable: Shortened duration of rotaviral illness and reduction in severity of diarrhea compared with controls, as well as decreased incidence of antibiotic-associated diarrhea. It may prove to be worthwhile to administer probiotics prophylactically to children in day care centers to reduce transmission of diarrheal illness.

Recurrent *Clostridium difficile* infection[26–29]
Improved digestion (lactose intolerance)[30–32]

> Symptoms of lactose intolerance are improved owing to delayed gastrointestinal transit time and through release of lactase (beta-galactosidase) upon destruction of bacterial cell walls.

Symptom improvement in inflammatory disorders (including juvenile rheumatoid arthritis and inflammatory bowel disease)[33–37]
Colon cancer chemoprevention[38–42]
Immunomodulatory effects (enhancement of local gastrointestinal and systemic immune function)[43–50]
Atopy and food allergies[51–54]
Dyslipidemias (equivocal data)[55–57]
Recurrent vaginal and urinary tract infections (equivocal data)[58–62]
Treatment of infection with *Helicobacter pylori* (very early rat data)[63]
Immunoadjuvant for oral vaccines[64]
Weight gain[65]

---

inflammatory bowel disease, rheumatic disorders, constipation, recurrent vaginitis, and urinary tract infections, and even in children with cystic fibrosis.[16, 17] Probiotics may prove beneficial for people with gastrointestinal infections, as a defense against illnesses associated with chemical and environmental toxins, in various inflammatory disorders, and when there is a need for enhanced nutrient absorption (Table 97–1).[18–65]

HOW SHOULD PROBIOTIC SUPPLEMENTS BE TAKEN?

To minimize exposure to gastric acid, it is generally recommended that probiotics be taken on an empty stomach. If taken in conjunction with antibiotics, probiotics should be started as soon as possible and continued for a few days after antibiotic therapy has been completed. Ingestion of the probiotic and the antibiotic should be separated by 3 to 4 hours to minimize interference. When taken in supplement form, be sure the capsules contain at least 1 billion organisms (1×10^{10}). Of all the probiotic products available, the organism with the most associated supportive data is *Lactobacillus GG* (Table 97–2).

Limited data are available regarding the appropriate length of therapy for various clinical conditions. Many practitioners have witnessed clinical improvement when patients ingest at least 1 billion colony-forming units (CFUs) daily for 10 to 14 days. Intermittent administration (every 2 to 3 days) thereafter may prove beneficial.

> **NOTE**
>
> *All strains do not act equally well for different situations. As an example, Lactobacillus GG appears to be more effective than Lactobacillus acidophilus in treating diarrheal disease.*

Table 97–2. Organisms with Probiotic Potential
....

Lactobacillus GG
Lactobacillus casei
Lactobacillus acidophilus
Lactobacillus plantarum 299V
Lactobacillus reuteri
Bifidobacterium bifidum/longum
Streptococcus thermophilus
Saccharomyces boulardii (yeast)

ARE THERE NATURAL FOOD SOURCES THAT PROVIDE PROBIOTIC EXPOSURE?

Yes, but not without a few caveats. European consumers have been enjoying the benefits of probiotics in functional foods for decades. The majority can be found in fermented and nonfermented products in the dairy case, including yogurt, milk, sauerkraut, kefir, and specific cheeses. The live cultures found in many yogurt products mainly include *Lactobacillus bulgaricus* and *Streptococcus thermophilus*, two organisms that may not survive passage through the gastrointestinal tract, as well as others. One must be certain that the organisms are added after the pasteurization process has taken place; otherwise, the bacteria are killed during pasteurization. Adequate refrigeration is also a concern so that the greatest number of viable probiotic bacteria is promoted. It is notable, however, that even the breakdown products of dead microorganisms can provide some probiotic benefits. Other products containing probiotics include soy products such as miso and tempeh, and some people may prefer such foods over dairy products owing to concerns about pasteurization and refrigeration, as well as the following:

• Perceived association with increased morbidity with cardiovascular disorders, atopy, and diabetes
• High saturated fat content

• Being rich in growth factors such as insulin-like growth factor-I (IGF-I), cow estrogens, and, perhaps, xenoestrogens

HOW SAFE ARE PROBIOTICS?

The paleolithic diet of our ancestors, including yogurts and fermented foods, provided for the intake of probiotics on a regular basis. No significant pathologic potential has yet been identified with such a diet.

In general, probiotics appear to be extremely safe.[66–70] Supplementation with probiotics raises a theoretical risk for people with compromised immune function, but reports of such adverse effects are few and far between. Still, with the lack of regulation in the industry, there is more than adequate reason for ongoing surveillance.

Caution is appropriate regarding the use of *Enterococcus faecium* as a probiotic. This organism has been implicated in infectious processes; also, antibiotic resistance is a growing problem with *E. faecium.*

References

1. Lilley DM, Stillwell RH: Probiotics: Growth promoting factors produced by microorganisms. Science 147:747–748, 1965.
2. Fuller R: Probiotics in man and animals. J Appl Bact 56:365, 1989.
3. Schrezenmeier J, de Vrese M: Probiotics, prebiotics, and synbiotics—approaching a definition. Am J Clin Nutr 73(Suppl):361S–364S, 2001.
4. Gibson GR, Roberfroid MB: Dietary manipulation of the human colonic microbiota: Introducing the concept of prebiotics. J Nutr 125:1401–1412, 1995.
5. Gibson GR: Dietary modulation of the human gut microflora using prebiotics. Br J Nutr 80(Suppl 2):S209–S212, 1998.
6. Coudray C, Bellanger J, Castiglia-Delavaud C, et al: Effect of soluble and partly soluble dietary fibre supplementation on absorption and balance of calcium, magnesium, iron and zinc in healthy young men. Eur J Clin Nutr 51:375–380, 1997.
7. Scholz-Ahrens KE, Schaafsma G, van den Heuvel EGHM, et al: Effects of probiotics on mineral metabolism. Am J Clin Nutr 73(Suppl):459S–464S, 2001.
8. Reddy BS, Hamid R, Rao CV: Effect of dietary oligofructose and inulin on colonic preneoplastic aberrant crypt foci inhibition. Carcinogenesis 18:1371–1374, 1997.
9. Rowlands IR, Rumney CJ, Coutts JT, et al: Effect of *Bifidobacterium longum* and inulin on gut bacterial metabolism and carcinogen-induced crypt foci in rats. Carcinogenesis 19:281–285, 1998.
10. Reddy BS: Prevention of colon cancer by pre- and probiotics: evidence from laboratory studies. Br J Nutr 80(Suppl 2):S219–S223, 1998.
11. Bengmark S: Bacteria for optimal health. Nutrition 16:611–615, 2000.
12. Hooper LV, Wong MH, Thelin A, et al: Molecular analysis of commensal host-microbial relationships in the intestine. Science, February 2, 2001.
13. Metchnikoff E: The Prolongation of Life. Optimistic Studies. London, William Heinemann, 1907.
14. Gronlund MM, Lehtonen OP, Eerola E, et al: Fecal microflora in healthy infants born by different methods of delivery: Permanent changes in intestinal flora after cesarean section. J Pediatr Gastroenterol Nutr 28:19–25, 1999.
15. Davidson GP, Butler RN: Probiotics in pediatric gastrointestinal disorders. Curr Opin Pediatr 12:477–481, 2000.

16. Vanderhoof JA: Probiotics and intestinal inflammatory disorders in infants and children. J Pediatr Gastroenterol Nutr 30:S34–S38, 2000.
17. Guarino A: Effects of probiotics in children with cystic fibrosis. Gastroenterol Int 11:91, 1998.
18. Gorbach SL: Efficacy of *Lactobacillus* in treatment of acute diarrhea. Nutr Today 31:19S–23S, 1996.
19. Hilton E, Kolakowski P, Singer C, et al: Efficacy of *Lactobacillus GG* as a diarrheal preventive in travelers. J Travel Med 4:41–43, 1997.
20. Isolauri E, Juntunen M, Routanen T, et al: A human *Lactobacillus* strain (*Lactobacillus casei* sp. Strain GG) promotes recovery from acute diarrhea in children. Pediatrics 88:90–97, 1991.
21. Silva M, Jacobus NV, Deneke C, et al: Antimicrobial substance from a human *Lactobacillus* strain. Antimicrob Agents Chemother 31:1231–1233, 1987.
22. Surawicz CM, Elmer G, Speelman P, et al: Prevention of antibiotic-associated diarrhea by *Saccharomyces boulardii:* A prospective study. Gastroenterology 9:981–988, 1989.
23. Marteau PR, de Vrese M, Cellier CJ, et al: Protection from gastrointestinal diseases with the use of probiotics. Am J Clin Nutr 73(suppl):430S–436S, 2001.
24. Shornikova A-V, Casas IA, Isolauri E, et al: *Lactobacillus reuteri* as a therapeutic agent in acute diarrhea in young children. J Pediatr Gastroenterol Nutr 24:399–404, 1997.
25. Ribiero H, Vanderhoof JA: Reduction of diarrheal illness following administration of *Lactobacillus plantarum* 299V in a daycare facility [abstract]. J Pediatr Gastroenterol Nutr 265:561, 1998.
26. Gorbach SL, Chang TW, Goldin B: Successful treatment of relapsing *Clostridium difficile* colitis with *Lactobacillus GG* [letter]. Lancet 2:1519, 1987.
27. McFarland LV: Biotherapeutic agents for *Clostridium difficile*-associated disease. In Elmer GW, McFarland LV, Surawicz CM (eds): Biotherapeutic Agents and Infectious Diseases. Totowa, NJ, Humana Press, 1999, pp 159–193.
28. Pochapin M: The effect of probiotics on *Clostridium difficile* diarrhea. Am J Gastroenterol 95(Suppl 1):511–513, 2000.
29. Biller JA, Katz AJ, Flores AF, et al: Treatment of recurrent *Clostridium difficile* colitis with *Lactobacillus GG.* J Pediatr Gastroenterol Nutr 21:224–226, 1995.
30. Kim HS, Gilliland SE: *Lactobacillus acidophilus* as a dietary adjunct for milk to aid lactose digestion in humans. J Dairy Sci 66:959–966, 1983.
31. Kolars JC, Levitt MD, Aoul M, et al: Yogurt—an autodigesting source of lactose. N Engl J Med 310:1–3, 1984.
32. de Vrese M, Stegelmann A, Richter B, et al: Probiotics—compensation for lactase insufficiency. Am J Clin Nutr 73(Suppl):421S–429S, 2001.
33. Gionchetti P, Rizzello F, Venturi A, et al: Probiotics in infective diarrhea and inflammatory bowel diseases. J Gastroenterol Hepatol 15:489–493, 2000.
34. Shanahan F: Probiotics and inflammatory disease: Is there a scientific rationale? Inflamm Bowel Dis 6:107–115, 2000.
35. Malin M, Verronen P, Mykkanen H, et al: Increased bacterial urease activity in faeces in juvenile chronic arthritis: Evidence of altered intestinal microflora? Br J Rheumatol 35:689–694, 1996.
36. Campieri M, Gionchetti P: Probiotics in inflammatory bowel disease: New insight into pathogenesis or a possible therapeutic alternative? Gastroenterology 116:1246–1249, 1999.
37. Nenonen MT, Helve TA, Rauma AL, et al: Uncooked, lactobacilli-rich, vegan food and rheumatoid arthritis. Br J Rheumatol 37:274–281, 1998.
38. Goldin BR, Gualtieri L, Moore RP: The effect of *Lactobacillus GG* on the initiation and promotion of dimethylhydrazine-induced intestinal tumors in the rat. Nutr Cancer 25:197–204, 1996.
39. Wollowski I, Rechkemmer G, Pool-Zobel BL: Protective role of probiotics and prebiotics in colon cancer. Am J Clin Nutr 73(suppl):451S–455S, 2001.
40. Brady LJ, Gallaher DD, Busta FF: The role of probiotic cultures in the prevention of colon cancer. J Nutr 130(Suppl 2):410S–414S, 2000.
41. Reddy BS: Prevention of colon cancer by pre- and probiotics: Evidence from laboratory studies. R J Nutr Suppl 2:S219–S223, 1998.

42. Rowlands IR, Rumney CJ, Coutts JT, et al: Effect of *Bifidobacterium longum* and inulin on gut bacterial metabolism and carcinogen-induced crypt foci in rats. Carcinogenesis 19:281–285, 1998.

43. Salminen S, Bouley C, Boutron-Ruault MC, et al: Functional food science and gastrointestinal physiology and function. Br J Nutr 80:S147–S171, 1998.

44. Isolauri E, Majamaa H, Arvola T, et al: *Lactobacillus casei* strain GG reverses increased gastrointestinal permeability induced by cow milk in suckling rats. Gastroenterology 105:1643–1650, 1993.

45. Sutas Y, Hurme M, Isolauri E: Downregulation of antiCD3 antibody-induced IL-4 production by bovine caseins hydrolysed with *Lactobacillus GG*–derived enzymes. Scand J Immunol 43:687–689, 1996.

46. Fukushima Y, Kawata Y, Hara H, et al: Effect of a probiotic formula on immunoglobulin A production in healthy children. Int J Food Microbiol 42:39–44, 1998.

47. Gaskins HR: Immunological aspects of host/microbiota interactions at the intestinal epithelium. In Mackie RI, White BA, Isaacson RE (eds): Gastrointestinal Microbiology. New York, International Thomson Publishing, 1997, pp 537–587.

48. Isolauri E, Sutas Y, Kankaanpaa P, et al: Probiotics: Effects on immunity. Am J Clin Nutr 73(Suppl):444S–450S, 2001.

49. Cunningham-Rundles S, Ahrne S, Bengmark S, et al: Probiotics and immune response. Am J Gastroenterol 95(Suppl 1):S22–S25, 2000.

50. Matsuzaki T, Chin J: Modulating immune responses with probiotic bacteria. Immunol Cell Biol 78:67–73, 2000.

51. Majamaa H, Isolauri E: Probiotics: A novel approach in the management of food allergy. J Allergy Clin Immunol 99:179–185, 1997.

52. Kalliomaki M, Salminen S, Arvilommi H, et al: Probiotics in primary prevention of atopic disease: A randomized placebo-controlled trial. Lancet 357:1076–1079, 2001.

53. Isolauri E, Arvola T, Sutas Y, et al: Probiotics in the management of atopic eczema. Clin Exp Allergy 30:1605–1610, 2000.

54. Wheeler JG, Shema SJ, Bogle ML, et al: Immune and clinical impact of *Lactobacillus acidophilus* on asthma. Ann Allergy Asthma Immunol 79:229–233, 1997.

55. Taylor GRJ, Williams CM: Effects of probiotics and prebiotics on blood lipids. Br J Nutr 80(Suppl 2):S225–S230, 1998.

56. Delzenne NM, Kok N: Effects of fructans-type prebiotics on lipid metabolism. Am J Clin Nutr 73(Suppl):456S–458S, 2001.

57. Agerholm-Larsen L, Raben A, Haulrik N, et al: Effect of 8 week intake of probiotic milk products on risk factors for cardiovascular diseases. Eur J Clin Nutr 54:288–297, 2000.

58. Reid G: Probiotic agents to protect the urogenital tract against infection. Am J Clin Nutr 73(Suppl):437S–443S, 2001.

59. McGroarty JA: Probiotic use of lactobacilli in the human female urogenital tract. FEMS Immunol Med Microbiol 6:251–264, 1993.

60. Hughes VL, Hillier SL: Microbiologic characteristics of *Lactobacillus* products used for colonization of the vagina. Obstet Gynecol 75:244–248, 1990.

61. Reid G, Bruce AW, Taylor M: Influence of three-day antimicrobial therapy and *Lactobacillus* suppositories on recurrence of urinary tract infections. Clin Ther 14:11–16, 1992.

62. Reid G, et al: Instillation of *Lactobacillus* and stimulation of indigenous organisms to prevent recurrence of urinary tract infections. Microecol Ther 65:3763–3766, 1995.

63. Kabir AMA, Aiba Y, Takagi A, et al: Prevention of *Helicobacter pylori* infection by lactobacilli in a gnotobiotic murine model. Gut 41:49–55, 1997.

64. Isolauri E, Joensuu J, Suomalainen H, et al: Improved immunogenicity of oral DxRRV reassortment rotavirus vaccine by *Lactobacillus casei* GG. Vaccine 13:310–312, 1995.

65. Robinson EL, Thompson WL: Effect on weight gain and the addition of *Lactobacillus acidophilus* to the formula of newborn infants. J Pediatr 41:395–398, 1952.

66. Naidu AS, Bidlack WR, Clemens RA: Probiotic spectra of lactic acid bacteria. In Clydesdale FM (ed): Critical Reviews in Food Science and Nutrition. Boca Raton, CRC Press LLC, 1999, pp 13–126.

67. Salminen S, von Wright A, Morelli L, et al: Demonstration of safety of probiotics—a review. Int J Food Microbiol 44:93–106, 1998.

68. Wagner RD, Warner T, Roberts L, et al: Colonization of congenitally immunodeficient mice with probiotic bacteria. Infect Immun 65:3345–3351, 1997.

69. Ishibashi N, Yamazaki S: Probiotics and safety. Am J Clin Nutr 73(Suppl):465S–470S, 2001.

70. Davidson GP, Butler RN: Probiotics in pediatric gastrointestinal disorders. Curr Opin Pediatr 12:477—481, 2000.

Selected Review Articles

Bengmark S: Ecological control of the gastrointestinal tract. The role of probiotic flora. Gut 42:2–7, 1998.

Collins MD, Gibson GR: Probiotics, prebiotics, and synbiotics: Approaches for modulating the microbial ecology of the gut. Am J Clin Nutr 69(Suppl):1052S–1057S, 1999.

de Roos NM, Katan MB: Effects of probiotic bacteria on diarrhea, lipid metabolism, and carcinogenesis: A review of papers published between 1988 and 1998. Am J Clin Nutr 71:405–411, 2000.

Macfarlane GT, Cummings JH: Probiotics and prebiotics: Can regulating the activities of intestinal bacteria benefit health? West J Med 171:187—190, 1999.

Orrhage K, Nord CE: Bifidobacteria and lactobacilli in human health. Drugs Exp Clin Res 26:95–111, 2000.

Saxelin M: *Lactobacillus GG*—a human probiotic strain with thorough clinical documentation. Food Rev Int 13:293–313, 1997.

Saavedra JM: Probiotics plus antibiotics: Regulating our bacterial environment. J Pediatr 135:535—537, 1999.

Vanderhoof JA: Probiotics and intestinal inflammatory disorders in infants and children. J Pediatr Gastroenterol Nutr 30:S34–S38, 2000.

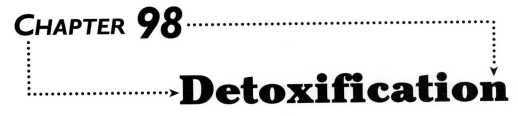

CHAPTER 98 ·········· Detoxification

Iris R. Bell, M.D., Ph.D., and Sharon McDonough-Means, M.D.

EXPOSURES/PATHOPHYSIOLOGY

Environmental toxicants can access the body via several routes (e.g., dermal, respiratory, gastrointestinal, and ocular) over time frames that can vary from acute to chronic to long term (>1 yr).[1] Air, water, and food are common environmental sources of toxicants. Chemical exposures can result from occupational, residential, or recreational use; other toxins such as fungi (e.g., *Penicillium, Cladosporium,* and *Alternaria*) and mycotoxins can also enter the body via air inhalation or food contamination in the diet.[1, 2] Especially vulnerable populations include fetuses, young and old persons, and individuals with inborn or acquired limitations of specific metabolic pathways. Epidemiologic and laboratory studies link environmental chemical exposures with a number of different disorders, including neurodevelopmental disorders, autoimmune disorders such as systemic lupus erythematosus, certain cancers, and Parkinson's disease.[3–6]

Although many agents undergo toxicity testing so that "safe" or acceptable exposure limits can be determined, there are relatively few data on real-world exposures to mixtures of multiple substances.[7] Table 98–1 lists common types of toxicants to which people can be exposed. Commonly cited statistics mention that more than 100,000 different chemicals are in commercial use in the United States, including more than 10,000 industrial chemicals that have not yet undergone appropriate risk assessment testing.[7] Chemical production escalated steeply after World

Table 98–1. Partial List of Types of Toxicant Exposures
··············

Pesticides, insecticides
Herbicides
Solvents
Other volatile organic compounds (VOCs)
Acids
Dioxins/polychlorinated biphenyls (PCBs)
Heavy metals (e.g., lead, mercury, cadmium)
Other toxic elements (e.g., arsenic, manganese, beryllium, aluminum, chromium)
Carbon monoxide
Radon
Fungi and mycotoxins
Food preservatives
Synthetic food dyes
Tobacco smoke
Asbestos

War II.[8] United States federal agencies with jurisdiction over these matters include the Occupational Safety and Health Administration (OSHA), the National Institute for Occupational Safety and Health, and the Environmental Protection Agency (EPA). Informational resources on toxicants also include regional or local poison control centers.

Toxicity is the state of being poisonous, locally or systemically. Conventional texts on environmental health point out that the toxic effects of a given agent depend on its physical and chemical properties. Conventional toxicology largely assumes (1) a linear dose-response mechanism (i.e., higher doses produce greater toxicity), and (2) a low dose below which no adverse effects occur. However, many substances have U-shaped or J-shaped dose-response curves, sometimes but not always due to toxic metabolic byproducts, or exhibit hormesis (bidirectional, opposite effects at low versus high doses).[9–11] Furthermore, the possibility of synergistic adverse effects of chemical mixtures[7, 12] is rarely considered in regulatory decisions.

It is important to note that "toxicity" and "detoxification" per se often encompass a different scope of issues in conventional versus alternative medical thinking. Generally, conventional clinical toxicology deems an individual to have a toxic state based on a history of higher dose exposure(s) to specific, identifiable agent(s) or a measurable biomarker of the presence (e.g., urinary heavy metal excretion) or effects (e.g., cholinesterase inhibition) of an agent in the person. Typically, the symptoms that the person reports coincide with documented patterns of symptoms characteristic of poisoning with a specific substance. Conventional medical care initiates detoxification procedures when an identifiable, toxicant-associated diagnosis is present (e.g., chelation therapy for lead poisoning).[1]

In contrast, several different but phenomenologically overlapping syndromes have raised much debate and controversy in recent years. These polysymptomatic, multisystem conditions include multiple chemical sensitivity (MCS), fibromyalgia (FM), chronic fatigue syndrome (CFS), and Gulf War Syndrome (GWS).[13, 14] MCS, FM, CFS, and GWS can include concomitant diagnoses of rhinitis, asthma, sinusitis, irritable bowel, and migraine headache, as well as multiple newly acquired food and drug intolerances. The primary symptom that presumptively links these syndromes is that of low-level chemical intolerance (CI), which occurs in all MCS patients, and in high proportions of FM, CFS, and GWS patients. Multiple epidemiologic studies also indicate that approximately 15% to 30% of the general population (depending on the phrasing of the question) also report CI per se, with approximately 4% to 5% experiencing it to a disabling degree.[15–17]

Multiple Chemical Sensitivity

Clinicians who treat MCS and related conditions acknowledge that the same low-level chemical exposure may trigger different symptoms in different patients; agents with no structural similarities can mobilize the same symptom responses, and patients may be relatively asymptomatic upon avoidance of triggering substances.[18] In some studies, more than one third of patients with currently severe chemical intolerances cannot identify a specific high-level chemical exposure that initiated their chronic difficulties with low-level chemicals.[19] In MCS patients who can identify an initiator, it is often pesticide application or remodeling (e.g., solvents, glues) at home or in the office.[20] Once ill, MCS patients report that multiple different substances, not just the original initiating exposure agent, now trigger symptom flares. Thus, MCS spectrum conditions do not meet criteria for classic toxicologic or immunologic disorders.

Early thinking on mechanisms of MCS focused on the immune system, but more recent research has found evidence for central, autonomic, and peripheral nervous system involvement. For example, replicated controlled laboratory studies on a neural sensitization model suggest that persons with CI are those who can sensitize their physiologic responses on a nonimmunologic basis, such as electroencephalographic alpha or diastolic blood pressure, to repeated, intermittent exposures to low-level chemicals.[14] Neural sensitization is a nonimmunologic amplification process in the host, with properties similar to those of MCS. Notably, animal studies have demonstrated that low-level formaldehyde can cross-sensitize with cocaine[21]; physical or psychological stress can cross-sensitize with stimulant drugs[22]; and other chemicals such as toluene[23] or certain pesticides[24] can initiate sensitization of behavioral and neurochemical patterns that manifest only in the presence of the triggering agent. Other data suggest that neurogenic inflammation involving C fibers in the peripheral nervous system may contribute to the multiple symptoms such as edema and muscle and joint pains seen in these patients.[25]

Complementary and Alternative Medicine Versus Conventional Medicine Approaches to Detoxification

Treatment approaches that some clinicians who treat MCS have adopted fall more into the complementary and alternative medicine (CAM)–derived methods than those of conventional medicine.[26] Moreover, beyond MCS spectrum problems within the larger field of CAM, many persons with a wide variety of conventional diagnoses and subclinical, undiagnosable conditions have received detoxification interventions. Many traditional healing systems, such as Ayurveda, traditional Chinese medicine, and Native American healing, consider detoxification both a preventive measure and a treatment option for various conditions.[27, 28] These healthcare systems developed long before the recent, exponential rise in environmental chemicals, but nonetheless, they perceived a need for periodic cleansing of the body.

Consequently, there is much debate between conventional and CAM providers over when to offer detoxification and for what type of patient, as well as which type of intervention to use. Conventional research has not found clinically reliable results from toxicity tests such as hair analysis,[29] although many CAM providers still include this test. Similarly, systematic research has not established a clinical benefit derived from mercury amalgam removal, but a subset of CAM providers still use this treatment strategy.[30] Possible links between conditions such as autism and mercury exposure are among the current clinical foci.[31] From the integrative perspective, the basic approach to detoxification encompasses three broad strategies[32]: (1) avoidance of, or reduction in, exposure; (2) improved metabolic handling of toxicants (e.g., activation of specific liver enzyme pathways); and (3) increased excretion from the body (e.g., from the skin or gastrointestinal tract). General support for improving host physiologic functioning is often part of the clinical strategy as well.[33]

Avoidance of, or Reduction in, Exposure

The simplest way to avoid becoming toxic is to avoid exposure in the first place. Take a basic occupational and environmental history emphasizing chronic, possibly elevated, exposures to chemicals at work, during hobbies (e.g., solvents), and at home (e.g., regular pesticide or herbicide spraying inside or around the home; type of heating and cooking fuel—gas or electric). Determine the relationship between time of onset of symptoms to any remodeling, including but not limited to new carpet and painting, at the office or at home. Principles for avoidance include finding occupations that do not involve routine toxicant exposures; using OSHA-recommended protective gear (e.g., goggles, respirators) when exposures occur; working in properly ventilated, ergonomically sound environments (30% of U.S. modern office buildings qualify as "sick" buildings, in which about one third of the occupants report mucous membrane irritation or other discomforts that resolve upon leaving the building)[34]; selecting nontoxic alternatives for pest and mold management at work and home[35–37]; and choosing less chemically contaminated foods for routine dietary intake. Professional industrial hygienists can systemically test business or residential sites for unacceptable levels of many toxicants. However, it often can be difficult to document a specific substance as the sole cause of air quality problems in a sick building.

Most people spend the greater part of the day indoors, and EPA studies have shown that indoor air is generally much more polluted than outdoor air by agents such as trichlorethane, xylene, benzene, and assorted pesticides.[38] In residences, one should check for lead-based paint and asbestos in older homes, as well as radon, pesticide residues, and carbon monoxide. One should use ceramic tile (secured by cement rather than glue) or hardwood floors and cotton scatter rugs, not wall-to-wall carpet and carpet pads. Electric-based over natural gas–based heating and cooking facilities are preferred in the home. Cotton-based clothing and bedding that has been less treated with chemicals are best. Scented personal hygiene products should be avoided, and dry-cleaned clothing should be aired out before it is worn or stored. When a new item emits a chemical odor, especially clothing, new beds, or furniture, one should wash clothing items repeatedly in unscented detergent and place larger items outdoors, or allow them to outgas or age for a time before introducing them into regular indoor use. Glass or stainless steel cooking utensils are preferred, as are glass or harder rather than softer plastic products for food storage.

The major risk of partial avoidance is that removing only some exposures from the patient's environment, can produce partial deprivation and expense without clinical improvement. On the other hand, the major risks of comprehensive avoidance can be social and physical isolation and crippling financial burdens that also raise concern for a reasonable risk/benefit ratio. One compromise that some physicians recommend is to focus avoidance efforts on cleaning up the potentially toxic exposures in the patient's bedroom, where they generally spend more than 8 hours per day. Note that more severely ill persons with MCS may not tolerate nutritional supplements, botanicals, or pharmaceutical drugs; for them, avoidance approaches and nondrug therapies (e.g., acupuncture, mind-body techniques, and massage) may be the best way to start treatment.

Diet/Nutrition

Purchase fresh foods as often as possible, choosing those with no additives or synthetic preservatives (see Chapter 82, How to Recommend an Elimination Diet). Some people find it necessary to use organic, whole food sources rather than processed commercial ones, which often add pesticide residues, waxes, synthetic dyes, and other xenobiotics at low levels into the diet. Many self-help books offer detailed suggestions for less toxic ways of

building, furnishing, and maintaining indoor environments, as well as instructions for growing and preparing organic foods. For persons who eat meat and fish, it is important to find and select sources that are chemically less contaminated. Although eating fish can be desirable from a nutritional standpoint, some sources provide excessive amounts of mercury over extended periods. For example, seafood sources such as shark or swordfish are more likely to accumulate toxins in their tissues because of their scavenger role in the ocean food chain. Tuna can also add a toxic load of mercury if consumed to excess. Fish from the Great Lakes can have various industrial contaminants that have been traced to developmental neurobehavioral problems in children whose mothers ingested the fish during pregnancy (see Chapter 5, Attention Deficit Disorder). The reader is also referred to the chapters on food intolerances (see Chapter 81, Food Allergies, and Chapter 82, How to Recommend an Elimination Diet) for further information on dietary management.

Resources for obtaining less toxic products include the American Environmental Health Foundation (800-428-AEHF; *www.aehf.com*), the Janice Corporation (1-800-526-4237; *www.janices.com*), and NEEDS (800-634-1380, www.needs.com). A nonprofit patient support group with informational newsletters and referral information is the Human Ecology Action League (HEAL: 404-248-1898; www. *HEALNatnl@aol.com*). Among many useful self-help books on MCS spectrum problems are Jacqueline Krohn's *The Whole Way to Allergy Relief and Prevention*; Doris Rapp's *Is This Your Child? Discovering and Treating Unrecognized Allergies in Children and Adults*; Sherry Rogers' *The EI Syndrome: A Treatment for Environmental Illness*; and Pamela Reed Gibson's *Multiple Chemical Sensitivity: A Survival Guide*.

Supplements

One company, HealthComm, Incorporated, manufactures a medical food supplement, UltraClear, which is specifically designed to foster detoxification processes. This product is distributed by Metagenics Ethical Nutrients, 971 Calle Regocio, San Clemente, CA, USA, 1-800-692-9400 or 1-714-366-0818. They report an advantage of this supplement over simple water or juice fasting, especially in medically complex patients. A major risk of water or juice fasting is loss of essential vitamins, minerals, and protein. UltraClear ingredients include specific macronutrients and micronutrients intended to support liver detoxification enzymes and provide antioxidant protection against free radicals generated during metabolism (see Fig. 98–1). Part of the concept is to facilitate the detoxification and excretion of substances that ordinary fasting could mobilize at increased levels into the circulation from fat and liver stores. This approach may reduce the unpleasant increases in symptoms that some individuals experience during fasts. Ingredients include rice

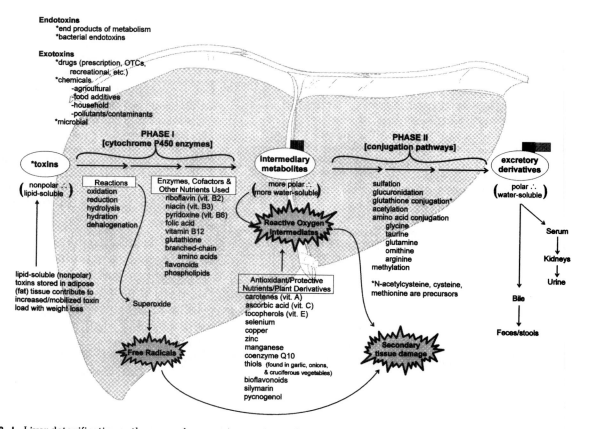

Figure 98–1. Liver detoxification pathways and supportive nutrients. (From Bland JS, Costarella L, Levin B, et al: Environment and toxicity. In Clinical Nutrition: A Functional Approach. Gig Harbor, Wash, Institute for Functional Medicine, 1999, p. 261.)

protein concentrate, rice syrup solids, magnesium citrate, dipotassium phosphate, calcium citrate, natural flavor, high oleic safflower oil, medium-chain triglycerides, vitamin C (esterized), vitamin A (beta-carotene), palmitate, vitamin E (tocopheryl, tocopherol), dicalcium phosphate, molybdenum amino acid chelate, zinc methionate, L-threonine, L-lysine hydrochloride, manganese gluconate, ferrous fumarate, L-glutathione, selenomethionine, copper gluconate, niacinamide, L-cysteine, N-acetylcysteine, pyridoxine hydrochloride, calcium pantothenate, riboflavin, thiamine hydrochloride, vitamin D, chromium polynicotinate, biotin, folic acid, potassium iodide, and cyanocobalamin.

Many clinicians use this food supplement in conjunction with a modified diet that emphasizes fresh organic foods, no food additives, many vegetables, and less contaminated sources of animal proteins such as certain fishes and turkey. One study showed a reduction in nonspecific symptom complaints after a 7-day program of this type in 25 disease-free persons, but no control group was evaluated.[32] The HealthComm, Incorporated research group has published a controlled study on a 10-week program comparing active intervention in 84 patients with chronic health problems but no life-threatening diseases, with 22 patients on a control diet (no placebo arm and no random assignment).[39] They found a significantly greater reduction in multiple symptoms

in the active than in the control arm (52% vs 22%, $P < .01$). They also reported some significant improvements in biochemical parameters after challenge tests in active versus control groups. They did not indicate any major adverse reactions to the treatment program. Much more research is required to establish the clinical and laboratory effectiveness and safety of this nutritional supplement in different patient populations, but at present the data are consistent with a possible short-term subjective and objective benefit in persons who fall within the subclinical-to-clinical range of symptoms within the MCS spectrum cluster of conditions.

It is also possible for patients to assemble their own program of nutritional supplement support with an understanding of the role of specific nutrients in detoxification and in interaction with one another.[40] Thus, it is important to consider combinations of supplements, rather than relying on single nutrients, to address detoxification processes. Basic suggestions would include:

- **Vitamin C:** 500 mg, two times per day. The body may absorb it more readily in powder form, but use what works best for the individual. People vary in their intestinal tolerance to vitamin C, so if the person experiences flatulence or loose stools, back down on the dosages. Tissue saturation can occur at 200 mg/day.

- **Vitamin E** (*d*-alpha tocopherol): 800 IU once daily, preferably in the form of natural vitamin E with mixed tocopherols per day. Because vitamin E is fat soluble, it is best absorbed when taken with a meal.
- **Selenium:** 200 micrograms per day. Selenium is a trace mineral with antioxidant and anticancer properties. Its absorption is enhanced when taken with vitamin E, but vitamin C inhibits its absorption, so take vitamin C at a separate time.
- **Mixed carotenes:** Beta-carotene is one of a family of pigmented compounds naturally found in yellow and orange fruits and vegetables and also dark, leafy greens. Consider supplementing the diet with 25,000 IU mixed carotenes (alpha- and beta-carotenes, lycopene, etc.) once daily. This type of supplement is now available in health food stores.
- **Green tea:** This contains catechins, a compound that current studies show has anticancer and antibacterial effects. Drinking 2 to 3 cups per day would be of benefit. Be aware that green tea does contain caffeine, although it has a smaller amount than coffee. It does come in a decaffeinated form.

Among a number of good resources for nutritional and botanical supplements (manufactured to avoid synthetic additives, toxicants, or common food allergens), including some combinations for detoxification purposes, are Thorne Research, Incorporated (800-228-1966; *www.thorne.com*) and Nordic Naturals (831-662-2852; *www.nordicnaturals.com*).

Botanicals

Milk Thistle (Silybum marianum)[41]

Milk thistle contains silymarin, which is a mixture of chemicals (flavonoids) that help protect the liver not only by reducing inflammation, but by promoting regeneration of the liver cells and helping them become more efficient at detoxifying the blood. The dose is based on the percent of silymarin, which should be at least 70%, with 140 to 210 mg taken three times per day. Nature's Way makes a good product called Thisilyn that can be bought at most health food stores. There is also a formulation called Silymarin phytosome that is better absorbed and needs to be taken at only 120 mg twice daily.

Schisandra (Schisandra chinensis)[42]

The berries of this plant contain lignans that help prevent liver damage from inflammation while lowering abnormal liver function tests and increasing the liver's ability to detoxify the blood. It is a nontoxic plant that is very safe. The usual dose is 500 mg to 1 g three times daily. One source of a dependable product is a company called Nuherbs in Oakland, California. Their telephone number is 1-800-233-4307.

Improved Metabolic Handling of Toxicants

Figure 98–1 summarizes the complex pathways and nutrient modulators involved in Phase I and Phase II detoxification pathways.[43] Phase I involves cytochrome-P450–related enzymes (e.g., Cyp3A4, Cyp1A1, Cyp1A2, Cyp2D6, and Cyp2C), which deal mainly with exogenous substances and endogenous steroid hormones. Phase I enzymes occur in the liver as well as several other types of tissues such as kidney, lung, intestinal mucosa, skin, adrenal cortex, and testis. Phase II involves conjugation reactions, including glucuronidation, sulfation, and glutathione and amino acid conjugation, that can form water-soluble products excreted in urine or bile. Phase II enzymes occur in the liver, kidney, lung, gastrointestinal system, and skin. It is beyond the scope of this chapter to delineate all of the specific mechanisms by which environmental factors can exert toxic effects. In general, these mechanisms can range from interference with normal cell functions (e.g., blocking normal ion movement into and out of cells, blocking receptors, or inhibiting respiratory enzymes) to DNA damage or initiation or promotion of cancer. Genetic polymorphisms can favor poor metabolic clearance of certain xenobiotics (foreign bodies) and thereby favor not only adverse pharmaceutical drug reactions, but also development of some disease states. Although much earlier toxicity testing undertaken to set safety standards considered primarily mortality, noncancer end-organ damage, cancer risk, and reproductive/developmental endpoints in animals and irritant thresholds in workers, emerging research has begun to focus on more subtle nervous system and immune system toxicity as well. Product testing for neurodevelopmental toxicity, however, is not required, and documentation of these types of adverse effects is on file for only 12 of 296 chemicals with such toxicity.[44]

Increased Excretion from the Body

Water Consumption

A primary preventive concept is intake of at least 6 to 8 glasses of good quality water per day. Products such as UltraClear® (discussed earlier) may also foster excretion, but water intake provides a vehicle for clearing toxins from the system. An essential caveat is that pregnancy contraindicates the various forms of fasting and excretion in that it is important for an expectant mother not to mobilize toxins from bodily stores that could cross the placenta and harm the fetus. Patients with medical conditions affecting electrolyte balance would also not tolerate fasting or increased excretion strategies.

Sauna Therapy

A primary modality from various traditions for increasing toxicant excretion is sauna to increase mobilization of toxicants from fat and liver stores and to excrete toxic products out through perspiration on the skin (i.e., via sauna treatments).[45] This type of approach has both modern and ancient roots (e.g., Ayurveda—see later). Heat stress detoxification induces release of fat-stored toxicants. There is no standardization for sauna procedures; temperatures, humidity, and duration of administration all vary greatly among different approaches. Regardless of procedural differences, both liver and kidney function must be monitored. Extreme heat activates sweating and increased circulation at the skin; it also increases metabolic rate, water and electrolyte losses, and heart rate.

One contemporary sauna-based detoxification program (Hubbard Program) involves multiple components: physical exercise; sauna; nutritional supplementation with niacin, as well as vitamins A, D, C, E, and B complex, calcium, magnesium, iron, zinc, manganese, copper, potassium, and iodine; water, salt, and potassium repletion; polyunsaturated oil; and a regular, balanced meal and sleep schedule.[46] Case-controlled data on a group of 14 firemen exposed to polychlorinated biphenyls (PCBs) and treated for 2 to 3 weeks in the previously described detoxification program indicated improvement in specific cognitive tests without changes in mood ratings.[47] However, measured levels of the toxicants did not correlate with degree of neurobehavioral impairment. This approach requires a great deal more controlled research to clarify its appropriate indications, risks, and benefits.

Colon Hydrotherapy

Colon hydrotherapy, a popular excretion strategy among certain MD and ND physicians,[48] involves the use of controlled cleansing of the colon to improve colon functioning and to remove waste products. Modern devices are FDA-approved and use filtered water, disposables, and EPA-approved sanitizing solutions. The International Association of Colon Hydrotherapy (210-366-2888; *wwwI-ACT.org*) issues standard operating procedures and guidelines and tests therapists for certification purposes. Indications include constipation, bowel training in paraplegics and quadriplegics, and preparation for diagnostic tests. Contraindications include uncontrolled hypertension, congestive heart failure, anemia, gastrointestinal hemorrhage, renal insufficiency, liver cirrhosis, and colon cancer. Sessions usually last less than 1 hour. Although it has not necessarily been supported by extensive research, some advocates of this method suggest that it is a beneficial adjunct for detoxification in a variety of conditions.

Biomechanical Methods

Many clinicians favor the use of massage as a modality to mobilize better blood and lymph circulation, as well as to assist in chronic pain management.[49] The type of massage should be recommended on the basis of individual patient needs and preferences. For example, some patients require the intensity of Rolfing, whereas others need the gentle rocking of Trager massage. Contact specific organizations for types of massage (see also American Massage Therapy Association, 847-864-0123; *www.amtamassage.org*).

Pharmaceuticals

For acute detoxification, physicians may use activated charcoal, urinary alkalinization, hemodialysis and hemoperfusion, plasmapheresis, drug antibodies, or exchange blood transfusion; their choice is dependent on the characteristics of the poison.[50] Conventional physicians reserve chelation interventions for specific documented cases of toxicity in which toxicants such as heavy metals are responsible for the symptomatology. They use oral agents such as 2,3-dimercaptosuccinic acid (DMSA) or intravenous medications such as dimercaptopropanesulfonate (DMPS),[51] both of which are purported to have less liver toxicity than earlier agents such as EDTA (ethylenediaminetetraacetic acid). However, in CAM, many providers have extended use of chelation techniques to a broad range of clinical disorders, including atherosclerosis in cardiovascular, cerebrovascular, and peripheral vascular diseases.[52] These individuals often employ intravenous chelation with drugs such as EDTA. The effectiveness and safety of CAM-type chelations still have not been established in mainstream journals, but much clinical research has previously been published on this topic.[52] Chelation therapy requires referral to an experienced provider. Be aware that chelation will remove not only potentially harmful, but also some necessary, minerals and that patients undergoing chelation will need supplementation for replacement (e.g., Heavy Metal Support from Thorne Research, Incorporated [see information previously provided]).

Patients with MCS spectrum disorders may suffer from concomitant depression or anxiety.[19] For them, conventional medications have some limited usefulness (e.g., serotonin reuptake inhibitors, anxiolytics [e.g., lorazepam], lithium, and gabapentin [Neurontin]). However, many of these patients do not tolerate medications well, and the drugs add another xenobiotic burden to an already sensitized system. Preliminary data suggest that acupuncture, for example, may offer a nondrug alternative therapy for depression in these situations.[53]

Mind-Body Therapy

For patients who have experienced toxic reactions (or perceived toxic reactions) to environmental substances, it is crucial that their sense of self-control, their capacity to do something to help themselves, be improved. These considerations are especially valid in clinical management of MCS spectrum disorders. Therefore, patient-centered interventions such as self-hypnosis, relaxation therapies, guided imagery (Academy for Guided Imagery, 415-389-9324 or 800-726-2070; *www.interactiveimagery.com*), meditation, and journaling can play a valuable adjunctive role in treatment.[54]

THERAPIES TO CONSIDER

Homeopathy

From the various schools of homeopathy, at least two intervention strategies should be considered: (1) animal studies suggest that isopathic use of homeopathic remedies (e.g., homeopathically prepared arsenic for arsenic poisoning) may increase excretion of the toxicant substance[55]; and (2) constitutional, classical homeopathic treatment for the individual on the basis of symptom patterns and essential nature of the person with the disease can be useful to strengthen the host. Particularly in MCS spectrum disorders, constitutional treatment (e.g., using the more gentle and flexibly dosed LM potencies [1/50,000 dilution factor] to accommodate patients' heightened sensitivity to all interventions) may be helpful.[56] In MCS, even when a chemical originally initiated the sensitization, the persistence of health problems may or may not derive from the persistence of a toxicant in the body. Referral information and educational programs in homeopathy are available from the National Center for Homeopathy (703-548-7790; *www.homeopathic.org*). Thus, the preferable strategy may be to reduce the host's sensitized state, a goal best accomplished by means of interventions such as constitutional homeopathy or acupuncture.

Traditional Chinese Medicine

Traditional Chinese medicine (TCM) offers a complete system of medicine that may provide a means by which to rebalance energetic disturbances in the system that manifest with symptoms of toxicity.[54] TCM draws on theories in which the individual is considered a microcosm of the larger natural environment (e.g., five elements of fire, earth, metal, water, wood, infused with a life energy called qi or chi). Yin (organ tissue) and yang (activity of an organ) are interactive concepts. Referral to an experienced expert in TCM is necessary (American Association of Acupuncture and Oriental Medicine, 888-500-7999; *www.aaom.org*). TCM encompasses acupuncture, individualized Chinese herbal mixtures, dietary changes, and exercise such as tai chi or qi gong. Different acupuncturists practice their field from a number of different theoretical and practical perspectives. For less individualized levels of prescribing, companies such as Health Concerns (telephone: 800-233-9355; *www.healthconcerns.com*) sell high-quality prepared Chinese herbal mixtures for particular indications to healthcare practitioners.

Ayurveda

Ayurvedic medicine is an ancient system of medicine derived from the Hindu tradition in India.[57] Among the treatments in Ayurveda is internal purification via Shodan cleansing (purvakarma, pradhanakarma, pashchatkarma), dependent on body type. Panchakarma (five actions) involves five main methods: (1) unction—intake of fat such as ghee (purified butter) by mouth or by anal administration, (2) purgation—use of a mixture of purgative plants to stimulate liver function and large intestine activity, (3) oil massage, (4) fomentation—sweating treatment to release toxins through the skin, via hot baths, hot herbalized steam environments, or ingestion of heat-generating foods such as ginger, pepper, and cardamom, and (5) enema (e.g., warm water or chamomile enema or oily/unctuous enema to cleanse the colon). Other cleansing approaches include nasal insufflation (medicinal oils and herbal mixtures are inhaled to drain the nasal passages and sinuses), emesis (voluntary vomiting to cleanse the upper part of the digestive tract), and blood cleansing (by blood donation). For referrals, contact the Maharishi Ayurveda Iowa organization (800-248-9050; *www.theraj.com*) or the Ayurvedic Institute (505-291-9698; *www.ayurveda.com*).

Energy Chelation

Finally, leading subtle energy healers such as Reverend Rosalyn Bruyere (*Wheels of Light*) perform processes to clear and activate an individual's energy fields from the feet upward, in a procedure called *energy chelation*.[58] Energy healers believe that disturbances in subtle energies precede physical manifestations of disease and that early intervention prevents expression at the physical level. Recent research evidence indicates that bona fide energy healers emit measurable pulses of biomagnetic fields, without physical contact with the patient's body, that exert effects on the function of biologic systems.[59]

THERAPEUTIC REVIEW

In summary, various methods, products, and theories address the issues of defining toxicity and of using detoxification interventions. Although many of these methods have thousands of years of tradition or some systematic research data to justify their use, definitive evidence of effectiveness and safety for a given modality in a given diagnostic condition is largely not yet available. General supportive measures for the individual include antioxidant mixtures, massage, and mind-body techniques; helpful nondrug therapies may include constitutional homeopathic treatment or acupuncture.

Avoidance
- *Clear home and work indoor environments of potential toxicants.*
- *Change diet—use organic, whole foods.*

Improved Metabolism of Toxicants
- *Add UltraClear® food supplement or comparable mixture of nutrient support, two scoops in 8 oz of water or juice for 7 to 14 days. (Detoxification may be enhanced if used with a modified fast. See Chapter 82, How to Recommend an Elimination Diet.) A 21-day supply costs about $75.00.*
- *Milk thistle, 140–210 mg tid.*
- *Schisandra, 500–1000 mg tid.*

Increased Excretion
- *Drink 6 to 8 glasses of water daily.*
- *Consider sauna therapy.*
- *Consider colon hydrotherapy.*

Pharmaceuticals
- *PO or IV chelating agents for identified toxins.*

ADDITIONAL RESOURCES

- Environmental Defense Fund Scorecard website: *www.scorecard.org.* Information on environmental toxins and their sources by geographic location (state and county), including superfund sites.
- Sanborn M, Abelson A: Environmental Health in Family Medicine Health Professions Task Force of the International Joint Commission, Canada Mortgage and Housing Corporation, and the Ontario College of Family Physicians Environmental Health Committee. *www.ijc.org/boards/hptf/modules/content.html*—downloaded free. Or by e-mail request: *houstonj@ottawa.ijc.org.* A six-module, peer-reviewed curriculum for the primary health care professional, including discussions of lead, indoor and outdoor air quality, pesticides, human health and water quality, and persistent organic pollutants. Included is information on taking an exposure history, as well as clues to appropriate resources and risk communication. Case studies (including those involving pediatrics and reproductive care) are provided.

ACKNOWLEDGMENT

The authors thank Peter Arambula for his assistance in researching source material for this chapter.

Supported in part by a grant from the Jennifer Altman Foundation, NIH K24 AT00057-01, R21 AT00315-01, and NIH P50 AT00008-02.

References

1. Van Ert MD, Crutchfield CD, Sullivan JB: Principles of environmental and occupational hazard assessment. In Sullivan JB, Krieger GR (eds): Clinical Environmental Health and Toxic Exposures. 2nd ed. Philadelphia, Lippincott Williams and Wilkins, 2001, pp 30–49.
2. Galvano F, Piva A, Ritieni A, Galvano G: Dietary strategies to counteract the effects of mycotoxins: A review. J Food Protect 64:120–131, 2001.
3. Darvill T, Londy E, Reihman J, et al: Prenatal exposure to PCBs and infant performance on the Fagan test of infant intelligence. Neurotoxicology 21:1029–1038, 2000.
4. D'Cruz D: Autoimmune diseases associated with drugs, chemicals, and environmental factors. Toxicol Lett 112–113:421–432, 2000.
5. Crinnion WJ: Environmental medicine, part 1: The human burden of environmental toxins and their common health effects. Altern Med Rev 5:52–63, 2000.
6. Semchuk KM, Love EJ, Lee RG: Parkinson's disease and exposure to agricultural work and pesticide chemicals. Neurology 42:1328–1335, 1992.
7. Dalefield RR, Oehme FW, Krieger GR: Principles of risk assessment. In Sullivan JB, Krieger GR (eds): Clinical Environmental Health and Toxic Exposures, 2nd ed. Philadelphia, Lippincott Williams and Wilkins, 2001, pp 77–92.
8. Ashford N, Miller C: Chemical Exposures. Low Levels and High Stakes. 2nd ed. New York, Van Nostrand Reinhold, 1998.
9. Calabrese EJ, Baldwin LA: A general classification of U-shaped dose-response relationships in toxicology and their mechanistic foundations. Hum Exp Toxicol 17:353–364, 1998.
10. NE Regional Environmental Public Health Center: University of Massachusetts School of Public Health. Biological Effects of Low Level Exposures Newsletter 9:1–47, 2001. (*www.BelleOnline.com*).
11. Calabrese EJ, Baldwin LA: Developing insights on the nature of the dose-response relationship in the low dose zone: Hormesis as a biological hypothesis. Biomed Ther 16:235–240, 1998.
12. Abou-Donia MB, Wilmarth KR, Jensen KF: Neurotoxicity result-

ing from coexposure to pyridostigmine bromide, DEET, and permethrin: Implications of Gulf War chemical exposures. J Toxicol Environ Health 48:35–56, 1996.

13. Bell IR, Baldwin CM, Schwartz GE: Illness from low levels of environmental chemicals: Relevance to chronic fatigue syndrome and fibromyalgia. Am J Med Suppl 105:74S–82S, 1998.

14. Bell IR, Baldwin CM, Fernandez M, Schwartz GER: Neural sensitization model for multiple chemical sensitivity: Overview of theory and empirical evidence. Toxicol Industr Health 15:295–304, 1999.

15. Meggs WJ, Dunn KA, Bloch RM, et al: Prevalence and nature of allergy and chemical sensitivity in a general population. Arch Environ Health 51:275–282, 1996.

16. Kreutzer R, Neutra RR, Lashuay N: Prevalence of people reporting sensitivities to chemicals in a population-based survey. Am J Epidemiol 150:1–12, 1999.

17. Bell IR, Miller CS, Schwartz GE, et al: Neuropsychiatric and somatic characteristics of young adults with and without self-reported chemical odor intolerance and chemical sensitivity. Arch Environ Health 51:9–21, 1996.

18. Miller CS: The compelling anomaly of chemical intolerance. Ann NY Acad Sci 933:1–23, 2001.

19. Fiedler N, Kipen HM, DeLuca J, et al: A controlled comparison of multiple chemical sensitivities and chronic fatigue syndrome. Psychosom Med 58:38–49, 1996.

20. Miller CS, Mitzel HC: Chemical sensitivity attributed to pesticide exposure versus remodeling. Arch Environ Health 50:119–129, 1995.

21. Sorg BA, Willis JR, See RE, et al: Repeated low-level formaldehyde exposure produces cross-sensitization to cocaine: Possible relevance to chemical sensitivity in humans. Neuropsychopharmacology 18:385–394, 1998.

22. Antelman SM: Time-dependent sensitization in animals: A possible model of multiple chemical sensitivity in humans. Toxicol Industr Health 10:335–342, 1994.

23. von Euler G, Ogren S, Eneroth P, et al: Persistent effects of 80 ppm toluene on dopamine-regulated locomotor activity and prolactin secretion in the male rat. Neurotoxicology 15:621–624, 1994.

24. Gilbert ME: Does the kindling model of epilepsy contribute to our understanding of multiple chemical sensitivity? Ann NY Acad Sci 933:68–91, 2001.

25. Bascom R, Meggs WJ, Frampton M, et al: Neurogenic inflammation: With additional discussion of central and perceptual integration of nonneurogenic inflammation. Environ Health Perspect 105(Suppl 2):531–537, 1997.

26. Rea WJ, Pan Y, Johnson AR, et al: Reduction of chemical sensitivity by means of heat depuration, physical therapy, and nutritional supplementation in a controlled environment. J Nutr Environ Med 6:141–148, 1996.

27. Verma V: Ayurveda. A Way of Life. York Beach, Maine, Samuel Weiser, Inc, 1995.

28. Cohen KBH: Native American medicine. Altern Ther Health Med 4(6):45–57, 1998.

29. Seidel S, Kreutzer R, Smith D, et al: Assessment of commercial laboratories performing hair mineral analysis. JAMA 285:67–72, 2001.

30. Ahlqwist M, Bengtsson C, Lapidus L, et al: Serum mercury concentration in relation to survival, symptoms, and diseases: Results from the prospective population study of women in Gothenburg, Sweden. Acta Odontol Scand 57:168–174, 1999.

31. Bernard S, Enayati A, Redwood L, et al: Autism: A novel form of mercury poisoning. Med Hypotheses 56:462–471, 2001.

32. MacIntosh A, Ball K: The effects of a short program of detoxification in disease-free individuals. Altern Ther Health Med 6:70–76, 2000.

33. Galland L: Power Healing. New York, Random House, 1997.

34. Seppanen OA, Fisk WJ, Mendell MJ: Association of ventilation rates and CO2 concentrations with health and other responses in commercial and institutional buildings. Indoor Air Internat J Indoor Air Qual Climate 9:226–252, 1999.

35. Randolph TG, Moss RW: An Alternative Approach to Allergies. New York, Harper and Row, 1989.

36. Crinnion WJ: Environmental medicine, part 2: Health effects of

and protection from ubiquitous airborne solvent exposure. Altern Med Rev 5:133–143, 2000.

37. Dadd-Redalia D: Home Safe Home: Protecting Yourself and Your Family from Everyday Toxics and Harmful Household Products in the Home. JP Tarcher, 1997.

38. Wallace L, et al: The TEAM study: Personal exposures to toxic substances in air, drinking water, and breath of 400 residents of New Jersey, North Carolina, and North Dakota. Environ Res 43:290–307, 1987.

39. Bland J, Barrager E, Reedy RG, Bland K: A medical food supplemented detoxification program in the management of chronic health problems. Altern Ther Health Med 1:62–71, 1995.

40. Pizzorno J: Total Wellness. Rocklin, Calif, Prima Publishing, 1996.

41. Pepping J: Milk thistle: Silybum marianum. Am J Health Syst Pharm 56:1195–1197, 1999.

42. Zhu M, Lin KF, Yeung RY, Li RC: Evaluation of the protective effects of Schisandra chinensis on phase I drug metabolism using a CCl4 intoxication model. J Ethnopharmacol 67:61–68, 1999.

43. Bland JS, Costarella L, Levin B, et al: Clinical Nutrition: A Functional Approach. Gig Harbor, Washington, Institute for Functional Medicine, Inc, 1999.

44. National Environmental Trust (NET), Physicians for Social Responsibility (PSR) and Learning Disabilities Association of America (LDA): Polluting Our Future: Chemical pollution in the US that affects child development and learning. September 2000.

45. McVicker M: Sauna Detoxification Therapy. Jefferson, NC, McFarland and Co, Inc, 1997.

46. Schnare DW, Denk G, Shields M, Brunton S: Evaluation of a detoxification regimen for fat stored xenobiotics. Med Hypotheses 9:265–282, 1982.

47. Kilburn KH, Warsaw RH, Shields MG: Neurobehavioral dysfunction in firemen exposed to polychlorinated biphenyls (PCBs): Possible improvement after detoxification. Arch Environ Health 44:345–350, 1989.

48. Walker M: Value of colon hydrotherapy verified by medical professionals. Townsend Lett 205–206:66–71, 2000.

49. Zanolla R, Monzeglio C, Balzarini A, Martino G: Evaluations of the results of three different methods of postmastectomy lymphedema treatment. J Surg Oncol 26:210, 1984.

50. Winchester JF: Active methods of detoxification. In Haddad LM, Shannon MW, Winchester JF (eds): Clinical Management of Poisoning and Drug Overdose, 3rd ed. Philadelphia, WB Saunders, 1998, pp 175–188.

51. Aaseth J, Jacobsen D, Andersen O, Wickstrom E: Treatment of mercury and lead poisonings with dimercaptosuccinic acid and sodium dimercaptopropanesulfonate. A review. Analyst 120:853–857, 1995.

52. Cranton EM (ed): A Textbook on EDTA Chelation Therapy, 2nd ed. Charlottesville, Va, Hampton Roads Publishing Co, 2001.

53. Allen JJB, Schnyer RN, Hitt SK: The efficacy of acupuncture in the treatment of major depression in women. Psychol Sci 9:397–401, 1998.

54. Jonas WB, Levin JS: Essentials of Complementary and Alternative Medicine. Philadelphia, Lippincott Williams & Wilkins, 1999.

55. Mitra K, Kundu SN, Khuda-Bukhsh AR: Efficacy of a potentized homeopathic drug (Arsenicum Album 30) in reducing toxic effects produced by arsenic trioxide in mice. I. On rate of accumulation of arsenic in certain vital organs. Complem Ther Med 6:178–184, 1998.

56. De Schepper L: LM potencies: One of the hidden treasures of the sixth edition of the Organon. Br Homeopath J 88:128–134, 1999.

57. Sharma HM, Nidich SI, Sands D, Smith DE: Improvement in cardiovascular risk factors through panchakarma purification procedures. J Res Educ Ind Med Oct–Dec:3–12, 1993.

58. Bruyere RL: Wheels of Light. New York, Simon and Schuster, 1994.

59. Oschman JL: Energy Medicine. The Scientific Basis. Edinburgh, Churchill Livingstone, 2000.

Strain and Counter-strain Manipulation Technique

Harmon L. Myers, D.O., and David Rakel, M.D.

WHAT IS IT?

Strain and counterstrain is a manipulative technique that has been found to be helpful in reducing pain and spasm in the myofascial system. It can act as an excellent therapeutic adjunct in the primary care setting to help facilitate relief of pain related to muscle and fascial layers. It is a safe, indirect technique that does not incorporate manipulation against mechanical barriers. It simply involves putting a muscle group in a position of relaxation that results in inhibition of the neurologic reflex cycle that may cause and maintain myofascial dysfunction and muscle spasm. The therapy is also known as positional release therapy.

HISTORY OF THE THERAPY

The therapy was originated by an osteopathic physician named Lawrence Jones who took pride in his ability to relieve pain with the use of manual techniques. He was given a challenging patient with severe low back pain with restricted movement. After multiple attempts to relieve the pain had failed, Jones decided to simply place the patient in a position of comfort so he could rest. After returning, Jones noticed that the patient's pain had significantly improved. The discovery resulted in the development of a therapy that focused on relieving myofascial pain by shortening muscles and placing them in positions of comfort.[1]

PATHOPHYSIOLOGY OF A TENDER POINT

Tender points of the myofascial system date back to the Chinese Tang dynasty of AD 618 when they were called Ah Shi points. Descriptions of these points in Western medicine have included terms such as *trigger points, fibrositis, muscle callus, chronic*

myositis, and *muscular nodules.* It appears that the underlying mechanism of pain and inflammation is the same. Tender points are the result of three mechanisms:

1. Neurologic (proprioceptive) response to acute muscle strain or injury.
2. Neurologic (nociceptive) response to visceral disease, muscle strain, or injury that persists owing to lack of response to treatment.
3. Reflex response to increased tone of the sympathetic nervous system that can result from anxiety and pain.

As a result, there is an accumulation of pro-inflammatory and vasoconstrictive chemical mediators, including histamine, prostaglandins, bradykinin, and potassium. These mediators team with an influx of calcium ions, resulting in overactivity of muscle stimulation, causing a neurologic reflex arc that creates taut bands of painful muscle. The underlying trigger of this phenomenon can be an acute injury, repetitive strain, imbalance of muscle use, visceral disease, or chronic stress and tension.

Strain-Counterstrain

Jones described the underlying pathophysiology of a tender point in regard to a strain on a pair of antagonistic muscles of a joint. Figure 99–1 depicts what happens with a misstep or injury and helps describe this theory. Two muscles (A and B) are present and a schematic shows electrical proprioceptor activation of the muscles. Section 2 shows a condition that results in strain of muscle A. The corresponding schematic of muscle A shows increased electrical (proprioceptive) activation when it is strained, which prompts the body to try to return the joint to the normal balanced state. At the same time, the hypershortened muscle (B) has decreased proprioceptive electrical activity. Muscle A is shortened in response to the strain and this results in a rebound stretching of muscle B. As muscle B quickly lengthens in response to the short-

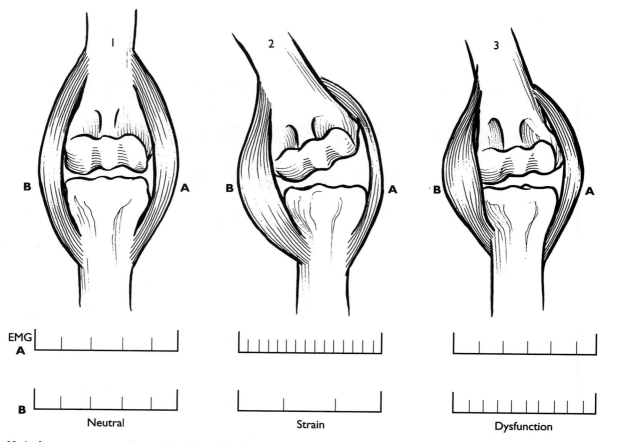

Figure 99–1. Jones neuromuscular model. (From D'Ambrogio KJ, Roth GB: Positional Release Therapy: Assessment and Treatment of Musculoskeletal Dysfunction. St. Louis, Mosby, 1997; modified from Jones LH: Strain and Counterstrain. Newark, Ohio, American Academy of Osteopathy, 1981).

ening of muscle A, the proprioceptive nerve endings in muscle B, which mainly respond to rate of length change, become overstimulated. This results in a theoretical massive nervous discharge that causes the muscle to register strain before it even reaches its resting length. This prevents the joint from returning to its neutral state, as is seen in section 3, which shows the status of the joint after injury with the tender point arising from the overstimulated muscle B. This becomes the primary source of persistent muscle dysfunction. An analogy that may make this concept easier to understand would be catching a ball of lead in your hand when you were expecting a ball of paper. It is the rebound contraction of the biceps muscle that pushes up against the weight that triggers the dysfunction in the triceps muscle, which is rapidly lengthened.

In treating the tender point in muscle B, the focus is on shortening this muscle to reduce the electrical activity that results in a disruption of the neuromuscular reflex arc that has kept the joint in an imbalanced state and the muscle in spasm. Shortening the muscle to reduce the inappropriate proprioceptor activity results in reduced pain and inflammation of the tender point and return of the joint to its normal state.

Occupational Repetitiveness

A sedentary lifestyle and occupational repetitiveness limit the number of muscles used on a regular basis. This leads to overuse of a small percentage of the body's muscles while others atrophy, resulting in a reduced ability to tolerate loads or strains. The chronically stressed tissues lead to tender points in muscle groups that have increased postural demands. Repeated microtrauma to these muscles results in a pain (nociceptive) response that affects the proprioceptor electrical stimuli similar to that described previously. An example of this may include pain in the trapezius, levator scapula, and suboccipital muscles in someone who spends most of the day sitting at a desk working on a computer. A regular exercise program can help keep a balanced tone in all muscle groups, helping prevent strain of atrophic muscles and tender points in chronically stressed muscles.

Tender Points Not Related to a Strain or Injury

Many trigger points are not related to a specific strain or injury, as can be seen in diseases such as fibromyalgia and trapezius discomfort related to tension. This clinical finding makes one appreciate the close association between the mind and the body and how stress and anxiety can act as triggers to this inflammatory cycle. It is well established that stress leads to an overactivity of the autonomic nervous system and sympathetic discharge. This is a key ingredient in myofascial dysfunction and pain. Attention should be given to any chronic condition that may have this as an underlying perpetuating factor so lifestyle and relaxation recommendations can be made to help prevent recurrence and reduce the pain threshold.

EVALUATING THE PATIENT FOR THERAPY

- Take a history of the length, severity, and location of the discomfort. Address a history of trauma, strain, occupational repetition, activity, and degree of stress and tension.
- Appreciate referral patterns. Location of pain may result from a referral pattern arising from a distant trigger point. With experience, the practitioner will learn of common referral patterns of tender points related to muscle groups.
- Learn what a tender point feels like. A nodule can often be palpated in involved muscle groups that will help guide therapy.
- Find what positions cause discomfort. Usually, stretching the dysfunctional muscle causes discomfort.

GENERAL GUIDELINES TO THERAPY[1]

- Move gently and slowly into and out of the position of treatment.
- Hold the position of treatment (comfort) for no less than 90 seconds.
- Anterior tender points are generally treated in a position of flexion.
- Posterior tender points are generally treated in a position of extension.
- More flexion or extension is used for tender points on or near the midline.
- More rotation and side bending are needed for points lateral to the midline.
- Tender points in the extremities are often found on the side opposite the side where the patient complains of pain.
- If there are multiple tender points, treat the most severe first.
- When tender points are in rows, treat the one in the middle first.
- Explain to the patient that she or he may be sore in 24 to 48 hours after a treatment.

STEPS IN THE TREATMENT OF TENDER POINTS[1]

1. Find a significant tender point.
2. Put the patient in a position of comfort.
3. Fine-tune the position to get maximum relief of the tender point as you monitor it with your finger (use the palpable response of the trigger point beneath your finger as well as the subjective response of pain relief from the patient to fine-tune the therapeutic position).
4. Release pressure while maintaining contact on the tender point during treatment.
5. Maintain the position of comfort for at least 90 seconds.
6. Slowly return to a neutral position.
7. Recheck the tender point. It should be at least 70% improved.

EXAMPLES OF THE TECHNIQUE

Two of the most common myofascial complaints seen in the primary care setting are neck pain (trapezius spasm, suboccipital neuralgia) and low back pain, particularly sciatica that involves posterior gluteal pain with referred pain down the back of the leg. To explain how this technique can be used in the primary care setting, we consider a group of muscles that are commonly involved in these complaints. It is important to realize that the practice of this technique involves a unique evaluation of each patient that may include numerous muscle groups that are not discussed here owing to space limitations.

Trapezius (Fig. 99–2)

The trapezius, a large muscle of the upper back, can have multiple trigger point locations, each with a different treatment. We focus on the most common two depicted by the X in Figure 99–2A.

Tender points: Located in the fibers of the upper part of the muscle at the junction of the neck and shoulder; can be medial or lateral.

Referral pattern: Pain can be located in the posterior neck, the suboccipital area, and the temporal area (see Fig. 99–2B).

Treatment position for more medial tender points: Place finger over trigger point and side-bend the cervical spine toward the side of pain until you feel the muscle relax (fold the neck over the tender point).

Treatment position for more lateral tender points: Bring the arms 150 to 170 degrees overhead as shown in Figure 99–2C and apply cephalic traction.

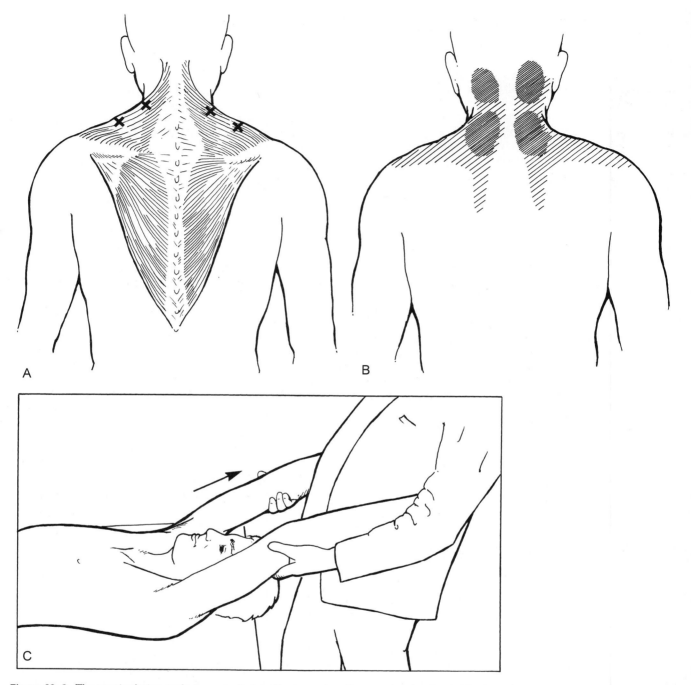

Figure 99–2. The manipulation technique applied to the trapezius. See text for details. *A*, Tender points. *B*, Pain referral pattern. *C*, Treatment position.

Levator Scapula (Fig. 99–3)

The levator scapula is a common source of pain that is seen in those with tension and anxiety (chronic shoulder shrug) or neck pain associated with holding a phone between the ear and the shoulder.

Tender point: At the superomedial aspect of the scapula between the scapula and the nape of the neck (see Fig. 99–3*A*).

Referral pattern: Pain at the junction of the neck and shoulder, extending to the midcervical area above and the spine of the scapula below (see Fig. 99–3*B*).

Treatment position: With the patient supine, adduct the arm approximately 30 degrees with the elbow flexed. Flex the shoulder slightly and apply a cephalic force through the shaft of the humerus to elevate the scapula. Side-bend the neck toward the side of the tender point. Imagine the patient holding an orange between the ear and the shoulder as you push the elbow toward the ear (see Fig. 99–3*C*).

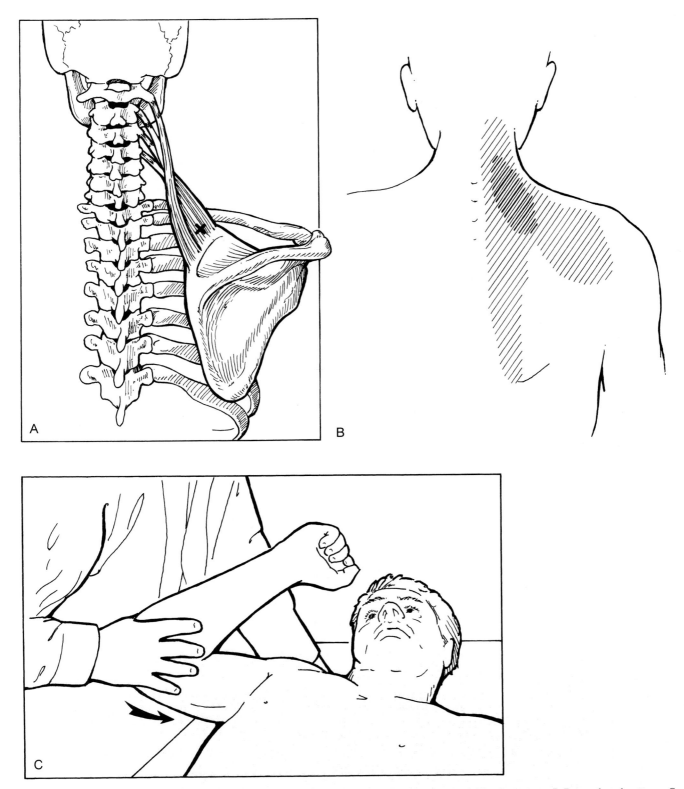

Figure 99–3. The manipulation technique applied to the levator scapula. See text for details. *A*, Tender points. *B*, Pain referral pattern. *C*, Treatment position.

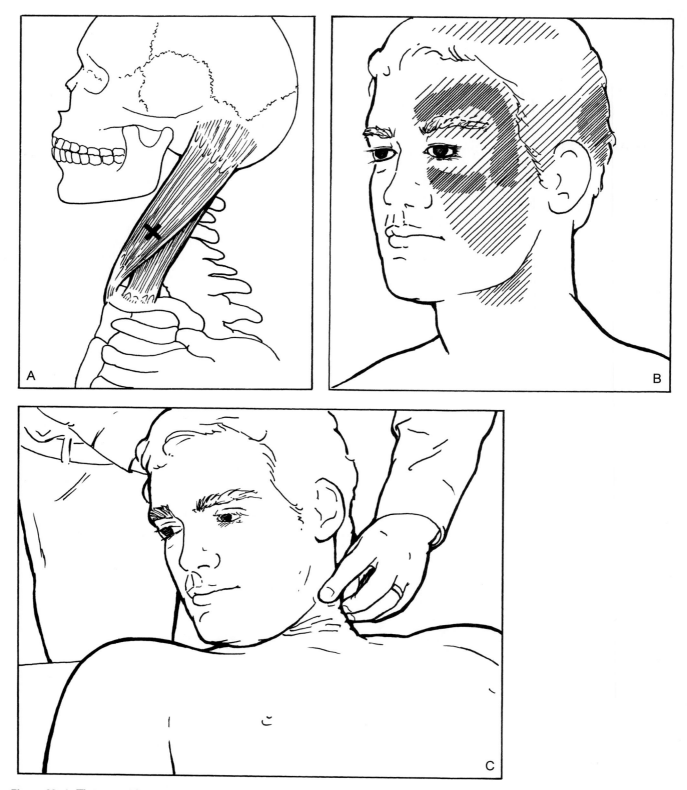

Figure 99–4. The manipulation technique applied to the sternocleidomastoid. See text for details. *A*, Tender points. *B*, Pain referral pattern. *C*, Treatment position.

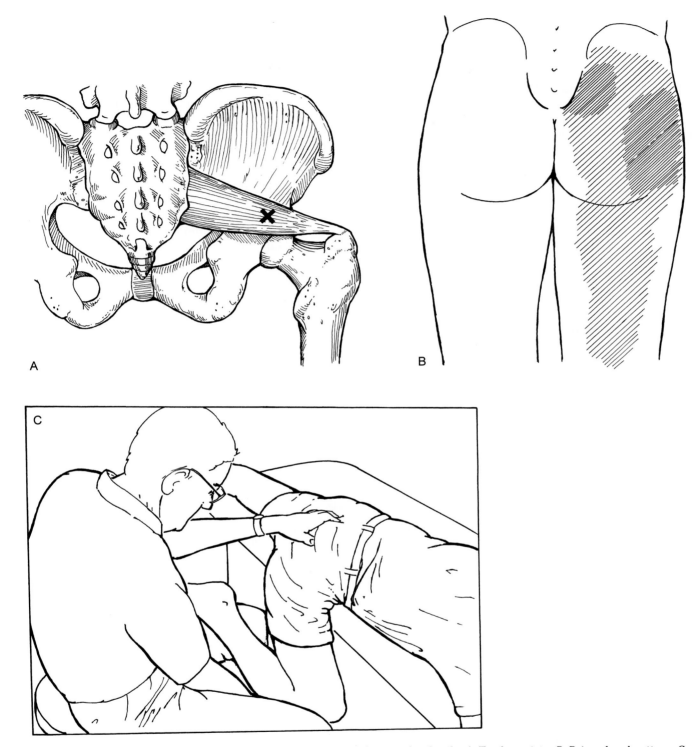

Figure 99-5. The manipulation technique applied to the piriformis. See text for details. *A*, Tender points. *B*, Pain referral pattern. *C*, Treatment position.

As you palpate the tender point, fine-tune with slight flexion/extension of the shoulder until you feel the tender point release.

Sternocleidomastoid (Fig. 99–4)

It is important to always check for tender points on the side of the body opposite where the pain is located. In this case, check for anterior pain along the sternocleidomastoid if the patient complains of posterior neck pain. As a rule, most patients will not complain of any discomfort in the anterior neck.

Tender point: Anywhere in the body of either the sternal or the clavicular division of the muscle. Squeeze the belly of the muscle with your thumb and index finger to help find the tender point. Most common area is two or three fingerbreadths above the sternoclavicular joint (see Fig. 99–4A).

Referral pattern: Pain into the suboccipital area, ear, temporomandibular joint, forehead, or eye (see Fig. 99–4B).

Treatment position: With the patient supine, support the head as you markedly flex the neck, side-bending toward and rotating away from the tender point. Imagine pushing the patient's ear toward the sternoclavicular joint (see Fig. 99–4C).

Fine-tune until you feel the tender point release or the patient reports subjective improvement.

Piriformis (Fig. 99–5)

The sciatic nerve and the piriformis muscle are in close proximity. In fact, in 5% of the population the nerve runs through or over the muscle, making irritation of the nerve much more likely when the muscle is inflamed. This is called *piriformis syndrome* and is a common cause of buttock pain with radiation of pain down the back of the thigh.

Tender point: Located in the piriformis muscle, which is 3 inches medial and slightly cephalic to the greater trochanter. Halfway between the midsacrum and the greater trochanter of the proximal femur (see Fig. 99–5A).

Referral pattern: Buttock and the back of the thigh (see Fig. 99–5B).

Treatment position: Patient is prone. Therapist sits on the same side as the tender point. The patient's leg on the tender point side is suspended off the table with the patient's anterior ankle resting on the therapist's thigh. Flex the hip 120 to 130 degrees, abduct the hip to tolerance, and slightly rotate the hip internally by gently pulling outward on the foot (see Fig. 99–5C).

BENEFITS OF THE THERAPY

- The therapy provides immediate relief of discomfort.

- It helps the body regain normal function and range of motion that may have been limited by chronic myofascial dysfunction.
- It is fun and rewarding to do.
- It enables you to touch the patient, increasing a sense of caring and rapport in a day in which technology is creating a barrier between practitioner and patient.
- The patient is always treated in a position of comfort.

LIMITATIONS OF THE THERAPY

- Pain relief can be transient with recurrence likely if a holistic understanding of why the pain may be continually triggered is not approached.
- A localized technique such as this may not be the best approach for someone with diffuse and disseminated tender points in conditions such as fibromyalgia.
- The technique is conceptually easy to learn but takes practice. Start with a few muscle groups and then progress from there. When able, practice on children. Their limited soft tissue mass allows for easy palpation of tender points and maneuverability for treatment positions.

Resources for Further Education

The Tucson Osteopathic Medical Foundation offers hands-on classes in Strain/Counterstrain taught by one of the authors (HM) twice a year. They are divided into the upper and lower aspects of the body. Call (520) 299-4545 for more information or go to www.tomf.org

Many courses in manual medicine including Strain/Counterstrain are offered annually by the American Academy of Osteopathy: www.aao.medguide.net

Books that provide further clinical information on positions of therapy include:

- *Jones Strain-Counterstrain.* By Lawrence H. Jones. Boise, Idaho, Jones Strain-Counterstrain, Inc., 1995.
- *Positional Release Therapy: Assessment and Treatment of Musculoskeletal Dysfunction.* By Kerry J. D'Ambrogio and George B. Roth. St. Louis, Mosby, 1997.
- *Myofascial Pain and Dysfunction: The Trigger Point Manual* by Janet G. Travell, M.D., and David G. Simons, M.D.

References

1. Jones LH: Jones Strain-Counterstrain. Boise, Idaho, Jones Strain-Counterstrain, Inc., 1995.
2. D'Ambrogio KJ, Roth GB: Positional Release Therapy: Assessment and Treatment of Musculoskeletal Dysfunction. St. Louis, Mosby, 1997.
3. Korr IM: Proprioceptors and somatic dysfunction. J Am Osteopath Assoc 74:638, 1975.
4. Levin SM: The importance of soft tissue for structural support of the body. Spine 9:357, 1995.
5. Lowe JC: Treatment-resistant myofascial pain syndrome. In Hammer WI (ed): Functional Soft Tissue Examination and Treatment by Manual Methods. Gaithersburg, Md, 1991.
6. Travell JF, Simons DG: Myofascial Pain and Dysfunction: The Trigger Point Manual. Baltimore, Williams & Wilkins, 1992.

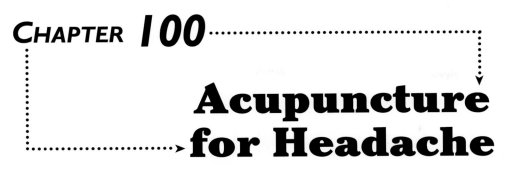

CHAPTER 100

Acupuncture for Headache

Malcolm Riley, B.D.S., F.D.S., M.R.D.

HEADACHE IN CHINESE MEDICINE

As in western medicine, the Chinese medicine approach to treatment of headache begins with the differential diagnosis, to identify any underlying disorders. The Chinese diagnosis is based on the state of energy (qi) flow within organ channels and collateral vessels, which constitutes the basis of Chinese medicine. In Chinese medicine, chronic headache is viewed as a blockage of qi in the yang meridians of the head. The qi blockage is usually caused by internal disturbances and rarely by external causes.

The number of acupuncture points used to treat headaches is rather large, and the particular points used depend on the specific Chinese diagnosis. The location of the pain is an important feature in determining which points are used. As headaches constitute a complex diagnostic problem in Chinese medicine, preliminary assessment of the patient by an experienced acupuncturist is recommended.

TECHNIQUE FOR ACUPUNCTURE TREATMENT OF HEADACHE

For symptomatic relief of headache, use of a group of specific acupuncture points has proved to be very effective in clinical practice (Figs. 100–1 to 100–5). These points are large intestine 4 (LI4), gallbladder 20 (GB20), liver 3 (LIV3), stomach 36 (ST36), and governor vessel 20 (GV20). These points are needled bilaterally, with the exception of GV20, which, being on a midline vessel, is a single point.

The points are needled to a maximum depth of 1 cm using a 2.5-cm stainless steel disposable acupuncture needle. An electrical acupuncture stimulator can be applied to either LI4 or ST36 bilaterally at a frequency of 2 to 4 Hz, which increases the effectiveness of the treatment.

Needles should be left in place for 20 minutes at each visit. Acupuncture in general has a cumulative action. At least four treatments should be given, to assess whether any benefit is obtained with this modality; the maximal effect occurs at around the sixth to eighth visit. In China, treatment is often given daily, but this approach is impractical in the United States, although for optimal benefit the first four treatments should be given within a 2-week period.

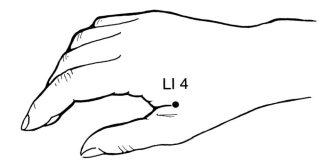

Figure 100–1. Acupuncture points: Large intestine 4 (LI4).

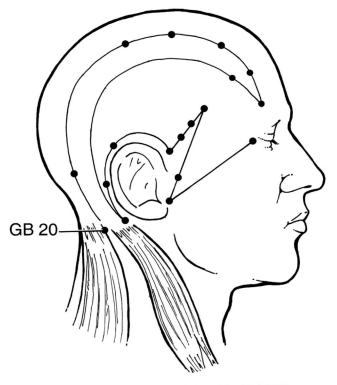

Figure 100–2. Acupuncture points: Gallbladder 20 (GB20).

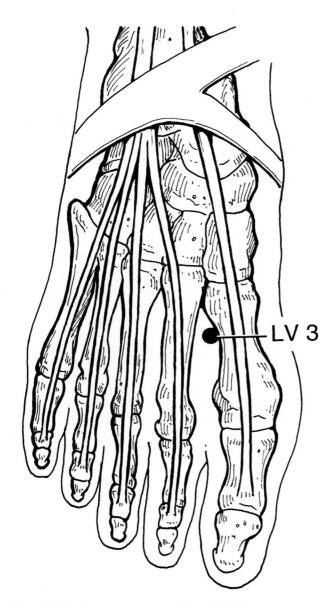

Figure 100–3. Acupuncture points: Liver 3 (LV3).

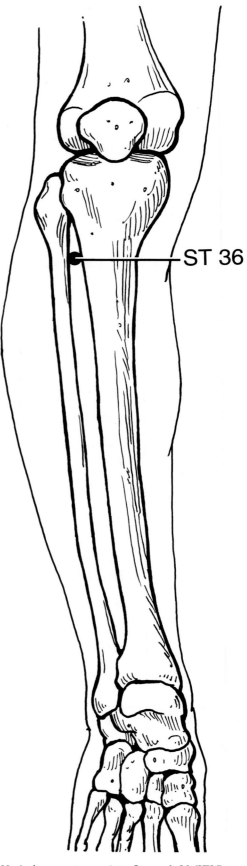

Figure 100–4. Acupuncture points: Stomach 36 (ST36).

Acupuncture should be considered a success if the number, frequency, and intensity of headaches are reduced and the need for medication is reduced or eliminated. In some instances acupuncture can completely resolve headaches. The formula presented here is for the *symptomatic* treatment of headaches, whereas an acupuncturist trained in traditional Chinese medicine would examine the patient for energy imbalances in the body and prescribe an individualized treatment to correct these imbalances, which is more likely to produce long-lasting results. With this approach, maintenance therapy is given every 6 to 12 weeks to maintain this energy balance.

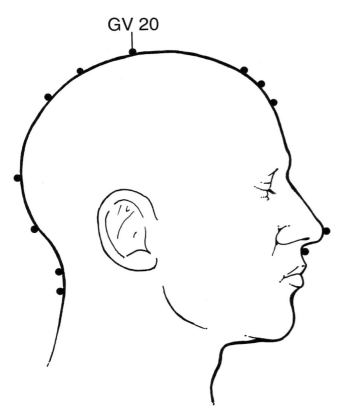

GV 20

Figure 100–5. Acupuncture points: Governor vessel 20 (GV20).

> ### NOTE
>
> *The formula presented here is one regimen for practical application of acupuncture in the treatment of headache. It should not be used unless further training has been pursued.*

LOCATION OF POINTS

The acupuncture points used in the treatment of headache are located as follows:

- Large intestine 4 (Li4)—located at the highest point of the adductor pollicis muscle observed when the index finger and thumb are abducted (see Fig. 100–1)
- Gallbladder 20 (GB20)—located between the origins of the sternocleidomastoid and the trapezius muscles (see Fig. 100–2)
- Liver 3 (LIV3)—located between the first and second metatarsals 2 Chinese inches (width of the thumb at the interphalangeal joint) from the web (see Fig. 100–3)
- Stomach 36 (ST36)—located in a depression between the tibia and fibula, lateral to the tibial tuberosity (see Fig. 100–4)
- Governor vessel 20 (GV20)—located in the midline on a line joining the highest points of the ears (see Fig. 100–5)

FINDING AN ACUPUNCTURIST

Many physicians have trained in acupuncture with the American Academy of Medical Acupuncture (AAMA). The AAMA web site provides information about the organization's training programs and also lists AAMA members:

http://www.medicalacupuncture.org/

Traditional chinese medicine practitioners are licensed in many states. There are several different styles of acupuncture, but a good benchmark to look for is certification from the National Certification Commission for Acupuncture and Oriental Medicine (NCCAOM). Information about state licensure and a searchable database of diplomates are available at

http://www.nccaom.org/

The clinician is advised to contact locally based practitioners to assess their interest in working with an integrative approach to patient care, before referring patients for treatment.

SUMMARY

The literature on the acupuncture treatment of headache is in general of rather poor quality, but in a recent review, Melchart and colleagues concluded: "Overall, the existing evidence suggests that acupuncture has a role in the treatment of recurrent headaches. However, the quality and amount of evidence [are] not fully convincing. There is urgent need for well-planned, large-scale studies to assess effectiveness and efficiency of acupuncture under real life conditions."

Reference

1. Melchart D, Linde K, Fischer P, et al: Acupuncture for recurrent headaches: A systematic review of randomized controlled trials. Cephalalgia 19:779–786, 1999.

CHAPTER 101

Acupuncture for Nausea and Vomiting

Malcolm Riley, B.D.S., F.D.S., M.R.D.

Acupuncture has been used to treat nausea and vomiting in Chinese medicine for several thousand years. Much of the evidence has been anecdotal, but in the past three decades a considerable amount of research has been devoted to this subject, particularly with the use of one acupuncture point—PC6 (Pericardium 6, Neiguan).

In traditional Chinese medicine, a fundamental constituent of life is called qi (pronounced chee). The qi of each organ is thought to have a direction associated with it. The qi of the healthy stomach moves downward and facilitates digestion and elimination. In cases of nausea, the natural flow of qi in the stomach is disrupted. In cases of vomiting, the natural flow of qi in the stomach is reversed. In acupuncture, it is qi that is manipulated with needles.

Each organ is associated with a meridian system where the qi of that organ is thought to flow through the body. It is along these meridians that many of the acupuncture points for that organ are located. Other organs and meridians are thought to influence each other in various ways. The stomach and spleen have a beneficial relationship. The liver and stomach have an antagonistic relationship. The meridian systems themselves also are thought to influence each other.

Acupuncture points that are commonly used in nausea and vomiting are usually associated with the stomach, spleen, and liver, such as stomach 36, bladder 20, and liver 3, or they are points that are thought to cause qi to descend, such as the large intestine 4 (LI4) (see Chapter 100 for diagrams of ST36, LV3 and LI4). Also, points on other influential meridians may be used, such as spleen 4 and PC6. And, last, points in the vicinity of the organ may be used, such as Conception Vessel 12. A trained acupuncturist selects from these and other points based on a Chinese diagnosis.

TECHNIQUES

The acupuncture point that has received the most attention recently in the treatment of nausea and vomiting is PC6 (Figs. 101–1 and 101–2). PC6 is located on the pericardium meridian, 2 cun (a "cun" is a Chinese inch, it is the width of the thumb across the interphalangeal joint) proximal to the wrist crease, between the tendons of the palmaris longus (medial) and the flexor carpi radialis (lateral)—the two most prominent tendons on the volar aspect of the wrist.

NOTE

Several acupuncture points are thought to cause qi to descend. It is important to note that during gestation, it is also qi that holds the fetus in place. Therefore, acupuncture should be used with caution or not at all in women who are at risk of miscarriage, particularly at the points that cause qi to descend (e.g., large intestine [LI4]).

Traditionally, PC6 is needled to a depth of 1 cm with a 2.5-cm acupuncture needle. When the median nerve is located at this point, minimal insertion to a depth of 2 to 3 mm is recommended (hypodermic needles should never be used for acupuncture). The needles are inserted for approximately 20 minutes. Traditionally, the needles are rotated back and forth on a 90-degree arc until the de qi sensation is felt (a

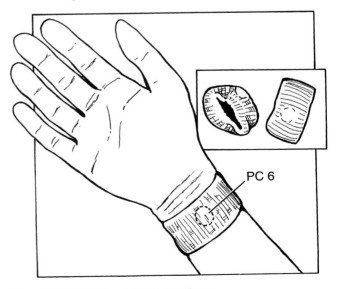

Figure 101–1. Sea-Band: PC, pericardium.

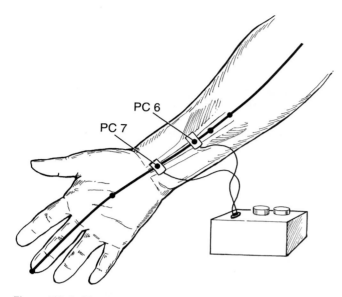

Figure 101–2. Transcutaneous electrical stimulation. PC, pericardium.

deep aching sensation). An alternative method of stimulation is with an electronic acupuncture stimulator attached to the needles. A frequency of 2 to 10 Hz is used and the intensity is such that the patient can feel a gentle tingling. The frequency of treatments depends on the patient's response, but with treatment for chemotherapy-induced nausea, daily treatment would be indicated. The effects of acupuncture treatment are cumulative, and the response to treatment is better judged around the time of the sixth treatment. If there is no response at this point, acupuncture will probably not be helpful; on the other hand, if a response is noticed, further treatment is likely to increase the response.

OTHER METHODS OF STIMULATION

Sea-Band

Manual stimulation of the points (acupressure), and a commercial elastic wristband (Sea-Band) (see Fig. 101–1) with a plastic stud, which is positioned over PC6, have been used with success in some studies. The Sea-Band was designed by internist Daniel Shu Jan Choy, M.D., in 1980, during the New York–Bermuda yacht race, and it is widely available. It is placed over PC6 and is effective for motion sickness and as a way of extending conventional acupuncture treatment between visits.

Transcutaneous Electrical Stimulation

Transcutaneous electrical stimulation (TCES) via surface electrodes provides a noninvasive and effective method of stimulation. Surface electrodes are positioned over PC6 and PC7 and are stimulated at a frequency of 2 to 10 Hz with sufficient current to elicit a tingling sensation (see Fig. 101–2).[1] This method of stimulation has the advantage of being simple and can also be applied by the patient; the disadvantage is the need for an electrical acupuncture stimulator. Acupuncture stimulators are slightly different from transcutaneous electrical nerve stimulators (TENS); TENS machines usually operate in the 80 to 200 Hz range, whereas acupuncture stimulators are generally adjustable between 1 and 100 Hz (some machines cover all of these frequencies). A study[2] in which conventional treatment was supplemented by minimal acupuncture electrostimulation, or no additional treatment, came to the conclusion that "… addition of daily electroacupuncture to an anti-emetic regimen may be superior to acupuncture or medication alone for emesis management in this study population, although the beneficial effect may be limited in duration."

NOTE

Electrical stimulation, either through needles or surface electrodes, should not be used in patients with cardiac pacemakers.

REVIEW OF LITERATURE

The literature on the use of acupuncture with nausea and vomiting has been focused on the following areas:

- Nausea of pregnancy
- Postoperative nausea and vomiting
- Nausea from chemotherapy
- Nausea from motion

Nausea of Pregnancy

Dundee[3] studied the effect of self-administered acupressure in 350 antenatal patients. The results showed a significant reduction of nausea compared with a dummy point or no treatment. The incidence of returned records was only 70%, which has led to some criticism of the study.

Hyde,[4] De Aloysio,[5] and Stainton[6] have used Sea-Bands, and the overall conclusion seems to be that they appear to be sufficiently effective to be recommended in routine practice with no side effects.

Carlsson,[7] in another study, demonstrated benefit with stimulation of PC6 in the treatment of hyperemesis gravidarum.

Postoperative Nausea and Vomiting

Dundee,[8] Sacco,[9] and Barsoum[10] have all shown

that stimulation of PC6 for the prevention of post-operative nausea and vomiting in adults seems to be beneficial. The studies in children are less conclusive. Yentis[11] found no benefit from acupuncture, droperidol (Inapsine), or both after strabismus surgery, which may be related to the high incidence of nausea usually associated with this procedure. A study using the Korean hand acupuncture[12] point K–K6 did show benefit when used before strabismus surgery.

A recent systematic analysis by Lee[13] came to the following conclusion: "This systematic review showed that nonpharmacologic techniques were equivalent to commonly used antiemetic drugs in preventing vomiting after surgery. Nonpharmacologic techniques were more effective than placebo in preventing nausea and vomiting within 6 hours of surgery in adults, but there was no benefit in children."

More studies are required to determine which method of stimulation is most appropriate and whether stimulation should be given before, during, or after surgery.

Nausea from Chemotherapy

Stimulation of PC6 with either needling or acupressure has been shown to reduce chemotherapy-induced nausea when used as an adjunct to standard antiemetic therapy. Self-applied acupressure can help prolong the effect and TCES applied every 2 hours has been found to be beneficial when applied by the patient.[11] One study showed benefit with magnets of 60 mT positioned over PC6.[14]

Nausea from Motion

The literature in this area is very sparse and limited to the use of Sea-Bands. Artificially induced nausea does not seem to improve with the Sea-Bands, but Bertolucci[15] did show benefit with a small sample size, and Hu[16] reported similar findings. There is a considerable amount of anecdotal evidence for the use of Sea-Bands.

CONCLUSION

The overall conclusion appears to be that acupuncture applied in various ways does have a role in the prevention and treatment of nausea and vomiting.[17]

References

1. Dundee JW, Yang J, Mc Millan C: Noninvasive stimulation of the PC6 (Neiguan) antiemetic acupuncture point in cancer chemotherapy. J R S Med 84:210–212, 1991.
2. Shen J, Wenger N, Glaspy J, et al: Electroacupuncture for control of myeloablative chemotherapy-induced emesis: A randomized controlled trial. JAMA 284:2755–2761, 2000.
3. Dundee JW, Milligan KR, McKay AC: The influence of intra-operative acupuncture and droperidol on postoperative emesis. Br J Anaesth 61:116–117, 1988.
4. Hyde E. Acupressure therapy for morning sickness. A controlled clinical trial. J Nurse-Midwifery 34:171–178, 1989.
5. De Aloysio D, Penacchioni P: Morning sickness control in early pregnancy by Neiguan point acupressure. Obst Gynecol 80:852–854, 1992.
6. Stainton MC, Neff EJ: The efficacy of Seabands for the control of nausea and vomiting in pregnancy. Health Care Woman Int 15:563–575, 1994.
7. Carlsson CP, Axemo P, Bodin A, et al: Manual acupuncture reduces hyperemesis gravidarum. A placebo-controlled, randomized, single blind, crossover study. J Pain Symptom Manage Oct; 20:273–279, 2000.
8. Dundee JW, Ghaly, RG, Fitzpatrick KTJ, et al: Acupuncture prophylaxis of cancer chemotherapy–induced sickness. J R Soc Med 82:268–271, 1989.
9. Sacco JJ, Grant WD, Luthringer DD, et al: The reduction of postoperative nausea and vomiting in patients receiving nitrous oxide. Anesthesiology 73:A15, 1990.
10. Barsoum G, Perry EP, Fraser IA: Postoperative nausea is relieved by acupressure. J R Soc Med 83:86–89, 1990.
11. Yentis SM, Bissonnette B: Ineffectiveness of acupuncture and droperidol in preventing vomiting following strabismus repair in childen. Can J Anaesth 39:151–154, 1992.
12. Schlager A, Boehler M, Puhringer F: Korean hand acupressure reduces postoperative vomiting in children after strabismus surgery. Br J Anaesth 85:267–270, 2000.
13. Lee A, Done ML: The use of nonpharmacologic techniques to prevent postoperative nausea and vomiting: A meta-analysis. Anesth Analg 88:1362–1369, 1990.
14. Liu S, Chen Z, Hou J, et al: Magnetic disk applied on Neiguan point for the prevention and treatment of cisplatin-induced nausea and vomiting. J Traditional Chinese Med 11:181–183, 1991.
15. Bertolucci LE, DiDario B: Efficacy of a portable acustimulation device in controlling seasickness. Aviat Space Environ Med 66:1155–1158, 1995.
16. Hu S, Stritzel R, Chandler A, Stern RM: Acupressure reduces symptoms of vection-induced motion sickness. Aviat Space Environ Med 66:631–634, 1995.

CHAPTER 102

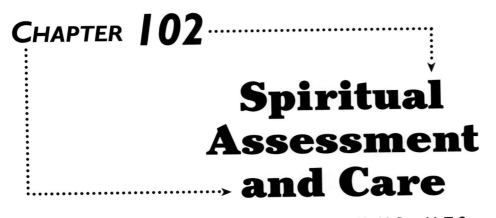

Spiritual Assessment and Care

Gregory A. Plotnikoff, M.D., M.T.S.

Spiritual and religious practices such as prayer represent the most prevalent complementary therapies in the United States. Nearly 80% of U.S. adults believe that religion, to a large extent, helps patients and families cope with illness.[1] Nearly 75% of the public believes that praying for someone else can help cure his or her illness. And 56% of adults state that faith has helped them recover from illness, injury, or disease.[2] Given these facts, it should be clear that one goal of holistic health care is to integrate the patient's spirituality into clinical encounters.

Spirituality is difficult to define or measure. As a formal definition, spirituality is a journey toward, or experience of, connection with the source of ultimate meaning. Spirituality includes connection with one's self, with others, with nature, and with a higher power. This connection is often with a greater story that makes sense of one's life. Spirituality may or may not involve formal religion. Spiritual concerns arise in clinical settings when these important connections are threatened or disrupted.

Spiritual beliefs demand professional attention. Sixty-three percent of American adults surveyed have stated that it is good for doctors to talk with patients about spirituality.[2] Seventy-seven percent of outpatients surveyed stated that physicians should address the patient's spiritual needs as part of routine medical care.[3] And 94% of outpatients surveyed who acknowledged spiritual or religious beliefs stated that physicians should inquire about their beliefs if they become ill.[4]

Physicians should be prepared to inquire and engage patients in discussions of spirituality. To ignore the patient's source of meaning, purpose, richness, and direction places the physician at risk for providing inefficient, ineffective, and unsatisfactory care.[5] The challenge is to identify the best means for doing so.

Multiple mnemonics exist to guide physicians in their interviews. These include FICA,[6] HOPE,[7] and SPIRIT,[8] which are outlined in Table 102–1. These mnemonics highlight content and provide questions that may lead to important insights on care for the patient and his or her family. For appropriate integration of spiritual assessment and care into clinical settings, this chapter identifies five practical goals. When these are addressed, three practical outcomes result: (1) improved diagnostic accuracy, (2) appropriately focused and directed resources, and (3) a strengthened therapeutic alliance.

THE FIVE CLINICAL GOALS OF SPIRITUAL ASSESSMENT AND CARE

Clinical Goal One: Anticipate the Presence of Religious and Spiritual Concerns in Both Adult and Pediatric Care

Spiritual and religious concerns in clinical care range from rituals or practices such as prayer to complex crises such as despair. Every illness is a potential spiritual crisis. This is true for the patient and family as well as for the care team. These crises can be found in both acute care and chronic care but may be most easily seen with end-of-life care. For example, common spiritual/religious concerns at that time include:

- Not being forgiven by God
- Not reconciling with others
- Dying alone or cut off from God
- Not having a blessing from a family member or clergy person
- Wondering whether anyone will miss you or remember you over time[9]

However, spiritual concerns can arise at any time. To recognize religious and spiritual concerns in others, one should be able to recognize them in oneself. Hence, all clinicians are challenged to develop self-awareness of their own spiritual history and perspectives.[10] In clinical care, the goal is to not to react to one's own spiritual needs or beliefs, but to

Table 102–1. Spiritual Assessment Tools

FICA—Pulchaski

F: **Faith or belief**—What is your faith or belief?

I: **Importance and influence**—Is it important in your life? How?

C: **Community**—Are you part of a religious community?

A: **Awareness and addressing**—What would you want me as your physician to be aware of? how would you like me to address these issues in your care?

HOPE—Anandarajah

H: **Hope**—What are your sources of hope, meaning, strength, peace, love, and connectedness?

O: **Organization**—Do you consider yourself part of an organized religion?

P: **Personal spirituality and practices**—What aspects of your spirituality or spiritual practices do you find most helpful?

E: **Effects**—How do your beliefs affect the kind of medical care you would like me to provide?

SPIRIT—Maugans

S: **Spiritual belief system**—What is your formal religious affiliation?

P: **Personal spirituality**—Describe the beliefs and practices of your religion or spiritual system that you personally accept/do not accept.

I: **Integration within a spiritual community**—Do you belong to a spiritual or religious group or community? What importance does this group have for you?

R: **Ritualized practices and restrictions**—Are there specific practices that you carry out as part of your religion/spirituality (e.g., prayer and meditation)? What significance do these practices or restrictions have to you?

I: **Implications for medical care**—What aspects of your religion/spirituality would you like me to keep in mind as I care for you?

T: **Terminal events planning**—As we plan for your care near the end of life, how does your faith impact on your decisions?

acknowledge and bracket them and then respond to the patient's spiritual concerns.

Both culture and spirituality can be implicit and unconscious. Both patients and physicians can be blind to the effects of their own perspective in clinical interviewing and decision making. For this reason, healthcare professionals should begin by conducting cultural and spiritual assessments of themselves before completing them on patients. The most effective interviewing allows deeply held beliefs to be both explicit and conscious.

The clinical challenge is to create a safe and conducive setting where concerns can be recognized and shared.

> **NOTE**
>
> *Spirituality is about questions, not answers. The challenge is for healthcare professionals to step out of their role as answer givers and into their role as listeners.*

When patients believe that they will not be judged, that someone will listen and not try to fix, dismiss, or deny their concerns, they will often freely share their

most private concerns. The sense of being heard is itself frequently therapeutic.

From an ethical viewpoint, physicians should maintain respect for their patients' beliefs and recognize patients' vulnerability to their own attitudes. No practitioner should impose his or her own religious, or antireligious, beliefs on patients.[11, 12] All practitioners need to recognize that their answers are their answers only.

To address spiritual and religious concerns does not require specifically religious or spiritual questions. Good open-ended questions include the following:

- How else do you hurt?
- Serious illness can affect lives in many unexpected ways. How has this illness affected your life?
- What do you miss most or fear most as a result of this illness?
- What are some of the things you wish you could talk about? Is there anyone you wish you could talk to?

The answers to such questions frequently reflect the patient's spiritual values and worldview in addition to identifying important connections that have been disrupted.

Clinical Goal Two: Comprehend How Patients Want Their Religious and/or Spiritual Beliefs and Community to be Seen as Resources for Strength and Recovery

Faith and related religious worldviews may be considered medically relevant only when they obstruct implementation of scientifically sound biomedical care.[13] However, this attitude is profoundly naïve. Every religion and cultural tradition has teachings, practices, and rituals that facilitate spiritual healing.[14]

> **NOTE**
>
> *The challenge is not to seek omnicultural and spiritual competency but to develop a humility that allows patients to teach about what is important to them.*

Patients often display many clues that can be keys to the beginning of a conversation. For example, "Mrs. Xiong, I see that you have white and red strings tied around your wrist. Could you share with me about their importance to you?" Such questioning would lead the healthcare professional into a deeper understanding of the patient's worldview and sources of strength. Such questioning would also prevent profound patient harm by accidental cutting and removal of sacred objects to make way for an IV placement or other biomedical intervention.

Related questions include:

- In the past, from where have you drawn the strength to cope with difficult situations?
- How can I be helpful regarding your spiritual concerns and practices?
- With regard to your care, what is most important to you?

The principal guideline in any such questioning is to listen for understanding rather than to express agreement or disagreement.

Clinical Goal Three: Understand Better Your Patients' Subjective Experiences and Diverse and Subjective Understanding of (Ultimate) Reality

Every effective healthcare professional is broadly familiar with the religious worldviews of the cultural groups within their patient population. Patients and their families can teach about the specifics. This is important because there is a significant danger in extrapolating the truth for one patient of one cultural group and making it the truth for all such patients. This constitutes practice by stereotype (e.g., this patient is Hmong; therefore. . . .). The challenge is to understand what *this* illness means for *this* patient.[15]

Seven concepts and questions that help guide clinician understanding include the following:

1. How is ultimate health understood?
2. How are affliction and suffering understood?
3. What are the different parts of a person?
4. How is the patient's illness/sickness or disease understood?
5. What interventions and/or care is believed necessary by the patient?
6. Who is seen as qualified to address the different parts that need healing?
7. What do the patient and family mean by efficacy or healing?[14]

Given the frequently implicit and unconscious nature of the answers to these questions, these should be seen only as prompts or guides. Healthcare professionals should ask themselves if they could answer these questions for their patient based on their interview(s). Doing so directs interviewing toward the clinically relevant meaning of the illness for the patient. The response to an open-ended question such as "What do you fear most about surgery?" often leads to a dialogue that may help answer these questions. Should this reveal a spiritual concern that cannot be addressed medically, further questioning can help identify the interventions that are needed and who should perform them.

Clinical Goal Four: Determine What Impact, Positive or Negative, Your Patients' Spiritual Orientation Has on Their Health Problems and Perceived Needs

Although spirituality is frequently seen in a positive light, there is, of course, a shadow side. The most recent Diagnostic and Statistical Manual (DSM-IV) has added a new axis IV concern—a religious or spiritual problem.[16] Examples cited include distressing experiences that involve loss or questioning of faith, problems associated with conversion to a new faith, or questioning of other spiritual values that may not necessarily be related to an organized church or religious institution.

When patients are asked about their sources of support, it is possible that what worked previously is not perceived to be working at present. For this reason, healthcare professionals are at risk for creating a sense of shame or guilt by denying, dismissing, or silencing doubts or theological challenges. Examples of valid spiritual suffering include:

Spiritual Alienation
"Where is God now when I need Him most?"
"Why isn't He listening?"
Spiritual Anxiety
"Will I ever be forgiven?"
"Am I going to die a horrible death?"
Spiritual Guilt
"I deserve this."
"I am being punished by God."
"I didn't pray hard enough."
Spiritual Anger
"I'm mad at God."
"I blame God for this."
"I hate God."
Spiritual Loss
"I feel empty."
"I don't care anymore."
Spiritual Despair
"There's no way God could ever care for me."
"I'm just a corpse waiting to happen."[5]

When spirituality is understood as including connections with one's self, with others, with nature, and with God or a higher power, then spiritual suffering can be seen as resulting from the loss of such connections—betrayal by one's body, loss of social roles, dependence on technology, and theological doubt or loss of faith. Healing, therefore, is the process of resolving such broken connections and recovering one's wholeness. The focus of healing is the human experience of illness. Healing can occur in any dimension: physical, emotional, social, and spiritual. Healing as the resolution of brokenness may or may not include curing disease. Healing is never quick or easy.

Spiritual healing begins with recognition and acknowledgment of spiritual pain. For this reason, the American Academy of Hospice and Palliative

Table 102–2. Spiritual Suffering Response Mnemonic
....

LET GO—American Academy of Hospice and Palliative Medicine
L—Listen to the patient's story.
E—Encourage the search for meaning.
T—Tell of your concern and acknowledge the pain of loss.
G—Generate hope whenever possible.
O—Own your own limitations, seek competence, and refer when appropriate.

Medicine's mnemonic LET GO can be quite helpful (Table 102–2).[17] The challenge here is to respond not as an expert with the answer(s), but as a fellow human being also struggling to make sense of tragedy. Listening, acknowledging, and validating are means for connecting at a deep level and are the most profound means of strengthening the therapeutic alliance. This connection between clinician and patient is the foundation for healing. Without this connection, without listening to the patient at a deep level, referral of patients to those with expertise in pastoral care and counseling may be perceived as abandonment by patients.

Generating hope whenever possible does not mean creating fake scenarios or deceiving patients. Generating hope means identifying what is important to the patient and working to achieve that. What constitutes hope and its shadow side, despair, change throughout the course of an illness.

NOTE

As with any medical referral, pastoral experts are available for assistance in understanding complex or difficult cases. Referrals can enhance the quality of care and, frequently, the patient's quality of life.

Clinical Goal Five: Determine Appropriate Referrals to Chaplains, Clergy, or Traditional Healers for Spiritual Care

Many spiritual concerns are addressed as a variation on the questions "Why? Why me? Why now?" Clearly, multiple members of the healthcare team can recognize the many varieties of such spiritual concerns in clinical settings. However, even if time allows, these are not questions that should be answered by healthcare professionals. To do so is to risk harming patients. For every such question, the best answers are found rather than given. The healthcare professional's role is to help give voice to such questions and to support the patient's search for answers.

Today, there is no need for any member of the healthcare team to be a self-sufficient virtuoso. This is especially true when Clinical Pastoral Education (CPE)–trained chaplains are available. Chaplains offer well-tuned skills in listening for, and responding to, spiritual concerns. Furthermore, they can help identify when a culture's spiritual healer (e.g., priest, pipe holder, or shaman) may be the most appropriate professional for a patient's spiritual concerns.

Care plans should identify a patient's spiritual resources, spiritual needs, and preferred spiritual care provider. Truly integrative medicine requires that a relationship be built between the physician and available chaplain services, leading to establishment of a network of local consultants and patient- or family-preferred spiritual care providers who can offer assistance.

THERAPEUTIC REVIEW

When spiritual assessment and care are integrated into clinical settings, three practical outcomes result: (1) improved diagnostic accuracy, (2) appropriately focused and directed resources, and (3) a strengthened therapeutic alliance. To achieve these outcomes, clinicians should consider integrating these eight summary points:

1. Mnemonics exist to guide inclusion of spirituality in clinical care. Expand the social history.
2. Spiritual needs can arise at any time or place. Anticipate them.
3. Spiritual healing begins with recognition and acknowledgment of spiritual pain. Listen intentionally.
4. Spirituality is about questions, not answers. Help voice the questions.
5. The best answers are found rather than given. Support the search.
6. Care plans should include patients' spiritual needs, resources, and preferred spiritual care providers. Identify them.
7. Every religious tradition has teachings, practices, and rituals that are resources for strength and recovery. Integrate these into the care plan.
8. Every illness is a potential spiritual crisis. Refer to pastoral care specialists for assistance.

References

1. Dujardin RC: Faith in medicine. Detroit Free Press, December 26, 1996:7D.

2. McNichol T: When religion and medicine meet: The new faith in medicine. USA Weekend, April 7, 1996:4.

3. King DE, Bushwick B: Beliefs and attitudes of hospital inpatients about faith healing and prayer. J Fam Pract 39:349–352, 1994.

4. Ehman JW, Ott BB, Short TH, et al: Do patients want physicians to inquire about their spiritual or religious beliefs if they become gravely ill? Arch Intern Med 159:1803–1806, 1999.

5. Plotnikoff GA: Should medicine reach out to the spirit? Postgrad Med 108:19–25, 2000.

6. Puchalski CM: Taking a spiritual history: FICA. Spirit Med Connect 3:1, 1999.

7. Anandarajah G, Hight E: Spirituality and medical practice: Using the HOPE questions as a practical tool for spiritual assessment. Am Fam Phys 63:81–88, 2001.

8. Maugans TA: The SPIRITual history. Arch Fam Med 5:11–16, 1996.

9. Nathan Cummings Foundation and the Fetzer Institute: Spiritual beliefs and the dying process: A report on a national survey, 1997. Available at *http://www.ncf.org/reports/rep_ fetzer_findings.html.* Accessed August 30, 2000.

10. Leonard BJ, Plotnikoff GA: Awareness: The heart of cultural competence. AACN Clin Issues 11:51–59, 2000.

11. Post SG, Puchalski CM, Larson DB: Physicians and patient spirituality: Professional boundaries, competency and ethics. Ann Intern Med 132:578–583, 2000.

12. Plotnikoff GA: Spirituality, religion, and the physician: New ethical challenges in patient care. Bioethics Forum 13:25–30, 1997.

13. Asser SM, Swan R: Child fatalities from religion-motivated medical neglect. Pediatrics 101:625–629, 1998.

14. Barnes LL, Plotnikoff GA, Fox K, Pendleton S: Spirituality, religion and pediatrics: Intersecting worlds of healing. Pediatrics 106:899–908, 2000.

15. Barnes LL, Plotnikoff GA: Fadiman and beyond—the dangers of extrapolation. Bioethics Forum 17:32–40, 2001.

16. American Psychiatric Association: Diagnostic and Statistical Manual of Mental Disorders, 4th ed. Washington, DC, American Psychiatric Press, Inc, 1994.

17. Storey P, Knight CF: UNIPAC 2: Alleviating Psychological and Spiritual Pain in the Terminally Ill. Gainesville, Florida, American Academy of Hospice and Palliative Medicine, 1997.

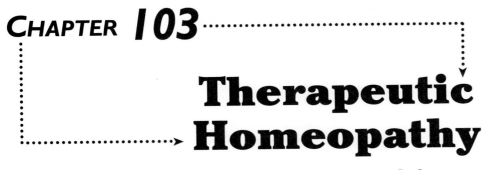

CHAPTER 103

Therapeutic Homeopathy

Mary Martin Bunker, D.O.

WHAT IS HOMEOPATHY?

Homeopathy is a safe, effective system of medicine that has been used by millions of people worldwide for more than 200 years. Homeopathic medicines are prepared from natural sources and are used in extremely small amounts. They are recognized as drugs by the U.S. Food and Drug Administration.[1] These medicines, called "remedies," are free from toxicity and can be used safely in patients of all ages, including infants and the elderly.

The homeopathic principle that "like cures like" was discovered and developed by Samuel Hahnemann in the late 18th century. It was first posited, however, by Hippocrates more than 2000 years ago. In his *Organon of Practical Medicine*, Hahnemann described this treatment by the Law of Similars: "To achieve a gentle and lasting cure, always choose a drug capable of provoking a disease similar (homion pathos) to the one it is to cure."[2]

HOW IS IT USED?

Imagine slicing a pungent red onion. Feel the copious watering of the eyes and the burning discharge from the nose. Just as the red onion can cause this characteristic discharge, so the homeopathic red onion, *Allium cepa*, can cure it. Whether illness results from the common cold, an upper respiratory infection, or a seasonal allergy, if the picture of the homeopathic remedy matches the patient's picture, the treatment can resolve the problem.

Homeopathy relies on the self-healing mechanism of the body. It views symptoms as expressions of these self-healing attempts and uses dilute doses of similar substances to stimulate this mechanism. For example, a cough is seen as the body's attempt to rid itself of an irritating substance, and the patient is treated with a matching remedy.

Such individually prescribed homeopathic treatment of acute childhood diarrhea was shown to significantly reduce both its duration and frequency in a randomized, double-blind, placebo-controlled trial reported in *Pediatrics*.[3]

HOW USEFUL IS IT?

This effective treatment modality is becoming increasingly popular with patients and physicians alike.

In a meta-analysis of 22 well-designed studies reported in the *British Medical Journal*, 15 demonstrated significantly positive results.[4] A 20-month International Data Collection Programme conducted by the Academic Departments of the Glasgow Homeopathic Hospital reported 68% efficacy in 1036 patient encounters.[5]

In a report of trends in alternative medicine used in the U.S. appearing in the November 1998 *Journal of the American Medical Association*, homeopathic treatment was one of the seven areas of greatest increase. Of the 42.1% of Americans using alternative medical therapies in 1997, the proportion using homeopathy had increased from 0.7 in 1990 to 3.4%.[6]

Two-year follow-up of a postgraduate physician education program found 78% of physicians continuing to integrate homeopathy into their practices.[7]

WHAT ABOUT ADVERSE EFFECTS?

Homeopathic medicines are dilute preparations of natural substances. Their use is associated with no contraindications, interactions, or adverse effects.

An acute, temporary exacerbation of symptoms, known as an *aggravation*, occasionally occurs during long-term prescribing. It occurs rarely in short-term treatment with remedies of low to mid potency.

HOW ARE THE MEDICINES PREPARED?

Homeopathic remedies must undergo a process of *potentization*, that is, serial *dilution* and *succussion* (shaking), according to stringent guidelines. The potencies commonly available are based on the decimal (X) and centesimal (C) systems. X potencies are diluted using one part of the mother tincture in nine parts of water; C potencies use one part in 99.

Table 103–1. Homeopathic Dosage Correlation with Injury Severity

Severity	Initially
Very acute	Every 5–10 minutes
Acute	Every 2–4 hours
Chronic	Once daily, weekly, monthly

After each dilution, the preparation is succussed. A 6X undergoes 1:9 dilution and succussion six times; a 30C, 1:99, 30 times.

NOTE

Remedies for oral use are available in tinctures, tablets, or pellets. For those used topically, these dosage forms can be added to 8 oz of water and applied externally.

HOW DO HOMEOPATHIC MEDICINES WORK?

Despite its 200 years of use worldwide, the exact mechanism of homeopathy remains unknown. Hahnemann recognized the paradox of greater potency in greater dilutions. However, 200 years of clinical experience have shown that homeopathy is effective. In a *Lancet* study comparing placebo versus homeopathic treatment in allergic asthma, the authors concluded that "homeopathy works, or the clinical trial does not."[8]

HOW ARE THE MEDICINES PRESCRIBED?

Homeopathic History

Homeopathic prescribing recognizes the totality of the individual as body, mind, and spirit, and thus requires an extensive history. Most physicians learned from DeGowin and DeGowin's *Bedside Diagnostic Examination* that the medical history "is an account of the events in the patient's life that have relevance to his mental and physical health."[9] In taking the homeopathic history, the physician can use DeGowin's PQRST mnemonic to sketch in the essential homeopathic details of symptom provocation—palliation, quality, region, severity, and temporal characteristics. A carefully elicited history draws a detailed patient picture, which enhances the physician's ability to prescribe accurately.

Homeopathic Prescription

Dosing correlates with illness or injury severity (Table 103–1).

- Acutely, evidence of a response should occur within the first 12 to 24 hours.
- Let the patient's response guide dosing: As acuteness diminishes, so does dosing frequency. With improvement, further dosing is required only if symptoms recur.
- The same dose can be given to all ages. Dose less frequently in the very frail.
- To begin integrating homeopathic therapeutics, always use the 30C potency.
- Choose homeopathic treatment only when a remedy matches the patient's presentation.

NOTE

Remedy handling: The remedies should not be touched. Use a 30C potency with a usual dose of 3 to 5 to tablets or pellets (or 5 drops of tincture); the dose should be placed under the tongue and left to dissolve. Ideally, no food or drink is taken within 15 to 30 minutes.

WHERE CAN HOMEOPATHIC TREATMENT BE USED?

Individuals can use homeopathy as over-the-counter treatment for first aid and acute care needs. Practitioners can use it to treat acute injury and illness. Classical homeopaths use constitutional prescribing to treat chronic disease.

Acute Injury

The two remedies *Arnica* and *Aconitum napellus* ("Aconite") "probably are indicated in 80% of accidents or emergencies, and many doctors have been converted to homeopathy following their initial experiments and successes with these two medicines."[10]

Shock

Aconitum napellus (Monkshood) is indicated in cases of sudden, intense shock, panic, or fear. Patients may experience collapse, hyperventilation, or palpitations. Onset of symptoms often occurs with such events as loss of a loved one and witness to trauma.

Table 103-2. Homeopathic Therapies for Traumatic Injuries
....

Strains, Sprains, and Bruises
  Arnica montana (Mountain daisy)
Wounds
  Cuts and scrapes—*Calendula* (Marigold), topically only
  Incised wounds—*Staphysagria* (Stavesacre)
  Deep cuts—*Hypericum* (St. John's wort)
  Puncture wounds—*Ledum* (Wild rosemary)
Burns
  Minor, first degree—*Calendula* (Marigold), topically only
  Minor, devoid of vesicles—*Urtica urens* (Stinging nettle)
  Second degree—*Hypericum* (St. John's wort) for burns with intact vesicles
  Extensive burns with bullae—*Cantharis* (Spanish fly)
  Electrical—*Phosphorus* (Phosphorus)

Strains, Sprains, and Bruises

Arnica montana (Mountain daisy) is the number one homeopathic first aid remedy for injuries and trauma and the most frequently prescribed homeopathic remedy in the U.S. and worldwide (Table 103–2). *Arnica* is indicated in soft tissue injury, sprains and strains, contusions, and concussions. It relieves muscle aches resulting from exercise and overuse, as well as postoperative pain and bruising.

NOTE

- *For ankle sprains, particularly recurrent, use* Ledum palustre *(Wild rosemary).*
- *For crush injuries and nerve pain, prescribe* Hypericum *(St. John's wort).*
- *For ligamentous injuries, choose* Ruta graveolens *(Rue-bitterwort).*
- *For fractures,* Symphytum *(comfrey or "Boneset") accelerates healing.*

Acute Illness

Homeopathic remedies can be used alone in conditions for which there is no conventional treatment, in which drug treatment is contraindicated or precluded by interactions or adverse effects, or when the patient chooses a safe alternative to drug treatment. Homeopathic therapy can be used as an adjunct to drug treatment, as when *Rhus toxicodendron* (Poison ivy) is integrated with conventional treatment of rheumatoid arthritis to relieve stiffness.

The common problems of early childhood exemplify ideal areas in which homeopathic therapeutics can be integrated. For conditions such as infant colic, teething pain, and childhood diarrhea, conventional medical therapy has little to offer. In otitis media, the high rate of recurrence and corresponding increase in antibiotic resistance have led to a prohibition against routine use of antibiotics. These conditions offer opportunities to enhance healing by integrating homeopathic medicines into the treatment plan.

Infant colic presents with paroxysmal intestinal cramping, associated with angry crying, legs drawn up, and passing gas. *Colocynthis* (Bitter cucumber) mirrors this spasmodic cramping in which the angry individual is doubled over in pain that is relieved with heat and pressure.

The **teething** child most commonly needs *Chamomilla* (German chamomile) for inconsolable pain. This child demands one thing after another, each time casting it aside, and is consoled only by being carried or rocked. This capricious child would need *Chamomilla* whether it was teething, colicky, suffering from ear pain, or ill with another malady.

Respiratory Disorders

Homeopathic alternatives to antibiotics avoid creating resistant strains (Table 103–3).

Otitis Media
- *Belladonna* (Deadly nightshade) is the picture of an acute infection, with its sudden onset of rubor, calor, and dolor.
- *Pulsatilla* (Windflower) is bland—mild in personality with bland discharges, often weepy but quite changeable.
- *Ferrum phosphoricum* (iron phosphate) is a good choice in the early stage of an infection when fever and symptoms are more diffuse than localized.

Conjunctivitis
- The patient needs *Apis mellifica* (Honeybee) when symptoms are similar to those from a bee sting: redness, stinging pain, and swelling that improve with applications of cold.
- The individual requiring *Arsenicum album* (White arsenic) experiences burning and watery discharge that improves with heat.
- The discharges of *Pulsatilla* (Windflower) are

Table 103-3. Homeopathic Therapies for Otitis Media
....

Remedy	Onset	Fever	Pain	Color
Belladonna	Sudden	High	Throbbing	Red
Pulsatilla	Slow	Moderate	Changeable	Pale, fair
Ferrum phosphoricum	Slow	Low	Nonlocalizing	Alternate red/pale

bland, copious, and thick. They may be yellow-white and purulent as well as pruritic.

- *Euphrasia* (Eyebright) has a long history of use as an herb for eye conditions. The patient who needs homeopathic *Euphrasia* presents with irritated, red eyes and tearing from copious acrid discharge. The individual is often photophobic and blinks frequently.

NOTE

Whether prescribing for conjunctivitis, colds, or allergies, one should select the remedy based on the characteristics of the patient's presentation.

Allergy

Treating the acute upper respiratory distress brought on by seasonal allergies such as hayfever or ragweed can be facilitated by noting the key characteristics of several homeopathic remedies (Table 103–4). Examples include the burning pains of *Arsenicum album* (White arsenic) and the bland nature of *Pulsatilla* (Windflower). The profuse watery discharge from the eyes and nose, as when an onion is sliced, depict *Allium cepa* (Red onion).

Sinusitis

- *Kali bichromicum* (Potassium bichromate) is the first choice in the treatment of sinus pain and congestion. The sinus headache begins at the root of the nose and behind the eyes. Mucous membranes may be congested with thick, stringy yellow discharge, and the nares may be crusty. The patient feels worse with motion, particularly stooping, and better with warmth.
- *Pulsatilla* (Windflower) may present with change-able symptoms, with diffuse and variable loci. Headache is often accompanied by gastrointestinal upset. Pulsatilla has a bland discharge, and patients may complain of a bad smell in the nose. Patients may weep with pain and are thirstless even with fever.
- *Bryonia* (Wild hops) may begin with a constant dull, throbbing frontal headache. It may radiate to the neck and stab over the eyes. The patient wants to avoid any movement even of the head or eyes, and feels better when firm pressure is applied. Mucous membranes are dry. Laryngitis and a dry cough may occur.

Table 103–4. Homeopathic Remedies for Seasonal Allergies

Remedy	Nasal Discharge	Eye Discharge
Arsenicum album	Burning	Burning
Pulsatilla	Bland	Bland
Euphrasia	Bland	Burning
Allium cepa	Burning	Bland[11]

Pharyngitis

- *Phosphorus* (Phosphorus) symptoms may include sore throat, dry cough, and chest congestion. Secretions may be blood-tinged, or epistaxis may occur. The throat may feel dry and sensitive, and the nose may feel dry, blocked, and sore. Hoarse-ness and a constant clearing of the throat are common. Cervical lymph nodes may be enlarged. The patient who needs *Phosphorus* is often hyper-sensitive, with complaints of hyperacusis, hyper-osmia, and hyperasthenia.
- *Belladonna* (Deadly nightshade) is most com-monly called for within the first 24 hours of the rapid onset of a red, swollen, sore throat and throbbing pain. The patient's countenance is red, and the skin is hot to the touch. Tonsils may be erythematous, edematous, and ulcerated, particu-larly on the right. The "strawberry tongue" of scarlet fever may be present.
- Patients with *Arsenicum* (White arsenic) have a burning sore throat and may be chilly, restless, and weak. Periodicity is key feature of *Arsenicum*, with recurrences at regular intervals, such as seasonally. The individual who needs *Arsenicum* feels better with warm drinks and worse with cold.
- *Apis* (Honeybee) causes stinging pains and swel-ling of the pharynx and tonsils. Blisters may form on the back of the tongue, and glossitis may rapidly evolve. The *Apis* sore throat is relieved by cold drinks and is aggravated by warmth.

Cough

- *Antimonium tartaricum* (Tartar emetic): A loose, rattling cough with chest congestion, frequently accompanied by nausea. It is improved with expec-toration and worsened by lying down.
- *Spongia* (Marine sponge): A croupy cough that sounds as if one is sawing through a log. It is better with warm drinks and is aggravated by talking. *Spongia* is the most commonly used remedy for a croupy cough.
- *Ipecacuanha* (Ipecac): A spasmodic cough with nausea and vomiting, often with rattling and wheezing.
- *Bryonia* (Wild hops): A dry cough, often following a cold or upper respiratory infection that has moved into the chest. It is characterized by dry mucous membranes and stitching pains. *Bryonia* is known as "the sleeping bear." One who needs this remedy is irritable and sluggish, wants only to lie still, and dislikes any movement.

Influenza

Gelsemium (Yellow jasmine) presents with the typical flu picture—aching, weakness, fever, chills, headache, and fatigue. Consequently, it is the most commonly prescribed homeopathic treatment for flu.

Rhus toxicodendron (Poison ivy) is achy with a

stiffness as if one is bruised that is improved by movement and a chilliness that is better for warmth.

Bryonia (Wild hops) is reluctant to move and prefers lying still. Movement, even of the eyes, is painful. Dryness, as in dry mucous membranes and dry cough, is significant and produces a great thirst.

NOTE

For influenza prophylaxis, prescribe Gelsemium 30C, 3 doses over 24 hours; then, once weekly during the flu season.

Gastrointestinal Disorders

Homeopathic remedies may be useful for gastrointestinal disorders (Table 103–5).

Nausea, Vomiting, Diarrhea, and Abdominal Pain

- In simultaneous upper and lower gastrointestinal tract involvement, as in food poisoning and gastroenteritis, think *Arsenicum* (White arsenic).
- Where severe nausea and vomiting predominate, consider *Ipecacuanha* (Ipecac).
- For cramping pain, think of both *Magnesia phosphorica* (Magnesium phosphate) and *Colocynthis* (Bitter cucumber). Both are improved with warmth, pressure, and bending over. To choose, note conditions that aggravate and the sensitivity of *Colocynthis* to anger and frustration.
- With an acute infection of sudden onset, for example, the patient is red, hot, and has throbbing pain, use *Belladonna* (Deadly nightshade). A gastrointestinal etiology is usually secondary.

NOTE

Homeopathic remedies should not be used prior to complete medical evaluation of symptoms that may warrant more aggressive therapy.

Dyspepsia, Peptic Ulcer

In the overworked, overstressed individual, consider two remedies. With either, the patient's symptoms are relieved with vomiting:

Argentum nitricum (Silver nitrate): Pains are epigastric, with onset after eating. Much flatulence and eructation occur, without relief. "Coffee-ground" emesis may also occur.

Nux vomica (Poison nut): Pain occurs 1 to 2 hours after eating and may radiate to the chest or between the scapulae. Dysphagia and reflux may occur, particularly after dietary indiscretions such as alcohol overuse.

Colitis

Colocynthis (Bitter cucumber): Cramping pain is noted with flatulence, distention, and urge to stool. Tenesmus and "currant-jelly" stool may be present. Symptoms are relieved by passing flatus and having bowel movements.

Cantharis (Spanish fly): Burning pains and burning stools may be accompanied by bloody diarrhea. Hematemesis may occur. Symptoms worsen with drinking liquids, particularly coffee, and improve with eructation and passing flatus.

Nux vomica (Poison nut): Pains are lancinating, and symptoms are brought on by overindulgence — in work, food, or alcohol. Constipation with urging is common. Colicky diarrhea may occur, as well as the passage of bright red blood.

Urogenital Conditions

Urinary Tract Infection, Cystitis

Cantharis (Spanish fly) is an important remedy for urinary burning, particularly with urgency and frequency. Burning pains may occur in the bladder or kidneys, and costovertebral angle tenderness may be present.

Urinary Retention/Incontinence

Causticum (Bisulphate of potash) is valuable in treating urinary retention and stress incontinence, as well as overflow incontinence following retention. It is often beneficial in nocturnal eneuresis.

Table 103–5. Homeopathic Remedies for Gastrointestinal Disorders

Remedy	Nausea/Vomiting	Diarrhea	Pain	Better with	Worse with
Arsenicum	With diarrhea	With vomiting	Burning	Heat	Food, drink
Ipecac	Extreme/continuous	With nausea		Rest	Food smells
Colocynthis	After intense pain	Cramps prior	Spasmodic	Doubling up	Rest
Mag phos	Unusual	Unusual	Cramping	Doubling up	Movement
Belladonna		With fever	Throbbing	Rest	Movement

Table 103–6. Homeopathic Remedies for Chronic Skin Disorders

Condition	Remedy	Eruption	Characteristic Physical	Characteristic Mental
Poison ivy	*Rhus tox*	Vesicular	Itching	None
Eczema	*Sulphur*	Atopic	Red, pruritic	Untidy, "ragged philosopher"
Impetigo	*Antimonium tart*	Pustular	Slow onset	Irritable, dislikes being touched
Shingles	*Arsenicum*	Vesicular	Burning	Fastidious, "type A"
Warts	*Thuja*	Excrescent		Preoccupied, very sensitive

Musculoskeletal Conditions

Arthritis

Use *Rhus toxicodendron* (Poison ivy) for "rusty gate" stiffness that improves with movement, as in rheumatoid arthritis.

Choose *Bryonia* (Wild hops) for pain that is worse with the slightest movement, as in osteoarthritis.

Alternate the two remedies as the characteristics of those better from movement and those worse from movement alternate in the patient. Both are better with heat.

Long-term Treatment

Dermatologic Problems

Although patients find skin lesions very disturbing, the homeopath views them as external manifestations of internal disorders (Table 103–6). The atopic patient whose disease manifestations alternate between eczema and asthma exemplifies this. Treating the whole patient by considering the totality of disease expression may require constitutional treatment by a homeopathic physician. *Constitution* means the inherited and acquired physical, emotional, and intellectual makeup of a person. It reveals itself in habits, the basic emotional and intellectual proclivities, and the way the individual reacts to internal and external stress factors.[12]

In homeopathic prescribing, pathognomonic symptoms common to all patients with a particular diagnosis are relatively unimportant in comparison to the peculiar symptoms unique to the individual's experience of the disease. Constitutional prescriptions are most often from the group of remedies known as *polycrests*. "To effect real cure in chronic illness, these broad, deep-acting remedies are essential—local prescribing will usually only palliate."[13] *Sulphur* (Brimstone), *Arsenicum* (White arsenic), and *Thuja* (Arbor vitae) are deep-acting *polycrests* and should be dosed infrequently as in chronic disease.

Psychiatric Disturbances

In homeopathy, mental symptoms are of greater import than are physical, as the direction of cure, according to Hering's Law, is seen to occur from the top downward and from within outward. The greatest precision in prescribing occurs in matching the patient's mental and emotional characteristics.

Anxiety/Panic

Aconitum napellus (Monkshood) is useful for sudden onset of abject panic or fear—of crowds, of going outdoors, of darkness, of death—even of indefinable fear.

Argentum nitricum (Silver nitrate) is beneficial in anticipatory anxiety in which the individual is filled with apprehension and the physiologic response is hypersympathetic.

Gelsemium (Yellow jasmine) is helpful for apprehension in which the individual is "paralyzed with fear," and the physiologic response is "weak in the knees" hypofunctioning.

THERAPEUTIC REVIEW

Homeopathy is an effective tool that can be easily integrated into a physician's armamentarium as monotherapy or as adjunctive treatment. It is not only free of adverse effects, but homeopathic treatment enhances immunity, leading to fewer illnesses, of shorter duration. Homeopathic medicines are inexpensive; the cost of an entire course of treatment is well under $10.

Practicing homeopathic medicine is rewarding for both the patient and the physician. Improved health and decreased treatment toxicity result for the patient, a broader array of tools and a more fulfilling practice are gained for the physician, and a more gratifying patient-physician relationship can occur for both.

THERAPEUTIC REVIEW *continued*

"As our understanding of the universe continues to evolve, it will become increasingly apparent that homeopathy is more consistent with emerging scientific theory than any other form of medicine, and that this holistic, humane, and natural approach to healing may well be the medicine of the future."[14]

Resources for further study

- *Studies of Homoeopathic Remedies* by Douglas Gibson is an insightful review of leading remedies that uses a systems approach and includes the pharmacology, physiology, and psychology of each.
- *Introduction to Homoeopathic Medicine* by Hamish Boyd is an excellent text for use by physicians who want to further integrate homeopathy into their practices. It includes sections on acute and chronic case history-taking and treatment.
- *Desktop Companion to Physical Pathology* by Roger Morrison is a valuable desk reference written to aid physicians in remedy selection during patient encounters.
- *Homeopathic Therapeutics* by Jacques Jouanny is a very useful reference of common conditions, particularly dermatologic exanthems depicted in photographs.
- *Portraits of Homeopathic Medicines* by Catherine Coulter is an exceptional three-volume set of psychosocial profiles of many important remedies for those interested in gaining greater insight into homeopathic remedy pictures and human psychology.
- *Everybody's Guide to Homeopathic Medicines: Taking Care of Yourself and Your Family with Safe and Effective Remedies,* by Stephen Cummings and Dana Ullman, is a valuable home care guide for patients.
- *Homeopathic Medicine at Home: Natural Remedies for Everyday Ailments and Minor Injuries,* by Maesimund Panos and Jane Heimlich, is another useful patient guide.
- *The National Center for Homeopathy,* at www.homeopathic.org, is an important homeopathic association and resource for homeopathic training, texts, and referrals.
- *The American Institute of Homeopathy,* at www.homeopathyusa.org, publishes a quarterly journal for practitioner members.

References

1. Homeopathy today. National Center for Homeopathy 21(1): 35, 2001.
2. Hahnemann S (Boericke W, trans): Organon of Practical Medicine. New Delhi, B. Jain Publishers, 1976.
3. Jacobs J, Jimenez M, Gloyd S, et al: Treatment of acute childhood diarrhea with homeopathic medicine. Pediatrics 93:719–725, 1994.
4. Kieijnen J, Knipschild P, ter Riet G: Clinical trials of homoeopathy. BMJ 302:316, 323, 1991.
5. Reilly D: The Foundations of Homeopathy, 15th ed. Glasgow Adhom Ltd, 1997.
6. Elsenberg D: Trends in alternative medicine use in the U.S., 1990–1997. JAMA 1280(18):1569–1975, 1998.
7. Reilly D: The Foundations of Homeopathy, 15th ed. Glasgow, Adhom Ltd, 1997.
8. Reilly D, Taylor M, Beattie N, et al: Is evidence for homeopathy reproducible? Lancet 344:1601–1606, 1994.
9. DeGowin RL: Bedside Diagnostic Examination, 5th ed. New York, Macmillan Publishing Co, 1987, p 15.
10. Boyd H: Introduction to Homoeopathic Medicine, 2nd ed. Beaconsfield, Bucks, England, Beaconsfield Publishers Ltd, 1997, p 76.
11. Reilly D: The Foundations of Homoeopathy. Section 21. Glasgow, Adhom Ltd, 1997.
12. Koehler G (Meuss A, trans): The Handbook of Homeopathy. Its Principles and Practice. Rochester, Vt, Healing Arts Press, 1989, p 176.
13. Boyd H: Introduction to Homoeopathic Medicine, 2nd ed. Beaconsfield, Bucks, England, Beaconsfield Publishers Ltd, 1989, p 31.
14. Wein M, Goss K: The Complete Book of Homeopathy. New York, Bantam, 1982.

CHAPTER 104

Functional Medicine

Hunter Yost, M.D.

Medicine is undergoing a revolution. . . . As healthcare providers move from a disease-focused model to health promotion and disease management based on patient uniqueness and evidence-based medicine, their tools will include improved understanding of the genetic uniqueness of the patient, the factors that modify disease expression, and the intercellular modulators of function that give rise to increased risk of age-related disease.

Jeffrey Bland, Ph.D.[1]

Most physicians, whether they are primary care or specialists, spend the majority of their time diagnosing and treating the gross manifestations of disease and acute illness. Using the large gauge filter of conventional diagnostic technology to rule in or out observable tissue pathology, blatant blood chemistry abnormalities, and signs of disease on physical examination, large numbers of individuals can be cycled through the daily office schedule and given either a clean bill of health or end up with no diagnosis to adequately explain their persistent symptoms. In one study, 74% of patients seen by general internists for various common complaints received no medical or psychiatric diagnosis to explain their complaints.[2] According to the National Center for Health Statistics, during the latter half of the 20th century, there was an increasing prevalence of chronic disorders. Seven of the ten leading causes of death, which account for 72% of deaths in the United States, are chronic in nature.[3]

Functional medicine has been defined as "the field of healthcare which employs assessment and early intervention into the improvement of physiological, cognitive/emotional, and physical functioning."[4] A central concept of functional medicine is that nutritional pharmacology can be used as an effective biologic response modifier for the restoration of homeodynamics/homeostasis in individuals with complex, chronic illness. Nutritional interventions interact with other biologic response modifiers to create a complex web of functioning. These biologic response modifiers are noted in Table 104–1.

Forward thinking practitioners of primary care medicine, biochemistry, and laboratory medicine began to ask different questions about how to better treat the chronically but not acutely ill patient who usually slips through the large-gauge filter of conventional medical diagnosis and treatment. "Could the evaluation of physiologic and biochem-

ical functioning be as important as the search for gross pathology?" "Could the assessment of triggers, antecedents, and mediators of illness processes be as important as the assessment of traditional signs and symptoms of disease?" During the early 1990s, a new medical field termed functional medicine was created to deal with the subtleties of illness and disease.[5–10] Basic principles and core physiologic and biochemical processes have been developed as have laboratory tests to assess functioning and organ reserve.

BASIC PRINCIPLES OF FUNCTIONAL MEDICINE

1. *Biochemical individuality* is determined by the nuclear and mitochondrial genome instead of statistical human data compiled from the bell-shaped curve.
2. *Health is positive vitality.* "Health is not only the absence of disease but also the presence of physical, mental, and social well-being."[11]
3. Functional health is maintained by balance within a *complex web* of physiologic, cognitive/emotional, and physical processes.
4. *Homeodynamics* is attained through a dynamic interaction between an individual's genome and his/her environment. For example, maintaining individual variations of blood pH or body temperature as opposed to the concept of homeostasis within a range of normal which obscures these individual variations.

The following core processes are the biochemical and physiological applications of the basic principals of functional medicine. They are not specific to any one disease or medical specialty, rather they

Table 104–1. Biologic Response Modifiers in Functional Medicine

Dietary nutrients and phytochemicals
Nutrient medical foods and supplements
Exercise
Oxygen/carbon dioxide modulation and balance
Pharmacologic substances
Environmental factors
Lifestyle factors
Structural factors
Energy
Surgery

underlie virtually all diseases and tend to blur the distinctions between specialties.

CORE FUNCTIONAL PROCESSES

1. *Gut function*: The barrier function of the gut is essential for maintaining the separateness of the internal environment of our bodies from the outside world. Since roughly 60% of the immune system is connected to the gut, the optimal balance of beneficial bacteria to potential pathogens is essential for proper immune system functioning. The gastrointestinal (GI) tract also has important nervous system functions because it contains 100 million neurons 1—about the same number as in the spinal cord. Also, gut receptors for more than 20 neurotransmitters with brain functions have been identified. Important GI functions such as dysbiosis (imbalanced gut flora) and intestinal permeability can be assessed through noninvasive tests.
2. *Liver functioning*: As the prime organ responsible for the detoxification of xenobiotics, pharmacologic agents, and internal metabolic byproducts, imbalances in the phase I-450 enzyme system and the phase II conjugation pathways of glucuronidation, glycination, glutathione conjugation, and sulfation are crucially important for the elimination of potential carcinogens, toxic substances, and hormonal balance. These processes can be assessed through a caffeine, salicylate, and acetaminophen challenge test.
3. *Mitochondrial dysfunction*: The basic biochemical processes of the Krebs energy cycle and oxidative phosphorylation essential to optimal energy production are relevant for chronic fatigue and pain conditions as well as neurologic conditions.
4. *Dysglycemia and dysinsulinism*: Considered by molecular geneticists to be the seminal process in aging, management of blood sugar, and insulin sensitivity. The gradual loss of insulin sensitivity and subsequent hyperinsulinemia result in type 2 diabetes, hypertension, cardiovascular disease, and obesity. Premature aging is accelerated by the formation of advanced glycosylated end products from persistently elevated blood sugars.
5. *Intercellular communication*: The relationship of cytokines (TNF, IL-2, IL-6, etc.), interleukins, leukotrienes, transcription factors (NF kappa B), and other mediators of inflammation and their influence on virtually every acute and chronic disease process.
6. *Oxidative Stress*: Involves free radical production and reactive oxygen species measured through saliva and urine levels of catechols; 2, 3 dihydroxybenzoate; reduced glutathione; and glutathione peroxidase, urine lipid peroxides, and superoxide dismutase involved in all degenerative processes, chronic illnesses, and inflammatory conditions.

Newer diagnostic laboratory tests, which have been developed since the early 1990s, are performed by various specialty laboratories around the country to assess functioning in all these areas. Imbalances in functioning are addressed through lifestyle, dietary changes, and specific nutritional protocols.

PATIENT-CENTERED FOCUS

To apply the basic principles of functional medicine, it is necessary to rethink the ICD-9 disease categories and to rethink the context of disease based on the experience of the individual. Galland[3] advocates a biographic versus a biologic description of individuals. In a biographic approach, disease is perceived as rising out of the ongoing narrative of a person's life experiences and not as an entry from outside. From this standpoint, the patient would say, "My disease arises out of the sum total of my life experiences as they interact with my genetic predispositions" rather than, "I have a disease that has been attached to me by some outside force or labeling process." Most indigenous systems of medicine outside of Western culture are innately biographic. The medical diagnostic schemas of the West are based on the botanical classification methodologies of the 18th and 19th centuries. They lend themselves well to reimbursement coding procedures but have little relevance to the experience of the individual.

ILLNESS AND DISEASE

To fully appreciate a functional medicine point of view, it is necessary to make important distinctions between illness and disease. According to Kleinman,[11] disease is a problem from the practitioner's perspective: "Disease is what the practitioner creates in the recasting of illness in terms of the theories of disorder. Disease is what practitioners have been trained to see through the theoretical lenses of their particular forms of practice." In the Western biomedical disease model, this means a disease is reconfigured only as an alteration in biologic structure or functioning. Kleinman defines illness as "the innately human experience of symptoms and suffering and refers to how the sick person and members of the family or wider social network perceive, live with, and respond to symptoms and disability."

Galland[3] defines disease as "nothing more than a pattern of signs, symptoms, behaviors, and tissue pathology occurring in individual human beings." A disease is not a "thing" and does not have an independent existence of its own outside an individual and the context of his or her life. Galland[3] has elaborated a conceptual schema of triggers, mediators, antecedents, signs, and symptoms to accommodate the complexity of the illness and the disease (Fig. 104–1).

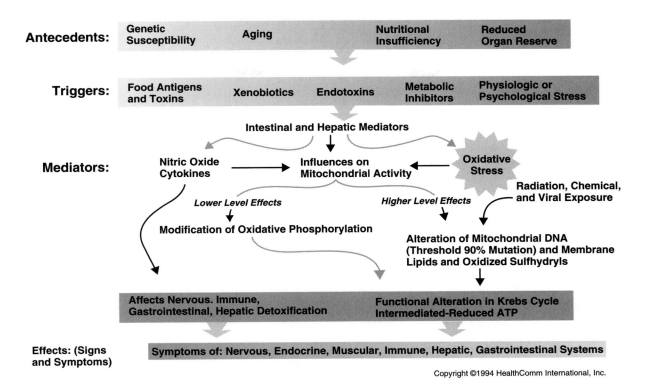

Figure 104–1. Modulators of mitrochondrial function and the etiology of functional health problems. (Copyright © 1994 HealthComm International, Gig Harbor, Wash.)

TRIGGERS

Triggers activate quiescent mediators in individuals. Sometimes, triggers are called "causes;" however, triggers can only activate mediators that are specific to the individual. This follows the concept of biologic structural determinism elaborated by Maturana.[12] Triggers usually are multiple and are not disease specific (Table 104–2).

Table 104–2. Common Triggers of Illness
···

Physical injury (concussion)
Repetitive injury (overuse syndromes)
Physical exercise (may trigger heart attacks)
Microbes (triggers of infectious disease)
  Bacteria
  Viruses
  Parasites
  Fungi
Drugs
  Therapeutic (aspirin)
  "Recreational" (alcohol or caffeine)
  Cigarette smoke
  Microbial (botulism)
Temperature extremes (may trigger asthma)
Adverse social interactions
Memories of previous sickness or distress
Feelings of anxiety (may trigger asthma or heart attacks)
Stressful life events (family illness)

MEDIATORS

A mediator is anything that produces symptoms, damages tissues of the body, or causes types of behaviors associated with being sick. Mediators contribute to illness because their activity is the main determinant of their function. Mediators are specific to the individual but not to any particular disease (Table 104–3).

Table 104–3. Common Mediators of Illness
···

Biochemical
  Stress hormones (adrenaline and cortisone)
  Neurotransmitters (serotonin)
  Neuropeptides (beta-endorphin, and substance P)
  Prostanoids
  Cytokines
  Free radicals
  Nitric oxide
Cognitive/emotional
  Fear of pain
  Fear of loss
  Beliefs about sickness
  Feelings about sickness (anxiety, depression)
  Poor self-esteem, low perceived self-efficacy
Social
  Rewards for being ill
  Behavioral conditioning
  Lack of resources (poverty, social isolation)
Subatomic
  Ions
  Electrons
  Electrical and magnetic energy fields

Table 104–4. Antecedents of Illness: Diathesis of Illness
....

Congenital Factors
  Genetic (sex and inherited traits)
  Acquired in the womb (resulting from maternal nutrition, toxic exposure [e.g., fetal alcohol syndrome])
Developmental Factors (those that develop over time)
  Effects of age
  Nutrition
  Traumatic events (physical or emotional)
  Effects of learning and conditioning
  Altered microbial ecology (e.g., depletion of normal intestinal bacteria)

ANTECEDENTS

The predisposition, or diathesis, to illness is the entire context of factors, congenital, biologic and social, that set the stage for illness to arise. An important belief in functional medicine is that genes are not destiny. The deterministic model of Mendelian genetics does not apply to human beings who have complicated multiple gene interactions and large discordance rates for diseases in identical twins. There are always multiple antecedents in any individual (Table 104–4).

Considering triggers, antecedents, and mediators, the practitioner can appreciate the complexity of the illness experience for purposes of evaluation and treatment interventions. Functional medicine offers great promise for a new paradigm in 21st century medicine. It can free us from the tendency to analyze a disease process outside the context of the individual for convenience in coding and for reimbursement requirements. Functional medicine also allows meaningful intervention into the illness process, restoration of optimal functioning, and improved quality of life for many chronic conditions.

An example of a functional approach to inflammatory bowel disease can be found in the following case study.

Case Study: Inflammatory Bowel Disease

A 52-year-old man with an established diagnosis of Crohn's disease over 15 years, taking sulfasalazine 4 g per day, has complaints of persistent loose stools, four to five bowel movements per day, accompanied by bloating and gas. He has previously taken many courses of metronidazole and prednisone at the direction of his gastroenterologist. He would like to avoid surgery and further use of steroids. He has not been following any special diet and admits to eating predominantly refined carbohydrates and lots of sweets, with low consumption of vegetables.

At the initial visit, he was given a special anti-inflammatory medical food powder designed for use in GI inflammation.

There are no significant laboratory or physical findings.

A comprehensive digestive stool analysis (CDSA), lactulose-mannitol assay, and food antibody profile were performed.

The CDSA shows 4+ Klebsiella pneumoniae, 3+ Citrobacter freundii, 0+ Lactobacillus, 1+ Bifidobacter, and 4+ Candida albicans. Long-chain fatty acids, fecal cholesterol, and total fecal fat were slightly elevated. Chymotrypsin was low. Total short-chain fatty acids and n-butyrate were low. Fecal lactoferrin was mildly elevated. Mucus was present but no blood.

Lactulose recovery by enzymatic method was 1.49 (.01–0.8) and lactulose/mannitol ratio was .208 (.01–.03), which suggests an increased permeability of the intestinal lining.

The food antibody profile showed 3+ IgG reactions for gluten, 2+ for corn, 2+ for tomatoes, 2+ for sugar, and 1+ for coffee.

Treatment
Remove: *The patient was placed on Cipro, 500 mg, twice daily for 7 days. All offending foods were removed from his diet.*
Replace: *Digestive enzymes with meals. A medical food with a high ratio of soluble/insoluble fiber, 2 scoops per day.*
Reinoculate: *Lactobacillus GG, 1 tablet, twice daily for 2 weeks and then once daily for 3 months.*
Repair: *Glutamine powder, 5000 mg, twice daily for 2 months.*

Four-Month Follow-up
The patient is now having solid, formed stools daily. There has been a significant decrease in gas and bloating. A repeat microbiology profile shows 1+ Citrobacter freundii, 4+ Lactobicillus, and 3+ Bifidobacterium. Lactobacillus and Bifidobacterium are beneficial intestinal flora. (see Chapter 97, Prescribing Probiotics). The lactulose/mannitol ratio is now within normal limits. He continues to take sulfasalazine as recommended by his gasteroenterologist.

1. The CDSA evaluates parameters of functional digestive health such as fecal triglycerides, chymotrypsin, isovalerate, isobutyrate, n-valerate, long-chain fatty acids, fecal cholesterol, total fecal fat, short-chain fatty acids, Lactobacillus, E. coli, Bifidus, possible pathogens, mycology, lactoferrin mucus, and occult blood.

2. The lactulose/mannitol assay shows intestinal permeability through urinary recovery of the ratio of these two sugars.

3. The IgE and IgG food antibody test assesses immediate and delayed reactions to common foods.

Laboratories Performing Functional Medicine Testing

Diagnos-Techs, 1-425-251-0596.
Doctor's Data, 1-708-231-3649.
Great Plains Laboratory, 1-913-341-8949.
Great Smokies Diagnostic Laboratories, 1-800-522-4762.
Immunodiagnostic Laboratories, 1-800-888-1113.
Immunosciences, 1-310-657-1077.
Meridian Valley Clinical Laboratory, 1-206-859-8700.
Metametrix, 1-800-466-3627.
Serammune PhysiciansLab, 1-800-553-5472.
SpectraCell Laboratories, 1-800-227-5227.

Further Resources

Institute of Functional Medicine, 5800 Soundview Drive, P.O. Box 1729, Gig Harbor, Wash., 98335; 1-800-228-0622; www.fxmed.com

References

1. Improving Intercellular Communication in Managing Chronic Illness: A Functional Medicine Approach to Regulating Biochemical Mediators. Seminar Series, Institute of Functional Medicine, 1999.
2. Kroenke K, Arrington ME, Mangelsdorff D: Common symptoms in ambulatory care: Incidence, evaluation, therapy, and outcome. Am J Med 86:262–266, 1989.
3. National Center for Health Statistics: Health, United States, 1995. Hyattsville, Md, Public Health Service, 1995.
4. Bland J: New Perspectives in Nutritional Therapies: Improving Patient Outcomes. HealthComm Seminar Series, Gig Harbor, Wash., 1996.
5. Galland L: The Four Pillars of Healing, aka Power Healing. New York, Random House, 1997.
6. Baker S: Detoxification and Healing: The Key to Optimum Health. New Canaan, Ct., Keats Publishing, 1997.
7. Bland J: The 20-Day Rejuvenation Diet Program. New Canaan, Ct., Keats Publishing, 1997.
8. Bland J: Genetic Nutritioneering. New Canaan, Ct., Keats Publishing, 1999.
9. Perlmutter D: Brain Recovery.com, 2000.
10. Jones D: Manager Care: High Stakes Health Care Poker, New Perspectives in Nutritional Therapies: Improving Patient Outcomes. Gig Harbor, Wash., HealthComm Seminar Series, 1996.
11. Constitution of the World Health Organization. In World Health Organization Handbook of Basic Documents, 5th ed. Geneva, Palais of Nations, 1952, pp 3–20.
12. Maturana H, Varela F: The Tree of Knowledge. New York, Shambhala Press, 1987.
13. Kleinman A: The Illness Narratives: Suffering, Healing and the Human Condition. New York, Basic Books, 1988.

Index

Note: Page numbers followed by the letter f refer to figures; those followed by the letter t refer to tables.